# Echocardiography

# ECHOCARDIOGRAPHY

## Harvey Feigenbaum, M.D.

*Distinguished Professor of Medicine*
*Director of Hemodynamic Laboratories*
*Indiana University School of Medicine*
*Senior Research Associate*
*Krannert Institute of Cardiology*
*Indianapolis, Indiana*

## 5th Edition

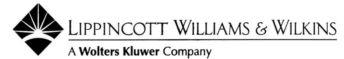

LIPPINCOTT WILLIAMS & WILKINS
A **Wolters Kluwer** Company
Philadelphia • Baltimore • New York • London
Buenos Aires • Hong Kong • Sydney • Tokyo

Williams & Wilkins
351 W. Camden Street
Baltimore, Maryland 21201-2436 USA

Rose Tree Corporate Center
1400 North Providence Road
Building II, Suite 5025
Media, Pennsylvania 19063-2043 USA

Executive Editor—R. Kenneth Bussy
Development Editor—Tanya Lazar
Project/Manuscript Editor—Frances M. Klass
Production Manager—Samuel A. Rondinelli

NOTE: Although the author(s) and the publisher have taken reasonable steps to ensure the accuracy of the drug information included in this text before publication, drug information may change without notice and readers are advised to consult the manufacturer's packaging inserts before prescribing medications.

**Library of Congress Cataloging-in-Publication Data**

Feigenbaum, Harvey.
    Echocardiography / Harvey Feigenbaum. — 5th ed.
        p.  cm.
    Includes bibliographical references and index.
    ISBN 0-8121-1692-5
    1. Ultrasonic cardiography.  I. Title.
    [DNLM: 1. Echocardiography.  WG 141.5.E2 F298e 1993]
    RC683.5.U5F44  1993
    616.1′207543—dc20
    DNLM/DLC
    for Library of Congress                          92-48436
                                                        CIP

First Edition, 1972
Second Edition, 1976
Third Edition, 1981
Fourth Edition, 1986

PRINTED IN THE UNITED STATES OF AMERICA

Print Number: 10  9  8  7  6

# Dedication

To the numerous outstanding scientists, engineers, and clinical investigators who have made echocardiography the excellent diagnostic tool that it is today.

# Preface

Numerous advances have occurred in echocardiography since the fourth edition. These advances include Doppler flow imaging or color Doppler, transesophageal echocardiography, new spectral Doppler applications, stress echocardiography, contrast echocardiography, intravascular ultrasound, and new computer techniques for capture, display, analysis, and 3D reconstruction of ultrasonic images. The field has expanded so greatly that it has been a tremendous challenge to try to include all of the major features of echocardiography and yet keep this book readable and at a reasonable size. Obviously, a great many compromises had to be made to meet these goals. Many readers of this book do not necessarily wish to be experts in the field of echocardiography and do not want to be burdened with excessive theory and experimental data. Therefore, as with previous editions, the discussion of technical details is limited and is found primarily in the first two chapters. The references, however, are voluminous and intended for those individuals who wish more detailed information about certain topics. The references are extensive but not exhaustive. It is obviously impossible to include the entire echocardiographic literature. An effort was made to provide multiple references on the same topic. Many new and unproven uses of echocardiography are mentioned, and those techniques with some promise are illustrated; however, the primary emphasis of this text is on clinically relevant and proven applications of echocardiography.

As with previous editions, the book is generously illustrated with over a thousand illustrations, many of which are in color. Many of these illustrations are taken from the literature in order to cover the field from multiple perspectives. In some ways, this book represents a collection of some of the best illustrations that have appeared in the echocardiographic literature. There are some new features concerning the illustrations. As mentioned there are far more color photographs than in the fourth edition. Many of the illustrations are from digital recordings and are displayed in a split or quad screen format. This technique makes it easy to have one figure demonstrate different views or multiple stages of a cardiac cycle. As in previous editions, illustrations are frequently duplicated so that the reader does not have to flip pages to see a figure that also appears in another chapter. Because of the numerous illustrations, the book can function as an atlas, and a serious effort has been made to keep the corresponding text and figures close to each other.

Many of the older M-mode recordings and discussions have been eliminated or reduced, permitting the introduction of newer information without greatly increasing the size of the book. On the other hand, considerable M-mode data are still included. Although M-mode echocardiography has been relegated to a lesser status, the technique still has more than historical value in the field. The temporal resolution exceeds any two-dimensional study. Thus, this capability still provides diagnostic information that is not available with a tomographic examination. For this reason, this edition still contains many discussions and illustrations pertaining to M-mode echocardiography.

Except for the first two chapters, the book is again organized according to clinical applications and not technology. When discussing a specific abnormality, the various echocardiographic examinations are integrated. An effort is made to inform the reader as to which echocardiographic studies are most appropriate for a given clinical problem.

Chapter 7 on Congenital Heart Disease has been written by my associate, Thomas Ryan. Tom has special training and interest in congenital heart disease. He runs an adult congenital heart disease clinic at Indiana University Medical Center. Tom is not a pediatrician, and the chapter is written from the perspective of caring primarily for adults and older children with congenital heart disease. For example, the topic of fetal echocardiography is only briefly mentioned. Tom and I would like to thank Randy Caldwell and Greg Ensing of the Department of Pediatrics at Indiana University School of Medicine for their assistance in providing some of the clinical material for the chapter on congenital heart disease.

As with the previous editions I am again indebted to the cardiac sonographers at the Indiana University Medical Center who performed the vast majority of the echocardiographic examinations from which many of the illustrations were obtained. These sonographers include Debbie Green Hess, Susan Swanson, Julie Kern, Patrick McClanahan, Jennifer Johnson, Melinda Huntley, Walter Klitsch, Amy Staab, and Cris Davis. I wish to thank the Illustration Department of Indiana University School of Medicine for again providing photographic assistance for this edition. Appreciation also goes to Donna Smith for typing many of the references. A special "thank you" is extended to my colleague, Doug Segar, who took the time to proofread this book. And lastly I wish to recognize the indispensible contribution of my secretary, Cheryl Childress. Cheryl again organized all of the references, typed the entire manuscript, and did much of the art work. This book would not be possible without her outstanding efforts.

Indianapolis, Indiana                    Harvey Feigenbaum

# Contents

## Chapter 1
### INSTRUMENTATION

## Chapter 2
### THE ECHOCARDIOGRAPHIC EXAMINATION

## Chapter 3
### ECHOCARDIOGRAPHIC EVALUATION OF CARDIAC CHAMBERS

## Chapter 4
## HEMODYNAMIC INFORMATION DERIVED FROM ECHOCARDIOGRAPHY

## Chapter 5
## ECHOCARDIOGRAPHIC FINDINGS WITH ALTERED ELECTRICAL ACTIVATION

## Chapter 6
## ACQUIRED VALVULAR HEART DISEASE

## Chapter 7
## CONGENITAL HEART DISEASE

# Chapter 8
## CORONARY ARTERY DISEASE

# Chapter 9
## DISEASES OF THE MYOCARDIUM

# Chapter 10
## PERICARDIAL DISEASE

# Chapter 11
## CARDIAC MASSES

## Chapter 12
### DISEASES OF THE AORTA

# 1

# Instrumentation

The instrumentation involved in echocardiography has become increasingly complex with the evolution from M-mode to two-dimensional echocardiography and with the introduction of various forms of Doppler, contrast, transesophageal, and now intravascular techniques. To understand completely the various aspects of the echocardiographic instrumentation, one should have a good background and understanding of physics and engineering. Fortunately, the empiric use of echocardiographic instruments does not absolutely require complete mastery of all the physical principles involved with echocardiographic information. Obviously, the more knowledgeable an individual is in these areas, the better his or her understanding in interpreting the clinical information.

Because this book is written principally for the clinician and sonographer using echocardiography for the examination of patients, an extensive description of the physics and engineering of echocardiography is beyond the scope of this text. Many of the physical principles have been simplified, and some important subtleties have been purposefully overlooked. Individuals who want a more detailed description are directed to the references at the end of this chapter.

## PHYSICAL PROPERTIES OF ULTRASOUND

By definition, ultrasound is sound having a frequency greater than 20,000 cycles per second,[1,2] that is, the sound is above the audible range. Actually, frequencies in the range of millions of cycles per second are used for medical diagnostic purposes. The principal advantages of high-frequency sound or ultrasound as a diagnostic tool are: (1) ultrasound can be directed in a beam, (2) it obeys the laws of reflection and refraction, and (3) it is reflected by objects of small size. The principal disadvantage of ultrasound is that it propagates poorly through a gaseous medium. The amount of ultrasound reflected depends on the acoustic mismatch. Thus, when the beam travels through tissue containing gases and solids, almost all of the sound is reflected and penetration is poor. A dense substance, such as bone, calcium, or metal, will also reflect almost all of the energy. Thus, lung, ribs, and prosthetic material offer distinct challenges for the echocardiographic examination. As a result, the ultrasound-producing element or transducer must have airless contact with the body during the examination of a patient. In addition, it is difficult to examine parts of the body that contain air.

When discussing any type of sound, one must understand the following terms: cycle, wavelength, velocity, and frequency.[3-5] Figure 1–1 demonstrates that a sound wave is a series of compressions and rarefactions. Such changes are frequently depicted as a sine wave with the peak of the hill representing the pressure maximum and the nadir of the valley the pressure minimum. The combination of one compression and one rarefaction represents one cycle, and the distance between the onset or peak compression of one cycle to the next is the wavelength. The velocity represents the speed at which sound waves travel through a particular medium. The frequency is the number of cycles in a given time. In other words, the velocity is equal to the frequency times the wavelength ($v = f \times \lambda$). Thus, frequency and wavelength are inversely related; the higher the frequency, the shorter the wavelength. The velocity at which sound travels through a medium depends on the density and elastic properties of that medium. For example, sound travels faster through a dense medium, such as a solid, than it does through a less dense substance, such as water. Velocity also depends on temperature. Because body temperature is relatively constant within a narrow range, however, changes in temperature are usually not an important factor in medical diagnostic work. The velocity of sound is fairly constant for human soft tissue: approximately 1,540 meters per second.[6] The difference in the velocity is significant if the sound passes through a solid structure such as bone.

How sound travels through a medium is frequently referred to as the acoustic impedance of that medium.[7] By definition, acoustic impedance is the density of the medium times the velocity that sound travels through that medium. For practical purposes, one may think of acoustic impedance in terms of the density of the medium. As a sound wave travels through a homogeneous medium, it essentially continues in a straight line. When the beam reaches an interface between two media with different acoustic impedances, it undergoes reflection and refraction. Figure 1–2 demonstrates the principles of reflection and refraction. As the sound wave travels through a relatively homogeneous medium (medium No. 1, Fig. 1–2), it is propagated essentially in a straight line. When it reaches an interface with a medium of different

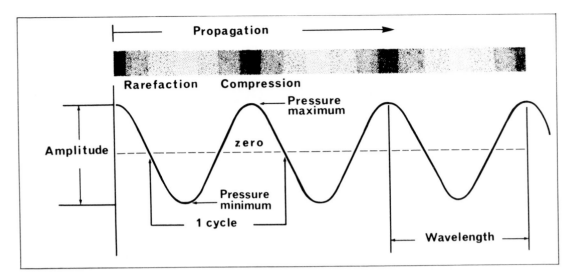

**Fig. 1–1.** A sound wave is a series of compressions and rarefactions. The combination of one compression and one rarefaction represents one cycle. The distance between the onset (peak compression) of one cycle to the next is the wavelength.

acoustic impedance or density (medium No. 2, Fig. 1–2), part of the beam is refracted and part is reflected. Almost all diagnostic ultrasound methods are based on the principle that ultrasound is reflected by an interface between media of different acoustic impedances. The amount of sound that is reflected depends on the degree of difference between the two media, i.e., the greater the acoustic mismatch, the greater the amount of sound reflected. For example, more sound is reflected from an interface between gaseous and solid media than from a liquid-solid interface.

When discussing ultrasonic echoes, it is important to distinguish between specular echoes and scattered echoes (Fig. 1–3). Specular echoes are produced by objects that are fairly large with respect to the wavelength and that present a relatively smooth surface to the ultrasonic beam. These objects regularly reflect the ultrasonic energy and are angle dependent. The angles of the echoes are predicted by the spatial orientation and the

shape of the reflecting object or interface. To date, echocardiography has been concerned principally with specular echoes originating from cardiac valves and walls.

With increasing use of cross-sectional or two-dimensional echocardiography as well as increasing interest in examining the myocardium has come a greater need for understanding scattered echoes. Such echoes originate from relatively small objects with irregular surfaces. The resultant echoes are reflected in multiple directions. Only a small percentage of the ultrasonic energy returns to the transducer. However small an amount, some energy does return to the transducer from scattered echoes. With specular echoes, if the angle is improper, virtually none of the ultrasonic energy returns to the transducer. Thus, although scattered echoes are difficult to record, they are ever present, are not angle dependent, and are important for visualizing objects essentially parallel to the ultrasonic beam, such as the lateral or medial walls of the left ventricle. With higher gain

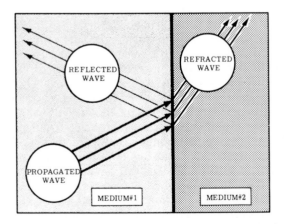

**Fig. 1–2.** Ultrasound is reflected and refracted by an interface between two media of different acoustic impedance.

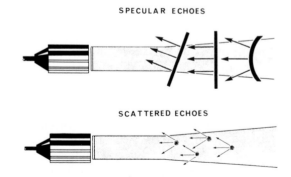

**Fig. 1–3.** Specular echoes originate from relatively large, strongly reflective, regularly shaped objects with smooth surfaces and are relatively intense and angle dependent. Scattered echoes originate from small, weakly reflective, irregularly shaped objects and are less angle dependent and less intense.

settings, higher frequency transducers, and better signal-to-noise ratio of instruments, echocardiography will be increasingly concerned with recording scattered echoes.

Whether the ultrasound is reflected by an interface also depends on the relative sizes of the mismatched media and the wavelength. If a solid object is submerged in water, whether the ultrasound is reflected from that object depends on the size of the solid object with respect to the wavelength of the ultrasound. The total thickness presented to the ultrasonic beam must be at least one fourth the wavelength of the ultrasound. Ultrasound having a higher frequency or a shorter wavelength can reflect sound from smaller objects. Thus, a higher frequency ultrasonic beam has greater resolving power, which is the ability to visualize objects or interfaces that are close to each other.[8] Echocardiography commonly uses ultrasound with a frequency of approximately 2,000,000 cycles per second or 2 megahertz (MHz). (Hertz or Hz is another term for cycles per second.) Sound with a frequency of 2 MHz permits the recording of distinct echoes from interfaces that are approximately 1 mm apart. Because high-frequency ultrasound is reflected by many small interfaces, a large percentage of the ultrasonic energy is reflected by these interfaces, and less energy is available to penetrate deeply into the body. Thus, penetration of the ultrasonic beam decreases as frequency increases.[1] Sonic absorption and scattering, which occurs even in a homogeneous medium, also determine how well ultrasound penetrates.[9] Again, ultrasound with higher frequencies has greater absorption and scattering, and thus poorer penetration. Naturally, the less homogeneous the medium, the more difficult it is for the ultrasound to penetrate, because reflection and refraction are important factors in diminishing the intensity of the beam as it travels through any nonhomogeneous medium.

The loss of ultrasound as it traverses a medium is known as attenuation, which is a combination of absorption and scattering. A term used to express the amount of absorption and attenuation of ultrasound in tissue is the "half-value layer,"[6] or "half-power distance."[4] These terms refer to the distance that ultrasound will travel in a particular tissue before its energy or amplitude is attenuated to half its original value. Table 1–1 gives the half-power distances for tissues and substances important in echocardiography. These values obviously depend on the frequency, and those listed in Table 1–1 are for a frequency of 2 MHz. As noted in this table, ultrasound can travel 380 cm in water before its power decreases to half its original value. The loss of power when ultrasound travels through blood, although considerably greater, is still relatively low considering the distances involved in echocardiography. As expected, the attenuation is greater for soft tissue and even higher for muscle. Thus, it is not surprising that a thick muscular chest wall would offer a significant obstacle to the transmission of ultrasound. Nonmuscular soft tissue, such as fat, has a longer half-power distance than muscle and is not quite as attenuating. The half-power distance for bone is still less than for muscle, which documents why

**Table 1–1**
Half-power Distances for Tissues and Substances Important in Echocardiography

| Material | Half-power Distance (CM) |
|---|---|
| Water | 380 |
| Blood | 15 |
| Soft tissue (except muscle) | 5 to 1 |
| Muscle | 1 to 0.6 |
| Bone | 0.7 to 0.2 |
| Air | 0.08 |
| Lung | 0.05 |

bone is such a barrier to ultrasound. Cartilage is not listed, but its attenuating properties are clearly less than those of bone. Air and lung have extremely short half-power distances and represent severe obstacles to the transmission of ultrasound.

The absorption or attenuation of ultrasound need not always be uniform throughout the recording.[10] A localized object that reflects or attenuates sound may impede the transmission of ultrasound only in that area. Such an object may produce an "acoustic shadow." Because little ultrasonic energy passes through this particular object, structures distant to or behind the "shadowing" object may not be recorded echographically. Acoustic shadowing is an important parameter in other areas of diagnostic ultrasound, especially in examinations of the abdomen or breast. This phenomenon occurs in echocardiography when examining dense structures, such as prosthetic valves or calcifications.

## TRANSDUCERS AND THE PRODUCTION OF ULTRASOUND BEAMS

The use of ultrasound became practical with the development of piezoelectric transducers.[11] Piezoelectric means "pressure-electric." Piezoelectric substances change shape under the influence of an electrical field;[3] quartz was one of the first elements noted to have this property. If one impresses an electrical current through a quartz crystal (Fig. 1–4), the shape of the crystal varies with the polarity. As the crystal expands and contracts, it produces compressions and rarefactions or sound waves. The reverse is also true; when the crystal is struck by a sound wave, it produces an electrical impulse. Such a piezoelectric element is the primary component of an ultrasonic transducer. Commercial transducers use ceramics, such as barium titanate or lead zirconate titanate, as the piezoelectric element. Figure 1–5 is a diagram of the essential components of a transducer showing the piezoelectric element with electrodes connected to an electrical source on both sides. Behind the piezoelectric element is some backing material, which absorbs sound energy directed backward and improves the shape of the forward energy.

Recent transducer design has made the thickness of the piezoelectric element one fourth the inherent wave-

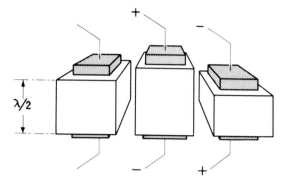

**Fig. 1–4.** Sketch of a crystal that has piezoelectric properties. The crystal changes shape as the surrounding electrical field is reversed. The wavelength (λ) of the emitted ultrasound is a function in the size of the crystal.

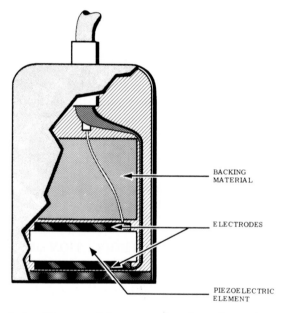

BACKING
MATERIAL

ELECTRODES

PIEZOELECTRIC
ELEMENT

**Fig. 1–5.** The essential components of an ultrasonic transducer.

length of the transmitted frequency. Designing the transducer in this fashion apparently has improved significantly the efficiency and sensitivity of the transducer. Transducer design is an evolving technology and is responsible for much of the image quality improvement in current instruments.

It is useful to have an understanding of the nature of the ultrasonic beam generated by the transducer. If one used a single small-element transducer, the ultrasonic waves would radiate from that transducer much as would the ripples created by a pebble dropped into water (Fig. 1–6). If one were to use a series of multiple small elements to produce the ultrasonic beam, then the individual curved waves or "ripples" would combine to form a linear wave front moving perpendicularly from the linearly arranged elements. Thus, if multiple small elements that fire simultaneously are used, a unidirectional ultrasonic beam can be generated. If a single large element is used, an infinite number of small elements would essentially result. The individual wave fronts form a compact linear wave front that moves perpendicularly away from the face of the transducer (see Fig. 1–6).

The principal sound waves produced by a transducer are longitudinal. These waves, which occur primarily in fluid, move parallel to the direction of the propagation of the sound waves. Other waves, such as sheer waves, move perpendicular to the propagation; however, these waves occur primarily in such solids as bone and play a relatively minor role in echocardiography. A more important secondary wave front presents the problem of "side lobes." As noted in Figure 1–6, the ultrasonic beam comprises multiple, circular wavelets that originate from each element, especially from the edges, and move in directions different from those of the principal longitudinal wave. This problem is greatest with a single small element and is least prominent with a single large element. Partially because of the increased number of edges, an ultrasonic beam generated by multiple small elements has more extraneous ultrasonic beams or side lobes than one formed from a single large element. These side lobes, which can produce artifactual information, will be discussed later in this chapter.

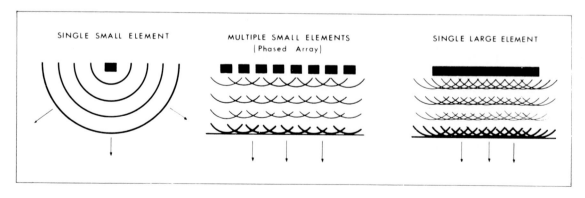

**Fig. 1–6.** Diagram demonstrating how longitudinal ultrasonic wave fronts are produced. The ultrasonic wavelets travel in a circular fashion from a single small element. With either multiple element or single large element transducer, the circular wavelets combine to produce a longitudinal wave front directed away from the face of the transducer.

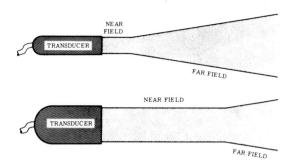

**Fig. 1–7.** Diagram demonstrating the influence of transducer size on the ultrasonic beam. The near field is shorter and divergence considerably greater when the transducer is smaller.

The series of longitudinal waves constitutes the ultrasonic beam. As the beam propagates, it remains essentially parallel for a given distance and then begins to diverge (see Fig. 1–7). That part of the beam closest to the transducer and parallel to it is known as the near field or Fresnel zone. When the beam begins to diverge, it is called the far field or Fraunhofer zone. The diagnostic use of ultrasound works best when the objects being examined are located in the near field because the beam is more parallel and the reflecting interfaces are more perpendicular to the transducer. One can detect many interfaces in the far field, although this becomes progressively more difficult the farther one goes into the far field.

The length of the near field (l) is a function of the radius of the transducer (r) and the wavelength (λ) and has been calculated as equal to the square of the radius divided by the wavelength $\left(1 = \dfrac{r^2}{\lambda}\right).$[12] Thus, to lengthen

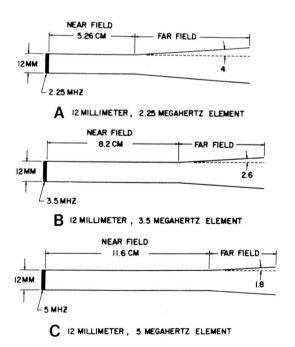

**A** 12 MILLIMETER, 2.25 MEGAHERTZ ELEMENT

**B** 12 MILLIMETER, 3.5 MEGAHERTZ ELEMENT

**C** 12 MILLIMETER, 5 MEGAHERTZ ELEMENT

**Fig. 1–8.** The effect of transducer frequency on the near field. Higher frequency transducers have longer near fields.

the near field, one would either decrease the wavelength or increase the size of the transducer. Figure 1–7 illustrates the effect of transducer size, and Figure 1–8 the effect of frequency on the length of the near field. Doubling the size of the transducer quadruples the near field (see Fig. 1–7). With a 12-mm diameter transducer, a 2.25-MHz transducer has a near field of 5.26 cm (see Fig. 1–8). A 3.5-MHz transducer with a 12-mm diameter has a near field of 8.2 cm. Increasing the frequency to 5 MHz increases the near field to 11.6 cm (see Fig. 1–8).

One can decrease the amount of diversion in the far field by using a focused transducer; such focusing is done by placing an acoustic lens on the surface of the transducer or by altering the curvature of the transducer itself. Using a lens with a concave surface or a transducer with a concave face, one brings the ultrasonic beam to a narrow zone at a predetermined distance from the transducer (Fig. 1–9). Narrowing the ultrasonic beam increases its intensity at the focal zone where the beam is narrowest and decreases the amount of divergence of the sound in the far field.

It is also possible to focus the ultrasonic beam electronically. By use of a transducer made up of multiple small elements, the wave front can be shaped according to the timing of the individual elements. Figure 1–10 shows a transducer composed of multiple small elements that are individually fired so that the ultrasonic beam is curved. By firing the outside elements, 1 and 7, first, then elements 2 and 6, 3 and 5, and 4, one can shape the ultrasonic beam so that it converges much as the beam would converge when an acoustic lens is used. The curve can be varied according to when the individual elements are fired, and thus the location of the focal zone can be changed. One can have a fixed-focus electronic beam or one can change the focal zone rapidly and generate a dynamically focused ultrasonic beam.[8,13,14,15] Such a transducer, which consists of multiple small elements fired individually in a controlled manner (in order to manipulate the ultrasonic beam), is known as a phased array transducer.

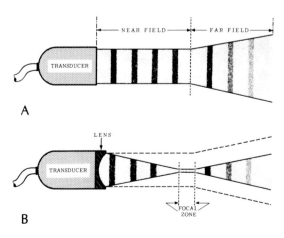

**Fig. 1–9.** Diagrams of the ultrasonic beam emitted by an unfocused (*A*) and a focused (*B*) transducer.

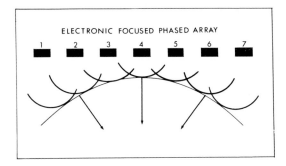

ELECTRONIC FOCUSED PHASED ARRAY

1    2    3    4    5    6    7

**Fig. 1–10.** Diagram demonstrating how a phased array transducer can focus the ultrasonic beam. By appropriate timing of the individual elements, the leading edges of the wavelets can produce a concentrically curved wave front so that the resultant ultrasonic beam focuses at a given point from the transducer.

It should be recognized that the ultrasonic beam is three-dimensional and not two-dimensional. Figure 1–11 illustrates the three-dimensional nature of the ultrasonic beam. When a transducer with a single, circular crystal is used, the beam is cylindric and is circular in cross-section. An ultrasonic beam generated by a phased array transducer made up of multiple, rectangular small elements produces an ultrasonic beam with a rectangular cross-section. The dimensions of the ultrasonic beam have been divided into axial (i.e., parallel to the direction of the ultrasonic beam) and lateral (i.e., perpendicular) to the ultrasonic beam. (Occasionally, axial is referred to as "linear" or "longitudinal" and lateral as "azimuthal."[5] In this text, the more common terms axial and lateral are used.) Because of the three-dimensional nature of the beam, the lateral dimension has been subdivided into y axis (vertical dimension) and x axis (horizontal dimension). With a single, circular crystal,

the x and y axes are equal; with a phased array rectangular beam, however, the x and y axes are frequently dissimilar.[16] Acoustic focusing using a lens or shaping of the ultrasonic element will change the x and y axes equally (Fig. 1–12A). Electronic focusing using the phased array principle and a transducer with multiple, rectangular elements decreases the x axis without influencing the y axis (see Fig. 1–12B and C).[17] A dynamically focused beam has a long focal zone (see Fig. 1–12C).[18] If the phased array elements were circles or a series of rings rather than a series of long, thin elements, then electronic focusing would decrease the y as well as the x axis (Fig. 1–12D). Such a phased array system is known as annular phased array.[19–22] The major feature of annular phased array is a reduction in the thickness or elevation of the two-dimensional or tomographic slice.

The ultrasonic beam is not absolute. The beam is greater in amplitude or intensity in the center, with decreasing intensity toward the edges of the beam (Fig. 1–13). Thus, one must recognize the relative nature of beam width or sound intensity profile. When the shape of the ultrasonic beam is diagrammed, one usually draws the edge of the beam to the half-value limit of the beam plot. Figure 1–14, which shows a transaxial beam plot, illustrates the relative nature of the beam width. At its

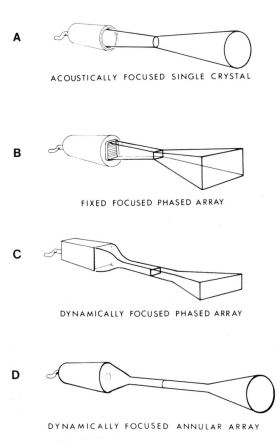

A

ACOUSTICALLY FOCUSED SINGLE CRYSTAL

B

FIXED FOCUSED PHASED ARRAY

C

DYNAMICALLY FOCUSED PHASED ARRAY

D

DYNAMICALLY FOCUSED ANNULAR ARRAY

**Fig. 1–12.** Diagram demonstrating the ultrasonic beams emitted by an acoustically focused single-crystal transducer (A), a fixed-focused phased array transducer (B), a dynamically focused phased array transducer (C), and a dynamically focused annular array transducer (D).

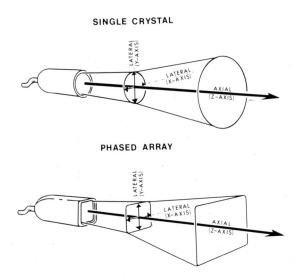

SINGLE CRYSTAL

LATERAL (Y-AXIS)
LATERAL (X-AXIS)
AXIAL (Z-AXIS)

PHASED ARRAY

LATERAL (Y-AXIS)
LATERAL (X-AXIS)
AXIAL (Z-AXIS)

**Fig. 1–11.** Three-dimensional presentation of the ultrasonic beam from a circular single-crystal transducer and from a phased array transducer demonstrating the various beam axes.

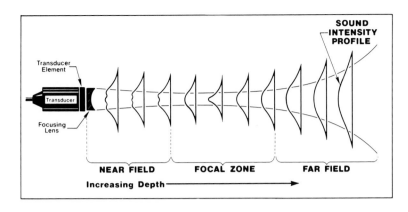

**Fig. 1–13.** The sound intensity profile of an acoustically focused transducer.

peak intensity, the beam may only be 1 mm wide. The beam width at its weakest intensity, however, is more than 12 mm wide. It is customary to measure the beam width at its half amplitude or intensity. In this particular example, the beam width of this ultrasonic beam would be 5.2 mm. It should be apparent that if one used a higher gain setting on the echograph, the weaker portion of the ultrasonic beam would be recorded and the beam width would be larger. Conversely, if one used a low gain setting and only the most intense portion of the ultrasonic beam were recorded, then the beam width would be narrowed. Understanding beam width is important because it is the cause for many potential artifacts in echocardiography.

## PRINCIPLES OF M-MODE AND TWO-DIMENSIONAL ECHOCARDIOGRAPHY

The instrument used to create an image using ultrasound is known as an echograph. Figure 1–15 shows a block diagram of an echograph. The essential components include the transducer, which is in contact with the tissue being examined and which both sends and receives the ultrasound. The transmitter regulates the sending of the ultrasound by the transducer by way of a timer that controls the duration and frequency of the ultrasonic pulses emitted by the transducer. The transducer converts the returning echoes to electrical impul-

**Instrumentation**

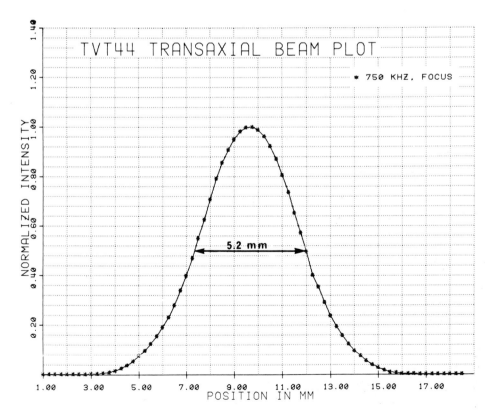

**Fig. 1–14.** Transaxial beam plot. The beam width or lateral resolution is a function of the intensity of the ultrasonic beam. The beam width is commonly measured at the half-intensity level.

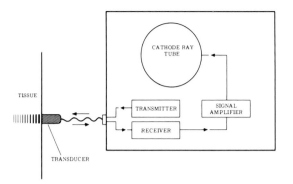

**Fig. 1–15.** Block diagram of the components of an ultrasonic echograph.

ses, which then go to the receiver and the signal amplifier. The returning echoes or impulses are processed so that they can be displayed on the cathode ray tube or oscilloscope.

Figure 1–16 demonstrates how one may use ultrasound to obtain an image of an object. Such acoustic imaging, sometimes called "echo ranging," depends primarily on the property of reflection together with pulsing of the ultrasonic beam.[23] The electric energy is fed intermittently into the transducer so that the piezoelectric

element sends out ultrasound for brief periods of time. The duration of each ultrasonic impulse, which may be as short as one microsecond, influences the shape of the ultrasonic pulse. Following the emission or burst of ultrasound, the transducer becomes a receiver waiting to record any reflected ultrasound waves or echoes. Following a relatively long period, another burst of ultrasound is emitted and the cycle is repeated. The rate with which the bursts of ultrasonic energy are emitted is the pulse repetition rate or pulse repetition frequency of the echograph. Commercial diagnostic echographs have repetition rates between 200 and 5000/sec. The M-mode examination has repetition rates of approximately 1000 to 2000/sec, whereas two-dimensional studies require repetition rates between 3000[24,25] and 5000/sec. Each burst of pulsed ultrasound may last only 1 to 2 μsec. Thus, the transducer functions as a receiver nearly 99% of the time. The commercial diagnostic echographs are extremely sensitive receivers and can detect a signal even when less than 1% of the ultrasonic energy is reflected.

In Figure 1–16, a transducer placed on the side of a beaker of water sends out short bursts of ultrasound at a given frequency. These bursts of ultrasound travel through the homogeneous water and are reflected by the interface between the water and the far side of the beaker. The reflected ultrasound or echo then retraces

## Instrumentation

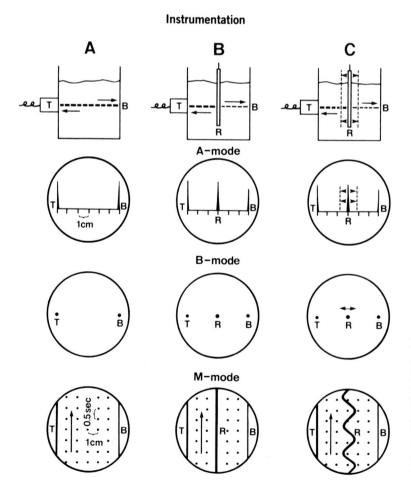

**Fig. 1–16.** Diagrams illustrating the principles of acoustic imaging using pulsed, reflected ultrasound (see text for details). T = transducer; B = beaker; R = rod. (From Feigenbaum, H. and Zaky, A.: Use of diagnostic ultrasound in clinical cardiology. J. Indiana State Med. Assoc., *59:* 140, 1966.)

its original path and strikes the transducer, which is now functioning as a receiver. An electrical signal is created as the sound hits the piezoelectric element and is registered on the oscilloscope of the echograph. If one knows the velocity of sound traveling through the medium being examined as well as the time it takes for the ultrasound to leave the transducer, strike the interface, and return as an echo, then calculating the distance of the reflecting interface from the transducer is simple. By calibrating the echograph for the velocity of sound of the medium being examined, time may be converted to distance automatically. Thus, instead of indicating how long it takes for a burst of ultrasound to leave the transducer and to return as an echo, the electrical signal generated by the returning echo is actually displayed on the oscilloscope of the echograph at a certain distance from the transducer. In this particular example (see Fig. 1–16A), the reflecting interface or the side of the beaker (B) is indicated as being 6.0 cm away from the transducer. A built-in electrical artifact (T) is used to indicate the position of the transducer.

If a rod (R, Fig. 1–16B) is placed in the center of the beaker, the ultrasound strikes the rod first. Since the rod is closer to the transducer than to the far side of the beaker, the echo reflected from this interface reaches the transducer earlier than it would from the far side of the beaker. The shorter time is converted to a shorter distance, and the echo from the rod is displayed on the oscilloscope as being only 3.0 cm from the transducer. Some ultrasonic energy will continue to move past the rod, strike the far side of the beaker, and return to the transducer as it did when the rod was absent. Thus, on the oscilloscope, the echo from the rod is indicated as being 3.0 cm from the transducer, and the echo from the far side of the beaker is 6.0 cm from the transducer.

If the rod is moving, its distance from the transducer is constantly changing (see Fig. 1–16C). When the first burst of ultrasonic energy hits the rod, it may be 4.0 cm from the transducer. The next burst may be 3.0 cm away, and the next 2.0 cm away. Thus, the oscilloscope shows that the position of the rod with respect to the transducer is constantly changing. How well this motion is visualized depends in part on the repetition rate or sampling rate of the echograph. With a repetition rate of approximately 1000/sec, this echo motion is almost continuous.

If the interface from which the echo is derived is constantly moving (see Fig. 1–16C), then the echo position changes constantly with reference to the transducer. The echo signal moves back and forth on the face of the oscilloscope. The motion could be recorded by filming or videotaping the oscilloscopic image. Another technique for displaying echo motion involves the use of intensity modulation. This type of modification converts the amplitude of the echo to intensity; the signal is converted from a spike (see Fig. 1–16, A-mode) to a dot (see Fig. 1–16, B-mode). Within limits, the taller the echo, the brighter the dot. This presentation is known as B-mode, the B standing for brightness. Having converted the signal to a dot, one now has another dimension available for the recording. Since the heart is a moving object,

one can record the motion by introducing time as the second dimension. For example, if the tracing is swept from bottom to top, as in the bottom diagram of Figure 1–16C, a wavy line is inscribed if the rod or interface is moving. If the object is stationary (bottom tracing, Fig. 1–16B), a straight line is inscribed. For calibration, one may use a grid or a series of dots that are 1 cm apart in one axis and 0.5 sec apart in the other. Because all interfaces of the heart constantly move, this type of display was the backbone of echocardiography for many years.

The term adopted for this type of echo presentation is "M-mode." M stands for motion. "Time motion" or TM is another name given to this presentation. The standard display that presents the echo as a spike is known as "A-mode." The A indicates the amplitude of the echo. The M-mode presentation may be recorded by taking a Polaroid photograph of the cathode ray tube. Such a photograph would be a time exposure as the intensity-modulated dots sweep from bottom to top to left to right across the oscilloscope. Most early commercial echographs had the oscilloscopic image sweep from bottom to top for the convenience of the A-mode presentation and Polaroid photography. Since an electrocardiographic tracing is usually displayed on the oscilloscope, and since the electrocardiogram is read from left to right rather than from bottom to top, one usually displays the echocardiogram as moving from left to right.

Figure 1–17 shows how the echocardiographic system can record an M-mode tracing of the heart. In this particular examination, the ultrasonic beam is directed at the heart in the vicinity of the left ventricular cavity. A small portion of the right ventricular cavity is also intersected by the ultrasonic beam. The actual M-mode recording was made on a strip chart recorder. As would be expected, the chest wall structures are not moving with cardiac motion and are exhibited as a series of straight lines. The echoes from the anterior right ventricular wall (ARV) are not visualized clearly and are a fuzzy band of echoes that are thicker in systole than in diastole. The relatively echo-free space between the right ventricular echo (ARV) and the right side of the interventricular septum (RS) is a segment of the right ventricular cavity transected by the ultrasonic beam. The interventricular septum (RS and LS) is represented by the band of echoes running through the middle of the tracing. The left side of the septum (LS) moves downward in systole and upward in diastole. The next major group of echoes originates from the posterior left ventricular wall with the endocardial (EN) echo having a greater amplitude during systole than the epicardial (EP) echo. The space between the two ventricular wall echoes represents the myocardium. The relatively echo-free space between the left side of the septum (LS) and the posterior left ventricular endocardium (EN) is the cavity of the left ventricle. Within the cavity, echoes from the mitral valve apparatus are visible occasionally.

If the spatial orientation of the transducer is tracked electronically, one could obtain a spatially oriented M-mode examination.[25–27] Spatial tracking of the ultrasonic beam is used more commonly to create a spatially

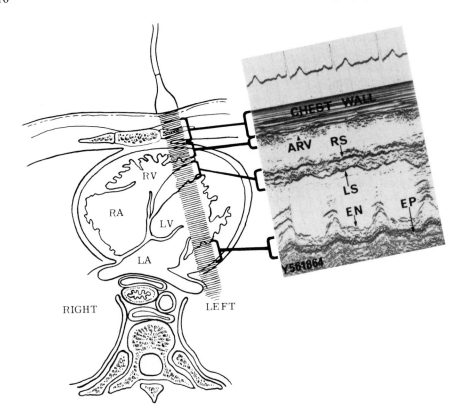

**Fig. 1–17.** Diagram and echocardiogram illustrating how echocardiography can obtain an "ice-pick" or one-dimensional view of the heart through the right and left ventricles. ARV = anterior right ventricular wall; RS = right septum; LS = left septum; EN = posterior left ventricular endocardium; EP = posterior left ventricular epicardium; RA = right atrium; RV = right ventricle; LV = left ventricle; LA = left atrium.

oriented B-mode or cross-sectional examination. Figure 1–18 diagrams how a spatially oriented B-mode scan can provide a cross-sectional or two-dimensional image of an object. When the ultrasonic transducer is close to the top of the beaker, it traverses the circular object at the point at which the walls are relatively close together (see Fig. 1–18A). As the transducer moves toward the bottom of the beaker, the beam transects the center of the circular object (see Fig. 1–18B). Now the two B-mode echoes from the walls are farther apart and in the center of the oscilloscope. Moving the transducer closer

to the bottom of the beaker causes the ultrasonic beam to again traverse the object at the point at which the walls are closer together (see Fig. 1–18C). The oscilloscope shows two B-mode dots closer together and nearer the bottom of the transducer. In combination, these dots reveal the shape and size of the object being examined (see Fig. 1–18D). If the object is motionless, one may take as much time as desired to move or scan the ultrasonic beam across the object. If the object is moving, however, then one should move the ultrasonic beam as rapidly as possible. A rapid B-mode scan is also

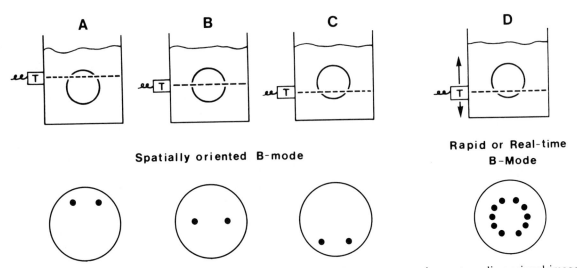

**Fig. 1–18.** Diagrams demonstrating how a spatially oriented B-mode scan can produce a two-dimensional image.

known as a "real-time" scan. A real-time B-mode scan of the heart is commonly called "cross-sectional" or "two-dimensional" echocardiography.

Unfortunately, the terminology for real-time B-mode scanning of the heart is confusing. The most popular terms are "cross-sectional" or "two-dimensional" echocardiography, or just "real-time" echocardiography. Many other terms, however, have been used in the literature. One of the first investigators called the technique "ultrasonic cinematography."[28] This particular technique used a mirror system on a rotating ultrasonic transducer in a water tank. Similar techniques have been proposed.[29] Other terms that have been used include "cine ultrasound cardiography,"[30] "ultrasonic tomography,"[31] "ultrasonocardiotomography,"[32] "cardiac ultrasonography,"[33] and "ultrasonic cardiokymography,"[26] The term "two-dimensional echocardiography" has been formally adopted by the American Society of Echocardiography. In keeping with an effort to standardize terminology, I use the term two-dimensional echocardiography in this text and only occasionally use cross-sectional echocardiography.

Ultrasonic scans can be obtained in various ways. Figure 1–19 demonstrates some types of scans available in medical diagnostic work. Figure 1–18 exemplifies a linear scan. Although linear scans of the heart are being done, sector scans are more popular. The principal advantage of a sector scan is that it functions better within the confines of the limited echocardiographic window that is frequently available for examining the heart.

Figure 1–20 compares the standard M-mode echocardiographic examination with a real-time two-dimen-

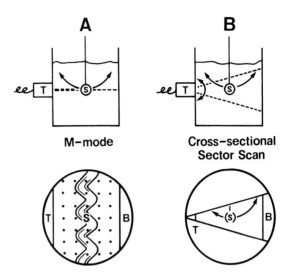

**Fig. 1–20.** Diagram comparing M-mode and cross-sectional sector scan of a spherical object moving as a pendulum in a beaker of water. (From Feigenbaum, H.: Echocardiography. *In* Heart Diseases. Edited by E. Braunwald. Philadelphia, W.B. Saunders Co., 1980.)

sional sector scan. The object in question is a sphere or ball moving as a pendulum within a beaker of water. When one is using the M-mode examination (see Fig. 1–20A), the oscilloscope shows a series of wavy lines principally from the leading and trailing edges of the sphere. Because of the beam width, one might see multiple secondary, less intense echoes from the leading and

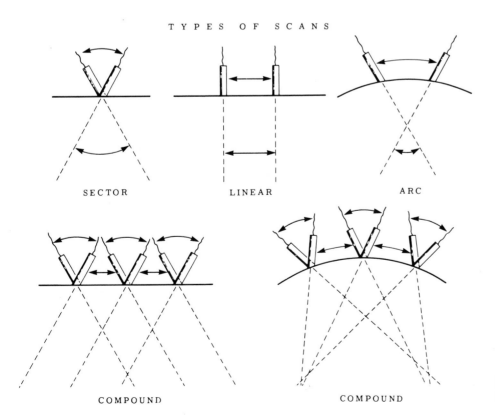

**Fig. 1–19.** Various types of scanning maneuvers.

trailing edges. The M-mode examination gives an excellent evaluation of the diameter of the object and the amount of motion in the axial direction. The examiner would have no appreciation of motion in the lateral direction (perpendicular to the ultrasonic beam) and would not understand the shape of the object being examined. From the M-mode examination, one could say that an object approximately 1 cm in diameter was moving approximately 1 cm in the axial direction.

With a cross-sectional or two-dimensional scan, the examiner would not appreciate that the object was spherical. One might not be able to see the entire circle of the object because part of the walls might be parallel to the ultrasonic beam and there would be echo dropout. It would be obvious, however, that the object was spherical and not rectangular. In addition, one could appreciate that the object was moving in an arc rather than in a straight line. Thus, the two-dimensional examination would provide the added information of lateral motion and shape.

There are two types of real-time two-dimensional scanners: mechanical and electronic (Fig. 1–21). Mechanical scanners move the ultrasonic beam by way of an electric motor, whereas electronic systems steer the ultrasonic beam electronically. The mechanical systems may use a probe with an oscillating transducer whereby the active element moves through a given angle.[24,25,32] A mechanical rotating transducer uses a series of active elements, usually three or four, mounted in a wheel located in a plastic housing filled with liquid. The principal advantage of the rotating transducer is that the active element is closer to the surface of the housing and theo-

retically can transmit and receive the ultrasonic beam with less interference from the ribs (see Fig. 1–21). The main advantages of the oscillating transducer are that only one ultrasonic element is required and the transducer is significantly less expensive. The oscillating transducer is also compatible with annular array transducers.

Another mechanical system that has played only a small role in echocardiography uses a mirror system.[28,29] One of the first real-time two-dimensional instruments used a rotating transducer that reflected the beam off of a parabolic mirror. One thus obtained a linear scan. A more novel mirror system was devised for echocardiography using a series of rotating transducers and a semitransparent mirror. This approach had some interesting theoretic advantages. In minimized the exit aperture because the apex of the sector beam actually was produced below the rib level. Using multiple transducers also offered some possibilities with regard to M-mode, two-dimensional, and Doppler examinations. Despite these advantages, thus far, this particular approach has not been commercially successful and is not currently available.

There are two basic electronic real-time scanners. The first such scanner uses a series of small elements that are fired sequentially (Fig. 1–22). The sequential firing of the transducers essentially moves the ultrasonic beam linearly.[34–37] This device, known as a multi-element linear array transducer, was probably the first commercially available, practical, real-time cardiac scanner and was responsible for much of the enthusiasm for two-dimensional echocardiography. Many improvements in this instrument have occurred. The beam can be improved by electronic focusing and by firing multiple elements for each ultrasonic line of information. Real-time linear array scanners are now popular in abdominal, pe-

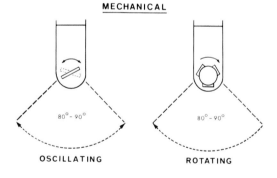

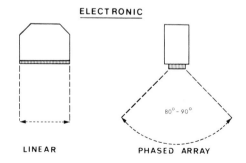

**Fig. 1–21.** Various types of real-time scanners.

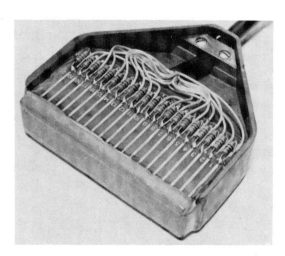

**Fig. 1–22.** Multi-element linear array transducer that provides an electronic scan of the heart. This particular probe consists of 20 piezoelectric elements. (From Bom, N.N., et al.: Multi-scan echocardiography. I, Technical description. *Circulation,* *48*:1066, 1973, by permission of the American Heart Association, Inc.)

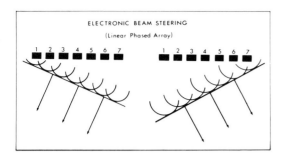

**Fig. 1–23.** Principles of electronic beam steering using linear phased array. By controlling the firing of the individual elements, one can alter the direction or the angle of wave front.

ripheral vascular, and small parts ultrasound examinations. For cardiac examinations, however, these scanners have the principal disadvantage of requiring a fairly large acoustic window. The large probe must overlie ribs and cannot be angled easily in the plane of the scan axis.

The most popular electronic real-time scanners use the phased array principle.[13–17] This type of scanner uses a multi-element transducer to create a single ultrasonic beam, the direction of which can be altered by controlling the timing when each element is fired. As noted in Figure 1–10, a multi-element transducer has the capability of electronic focusing by firing the individual elements so that a curved or focused wave front is formed. A similar technique can be used to change the direction of the angle of the wave front with a phased array system (Fig. 1–23). In this example, the ultrasonic wave front created by the multi-element, phased array transducer can be directed at a given angle and direction by firing each element individually, that is, elements one, two, three, four, and so on. Thus, the leading edge of the wave front from the first transducer is farther away from the face of the probe than is that part of the wave front contributed by firing the seventh element. The resultant ultrasonic beam moves perpendicularly to the wave front. Changing the sequence of the firing of each element alters the direction of the wave front. Thus, by using a computer or microprocessor to control the firing of each element, it is possible to control the direction of the ultrasonic beam rapidly and randomly.

An important factor in scanning the heart is the relationship of the surface area and shape of that part of the transducer in contact with the patient. This feature is called the aperture or footprint of the transducer. The relationship of the aperture and the available echocardiographic window can be critical in a given patient. In this regard, the rotating mechanical transducer has a slight advantage over the oscillating mechanical transducer (see Fig. 1–21). The phased array transducer theoretically has an advantage over both mechanical systems. If the phased array transducer is small enough to fit within the intercostal spaces, the aperture can be quite small, with minimum interference from the ribs. It must be recognized, however, that all the elements of the phased array transducer must be in contact with the skin to obtain a proper scan. If the entire face of the

transducer is not in contact or if part of it is overlying the rib, then greater distortion may occur with the phased array than with the mechanical approach. The apertures of some phased array transducers are larger than with mechanical systems.

As already discussed, phased array systems have the advantage of electronically focusing the beam, either at some fixed distance or dynamically to give a relatively long focal zone (see Fig. 1–12C). Electronic focusing not only permits shaping of the beam, but also one can focus the received echoes by controlling the timing in a manner opposite from that used in creating the focused beam. Thus, phased array systems can focus the beam in the y axis by focusing the transmitted beam and the returning echoes.

Mechanical sector scanners usually do not have electronic focusing. Annular array transducers, however, can electronically focus the beam in the x axis as well as in the y axis (Fig. 1–12D). It would be extremely difficult, if not impossible, for current phased array systems to use annular phased array transducers because of the complexity in electronically steering an annular array beam. Moving the annular array transducer mechanically would be far easier.

Side lobes are discussed in more detail later. This potential artifact presents a greater problem with phased array systems than it does with mechanical scanners.

Some advantages to using higher frequency transducers are obvious. The most immediate need for such high-frequency systems is in examinations of small children or infants. The resolution is significantly better and, as already noted, so is the beam shape. Because of the manner in which phasing is accomplished to steer the ultrasonic beam, creating phased array transducers in excess of 5.0 MHz is difficult and only recently has been commercially available.

The computer, or microprocessor, necessary for controlling the sequence of firing of phased array systems adds to the physical bulk of the system. As a result, phased array echocardiographs have traditionally been larger than mechanical systems. Significant progress has occurred in miniaturizing the electronics necessary for phased array technology. Thus, the current instruments are considerably smaller and more portable than earlier models. They are still larger, however, than the mechanical systems, which have also become smaller. In fact, some mechanical systems are truly portable; they can fit in a large suitcase and can be hand carried. Thus, cost and portability will remain an advantage of the mechanical system for some time.

Another advantage of the phased array system is that the active elements are in direct contact with the surface of the skin, and the ultrasonic beam does not have to travel through a liquid medium and a plastic housing. Thus, attenuation of the beam should be minimal. In addition, the plastic housing offers the opportunity for reverberation artifacts.

Electronic and mechanical sector scanners have several minor disadvantages. One disadvantage of the phased array system is that the ultrasonic beam varies somewhat with the angle. The beam profile is not exactly the same with the beam perpendicular to the face of the transducer as when it is 45° from the center. To what extent this difference alters the image has not been demonstrated. A minor disadvantage of the mechanical system is that the transducer is constantly moving and is therefore in a slightly different location when it sends and receives a given burst of ultrasound. The angle of the transducer changes slightly when the returning echoes hit the transducer. The importance of this difference is probably minor and does not significantly alter the image.

## VARIABLES INVOLVED IN REAL-TIME SECTOR SCANNING

To understand the nature of real-time sector scanning, one must appreciate the variables involved in obtaining such images. One must remember that we are creating images by relatively slow-moving means—with sound. Although two-dimensional echocardiograms are similar to angiograms or to photographs, one does not use fast-moving energy sources such as x rays or light to obtain these images. The speed of sound is considerably slower. Thus, the limiting factor is the speed of sound in soft tissue, and compromises must be made when generating a real-time two-dimensional image.

The variables and compromises to consider are the depth of the examination desired, the line density, the pulse repetition frequency, the angle of the sweep, and the sweep or frame rate. Because the terms sweep, field, and frame are frequently used interchangeably, they can be confusing. A sweep indicates the movement of the ultrasonic beam through the desired angle. Field and frame usually refer to the television system on which most of these recordings are made. Television is made up of fields, each of which is one-sixtieth of a second. Two fields are interlaced; the lines are laid down between each other to improve line density. Two interlaced $\frac{1}{60}$-sec "fields" produce one $\frac{1}{30}$-sec "frame." Thus, if the sector scanner is sweeping at a rate of 60 times/sec, then each sweep is comparable to a single field, and two sweeps can be interlaced to produce one television frame. The frame rate, therefore, would be 30/sec, whereas the field or sweep rate would be 60/sec.

Table 1–2 presents some examples of how these variables interact in creating a real-time cross-sectional image. If the examination is to include 20 cm of depth, then each ultrasonic line must travel 40 cm as the impulse leaves the transducer and returns as an echo. Because the velocity of ultrasound is 1540 M/sec, it would take 0.28 msec for each ultrasonic line when one includes 0.02 msec for fly-back time. If the sweep rate is 60/sec, then 17 msec are available for each sweep of the ultrasonic beam. The lines per sweep are determined by the time available for one sweep and the time necessary for each ultrasonic line to be generated. In this particular case, one would have approximately 60 lines of ultrasonic information available for every sweep of the beam. The pulse repetition frequency that would be necessary to generate the necessary lines per sweep and the sweeps per second would be 3600 pulses/sec, a result obtained by multiplying the sweep rate by the lines per sweep. If one desires a 30° scan angle, two lines per degree would be available for line density. If all variables remain constant, except for the scan angle, which is increased from 30 to 90° (Table 1–2, column 2), only the line density changes. It would move from two lines per

**Table 1–2**
Variables in Real-Time Sector Scanning

| Variables | Possible Combinations | | | |
|---|---|---|---|---|
| Dept of examination (cm) | 20 | 20 | 20 | 10 |
| Time for each ultrasonic line (total distance traveled by ultrasound divided by velocity of sound plus fly-back time) | (40 cm or 0.4 m ÷ 1540 m/sec = 0.26 msec + 0.02 msec fly-back time = 0.28 msec) | (40 cm or 0.4 m ÷ 1540 m/sec = 0.26 msec + 0.02 msec fly-back time = 0.28 msec) | (40 cm or 0.4 m ÷ 1540 m/sec = 0.26 msec + 0.02 msec fly-back time = 0.28 msec) | (20 cm or 0.2 m ÷ 1540 m/sec = 0.13 msec + 0.02 msec fly-back time = 0.14 msec) |
| Sweep rate (sweeps per second) | 60 | 60 | 30 | 60 |
| Time for each sweep (msec) | 17 | 17 | 34 | 17 |
| Lines per sweep time/sweep ÷ time/line | 60 17 msec ÷ 0.28 msec | 60 17 msec ÷ 0.28 msec | 120 34 msec ÷ 0.28 msec | 120 17 msec ÷ 0.14 msec |
| Pulse repetition frequency (pulses/sec) lines/sweep × sweeps sec | 3,600 60 × 60 | 3,600 60 × 60 | 3,600 120 × 60 | 7,200 120 × 60 |
| Angle | 30° | 90° | 90° | 90° |
| Line density (lines/degree) lines/sweep-angle | 2 60–30° | 0.67 60–90° | 1.33 120–90° | 1.33 120–90° |

degree with a 30° scan to 0.67 lines per degree using a 90° examination. Thus, degradation of line density and image quality would be significant.

Some loss in line density could be recovered by decreasing the sweep rate (Table 1–2, column 3). By sweeping the ultrasonic beam 30 rather than 60 times/sec, the time for each sweep would double, the lines per sweep would double, and the line density would be 1.33 lines per degree or twice that when recording at a rate of 60 sweeps/sec. The line density could also be improved by decreasing the depth of the examination (Table 1–2, column 4). If one were satisfied with examining only 10 cm of depth, one could again have twice the number of lines per sweep available and a line density of 1.33 lines per degree. Thus, multiple combinations could be used depending on the desired information and on the compromises one is willing to make.

Because almost all current two-dimensional echocardiographs use scan converters and digital manipulation of the images, one cannot appreciate how the instrument is actually sweeping and processing the ultrasonic information. The individual ultrasonic lines, or raster lines, are eliminated by digital manipulation so that one does not see still pictures as consisting of a series of radial spokes, as with some of the early two-dimensional instruments. The instruments are "playing games," however, to eliminate the distractions. Some of the information is repeated to fill in the missing gaps. Although this manipulation does not interfere with the real-time images, one can see occasional distorted still frames (Fig. 1–24). Among other findings, one might observe serial still frames that are identical because they are repeated.

This discussion brings out a fundamental principle of echocardiographic instrumentation. Echocardiographic technology is filled with compromises and "trade-offs." If one wants a faster frame rate, then the angle or depth must be reduced. As will be mentioned, if one wants a 128-element transducer or a lower frequency transducer, the aperture or footprint of the transducer must be larger. Similar compromises are evident when Doppler principles and digital storage and retrieval of images are discussed later.

## SIGNAL PROCESSING

When the ultrasonic energy returns as an echo and strikes the piezoelectric element of the transducer, an electrical impulse is created and transmitted back to the echograph. This impulse is in the form of a radio frequency or RF signal. The RF presentation is seen on the oscilloscope as a burst of signals rising above and below the baseline on the oscilloscope (Fig. 1–25A). A better method of presenting this information is by video display. With this method, the RF signal is processed so that merely the envelope or the outline of the upper half of an electric signal is presented on the face of the oscilloscope (Fig. 1–25B). The most common display used in all routine echographs, video display may be further modified by accentuating the leading edge of the echo. This modification is accomplished by taking the first derivative of the video signal (Fig. 1–25C), which converts the echo to a thinner signal. Also, a small negative echo follows the initial spike. This negative signal, in association with DC restoration, further accentuates the leading edge of the signal. This type of differentiation, sometimes called "fast-time constant" or "leading-edge enhancement," helps to accentuate individual echoes and to differentiate echoes that are closer together. This type of signal processing is commonly used with M-mode echocardiography because the manipulation influences axial resolution only. Leading edge enhancement is not

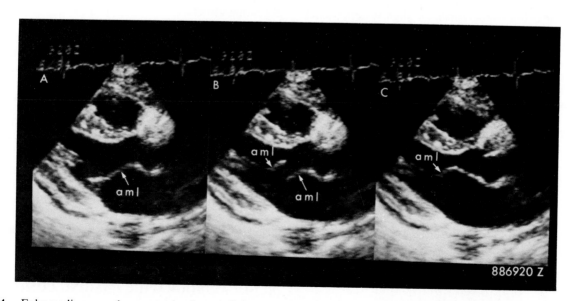

**Fig. 1–24.** Echocardiograms demonstrating how a digital scan converter can distort individual still frames. Echocardiogram *B* shows an artifactual anterior mitral leaflet (aml) as a scan converter displays an image that is halfway between echogram *A* and echogram *C*.

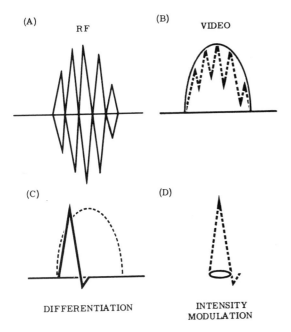

(A) RF

(B) VIDEO

(C) DIFFERENTIATION

(D) INTENSITY MODULATION

**Fig. 1–25.** Ways of processing the returning ultrasonic echo. *A* represents the RF or radio frequency type of echo display. The video display in *B* represents the average height of the upper half of the RF signal. The differentiation in *C* is obtained by taking the first derivative of the video display. Intensity modulation in *D* represents the conversion of signal amplitude to intensity and changing the signal from a spike to a dot.

as useful with two-dimensional echocardiography because it has no effect on the lateral resolution. In addition, the dot size on the two-dimensional image becomes distorted with the axial dimension becoming narrower than the lateral dimension. Thus, most instruments have different circuits for M-mode and two-dimensional imaging. The presence of leading-edge enhancement explains why M-mode echocardiograms have slightly better axial resolution.

A concept that is becoming increasingly important with advances in instrumentation is that of dynamic range (see the diagram in Fig. 1–26). In essence, the dynamic range is the range of useful ultrasonic signals that can be recorded. It is usually expressed in decibels

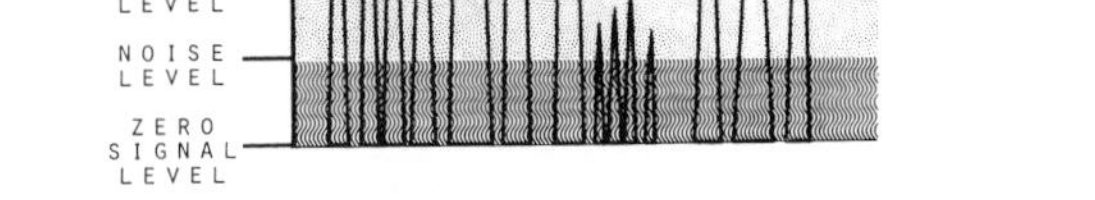

(db) as a ratio between the largest and smallest signals measured at the point of input to the display. As indicated in Figure 1–26, the dynamic range does not include all available signals. Some signals represent noise and some represent undesired echoes that are eliminated using reject control. Signals also exist beyond the saturation level of the recording system. Because a large dynamic range is desirable, one strives to keep the noise level and undesired echoes requiring reject control to a minimum.

The recording of all available signals is limited by the ability of the cathode ray tube to record these echoes. For example, usually about 100 db of ultrasonic information is available, but the cathode ray tube can only record about 30 db. As a result, many weak echoes were eliminated in early echocardiographs. The M-mode systems were principally concerned with recording specular echoes originating from valves and leading edges of heart walls. As a result, the systems were adjusted to record merely the strong, dominant specular echoes. As interest in two-dimensional echocardiography increased, so did concern over weaker echoes, especially those arising from the myocardium. These echoes are primarily scattered and are weak compared with the specular valvular echoes.

One method for recording all ultrasonic information, both strong specular echoes and weak echoes, or, in other words, a method for increasing the dynamic range of the system, involves logarithmic compression. Figure 1–27 attempts to explain the logarithmic compression system. An input dynamic range of 100 db, which has a 100,000 to 1 input signal range, is beyond the capability of the cathode ray tube. Thus, the 100-db range is logarithmically compressed to a 30-db range with a 32 to 1 output signal range. Every 3.3 db on the input is mapped into 1 db on the output. Needless to say, this description oversimplifies a fairly complicated means of signal processing. There are many different ways of accomplishing the same effect.

A wide dynamic range is necessary for recording gray scale. Gray scale indicates the ability of a display to record both bright and weak echoes in varying shades of gray. The number of gray scale levels is a measure of the dynamic range. Early echocardiographs had little gray scale because the primary interest was locating specular echoes and mapping their motion. Now, with considerably more interest in judging the brightness of echoes as well as their location and motion, gray scale and dynamic range are becoming increasingly important. Figure 1–28*B* shows a two-dimensional image with gray scale, and Figure 1–28*A* has minimal or no gray scale. The differences in brightness in the recordings that have gray scale is readily apparent. The echocardiogram in Figure 1–28*B* uses digital processing, which helps to enhance or accentuate the gray scale.

## ECHOCARDIOGRAPHIC IMAGING CONTROLS

A variety of controls modify the echocardiogram on all commercial echocardiographs. These controls can

SCHEMATIC DEFINITION OF DYNAMIC RANGE

SIGNAL SATURATION LEVEL

ULTRASONIC SIGNALS

DYNAMIC RANGE

REJECT LEVEL

NOISE LEVEL

ZERO SIGNAL LEVEL

**Fig. 1–26.** Schematic definition of dynamic range.

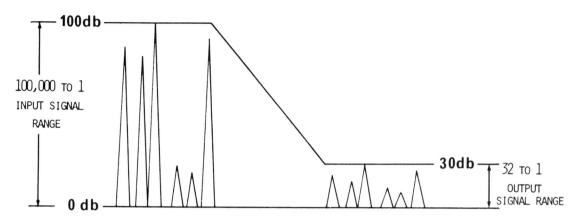

(EVERY 3.3db ON THE INPUT IS MAPPED INTO 1db ON THE OUTPUT)

**Fig. 1–27.** Logarithmic dynamic range compression: linear scheme. This diagram demonstrates how 100 db of ultrasonic information can be compressed to a 30-db output using logarithmic compression.

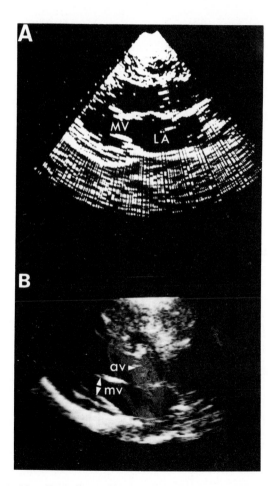

**Fig. 1–28.** Two-dimensional echocardiograms without (*A*) and with (*B*) gray scale. MV, mv = mitral valve; LA = left atrium; av = aortic valve.

greatly influence the echo display and, as will be demonstrated, are vitally important in recording specific cardiac echoes. First, since ultrasound is attenuated and decreases in intensity as it travels through the body, some mechanism for enhancing the distant echoes is necessary. All commercial echocardiographs have a circuit for suppressing near-field echoes and for enhancing far-field echoes. Such a device appears under many names, including "time-gain-compensation" (TCG), "depth compensation," or "electronic distance compensation."[38] A representation of the compensating wave form is frequently displayed as a break in the base line with a variable slope (Fig. 1–29). Both the beginning of this compensating mechanism, or "ramp," and the slope of the ramp may be varied. All echoes to the left of the ramp are suppressed (see Fig. 1–29). The ramp itself represents increasing depth compensation. Maximal depth compensation is reached at the plateau to the right of the ramp. Figure 1–29 shows how this form of depth compensation is used to suppress near-field echoes and to enhance far-field echoes. The exact way in which this depth compensation mechanism is used varies in several commercial echocardiographs. Near-field gain may be altered by a control called "near-gain." Other instruments may have a control that increases or reduces the ramp on the depth compensation and thus influences the near-field echoes. Several commercial echocardiographs have a variable depth-compensation control that consists of a series of levers that alter the relative gain throughout the entire tracing (Fig. 1–30). Figure 1–31 demonstrates how the depth compensation can be varied with this system.

The depth-compensation control is undoubtedly the most confusing and frequently the most difficult to use for the echocardiographer. One can distort the recording by varying this particular control. If one remembers that the purpose of this device is to compensate for the loss of ultrasonic energy or attenuation as the beam enters

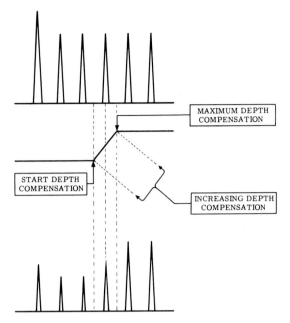

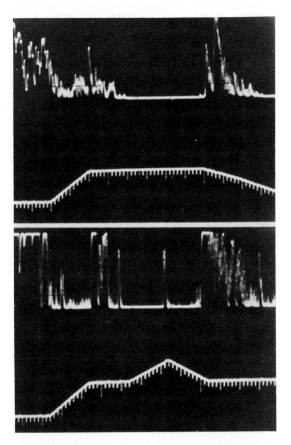

**Fig. 1–29.** Diagram illustrating how depth compensation reduces the amplitude of the near field echoes and enhances those originating from interfaces in the far field.

the body, then one better understands how the control should be used. The general purpose is to enhance the far echoes and to suppress the near echoes. Where one places the ramp depends in part on that portion of the recording to be suppressed or enhanced. This topic is discussed further in the chapter on the echocardiographic examination.

Most echocardiographs have sensitivity transmit or gain controls that merely increase or amplify the height or intensity of the echoes as they are received or the amount of ultrasonic energy transmitted. As mentioned

**Fig. 1–31.** Echocardiograms demonstrating how the multiple depth compensation controls in Figure 1–33 can influence the gain. In the lower recording, the gain has been increased at 8 cm and helps to bring out an echo that is not visible in the above tracing.

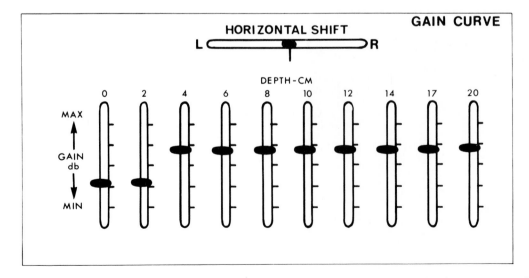

**Fig. 1–30.** Illustration of depth compensation control whereby each lever controls the gain of a given segment of the echocardiogram.

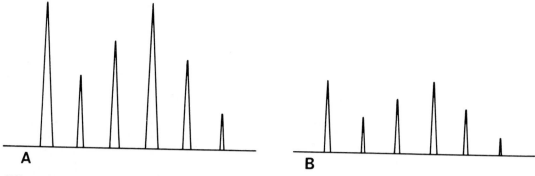

**Fig. 1–32.** Effect of damping or overall gain control. A decrease in gain or an increase in damping (*B*) will uniformly lower the amplitude of all echoes.

previously, some echocardiographs permit one to selectively control the near field, that area to the left of the depth compensation ramp, as well as the overall gain of the entire display. Turning up a gain control increases the amplitude and number of echoes recorded. Some commercial instruments use an attenuator whereby an increase in that control actually reduces the number of echoes displayed. The damping control present on some instruments functions in a manner similar to an attenuator in that the higher the control the fewer the echoes; however, the "damping" control regulates the ringing of the transducer and influences the amount of ultrasonic energy entering the body rather than modifying the received signals. Damping may also enhance the resolution by decreasing the amount of ringing of the element and the size of the pulse.

Whether one uses a gain, attenuator, or damping control, one uniformly increases or decreases the number of echoes being displayed (Fig. 1–32). On the other hand, the reject control (Fig. 1–33) selectively eliminates the recording of echoes according to the reject level. This control varies the threshold necessary for an echo to be displayed; those echoes below the threshold necessary for display are totally eliminated. Figure 1–33 shows how elevating the threshold by increasing the reject control eliminates the recording of weaker echoes. Some echocardiographs also have a control that regulates the dynamic compression and may be called a "compress" control. This factor will affect gray scale and overall gain. Depth is always an option and is usually

gained at the expense of frame rate. The angle of the sector scan is also a variable and influences frame rate.

With the advent of scan converters and digital processing of two-dimensional images, manipulation of the gray scale is available in almost all commercial instruments. Figure 1–34 shows how one can alter the amplitude gray-scale curve to enhance or suppress certain echoes. Post-processing curve 1 has a 1:1 ratio between amplitude and gray scale. In post-processing curve 2, the weaker gray scale echoes are increased in amplitude. On the two-dimensional image, one sees an increased number of echoes, especially the weaker myocardial and intracavitary echoes. The reverse curve is seen in post-processing 3. Now the weaker echoes are suppressed, and the myocardial echoes are barely apparent. No intracavitary echoes are present. Another way of suppressing the low-level echoes is to merely eliminate those echoes (post-processing 4). This type of curve has an effect similar to that of a reject control. Such manipulation of the gray scale can be done on-line or off-line using digital analyzers.

## FACTORS INFLUENCING RESOLUTION

Resolution or resolving power is the ability to distinguish or identify two objects that are close together. If two objects are a millimeter apart and one can identify both objects as distinctly separate entities, then the system has a 1-mm resolution. If the objects need to be 2

**Instrumentation**

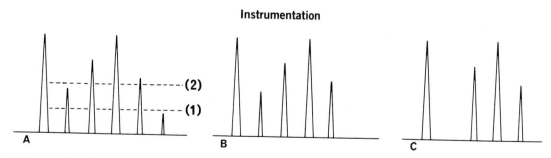

**Fig. 1–33.** Diagram showing the effects of reject control. By elevating the reject control to level 1, the smallest echo in *A* is eliminated (*B*). When the reject control is elevated to level 2, the next smallest echo that is below this threshold is also eliminated (*C*). The remaining echoes retain their full amplitude.

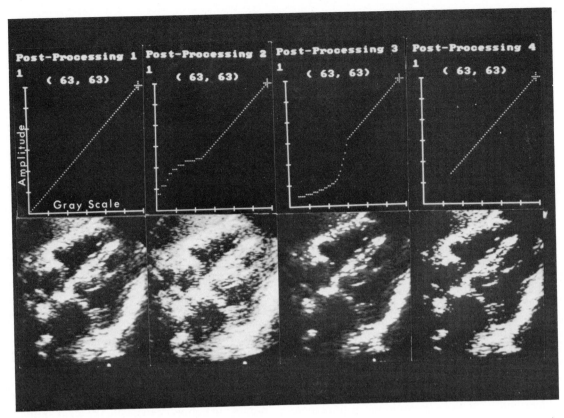

**Fig. 1–34.** Gray scale manipulation of a two-dimensional echocardiogram. The gray scale curves and the resultant images with a variety of post-processing possibilities are presented. Post-processing 1 provides a 1:1 relationship for gray scale and echo amplitude. In post-processing 2, the echoes with low gray scale are enhanced. Post-processing 3 suppresses the low gray level echoes. In post-processing 4, the low gray level echoes are eliminated.

mm apart before they can be identified as distinct entities, then the system has 2-mm resolution. Multiple factors affect resolution.

The frequency or wavelength of the ultrasonic beam is one of the important determinants in axial resolution. To identify or record small objects, one needs a small wavelength. In addition, the manner in which the returning echo signal is processed influences the axial resolution. Figure 1–35 shows echoes in both the A-mode and the M-mode recorded on two echocardiographic systems from the same test block. In the A-mode presentation (*A* and *B*), both systems record two strong echoes that are close together and a third, weaker echo farther away from the transducer. In the M-mode recording (*A'* and *B'*), one can again distinguish all three echoes with the left-hand system (*A'*), but on the right (*B'*), the two echoes that are close together now appear as one broad, thick echo. One cannot determine how many echo-producing interfaces are present in this thick echo. Thus, the echocardiographic system on the left has better resolution than that on the right. The reasons for the poor resolution with the right-hand system are, first, the echocardiograph did not differentiate the returning echoes so that the signals or echoes were not as narrow initially. Second, the M-mode recording on the right was taken with a non-gray-scale storage oscilloscope. With-

out gray scale, the individual echo was either all black or all white.

Ideally, the ultrasonic beam should be extremely narrow so that one can obtain an "ice pick" view or "slice" of the heart. But, as already described, the beam has a finite width and tends to widen further or to diverge as it enters the body. The amount of divergence is a function of frequency and size of the transducer. Efforts at decreasing the size of the beam width have already been discussed. In keeping with the principles of the ultrasonic beam, Figure 1–36 shows the interplay between the size of the beam, its relative intensity, and the relative acoustic properties of the reflecting object. The intensity of the ultrasonic beam obviously varies; the center of the beam is more intense than are the edges (Fig. 1–36). If the center of the ultrasonic beam (*dark area*) intersects a strong reflecting object (*black dots*) or a weak reflecting object (*gray dots*), one records an echo from both objects with the stronger reflecting object transmitting a stronger signal. On the other hand, if these objects are being intersected by the edges of the ultrasonic beam (*light area*), then only the stronger reflecting objects (*black dots*) may produce a signal. Less ultrasonic energy at the edge of the beam may be insufficient to produce an echo from a weaker object (*gray dots*). In addition, the returning echo from the strong object

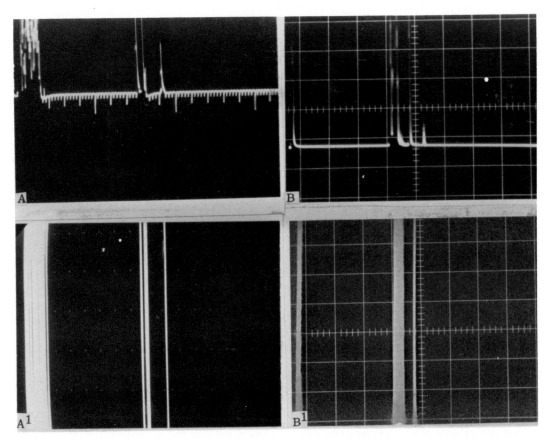

**Fig. 1–35.** Echocardiograms illustrating variations in resolving power of two different echographs. In the A-mode presentation, both systems demonstrate two strong echoes close together and a weaker third echo slightly farther away from the transducer, *A* and *B*. With the M-mode presentation, the system in *A'* again shows three separate echoes. However, in *B'* the initial two echoes, which are close together, fuse into one broad echo, and one cannot clearly identify two separate echo-producing structures.

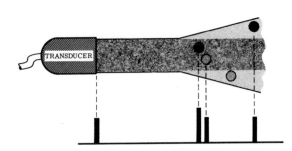

**Fig. 1–36.** Diagram illustrating the interrelationship between the intensity of the ultrasonic beam and the acoustic impedance of objects being examined. The center of the beam has a greater intensity (*dark area*) than do the edges of the beam (*light area*). Whether or not an echo is produced and with what amplitude it is recorded depend on the relationship between the intensity of the beam and the acoustic mismatch of the object being examined. Objects with high acoustic impedance (*black dots*) produce echoes even at the edges of the ultrasonic beam. Weak echo-producing objects (*gray dots*) only produce echoes of reduced amplitude in the center of the beam.

(*black dots*) is weaker when intersected by the edge of the beam than when intersected by the center of the beam.

Figure 1–37 shows some of the distortion that can be produced by the width of the ultrasonic beam. This illustration shows how two point objects (A and B) that are primarily side by side appear as if one is behind the other (A' and B') if both are in the path of the ultrasonic beam. The distortion produced by the beam width has led to many confusing echocardiograms and is an important factor that must be kept in mind when interpreting echocardiograms.[39]

Beam width artifacts in M-mode echocardiography can produce confusing echoes and hence misinterpretations because echoes seem to appear in certain areas where they actually do not exist. With two-dimensional echocardiography, beam width artifact is probably even more important because it actually distorts the basic image. Probably the most important point with regard to beam width in two-dimensional echocardiography is that it is the primary determining factor of lateral resolution. Figure 1–38 illustrates an attempt to determine lateral resolution using a two-dimensional scanner. The test object is a series of small wires in a tank of water. In Figure

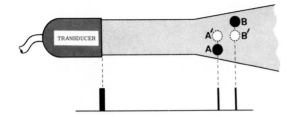

**Fig. 1–37.** Diagram illustrating how beam width can distort interpretation of the returning echoes. Objects A and B are essentially side by side. Although object B is farther away from the transducer than object A, they are not directly behind each other. Because of the width of the ultrasonic beam, both objects are recorded simultaneously. The resulting echoes suggest that the two objects are directly behind each other (A′ and B′) rather than side by side.

1–38A, one can clearly identify 12 reflecting objects that are a certain distance apart. Although this system was adjusted for the best possible resolution, it is clear that the lateral resolution is not as good as the axial resolution. Although the wires were equal in all directions, one records a series of lines rather than small dots. Thus, the axial resolution is inherently better than the lateral resolution in virtually all cross-sectional systems. Figure 1–38B demonstrates that the lateral resolution is also dependent on the gain. As one increases the gain, the lines become wider, and one can no longer even distinguish that 12 individual wires are being examined. As predicted from Figure 1–36, as one increases the gain, more of the available ultrasonic beam is recorded, the beam width increases, and lateral resolution decreases.

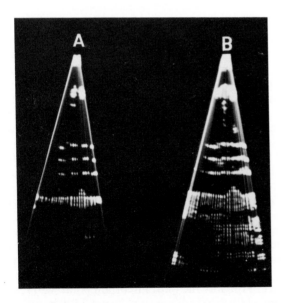

**Fig. 1–38.** Effect of gain on lateral resolution of a two-dimensional sector scan (*A*). With an increase in gain, the individual echoes from the wires in the water tank blend into continuous horizontal lines (*B*). One cannot identify the individual wires. Gain does not significantly alter axial resolution in this echocardiograph.

Thus, to enhance lateral resolution, one should attempt to use a minimum amount of gain.[40,41] Figure 1–39 shows a clinical example of how gain setting can drastically alter lateral resolution. In this recording of a stenotic mitral valve, one can identify two different mitral valve orifices with two different gain settings. With a low gain setting (Fig. 1–39A), one sees an orifice (*white arrow*) that is significantly larger than when the gain is increased (Fig. 1–39B, *black arrow*). It should be noted that this particular echocardiograph had both gain-sensitive axial and lateral resolution. The echoes became fatter as well as wider with an increase in gain. The echocardiographic system demonstrated in Figure 1–38 showed gain-sensitive lateral resolution, but because of more differentiation of the echo signals, the axial resolution did not change appreciably with an increase in gain.

Figure 1–40 demonstrates how the beam width is important in the basic configuration of the two-dimensional image. If one scans a series of objects that represent small dots, the beam width displays these dots as a series of lines depending on the size of the beam. A nonfocused ultrasonic beam gives a series of increasingly longer lines (Fig. 1–40A). Focusing the ultrasonic beam improves the situation and diminishes the size of the lines so that they more appropriately reproduce the actual objects, which would appear as a series of dots (Fig. 1–40B).

## POTENTIAL ARTIFACTS

### Side Lobes

Side lobes were recognized primarily with the increasing use of two-dimensional echocardiography. These extraneous beams of ultrasound are generated from the edges of the individual transducer elements and are not in the direction of the main ultrasonic beam. Although all transducers generate side lobes, the problem is somewhat greater with phased array transducers.

Figure 1–41 illustrates how side lobes can produce artifactual information. If the main ultrasonic beam is directed at the object in question (Fig. 1–41A) then an echo from the object is displayed on the oscilloscope. If the main ultrasonic beam is directed away from the object (Fig. 1–41B) then no echoes are generated by the main beam. The side lobe may be hitting the object, however, and producing echoes from it. Those echoes again hit the transducer, and the echocardiograph displays the resultant echoes as though they were generated by the main beam. The echocardiographic system does not know the location of the side lobes. All returning signals are interpreted as if they originated from the main beam. Thus, an echo of probably weaker intensity is recorded on the oscilloscope in the direction of the main beam. In fact, no such echo exists at this location. If the beam is oscillating rapidly, as in Figure 1–41C, then the multiple artifactual echoes produced by the side lobes are displayed as a curved line at the same level as the true object.

It should be emphasized that the side lobes are consid-

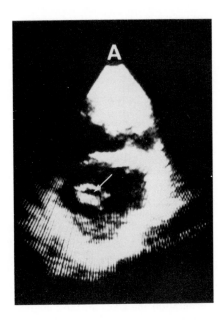

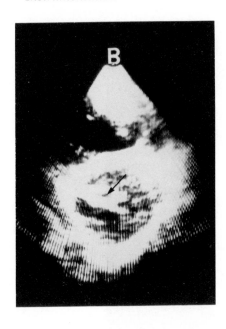

**Fig. 1–39.** Two-dimensional echocardiograms illustrating how lateral and axial resolution is impaired by an increase in gain. The mitral valve orifice (*arrows*) is much smaller with an increase in gain (*B*).

erably weaker than the main beam; thus, the returning echoes are clearly weaker than the dominant, real echoes. In fact many side lobe echoes are not actually seen because they are overshadowed by true echoes in the same vicinity. Side lobes usually become evident when they do not conflict with real echoes. For example, in Figure 1–42, the large, relatively echo-free left atrium provides an opportunity for the side lobes to be displayed within the cavity of the left atrium. If the left atrium had been of normal size, then the side lobe would be masked by the echoes from the posterior left atrial wall and lung. Another prerequisite for a dominant side lobe artifact is that the artifactual echoes must originate from a fairly strong reflecting surface. The atrioventricular groove and the fibrous skeleton of the heart represent good sources for side lobe echoes. If these artifactual echoes are not recognized, one can easily see how misinterpretations could occur. In Figure 1–42, considerable confusion could arise concerning the size of the left atrium or whether the left atrium is divided into two sections. Lesser degrees of side lobe artifact can merely

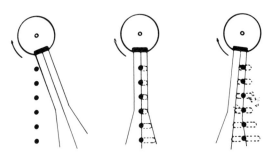

**A** POINT SPREAD FUNCTION PRODUCED BY A NON-FOCUSED BEAM OF ULTRASONIC ENERGY

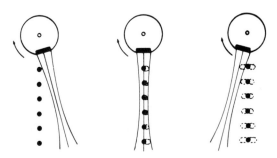

**B** POINT SPREAD FUNCTION PRODUCED BY A FOCUSED BEAM OF ULTRASONIC ENERGY

**Fig. 1–40.** Diagrams demonstrating how beam width distorts the image with a two-dimensional sector scan (*A*) and how a focused beam can reduce the distortion (*B*). The true image should be a series of dots; beam width, however, distorts the image into a series of lines.

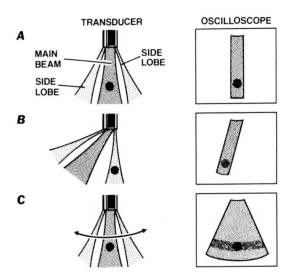

**Fig. 1–41.** Diagram demonstrating how side lobes produce artifacts on two-dimensional echocardiograms (see text for details).

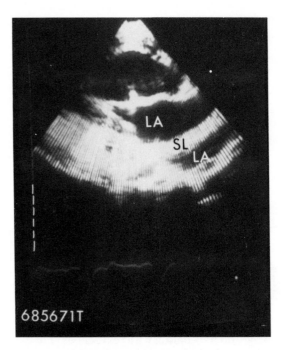

**Fig. 1–42.** Two-dimensional echocardiogram demonstrating a side lobe (SL) within a dilated left atrium (LA).

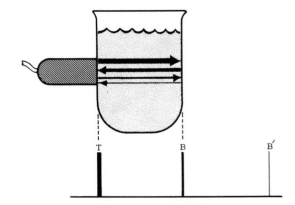

**Fig. 1–43.** Diagram of the origin of reverberations. The ultrasonic beam leaves the transducer, strikes the side of the beaker, and returns to the transducer. The returning ultrasound produces echo B. Some ultrasound is also reflected by the transducer and returns to the side of the beaker. Returning to the transducer a second time, it produces a weaker echo (B′). Echo B′ is a reverberation and gives the false impression of a second interface twice as far from the transducer as the side of the beaker.

increase the general noise level of the system and thus decrease the dynamic range. One may need to increase the reject level or to decrease the gain to eliminate some of these artifacts, but in so doing, one decreases the dynamic range.

### Reverberations

Reverberations are another important potential artifact. Figure 1–43 illustrates the principle of reverberations. The ultrasonic beam travels through the homogeneous water, strikes the opposite side of the beaker, returns to the transducer, and the echocardiograph displays a signal or echo at point B. It is still possible, however, that the near side of the beaker or the transducer may function as another reflecting surface and that the ultrasonic beam will retrace itself, hit the far side of the beaker again, and then return to the transducer. This added distance traveled by the same burst of ultrasound produces another signal (B′) at twice the distance from the transducer as does the original echo (B). The second echo or reverberation may be weaker than the original echo. If the echo is moving, the amplitude of motion may be twice as great as that of the original echo. This type of echo is an artifact known as a reverberation; reverberations can be troublesome if not understood. Such artifacts not only may result from the ultrasonic beam reflecting from the transducer, but also they may originate from some other echo-producing structures within the heart or chest.

Figure 1–44 demonstrates a catheter (*arrow*) in the right ventricle (RV). A series of linear echoes spreads from the catheter into the left ventricle (LV). These echoes (*arrowheads*) represent reverberation from the catheter.

Figure 1–45 shows a reverberation behind the left ven-

tricle. The desired echoes from the heart are primarily from the left ventricular cavity, which is bordered by the left side of the septum (LS) and the posterior left ventricular endocardium (EN). An echo from the anterior mitral valve leaflet (AMV) is seen toward the right-hand portion of the recording. In addition, a moving echo is behind the posterior left ventricular wall. The motion of this echo is clearly from the mitral valve; however, nothing is on the original recording that entirely resembles this extra posterior mitral valve echo. This posterior echo is clearly a reverberation and most likely originates from the posterior mitral leaflet; it is thus labeled PMV′. As can be noted, the amplitude of motion is greater than it was for the original posterior mitral valve echo. In fact, the primary posterior mitral valve leaflet is not well recorded within the actual left ventricular cavity. This illustration demonstrates how confus-

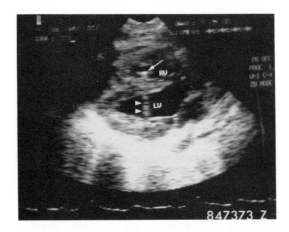

**Fig. 1–44.** Echocardiogram demonstrating reverberations (*arrowheads*) from a catheter in the right ventricle (*arrow*). RV = right ventricle; LV = left ventricle.

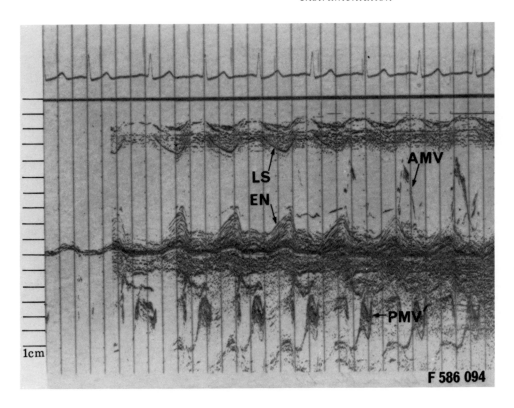

**Fig. 1–45.** An M-mode echocardiogram demonstrating a reverberation. The left septal (LS) and posterior end (EN) echoes are clearly identified as is the faint echo from the anterior mitral leaflet (AMV). Below the borders of the heart one can again see signals that have cardiac motion. This motion suggests that the echoes originate from the mitral valve. Although their exact origin is unclear, the signals probably represent reverberations from echoes originating from the posterior mitral valve leaflet (PMV'). The pattern of motion is correct, and the amplitude is much greater. Thus, reverberations can be seen from structures that do not produce primary echoes on the echocardiogram.

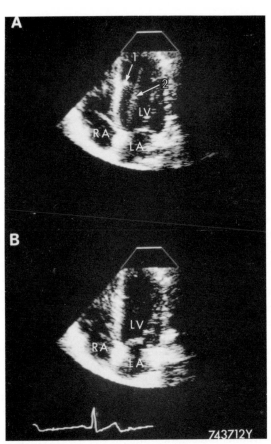

**Fig. 1–46.** Reverberations in a two-dimensional echocardiogram. *A*, Reverberation 1 oscillated in real time. Reverberation 2 probably originates from the plastic that surrounds the transducer. *B*, Both reverberation artifacts could be eliminated by readjusting the angle of the transducer.

ing reverberations can be and how one must be careful not to attempt a diagnosis based on echoes that appear outside the true cardiac border.

Sometimes the reverberations may occur within the cardiac recording, and their origin may not be obvious.[42] Such reverberations may be particularly troublesome. Some of the new instruments, especially those that use plastic housing, have introduced new potential reverberations, many of which may appear within the cardiac echoes. Figure 1–46 illustrates artifacts within the cardiac image owing to reverberations. Figure 1–46A demonstrates two such artifacts. A small bright dot oscillates in real time (Fig. 1–46A-1). A second long echo is in the center of the left ventricular cavity (Fig. 1–46A-2). By readjusting the angle, depth, or frequency of the transducer (Fig. 1–46B), these artifacts can be eliminated. Whenever one sees confusing unidentifiable echoes, the possibility that they represent reverberations must be considered.

### Shadowing

With greater interest in examining structures with high density, such as calcium or prosthetic valves, the artifact of acoustic shadowing is important to recognize. Shadowing can be a problem when trying to visualize something behind a strong reflector. Figure 1–47 is a two-dimensional echocardiogram of a patient with a Starr-Edwards prosthetic mitral valve. The prosthetic valve is indicated by the bright echoes from the leading edge of the prosthesis (*arrowheads*). The complete outline of the valve is not seen. Posterior to the prosthesis, the echoes from the posterior left atrium are weak, and directly behind the valve, they are actually absent (XX). This loss of echoes behind the strong reflector repre-

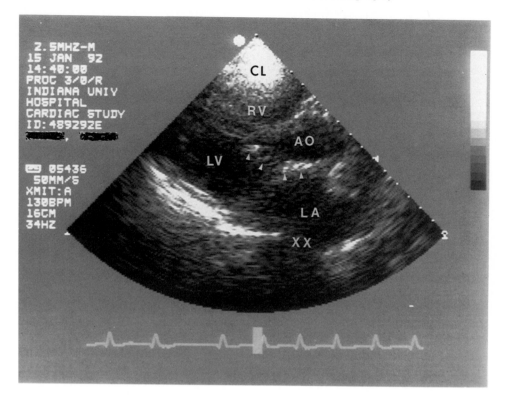

**Fig. 1–47.** Two-dimensional echocardiogram of a patient with a prosthetic mitral valve. The valve produces strong, highly reflective echoes (*arrowheads*). This end reduces the amount of energy available to record structures behind the valve. As an example, the posterior left atrial wall (XX) is not visualized because of this acoustic "shadowing." There is also near field clutter (CL). RV = right ventricle; AO = aorta; LV = left ventricle; LA = left atrium.

sents shadowing. This artifact can be useful in identifying a strong reflector such as calcium.

### Near Field Clutter

Many instruments, especially phased array systems, have acoustic noise near the transducer called "near field clutter" or "ring-down artifact." The problem arises from high amplitude oscillations of the piezoelectric elements. This artifact is troublesome when trying to identify an echogenic mass or structure in the near field. In Figure 1–47, the right ventricular wall and cavity are indistinct because of near field clutter (CL). As will be discussed later, intravascular transducers are inherently troubled with this problem.

## PRINCIPLES OF DOPPLER ECHOCARDIOGRAPHY

Doppler echocardiography is an integral part of almost every ultrasonic examination of the heart. Thus, knowledge of Doppler principles is essential for anyone involved with echocardiography.[43–47] The way in which the ultrasonic energy is used and the type of information obtained from a Doppler examination are vastly different from those findings in M-mode and two-dimensional cardiac imaging. With the Doppler approach, one is primarily interested in gleaning information from moving targets. In most cases, these targets represent red blood cells. Thus, Doppler echocardiography is primarily a technique for recording the manner in which blood moves within the cardiovascular system.

The Doppler examination is based on the Doppler effect first described by Christian Johann Doppler in 1842.

If a source of sound is stationary, then the wavelength and frequency of the sound emanating from that source are constant (Fig. 1–48*A*). If, however, the source of the sound is moving toward one's ear, then the wavelength is decreasing and the frequency is increasing (Fig. 1–48*B*). If the source of sound moves away from the ear (Fig. 1–48*C*), then the wavelength is increasing and the frequency is decreasing. The classic example of this phenomenon is the sound originating from a moving train. As the train moves toward an individual, the sound coming from the train whistle is increasing in pitch or frequency. As the train passes the individual and moves away, the whistle from the train decreases in frequency or pitch.

Figure 1–49 demonstrates how one can use reflected sound to determine the motion of a target that reflects the ultrasonic energy. If one has two transducers, a transmitting transducer (t) and a receiving transducer (r), an ultrasonic beam can be directed at a target. The receiving transducer can record the reflected echoes. If the target is stationary, then the frequency of the transmitted ultrasonic beam and the frequency of the reflected ultrasonic beam are identical (Fig. 1–49*A*). If the target reflecting the ultrasonic energy is moving toward the transducers (Fig. 1–49*B*), then the frequency of the ultrasonic beam is distorted and the received frequency is increased. The reverse situation occurs if the target is moving away from the transducers (Fig. 1–49*C*). Under these circumstances, the frequency of the received ultrasonic beam ($f_r$) is less than the transmitted frequency ($f_t$). The Doppler shift, or frequency, represents the difference between the received and the transmitted frequencies.

## DOPPLER EFFECT

**A** Source of sound stationary

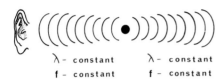

$\lambda$ – constant  $\lambda$ – constant
f – constant  f – constant

**B** Source of sound moving toward ear

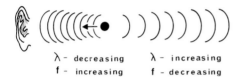

$\lambda$ – decreasing  $\lambda$ – increasing
f – increasing  f – decreasing

**C** Source of sound moving away from ear

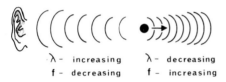

$\lambda$ – increasing  $\lambda$ – decreasing
f – decreasing  f – increasing

**Fig. 1–48.** Diagram illustrating the Doppler effect. When a source of sound is stationary (*A*), the wavelength ($\lambda$) and frequency (f) are constant. If the source of sound moves toward the ear (*B*), the wavelength is decreasing and the frequency is increasing. When the source of sound moves away from the ear (*C*), the sound heard by the ear has an increasing wavelength or decreasing frequency.

## DOPPLER EFFECT

### REFLECTED SOUND FROM TARGET

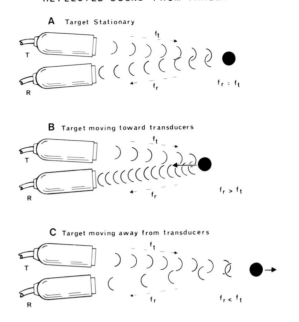

**A** Target Stationary

**B** Target moving toward transducers

**C** Target moving away from transducers

DOPPLER SHIFT OR FREQUENCY $(f_d) = f_r - f_t$

**Fig. 1–49.** Drawings demonstrating the Doppler effect using reflected sound from a target. The reflected frequency ($f_r$) is greater than the transmitted frequency ($f_t$) when the target is moving toward the transducers (*B*). The reflected frequency is smaller than the transmitted frequency when the target moves away from the transducer (*C*). The Doppler shift or frequency ($f_d$) is the difference between the transmitted and reflected frequencies.

Figure 1–50 shows the mathematical relationship between the velocity of the target and the Doppler frequency. As noted in the Doppler equations, the velocity of the moving target (v) is a function of the Doppler frequency, the velocity of sound in the medium being examined, the transmitted frequency, and the angle ($\theta$) between the ultrasonic beam and the path of the moving target. Since the velocity of sound in the medium is known and is reasonably constant, and the transmitted frequency is also known, then velocity is a function of the Doppler frequency and the angle. The equation denotes that the relationship between the Doppler frequency and velocity is a function of the cosine of the angle. Figure 1–51 shows the relationship of the angle to the cosine of the angle.[43] The graph demonstrates that as long as the angle is 20° or less, the cosine is close to one. Under these circumstances, the angle can almost be ignored. Once the angle exceeds 20°, however, then the cosine becomes significantly less than one. Under these circumstances, the angle is critical if one wishes to calculate the velocity from the Doppler frequency. This graph also illustrates that if the angle is 90°, then the cosine of the angle is zero and there is no Doppler shift. Thus, the best Doppler information is obtained when the ultrasonic beam is parallel to the moving tar-

### DOPPLER EQUATIONS

$$f_d = f_r - f_t$$

$$f_d = 2 f_t \frac{v \cdot \cos \theta}{c}$$

$$v = \frac{f_d \cdot c}{2 f_t (\cos \theta)}$$

c = velocity of sound

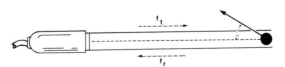

**Fig. 1–50.** Doppler equations relating Doppler frequency ($f_d$), received frequency ($f_r$), transmitted frequency ($f_t$), and the angle ($\theta$) between the direction of the moving target and the path of the ultrasonic beam.

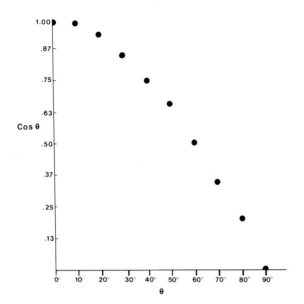

RELATIONSHIP OF ANGLE (θ) TO COSINE OF ANGLE

**Fig. 1–51.** Graph demonstrating the relationship between an angle and the cosine of an angle. The cosine of an angle is close to unity provided the angle is 20° or less. The cosine becomes markedly less than unity as the angle increases.

get. It is important to remember that this relationship is just the opposite of that for imaging with M-mode or two-dimensional echocardiography. The best quality images are obtained when the objects are essentially perpendicular or 90° to the ultrasonic beam. Thus, it is usually difficult to obtain an excellent Doppler examination and

an excellent cardiac image simultaneously. The best examination for a Doppler recording is rarely the best examination for a two-dimensional or M-mode image.

As noted with the Doppler equation, the velocity is also a function of the transmitted or carrier frequency. As noted later, high velocities are clinically important. The graph in Figure 1–52 demonstrates that it is easier to record a high velocity, such as 6 M/sec, with a 1-MHz transducer than with a 2-MHz transducer. In fact, it is virtually impossible to obtain such a high velocity using the Doppler approach and a 5-MHz transducer. Thus, the best Doppler information occurs with lower frequency transducers than with higher frequency transducers. This situation is just the reverse of what is preferred for M-mode or two-dimensional imaging. The best images with the greatest resolution occur with higher frequency transducers. This fact demonstrates another of the many differences between ultrasonic imaging and ultrasonic Doppler examinations.

Figure 1–49 illustrates the principle of continuous wave Doppler ultrasound. One uses two transducers, a transmitter and a receiver, or a transducer with both transmitter and receiver elements (Fig. 1–53). Both transducers are constantly functioning in their respective capacities. This Doppler approach is the same as that used for examining peripheral vessels for many years. Since the ultrasonic beam is constant, all the moving targets within the beam produce Doppler signals. One has no way of knowing where the individual target might be with relation to the transducer. In addition, one cannot determine whether there is more than one moving target. One has no "range" definition with a continuous wave system. To overcome this problem,

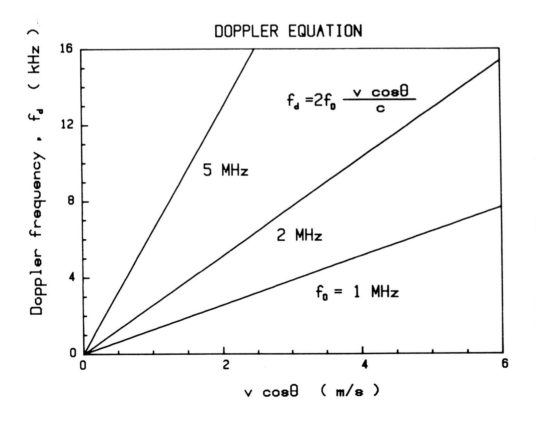

$$f_d = 2f_0 \frac{v \cos\theta}{c}$$

**Fig. 1–52.** Graph demonstrating the relationship between Doppler frequency, velocity of cosine theta (v cos θ), and the transmitted or carrier frequency ($F_0$). Lower carrier frequency transducers can detect higher velocities. (From Hatle, L. and Angelsen, B.: Doppler Ultrasound in Cardiology: Physical Principles and Clinical Applications, 2nd ed. Philadelphia, Lea & Febiger, 1985.)

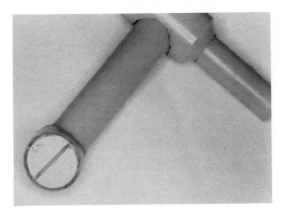

**Fig. 1–53.** A continuous-wave Doppler ultrasound transducer. The round transducer element is split into two semicircles. The semicircular elements act as sending and receiving transducers, respectively.

especially when examining the heart, a range-gated Doppler system was needed so that specific areas of the heart were interrogated. The solution to this problem was pulsed Doppler.[48–52] Figure 1–54 demonstrates that one can obtain Doppler information using a pulsed transducer. By sending a short burst of ultrasound, the frequency of that burst is distorted if the target from which it is reflected is moving. In Figure 1–54, the target is moving toward the transducer, and thus the frequency of the received burst of ultrasound ($f_r$) is higher than the transmitted frequency ($f_t$). The difference in the received and transmitted frequencies again produces a

**PULSED DOPPLER**

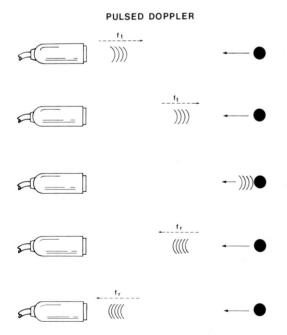

**Fig. 1–54.** Drawings demonstrating the principle of pulsed Doppler echocardiography. If the object reflecting the pulses of ultrasound is moving toward the transducer, then the frequency of the received pulse ($f_r$) is greater than the transmitted frequency ($f_t$).

Doppler shift. One can determine velocity just as with the continuous wave approach. The advantage of the pulsed Doppler system is that one now has the ability to obtain an M-mode or two-dimensional image as with any other pulsed ultrasonic device. Thus, pulsed Doppler permits one to obtain a Doppler signal from a specific area of the cardiovascular system. The introduction of pulsed Doppler was one of the major developments that made Doppler echocardiography a clinically useful tool.

As might be expected, pulsed Doppler has its disadvantages as well as its advantage. The major disadvantage of pulsed Doppler is that the velocity one can measure is limited. The pulsed system inherently has a pulsed repetition frequency or PRF. The PRF determines how high a Doppler frequency the pulse system can detect. In Figure 1–55, the darker sine wave ($\lambda$ 1 and $f_d$ 1) is easily identified by the sampling sites (*squares*) in this pulsed system. This echograph, however, does not sample rapidly enough, i.e., the PRF is not high enough to identify the frequency and wavelength of the higher Doppler frequency ($\lambda$ 2 and $f_d$ 2). The inability of a pulsed Doppler system to detect high-frequency Doppler shifts is known as "aliasing."[45,53] The upper limit of frequency that can be detected with a given pulsed system is known as the "Nyquist" limit or number. This limit is defined as one half the pulse repetition frequency. In the example in Figure 1–55, the pulse repetition frequency is 7 per given time "t." For the lower Doppler frequency ($f_d$ 1), there are two cycles per "t." The Nyquist limit for this system would be 3.5, and thus the lower frequency would be easily detected with this system. The frequency ($f_d$ 2) has 8 cycles per given time "t." The Nyquist limit of 3.5 is insufficient to identify the higher frequency in this illustration. Thus, pulsed Doppler has a limitation as to how high a frequency or velocity it can detect.

Figure 1–56 demonstrates a pulsed Doppler recording flow within the descending aorta. Although there is essentially systolic flow away from the transducer, the Nyquist limit for forward flow in this particular recording was 65 cm/sec. The flow exceeded this limit and was recorded as flow above the baseline, as if it were moving toward the transducer. This phenomenon is commonly called "wrap around," where the flow that exceeds the Nyquist limit appears as if it were flowing in the opposite direction.

Figure 1–57 shows a sample volume in the left ventricular outflow tract in a patient with aortic regurgitation. High velocity flow is occurring in diastole toward the transducer. Because the velocity exceeds 82 cm/sec, the Doppler signal wraps around and appears in diastole below the baseline as if it were moving away from the transducer. Aliasing introduces confusion as to the direction of the flow and also prohibits one from measuring the maximal velocities.

Figure 1–58 shows that the ability of a pulsed Doppler system to detect velocity is a function of both range or depth of examination, determined to a large extent by the PRF, and also the frequency of the transducer. As with the continuous wave system, the lower frequency transducers can detect a higher velocity at a given range.

## PULSED DOPPLER ALIASING

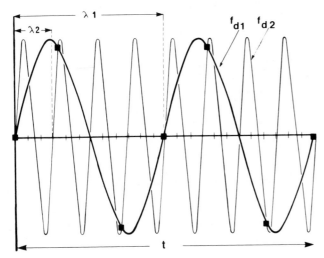

$$PRF = \frac{7}{t}$$

$$f_{d1} = \frac{2}{t}$$

$$f_{d2} = \frac{8}{t}$$

Aliasing occurs when $f_d > \frac{1}{2}$ PRF

Nyquist limit $= \dfrac{PRF}{2}$

**Fig. 1–55.** Drawing illustrating the principle of aliasing with pulsed Doppler. $\lambda 1$ = wavelength 1; $\lambda 2$ = wavelength 2; $f_{d1}$ = Doppler frequency 1; $f_{d2}$ = Doppler frequency 2; PRF = pulse repetition frequency (see text for details).

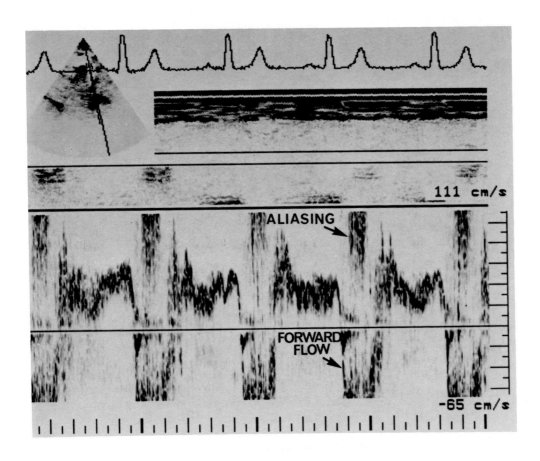

**Fig. 1–56.** Doppler echocardiogram demonstrating aliasing with the forward flow, which is moving away from the transducer, wrapping around, and appearing above the baseline. This type of aliasing can be overcome by merely shifting the baseline or zero line upward so the entire Doppler recording can be displayed below the baseline.

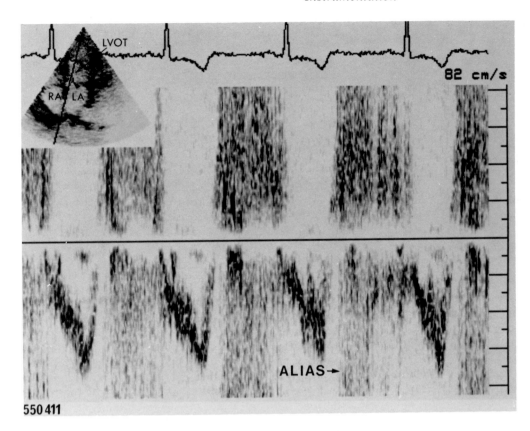

**Fig. 1–57.** Another example of aliasing whereby the flow velocity is so high that the Doppler signals wrap around many times. One cannot detect the peak velocity even by shifting the baseline in a patient with velocity exceeding the capability of this pulsed Doppler system.

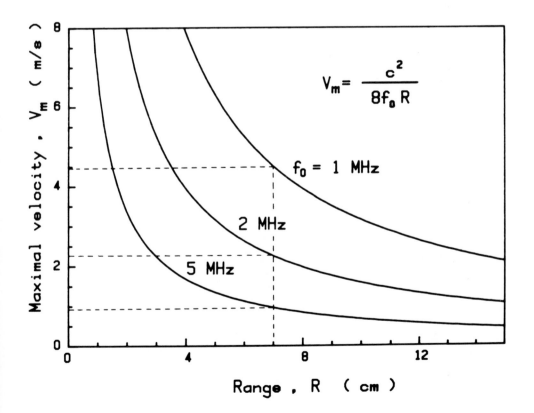

$$V_m = \frac{c^2}{8 f_0 R}$$

**Fig. 1–58.** Graph demonstrating the relationship between maximal velocity and range. Pulsed Doppler transducers utilizing lower frequencies can detect high velocities at greater ranges. $V_m$ = maximum velocity; $c$ = velocity of sound; $f_0$ = transmitted or carrier frequency; $R$ = range. (From Hatle, L. and Angelsen, B.: Doppler Ultrasound in Cardiology: Physical Principles and Clinical Applications, 2nd ed. Philadelphia, Lea and Febiger, 1985.)

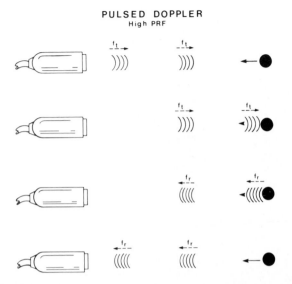

**PULSED DOPPLER**
High PRF

**Fig. 1–59.** Diagram demonstrating the principle of high pulse repetition frequency (PRF) pulsed Doppler (see text for details).

For example, at 4 cm depth, a 2-MHz transducer can detect about 4 M/sec, whereas the 5-MHz transducer can detect less than 2 M/sec.

A potential solution to aliasing with pulsed Doppler is to use high PRF pulsed Doppler. By increasing the pulse repetition rate by two (Fig. 1–59), one essentially raises the Nyquist limit by two and increases the ability to obtain high frequency Doppler. One could obviously insert three, four, or more gates to improve the Nyquist limit even further, but technical problems are associated with this approach. Some range ambiguity is introduced because the system does not know specifically which

gate is where. In some respects, this approach is somewhere between pulsed Doppler and continuous wave Doppler. Although commercial versions of this approach are available, its clinical utility is somewhat limited.

## DOPPLER DISPLAY

Two forms of Doppler display are used in echocardiography. The first of these displays is spectral Doppler. Using a fast Fourier transform technique, the Doppler velocities are displayed graphically against time. Gray scale is used to judge the intensity or, to some extent, the number of red cells in the moving column of blood being interrogated.

Basically two flow patterns can be detected with spectral Doppler echocardiography (Fig. 1–60).[46,47] The first of these patterns is laminar flow. Under these circumstances, the reflecting red cells are all traveling in the same direction and with little difference in velocities. The blood in the center of the vessel or chamber is moving somewhat more rapidly than those cells along the walls; some viscous friction slows the flow along the walls. The Doppler signals from such flow indicate a narrow velocity band or small amount of spectral spread. The second type of flow is turbulent or disturbed. This situation occurs when blood is flowing across an obstruction or narrowed area in the cardiovascular system. Turbulent flow might occur with valvular stenosis whereby blood is flowing across a narrowed orifice. A similar situation might be present if blood is flowing through a defect between the two sides of the heart, such as a ventricular septal defect. Disturbed or turbulent flow would also be present if the blood is flow-

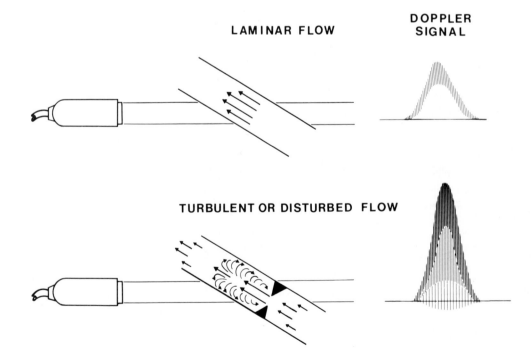

**LAMINAR FLOW**

**DOPPLER SIGNAL**

**TURBULENT OR DISTURBED FLOW**

**Fig. 1–60.** Doppler signals recorded from laminar flow and turbulent or disturbed flow. With laminar flow, all the velocities are similar. The Doppler signal produces a relatively thin wave form with minimal spectral broadening. When blood flows across an area with a significant change in the caliber of the vessel, flow with multiple velocities and different directions is produced. Such disturbed flow produces a Doppler signal with multiple frequencies and marked spectral broadening.

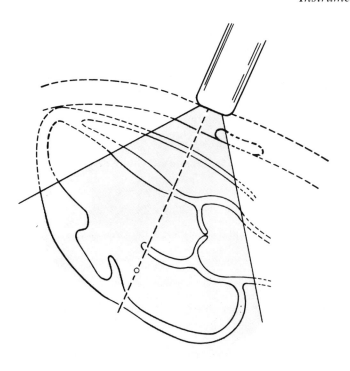

**Fig. 1–61.** Diagram demonstrating how one can place a single Doppler sample (*arrow*) within a two-dimensional echocardiographic image. (From Feigenbaum, H.: Doppler Color Flow Imaging. *In* Heart Disease Update. Edited by E. Braunwald. Philadelphia, W.B. Saunders Co., 1988).

ing through a regurgitant valve. Under these circumstances, several phenomena occur that are important to the examination. The flow of blood distal to the narrowed area is no longer laminar because the direction of the flow becomes variable. Some of the blood cells move in divergent directions with varying velocities. In addition, the central column of blood passing through the narrowed orifice increases its velocity significantly. Thus, the Doppler signal indicates multiple frequencies that produce a wide spectral spread (Fig. 1–60). In addition, the peak or maximum velocity of the central column of blood passing through the narrowed orifice is increased.

One of the features of pulsed Doppler is that the pulsing of the ultrasonic beam permits simultaneous cardiac imaging and Doppler recording. Figure 1–61 shows how a pulsed Doppler sample can be placed within the cardiovascular system. Such an examination permits the spectral display of blood flow from a specific site in the heart. Figure 1–62 shows the spectral pulsed Doppler display of blood through the mitral orifice.

Multiple Doppler samples can be placed along the scan or rastor line (Fig. 1–63). This examination produces a flow image analogous to an M-mode recording and was originally called "M/Q" Doppler.[54,55] The Doppler flow imaging display is superimposed on the M-mode echocardiogram. To identify the direction of flow, color is introduced. The common system used is to encode flow toward the transducer in red and that going away from the transducer in blue (BART-blue away, red toward). Figure 1–64 demonstrates an M-mode color flow image at the level of the mitral valve demonstrating red flow passing through the mitral valve in early dias-

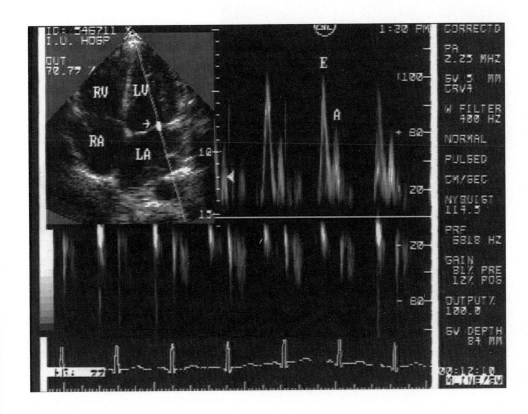

**Fig. 1–62.** Pulsed Doppler examination with the sample volume at the orifice of the mitral valve. Normal mitral flow produces a tall E wave in early diastole and a shorter A wave with atrial systole. RV = right ventricle; RA = right atrium; LV = left ventricle; LA = left atrium.

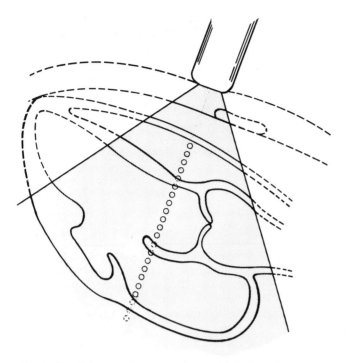

**Fig. 1–63.** Diagram demonstrating multiple Doppler samples (*small circles*) linearly arranged along a stationary ultrasonic beam. These multiple sampling sites permit the recording of blood flow along the ultrasonic beam. (From Feigenbaum, H.: Doppler Color Flow Imaging. *In* Heart Disease Update. Edited by E. Braunwald. Philadelphia, W.B. Saunders Co., 1988).

tole and blue flow above the valve in the left ventricular outflow tract in mid-diastole. Diastolic flow in the right ventricle is red.

Two-dimensional Doppler flow imaging is produced by introducing multiple[47,56–60] rastor or scan lines with numerous sampling sites, as depicted in Figure 1–65. The Doppler flow is superimposed on the two-dimensional cardiac image. Figure 1–66 demonstrates a two-dimensional Doppler flow image echogram showing blood flow through the mitral valve displayed in red and flow going out the left ventricular outflow tract in blue. The velocity is displayed in varying hues, with the brighter colors representing faster velocity.[61–63]

Color flow imaging is pulsed Doppler and therefore is limited in its ability to measure high velocities. In fact, the Nyquist limit of color flow Doppler imaging is usually lower than ordinary pulsed, spectral Doppler. Thus, as velocity increases, aliasing occurs. The aliasing is displayed on color flow Doppler as a reversal of color. If the velocity is high, one may see multiple bands of reversed color. Figure 1–67 shows flow in a left ventricular outflow tract in which the velocity is accelerating beyond the Nyquist limit and one can detect changes in color.

Laminar flow is displayed in pure shades of blue or red. Turbulent flow can be identified in several different ways. One can use multiple colors to indicate the multiple velocities inherent in turbulent flow. Another technique is to colorize the flow in shades of green when the instrument recognizes a spread or "variance" in veloci-

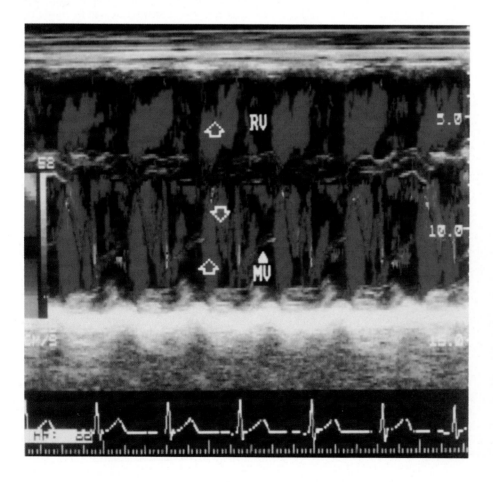

**Fig. 1–64.** M-mode color flow recording (M/Q) at the level of the mitral valve. When the valve opens, blood flows toward the transducer and is encoded in red (*up arrow*). In early diastole, the blood moves away from the transducer and is recorded in blue (*down arrow*). Tricuspid valve flow passing through the right ventricular inflow tract in diastole is shown within the right ventricle as a red-encoded Doppler signal (*up arrow*). RV = right ventricle; MV = mitral valve.

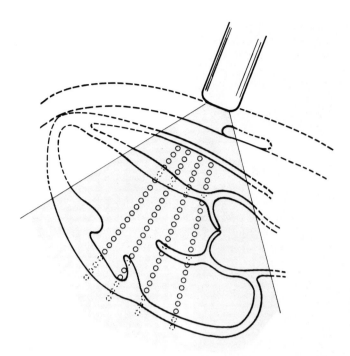

**Fig. 1–65.** Diagram illustrating the use of multigate sampling to create a two-dimensional display within the cross-sectional ultrasonic image. (From Feigenbaum, H.: Doppler Color Flow Imaging. *In* Heart Disease Update. Edited by E. Braunwald. Philadelphia, W.B. Saunders Co., 1988.)

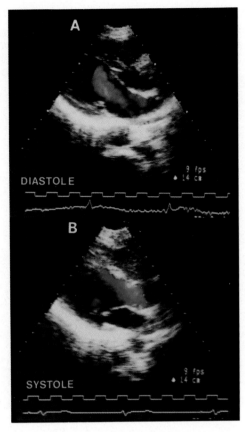

**Fig. 1–66.** Long-axis color flow Doppler image showing flow through the mitral valve in diastole (*A*) and flow out the left ventricular outflow tract in systole (*B*). Mitral valve inflow is directed toward the transducer and is encoded in red. Flow out the left ventricular outflow tract is away from the transducer and is blue. Different hues indicate differences in velocity. The brighter colors are faster velocities. (From Feigenbaum, H.: Doppler color flow imaging. *In* Heart Disease Update. Edited by E. Braunwald. Philadelphia, W.B. Saunders Co., 1988).

ties that exceeds an arbitrary value. Thus, shades of green will also be indicative of turbulent flow. Figure 1–68 shows four different color maps or displays available from the same instrument in a patient with turbulent mitral regurgitation flow. Figure 1–68A has no variance. The color bar is not split vertically and the colors range from bright yellow to light blue. The other three color maps have variance introduced. The color bar is now split with red-yellow on the top and blue-green on the bottom. The decision as to which color map to use is primarily aesthetic and is based on personal preference.

Because color is such a characteristic feature of Doppler flow imaging, it is commonly referred to as color flow Doppler or just color Doppler. The flow of course can be displayed in shades of black and white whereby turbulent flow is speckled and laminar flow is smooth. The direction of flow is determined by the physiologic motion of the moving flow. Figure 1–69 shows a color flow image in black and white. For a variety of reasons, Doppler flow imaging displaying color is more informative and is obviously more popular; however, in this text, some black and white Doppler flow images are displayed.

## PHYSIOLOGIC INFORMATION OBTAINED WITH DOPPLER ECHOCARDIOGRAPHY

With laminar flow it becomes possible to measure blood flow, as well as velocity, using Doppler echocardiography.[45,64–67] If one can determine the mean velocity

passing through a vessel or orifice, one need only know the area of the vessel or orifice to calculate blood flow (Fig. 1–70). At least theoretically, the area of the vessel or orifice could be calculated by either M-mode or two-dimensional echocardiography, and the area can be combined with the Doppler velocity measurement to calculate flow. This topic is discussed further in the chapter on hemodynamics, but ample data indicate that such measurements are feasible under certain circumstances.

The development that probably has been most instrumental in increasing the interest in Doppler echocardiography is the use of Doppler velocity measurements to estimate a pressure gradient or pressure drop across an orifice.[68–70] By modifying the Bernoulli equation, one can relate the velocity distal to a narrowed orifice to the pressure gradient across that orifice.[69–72] Figure 1–71 demonstrates the rationale and theory behind this approach. Several assumptions must be made to develop such a simple equation as $\Delta p = 4 V 2^2$. The assumptions are that the flow acceleration and viscous friction are

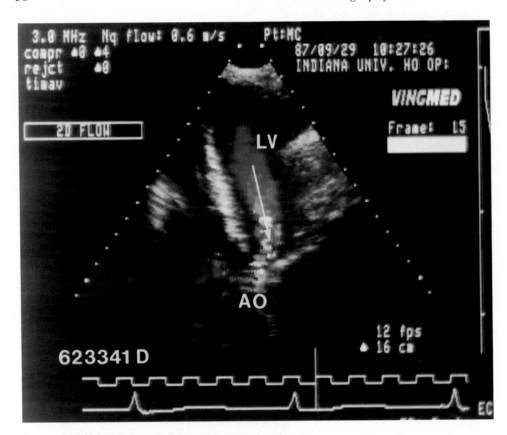

**Fig. 1–67.** Two-dimensional Doppler flow image of a patient with left ventricular outflow obstruction. The relatively low velocity left ventricular outflow is encoded in blue. As the area of narrowing is approached, the velocity increases, aliasing occurs, and the flow signal changes to red. At the site of the obstruction is a relatively narrow turbulent flow recording. LV = left ventricle; AO = aorta. (From Feigenbaum, H.: Doppler Color Flow Imaging. *In* Heart Disease Update. Edited by E. Braunwald. Philadelphia, W.B. Saunders Co., 1988).

not relevant under clinical circumstances. It also assumes that the velocity distal to the obstruction is significantly higher than the proximal velocity, and thus the proximal velocity can be ignored. As discussed later in the chapter on valvular heart disease, these assumptions seem to be reasonable. Thus, the empiric observation relating velocity to pressure gradient seems to have some value. Since velocity across obstructed semilunar valves is usually quite high, the inability of pulsed Doppler to record high velocities represents a major deficiency in its ability to evaluate stenotic semilunar valves.

Another fundamental Doppler principle is the use of the continuity equation.[73] This principle essentially combines the ability of Doppler imaging to measure blood flow and pressure gradient. The continuity equation permits one to calculate the area of a stenotic orifice. Figure 1–72 demonstrates the theory behind the continuity equation. If one knows the cross-sectional area of the vessel or vascular container proximal to an obstruction ($A_1$) as well as the mean velocity passing through that area, one can calculate the blood flow. The velocity across the obstructed area can be measured with continuous wave Doppler. The continuity equation states that the blood flowing through different areas of a continuous, intact vascular system must be equal. Thus the blood flow proximal to a narrowed area ($A_1 \times V_1$) should equal that at the stenosis ($A_2 \times V_2$). With this equation, the unknown variable is $A_2$, which can be calculated from the measured $A_1$, $V_1$, and $V_2$.

Another basic principle of Doppler flow is illustrated

in Figure 1–73. As blood is flowing toward, through, and past an obstruction, the pattern and velocities change.[74,75] As already indicated, the flow downstream from an obstruction becomes turbulent with multiple velocities and multiple directions. Color flow imaging displays this turbulence in a variety of shades of color.[76,77] In this diagram, the disturbed turbulent flow is illustrated in green. In addition, as blood is flowing toward a narrowed orifice, the velocity accelerates. Because color Doppler is pulsed and aliases easily, one sees changes in color or aliasing proximal to a narrowed orifice (Fig. 1–74).[78–80] Concentric, circular bands of red and blue are evident proximal to an obstruction. This convergence acceleration has diagnostic value, and some data suggest that one can use this phenomenon to quantitate the amount of blood flowing through a narrowed orifice.[78,79]

## DOPPLER CONTROLS

Several controls on the echocardiographs are specifically for the Doppler recording. With pulsed Doppler, one needs a mechanism for positioning the sample volume in the desired location. The manner in which this operation is performed varies with different instruments. Some manufacturers utilize a joystick, others use a series of directional buttons that need to be pressed individually, and another technique is the use of a track ball. Differences in the ease with which one can move the sample volume may be significant. Since the Doppler

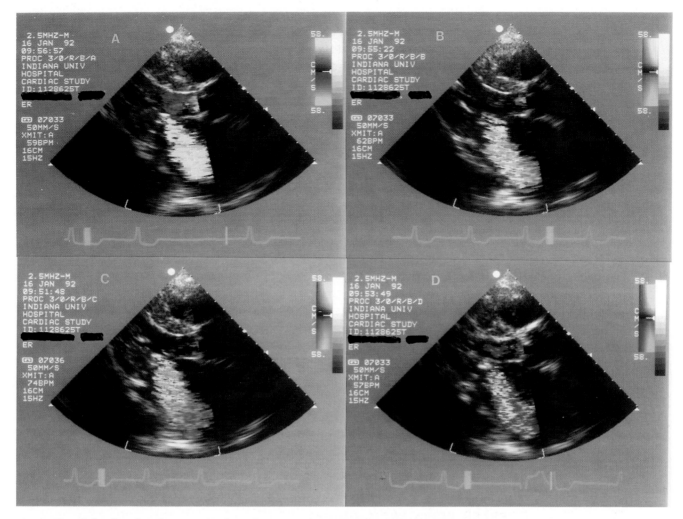

**Fig. 1–68.** Color flow imaging examinations demonstrating the various color maps that can be used to display regurgitant flow. A variance form of color map was used in *B*, *C*, and *D*.

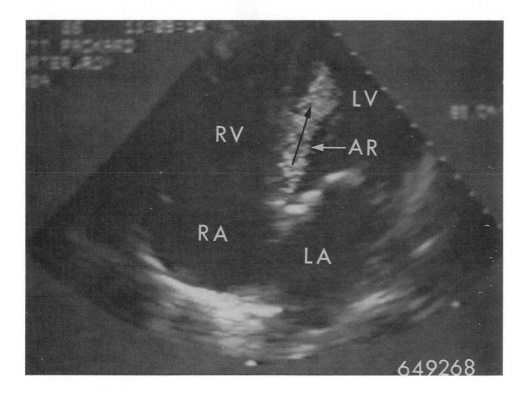

**Fig. 1–69.** Doppler flow echocardiogram in which the flow is displayed in black and white rather than in color. The turbulent aortic regurgitant jet (AR) is recorded as a bright band of echoes within the left ventricle (LV). RV = right ventricle; RA = right atrium; LA = left atrium.

37

## DOPPLER ECHOCARDIOGRAPHY

### BLOOD FLOW MEASUREMENT          DOPPLER SIGNAL

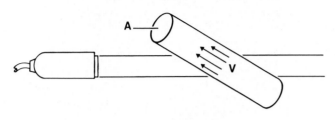
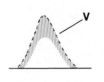

CO = A x V x HR

CO = Cardiac Output

A = Area of Vessel or Orifice

V = Integrated Flow Velocity

HR = Heart Rate

**Fig. 1–70.** Diagram demonstrating how Doppler echocardiography can measure blood flow if one knows the mean velocity of flow (V) and the cross-sectional area (A) of the vessel or orifice through which the blood is flowing.

examination can be fairly tedious, the ability to position the sample volume easily is a major advantage. Steerable continuous wave Doppler is available on most instruments as well.

The zero velocity line is the dividing point between the display of flow toward or away from the transducer. It is practical to be able to move the zero velocity line either upward or downward. Almost all the current instruments have a control that performs this function.

It is frequently advisable to filter out low frequency signals, many of which occur from the motion of cardiac walls. These so-called wall filters are essentially reject controls for eliminating unwanted "noise."

The size of the sample volume can be altered on many instruments. One may calculate angle θ between the ultrasonic beam and the presumed path of the blood flow. Once the angle is known, the instruments usually automatically calculate the velocity based on the angle.

## DOPPLER ECHOCARDIOGRAPHY

### PRESSURE DROP OR GRADIENT MEASUREMENT

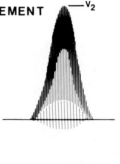
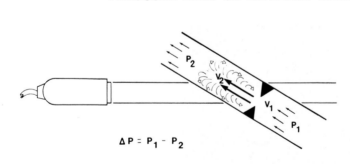

$\Delta P = P_1 - P_2$

### BERNOULLI EQUATION

$$P_1 - P_2 = \frac{1}{2}\rho(V_2^2 - V_1^2) + \rho\int_1^2 \frac{\overrightarrow{DV}}{DT} DS + R(\overrightarrow{V})$$

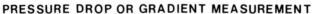

CONVECTIVE      FLOW      VISCOUS
ACCELERATION  ACCELERATION  FRICTION

$$P_1 - P_2 = \frac{1}{2}\rho(V_2^2 - V_1^2)$$

$V_1$ MUCH $< V_2$ ∴ IGNORE $V_1$

$\rho$ = MASS DENSITY OF BLOOD = $1.06 \cdot 10^3$ KG/M$^3$

∴ $\Delta P = 4V_2^2$

**Fig. 1–71.** Principles of using a modification of the Bernoulli equation to measure a pressure drop or gradient utilizing Doppler echocardiography. $P_2$ = pressure distal to an obstruction; $P_1$ = pressure proximal to an obstruction; $V_2$ = velocity distal to an obstruction; $V_1$ = velocity proximal to an obstruction; $\Delta P$ = difference in pressures across an obstruction.

### DOPPLER ECHOCARDIOGRAPHY
### CONTINUITY EQUATION

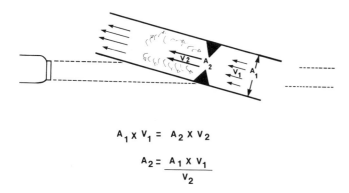

$$A_1 \times V_1 = A_2 \times V_2$$

$$A_2 = \frac{A_1 \times V_1}{V_2}$$

**Fig. 1–72.** Diagram illustrating the principles of using Doppler echocardiography and the continuity equation for calculating the area of a stenotic orifice. $A_1$ = area proximal to the stenosis; $A_2$ = area of the stenosis; $V_1$ = velocity proximal to the stenosis; $V_2$ = velocity through the stenosis. (From Feigenbaum, H.: Echocardiography. *In* Heart Disease, 4th ed. Edited by E. Braunwald. Philadelphia, W.B. Saunders, Co., 1992.)

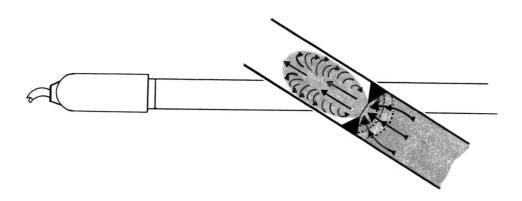

**Fig. 1–73.** Diagram demonstrating how blood flowing toward a narrowed orifice accelerates as it approaches the narrowing. The Doppler recording will produce aliasing as the velocity increases and one obtains a band of red-blue colors as the blood increases in velocity proximal to the orifice.

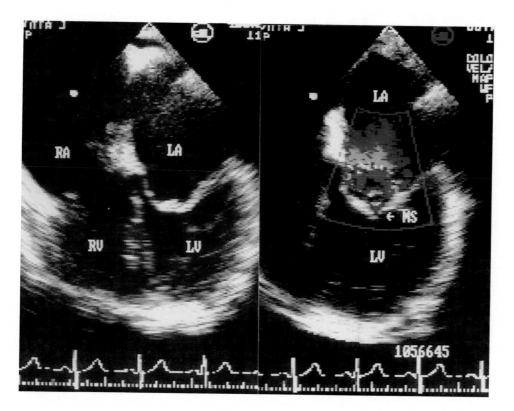

**Fig. 1–74.** Transesophageal echocardiogram of a patient with mitral stenosis. The color flow study on the right shows proximal flow acceleration with bands of aliasing color on the left atrial side of the mitral orifice. LA = left atrium; MS = mitral stenosis; LV = left ventricle; RA = right atrium; RV = right ventricle.

Because the Doppler signal is audible, a control of the speakers is needed to increase or decrease the volume. Headsets can also be used for the operator so that the Doppler sounds do not fill the entire laboratory. Having several Doppler studies performed in the same room simultaneously can produce quite a racket. Because M-mode and two-dimensional imaging are done best with a higher frequency transducer and Doppler imaging requires a lower frequency transducer, dual frequency transducers are now becoming available.

Doppler flow imaging has several unique controls. Figure 1–75 is a photograph of a Doppler flow set-up menu illustrating the many control options available on commercial instruments. The color flow image usually displays velocity, although one option is to record the Doppler power mode.[81] This mode essentially records the intensity of the moving column of blood. To some extent, this value relates to the number of red cells that are flowing. The power mode is useful in detecting low velocity flow.[82] Most other applications are probably best used with the velocity mode. Controls are available that minimize the overlap of tissue and flow mapping. One does not necessarily want the color Doppler effect on fast moving tissue, so certain controls and filters are designed to make certain that the flow does not map tissue rather than moving red cells. Various techniques try to record low velocity flow. As already indicated, various color maps are available for displaying turbulence.

The frame rate with color flow imaging is relatively slow because of all of the electronic manipulations that must be carried out.[75,83] One can increase the frame rate by decreasing the size of the color sampling. In addition, the size of the black and white display can also be reduced to enhance frame rate. The color image can be altered by wall filters or smoothing algorithms, which give a continuous type of display to the color. Some instruments have the ability to alter the density of the color lines to enhance the color image. This technique is sometimes referred to as high definition or high density color.

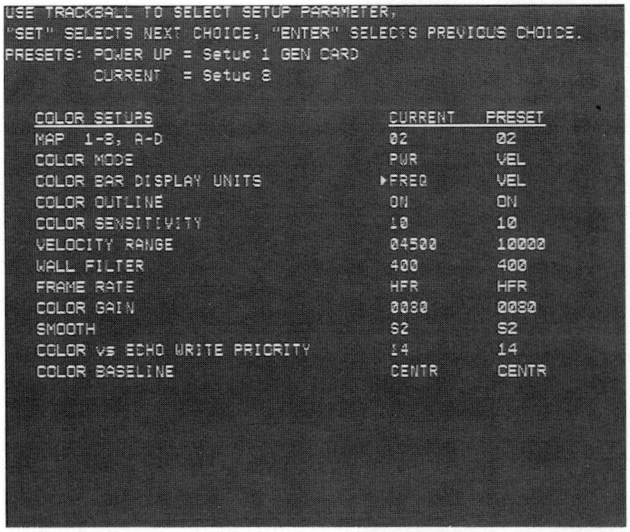

## TECHNICAL LIMITATIONS OF DOPPLER FLOW IMAGING

Needless to say, the technology involved with color flow imaging is complex. The ability to sample multiple sites in real time is a major technologic feat. Many compromises had to be introduced to accomplish this task with a slow moving medium such as sound. One of the principle techniques used is autocorrelation whereby the phase differences from successive echoes of the same site are analyzed in order to identify the velocities. The result is a display of mean velocity of each sample on the two-dimensional image. The amount of electronic manipulation is so great that it is difficult to find two manufacturers who accomplish the feat in the same fashion. Thus, one of the numerous limitations to color flow imaging is the fact that images from one instrument cannot necessarily be compared directly with those of another.

Other problems have arisen with color flow imaging.[84–89] Changes in the color can be confusing. Blood flowing in the same direction will change color merely because of the relationship of the column of blood and the transducer. Figure 1–76 shows how a column of blood can go from red to blue as it passes from left to right across the sector. When the ultrasonic beam is ex-

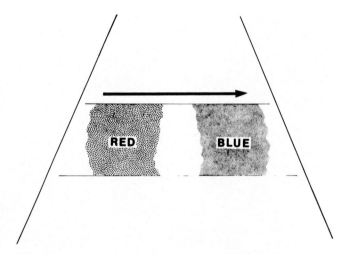

**Fig. 1–76.** Diagram of a color flow image of blood flowing through a tubular structure as perpendicular to the ultrasonic beam. On the left, blood is flowing toward the transducer and is displayed in red. In the center of the record, flow is perpendicular to the ultrasonic beam, and no Doppler signal is recorded. As the flow moves away from the transducer, on the right, the velocities are now inscribed in blue. (From Feigenbaum, H.: Doppler Color Flow Imaging. *In* Heart Disease Update. Edited by E. Braunwald. Philadelphia, W.B. Saunders Co., 1988.)

```
USE TRACKBALL TO SELECT SETUP PARAMETER,
"SET" SELECTS NEXT CHOICE, "ENTER" SELECTS PREVIOUS CHOICE.
PRESETS: POWER UP = Setup 1 GEN CARD
         CURRENT   = Setup 8

COLOR SETUPS                      CURRENT    PRESET
  MAP 1-8, A-D                    02         02
  COLOR MODE                      PWR        VEL
  COLOR BAR DISPLAY UNITS        ►FREQ       VEL
  COLOR OUTLINE                   ON         ON
  COLOR SENSITIVITY               10         10
  VELOCITY RANGE                  04500      10000
  WALL FILTER                     400        400
  FRAME RATE                      HFR        HFR
  COLOR GAIN                      0030       0030
  SMOOTH                          S2         S2
  COLOR vs ECHO WRITE PRIORITY    14         14
  COLOR BASELINE                  CENTR      CENTR
```

**Fig. 1–75.** A listing of some of the options available in doing a color Doppler study.

actly perpendicular to the blood flow, no flow or color is recorded. As already indicated, color flow imaging is a form of pulsed Doppler with a low Nyquist limit. As a result aliasing occurs fairly easily. As the color flow image aliases, the color changes from blue to red, and so on. Another limitation is that the time required to create the color image reduces the frame rate. One must make numerous compromises in the sector angle, the size of the color sample, and the amount of black and white image displayed to try to increase the frame rate. Rapidly moving structures, such as valves, can also produce flashes of color or "ghosting."

One of the major functions of color Doppler imaging is to identify abnormal flow patterns, such as valvular regurgitation or shunts. The color flow image resembles contrast angiography. Thus, there is a tendency to relate color Doppler valvular regurgitation to that seen on an angiogram. Unfortunately, these two technologies have many significant differences. First, the angiogram records the shadow produced by iodinated contrast medium as it regurgitates through an incompetent valve. If an iodinated medium is injected in the left ventricle of a patient with mitral regurgitation, whatever contrast material is seen in the left atrium had to come from the left ventricle. Doppler imaging, however, only records moving cells with a velocity rapid enough to be detected by the color system. Those red cells need not all originate from the left ventricle. Figure 1–77 tries to illustrate this point. In the upper part of the diagram, all the red cells in the left ventricle are illustrated as circles. Those in the left atrium are indicated as stars. With mitral regurgitation, left ventricular red cells (*circles*) move into the left atrium with sufficient velocity to be detected by the Doppler (*black circles*). In addition, as this column of blood enters the left atrium, they act as a cue ball on a billiard table and strike red cells already in the left atrium. These moving red cells are also seen on the Doppler image (*black stars*). Thus, the moving red cells seen in the left atrium in a patient with mitral regurgitation are not all originating from the left ventricle but are energized by the regurgitant blood. This phenomenon is occasionally called the "billiard ball effect."

One of the techniques for estimating the amount of valvular regurgitation is to measure the size of the regurgitant, turbulent flow, or "spray."[90,91] One must again remember that the Doppler study measures velocity and not blood flow. Figure 1–78 shows that the velocity is inversely related to the regurgitant orifice size. Theoretically, a larger regurgitant orifice produces a larger regurgitation flow. Thus, we would like the regurgitant Doppler flow area to be larger with a larger regurgitant orifice. Unfortunately, the velocity actually increases as the size of the regurgitant orifice decreases (Fig. 1–78*B*). The analogy is when one partially occludes the outlet of a garden hose, the resultant water spray is faster, farther, and wider. As the orifice decreases further, then the regurgitant volume will decline to the point that the downstream velocity and spray will also decrease (Fig. 1–78*C*).

Another important factor that influences the size of a regurgitant jet is its location with regard to the chamber

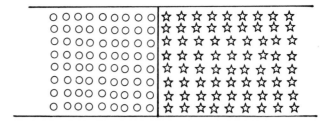

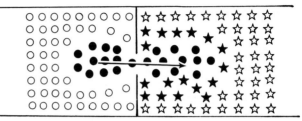

**Fig. 1–77.** Diagram showing how red cells moving from one compartment to another can influence a color Doppler image. On the top of the diagram, one has red cells in the left hand compartment inscribed as circles and in the right hand compartment as stars. If there is a communication between the compartments and the circular red cells flow from left to right, the moving red cells (*black circles*) can be seen within the right hand chamber. The moving red cells from the left hand chamber, however, cause some of the red cells in the right chamber (*black stars*) to move. This effect is sometimes referred to as "billiard ball phenomenon." Doppler flow imaging only records moving red cells. The Doppler study cannot distinguish whether the moving red cells came from the left hand chamber or are just energized red cells that were always in the right hand chamber.

into which it flows.[92] In Figure 1–79*A*, the jet is flowing into the center of a chamber ("free jet") and essentially fills the chamber. In Figure 1–79*B*, the regurgitant orifice size and volume are the same, although the jet is eccentric so that it is directed at one of the walls of the chamber ("wall jet"). Under these circumstances, the flow will cling or is "entrained" to the wall and will not fill the entire chamber. Thus, the area of the turbulent flow will be considerably less than that in Figure 1–79*A* despite the fact that the size of the regurgitant orifice and the volume of regurgitant blood are the same.

Lastly, the size of the regurgitant blood flow is instrument dependent.[86–88] One can vary the amount of turbulent flow depending on multiple controls available on a color Doppler system. The interrogating or carrier frequency, the sector width, the specific color map, the PRF, the number of sampling sites or ensemble length along a scan line, and filter settings can all influence the size of the jet.

Certain physiologic factors must be considered when quantitating valvular regurgitation. The jet is a three-dimensional phenomenon and one must use multiple planes to get a true appreciation of the size of the regurgitant velocities. Physiologic factors such as afterload, the pressure gradient, and compliance of the various chambers influence the degree of regurgitant volume or fraction.

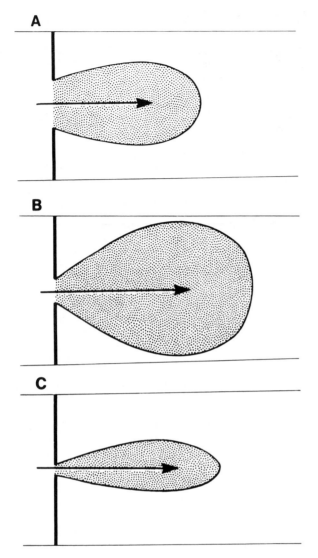

**Fig. 1–78.** Diagram demonstrating how the turbulent downstream spray from fluid passing through a narrowed orifice varies with the size of the orifice. The velocity increases as the orifice becomes smaller. Thus, the jet in *B* can produce a larger velocity map than in *A*. When the orifice is small (*C*), the spray area may in fact be smaller.

Despite these problems, clinical and "intuitive" data indicate that the size of the regurgitant spray is related to the severity of the regurgitation. Better techniques, however, using the proximal convergence acceleration (Fig. 1–73) or measure of regurgitant energy or momentum, are under investigation using Doppler imaging. Other echocardiographic techniques for quantitating valvular regurgitation are discussed in chapter 6, Valvular Heart Disease.

## TRANSTHORACIC TRANSDUCERS

Figure 1–80 illustrates two commercially available phased array and two mechanical transducers. The phased array transducers have a flat surface and no visi-

ble moving parts. The only difference between the transducers is the size of the aperture or the surface of the transducer that is in contact with the body. Phased array transducers vary with frequency and the number of elements in the transducer. The frequency may range from 2.0 to 7.5 MHz. The higher frequency transducers are usually smaller. The number of elements may range from 32 to 128. Again, the transducer with more elements is usually larger. The various frequencies and elements have their advantages and disadvantages. As already mentioned, lower frequency transducers have better penetration and produce better Doppler recordings. The higher frequency transducers give better resolution and finer image quality. Some transducers have dual frequency features whereby one creates images with a higher frequency for better resolution while a lower frequency is available for Doppler interrogation. Broad band transducers that have a range of frequencies, such as 2 to 4 MHz or 3 to 6 MHz, are also being used.

The two mechanical transducers depicted in Figure 1–80 have rounded plastic housings, which are filled with fluid and contain a moving transducer. The transducer on the right is a rotating transducer. Three rotating elements fire in sequence. This transducer has a smaller curvature and acoustic footprint. The slightly larger mechanical transducer has an oscillating single element. This particular transducer has an annular array element. The trade-off is that the annular array provides higher resolution with better lateral beam profiles, but the

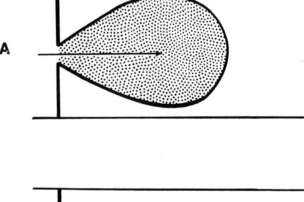

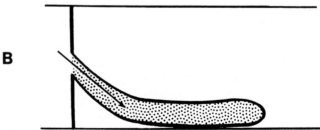

**Fig. 1–79.** Drawing showing that a regurgitant jet with the same orifice and volume can have different spray areas depending on whether the regurgitant flow is into the center of the receiving chamber (free jet) (*A*) or against one of the walls (wall jet) (*B*).

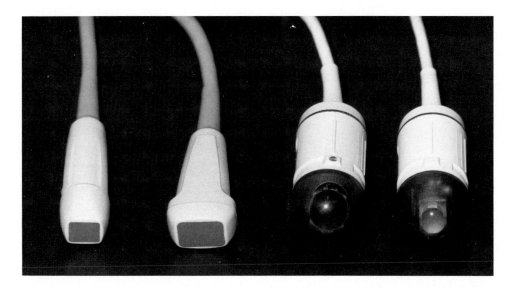

**Fig. 1–80.** Four types of commercially available transthoracic ultrasonic transducers. The two transducers on the left are phased array devices of two different frequencies. The two mechanical probes on the right demonstrate a rotating type of mechanical transducer (far right) and an oscillating annular array transducer (second from the right).

acoustic footprint is larger and the frame rate is somewhat slower.

## TRANSESOPHAGEAL TRANSDUCERS

One of the versatilities of ultrasonic imaging is that the transducers can be of almost any size. Thus, they can be placed on endoscopic instruments, or as will be noted, even on intravascular catheters. Figure 1–81 demonstrates a commercially available transesophageal echocardiographic probe. The ultrasonic transducer is placed at the tip of a standard endoscope. The transducer can be either mechanical[93] or phased array. The diagrams in Figure 1–82 illustrate several phased array, transesophageal echocardiographic transducers. Initially, the probes had a single phased array transducer, which produced a tomographic slice that was perpendicular to the endoscope.[94–97] More recently, devices are available that have two phased array crystals, one that scans horizontally and the other that scans longitudinally.[98–102a] At least one company is making a matrix-type array esophageal probe so that a single transducer can produce both horizontal and longitudinal examinations.[103,104] With the usual biplane probe, the horizontal and longitudinal slices are separated by a few millimeters. The matrix biplane produces two simultaneous scans from the same point. Another manufacturer obtains simultaneous biplane images with two crystals that have independent beam formers.

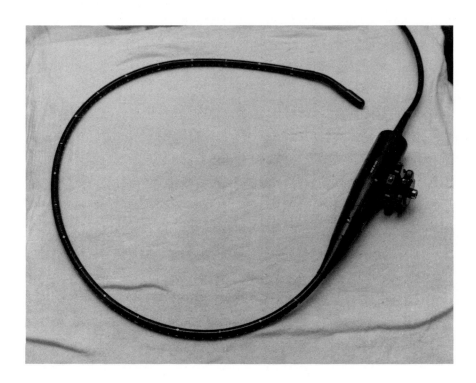

**Fig. 1–81.** A commercially available transesophageal echocardiographic probe.

## PROGRESS IN TEE PROBE
## FOR ADULT

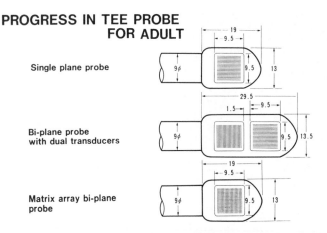

Single plane probe

Bi-plane probe
with dual transducers

Matrix array bi-plane
probe

**Fig. 1–82.** Diagrams demonstrating single plane, bi-plane, and matrix array bi-plane transesophageal probes. (From Omoto, R., et al.: New direction of biplane transesophageal echocardiography with special emphasis on real-time, biplane imaging and matrix phased array biplane transducer. Echocardiography, *7*:691, 1990.)

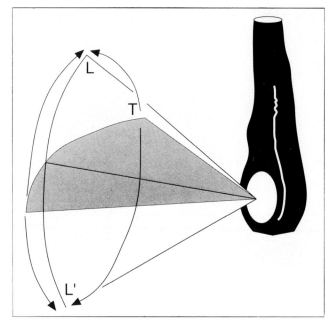

**Fig. 1–84.** Diagram of an omniplane transesophageal probe illustrating how the examining plane can be rotated from the longitudinal to the transverse views. (From Roelandt, J., et al.: Multiplane transesophageal echocardiography with a vari-oplane transducer system. Thoraxcentre Journal, *4*:38, 1992.)

Figure 1–83 shows the transducers in some of the commercially available transesophageal echocardiographic probes. The top transducer is a single plane probe with 32 elements. The second probe also has a single plane but it has 64 elements. The third probe is a biplane with each transducer having 32 elements. The last probe is a matrix-type transducer that has 32 × 32 elements. All of these probes have 5-MHz transducers.

The interest in transesophageal echocardiography is great because of the high quality of imaging that can be obtained through the esophagus. The esophageal window provides an unobstructed view of the heart; the ribs, muscle, and lungs do not obscure the picture. As a result, a host of new transesophageal probes are being developed. Small pediatric probes are now avail-

able.[105–107a] Several multiplane or omniplane transducers are also being used.[107b,107c] Both mechanical and phased array devices are utilized. Phased array devices may have transducers of various shapes that mechanically rotate from horizontal to longitudinal tomographic views. Figure 1–84 demonstrates how an omniplane transesophageal transducer rotates between the longitudinal and transverse planes.

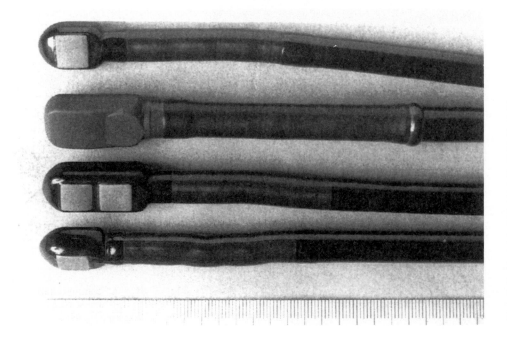

**Fig. 1–83.** Various types of transesophageal probes. The top is a single plane probe with 32 elements. The second from the top is a single plane 64-element transducer. The third probe is a bi-plane probe with 32 elements each. The bottom probe is a matrix bi-plane device. (From Omoto, R., et al.: New direction of biplane transesophageal echocardiography with special emphasis on real-time, biplane imaging and matrix phased array biplane transducer. Echocardiography, *7*:691, 1990.)

Multiplane TEE (Transesophageal Views)

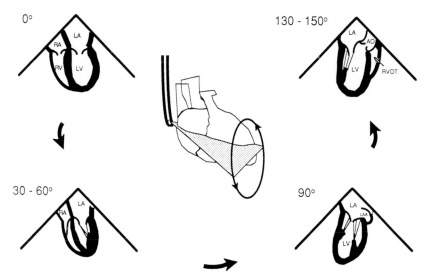

**Fig. 1–85.** Another diagram of an omiplane or multiplane transesophageal examination showing how rotation of the transducer can produce different tomographic views of the heart. The horizontal plane is at zero degrees (upper left) and the longitudinal examination is depicted by the 90° examination (right lower). One can see how intermediate angles (30 to 60°) produce an intermediate image. Rotating the transducer beyond 90° (130 to 150°) reverses the images and shows the right ventricle on the opposite side of the left ventricle. RA = right atrium; LA = left atrium; RV = right ventricle; LV = left ventricle; AO = aorta; RVOT = right ventricular outflow tract; LAA = left atrial appendage. (From Pandian, N.G., et al.: Multiplane transesophageal echocardiography: Imaging planes, echocardiographic anatomy, and clinical experience with a prototype phased array omniplane probe. Echocardiography, 9:649, 1992.)

The diagram in Figure 1–85 shows how an omniplane or multiplane study produces varying tomographic views of the heart. The transverse or horizontal plane is depicted as zero degree rotation (upper left). Ninety-degree rotation of the transducer is equivalent to a longitudinal examination (lower right). An intermediate angle (30 to 60°) shows a tomographic image that is in between the longitudinal and transverse examinations. Rotating the transducer beyond 90° essentially reverses the image (130 to 150°) and records the right ventricle on the other side of the left ventricle.

In addition to multiplane esophageal imaging, wide angle esophageal probes are also available.[108,109] Figure 1–86 shows the schematic drawing of a panoramic transesophageal probe. The transducer rotates mechanically. Figure 1–87 shows a standard horizontal transesophageal, two-dimensional echocardiographic image. Figure 1–87 demonstrates a wide-field tomographic esophageal image.

## INTRAVASCULAR TRANSDUCERS

As already indicated, ultrasonic transducers can be placed on an intravascular catheter of almost any size.[110–112] Five-French (1.8 mm) and larger catheters with ultrasonic transducers at the tip are currently available. It is anticipated that even smaller catheters (3.5F, 1.2 mm) will be available shortly. Ultrasonic transducers can be used at the tip of a small catheter in at least three different ways.[113] Figure 1–88 shows a mechanically rotating ultrasonic transducer. A mechanical shaft through the catheter rotates the transducer.[114–118] The transducer may be at a slight forward angle so that the slice is slightly in front of the tip of the catheter. Obviously, the shaft must be flexible, and electric wires are contained within it to operate the transducer. Another

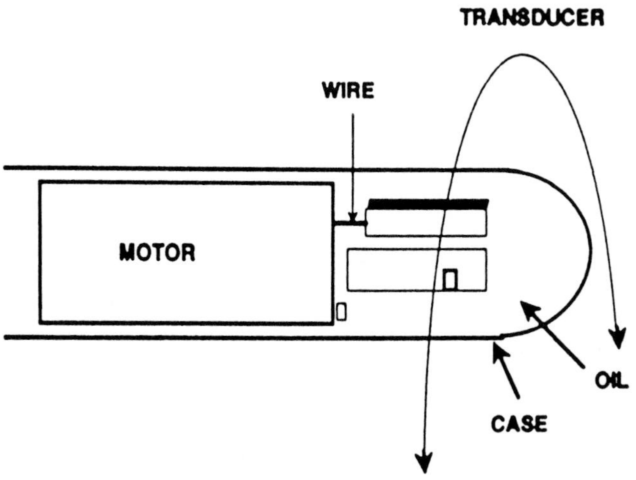

**Fig. 1–86.** Schematic drawing showing the basic design of a panoramic transesophageal probe tip. (From Shu, T.L., et al.: Panoramic transesophageal echocardiography. Echocardiography, 8:677, 1991.)

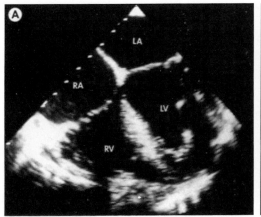
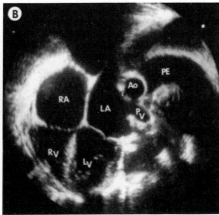

**Fig. 1–87.** Comparison of a two-dimensional transesophageal echocardiogram (*A*) and a wide field tomographic (*B*) study in a patient with bronchogenic carcinoma. E = esophagus; LV = left ventricle; RV = right ventricle. (From Seward, J.B., et al.: Wide field transesophageal echocardiographic tomography: Feasibility study. Mayo Clin. Proc., *65*:31, 1990.)

method is to have a stationary transducer housed with a rotating mirror (Fig. 1–89).[119–121] One of the advantages of the mirror device is the longer distance from the transducer to the tissue being interrogated, which minimizes some of the near field clutter or ring-down artifact that is inherent in all ultrasonic imaging. The third method for intravascular ultrasonic imaging is to use an electronically switched phased array system.[122,123] Figure 1–90 demonstrates such a device, which has a series of elements arranged circularly around the tip of a transducer.

Interest in intravascular ultrasound is extremely high and the technology is advancing rapidly.[124,125] Spectacular images of intraarterial structures have been reported and are redefining our understanding of atherosclerosis.[126–126b] Figure 1–91 demonstrates an intravascular ultrasonic catheter in a coronary artery. The resultant ultrasonic image shows an atherosclerotic plaque (*arrows*) in the left anterior descending artery. The frequencies used in intraarterial vascular catheters are usually 20 to 40 MHz. Obviously, one obtains excellent resolution but poor penetration. Catheters with intravascular ultrasound and balloons for angioplasty have been developed.[127]

The use of intravascular ultrasonic devices for intracardiac examinations has also generated interest.[128–131]

These catheters are considerably larger and are placed in large vessels or directly within the heart. The frequency is lower so that penetration is better. Figure 1–92 demonstrates some cardiac images that can be obtained with an intravascular ultrasonic probe within the left side of the heart.

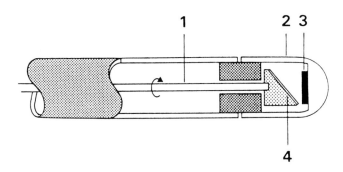

**Fig. 1–89.** Drawing showing a mechanically driven shaft (1) that rotates a mirror (4). The mirror reflects the ultrasonic beam generated from the transducer (3). (From Bom, N., et al.: Early and recent interluminal ultrasound devices. *In* Intravascular Ultrasound. Edited by N. Bom and J. Roelandt. Dordrecht, Netherlands, Kluwer Academic Publishers, 1989.)

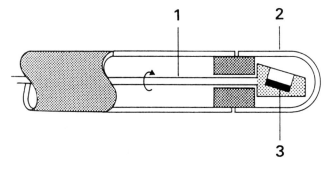

**Fig. 1–88.** Diagram illustrating an intravascular ultrasonic probe that uses a rotating shaft (1), a transparent dome (2), and an echo element (3) in a catheter tip system. (From Bom, N., et al.: Early and recent interluminal ultrasound devices. *In* Intravascular Ultrasound. Edited by N. Bom and J. Roelandt. Dordrecht, Netherlands, Kluwer Academic Publishers, 1989.)

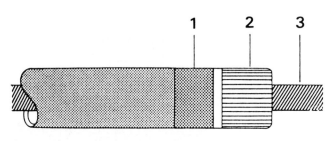

**Fig. 1–90.** Intravascular ultrasound device using a switched phased array catheter tip. The guidewire (3) passes through the catheter (1), which contains the multiple elements (2). (From Bom, N., et al.: Early and recent interluminal ultrasound devices. *In* Intravascular Ultrasound. Edited by N. Bom and J. Roelandt. Dordrecht, Netherlands, Kluwer Academic Publishers, 1989.)

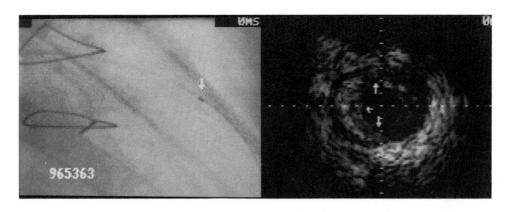

**Fig. 1–91.** An intravascular ultrasonic device in the left anterior descending coronary artery of a patient with coronary atherosclerosis. The coronary angiogram shows the device (*arrow*) within the artery. The ultrasonic examination on the right shows a thickened, crescent-shaped band of echoes (*arrows*) along the left hand side of the arterial wall.

Doppler transducers can also be placed on catheters. Such probes have been used to measure coronary or pulmonary artery velocities.[132–135a] Figure 1–93 illustrates an example of one of these intravascular Doppler transducers.[135b] A Doppler catheter has also been devised for guiding retrograde aortic catheterization.[135c]

## OTHER TRANSDUCERS

A variety of other transducers have been designed. At least two types of hand-held transducers have been described. The first was a linear scanner shaped like an hour glass.[136,137] More recently, a small mechanical sector scanner has been used in a "hand held" manner.[138]

Ultrasonic transducers with transponders have also been built.[139] The transponder sends out a sonic signal that shows up on the echogram. By placing it at the tip of a needle or catheter, the transponder allows the examiner to know exactly where the tip is located.

Transducers have also been designed for use in the operating room for epicardial examination.[140–142] These high frequency devices are held by the surgeon and placed directly on the heart. Epicardial scanning is largely being replaced by transesophageal monitoring during surgery.

## CONTRAST ECHOCARDIOGRAPHY

Early in the history of echocardiography, it was discovered that whenever a liquid was injected within the cardiovascular system tiny suspended bubbles produced

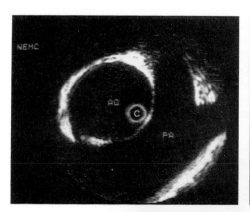

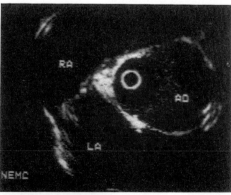

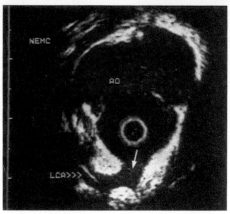

**Fig. 1–92.** Cardiac images taken with an intravascular ultrasonic probe placed in the aortic root. AO = aorta; PA = pulmonary artery; C = catheter; RA = right atrium; LA = left atrium; LCA = left coronary artery. (From Pandian, N.G., et al.: Real-time, intracardiac, two-dimensional echocardiography. Echocardiography, *8*:407, 1991.)

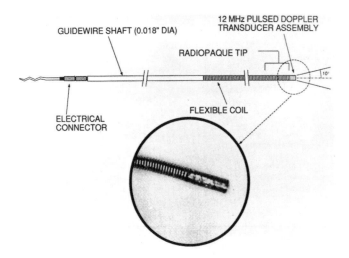

**Fig. 1–93.** Diagram of a Doppler guidewire. The Doppler transducer is mounted at the tip of a flexible coil to be placed within the arterial tree. (From Doucette, J.W., et al.: Validation of a Doppler guide wire for intravascular measurement of coronary artery flow velocity. Circulation, *85*:1899, 1992, by permission of the American Heart Association, Inc.)

a cloud of echoes. This phenomenon was first recognized with the use of indocyanine green dye during cardiac catheterization.[143–145] Almost any liquid with suspended bubbles gives the same effect. The cloud of echoes varies somewhat with the size and quantity of the bubbles. At present, contrast agents commonly used include saline that has been agitated with a small amount of air. Sonication of agents such as iodinated contrast or albumen gives a high quality contrast effect.[146–148] More recently, contrast agents that contain tiny bubbles have been commercially manufactured.[149] Two agents produce contrast in slightly different fashions. One agent has a saccharide particle that either has a bubble trapped or generates a bubble in vivo.[150,151] The other agent uses sonicated albumen, which produces tiny bubbles.[152,153]

The unique feature of these two agents is that the bubbles are small enough to pass through capillaries.[154,155] The bubbles usually produced by agitated saline or sonicated Renografin (diatrizoate meglumine) will not pass through capillaries. Figure 1–94 demonstrates an intravenous injection of sonicated albumen that lights up the right ventricle, passes through the pulmonary capillaries, and opacifies the cavity of the left ventricle. The new commercial microbubbles are 2 to 12 μm in diameter. Only those less than 10 μm pass through the lungs and only those greater than 6 μm are visualized ultrasonically. Thus, the ideal bubble is between 6 and 8 μm in diameter.

Contrast echocardiography has been used for a variety of clinical diagnoses. The most common indication is for right-to-left shunting.[156] The technique is a sensitive means of finding small shunts. In addition, a considerable amount of work has gone into using contrast echocardiography for myocardial opacification to identify perfusion.[157–160] Under these circumstances, the contrast material is injected directly into the coronary arteries or at the root of the aorta. Both of these applications will be discussed in their appropriate chapters. Contrast medium is also being used to enhance both spectral and color Doppler examinations.[161–164]

A contrast effect may be seen within an echocardiogram spontaneously. The opacification of the blood usually appears as a swirling, "smoke-like" cloud. This phenomenon has been recognized for many years and occurs primarily with evidence of stagnant blood. It has been seen in patients with dilated, poorly contracted left ventricles or apical aneurysms (Fig. 1–95). More recently, the phenomenon has been seen regularly with dilated left atria resulting from mitral valve disease.[165,166] The spontaneous echoes in the left atrium are seen best with transesophageal echocardiography and in the left ventricle with a 5.0-MHz transthoracic transducer. Various theories have been proposed concerning the etiology of spontaneous contrast. Erythrocyte rouleaux formation[166a] and interaction of erythrocytes and

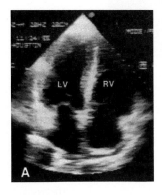
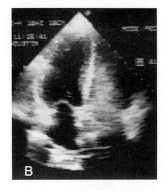
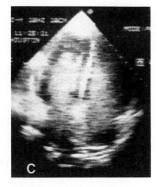

**Fig. 1–94.** Apical four-chamber echocardiogram showing the contrast effect with an intravenous injection of sonicated albumin microspheres. The contrast is seen initially in the right ventricle (*B*). Later, the microspheres pass through the lungs and appear in the left ventricle (*C*). LV = left ventricle; RV = right. Reprinted with permission of the American College of Cardiology. (From Feinstein, S.B., et al.: Safety and efficacy of a new transpulmonary ultrasound contrast agent: Initial multicenter clinical results. J. Am. Coll. Cardiol., *16*:316, 1990.)

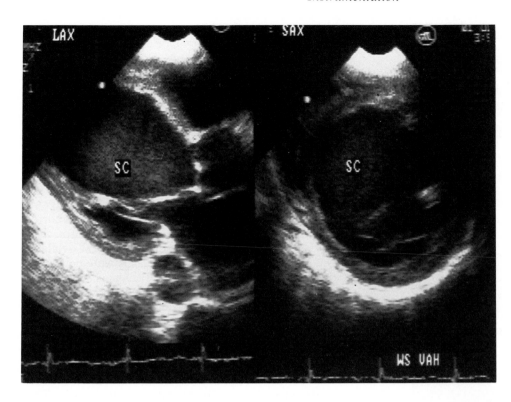

**Fig. 1–95.** Spontaneous contrast (SC) in the left ventricle of a patient with a dilated cardiomyopathy. LAX = long axis; SAX = short axis.

plasma proteins modulated by shear forces[166b] are among them.

## DIGITAL ECHOCARDIOGRAPHY

The usual history of echocardiography begins with M-mode echocardiography and goes on to two-dimensional, Doppler, color flow Doppler, and transesophageal imaging. There is a parallel history of the recording of echocardiographic information. In the early years, many echocardiographers recorded the M-mode tracings on Polaroid film. A major breakthrough was the development of strip chart recorders, which permitted an easier and more valuable recording of M-mode tracings. With the advent of two-dimensional echocardiography came the need for a real-time, two-dimensional recording. Some investigators used movie film. Then, almost everyone began using videotape. A variety of different types of videotape recordings have been used, and this medium remains the backbone of two-dimensional echocardiography. Because of many inconveniences of having large reams of strip chart paper, videotape is used in many echocardiographic laboratories for all recordings, both M-mode and Doppler, as well as for two-dimensional and color flow studies.

Although videotape is an extremely versatile and cost-effective means of recording and storing echocardiographic images, there are significant limitations. One problem is the tendency to record excessive amounts of information. A full study, including two-dimensional, M-mode, spectral Doppler, and color flow imaging may take 10 to 20 minutes of videotape. One of the major disadvantages of this approach is that the clinician fre-

quently does not have the patience to view that much videotape. Furthermore, the tape may not be easily accessible to the referring clinician; it may still be in the instrument or it may be on a shelf along with studies of 10 or 20 other patients on a 2-hour videotape. Merely finding a specific patient on a tape may be too time consuming for the average physician. As a result, relatively few clinicians who have no special interest in echocardiography take the time to look at echocardiograms on videotape. It is also difficult to show videotapes at conferences because an unedited videotape is lengthy. One of the consequences of this difficulty is that many cardiologists are not adequately familiar with echocardiography and clearly do not look at the echocardiograms of their patients.

Another deficiency of videotape is trying to use this medium for serial studies. Echocardiography is an ideal technique for doing multiple studies of a given patient. The examination is virtually painless, does no harm that we can detect, and is less costly than other sophisticated imaging examinations. Trying to view more than one study, however, is difficult. One usually looks at the current examination and merely compares it with a previous report. One would have to get an old tape, view it, look at the current tape, and make a mental comparison; the studies are not viewed side-by-side. Using this technique to compare more than two examinations would be out of the question.

An alternative way of recording and storing echocardiograms is to use a digital technique with computer storage.[167] One can use frame grabbers to digitally capture individual cardiac cycles and store them in a variety of different fashions. Figure 1–96 shows a standard echocardiograph with a commercially available frame

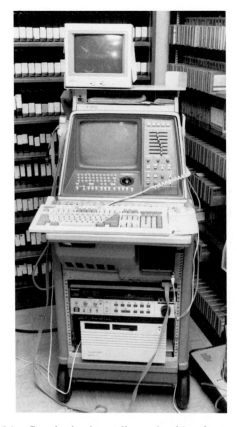

**Fig. 1–96.** Standard echocardiograph with a frame-grabbing computer below the tape recorder. The computer monitor is on top. The keyboard is on the handles and can be placed in the compartment on the top during transport.

grabber inserted below the tape recorder. The computer monitor is mounted on top. One can digitize and display a single full image, two views as a split image, or four examinations as a quad screen. Four views can be displayed simultaneously. Newer digital systems can display as many as 16 images on one screen. Digital recordings overcome many of the deficiencies of videotape. They make the examination readily accessible for the clinician to review. Individual studies can be retrieved in 10 to 30 seconds. One can look at the study as long as is necessary without rewinding the videotape. The digital approach is ideal for analyzing serial studies. One can easily compare two, three, or four studies simultaneously to see whether or not any changes have occurred. Furthermore, with the study in the digital form, all of the versatility of digital technology becomes available. Quantitation using computers is easier. Automatic quantitation is feasible. Networking the images is a viable option, as is sending images by modem.[168] Higher quality hard copy images are easier with digital recordings. Most of the newer illustrations in this book are from digitally recorded echocardiograms. Figure 1–97 shows a quad screen, digital echocardiogram. The parasternal long-axis, short-axis, and apical four-chamber and two-chamber views can be analyzed at the same time. The views were not actually obtained simultaneously. They were captured sequentially by triggering off the electrocardiogram and then displaying them synchronously.

Digital retrieval and storage of echocardiograms again raises the issue of compromise. One has to decide what is important in the digital recordings. Table 1–3 demonstrates some of the factors to consider when storing digi-

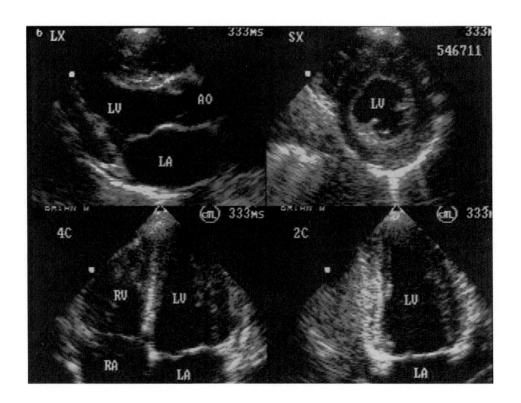

**Fig. 1–97.** Digitally acquired two-dimensional echocardiographic images displayed in a quad screen format. LX = long axis; SX = short axis; 4C = four chamber; 2C = two chamber; LV = left ventricle; AO = aorta; LA = left atrium; RV = right ventricle; RA = right atrium.

**Table 1–3**
Factors Involved in Digital Echocardiography

A. Video signal and monitor
  1. Off-line, videotape
  2. On-line, live
    a. Composite video
    b. R G B
B. Resolution
  1. 512 × 512 (512 × 480)
  2. 512 × 256 (512 × 240)
  3. 256 × 256 (256 × 240)
C. Electrocardiographic triggering
  1. Internal trigger
  2. External trigger
  3. On-line
  4. Off-line
D. Number of frames or cells per cardiac cycle
E. Interval or interim delay
F. Start delay
G. Playback delay
H. Storage
  1. Normal
  2. Compressed
I. Storage medium
  1. RAM
  2. Hard disk
  3. Floppy disk
  4. Optical disk
  5. Network
  6. Modem

tal echocardiograms. First, one needs to identify the video signal. This signal could be a composite video or RGB. RGB stands for red, green, blue and is the preferred signal, especially for color recordings. The video source could be tape or, preferably, a live, on-line examination. The on-line recording is of higher quality. The digital resolution that is stored can vary. Obviously, the highest quality images are obtained with the highest resolution. Electrocardiographic triggering is critical for capturing the images. Another major issue is how many frames or cells per cardiac cycle will be stored. Then, the interval or interim delay between each cardiac cell is determined. An option is whether or not a start delay is introduced. The playback delay is also a variable. And lastly, the storage can be normal or compressed to conserve space on the digital medium. The next issue is where to store the images. Options include floppy disks, hard disks, optical disks, and networks.

Ideally, one would want the highest resolution, the most frames per cardiac cycle, and normal storage. As with all echocardiography, however, compromises are frequently necessary. For example, one has to decide what type of permanent storage medium to use. One cardiac cycle with 512 × 512 pixel resolution, 30 frames per second, and normal storage requires 7.5 megabytes of storage. A color image will be two to three times that much. Current standard, inexpensive floppy disks have only 1.2 to 1.4 megabytes of storage. Hard disks of several hundred megabytes are readily available. But even several hundred megabytes will not store studies of

many patients for long periods. Thus, hard disk storage would be temporary. Optical disks store more studies, but they must be played back on an optical disk system, which is fairly expensive. Usually, multiple studies are on a given optical disk and many people may want access to that optical disk simultaneously. The ability of clinicians to see their studies and to conduct serial reviews, the principle reasons for digital echocardiography, may not be practical if everything is on one optical disk in one playback system.

Probably the ideal approach is to have a network whereby multiple examinations are stored permanently on a multiple optical disk jukebox. But even an optical disk jukebox has a finite limit as to how much memory one can practically use per study. Using more than 2 to 3 megabytes per study would seriously limit even a network with optical disks. As a result, the most practical approach is to keep the amount of memory to a minimum. Not only would one save on the amount of storage memory needed, but also the retrieval time would be reduced. A clinician is busy and has a limited attention span. Retrieving a 30-frame, 512 × 512 study could easily take several minutes if stored on an optical disk.

A scheme that has been used at our institution for many years involves two-dimensional echocardiographic resolution of 256 × 256 and eight cells per cardiac cycle. All two-dimensional images, including color, are usually captured as a quad screen (see Fig. 1–97) to maximize the amount of information per digital memory. Furthermore, the images are stored with nondestructive compression and 64 shades of gray. Color images obviously require more memory but the resolution is the same. Only five bit color is usually stored. Doppler and M-mode images are captured at 512 × 240 resolution and stored using a compression algorithm. As computer technology, storage medium, and compression algorithms improve, this scheme may also change. But for the time being, this approach has been extremely useful and provides the necessary information in most cases.

The digital recording functions as a brief review or abstract of the total case. The digital approach does not have sufficient information to replace videotape at this time. With the rapid advances in digital technology, however, this situation may change in the near future.

## COMPUTER MANIPULATION OF ECHOCARDIOGRAPHIC RECORDINGS

Besides capturing and storing echocardiographic images digitally, computers can manipulate the data to enhance the quality or the interpretation of the examination. Image quality has always been a major goal of ultrasonic examinations. Echocardiography is obtained in a somewhat hostile environment and the signal-to-noise ratio is not always optimal. The manufacturers digitally "massage" the data extensively before it is seen on the ultrasonic monitor. There are efforts to go beyond what the manufacturers provide to try to improve the image even further.[169,170] For example, it is possible to digitally average several cardiac cycles to

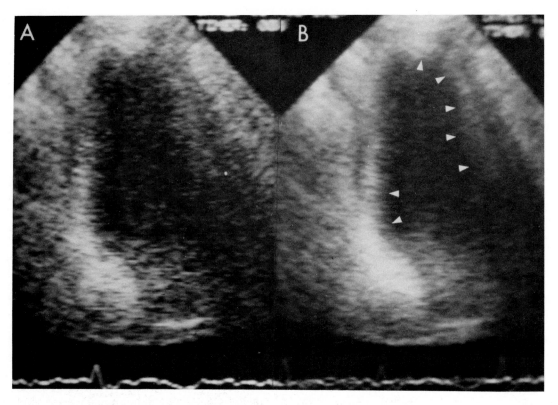

**Fig. 1–98.** Echocardiogram demonstrating the effect of digital averaging. The image in *B* is a composite of three similar echograms taken from different cardiac cycles. The three images are digitally averaged. This technique improves the signal-to-noise ratio. Intracavitary echoes are suppressed, and myocardial echoes are enhanced. The myocardium blood pool interface (*arrowheads*) is better seen with the digitally processed image.

improve the signal-to-noise ratio.[171] Figure 1–98 shows how one can improve myocardial definition by digitally averaging three cardiac cycles. Certainly motion artifact needs to be eliminated to minimize artifact.

The echocardiographic images can be converted to color. This so-called "B color" or pseudocolor converts gray scale to different shades of color.[172–175] Figure 1–99 demonstrates one of the early efforts at colorizing a two-dimensional echocardiogram. The dense fibrous areas are colorized in shades of red for easier identification. Figure 1–100 shows newer efforts at colorizing two-dimensional images. This technique is intended to enhance the perception of the endocardial edges.

Figure 1–101 shows another way of using colorized two-dimensional imaging to enhance the visualization of cardiac motion. The diastolic image is encoded in blue with all of the other images in shades of red. Those walls that are moving are identified as a thick rim of red. If there is minimal or no motion, there is minimal or no red rim (*arrowheads*).

Investigators have been interested in automatically identifying the endocardial edge so that quantification of ventricular function can be improved.[176–180] One of the latest techniques produces automatic edge detection, which is based on identifying the endocardial-blood interface (Fig. 1–102).[181] The technique analyzes the radio frequency signal and is obtained in real time. Once the

endocardial outline is identified, one can place a cursor around the cavity and a real-time graph of cavity area is displayed (Fig. 1–103). Because of lateral myocardial dropout, the system also has a lateral gain control to enhance the automatic edge detection technique (Fig. 1–104).[181a] Unfortunately, this lateral gain can also produce artifact, and thus it needs to be used carefully. For example, in Figure 1–104, the apical dilatation is not obvious in the lateral gain enhanced four-chamber view.

A relatively new technique of looking at phase analysis of digitized two-dimensional echocardiograms is being suggested as a sensitive way for looking at wall motion.[182]

## TISSUE IDENTIFICATION USING ULTRASOUND

Ultrasound has been used for tissue identification for many years. Investigators have used various techniques to recognize tissue types from a variety of different organs. Experimental data indicate that the reflected sound is different from various tissue types.[183–187] Most of the current work involves interrogation of the integrated spectral backscatter, which is done by using the raw radio frequency signal before digital and video manipulation. Figure 1–105 shows an M-mode echocardiogram whereby tissue identification is performed. The

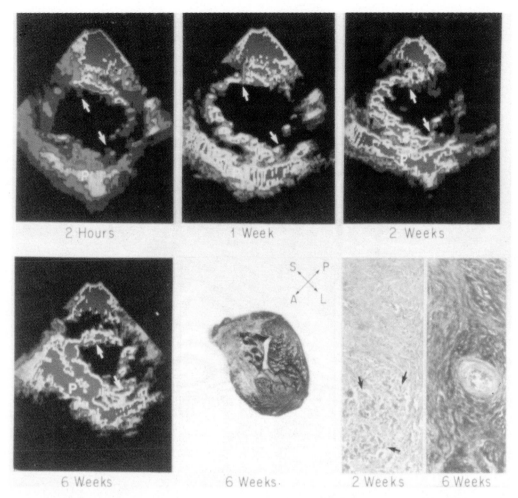

**Fig. 1–99.** Color-encoded two-dimensional echocardiogram using color to enhance visualization of echo amplitudes. This series of echocardiograms demonstrates the development of high-intensity echoes from fibrosis as collagen is laid down in this experimental myocardial infarction. The high-intensity echoes are depicted in the red colors. (From Parisi, A.F., et al.: Enhanced detection of the evolution of tissue changes after acute myocardial infarction using color encoded two-dimensional echocardiography. Circulation, *66*:64, 1982, by permission of the American Heart Association, Inc.)

real-time, backscatter, M-mode echocardiographic recording is analyzed by placing a cursor within the middle of the myocardium. Cyclic variation of the backscatter has been observed in the normal individual.[188] If the myocardium is ischemic, no cyclic variation is noted.[189-191] This work is under active investigation and is discussed further in the chapter on coronary artery disease.

Techniques have been explored to try to distinguish clot from tissue or tumors.[187-192] Other efforts have been directed toward identifying such tissue types as amyloidosis[191] or hypertrophic cardiomyopathy.[183-186]

## THREE-DIMENSIONAL ECHOCARDIOGRAPHY

Shortly after the introduction of two-dimensional echocardiography, investigators began working on efforts to produce three-dimensional cardiac ultrasonic images.[193-197] Most of the efforts thus far involve reconstruction of two-dimensional scanning.[198] If one knows the spatial position of the ultrasonic transducer,[199,199a] and if the endocardial borders are digitized, one can produce a three-dimensional reconstruction of the left ventricular cavity. Figure 1–106 is one of the early efforts at this type of investigation. Numerous techniques have been devised since these early attempts.[200-202] The newer examinations are far more sophisticated and more accurate but are basically founded on the same technique. Because of the high quality of imaging derived from the transesophageal approach, considerable interest has been generated in three-dimensional reconstruction of the heart using transesophageal imaging.[203]

Figure 1–107 shows a three-dimensional reconstruction of a transesophageal echocardiographic study using a multiplane transducer.[203a] By obtaining tomographic slices of the heart at multiple angles, one can record sufficient information to permit three-dimensional re-

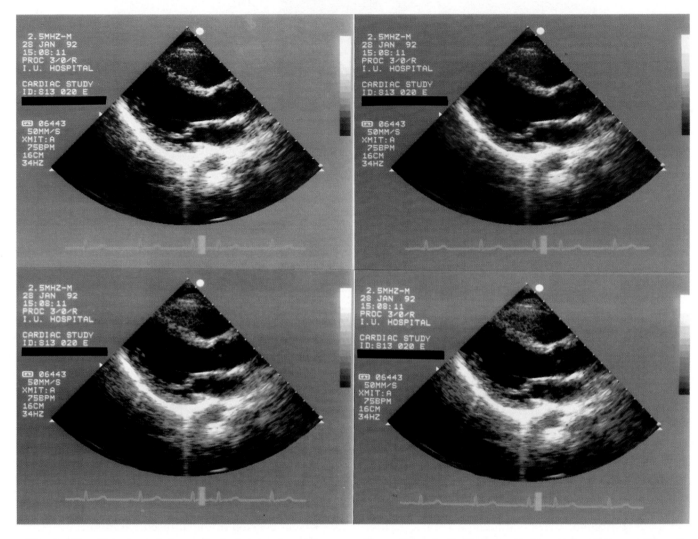

**Fig. 1–100.** Color-encoded two-dimensional echocardiograms. These "B color" displays can be produced in a variety of different colors and shades.

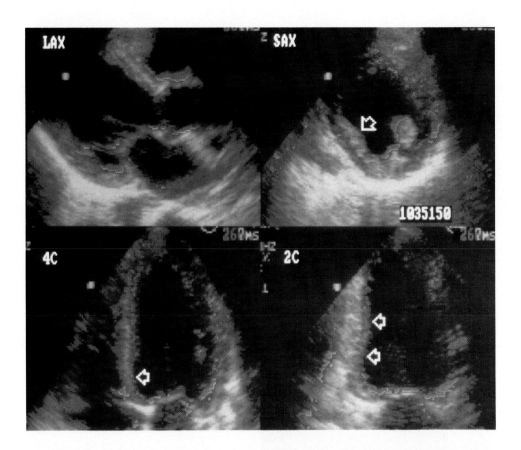

**Fig. 1–101.** A colorized two-dimensional echocardiogram with images of diastole (light blue) and systole (red). Superimposing the colors shows wall motion as rims of red. No red rim (*arrowheads*) indicates no or minimal wall motion.

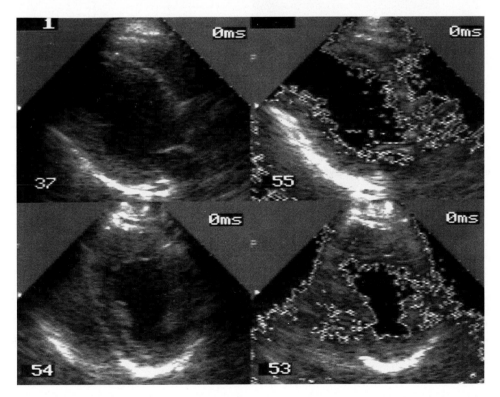

**Fig. 1–102.** Two-dimensional echocardiogram demonstrating an edge detection technique for identifying the blood-endocardial interface. This detection is performed in real-time.

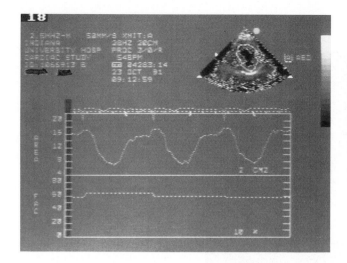

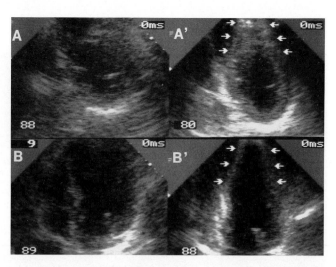

**Fig. 1–103.** This illustration demonstrates how the real-time edge detection device can produce a display of the cyclic variation in the area of the left ventricle. An area of interest is drawn around the left ventricular cavity and the instrument automatically determines the area on a frame-to-frame basis. The graphic display shows the change in area and the fractional area change (FAC).

**Fig. 1–104.** Two-dimensional echocardiogram demonstrating an effort at enhancing lateral gain on two-dimensional images. The lateral gain of the short-axis view (*A′*) clearly improves the visualization of the endocardial border. The lateral gain, however, when used in the four-chamber view (*B′*), can produce an artifactual apex (*arrows*). The lateral gain would indicate a narrowed apex where in fact the apex is dilated (*B*).

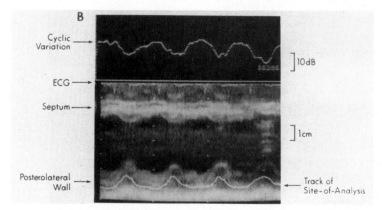

**Fig. 1–105.** M-mode echocardiogram showing how one can track the integrated backscatter of the posterior left ventricular wall. The cyclic variation of the backscatter is demonstrated graphically at the top of the recording. (From Milunski, M.R., et al.: Ultrasonic tissue characterization with integrated back scatter. Circulation, *80*:491, 1989, by permission of the American Heart Association, Inc.)

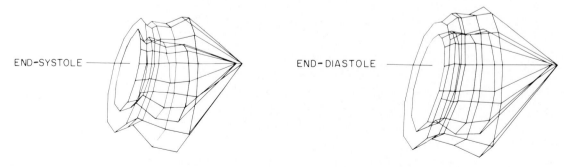

**Fig. 1–106.** A computer-generated display of a three-dimensional echocardiogram of the left ventricle at end-diastole and end-systole. (From Geiser, E.A., et al.: Dynamic three-dimensional echocardiographic reconstruction of the intact left ventricle: Technique and initial observation in patients. Am. Heart J., *103*:1056, 1982.)

construction of the examination. Once the information is in the computer, the display can be manipulated. The structures can be viewed in multiple ways. Figure 1–108 shows another effort at three-dimensional reconstruction using transesophageal echocardiography. In this case, one uses a single transesophageal plane and gradu-

ally withdraws the transducer using a mechanical system, thereby obtaining multiple tomographic views of the heart.[203b] The recordings can then be reconstructed. All of these reconstruction techniques require the superimposition of multiple cardiac cycles. Respiration has to be controlled or gated to minimize artifact.

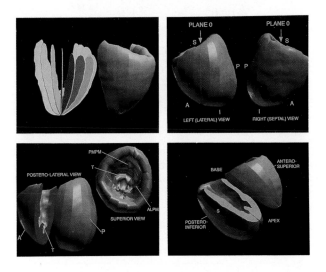

**Fig. 1–107.** Three-dimensional display of a reconstructed transesophageal examination. The study was obtained with multiple transesophageal echocardiographic images. The transducer is rotated through various angles to obtain the multiple views. This illustration demonstrates some of the ways that the three-dimensional image can be displayed. S = ventricular septum; T = trabeculation; A = anterior lateral wall; ALPM = anterior lateral papillary muscle; I = inferior wall; LW = lateral wall; P = posterior wall; PMDM = posterior medial papillary muscle. (From Nanda, N.C., et al.: Multiplane transesophageal echocardiographic imaging in three-dimensional reconstruction: A preliminary study. Echocardiography, 9:667, 1992.)

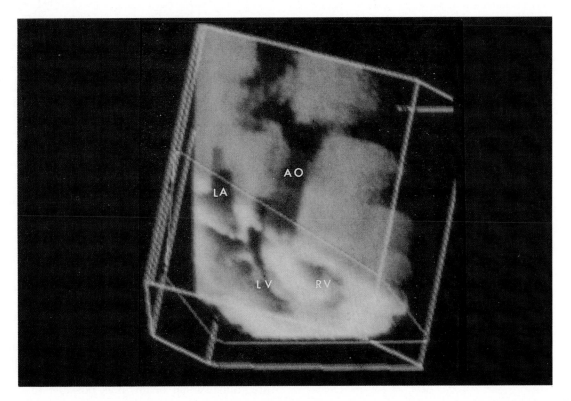

**Fig. 1–108.** Another effort at obtaining three-dimensional reconstruction of a transesophageal echocardiographic study. In this example, the transducer is mechanically withdrawn within the esophagus to create multiple linear tomographic slices of the heart. LA = left atrium; AO = aorta; LV = left ventricle; RV = right ventricle. (From Pandian, N.G., et al.: Three-dimensional and four-dimensional transesophageal echocardiographic imaging of the heart and aorta in humans using computed tomographic imaging probe. Echocardiography, 9:677, 1992.)

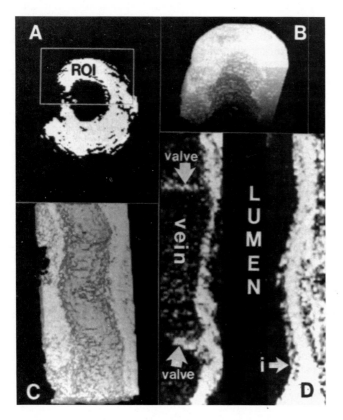

**Fig. 1–109.** Three-dimensional reconstruction of an intravascular ultrasonic examination of an artery. *A* is the region of interest (ROI), which is then displayed three-dimensionally in *B*. The cylindric image can be rotated to display the inner surface (*C*). One can also recreate a sagittal view of the lumen (*D*). (From Rosenfield, K., et al.: Three-dimensional reconstruction of human coronary and peripheral arteries from images recorded during two-dimensional intravascular ultrasound examination. Circulation, *84*:1938, 1991, by permission of the American Heart Association, Inc.)

## Pyramidal Scan

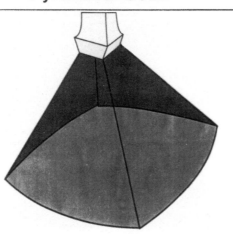

**Fig. 1–110.** Schematic diagram of a three-dimensional pyramidal scan. (From Sheikh, K.H., et al.: Real-time three-dimensional echocardiography: Feasibility and initial use. Echocardiography, *8*:119, 1991.)

## C-Scan

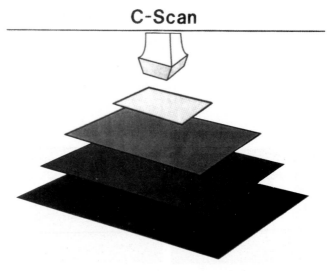

**Fig. 1–111.** Schematic diagram of a C-scan presentation. The images are displayed parallel rather than perpendicular to the transducer. (From Sheikh, K.H., et al.: Real-time three-dimensional echocardiography: Feasibility and initial use. Echocardiography, *8*:119, 1991.)

## Three-dimensional Volume

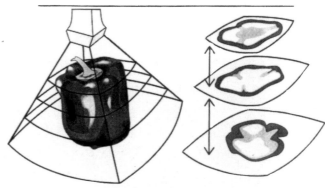

**Fig. 1–112.** Schematic diagram demonstrating how one could create three-dimensional volumes with serial parallel cuts through an object. (From Sheikh, K.H., et al.: Real-time three-dimensional echocardiography: Feasibility and initial use. Echocardiography, *8*:119, 1991.)

Intravascular imaging offers further opportunities for three-dimensional reconstruction.[204] Figure 1–109 demonstrates a reconstruction type of examination of a coronary artery using intravascular ultrasound. Different ways to display three-dimensional images exist.

There are a few investigators looking at real-time three-dimensional imaging.[207,208] Using matrix type phased array scanners and parallel processing one can produce a "pyramidal" scan (Fig. 1–110). With a truly three-dimensional beam, it is possible to create two-dimensional scans in almost any plane, including C-scans (Fig. 1–111). These C-scans are essentially frontal planes or planes which are parallel to the transducer's surface. Figure 1–112 demonstrates how one might create a three-dimensional volume of an object using C-scans.[205,206]

## BIOLOGIC EFFECTS OF ULTRASOUND

One of the principal reasons for the popularity of and interest in echocardiography is that the examination is presumed to pose no hazard to the patient. In contrast to the usual invasive techniques that require catheterization and angiography, the risk to the patient is virtually negligible. Even the avoidance of ionizing radiation is an advantage of ultrasound. Ultrasonic examinations of all parts of the body, including such sensitive tissues as a pregnant uterus and the eye, have been performed on thousands of patients all over the world without reports of a single untoward reaction. The question of safety of this external energy source, however, must still be constantly reviewed since there are obvious biologic effects of ultrasound.[207–215,215a] Furthermore, newer applications and instruments with higher energy are being introduced. For example, some Doppler systems have very high energy, raising concern about examining the fetus under these conditions.

When discussing the safety or biologic effects of diagnostic ultrasound, it is necessary to understand some of the terms used. Any biologic effect of ultrasound depends on the energy in question. The amount of acoustic energy (capacity to do work or to produce a biologic effect) is measured in joules.[216] A joule is the amount of heat generated by the energy in question, in this case, ultrasound. A joule is equal to 0.239 calories. A calorie is the amount of heat energy required to raise the temperature of 1 g of water 1°C. Acoustic power is the amount of acoustic energy per unit time. For example, the power is one watt (1 W) if 1 joule of energy is produced per second. A milliwatt (mW) is 0.001 W and the kilowatt (kW) is 1000 W. The biologic effects of ultrasound are usually discussed in terms of power, and the units of power are in the milliwatt range.[216]

Another term used to describe the amount of energy used in diagnostic ultrasound is intensity. Intensity may also be called "power density," and is the concentration of power within an area usually expressed as watts per meter squared ($W/m^2$) or in milliwatts per centimeter squared ($mW/cm^2$). As previously discussed in this chapter, ultrasonic intensity varies spatially within the ultrasonic beam. For example, if one uses a continuous wave ultrasonic beam, the average intensity, frequently called the spatial average (SA) intensity, is obtained by dividing the total power emitted by the transducer by the surface area of the face of the transducer. If the power output of the transducer were 2.0 mW and the radiating surface of the transducer were 1.0 cm², then the spatial average intensity would be 2.0 mW/cm². Since the shape and amplitude of the ultrasonic beam vary (see Fig. 1–13), so does the intensity of the ultrasonic energy. Thus, the peak or spatial peak (SP) intensity varies at different locations within the ultrasonic beam. As expected, the SP intensity is greater in the center of the beam than at the periphery. The peak or spatial peak intensity can be measured by using a small thermocouple temperature sensor to detect minuscule rises in temperature in certain areas of the sound field. One may also measure intensity by using a second tiny receiving piezoelectric transducer and noting the resultant voltage changes within the beam.

Evaluating the intensity of the ultrasonic beam with a pulsed system is more complicated. The intensity of the ultrasound now varies not only with the spatial pattern of the beam, but also according to the temporal pattern of the pulsing. To make the necessary calculations, one must know the pulse repetition frequency or pulse repetition rate. The duration of the pulse must also be known. For M-mode echocardiography, a pulse repetition rate of 1000/sec and a pulse duration of 1.5 μsec, are fairly common. To calculate the energy from a pulsed ultrasonic beam, one must know the duty factor, which represents that fraction of time during which the transducer emits ultrasound. If the pulse duration is 1.5 μsec and the pulse repetition rate is 1000/sec, then the pulse repetition period, i.e., the time between the onset of each pulse, would be 1000 μsec or 1 msec. Thus, the duty factor would be 1.5 divided by 1000 or 0.0015 (0.15%). The duty factor must be known to calculate power or intensity of pulsed ultrasonic systems. The average power of a pulsed echocardiograph would be the peak power multiplied by the duty factor. For example, if the peak power were about 10 W and the duty factor were 0.0015, then the average power would be 0.015 W or 15 mW.

When discussing intensity for pulsed mode systems, one must discuss not only spatial average (SA) intensity and spatial peak (SP) intensity, but also temporal average (TA) intensity and temporal peak (TP) intensity.[217] The spatial average, temporal average (SATA) intensity is obtained by measuring the average power of a transducer and dividing it by the surface area of the transducer. This measure, frequently quoted by manufacturers, is the lowest of the various intensities measured with a pulsed system. The spatial average, temporal peak (SATP) intensity is the spatial average value of intensity during a given pulse and is calculated by taking the SATP intensity and dividing it by the duty factor. This calculation allows for the fact that the transducer is transmitting pulsed and not continuous ultrasound. One can, of course, calculate the intensity by using the SP intensity and the TA intensity, which would result in a measurement that indicates the intensity in the center of the beam rather than at the edges. There is a spatial peak (SP)/spatial average (SA) factor. This factor divides the measured peak intensities in the center of the ultrasonic beam by the average intensities over the entire ultrasonic beam. The SP intensity is usually two to three times greater than the SA intensity. The highest possible intensity within a pulsed ultrasonic beam would be calculated using the spatial peak and temporal peak measurements. The spatial peak, temporal peak (SPTP) intensity would be calculated by multiplying the spatial average intensity by the SP/SA factor and then dividing it by the duty factor. For example, if one had a pulsed ultrasonic system with a spatial average, temporal average intensity of 3 mW/cm², with a duty factor of 0.001, and an SP/SA factor of 3, then the SATA intensity would be 3 mW/cm², SATP intensity 3000 mW/cm² or 3 W/cm², SPTA (spatial peak/temporal average) intensity 9 mW/cm², and SPTP intensity 9000 mW/cm² or 9 W/cm².

Commercial ultrasonic instrument companies offer various pulsed ultrasonic devices that have SPTA intensities in the range of 0.001 to 200 mW/cm².[218] Pulsed Doppler, however, may have a SPTA of 1900 mW/cm², which is considerably higher than 100 mW/cm², a level that has been studied extensively and has never produced any biologic effect.[215] The higher intensities have been evaluated as well, but still have not produced any demonstrably deleterious effect.

One of the biologic effects of ultrasound is the production of heat, which is a principal goal of ultrasonic therapy. With the pulsed ultrasound used in echocardiography, it is extremely unlikely that the duty factor is long enough for any heat to be generated within the body.[219] The evidence available at present indicates that the brief pulses of ultrasound used in echocardiography are not likely to cause any cumulative damage.[220–222] The pulse repetition rate of two-dimensional echocardiography is higher; hence, the duty factor is higher. The beam is constantly moving, however, so that, except for the skin surface, the heart actually receives less ultrasonic energy. Even the higher average intensities used with continuous ultrasound, such as continuous wave Doppler, probably are too low to produce any heat in in vivo tissues.[219]

Transesophageal echocardiography has a unique potential problem with heat generation because of its proximity to the esophagus and the fact that the probe may be left in place for long periods of time when monitoring a patient during surgery. As a result, the manufacturers have inserted a heat-sensing device that automatically shuts off the transducer if a certain temperature is reached. If the patient has a high fever, the sensing device may shut off the probe for the wrong reason.

Another physical effect of ultrasound is cavitation.[223] This effect is apparently produced by gaseous cavitations formed during the negative phase of the sound wave cycle. Unfortunately, there are no accurately sensitive techniques for detecting cavitation in vivo. It is highly unlikely, however, that such an effect could occur in blood or soft tissue because of the relatively high viscosity of these substances.

Cavitation, however, will affect highly compressible bodies of gas or bubbles. Thus, this biologic effect is enhanced when microbubbles are introduced as with contrast echocardiography. The ultrasound also causes the bubble to increase cyclically and decrease its diameter or resonate. This effect depends on the relationship between the size of the bubble and the frequency of the ultrasound. The resultant vibration may cause the bubble to absorb more energy, which may be released as heat. With the arrival of commercial contrast agents, which consist of bubbles, has come investigation of these bioeffects.

A variety of other physical forces might be produced by ultrasonic energy, including oscillatory, sheer, and Oseen forces, radiation, pressure, Venoulli effect, and microstreaming. All these effects have been demonstrated in vitro, but few are fully understood. No evidence of any of these physical effects has been demonstrated in any experimental animal or in any patients. Many investigators have attempted to study the safety of ultrasonic procedures in various laboratory settings. Despite numerous approaches, virtually no consistent biologic effects have been demonstrated using ultrasound at diagnostic power levels. A few reports have suggested that some change might occur at the chromosomal level that affects fetal behavior and movement.[223–225] These observations caused considerable concern for individuals using Doppler devices in obstetrics. Several investigators, however, have had difficulty duplicating these studies. Thus, there are still no confirmed reports of deleterious effects produced by ultrasound in experimental animals, using the dosage parameters of current clinical applications.[226]

Research is continuing in this area. All findings thus far indicate that diagnostic ultrasound, particularly that used in echocardiography, is an extremely safe tool with no known deleterious effects, even with the introduction of newer techniques such as Doppler, transesophageal, epicardial, and contrast examinations and use of more powerful instruments. Despite this reassurance, we must never let our desire for more and better information cause us to overlook possible hazardous biologic effects from the examination. Thus, a constant reassessment of the safety of echocardiography will always be with us.

## REFERENCES

1. Wells, P.N.T.: Biomedical Ultrasonics. London, Academic Press, 1977.
2. Kossoff, G.: Diagnostic applications of ultrasound in cardiology. Australas Radiol., 10:101, 1966.
3. Wells, P.N.T.: Absorption and dispersion of ultrasound in biological tissue. Ultrasound Med. Biol., 1:369, 1975.
4. Wells, P.N.T.: Physics: An Introduction to Echocardiography. Edited by G. Leech and G. Sutton. London, Medi-Cine Ltd., 1978.
5. Eggleton, R.C.: Interim AIUM Standard Nomenclature. Reflections, 4:275, 1978.
6. Goldman, D.E. and Jueter, T.F.: Tabular data of the velocity and absorption of high-frequency sound in mammalian tissues. J. Acoust. Soc. Am., 28:35, 1956.
7. Gregg, E.C. and Palogallo, G.L.: Acoustic impedance of tissue. Invest. Radiol., 4:357, 1969.
8. Reid, J.: A review of some basic limitations in ultrasonic diagnosis. In Diagnostic Ultrasound. Edited by C.C. Grossman, J.H. Holmes, C. Joyner, and E.W. Purnell. Proceedings of the First International Conference, University of Pittsburgh, 1965. New York, Plenum Press, 1966.
9. Fry, W.J.: Mechanism of acoustic absorption in tissue. J. Acoust. Soc. Am., 24:412, 1952.
10. Goss, S.A., Frizzell, L.A., and Dunn, F.: Ultrasonic absorption and attenuation in mammalian tissues. Ultrasound Med. Biol., 5:181, 1979.

11. Mason, W.P.: Piezoelectric crystals and their application to ultrasonics. New York, Van Nostrand, 1950.

12. Hertz, C.H.: Ultrasonic engineering in heart diagnosis. Am. J. Cardiol., *19*:6, 1967.

13. Morgan, C. L., Trought, W.S., Clark, W.M., Von-Ramm, O.T., and Thurstone, F.L.: Principles and applications of a dynamically focused phased array real time ultrasound system. JCU, *6*:385, 1978.

14. VonRamm, O.T. and Thurstone, F.L.: Thaumascan: Design considerations and performance characteristics. *In* Ultrasound in Medicine. Edited by D. White. New York, Plenum Press, 1975.

15. Kisslo, J.A., VonRamm, O.T., and Thurstone, F.L.: Dynamic cardiac imaging using a focused, phased-array ultrasound system. Am. J. Med., *63*:61, 1977.

16. Eggleton, R.C. and Johnston, K.W.: Real-time mechanical scanning system compared with array techniques. I.E.E.E. Proc. Sonics Ultrasonics, Cat. No. 74-CH 0896-1, 1974, p. 16.

17. VonRamm, O.T. and Thurstone, F.L.: Cardiac imaging using a phased array ultrasound system. Circulation, *53*: 258, 1976.

18. Vogel, J., Bom, N., Ridder, J., and Lancee, C.: Transducer considerations in dynamic focusing. Ultrasound Med. Biol., *5*:187, 1979.

19. Melton, H.E., Jr., and Thurstone, F.L.: Annular array design and logarithmic processing for ultrasonic imaging. Ultrasound Med. Biol., *4*:1, 1978.

20. Kossoff, G., Garrett, W.J., Dadd, M.J., Paoloni, H.J., and Wilcken, D.E.L.: Cross-sectional visualization of the normal heart by the UIOCTOSON. J. Clin. Ultrasound, *6*:3, 1978.

21. Foster, F.S., Larson, J.D., Pittaro, R.J., Corl, P.D., Greenstein, A.P., and Lum, P.K.: A digital annular array prototype scanner for real-time ultrasound imaging. Ultrasound Med. Biol., *15*:661, 1989.

22. Ryan, T., Armstrong, W.F., Feigenbaum, H.: Annular Array Technology: Application to Cardiac Imaging. Echocardiography, *4*:203, 1987.

23. Feigenbaum, H. and Zaky, A.: Use of diagnostic ultrasound in clinical cardiology. J. Indiana State Med. Assoc., *59*:140, 1966.

24. Griffith, J.M. and Henry, W.L.: A sector scanner for real time two-dimensional echocardiography. Circulation, *49*: 1147, 1974.

25. Eggleton, R.C., et al.: Visualization of cardiac dynamics with real-time B-mode ultrasonic scanner. *In* Ultrasound in Medicine. Edited by D. White. New York, Plenum Press, 1975.

26. Nagayama, T., Nakamura, S., Hayakawa, K., and Komo, Y.: Ultrasonic cardiokymogram. Acta Med. U. Kagoshima, *4*:229, 1962.

27. Matsumoto, M., Matsuo, H., Ohara, T., and Abe, H.: Use of kymo-two-dimensional echocardiography for the diagnosis of aortic root dissection and mycotic aneurysm of the aortic root. Ultrasound Med. Biol., *3*:153, 1977.

28. Asberg, A.: Ultrasonic cinematography of the living heart. Ultrasonics, *6*:113, 1967.

29. Hertz, C.H. and Lundstrom, K.: A fast ultrasonic scanning system for heart investigation. 3rd International Conference on Medical Physics. Gotenburg, Sweden. August 1972.

30. Gramiak, R., Waag, R., and Simon, W.: Cine ultrasound cardiography. Radiology, *107*:175, 1973.

31. Kratochwil, A., Jantsch, C., Mosslacher, H., Slany, J., and Wenger, R.: Ultrasonic tomography of the heart. Ultrasound Med. Biol., *1*:275, 1974.

32. Ebina, T., et al.: The ultrasono-tomography of the heart and great vessels in living human subjects by means of the ultrasonic reflection technique. Jpn. Heart J., *8*:331, 1967.

33. King, D.L.: Cardiac ultrasonography: Cross-sectional ultrasonic imaging of the heart. Circulation, *47*:843, 1973.

34. Bom, N., Lancee, C.T., Honkoop, J., and Hugenholtz, P.C.: Ultrasonic viewer for cross-sectional analyses of moving cardiac structures. Biomed. Eng., *6*:500, 1971.

35. Bom, N., Lancee, C.T., Van Zwieten, G., Kloster, F.E., and Roelandt, J.: Multi-scan echocardiography. I. Technical description. Circulation, *48*:1066, 1973.

36. Yoshikawa, J., et al.: Electroscan echocardiography: Application to the cardiac diagnosis. J. Cardiogr., *7*:33, 1977.

37. Pedersen, J.F. and Northeved, A.: An ultrasonic multitransducer scanner for real-time heart imaging. JCU, *5*: 11, 1977.

38. Pye, S.D., Wild, S.R., and McDicken, W.N.: Adaptive time gain compensation for ultrasonic imaging. Ultrasound Med. Biol., *18*:205, 1992.

39. Roelandt, J., Van Dorp, W.G., Bom, N., Laird, J.D., and Hugenholtz, P.G.: Resolution problems in echocardiography: A source of interpretation errors. Am. J. Cardiol., *37*:256, 1976.

40. Martin, R.P., Rokowski, H., Kleiman, J.H., Beaver, W., London, E., and Popp, R.L.: Reliability and reproducibility of two-dimensional echocardiographic measurements of the stenotic mitral valve orifice area. Am. J. Cardiol., *43*:56, 1979.

41. Latson, L.A., Cheatham, J.P., and Gutgesell, H.P.: Resolution and accuracy in two-dimensional echocardiography. Am. J. Cardiol., *48*:106, 1981.

42. Yeh, E.: Reverberations in echocardiograms. J. Clin. Ultrasound, *5*:84, 1977.

43. Rushmer, R.F., Baker, D.W., and Stegall, H.F.: Transcutaneous Doppler flow detection as a nondestructive technique. J. Appl. Physiol., *21*:554, 1966.

44. Yoshida, T., et al.: Study of examining the heart with ultrasonics. III. Kinds of Doppler beats. IV. Clinical applications. Jpn. Circ. J., *20*:228, 1956.

45. Hatle, L. and Angelsen, B.: Doppler Ultrasound in Cardiology: Physical Principles and Clinical Applications, 2nd ed. Philadelphia, Lea & Febiger, 1984.

46. Burns, P.N.: The physical principles of Doppler and spectral analysis. JCU, *15*:567, 1987.

47. Nanda, N.C.: Textbook of Color Doppler Echocardiography. Edited by N.C. Nanda, Philadelphia, Lea & Febiger, 1989.

48. Baker, D.W., Rubenstein, S.A., and Lorch, G.S.: Pulsed Doppler echocardiography: Principles and applications. Am. J. Med., *63*:69, 1977.

49. Pearlman, A.S.: Doppler echocardiography. Int. J. Cardiol., *3*:81, 1983.

50. Baker, D.W.: Pulsed ultrasonic Doppler blood-flow sensing. I.E.E.E. Trans. Sonics Ultrasonics, SU-17, No. 3, July 1970.

51. Kalmanson, D., Veyrat, C., Bouchareine, F., and Degroote, A.: Non-invasive recording of mitral valve flow velocity patterns using pulsed Doppler echocardiography. Application to diagnosis and evaluation of mitral valve disease. Br. Heart J., *39*:517, 1977.

52. Schwartz, M.D. and DeCristofaro, D.: Review and evaluation of range-gated, pulsed, echo-Doppler. J. Clin. Eng., *3*:153, 1978.

53. Bom, K., de Boo, J., and Rijsterborgh, H.: On the

aliasing problem in pulsed Doppler cardiac studies. JCU, *12*:559, 1984.

54. Brandestini, M.A., Eyer, M.K., and Stevenson, J.G.: M/Q-mode echocardiography. The synthesis of conventional echo with digital multigate Doppler. *In* Echocardiography. Edited by C.T. Lancee. The Hague, Martinus Nijhoff, 1979.

55. Eyer, M.K., Brandestini, M.A., Phillips, D.J., and Baker, D.W.: Color digital echo/Doppler image presentation. Ultrasound Med. Biol., *7*:21, 1981.

56. Omoto, R.: Color Atlas of Real-Time Two-Dimensional Doppler Echocardiography. Tokyo, Shindan-To-Chiryo Co., Ltd., 1984.

57. Miyatake, K., Okamoto, M., Kinoshita, N., Izumi, S., Owa, M., Takao, S., Sakakibara, H., and Nimura, Y.: Clinical applications of a new type of real-time two-dimensional Doppler flow imaging system. Am. J. Cardiol., *54*:857, 1984.

58. Khandheria, B.K., Tajik, A.J., Reeder, G.S., Callahan, M.J., Nishimura, R.A., Miller, F.A., and Seward, J.B.: Doppler color flow imaging: A new technique for visualization and characterization of the blood flow jet in mitral stenosis. Mayo Clin. Proc., *61*:623, 1986.

59. Merritt, C.R.B.: Doppler color flow imaging. JCU, *15*:591, 1987.

60. Yoganathan, A.P., Cape, E.G., Sung, H-W., Williams, F.P., and Jimoh, A.: Review of hydrodynamic principles for the cardiologist: Applications to the study of blood flow and jets by imaging techniques. J. Am. Coll. Cardiol., *12*:1344, 1988.

61. Aggarwal, K.K., Moos, S., Philpot, E.F., Jain, S.P., Helmcke, F., and Nanda, N.C.: Color velocity determination using pixel color intensity in Doppler color flow mapping. Echocardiography, *6*:473, 1989.

62. Fan, P., Nanda, N.C., Cooper, J.W., Cape, E., and Yoganathan, A.: Color Doppler assessment of high flow velocities using a new technology: In vitro and clinical studies. Echocardiography, *7*:763, 1990.

63. Tamura, T., Yoganathan, A., and Sahn, D.J.: In vitro methods for studying the accuracy of velocity determination and spatial resolution of a color Doppler flow mapping system. Am. Heart J., *114*:152, 1987.

64. Huntsman, L.L., Gams, E., Johnson, C.C., and Fairbanks, E.: Transcutaneous determination of aortic blood flow velocities in man. Am. J. Heart, *89*:605, 1975.

65. Light, L.H.: Transcutaneous observation of blood velocity in the ascending aorta in man. Biol. Cardiol., *26*:214, 1969.

66. Griffith, J.M. and Henry, W.L.: An ultrasound system for combined cardiac imaging and Doppler blood flow measurement in man. Circulation, *57*:925, 1978.

67. Alverson, D.C., Eldridge, M., Dillon, T., Yabek, S.M., and Berman, W., Jr.: Noninvasive pulsed Doppler determination of cardiac output in neonates and children. J. Pediatr., *101*:46, 1982.

68. Holen, J. and Simonsen, S.: Determination of pressure gradient in mitral stenosis with Doppler echocardiography. Br. Heart J., *41*:529, 1979.

69. Hatle, L., Brubakk, A., Tromsdal, A., and Angelsen, B.: Noninvasive assessment of pressure drop in mitral stenosis by Doppler ultrasound. Br. Heart J., *40*:131, 1978.

70. Hatle, L., Angelsen, B., and Tromsdal, A.: Noninvasive assessment of aortic stenosis by Doppler ultrasound. Br. Heart J., *43*:284, 1979.

71. Stam, R.B. and Martin, R.P.: Quantification of pressure gradients across stenotic valves by Doppler ultrasound. J. Am. Coll. Cardiol., *2*:707, 1983.

72. Berger, M., Berdoff, R.L., Gallerstein, P.E., and Goldberg, E.: Evaluation of aortic stenosis by continuous wave Doppler ultrasound. J. Am. Coll. Cardiol., *3*:150, 1984.

73. Taylor, R.: Evolution of the continuity equation in the Doppler echocardiographic assessment of the severity of valvular aortic stenosis. J. Am. Soc. Echocardiogr., *3*:326, 1990.

74. Thomas, J.D., O'Shea, J.P., Rodriquez, L., Popovic, A.D., Svizerro, T., and Weyman, A.E.: Impact of orifice geometry on the shape of jets: An in vitro Doppler color flow study. J. Am. Coll. Cardiol., *17*:901, 1991.

75. Utsunomiya, T., Ogawa, T., King, S.W., Sunada, E., Lobodzinski, S.M., Henry, W.L., and Gardin, J.M.: Pitfalls in the display of color Doppler jet areas: Combined variability due to Doppler angle, frame rate, and scanning direction. Echocardiography, *7*:739, 1990.

76. Gardin, J.M. and Lobodzinski, S.M.: Do Doppler color flow algorithms for mapping disturbed flow make sense? J. Am. Soc. Echocardiogr., *3*:310, 1990.

77. Hoit, B.D., Jones, M., Eidbo, E.E., Elias, W., and Sahn, D.J.: Sources of variability for Doppler color flow mapping of regurgitant jets in an animal model of mitral regurgitation. J. Am. Coll. Cardiol., *13*:1631, 1989.

78. Levine, R.A.: Doppler color mapping of the proximal flow convergence region: A new quantitative physiologic tool. J. Am. Coll. Cardiol., *18*:833, 1991.

79. Utsunomiya, T., Ogawa, T., Doshi, R., Patel, D., Quan, M., Henry, W.L., and Gardin, J.M.: Doppler color flow: "Proximal isovelocity surface area" method for estimating volume flow rate: Effects of orifice shape and machine factors. J. Am. Coll. Cardiol., *17*:1103, 1991.

80. Baumgartner, H., Schima, H., and Kuhn, P.: Value and limitations of proximal jet dimensions for the quantitation of alvular regurgitation: An in vitro study using Doppler flow imaging. J. Am. Soc. Echocardiogr., *4*:57, 1991.

81. Yagi, T., Yoshikawa, J., Yoshida, K., Akasaka, T., Syakudo, M., Fukaya, T., Maenishi, F., Kato, H., and Jyo, Y.: The usefulness and limitation of power-mode imaging in two-dimensional Doppler color flow mapping. Jpn. J. Med. Ultrasonics, *14*:1, 1987.

82. von Bibra, H., Stempfle, H-U, Poll, A., Scherer, M., Bluml, G., and Blomer, H.: Limitations of low detection by color Doppler: In vitro comparison to conventional Doppler. Echocardiography, *8*:633, 1991.

83. Goldberg, S.J.: Relation between color Doppler-detected directional flow in a ventricular septal defect and frame rate. J. Am. Coll. Cardiol., *16*:1445, 1990.

84. Rao, S.R., Richardson, S.G., Simonetti, J., Katz, S.E., Caldeira, M., and Pandian, N.G.: Problems and pitfalls in the performance and interpretation of color Doppler flow imaging. Echocardiography, *7*:747, 1990.

85. Smith, M.D., Grayburn, P.A., Spain, M.G., DeMaria, A.N., Kwan, O.L., and Moffett, C.B.: Observer variability in the quantitation of Doppler color flow jet areas for mitral and aortic regurgitation. J. Am. Coll. Cardiol., *11*:579, 1988.

86. Baumgartner, H., Schima, H., and Kuhn, P.: Importance of technical variables for quantitative measurements by color Doppler imaging. Am. J. Cardiol., *67*:314, 1991.

87. Utsunomiya, T., Ogawa, T., King, S.W., Sunada, E., Moore, G.W., Henry, W.L., and Gardin, J.M.: Effect of machine parameters on variance display in Doppler color flow mapping. Am. Heart J., *120*:1395, 1990.

88. Stewart, W.J., Cohen, G.I., and Salcedo, E.E.: Doppler color flow image size: Dependence on instrument settings. Echocardiography, 8:319, 1991.

89. Sahn, D.J.: Instrumentation and physical factors related to visualization of stenotic and regurgitant jets by Doppler color flow mapping. J. Am. Coll. Cardiol., 12:1354, 1988.

90. Krabill, K.A., Sung, H-W, Tamura, T., Chung, K.J., Yoganathan, A.P., and Sahn, D.J.: Factors influencing the structure and shape of stenotic regurgitant jets: An in vitro investigation using Doppler color flow mapping and optical flow visualization. J. Am. Coll. Cardiol., 13:1672, 1989.

91. DeMaria, A.N., Smith, M.D., and Harrison, M.R.: Clinical significance of in vitro and in vivo experimental findings regarding Doppler flow velocity recordings. J. Am. Coll. Cardiol., 13:1682, 1989.

92. Cape, E.G., Yoganathan, A.P., Weyman, A.E., and Levine, R.A.: Adjacent solid boundaries alter the size of regurgitant jets on Doppler color flow maps. J. Am. Coll. Cardiol., 17:1094, 1991.

93. Reichert, S.L.A., Visser, C.A., Koolen, J.J., Chapman, J.V., Angelsen, B.A.J., Meyne, N.G., and Dunning, A.J.: Transesophageal examination of the left coronary artery with a 7.5 MHz annular array two-dimensional color flow Doppler transducer. J. Am. Soc. Echocardiogr., 3:118, 1990.

94. Schluter, M. and Hanrath, P.: Transesophageal echocardiography: Potential advantages and initial clinical results. Practical Cardiol., 9:149, 1983.

95. Hisanaga, K., Hisanaga, A., Nagata, K., and Ichie, Y.: Transesophageal cross-sectional echocardiography. Am. Heart J., 100:605, 1980.

96. Schluter, M., et al.: Transesophageal cross-sectional echocardiography with phased array transducer system. Technique and initial clinical results. Br. Heart J., 48:67, 1982.

97. Seward, J.B., Khandheria, B.K., Oh, J.K., Hughes, R.W., Edwards, W.D., Nichols, B.A., Freeman, W.K., and Tajik, A.J.: Transesophageal echocardiography: Technique, anatomic correlations, implementation, and clinical applications. Mayo Clin. Proc., 63:649, 1988.

98. Omoto, R., Kyo, S., Matsumura, M., Maruyama, M., and Yokote, Y.: Future technical prospects in biplane transesophageal echocardiography: Use of adult and pediatric biplane matrix probes. Echocardiography, 8:713, 1991.

99. Nanda, J.C., Pinheiro, L., Sanyal, R.S., and Storey, O.: Transesophageal biplane echocardiographic imaging: Technique, planes and clinical usefulness. Echocardiography, 7:771, 1990.

100. Bansal, R.C., Shakudo, M., Shah, P.M., and Shah, P.M.: Biplane transesophageal echocardiography: Technique, image orientation, and preliminary experience in 131 patients. J. Am. Soc. Echocardiogr., 3:348, 1990.

101. Pearson, A.C. and Pasierski, T.: Initial clinical experience with a 48 by 48 element biplane transesophageal probe. Am. Heart J., 122:559, 1991.

102. Richardson, S.G., Weintraub, A.R., Schwartz, S.L., Simonetti, J., Caldeira, M.E., and Pandian, N.G.: Biplane transesophageal echocardiography utilizing transverse and sagittal imaging planes. Echocardiography, 8:293, 1991.

102a. Omoto, R., Kyo, S., Matsummura, M., Shah, P.M., Adachi, H., Yokote, Y., and Kondo, Y.: Evaluation of biplane color Doppler transesophageal echocardiography in 200 consecutive patients. Circulation, 85:1237, 1992.

103. Omoto, R., Kyo, S., Matsumura, M., Adachi, H., Maruyama, M., and Matsunaka, T.: New direction of biplane transesophageal echocardiography with special emphasis on real-time biplane imaging and matrix phased-array biplane transducer. Echocardiography, 7:691, 1990.

104. Omoto, R., Kyo, S., Matsumura, M., Maruyama, M., and Yokote, Y.: Future technical prospects in biplane transesophageal echocardiography: Use of adult and pediatric biplane matrix probes. Echocardiography, 8:713, 1991.

105. Roberson, D.A., Muhiudeen, I.A., and Silverman, N.H.: Transesophageal echocardiography in pediatrics: Technique and limitations. Echocardiography, 7:699, 1990.

106. Ritter, S.B.: Pediatric transesophageal color flow imaging 1990: The long and short of it. Echocardiography, 7:713, 1990.

107. Helmcke, F., Mahan, E.F. III, Nanda, N.C., Cooper, J.W., and Sanyal, R.: Use of the smaller pediatric transesophageal echocardiographic probe in adults. Echocardiography, 7:727, 1990.

107a. Weintraub, R., Shiota, T., Elkadi, T., Golebiovski, P., Zhang, J., Rothman, A., Ritter, S.B., and Sahn, D.J.: Transesophageal echocardiography in infants and children with congenital heart disease. Circulation, 86:711, 1992.

107b. Pandian, N.G., Hsu, T-L., Schwartz, S.L., Weintraub, A., Cao, Q-L., Schneider, A.T., Gordon, G., England, M., and Simonetti, J.: Multiplane transesophageal echocardiography. Echocardiography, 9:649, 1992.

107c. Roelandt, J., Brommersma, P., Bom, N., Vletter, W.B., Taams, M., Ten Cate, F.J., and Linker, D.T.: Multiplane transesophageal echocardiography with a varioplane transducer system. Thoraxcentre J., 4:38, 1992.

108. Seward, J.B., Khandheria, B.K., and Tajik, A.J.: Widefield transesophageal echocardiographic tomography: Feasibility study. Mayo Clin. Proc., 65:31, 1990.

109. Hsu, T-L., Weintraub, A.R., Ritter, S.B., and Pandian, N.G.: Panoramic transesophageal echocardiography. Echocardiography, 8:677, 1991.

110. Glassman, E. and Kronzon, I.: Transvenous intracardiac echocardiography. Am. J. Cardiol., 47:1255, 1981.

111. Pandian, N.G.: Intravascular and intracardiac ultrasound imaging. Circulation, 80:1091, 1989.

112. Bom, N. and Roelandt, J.: Intravascular Ultrasound. Techniques, Developments, Clinical Perspectives. Edited by N. Bom and J. Roelandt. Dordrecht, Kluwer Academic Publishers, 1989.

113. Bom, N., tenHoff, H., Lancee, C.T., Gussenhoven, W.J., and Bosch, J.G.: Early and recent intraluminal ultrasound devices. Int. J. Cardiac Imaging, 4:79, 1989.

114. Sheikh, K.H., Davidson, C.J., Kisslo, K.B., Harrison, J.K., Himmelstein, S.I., Kisslo, J., and Bashore, T.M.: Comparison of intravascular ultrasound, external ultrasound and digital angiography for evaluation of peripheral artery dimensions and morphology. Am. J. Cardiol., 67:817, 1991.

115. Pandian, N.G., Kreis, A., Brockway, B., Isner, J.M., Salem, D., Sacharoff, A., Boleza, E., and Caro, R.: Ultrasound angioscopy: Feasibility and potential. Echocardiography, 6:1, 1989.

116. Roelandt, J.R., Bom, N., Werruys, P.W., Gussenhoven, E.J., Lancee, C.T., and Sutherland, G.R.: Intravascular high-resolution real-time cross-sectional echocardiography. Echocardiography, 6:9, 1989.

117. Davidson, C.J., Sheikh, K.H., Harrison, J.K., Himmelstein, S.I., Leithe, M.E., Kisslo, K.B., and Bashore, T.M.: Intravascular ultrasonography versus digital subtraction angiography: A human in vivo comparison of vessel size and morphology. J. Am. Coll. Cardiol., *16*: 633, 1990.

118. Tobis, J.M., Mallery, J.A., Gessert, J., Griffith, J., Mahon, D., Bessen, M., Moriuchi, M., McLeay, L., McRae, M., and Henry, W.L.: Intravascular ultrasound cross-sectional arterial imaging before and after balloon angioplasty in vitro. Circulation, *80*:873, 1989.

119. Yock, P.G., Fitzgerald, P.J., Linker, D.T., and Angelsen, B.A.J.: Intravascular ultrasound guidance for catheter-based coronary interventions. J. Am. Coll. Cardiol., *17*:39B, 1991.

120. Yock, P.G., Linker, D.T., and Angelsen, B.A.J.: Two-dimensional intravascular ultrasound: Technical development and initial clinical experience. J. Am. Soc. Echocardiogr., *2*:296, 1989.

121. Nishimura, R.A., Edwards, W.D., Warnes, C.A., Reeder, G.S., Holmes, D.R., Jr., Tajik, A.J., and Yock, P.G.: Intravascular ultrasound imaging: In vitro validation and pathologic correlation. J. Am. Coll. Cardiol., *16*: 145, 1990.

122. Valdes-Cruz, L.M., Sideris, E., Sahn, D.J., Murillo-Olivas, A., Knudson, O., Omoto, R., Kyo, S., and Gulde, R.: Transvascular intracardiac applications of a miniaturized phased-array ultrasonic endoscope. Circulation, *83*: 1023, 1991.

123. Nissen, S.E., Grines, C.L., Gurley, J.C., Sublett, K., Haynie, D., Kiaz, C., Booth, D.C., and DeMaria, A.N.: Application of a new phased-array ultrasound imaging catheter in the assessment of vascular dimensions. Circulation, *81*:660, 1990.

124. Potkin, B.N., Bartorelli, A.L., Gessert, J.M., Neville, R.F., Almagor, Y., Roberts, W.C., and Leon, M.B.: Coronary artery imaging with intravascular high-frequency ultrasound. Circulation, *81*:1575, 1990.

125. Moriuchi, M., Tobis, J.M., Mahon, D., Gessert, J., Griffith, J., McRae, M., Moussabeck, O., and Henry, W.L.: The reproducibility of intravascular ultrasound imaging in vitro. J. Am. Soc. Echocardiogr., *3*:444, 1990.

126. Nissen, S.E., Gurley, J.C., Grines, C.L., Booth, D.C., McClure, R., Berk, M., Fischer, C., and DeMaria, A.N.: Intravascular ultrasound assessment of lumen size and wall morphology in normal subjects and patients with coronary artery disease. Circulation, *84*:1087, 1991.

126a. DiMario, C., The, S.H.K., Madretsma, S., Van Suylen, R.J., Wilson, R.A., Serruys, P.W., Gussenhoven, E.J., Roelandt, J.R.T.C., Zhong, Y., and Wenguang, L.: Detection and characterization of vascular lesions by intravascular ultrasound: An in vitro study correlated with histology. J. Am. Soc. Echocardiogr., *5*:135, 1992.

126b. Ge, J., Erbel, R., Gorge, G., Gerber, T., Brennecke, R., Seidel, I., Reichert, T., and Meyer, J.: Intravascular ultrasound imaging of arterial wall architecture. Echocardiography, *9*:475, 1992.

127. Isner, J.M.: Combination balloon-ultrasound imaging catheter for percutaneous transluminal angioplasty. Validation of imaging, analysis of recoil, and identification of plaque fracture. Circulation, *84*:739, 1991.

128. Pandian, N.G., Weintraub, A., Kreis, A., Schwartz, S.L., Konstam, M.A., and Salem, D.N.: Intracardiac, intravascular, two-dimensional, high-frequency ultrasound imaging of pulmonary artery and its branches in humans and animals. Circulation, *81*:2007, 1990.

129. Pandian, N.G., Kreis, A., Weintraub, A., Motarjeme, A., Desnoyers, M., Isner, J.M., Konstam, M., Salem, D.N., and Millen, V.: Real-time intravascular ultrasound imaging in humans. Am. J. Cardiol., *65*:1392, 1990.

130. Pandian, N.G., Kumar, R., Katz, S.E., Tutor, A., Schwartz, S.L., Weintraub, R., Gillam, L.D., McKay, R.G., Konstam, M.A., Salem, D.N., and Aronovitz, M.: Real-time, intracardiac, two-dimensional echocardiography. Echocardiography, *8*:407, 1991.

131. Seward, J.B., Khandheria, B.K., McGregor, C.G.A., Locke, T.J., and Tajik, A.J.: Transvascular and intracardiac two-dimensional echocardiography. Echocardiography, *7*:457, 1990.

131a. Coy, K.M., Maurer, G., and Siegel, R.J.: Intravascular ultrasound imaging: A current perspective. J. Am. Coll. Cardiol., *18*:1811, 1991.

132. Segal, J., Pearl, R.G., Ford, A.J., Stern, R.A., and Gehlbach, S.M.: Instantaneous and continuous cardiac output obtained with a Doppler pulmonary artery catheter. J. Am. Coll. Cardiol., *13*:1382, 1989.

133. Sibley, D.H., Millar, H.D., Hartley, C.J., and Whitlow, P.L.: Subselective measurement of coronary blood flow velocity using a steerable Doppler catheter. J. Am. Coll. Cardiol., *8*:1332, 1986.

134. Wilson, R.F. and White, C.W.: Measurement of maximal coronary flow reserve: A technique of assessing the physiologic significance of coronary arterial lesions in humans. Herz., *12*:163, 1987.

135. Segal, J., Nassi, M., Ford, Jr., A.J., and Schuenemeyer, T.D.: Instantaneous and continuous cardiac output in humans obtained with a Doppler pulmonary artery catheter. J. Am. Coll. Cardiol., *16*:1398, 1990.

135a. Segal, J., Kern, M.D., Scott, N.A., King, III, S.B., Doucette, J.W., Heuser, R.R., Ofili, E., and Siegel, R.: Alterations of phasic coronary artery flow velocity in humans during percutaneous coronary angioplasty. J. Am. Coll. Cardiol., *20*:276, 1992.

135b. Doucette, J.W., Corl, D., Payne, H.M., Flynn, A.E., Goto, M., Nassi, M., and Segal, J.: Validation of a Doppler guide wire for intravascular measurement of coronary artery flow velocity. Circulation, *85*:1899, 1992.

135c. Frazin, L.J., Vonesh, M.J., Khasho, F., Lanza, G., Chandran, K.B., Talano, J.V., and McPherson, D.D.: A Doppler guided retrograde catheterization system. Cathet. Cardiovasc. Diagn., *26*:41, 1992.

136. Ligtvoet, C., Rijsterborgh, H., Kappen, L., and Bom, N.: Real-time ultrasonic imaging with a hand-held scanner. I. Technical description. Ultrasound Med. Biol., *4*: 91, 1978.

137. Roelandt, J., Wladimiroff, J.W., and Baars, A.M.: Ultrasonic real-time imaging with a hand-held scanner. Ultrasound Med. Biol., *4*:93, 1978.

138. Schwarz, K.Q. and Meltzer, R.S.: Experience rounding with a hand-held two-dimensional cardiac ultrasound device. Am. J. Cardiol., *62*:157, 1988.

139. Landzberg, J.S., Franklin, J.O., Langberg, J.J., Herre, J.M., Scheinman, M.M., and Schiller, N.B.: The transponder system: A new method of precise catheter placement in the right atrium under echocardiographic guidance. J. Am. Coll. Cardiol., *12*:753, 1988.

140. Matsuwaka, R., Matsuda, H., Nakano, S., Hirata, N., Nishimura, M., Mitsuno, M., and Kawashima, Y.: A new angled transducer for intraoperative epicardial echocardiography. Echocardiography, *8*:341, 1991.

141. Smyllie, J., van Herwerden, L.A., Brommersma, P., de Jong, N., Bom, N., Bos, E., Gussenhoven, E., Roelandt,

J., and Sutherland, G.R.: Intraoperative epicardial echocardiography: Early experience with a newly developed small surgical transducer. J. Am. Soc. Echocardiogr., *4*: 147, 1991.

142. Haratzka, L.F., McPherson, D.D., Lamberth, W.C., Brandt, B., Armstrong, M.L., Schroder, E., Hunt, M., Kieso, R., Megan, M.D., Tompkis, P.K., Marcus, M.L., and Kerber, R.E.: Intraoperative evaluation of coronary artery bypass graft anastomoses with high-frequency epicardial echocardiography: Experimental validation and initial studies. Circulation, *73*:1199, 1986.

143. Gramiak, R., Shah, P.M., and Kramer, D.H.: Ultrasound cardiography: Contrast studies in anatomy and function. Radiology, *92*:939, 1969.

144. Feigenbaum, H., Stone, J.M., Lee, D.A., Nasser, W.K., and Chang, S.: Identification of ultrasound echoes from the left ventricle using intracardiac injections of indocyanine green. Circulation, *41*:615, 1970.

145. Seward, J.B., Tajik, A.J., Spangler, J.G., and Ritter, D.G.: Echocardiographic contrast studies: Initial experience. Mayo Clin. Proc., *50*:163, 1975.

146. Sanders, W.E., Cheirif, J., Desir, R., Zoghbi, W.A., Hoyt, B.D., Schulz, P.E., and Quinones, M.A.: Contrast opacification of left ventricular myocardium following intravenous administration of sonicated albumin microspheres. Am. Heart J., *122*:1660, 1991.

147. Feinstein, S.B., Keller, M.W., Kerber, R.E., Vandenberg, B., Hoyte, J., Kutruff, C., Bingle, J., Fraker, T.D., Jr., Chappell, R., and Welsh, A.H.: Sonicated echocardiographic contrast agents: Reproducibility studies. J. Am. Soc. Echocardiogr., *2*:125, 1989.

148. Reisner, S.A., Ong, L.S., Lichtenberg, G.S., Amico, A.F., Shapiro, J.R., Allen, M.N., and Meltzer, R.S.: Myocardial perfusion imaging by contrast echocardiography with use of intracoronary sonicated albumin in humans. J. Am. Coll. Cardiol., *14*:660, 1989.

149. Feinstein, S.B.: New developments in ultrasonic contrast techniques: Transpulmonary passage of contrast agents and diagnostic implications. Echocardiography, *6*:27, 1989.

150. Rovai, D., Lombardi, M., Cini, G., Morales, M.A., Colonna, M., Bechelli, G., Marino, P., Zanolla, L., Prioli, M.A., Nicolosi, G.L., Pavan, D., Zanuttini, D., Iliceto, S., Izzi, M., Rizzon, P., and L'Abbate, A.: Echocardiographic contrast imaging of the human right heart: A multicenter study of the efficacy, safety, and reproducibility of intravenous SHU-454. JCU, *19*:523, 1991.

151. Williams, A.R., Kubowicz, G., Cramer, E., and Schlief, R.: The effects of the microbubble suspension SHU-454 (Echovist) on ultrasound-induced cell lysis in a rotating tube exposure system. Echocardiography, *8*:423, 1991.

152. Keller, M.W., Glasheen, W., and Kaul, S.: Albunex: A safe and effective commercially produced agent for myocardial contrast echocardiography. J. am. Soc. Echocardiogr. *2*:48, 1989.

153. Feinstein, S.B., Cheirif, J., Ten Cate, F.J., Silverman, P.R., Heidenreich, P.A., Dick, C., Desir, R.M., Armstrong, W.F., Quinones, M.A., and Shah, P.M.: Safety and efficacy of a new transpulmonary ultrasound contrast agent: Initial multicenter clinical results. J. Am. Coll. Cardiol., *16*:316, 1990.

154. Keller, M.W., Feinstein, S.B., and Watson, D.D.: Successful left ventricular opacification following peripheral venous injection of sonicated contrast agent: An experimental evaluation. Am. Heart J., *114*:570, 1987.

155. Smith, M.D., Elion, J.L., McClure, R.R., Kwan, O.L.,

DeMaria, A.N., Evans, J., and Fritzsch, T.H.: Left heart opacification with peripheral venous injection of a new saccharide echo contrast agent in dogs. J. Am. Coll. Cardiol., *13*:1622, 1989.

156. Shub, C., Tajik, A.J., Seward, J.B., and Dines, D.E.: Detecting intrapulmonary right-to left shunt with contrast echocardiography. Mayo Clin. Proc., *51*:81, 1976.

157. Jayaweera, A.R., Matthew, T.L., Sklenar, J., Spotnitz, W.D., Watson, D.D., and Kaul, S.: Method for the quantitation of myocardial perfusion during myocardial contrast two-dimensional echocardiography. J. Am. Soc. Echocardiogr., *3*:91, 1990.

158. Lichtenberg, G.S. and Meltzer, R.S.: Myocardial perfusion studies by contrast echocardiography. J. Am. Soc. Echocardiogr., *3*:170, 1990.

159. Kemper, A., Force, T., Filfoil, M., Perkins, L.A., and Parisi, A.F.: Topographic correspondence of contrast echocardiographic perfusion mapping and myocardial infarct extent after varying durations of coronary occlusion. J. Am. Soc. Echocardiogr., *1*:104, 1988.

160. Armstrong, W.F. and Gage, S.W.: Evaluation of reperfusion hyperemia with myocardial contrast echocardiography. J. Am. Soc. Echocardiogr., *1*:322, 1988.

161. Von Bibra, H., Stempfle, H-U, Poll, A., Schlief, R., and Emslander, H.: Echo contrast agents improve flow display of color Doppler. Echocardiography, *8*:533, 1991.

162. Beard, J.T. and Byrd, B.F.: Saline contrast enhancement of trivial Doppler tricuspid regurgitation signals for estimating pulmonary artery pressure. Am. J. Cardiol., *62*:486, 1988.

163. Wagonner, A.D., Brazilai, B., and Perez, J.E.: Saline contrast enhancement of tricuspid regurgitant jets detected by Doppler color flow imaging. Am. J. Cardiol., *65*:1368, 1990.

164. Himelman, R.B., Stulbarg, M.S., Lee, E., Kuecherer, H.F., and Schiller, N.B.: Noninvasive evaluation of pulmonary artery systolic pressures during dynamic exercise by saline-enhanced Doppler echocardiography. Am. Heart J., *119*:685, 1990.

165. Smith, M.D., Elion, J.L., McClure, R.R., Kwan, O.L., DeMaria, A.N., Evans, J., and Fritzsch, T.H.: Left heart opacification with peripheral venous injection of a new saccharide echo contrast agent in dogs. J. Am. Coll. Cardiol., *13*:1622, 1989.

166. Daniel, W.G., Nellessen, U., Schroder, E., Nonnast-Daniel, B., Bednarski, P., Nikutta, P., and Lichtlen, P.R.: Left atrial spontaneous echo contrast in mitral valve disease: An indicator for an increased thromboembolic risk. J. Am. Coll. Cardiol., *11*:1204, 1988.

166a. Wang, X-F., Liu, L., Cheng, T.O., Li, Z-A., Deng, Y-B., and Wang, J-E.: The relationship between intracardiovascular smoke-like echo and erythrocyte rouleaux formation. Am. Heart J., 124:*961*, 1992.

166b. Merino A, Hauptman P, Badimon L, Badimon JJ, Cohen M, Fuster V, Goldman M: Echocardiographic "smoke" is produced by an interaction of erythrocytes and plasma proteins modulated by shear forces. *20*:1661–1168, 1992. Dec No. 7 J Am Coll Cardiol.

167. Collins, S.M. and Skorton, D.J.: Computers in cardiac imaging. J. Am. Coll. Cardiol., *9*:699, 1987.

168. Finley, J.P., Human, D.G., Nanton, M.A., Roy, D.L., Macdonald, R.G., Marr, D.R., and Chiasson, H.: Echocardiography by telephone—evaluation of pediatric heart disease at a distance. Am. J. Cardiol., *63*:1475, 1989.

169. Skorton, D.J., McNary, C.A., Child, J.S., Newton, F.C., and Shah, P.M.: Digital imaging processing of two-

dimensional echocardiograms. Identification of the endocardium. Am. J. Cardiol., *48*:479, 1981.

170. Sinclair, R.B.L., Oldershaw, P.J., and Gibson, D.G.: Computing in echocardiography. Prog. Cardiovasc. Dis., *25*:456, 1983.

171. Petrovic, O., Feigenbaum, H., Armstrong, W.F., Ryan, T., West, S.R., Green-Hess, D., Stewart, J., Mattson, J.L., Fineberg, N.S.: Digital averaging to facilitate two-dimensional echocardiographic measurements. J.C.U. *14*:367–372, 1986.

172. Flinn, G.S.: Color encoded display of M-mode echocardiograms. J. Clin. Ultrasound, *4*:339, 1976.

173. Parisi, A.F., et al.: Enhanced detection of the evolution of tissue changes after acute myocardial infarction using color-encoded two-dimensional echocardiography. Circulation, *66*:764, 1982.

174. Logan-Sinclair, R., Wong, C.M., and Gibson, D.G.: Clinical application of amplitude processing of echocardiographic images. Br. Heart J., *45*:621, 1981.

175. Comess, K.A., Beach, K.W., Hatsukami, T., Strandness, D.E., Jr., and Daniel, W.: Pseudocolor displays in B-mode imaging applied to echocardiography and vascular imaging: An update. J. Am. Soc. Echocardiogr., *5*:13, 1992.

176. Melton, H.E., Jr., Collins, S.M., and Skorton, D.J.: Automatic real-time endocardial edge detection in two-dimensional echocardiography. Ultrasonic Imaging, *5*:300, 1983.

177. Collins, S.M., Skorton, D.J., Geiser, E.A., Nichols, J.A., Conetta, D.A., Pandian, N.G., and Kerber, R.E.: Computer-assisted edge detection in two-dimensional echocardiography: Comparison with anatomic data. Am. J. Cardiol., *53*:1380, 1984.

178. Klingler, J.W., Begeman, M.S., Fraker, T.D., and Andrews, L.T.: Automatic detection of inter-frame motion in echocardiographic images. Ultrasound Med. Biol., *15*:683, 1989.

179. Geiser, E.A., Oliver, L.H., Gardin, J.M., Kerber, R.E., Parisi, A.F., Reichek, N., Werner, J.A., and Wayman, A.E.: Clinical validation of an edge detection algorithm for two-dimensional echocardiographic short-axis images. J. Am. Soc. Echocardiogr., *1*:410, 1988.

180. Vandenberg, B.F., Rath, L.S., Stuhlmuller, P., Melton, Jr., J.E., and Skorton, D.J.: Estimation of left ventricular cavity area with an on-line, semiautomated echocardiographic edge detection system. Circulation, *86*:159, 1992.

181. Perez, J.E., Waggoner, A.D., Barzilai, B., Melton, Jr., H.E., Miller, J.G., and Sobel, B.E.: On-line assessment of ventricular function by automatic boundary detection and ultrasonic backscatter imaging. J. Am. Coll. Cardiol., *19*:313, 1992.

181a.Perez, J.E., Klein, S.C., Prater, D.M., Fraser, C.E., Cardona, H., Waggoner, A.D., Holland, M.R., Miller, J.G., and Sobel, B.E.: Automated, on-line quantification of left ventricular dimensions and function by echocardiography with backscatter imaging and lateral gain compensation. Am. J. Cardiol., *70*:1200, 1992.

182. Kuecherer, H.F., Abbott, J.A., Botvinick, E.H., Scheinman, E.D., O'Connell, J.W., Scheinman, M.M., Foster, E., and Schiller, N.B.: Two-dimensional echocardiographic phase analysis. Circulation, *85*:130, 1992.

183. Lattanzi, F., Spirito, P., Picano, E., Mazzarisi, A., Landini, L., Distante, A., Vecchio, C., and L'Abbate, A.: Quantitative assessment of ultrasonic myocardial reflectivity in hypertrophic cardiomyopathy. J. Am. Coll. Cardiol., *17*:1085, 1991.

184. Sagar, K.B., Pelc, L.R., Rhyne, T.L., Komorowski,

R.A., Wann, L.S., and Warltier, D.C.: Role of ultrasonic tissue characterization to distinguish reversible from irreversible myocardial injury. J. Am. Soc. Echocardiogr., *3*:471, 1990.

185. Vandenberg, B.F., Stuhlmuller, J.E., Rath, L., Kerber, R.E., Collins, S.M., Melton, H.E., and Skorton, D.J.: Diagnosis of recent myocardial infarction with quantitative backscatter imaging: Preliminary studies. J. Am. Soc. Echocardiogr., *4*:10, 1991.

186. Skorton, D.J. and Collins, S.M.: Clinical potential of ultrasound tissue characterization in cardiomyopathies. J. Am. Soc. Echocardiogr., *1*:69, 1988.

187. Vandenberg, B.F., Kieso, R.A., Fox-Eastham, K., Kerber, R.E., Melton, H.E., Collins, S.M., and Skorton, D.J.: Characterization of acute experimental left ventricular thrombi with quantitative backscatter imaging. Circulation, *81*:1017, 1990.

188. Stuhmuller, J.E., Skorton, D.J., Burns, T.L., Melton, Jr., H.E., and Vandenberg, B.F.: Reproducibility of quantitative backscatter echocardiographic imaging in normal subjects. Am. J. Cardiol., *69*:542, 1992.

189. Eaton, M.H., Lappas, D., Waggoner, A.D., Perez, J.E., Miller, J.G., and Barzilai, B.: Ultrasonic myocardial tissue characterization in the operating room: Initial results using transesophageal echocardiography. J. Am. Soc. Echocardiogr., *4*:541, 1991.

190. Van Der Steen, A.F.W., Rijsterborgh, H., Mastick, F., Lancee, C.T., Van Hoorn, W.M., and Bom, N.: Influence of attenuation of measurements of ultrasonic myocardial integrated backscatter during cardiac cycle (an in vivo study). Ultrasound Med. Biol., *17*:869, 1991.

191. Perez, J.E., Miller, J.G., Barzilai, B., Wickline, S.M., Mohr, G.A., Wear, K., Vered, Z., and Sobel, B.E.: Progress in quantitative ultrasonic characterization of myocardium: From the laboratory to the bedside. J. Am. Soc. Echocardiogr., *1*:194, 1988.

192. McPherson, D.D., Knosp, B.M., Kieso, R.A., Bean, J.A., Kerber, R.E., Skorton, D.J., and Collins, S.M.: Ultrasound characterization of acoustic properties of acute intracardiac thrombi: Studies in a new experimental model. J. Am. Soc. Echocardiogr., *1*:254, 1988.

193. Ghosh, A., Nanda, N.C., and Maurer, G.: Three-dimensional reconstruction of echo-cardiographic images using the rotation method. Ultrasound Med. Biol., *8*:655, 1982.

194. Nixon, J.V., Saffer, S.I., Kipscomb, K., and Blomqvist, C.G.: Three-dimensional echoventriculography. Am. Heart J., *106*:435, 1983.

195. Geiser, E.A., Ariet, M., Conetta, D.A., Lupkiewics, S.M., Christie, L.G., and Conti, C.R.: Dynamic three-dimensional echocardiographic reconstruction of the intact human left ventricle: Technique and initial observations in patients. Am. Heart J., *103*:1056, 1982.

196. Matsumoto, M., Inoue, M., Tamura, S., Tanaka, K., and Abe, H.: Three-dimensional echocardiography for spatial visualization and volume calculation of cardiac structures. J.C.U., *9*:157, 1981.

197. Nikravesh, P.E., Skorton, D.J., Chandran, K.B., Attarwala, Y.M., Pandian, N., and Kerber, R.E.: Computerized three-dimensional finite element reconstruction of the left ventricle from cross-sectional echocardiograms. Ultrasonic Imaging, *6*:48, 1984.

198. Gopal, A.S., King, D.L., Katz, J., Boxt, L.M., King, Jr., D.L., Shao, M.Y-C.: Three-dimensional echocardiographic volume computation by polyhedral surface reconstruction: In Vitro validation and comparison to magnetic resonance imaging. J. Am. Soc. Echocardiogr., *5*: 115, 1992.

199. Geiser, E.A., Christie, Jr., L.G., Conetta, D.A., Conti, C.R., and Gossman, G.S.: A mechanical arm for spatial registration of two-dimensional echocardiographic sections. Cathet. Cardiovasc. Diagn., *8*:89, 1982.

199a.King, D.L., Harrison, M.R., King, D.L., Jr., Gopal, A.S., Kwan, O.L., and DeMaria, A.N.: Ultrasound beam orientation during standard two-dimensional imaging: Assessment by three-dimensional echocardiography. J. Am. Soc. Echocardiogr., *5*:569, 1992.

200. Raichlen, J.S., Trivedi, S.S., Herman, G.T., St. John, Sutton, M.G., Reichek, N.: Dynamic three-dimensional reconstruction of the left ventricle from two-dimensional echocardiograms. J. Am. Coll. Cardiol., *8*:364, 1986.

201. Geiser, E.A.: Three-dimensional echocardiographic reconstruction: how does it stack up? Int. J. Cardiol., *7*: 77, 1985.

202. Thomas, J.D., Hagege, A.A., Choong, C.Y., Chir, B., Wilkins, G.T., Newell, J.B., Weyman, A.E.: Improved accuracy of echocardiographic endocardial borders by spatiotemporal filtered Fourier reconstruction: description of the method and optimization of filter cutoffs. Circulation, *77*:415, 1988.

203. Kuroda, T., Kinter, T.M., Seward, J.B., Yanagi, H., Greenleaf, J.F.: Accuracy of three-dimensional volume measurement using biplane transesophageal echocardiographic probe: In vitro experiment. J. Am. Soc. Echo., *4*:475, 1991.

203a.Nanda, N.C., Pinheiro, L., Sanyal, R., Rosenthal, S., and Kirklin, J.K.: Multiplane transesophageal echocardiographic imaging and three-dimensional reconstruction. Echocardiography, *9*:667, 1992.

203b.Pandian, N.G., Nanda, N.C., Schwartz, S.L., Fan, P., Cao, Q-L., Sanyal, R., Hsu, T-L., Mumm, B., Wollschlager, H., and Weintraub, A.: Three-dimensional and four-dimensional transesophageal echocardiographic imaging of the heart and aorta in humans using a computed tomographic imaging probe. Echocardiography, *9*: 677, 1992.

204. Burrell, C.J., Kitney, R.I., Rothman, M.T.: Intravascular ultrasound imaging and three-dimensional modeling of arteries. Echocardiography, *7*:475, 1990.

205. Sheikh, K.H., Smith, S.W., Von Ramm, O., Kisslo, J.: Real-time three-dimensional echocardiography: feasibility and initial use. Echocardiography, *8*:119, 1991.

206. Snyder, J.E., Kisslo, J., vonRamm, O.T.: Real-time orthogonal mode scanning of the heart. I. System design, J. Am. Coll. Cardiol., *7*:1279, 1986.

207. Veluchamy, V.: Medical ultrasound and its biological effects. J. Clin. Eng., *3*:162, 1978.

208. Erdmann, W.A., Johnson, L.K., and Baird, A.I.: Ultrasonic toxicity study. Ultrasound Med. Biol., *3*:351, 1978.

209. Galperin-Lemaitre, H.: Safety threshold of ultrasound in medical use? Am. Heart J., *94*:260, 1977.

210. Frizzell, L.A. and Lizzi, F.L.: AIUM Bioeffects Committee. J. Ultrasound Med., *2*:R14, 1983.

211. Baker, M.L. and Dalrymple, G.V.: Biological effects of diagnostic ultrasound: A review. Radiology, *126*:479, 1978.

212. Pizzarello, D.J., Vivino, A., Newall, J., and Wolsky, A.: Effect of pulsed low-power ultrasound on growing tissues. II. Malignant tissues. Exp. Cell Biol., *46*:240, 1978.

213. Velchamy, V.: Medical ultrasound and its biological effects. J. Clin. Eng., *3*:162, 1978.

214. Stewart, H.D., Stewart, H.F., Moore, R.M. and Garry, J.: Compilation of reported biological effects data and ultrasound exposure levels. JCU, *13*:167, 1985.

215. Skorton, D.J., Collins, S.M., Greenleaf, J.F., Meltzer, R.S., O'Brien, Jr., W.D., Schnittger, I., and von Ramm, O.T.: Ultrasound bioeffects and regulatory issues: An introduction for the echocardiographer. J. Am. Soc. Echocardiogr., *1*:240, 1988.

215a.Carstensen, E.L., Duck, F.A., Meltzer, E.S., Schwarz, K.Q., and Keller, B.: Bioeffects in echocardiography. Echocardiography, *9*:605, 1992.

216. Who's afraid of a hundred milliwatts per square centimeter (10 mW/cm$^2$, SPTA)? Prepared by the American Institute of Ultrasound in Medicine Bioeffects Committee. American Institute of Ultrasound in Medicine, 1979.

217. Barnett, S.B. and Kossoff, G.: Temporal peak intensity as a critical parameter in ultrasound dosimetry. J. Ultrasound Med., *3*:385, 1984.

218. Nyborg, W.L., Buxbaum, C., Carson, P.L., Carstensen, E.L., O'Brien, W.D., Jr., Rooney, J.A., Stratmeyer, M.E., and Taylor, K.J.W.: Should there be upper limits to intensities for diagnostic ultrasound equipment? A panel discussion. Reflections, *4*:293, 1978.

219. Taylor, K.J.W.: Current status of toxicity investigation. JCU *2*:149, 1974.

220. Edler, I., Gustafson, A., Karlefors, T., and Christensson, B.: Ultrasound cardiography. Acta Med. Scand. (Suppl.), *370*:68, 1961.

221. Huter, T.F., Ballantine, H.T., Jr., and Coller, W.C.: Production of lesions in the central venous system with focused ultrasound: A study of dosage factors. J. Acoust. Soc. Am., *28*:192, 1956.

222. Lehmann, J.: The biophysical basis of biological ultrasonic reactions with special reference to ultrasonic therapy. Arch. Phys. Med. Rehabil., *34*:139, 1953.

223. Flynn, H.G.: Physics of acoustic cavitation in liquids. *In* Physical Acoustics. Edited by W.P. Mason. New York, Academic Press, 1964.

224. Macintosh, I.C.C. and Davey, D.A.: Relationship between intensity of ultrasound and induction of chromosome aberrations. Br. J. Radiol., *45*:320, 1972.

225. Murai, N., Hoshi, K., and Nakamura, T.: Effects of diagnostic ultrasound irradiated during fetal state on development of orienting behavior and reflex ontogeny in rats. Tohoku J. Exp. Med., *47*:640, 1976.

226. David, H., Weaver, J.B., and Pearson, J.F.: Doppler ultrasound and fetal activity. Br. Med. J., *2*:62, 1975.

# 2

# The Echocardiographic Examination

The ability to obtain a high-quality echocardiographic recording is probably the most important factor in determining how useful an echocardiographic examination will be. No matter how expertly one interprets echocardiograms, it is not possible to obtain useful information from an inadequate tracing. The technical details involved in getting a high-quality echocardiogram are somewhat unique to this particular type of examination. Unfortunately, examinations must be customized for each patient. One cannot place the transducer in routine positions over the chest as one does electrocardiographic leads and hope that the recording will be comparable from one patient to another. The examination is considered adequate when the one performing the study records what he or she recognizes and feels is necessary for that individual patient. Thus, the echocardiographic examination has become a highly sophisticated technique that requires experience, skill, and an understanding of the requirements for an adequate echocardiogram.

## SELECTION OF TRANSDUCERS

As noted in chapter 1, a variety of transducers are available for the routine or transthoracic echocardiographic examination. Invasive echocardiographic studies using transesophageal, intravascular, and epicardial examinations are discussed subsequently. Whether one uses a mechanical or a phased array transducer is dictated by the instrument available. Few instruments can use both types of transducers. Almost all examinations are done with the expectation of performing a full examination, which includes cardiac imaging as well as Doppler studies. As indicated in Chapter 1, higher definition cardiac images are obtained with higher frequency transducers, although penetration is relatively poor. Furthermore, the best Doppler studies are obtained with lower frequency transducers. Some of the newer instruments have dual frequency transducers, which avoid some of this difficulty. One may not need to change the transducer and can switch from one frequency to another. The frequency of the transducer for cardiac imaging depends to a large extent on the body habitus of the patient. With a young child or thin adult, one would prefer a 3.5-MHz or even a 5-MHz transducer; however, with a thick-chested individual, a 2.0 to 2.5-MHz transducer

is necessary for adequate penetration. A neonate may be best imaged with a 7 or 7.5-MHz transducer.

The size or "footprint" of the transducer can be a major factor in the quality of the study. Examinations in patients who have relatively narrow intercostal spaces and whose ribs are calcified can be difficult. Ideally, one would like the smallest possible transducer. On the other hand, the smaller surface also produces a larger beam width and poorer penetration. In practice, the size of the transducer is usually dictated by the frequency. The manufacturer rarely has the same frequency transducers with different sizes. Thus, one usually selects the frequency of the transducer and does not have an option in varying the size. With a mechanical system, the size of the transducers may vary depending on whether one uses an annular phased array, rotating transducer, or a single oscillating crystal (see Chapter 1).

Almost all echocardiographic studies are done with two-dimensional echocardiographic orientation. A stand-alone M-mode echocardiogram is virtually never performed, although it is still occasionally useful to do a nonimaging Doppler study, especially with continuous wave Doppler. Thus, a Pedoff continuous wave Doppler transducer is still being used because of its versatility and the high quality Doppler recording that it provides (Fig. 2–1).

Some examination locations, such as the suprasternal notch, may be somewhat difficult and occasionally specialized transducers are required for that particular examination.

## POSITION OF THE PATIENT

Almost all echocardiographic examinations are done with the patient in some variation of the supine position. Occasionally, the patient is flat, but more often he or she is in the left lateral decubitus position and, occasionally, in the right lateral decubitus position. This left lateral approach uses gravity, bringing more of the heart to the left of the sternum and facilitating the recording of most intracardiac echoes. The degree to which the patient rotates to the left varies from one individual to another. Figure 2–2 demonstrates a transthoracic echocardiographic examination with the patient in the left lateral position. Whether one uses the right or left hand to hold the transducer is a matter of preference. Some

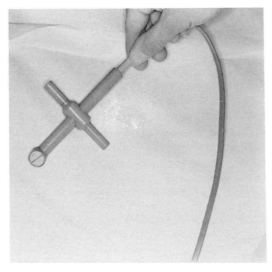

**Fig. 2–1.** Pedoff continuous wave Doppler transducer.

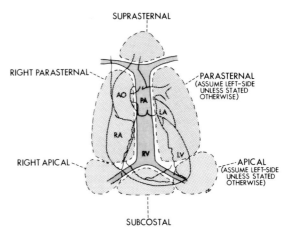

NOMENCLATURE FOR TRANSDUCER LOCATION

**Fig. 2–3.** Diagram demonstrating the various transducer locations for echocardiography. AO = aorta; PA = pulmonary artery; LA = left atrium; RA = right atrium; RV = right ventricle; LV = left ventricle. (From Henry, W.L., et al.: Report of the American Society of Echocardiography Committee on Nomenclature and Standards in Two-dimensional Echocardiography. Circulation, *62*:212, 1980, by permission of the American Heart Association, Inc.)

of the transducers can be relatively heavy, and it is easier to support the weight of the transducer with four fingers rather than with the thumb. In addition, the cable leading from the transducer to the instrument must also be supported by the left thumb when examining from the left side. On the other hand, examining with the right hand requires reaching across the patient, and this is not always easily done.

## PLACEMENT OF THE TRANSDUCER

Figure 2–3 illustrates the various locations for placement of a transthoracic transducer during examination

of the heart and great vessels.[1] The most common place to begin an examination is along the left sternal border, which has been designated left parasternal or just parasternal. Figure 2–2 demonstrates such a transducer position. The second most common location is with the transducer over the apex (Fig. 2–4). Both of these examinations are best done with the patient in the left lateral decubitus position.

With the patient in the left lateral decubitus position

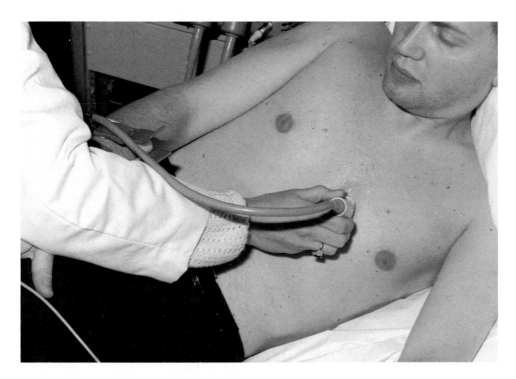

**Fig. 2–2.** Echocardiographic examination with the transducer in the left parasternal location.

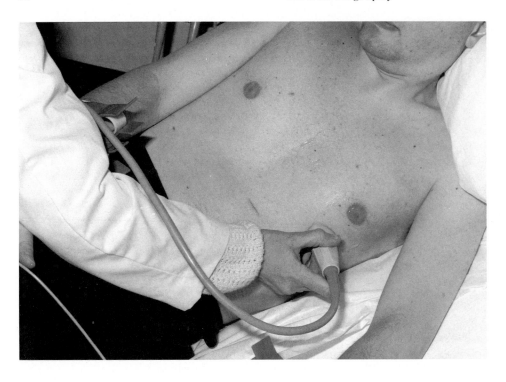

**Fig. 2–4.** Echocardiographic transducer placed at the apical position.

and the transducer over the apex, the surface of the bed or examining table may interfere. As a result, a cutaway table or mattress is available to facilitate the apical examination (Fig. 2–5).

The subcostal approach (Fig. 2–6) is particularly useful in patients who have low diaphragms and hyperinflated lungs.[2] The subcostal examination also is necessary for viewing the inferior vena cava and hepatic veins[3,4] as well as many congenital anomalies.[5,6] The suprasternal approach (Fig. 2–7) gives a view of the base of the heart and great vessels.[7,8] Both imaging and Doppler studies are frequently performed with this examination.[9] The subcostal and suprasternal studies are best done with the patient flat on his or her back.

The right parasternal window can be particularly helpful in looking at the aorta[10,11] or the interatrial septum.[12] When examining from the right side of the sternum, the patient is best positioned in the right lateral decubitus (Fig. 2–8). This approach is commonly used when recording blood flow across the aortic valve.

Lesser used windows include the right apical, the right supraclavicular fossa, and even the back.[13,14] The right

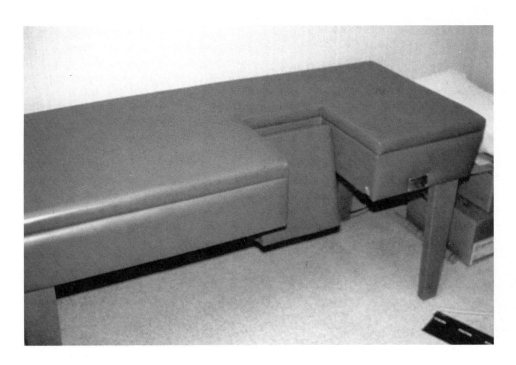

**Fig. 2–5.** Examining table with a dropout component to facilitate placement of the transducer in the apical position.

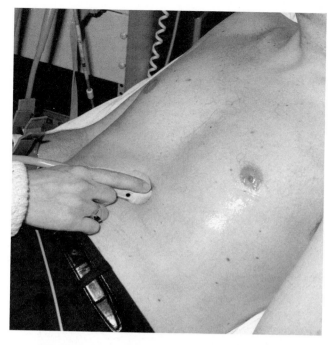

Fig. 2–6.  Transducer in the subcostal position.

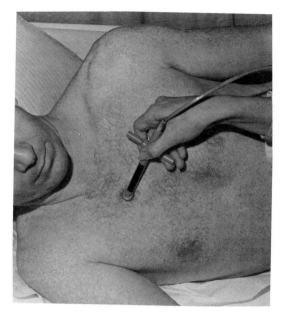

Fig. 2–8.  Transducer location for obtaining ascending aortic flow from the right sternal border. The patient is best examined while in the right lateral decubitus position.

apical view may give a good opportunity to interrogate the inferior vena and hepatic veins. The right supraclavicular examination is the transducer position of choice for recording the superior vena cava. With a large pleural effusion, the fluid can be used as an acoustic window. Thus, the transducer may be placed in the back or even in the midaxillary line while the heart is visualized through the pleural fluid. A right paraspinal examination can occasionally be used to look at the descending aorta, especially when looking for dissection.[14]

## TWO-DIMENSIONAL EXAMINATION

Two-dimensional echocardiography is the backbone of cardiac ultrasound.[15] Almost all studies are done with reference to the two-dimensional image. Doppler and M-mode examinations are obtained after first having a reference from the two-dimensional examination. Thus, the initial approach to the cardiac examination begins with the two-dimensional study. Figure 2–9 illustrates the three basic orthogonal views used for two-dimensional imaging.[1] The long-axis plane runs parallel to the heart or left ventricle. The short-axis plane is perpendicular to the long axis. The four-chamber plane is orthogonal to the other two and somewhat represents a frontal plane.

Figure 2–10 shows the approximate transducer location for long-axis and short-axis studies of the root of the aorta. The long-axis examination (Fig. 2–10, plane one), provides a long-axis view of the aorta, aortic valve, left atrium, and left ventricular outflow tract (Fig. 2–11). Although the mitral valve may be seen in this examination, this valve is best examined in a slightly different plane. The aortic valve can be seen opening as two parallel echoes running near the walls of the aorta in systole (Fig. 2–11A). The leaflets close in diastole and one sees a dominant echo where the leaflets meet (Fig. 2–11B). Faint echoes may also come from the body of the leaflets. These echoes are usually recorded only when the valve is thickened or when the patient is unusually easy to examine.

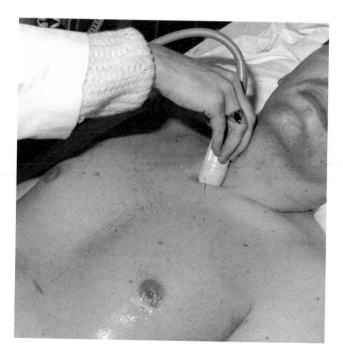

Fig. 2–7.  Echocardiographic examination with the transducer in the suprasternal notch.

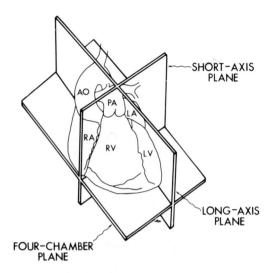

## TWO-DIMENSIONAL ECHOCARDIOGRAPHIC IMAGING PLANES

**Fig. 2–9.** Diagram demonstrating the three orthogonal planes for two-dimensional echocardiographic imaging. AO = aorta; PA = pulmonary artery; LA = left atrium; RA = right atrium; RV = right ventricle; LV = left ventricle. (From Henry, W.L., et al.: Report of the American Society of Echocardiography Committee on Nomenclature and Standards in Two-dimensional Echocardiography. Circulation, *62*:212, 1980, by permission of the American Heart Association, Inc.)

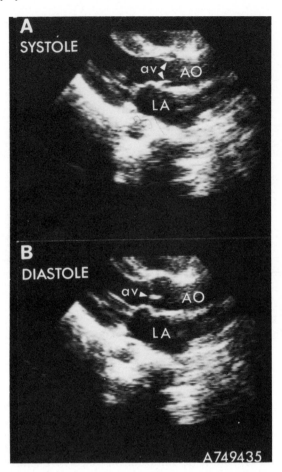

**Fig. 2–11.** Systolic (*A*) and diastolic (*B*) parasternal long-axis echocardiograms through the aorta (AO), aortic valve (av), and left atrium (LA).

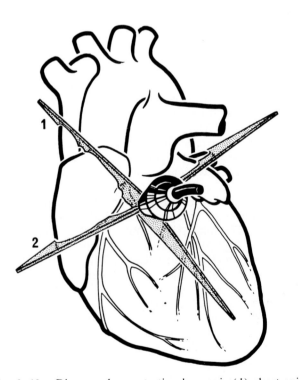

**Fig. 2–10.** Diagram demonstrating long-axis (*1*) short-axis (*2*) sector scans of the root of the aorta. Note approximate transducer location.

The short-axis view through the aorta and base of the heart (Fig. 2–10, plane two), is approximately 90° to the long-axis aortic examination. Figure 2–12 demonstrates the many cardiac structures that can be seen with this two-dimensional short-axis view. These structures include the aorta, left atrium, right atrium, right ventricle, aortic valve (AV), pulmonary valve (PV), tricuspid valve (TV), interatrial septum (IAS), and left main coronary artery (LMCA). Figure 2–13 is a short-axis examination of the aorta in a patient with well-defined aortic leaflets. The right (r), left (l), and noncoronary (n) cusps of the aortic valve in this patient can be readily identified in both diastole and systole.

Figure 2–14 demonstrates that with a slight change in angulation of the transducer, it is also possible to record the length of the pulmonary artery to the point of its bifurcation. Figure 2–15 shows a diastolic and systolic short-axis examination through the base of the heart. During diastole (Fig. 2–15*A*), the pulmonary valve (PV) and proximal portion of the pulmonary artery (PA) are seen. With ventricular systole, the heart moves into a position that reveals the echo-free space from the pulmonary artery and its two major branches (Fig. 2–15*B*). This echocardiogram provides a good appreciation of

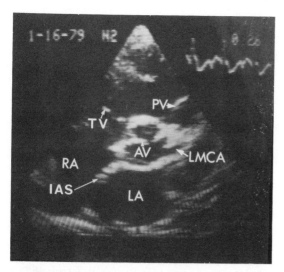

**Fig. 2–12.** Two-dimensional short-axis echocardiogram of the base of the heart demonstrating the aortic valve (AV) within the aorta, the pulmonary valve (PV), the tricuspid valve (TV), the right atrium (RA), the interatrial septum (IAS), the left atrium (LA), and the left main coronary artery (LMCA).

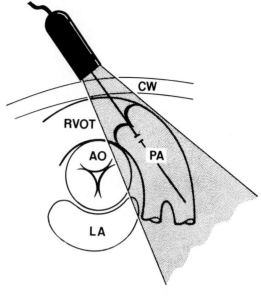

**Fig. 2–14.** Diagram demonstrating how the pulmonary artery (PA) can be visualized with a parasternal short-axis examination. CW = chest wall; RVOT = right ventricular outflow tract; AO = aorta; LA = left atrium.

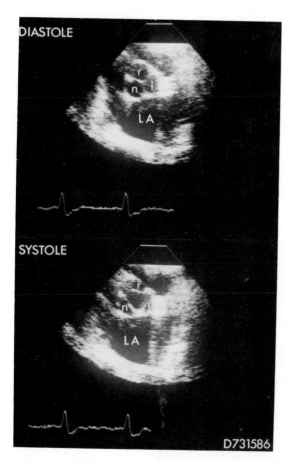

**Fig. 2–13.** Diastolic and systolic short-axis echocardiograms of the aortic valve showing right coronary (r), left coronary (l), and noncoronary (n) aortic valve leaflets. The patient had a low cardiac output; thus the aortic valve orifice is not circular in systole. LA = left atrium.

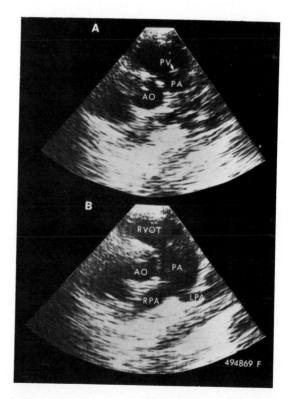

**Fig. 2–15.** Diastolic (*A*) and systolic (*B*) short-axis echocardiographs at the levels of the aorta and pulmonary artery. With systole, the pulmonary artery and its two major branches can be visualized. PV = pulmonary valve; PA = pulmonary artery; AO = aorta; RPA = right pulmonary artery; LPA = left pulmonary artery; RVOT = right ventricular outflow tract.

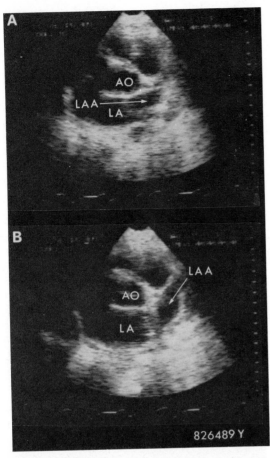

how the pulmonary artery curves around the aorta and bifurcates posteriorly. The parasternal short-axis view also permits one to identify the left atrial appendage. Figure 2–16 shows the location of the left atrial appendage (LAA) with relation to the body of the left atrium (LA). As noted later, the left atrial appendage is seen better with transesophageal echocardiography.

Between the pulmonary artery and left atrium lies the left coronary artery. Figure 2–17 demonstrates the left main coronary artery (lm) coming off of the aorta (AO). The division of bifurcation of the artery into its left anterior descending (lad) and left circumflex (lcx) branches can be noted. In this particular recording, it is also possible to see the first diagonal branch (dg) of the left anterior or descending artery. Figure 2–18 illustrates the proximal right coronary artery (rca), as well as the left main (lm) in the short-axis view. Communication of the right coronary artery with the aorta is noted in Figure 2–18. Several views in addition to the short-axis view have been used to visualize the coronary arteries. These views are discussed in Chapter 8, Coronary Artery Disease.

The parasternal long-axis view of the body of the left ventricle is in a slightly different plane than that of the left ventricular outflow tract and aorta. The body of the left ventricle is best recorded using the transducer position shown in Figure 2–19, plane one. The transducer is almost perpendicular to the surface of the chest. This is the best view for recording the long axis of the mitral valve. Figure 2–20 shows four frames from a two-dimensional study of the mitral valve with the valve at end diastole (Fig. 2–20A), end systole (Fig. 2–20B), early diastole (Fig. 2–20C), and mid-diastole (Fig. 2–20D). Figure 2–21 shows a long-axis parasternal view through the body of the left ventricle and the mitral valve showing an "apparent apex." This rounded apical segment of the body of the left ventricle is probably a truncated view created by the ultrasonic beam transecting the me-

**Fig. 2–16.** Short-axis two-dimensional echocardiograms through the base of the heart illustrating the location of the left atrial appendage (LAA). AO = aorta; LA = left atrium.

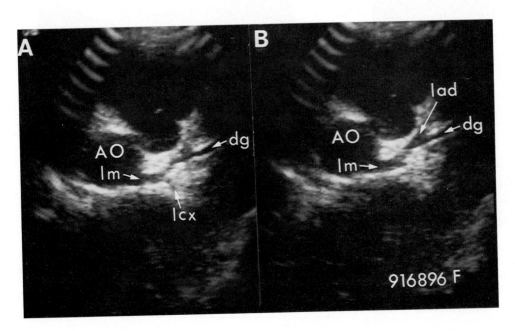

**Fig. 2–17.** Short-axis two-dimensional echocardiographic examination of the aorta (AO) and the proximal left coronary arteries. lm = left main coronary artery; dg = diagonal; lcx = left circumflex; lad = left anterior descending. (From Feigenbaum, H.: Echocardiography. *In* Heart Disease, 4th ed. Edited by E. Braunwald. Philadelphia, W.B. Saunders Co., 1992.)

ventricular echocardiogram. The first short-axis view (Fig. 2–24*A*), at the level of the mitral valve, is produced by examining plane one in Figure 2–23. The mitral valve is visible within the circular left ventricular cavity. Transducer position two is a short-axis view at the level of the papillary muscles. The echoes from the papillary muscles can be seen encroaching on the cavity of the left ventricle. The short-axis examination resulting from examining plane three in Figure 2–23 is at the level of the cardiac apex. Neither the mitral valve nor the papillary muscles are visible.

The short-axis left ventricular examination provides an opportunity for a short-axis study of the mitral valve. Figure 2–25*A* shows the mitral valve in its open position. Figure 2–25*B* illustrates a partially closed mitral valve, and a completely closed mitral valve is shown in Figure 2–25*C*. Because the mitral valve and mitral annulus are constantly moving in a superior-inferior direction, recording the mitral valve throughout the cardiac cycle in one short-axis plane is not always easy. To best see the valve in diastole may require one plane, whereas mitral valve closure may be best recorded in a slightly different plane. The mitral valve and annulus move toward the apex with systole and in the reverse direction in diastole.

The right ventricle and tricuspid valve can also be

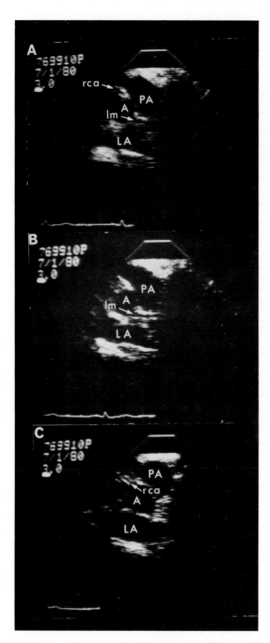

**Fig. 2–18.** Short-axis echocardiograms illustrating the locations of the right (rca) and left main (lm) coronary arteries. PA = pulmonary artery; A = aorta; LA = left atrium.

dial wall of the left ventricle. To truly record the left ventricular apex, the transducer should be moved to a lower interspace and directed somewhat laterally (Fig. 2–19, plane two). As the transducer is placed over the apex, one obtains an apical long-axis view. Figure 2–22 illustrates how one can obtain long-axis views from either the apical, parasternal, or suprasternal windows.

Figure 2–23 shows three transducer positions for short-axis examinations of the left ventricle. The interspace is the same for planes one and two. One merely changes the angle of the transducer. Examining plane three requires moving the transducer to a lower interspace. Figure 2–24 shows the resultant short-axis left

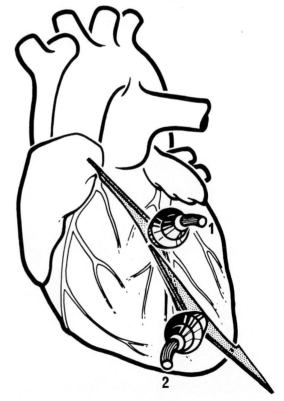

**Fig. 2–19.** Diagram demonstrating the transducer position and the direction of the ultrasonic beam for parasternal long-axis examinations of the left ventricle and mitral valve. Both the transducer location and the direction of the beam for examining the mitral valve and body of the left ventricle (*position 1*) are different than those for the apical portion of the left ventricle (*position 2*).

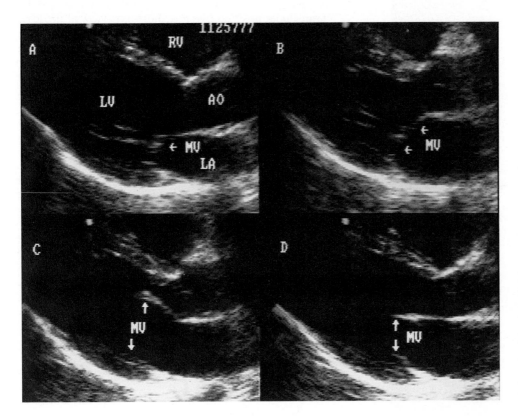

Fig. 2–20. Serial frames from a two-dimensional echocardiogram showing the position of the mitral valve (MV) at end-diastole (*A*), end-systole (*B*), early diastole (*C*), and mid-diastole (*D*). LV = left ventricle; RV = right ventricle; AO = aorta; LA = left atrium.

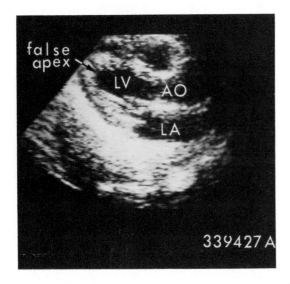

Fig. 2–21. Long-axis parasternal examination of the left ventricle showing a "false apex." The apparent apex probably originates from the medial wall of the left ventricle. LV = left ventricle; AO = aorta; LA = left atrium.

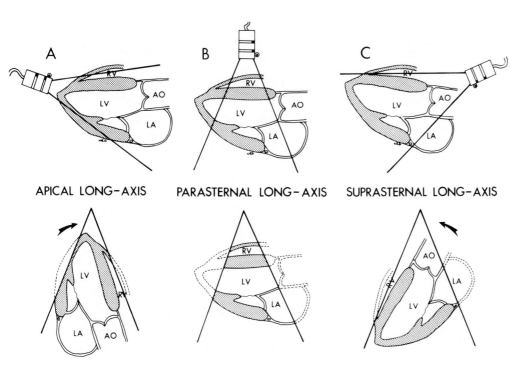

APICAL LONG-AXIS    PARASTERNAL LONG-AXIS    SUPRASTERNAL LONG-AXIS

**Fig. 2–22.** Diagrams indicating how one can obtain a long-axis examination of the heart from the following transducer positions: *A*, apical, *B*, parasternal, and *C*, suprasternal. The suprasternal long-axis examination is more theoretical than actual since such an examination is difficult to obtain in most patients. RV = right ventricle; LV = left ventricle; LA = left atrium; AO = aorta. (From Henry, W.L., et al.: Report of the American Society of Echocardiography Committee on Nomenclature and Standards in Two-dimensional Echocardiography. Circulation, *62*:212, 1980, by permission of the American Heart Association, Inc.)

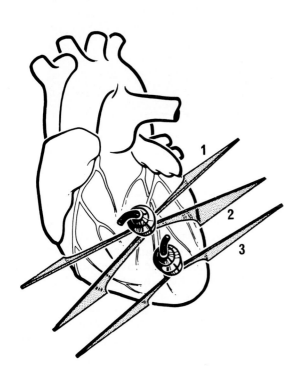

**Fig. 2–23.** Transducer positions for short-axis examinations of the left ventricle. Plane 1 passes through the mitral valve, plane 2 through the papillary muscles, and plane 3 through the left ventricular apex.

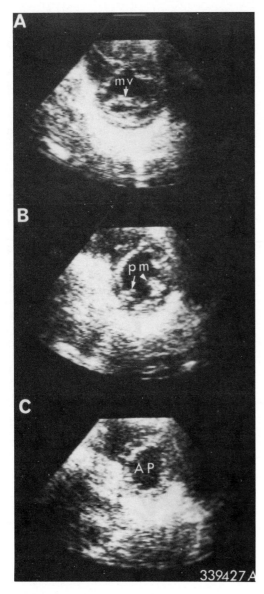

**Fig. 2–24.** Short-axis parasternal echocardiograms. *A,* The mitral valve (mv); *B,* the papillary muscles (pm); and *C,* the left ventricular apex (AP).

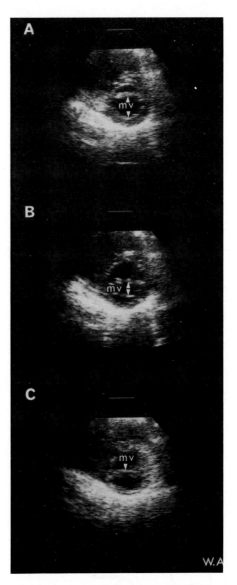

**Fig. 2–25.** Short-axis parasternal echocardiograms of the mitral valve (mv) in early diastole (*A*), mid-diastole (*B*), and systole (*C*).

recorded with the transducer in the parasternal position (Fig. 2–26). The plane of the examination does not exactly fit either the long axis or short axis. It is important to note that the three basic planes—long axis, short axis, and four chamber—are only approximations. The right ventricular inflow, parasternal view is one of many modifications of these three basic planes. Figure 2–27 shows the right ventricular inflow tract and right atrium by way of such a parasternal examination. This study provides an opportunity to record the motion of the tricuspid valve. Figure 2–28 shows diastolic and systolic frames of the tricuspid valve in the long axis.

Figure 2–29 diagramatically illustrates the two commonly used two-dimensional echocardiographic views with the transducer placed at the cardiac apex. Exami-

nation plane one demonstrates the apical four-chamber view of the heart. Figure 2–30A shows an example of a four-chamber apical echocardiogram. With slight angulation of the transducer, one can record the root of the aorta from the apical four-chamber view. Figure 2–31A demonstrates another four-chamber apical examination. By tilting the transducer slightly anteriorly, one can record the aorta (Fig. 2–31B). The four-chamber view plus aorta is commonly referred to as the "five-chamber view."

As noted in Figure 2–22, it is possible to obtain an apical view of the long axis of the heart similar to that seen from the parasternal view. Such an examination includes portions of the right ventricle and the aorta. A more common examination from the apex is the apical two-chamber view (Fig. 2–29, plane two). This examina-

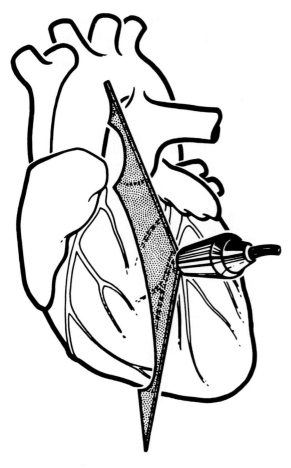

**Fig. 2–26.** Transducer position for a long-axis parasternal examination of the tricuspid valve, right atrium, and right ventricular inflow tract.

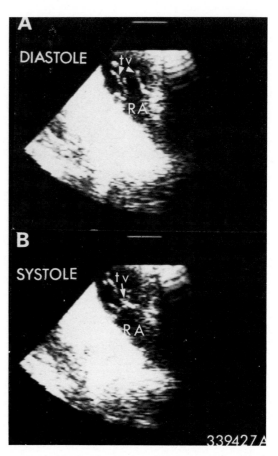

**Fig. 2–28.** Diastolic (*A*) and systolic (*B*) long-axis echocardiograms of the tricuspid valve (tv). RA = right atrium.

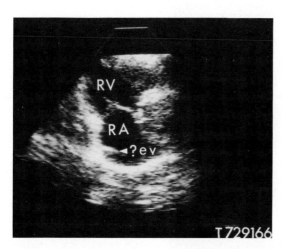

**Fig. 2–27.** Two-dimensional echocardiogram of the right atrium (RA) and right ventricular inflow tract (RV). ev = eustachian valve.

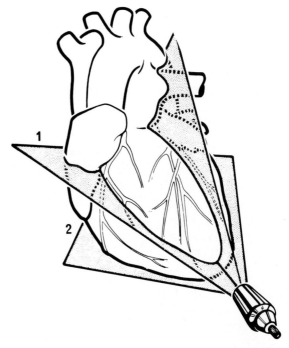

**Fig. 2–29.** Transducer position and examining planes for apical, two-dimensional echocardiograms. Plane 1 passes through the four-chamber plane of the heart. Plane 2 represents the path of the ultrasonic beam for the two-chamber apical examination.

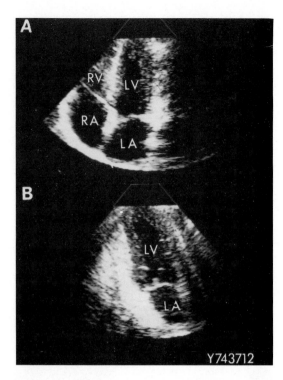

**Fig. 2–30.** Four-chamber (*A*) and two-chamber (*B*) apical two-dimensional echocardiograms. RV = right ventricle; LV = left ventricle; RA = right atrium; LA = left atrium.

four-chamber view to the two-chamber view by rotating the transducer at the apex counterclockwise approximately 90°.

Figure 2–32 shows the interrelationship between the two-chamber, four-chamber, long-axis, and the short-axis examinations. As this diagram illustrates, the long-axis and four-chamber views are not exactly orthogonal to each other. In fact, the two-chamber, long-axis, and four-chamber planes, which can be considered longitudinal views, essentially divide the short-axis into six components. This fact becomes important when dividing the left ventricle into segments for regional wall analysis.

The subcostal transducer location produces examinations approximating the four-chamber and short-axis views. The ultrasonic plane indicated in Figure 2–33*A* is similar to examining plane one in Figure 2–29. The resultant subcostal four-chamber echocardiogram appears in Figure 2–34*A*. Figure 2–33*B* shows how the transducer can be rotated 90° to provide a subcostal short-axis examination of the heart.[16] The resultant echocardiogram is illustrated in Figure 2–34*B*. The subcostal four-chamber view is particularly helpful in examining the interatrial and interventricular septa.[5,6] By directing the transducer in a slightly modified short-axis examination (Fig. 2–35*A*), one can obtain an excellent view of the right side of the heart (Fig. 2–36). This study may be particularly helpful when looking at the right ventricular outflow tract in patients with congenital heart disease. The subcostal location also permits an opportunity to direct the ultrasonic beam through the inferior vena cava and hepatic vein (Fig. 2–35*B*). Two-dimensional echocardiographic views of the inferior vena cava and hepatic vein are noted in Figure 2–37. One feature of this study is the normal collapse of the inferior vena cava with inspiration.

tion is characterized by visualizing the left atrium and left ventricle (Fig. 2–30*B*). The aorta is absent. The examination is comparable to the right anterior oblique, left ventricular angiogram commonly obtained at cardiac catheterization. Thus, the two-chamber view is also known as the "RAO equivalent." One can go from the

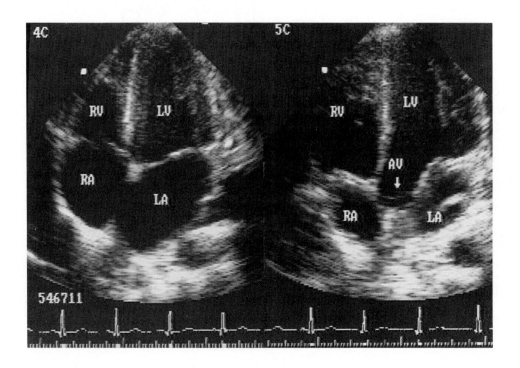

**Fig. 2–31.** Apical four-chamber (4C) and five-chamber (5C) views. RV = right ventricle; LV = left ventricle; RA = right atrium; LA = left atrium; AV = aortic valve.

Relationship of Long-Axis, Four-Chamber

and Two-Chamber Views To Short-Axis

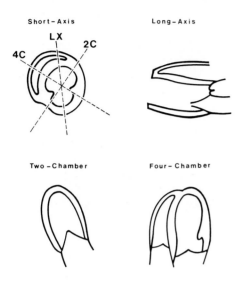

**Fig. 2–32.** Diagram demonstrating the relationship between the short-axis, long-axis (LX), two-chamber (2C), and four-chamber (4C) views of the heart.

The two examining planes with the transducer in the suprasternal notch are depicted in Figure 2–38. The ultrasonic view in Figure 2–38*A* is approximately equivalent to that of a four-chamber plane, and the view in Figure 2–38*B* is somewhat comparable to that of a long-axis plane. It is probably best, however, to orient the ultrasonic beam with regard to the arch of the aorta rather than to the heart because one does not record much of the heart with the transducer in this position, especially in the adult. In addition, the planes are different than with the transducer at the apex or subcostal region. Thus, better terminology with regard to examining planes from the suprasternal location would be *parallel* or *perpendicular* to the arch of the aorta. Figure 2–39 shows a suprasternal examination parallel to the arch of the aorta. In this view, note the aorta (AO), the pulmonary artery (P), and the left atrium (LA). With adjustment of the scanning plane, one can frequently identify the innominate (I), the left carotid (LC), and the left subclavian (SC) arteries (Fig. 2–40). A short-axis suprasternal examination of the arch of the aorta reveals a circular aorta, the pulmonary artery, and part of the left atrium (Fig. 2–41). Note also the bifurcation of the pulmonary artery.

Less frequently considered cardiac structures can also be seen in the various two-dimensional views already discussed. In the parasternal long-axis view of the left ventricle, it is possible to record an echo-free space in the coronary sinus (Fig. 2–42*A*). The structure is seen

**A**          **B**

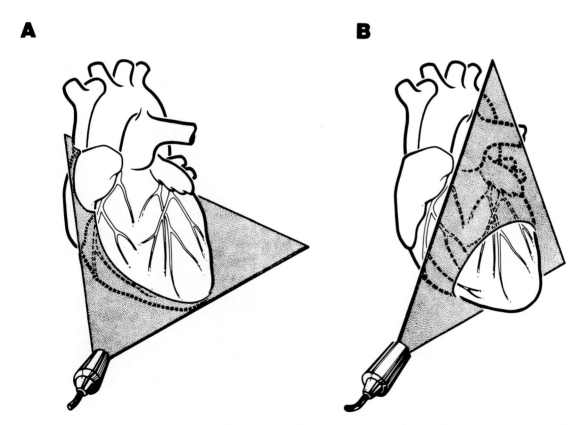

**Fig. 2–33.** Diagrams showing the transducer position and examining planes for a subcostal four-chamber examination (*A*) and a subcostal short-axis examination (*B*).

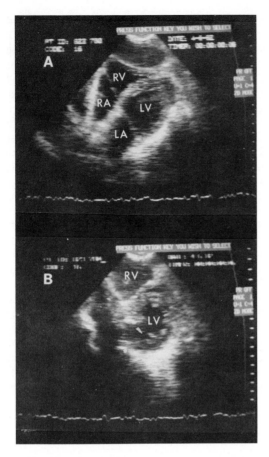

Fig. 2–34. Subcostal two-dimensional echocardiogram in the four-chamber plane (*A*) and the short-axis plane (*B*). RV = right ventricle; RA = right atrium; LA = left atrium; LV = left ventricle.

at the junction of the left ventricle and left atrium. It is important to note that this echo-free space moves with the atrioventricular groove. The curved nature of the coronary sinus can be appreciated with a short-axis examination (Fig. 2–42). Another echo-free space poste-

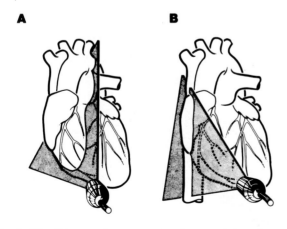

Fig. 2–35. Diagram demonstrating the examining planes and transducer positions for the subcostal examination of the right side of the heart (*A*) and the inferior vena cava (*B*).

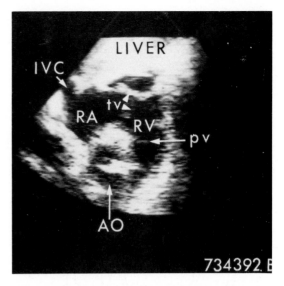

Fig. 2–36. Subcostal two-dimensional echocardiogram of the right side of the heart demonstrating the inferior vena cava (IVC), right atrium (RA), tricuspid valve (tv), right ventricle (RV), and pulmonary valve (pv). AO = aorta.

rior to the heart originates from the descending aorta. Figure 2–43 illustrates the descending aorta as seen in a parasternal long-axis study. If one rotates the transducer so that the examining plane is parallel to the descending aorta, then two long parallel echoes can be recorded (Fig. 2–43*B*).

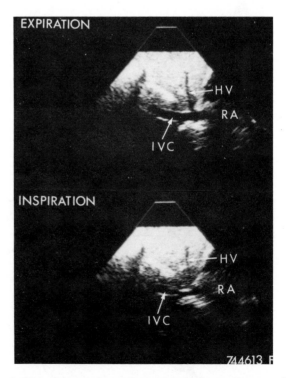

Fig. 2–37. Subcostal two-dimensional echocardiogram of the inferior vena cava (IVC) and hepatic veins (HV). The inferior vena cava decreases in size with inspiration. RA = right atrium.

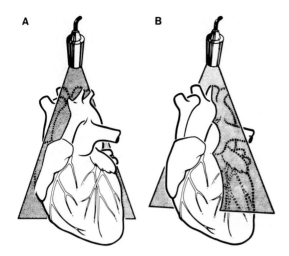

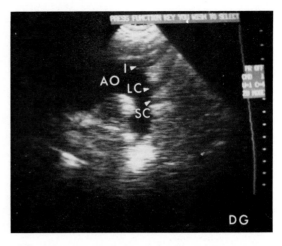

**Fig. 2–38.** Transducer position and examining plane for the suprasternal examination parallel to the arch of the aorta (*A*) and perpendicular to the arch of the aorta (*B*).

**Fig. 2–40.** Suprasternal echocardiogram of the aorta showing the innominate (I), left common carotid (LC), and left subclavian (SC) arteries. AO = aorta.

The descending aorta can also be visualized from the apical window. Figure 2–44 shows the descending aorta (DA) behind the left atrium (LA) in an apical four-chamber examination. With rotation of the transducer, the length of the descending aorta can be visualized from this transducer position (Fig. 2–44*B*).

Unusual echocardiographic windows are necessary periodically. The right parasternal window is commonly used for evaluating the aorta and occasionally the interatrial septum.[12] In patients who have thoracic surgery with displacement of the heart, the same window may be necessary for the entire echocardiographic examination. The right apical window may be analogous to a standard left apical window in a patient with right cardiac displacement or dextracardia.

On rare occasions, a patient with cephalad displacement of the heart, as might occur with abdominal distention, massive ascites, or massive obesity, a high interspace may be necessary to view the heart. Such a high interspace may also be helpful in looking at some of the great vessels.

The left axillary approach is a rare window that may be necessary for imaging a patient with horizontal orientation of the heart. If one has a large left pleural effusion, a new echocardiographic window becomes available. Now, a posterior lateral transducer location may be useful. Under these circumstances, rotating the patient to the right lateral decubitus position will open up the window for visualizing the heart.

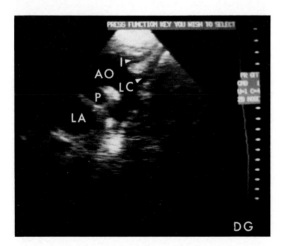

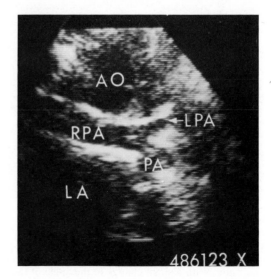

**Fig. 2–39.** Suprasternal two-dimensional echocardiogram of the arch of the aorta (AO), pulmonary artery (P), and left atrium (LA). I = innominate artery; LC = left common carotid artery. (From Feigenbaum, H.: Echocardiography. *In* Heart Diseases, 2nd ed., Edited by E. Braunwald. Philadelphia, W.B. Saunders, Co., 1984.)

**Fig. 2–41.** Suprasternal echocardiogram perpendicular to the arch of the aorta demonstrating a circular aorta (AO) and a more horizontal right pulmonary artery (RPA). A somewhat distorted view of the main pulmonary artery (PA) and left pulmonary artery (LPA) is also visible. LA = left atrium.

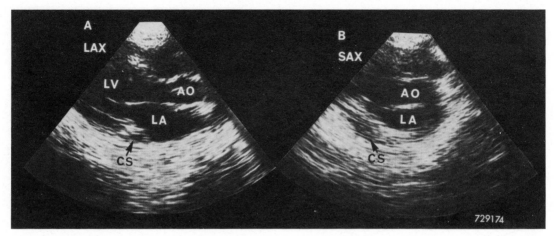

**Fig. 2–42.** Long-axis (LAX) and short-axis (SAX) parasternal two-dimensional echocardiogram demonstrating the coronary sinus (CS). LV = left ventricle; LA = left atrium; AO = aorta.

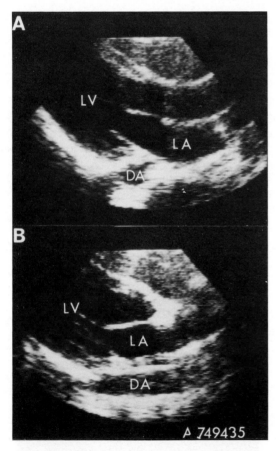

**Fig. 2–43.** Parasternal two-dimensional echocardiograms of the descending aorta. In the usual long-axis view of the left ventricle and left atrium (*A*), the descending aorta appears as a circular, echo-free space posterior to the left ventricular and left atrial walls. With a slight change in the angle of the beam rendering the examining plane parallel to the descending aorta (*B*), the length of the descending aorta can be recorded. LV = left ventricle; LA = left atrium; DA = descending aorta.

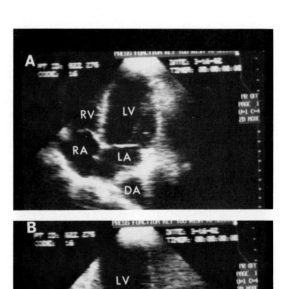

**Fig. 2–44.** Echocardiograms demonstrating how the descending aorta (DA) can be seen posterior to the left atrium (LA) with the transducer at the apex. RV = right ventricle; LV = left ventricle; RA = right atrium.

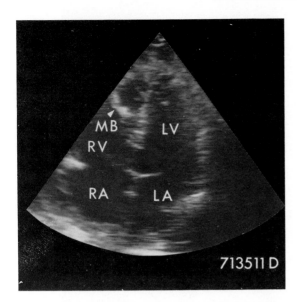

**Fig. 2–45.** Apical four-chamber echocardiogram demonstrating a prominent moderator band (MB) in the right ventricle (RV). LV = left ventricle; RA = right atrium; LA = left atrium.

### Normal Variants

A number of normal variants must be recognized on the two-dimensional echocardiogram. A prominent moderator band is a frequent finding in the right ventricle (Fig. 2–45).[17] A less frequent, but somewhat similar, finding can be noted in the left ventricle. A finer filamentous structure traverses the left ventricular cavity (Fig. 2–46). This structure is thought to represent false chordae tendineae and is of no pathologic significance.[18–22] A prominent eustachian valve is commonly

seen in the right atrium at the junction of the inferior vena cava and the right atrium (see Fig. 2–27).[23] Figure 2–47 shows a patient with an unusually large eustachian valve. This structure can be visualized from the parasternal long-axis, the apical four-chamber, and the subcostal four-chamber views. In this particular patient, the inferior vena cava was also dilated, suggesting the presence of partial obstruction to blood flow by this eustachian valve. The patient was otherwise totally asymptomatic, and the echocardiographic findings did not represent any significant clinical problem.

Filamentous echoes within the right atrium can originate from residual tissue thought to represent the Chiari network (Fig. 2–48).[24] These echoes are mobile, are nonpathologic, and represent interesting curiosities.

The shape of the interventricular septum and left ventricular outflow tract may change with age (Fig. 2–49).[25,26] The septum becomes "S"-shaped or "sigmoid" with bulging (*arrowhead*) into the outflow tract. This development is probably responsible for many of the systolic ejection murmurs heard in elderly patients.[27] Normal variants are discussed again in the chapter on cardiac masses.

### Terminology for Two-Dimensional Echocardiography

The echocardiographic literature uses numerous terms for the same two-dimensional views. Long-axis examinations are also called "sagittal" or "longitudinal;" short-axis parasternal examinations are "horizontal," "transverse," or "cross-sectional;" and the apical four-chamber view is "frontal." To minimize confusion, these terms are not used in this text in favor of following as closely as possible the terminology of the American Society of Echocardiography.

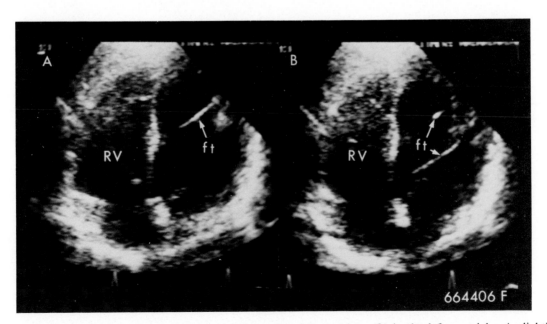

**Fig. 2–46.** Apical four-chamber echocardiograms demonstrating false tendons (ft) in the left ventricle. A slightly different examining plane (*B*) records additional false tendons. RV = right ventricle.

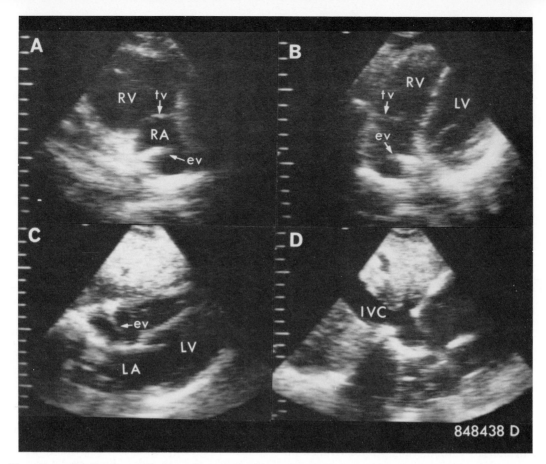

**Fig. 2–47.** Two-dimensional echocardiogram of a patient with an unusually large eustachian valve (ev). The valve can be seen in the long-axis view of the right ventricular inflow tract (*A*), the apical four-chamber view (*B*), and the subcostal four-chamber view (*C*). The inferior vena cava (IVC) is dilated (*D*). RV = right ventricle; tv = tricuspid valve; RA = right atrium; LV = left ventricle; LA = left atrium.

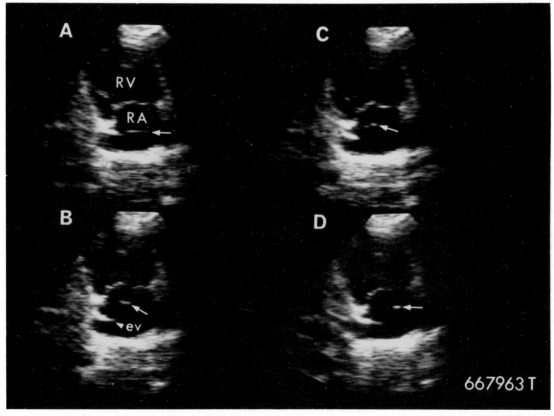

**Fig. 2–48.** Two-dimensional echocardiograms of a patient with a Chiari network. The echoes originating from the filamentous structures (*arrows*) move randomly within the right atrium (RA). RV = right ventricle; ev = eustachian valve.

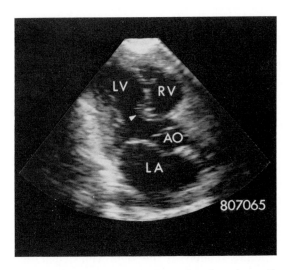

**Fig. 2–49.** Long-axis two-dimensional echocardiogram showing the base of the interventricular septum (*arrowhead*) bulging into the left ventricle outflow tract between the left ventricle (LV) and aorta (AO). RV = right ventricle; LA = left atrium.

## Orientation of Two-Dimensional Images

The orientation of two-dimensional echocardiographic images may vary with different investigators. A few echocardiographers orient the parasternal long-axis views with the aorta on the left (Fig. 2–50B), as opposed to the usual orientation (Fig. 2–50A). A more common left-right variation is to switch the left and right orientation of the apical four-chamber view (Fig. 2–51A and B).[15] Yet another variation is to invert the two-dimensional image, especially when using an apical or subcostal examination. Figure 2–51C shows an inverted four-chamber examination in which the position of the transducer is at the bottom of the illustration with the atria above the ventricles. Most pediatric echocardiographers prefer these inverted or sector apex-down presentations for the apical and subcostal views. As a result, there will

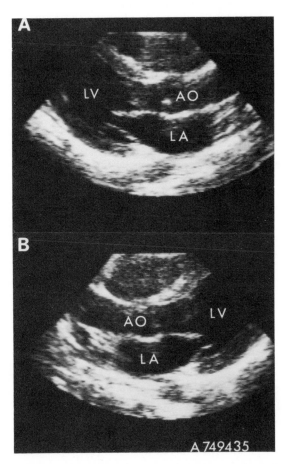

**Fig. 2–50.** Parasternal long-axis examinations of the left ventricle (LV), aorta (AO), and left atrium (LA), using two different orientations. *A*, The cardiac apex is toward the left and the base of the heart toward the right. *B*, The reverse orientation.

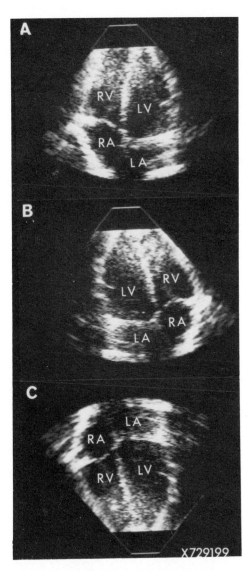

**Fig. 2–51.** Echocardiograms demonstrating three orientations for apical four-chamber views. *A*, The four-chamber view used primarily in this text. *B*, Four-chamber view reversed. *C*, Inverted image of *A*. RA = right atrium; RV = right ventricle; LA = left atrium; LV = left ventricle.

be many illustrations with this presentation in Chapter 7, Congenital Heart Disease.

Because of the confusion in the literature, the American Society of Echocardiography has recommended a standardized orientation of two-dimensional images.[1] The Society suggests that all two-dimensional imaging transducers have an index mark that indicates the edge of the imaging plane, i.e., the direction in which the ultrasonic beam is swept (Fig. 2–52). The index mark should be located on the transducer to indicate the edge of the image to appear on the right side of the display. For example, in a parasternal long-axis examination, the index mark should point in the direction of the aorta, making the aorta appear on the right side of the image display. In addition, the index mark should point in the direction of either the patient's head or his or her left side. With this recommended transducer orientation, the long-axis parasternal view shows the aorta on the right, the short-axis parasternal view shows the left ventricle on the right, the apical four-chamber view shows the left ventricle on the right, and the subcostal four-chamber view shows the two ventricles on the right. The Society is leaving inversion of the image as a possible option. Unfortunately, despite this recommendation, some laboratories display the apical four- and two-chamber views reversed from right to left (Fig. 2–51*B*).

### Identification of Myocardial Wall Segments

The American Society of Echocardiography has adopted a set of standards for the identification of left ventricular myocardial segments.[28,29] The scheme that was adopted begins by dividing the ventricles into thirds along their length (Fig. 2–53). The base and tip of the papillary muscles represent the border between the apical and basal thirds. The Society also identified the left and right ventricular outflow tracts. From a functional point of view, the left ventricular outflow tract extends from the free edge of the anterior mitral leaflet to the aortic valve annulus (Fig. 2–54*A*). The right ventricular outflow tract extends cephalad and in a leftward direction from the anteromedial portion of the tricuspid valve annulus to the pulmonary valve annulus (Fig. 2–54, bottom panel). The anterior border is the anterior right ventricular free wall. The posterior boundary is the anteromedial portions of the aortic root. In normal hearts, the crista supraventricularis is an anatomically identifiable structure related to the right ventricular outflow tract.

Having divided the length of the ventricles in thirds, the Society then divided the short axis by eight[28] and then changed to dividing the short axis into six segments (Fig. 2–55).[29] The eight-segment divisions were originally developed on the basis of anatomic landmarks; however, with the increasing importance of coronary artery disease and with an attempt to relate the longitudinal views (long axis, four chamber, and two chamber), to the short axis, a scheme dividing the short axis into six segments became more practical. As indicated in Figure 2–32, the longitudinal views essentially divide the short axis into six segments. Furthermore, as noted in the chapter on coronary artery disease, this type of division

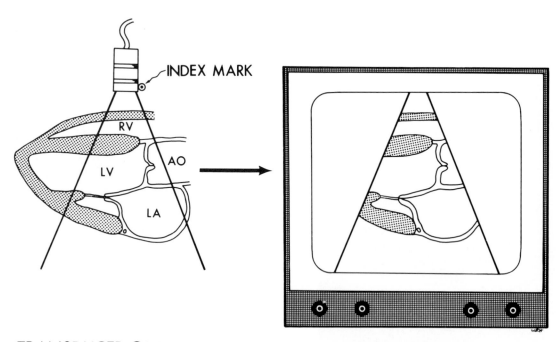

## TRANSDUCER ORIENTATION                    IMAGE DISPLAY

**Fig. 2–52.** Illustration of the relation between transducer orientation (indicated by the direction of the index mark) and that of the resulting image on display. RV = right ventricle; LV = left ventricle; AO = aorta; LA = left atrium. (From Henry, W.L., et al.: Report of the American Society of Echocardiography Committee on Nomenclature and Standards in Two-dimensional Echocardiography. Circulation, *62*:212, 1980, by permission of the American Heart Association, Inc.)

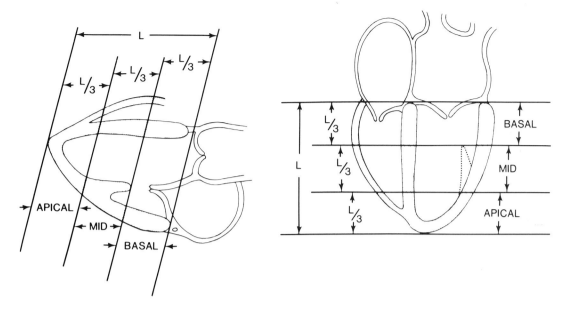

APICAL FOUR—CHAMBER

**Fig. 2–53.** Diagrams demonstrating how the left and right ventricles are divided into thirds along the long axis of the ventricles. (From Henry, W.L., et al.: Report of the American Society of Echocardiography, Committee on Nomenclature and Standards: Identification of Myocardial Wall Segments. American Society of Echocardiography, Raleigh, N.C., Nov., 1982.)

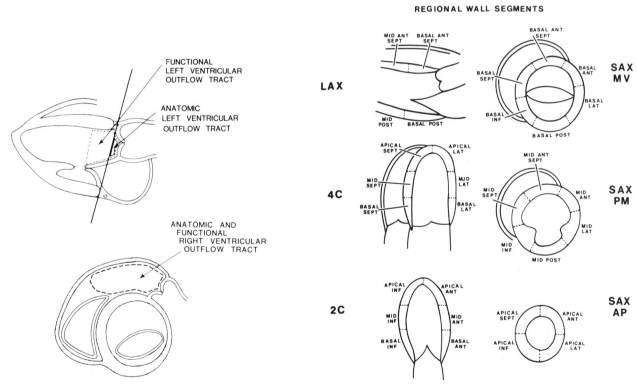

**Fig. 2–54.** The location of the left and right ventricular outflow tracts. (From Henry, W.L., et al.: Report of the American Society of Echocardiography, Committee on Nomenclature and Standards: Identification of Myocardial Wall Segments. American Society of Echocardiography, Raleigh, N.C., Nov., 1982.)

**Fig. 2–55.** Diagram showing how the left ventricle can be divided into 16 segments. The 16 segments can be identified in the longitudinal views (long-axis = LAX, four-chamber = 4C, and two-chamber = 2C). The same segments can be recorded in serial short-axis (SAX) views at the mitral valve (MV), papillary muscle (PM), and apical (AP) levels.

correlates better with the coronary artery anatomy. The basal and middle thirds are divided into six segments, as indicated in Figure 2–55. The apical third is divided into four segments. The longitudinal views are compatible with this scheme. Because the parasternal long-axis view does not visualize the apex, it does not contribute to the scoring. Thus, the four apical segments are derived from the apical four-chamber and two-chamber views. The 16-segment approach can be appreciated with either the three longitudinal or three serial short-axis views, because the segments overlap. Such a left ventricular regional wall scheme is the basis for evaluating segmental wall motion by generating a regional score index. This topic is discussed further in Chapters 3 and 8.

## M-MODE EXAMINATION

A free-standing M-mode examination is no longer performed. The M-mode echocardiogram has become an ancillary study to the basic two-dimensional examination. Stand-alone transducers are no longer produced. Figure 2–56 demonstrates how one can place a cursor through a rastor or scan line through the two-dimensional echocardiogram and obtain an M-mode recording. As noted in Chapter 1, one of the hallmarks of M-mode echocardiography is high temporal resolution. Distance or depth is along the vertical axis and time is on the horizontal axis. The major feature of an M-mode study is the rapid sampling rate and the ability to see subtle changes in wall or valve motion.

Figure 2–57 illustrates four M-mode positions that can be obtained with a parasternal long-axis examination. Figure 2–58 diagramatically shows the M-mode recording that would correspond to the four positions. Position number two is comparable to that illustrated in Figure 2–56. The ultrasonic beam crosses the left ventricular chamber at the level of the edges of the mitral valve leaflets (AMV, PMV) or the chordae. The beam passes through a small portion of the right ventricle (RV). The interventricular septum, which is the structure between the right and left ventricles, has a fairly characteristic pattern of motion, basically downward or toward the left ventricle in systole and upward toward the right ventricle in diastole. The posterior left ventricular free wall (PLV) moves in the opposite direction. The posterior left ventricular wall is represented by an endocardial echo (EN), which borders the cavity of the left ventricle, and an epicardial echo (EP), which borders the pericardium (PER). The anterior mitral leaflet has an M-shaped appearance in diastole with the opposing posterior leaflet assuming the letter W. The anterior right ventricular wall is thinner than the left ventricular wall and moves downward in systole and upward in diastole. There may or may not be a small echo-free space between the chest wall and the right ventricular wall.

As the M-mode cursor is directed toward the apex (position one, Figs. 2–57 and 2–58), the mitral valve structures are no longer visible, and one may see a band

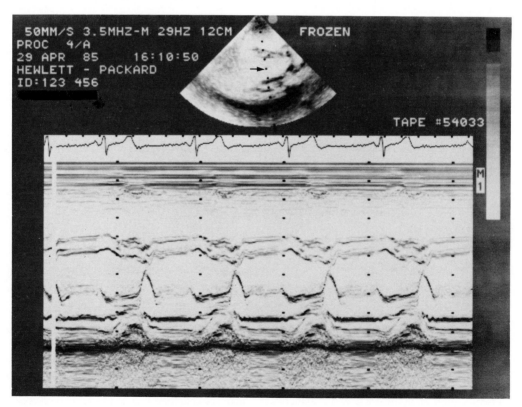

**Fig. 2–56.** Simultaneous two-dimensional and M-mode echocardiogram utilizing a phased array system. The M-mode cursor (*arrow*) on the two-dimensional recording indicates where the M-mode examination is obtained.

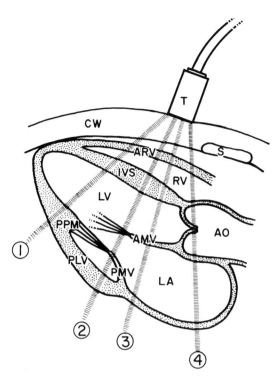

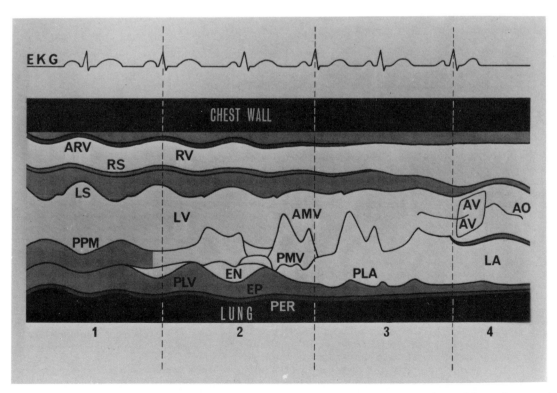

**Fig. 2–57.** A cross-section of the heart showing the structures through which the ultrasonic beam passes as it is directed from the apex toward the base of the heart. CW = chest wall; T = transducer; S = sternum; ARV = anterior right ventricular wall; RV = right ventricular cavity; IVS = interventricular septum; LV = left ventricle; PPM = posterior papillary muscle; PLV = posterior left ventricular wall; AMV = anterior mitral valve leaflet; PMV = posterior mitral valve leaflet; AO = aorta; LA = left atrium. (From Feigenbaum, H.: Clinical applications of echocardiography. Prog. Cardiovasc. Dis., *14*: 531, 1972.)

**Fig. 2–58.** Diagrammatic presentation of the M-mode echocardiogram as the transducer is directed from the apex (*position 1*) to the base of the heart (*position 4*). The areas between the dotted lines correspond to the transducer position as depicted in Figure 2–19. LS = left septum; RS = right septum; EN = endocardium of the left ventricle; EP = epicardium of the left ventricle; PER = pericardium; PLA = posterior left atrial wall. For explanation of other symbols see Figure 2–19. (From Feigenbaum, H.: Clinical applications of echocardiography. Prog. Cardiovasc. Dis., *14*:531, 1972.)

of echoes originating from the posterior papillary muscle (PPM). Moving the M-mode cursor toward the aorta, the ultrasonic beam reaches position three. At this point, the posterior mitral leaflet is no longer visible. The posterior left ventricular wall becomes the posterior left atrial wall (PLA). The posterior left atrial wall is characterized by a lack of systolic anterior motion. The wall is thinner and the motion is primarily in diastole. Moving the cursor to the aorta and aortic valve (position four) records the aortic valve (AV), the aorta (AO), and the body of the left atrium (LA). The aorta is represented by two parallel echoes that basically move anteriorly with systole and posteriorly with diastole. The aortic valve produces a box-like configuration in systole and a linear echo in diastole. The posterior left atrial wall has relatively little motion at this location.

Figure 2–59 is an M-mode tracing showing an actual echocardiogram as the M-mode cursor passes from the area of the papillary muscles (position one) to the aorta and aortic valve (position four). This tracing was actually obtained with a stand-alone M-mode transducer with which one can make some fine adjustments. It would not be quite as easy to obtain this type of recording with a two-dimensional echocardiogram because the examining plane is not exactly identical (Fig. 2–60). The best mitral valve recording is obtained at a slightly different plane than that for the best aortic valve recording. Thus, one would have to move the plane of the transducer as well as the M-mode cursor to make this type of recording.

Figure 2–12 shows a short-axis two-dimensional echocardiogram whereby the aortic valve, pulmonary valve,

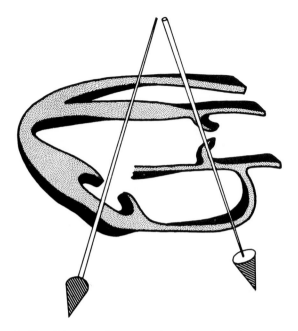

**Fig. 2–60.** Diagram demonstrating that the left ventricular outflow tract and the cardiac apex are not in the same plane. When one is examining the base of the heart in the vicinity of the aortic valve, the ultrasonic transducer is directed medially and superiorly. As the angle of the transducer is tilted toward the cardiac apex, the direction changes inferiorly and laterally.

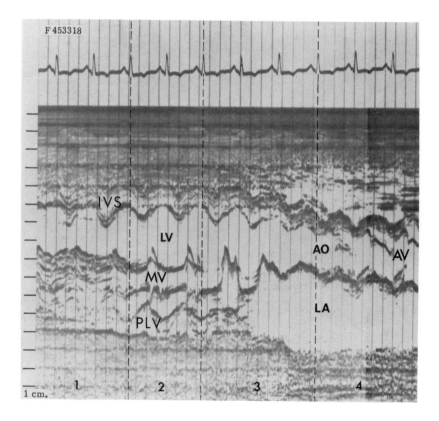

**Fig. 2–59.** M-mode echocardiographic scan of the heart. The areas between the dotted lines correspond to those in Figure 2–58. IVS = interventricular septum; LV = left ventricular cavity; MV = mitral valve; PLV = posterior left ventricular wall; AV = aortic valve; AO = aorta; LA = left atrium. (From Feigenbaum, H.: Clinical applications of echocardiography. Prog. Cardiovasc. Dis., *14*: 531, 1972.)

and tricuspid valve can be seen in the same view. Figures 2–61 and 2–62 show the M-mode relationship between the aortic, the tricuspid (Fig. 2–61), and the pulmonary (Fig. 2–62) valves. Usually, only a single leaflet of both tricuspid and pulmonary valves are visible on the M-mode echocardiogram. The anterior tricuspid valve leaflet (ATV, Fig. 2–61), resembles the anterior leaflet of the mitral valve. The single leaflet of the pulmonary valve seen with the M-mode recording is a posterior leaf-

let and resembles the posterior leaflet of the aortic valve.

Figure 2–63 shows how the M-mode recording of the mitral valve is usually labeled. The end of systole, immediately before the opening of the valve, is designated D. As the anterior leaflet opens, it peaks at E. The nadir of the initial diastolic closing is labeled F. There may or may not be another upward motion of the mitral leaflet in mid-diastole, depending on the length of diastole. This interval is not given any specific label. In atrial systole,

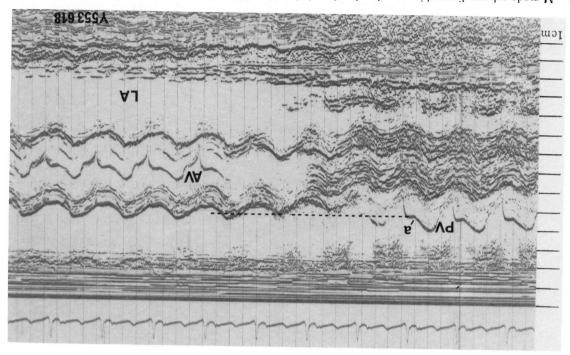

**Fig. 2–62.** M-mode echocardiographic scan showing the relationship of the pulmonary valve (PV) to the aortic valve (AV). LA = left atrium. (From Chang, S.: Echocardiography: Techniques and Interpretation, ed. 2. Philadelphia, Lea & Febiger, 1981.)

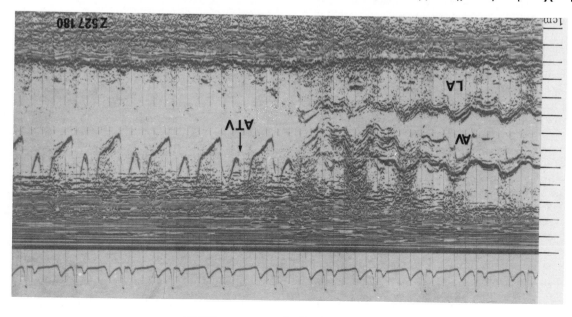

**Fig. 2–61.** M-mode echocardiographic scan from the aortic valve to the anterior tricuspid valve leaflet (ATV). The echo resembles that of the anterior mitral valve leaflet. AV = aortic valve; LA = left atrium.

curs after the onset of ventricular systole at C. During systole, the leaflet gradually moves upward until the onset of mitral valve opening again occurs at D. The posterior mitral leaflet is a virtual mirror image of the anterior leaflet, except that the amplitude of motion is usually less. Specific letters are not assigned to the posterior leaflet, although occasionally those given to the anterior leaflet are used, with the addition of a prime, for example, E', F', A', and so on. The slope between the E and F points is not necessarily straight, and occasionally an $F_0$ is indicated where a break in the diastolic E to F slope occurs.

Specific labels are not assigned to the aortic valve; however, labeling similar to that for the mitral valve is given to the tricuspid and pulmonary valves. Figure 2-64 shows the tricuspid valve echocardiogram with the appropriate labels. The tricuspid valve is similar in appearance to the mitral valve and the labels are also similar.

Figure 2-65 shows the labels commonly given to the pulmonary valve.[30] The letters essentially correspond to those used for the mitral valve. For example, the downward motion, labeled a, follows atrial contraction and coincides with the A wave of the mitral valve. The b point represents the onset of ventricular systole. With ejection of blood through the pulmonary valve, the leaflet opens to its maximum downward position noted at c. During systole, the leaflets move gradually anteriorly to point d, at which time closure begins. Closure is completed at point e. Configuration of diastole varies. The point immediately prior to the next a wave is the f point. An early diastolic upward motion may occur after the point designated e. In adults, it is unusual to record any

blood is propelled through the mitral orifice, and the mitral leaflets reopen. The peak of this phase of mitral valve motion is indicated as A. The valve begins to close with atrial relaxation. Ventricular systole begins during the downslope of the mitral leaflet and may produce a slight interruption in closure at B. Complete closure oc-

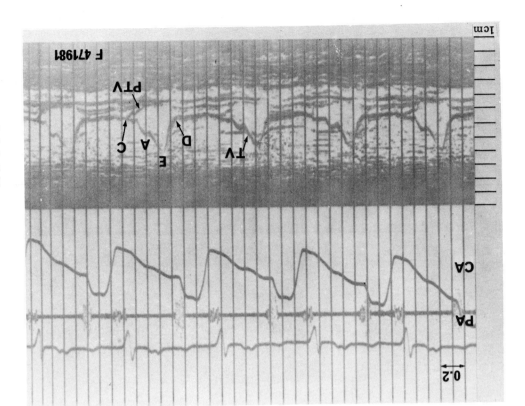

**Fig. 2-64.** Labeling of the tricuspid valve M-mode echocardiogram. PA = phonocardiogram in pulmonary area; CA = carotid artery pulse; TV = anterior tricuspid valve leaflet; PTV = posterior tricuspid valve leaflet. (From Chang, S.: Echocardiography: Techniques and Interpretation, ed. 2. Philadelphia, Lea & Febiger, 1981.)

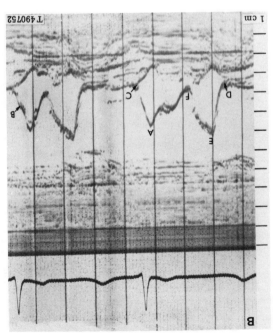

**Fig. 2-63.** Labeling of the mitral valve M-mode echocardiogram.

more than the posterior leaflet of the pulmonary valve (Fig. 2–65). In children or in patients with unusually large pulmonary arteries, one may also record an anterior leaflet. In fact, one rarely can record the entire excursion of the pulmonary valve throughout the cardiac cycle in adults. One more likely sees the diastolic and early systolic components of the pulmonary valve, as in Figure 2–65B. One can usually identify the e to f interval, the a dip, and the b to c opening.

## DOPPLER ECHOCARDIOGRAPHY

There are many important differences between the Doppler echocardiographic examination and M-mode and two-dimensional techniques. The Doppler examination is frequently done best with a lower frequency transducer. On the other hand, one attempts to obtain the best imaging resolution with M-mode and two-dimensional echocardiography by using higher frequency transducers. Probably the most important difference between the Doppler and imaging techniques is the orientation of the ultrasonic beam and the structure being examined. One attempts to have the beam as perpendicular as possible to the cardiac walls and valves when obtaining M-mode and two-dimensional examinations. The more parallel the structure is to the ultrasonic beam, the poorer is the M-mode and two-dimensional image. The reverse is true with Doppler echocardiography. The Doppler examination requires that the ultrasonic beam be as parallel to the moving column of blood as possible. As the angle increases, the accuracy of measuring velocity falls dramatically. As the relationship between the path of the red cells and the ultrasonic beam approaches 90°, the Doppler signal drops to zero. Thus, one rarely

obtains excellent quality M-mode or two-dimensional images and Doppler recordings simultaneously. The best Doppler recordings are usually obtained when the ultrasonic image is poor and vice versa.

Figure 2–66 shows a pulsed Doppler examination of mitral valve flow. The transducer is at the apex and the two-dimensional echocardiogram is an apical four-chamber view. The Doppler flow through the mitral valve resembles the motion of the anterior leaflet of the mitral valve as seen on an M-mode echocardiogram. A rapid upstroke in early diastole to a peak (E) is followed by a fall in velocity. After atrial systole, velocity again increases to a peak (A) and then decreases before the onset of ventricular systole. This illustration also demonstrates the difference between Doppler and cardiac imaging. The examination was optimized for the best imaging. As a result, the two-dimensional possible Doppler recording may be less than satisfactory.

Figure 2–67 diagrammatically shows the characteristic Doppler flow patterns in the central circulation. Flow through an atrioventricular valve or ventricular inflow, as illustrated in Figure 2–66, is characterized by rapid increase in velocity in early diastole to a peak, followed by a fairly rapid cessation of flow. In mid-diastole, there may be no flow. With atrial systole, flow again increases. It reaches a peak and begins to recede with atrial relaxation before ventricular systole. The flow passing through a semilunar valve or ventricular outflow has a single phase in systole. The Doppler recording shows rapid acceleration of flow in early systole, reaching a peak in mid-systole and then receding in the later half of systole. No flow is noted during diastole. Venous flow has both systolic and diastolic phases. During systole, blood flows toward the atrium and then subsides in the latter half of systole. In diastole, there is another,

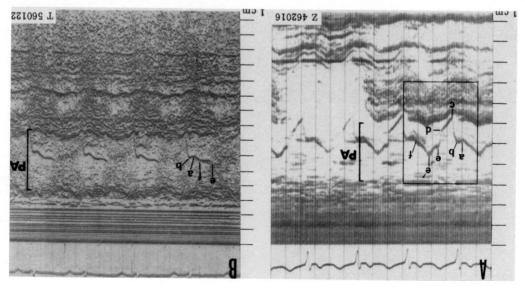

**Fig. 2–65.** Labeling of the pulmonary valve echocardiogram. A shows a fairly complete M-mode recording of a posterior pulmonary valve leaflet. Usually only diastolic and early systolic motion can be detected (B). (From Weyman, A.E., Dillon, J.C., Feigenbaum, H., and Chang, S.: Echocardiographic patterns of pulmonic valve motion with pulmonary hypertension. Circulation, 50:905, 1974, by permission of the American Heart Association, Inc.)

Figure 2-68 demonstrates normal flow in the ascending aorta, descending aorta, and left ventricular outflow tract. A similar flow pattern but lower velocity is recorded across the pulmonary valve (Fig. 2-69). Normal mitral valve flow is seen in Figure 2-66 with corresponding tricuspid flow shown in Figure 2-70. Flow in and out of the ventricles is not entirely unidirectional. Side currents do occur; for example, atrial systolic flow may be transmitted into the left ventricular outflow tract, especially near the apex. These "J" waves (Fig. 2-71) relate to the vigor of atrial contraction. They also tend to disappear when the ventricle is dilated. Doppler flow within the left ventricle, especially near the apex, may also occur with isovolumic relaxation. This finding primarily occurs in patients with small left ventricular systolic volumes, such as occurs with hypertrophic cardiomyopathy and with rapid relaxation. The main significance of this finding is the need to not confuse it with true mitral inflow.[31] Venous flow is not recorded as easily and unusual views are required, especially with the transthoracic examination.[32,33] Systemic venous flow is obtained from a subcostal examination of the hepatic vein (Fig. 2-72). Superior vena caval flow can be recorded from the right supraclavicular fossa (Fig. 2-73). Systemic venous flow can also be recorded with the transesophageal approach.[34,35]

Figure 2-74 diagrammatically shows some of the systemic venous flow patterns that can be obtained with spectral Doppler examinations.[36] This diagram shows the

usually lesser degree of flow, toward the atrium. Atrial contraction is associated with reverse flow away from the atrium.

This basic scheme is appropriate for both the right and the left sides of the heart. Certainly, variations in amplitude occur. The velocity of flow through the aorta is considerably higher than that through the pulmonary

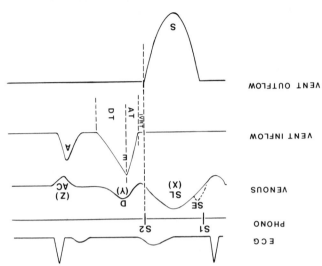

**Fig. 2-67.** Diagram showing the relationship between the electrocardiogram (ECG), phonocardiogram (PHONO), Doppler venous, ventricular inflow, and ventricular outflow velocities. SE = early systole; SL = late systole; D = diastole; AC = atrial contraction; IVRT = isovolumic relaxation time; AT = acceleration time; DT = deceleration time.

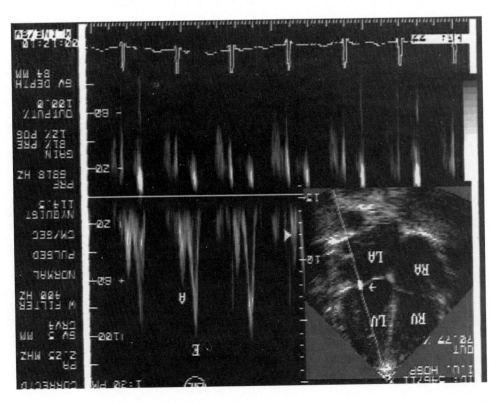

**Fig. 2-66.** Pulsed Doppler examination with a sample volume at the orifice of the mitral valve. Normal mitral flow produces a tall E wave in early diastole and a shorter A wave with atrial systole. RV = right ventricle; RA = right atrium; LV = left ventricle; LA = left atrium.

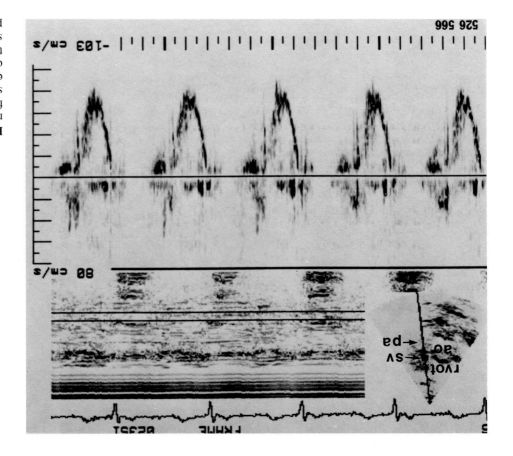

**Fig. 2-69.** Pulsed Doppler recording of pulmonary artery flow. The two-dimensional scan is a parasternal short-axis examination through the base of the heart. rvot = right ventricular outflow tract; sv = sample volume; ao = aorta; pa = pulmonary artery.

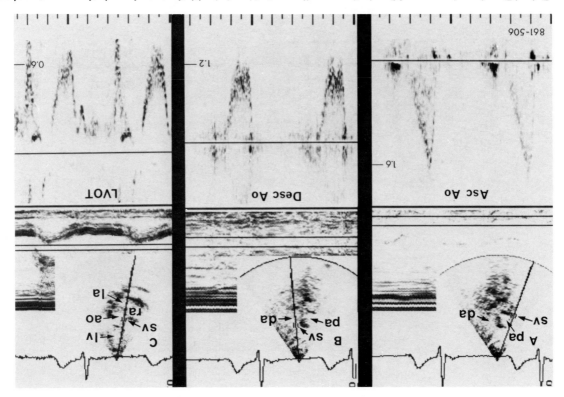

**Fig. 2-68.** Pulsed Doppler echograms of flow in the ascending aorta (Asc Ao) with the transducer in the suprasternal notch (A), flow in the descending aorta (Desc Ao) with the transducer in the suprasternal notch (B), and Doppler flow in the left ventricular outflow tract (LVOT) with the transducer at the apex (C). pa = pulmonary artery; sv = sample volume; da = descending aorta; lv = left ventricle; ao = aortic root; ra = right atrium; la = left atrium.

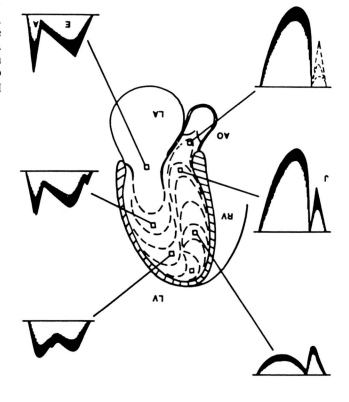

**Fig. 2-71.** Diagram demonstrating the flow patterns in and out of the normal left ventricle. Pulsed Doppler sampling of the left ventricular outflow tract near the apex shows a "J" wave, which is due to atrial systole. (From Jaeyer, K.W., et al.: Doppler characteristics of late diastolic flow in the left ventricular outflow tract. J. Am. Soc. Echocardiogr., 3:179, 1990.)

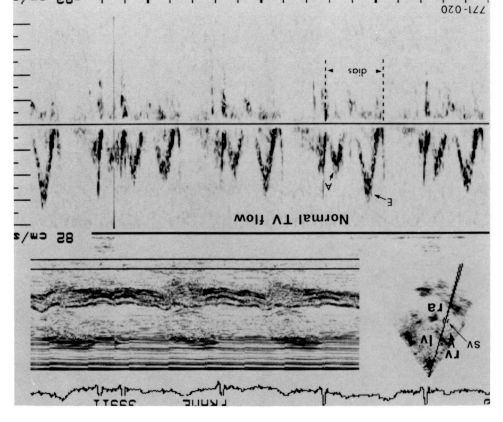

**Fig. 2-70.** Pulsed Doppler echocardiogram illustrating flow through a normal tricuspid valve (TV). rv = right ventricle; lv = left ventricle; sv = sample volume; ra = right atrium.

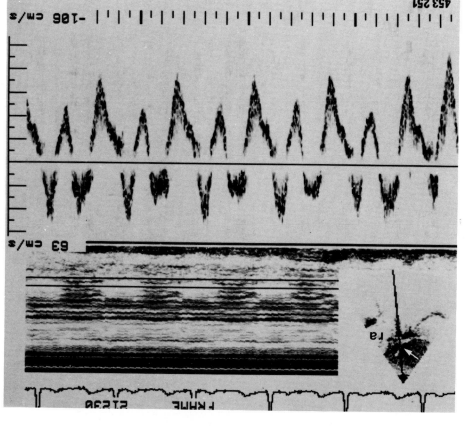

**Fig. 2-72.** Doppler flow recording with the sample volume (*arrow*) in the hepatic vein. The transducer is in the subcostal position. ra = right atrium.

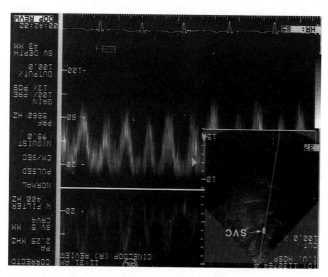

**Fig. 2-73.** Pulsed Doppler velocity from the superior vena cava (SVC).

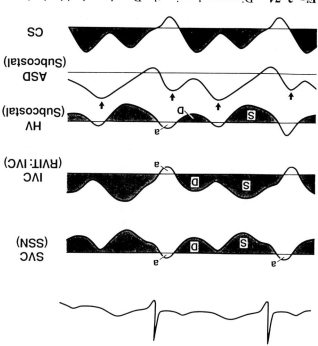

CS

ASD
(Subcostal)

HV
(Subcostal)

IVC
(RVIT:IVC)

SVC
(SSN)

**Fig. 2-74.** Diagram showing the Doppler velocities in the superior vena cava (SVC), the inferior vena cava (IVC), hepatic vein (HV), atrial septal defect (ASD), and coronary sinus (CS). SSN = suprasternal notch; RVIT = right ventricular inflow tract. (From Reynolds, T., et al.: Doppler flow velocity pattern of the superior vena cava, inferior vena cava, hepatic vein, coronary sinus, and atrial septal defect: A guide for the echocardiographer. J. Am. Soc. Echocardiogr., 4:503, 1991.)

normal patterns from the superior vena cava, inferior vena cava, hepatic vein, an uncomplicated atrial septal defect, and the coronary sinus. In Figure 2–75, the various components of hepatic venous flow are labeled and the effect of inspiration is noted.[37]

Pulmonary venous flow is technically even more difficult to record from the chest.[38] One usually records one of the pulmonary veins using the apical four-chamber view. It is easier to visualize the left atrium and the pulmonary veins using transesophageal echocardiography.[39-44] Most of the pulmonary venous recordings are obtained by using this approach. The systolic component may be monophasic (Fig. 2–76) or biphasic (2–77).

The pulsed Doppler recording of the mitral valve can vary depending on the position of the sample volume.[45-49] A recording with the sampling at the mitral annulus will produce a relatively tall A wave (Fig. 2–78). When the sample volume is at the tips of the mitral leaflets, the A wave is reduced relative to the E wave (Fig. 2–78). Because the relative height of the E and A waves has clinical significance, the exact location of the sample volume is important. Both mitral and tricuspid flow patterns vary with the age of a patient.[50-52] In a young individual, the E wave is considerably taller than the A wave. The E to A ratio may reverse with the normal aging process (Fig. 2–79).

The Doppler tracings illustrated thus far were obtained with pulsed Doppler. Continuous wave Doppler gives similar flow patterns, although all of the velocities along the ultrasonic beam are recorded. As a result, a continuous wave recording is broader than that obtained with pulsed Doppler. Figure 2–80 demonstrates a pulsed Doppler mitral flow (A) compared with a continuous wave recording (B) of the same patient.

Table 2–1 demonstrates the peak velocity through the four valvular orifices in normal adults. Thus far, the discussion of the Doppler examination has been limited to analyzing the hard copy spectral recording. It must be remembered, however, an audible Doppler signal is also important in performing the examination. One should become accustomed to the sounds of the various types

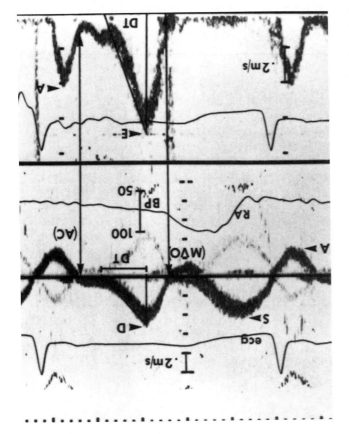

Fig. 2–76. Recording of a pulmonary vein velocity curve (*top*) aligned with a mitral valve velocity (*bottom*) demonstrating the Doppler measurements as well as the temporal relationships between the tracings, S = systole; D = diastole; AC = atrial contraction. (From Nishimura, R.A., et al.: Relation of pulmonary vein to mitral flow velocities by transesophageal Doppler echocardiography. Circulation, 81:1488, 1990, by permission of the American Heart Association, Inc.)

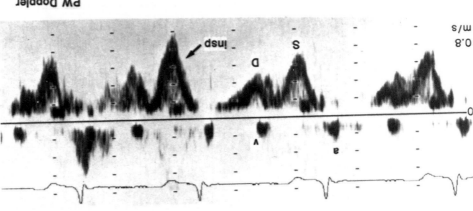

Fig. 2–75. Doppler recordings of a normal hepatic vein. The systolic (S) wave is larger than the diastolic wave (D) and both components increase with inspiration (INSP). PW = pulsed wave Doppler. (From Reynolds, T., et al.: Doppler flow velocity patterns of the superior vena cava, inferior vena cava, hepatic vein, coronary sinus, and atrial septal defect: A guide for the echocardiographer. J. Am. Soc. Echocardiogr., 4:503, 1991.)

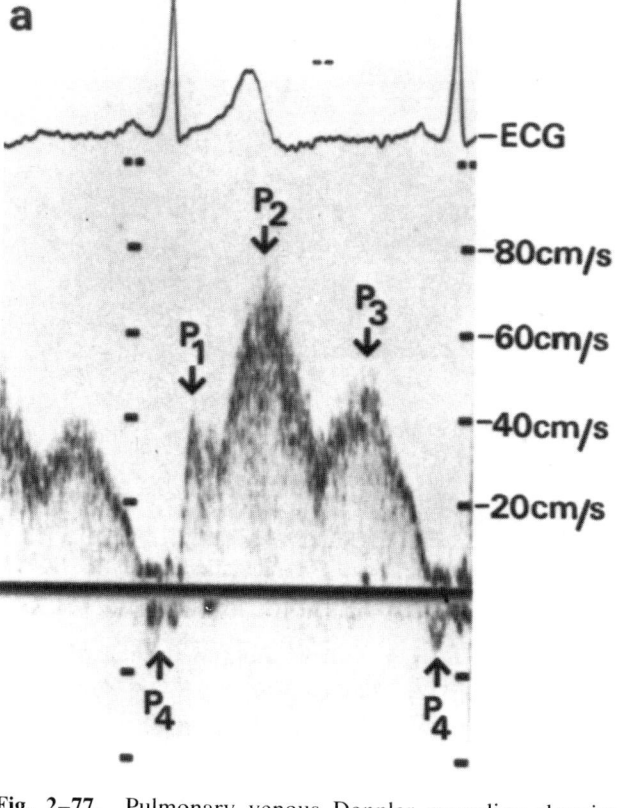

Fig. 2–77. Pulmonary venous Doppler recording showing two systolic components (P1, P2) as well as early diastolic (P3) and late systolic reversal (P4) waves. (From Bartzokis, T., et al.: Transesophageal echo-Doppler echocardiographic assessment of pulmonary venous flow patterns. J. Am. Soc. Echocardiogr., 4:457, 1991.)

of flow. The sound of laminar flow has a totally different quality than that of disturbed or turbulent flow. In addition, the sound generated by wall motion and/or valve opening and closure are distinctive and should be recognized.

### Doppler Flow Imaging

As discussed in Chapter 1, Doppler flow imaging is a fairly complex technology, which therefore can be influenced by many technical factors. To provide a two-dimensional display of Doppler flow superimposed on the cardiac image, fairly sophisticated instrumentation had to be developed. The usual spectral analysis of the Dop-

pler signal would be too slow to provide a real-time display of two-dimensional flow. As a result, a technique called autocorrelation was developed. Autocorrelation normalizes the Doppler signal from multiple echoes of the same site and analyzes the phases of each signal to determine the velocity. As many as 15,000 data points may be analyzed in this fashion; thus, the Doppler flow study is inherently slow. To achieve a reasonable frame rate, many compromises are necessary. The complexity of the technology also introduces multiple factors that can influence the appearance of the Doppler image.

Figure 2–81 shows some of the variables that need to be addressed when setting up an instrument to do a color Doppler study. Several color maps display the Doppler flow differently. Figure 2–82 demonstrates how the various maps can influence the recording. In this patient with mitral regurgitation, the regurgitant flow is presented in a variety of color displays. The color mode determines whether one will record the velocity or power output of the Doppler signal. Velocity is the more common way of recording the Doppler signal. The power mode is an option that essentially records the number of moving red cells.

Turbulent flow is usually recorded as multicolored with excessive aliasing. If one chooses a variance mode,

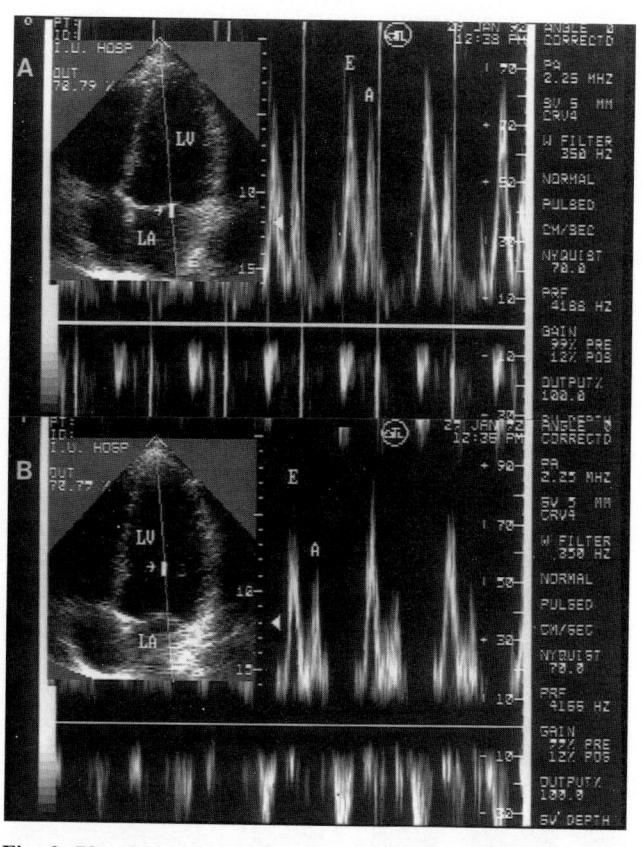

Fig. 2–78. Pulsed Doppler mitral valve flow showing the effect of sample volume site. With the sample volume at the mitral annulus (A), the E wave is slightly greater than the A wave. With the sample volume deeper in the left ventricle near the tips of the mitral leaflet (B), the E to A ratio is increased. LV = left ventricle; LA, left atrium.

**Table 2–1**
$V_{max}$ in Normal Adults

| Valve | Flow Velocity (m/sec) |
| --- | --- |
| Mitral | 0.6–1.3 |
| Tricuspid | 0.3–0.7 |
| Pulmonary | 0.5–1.0 |
| Aortic | 0.9–1.7 |

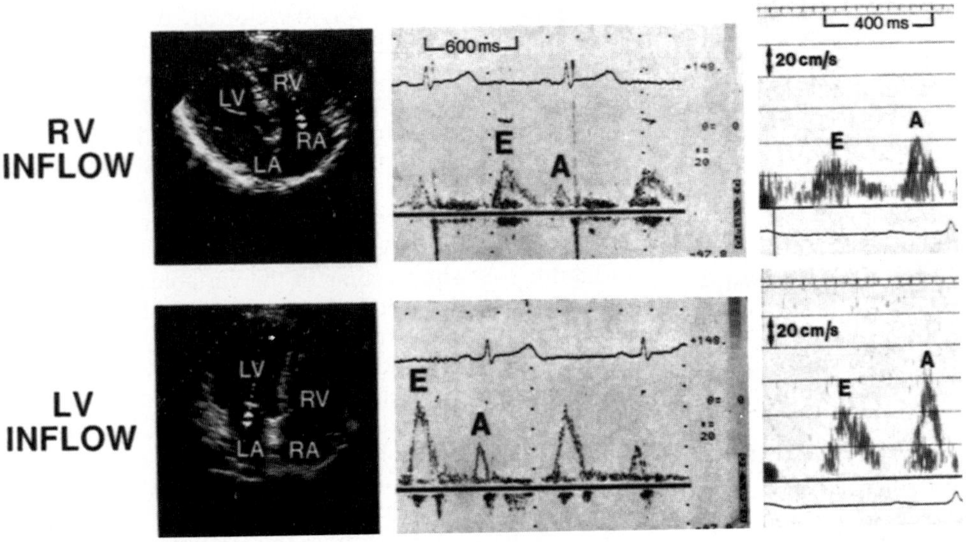

28 y.o. man          66 y.o. man

**RV
INFLOW**

**LV
INFLOW**

**Fig. 2–79.** Right ventricular (RV) and left ventricular (LV) inflow velocities in a 28- and a 66-year-old man with no evidence of heart disease. The E to A ratios are reversed in the older subject. (From Soghbi, W.A., et al.: Doppler assessment of right ventricular filling in a normal population. Circulation, *82*:1316, 1990, by permission of the American Heart Association, Inc.)

the turbulent flow will be displayed in a different color. Figure 2–83 shows another patient with mitral regurgitation. The turbulent, regurgitant flow is illustrated as shades of blue and white. Using a different instrument and the variance option, mitral regurgitation is now displayed in combinations of blue and yellow or green (Fig. 2–84).

Some of the other variables, as listed in Figure 2–81, alter the amount of color flow seen on an image.[53] Changing the gain can increase the overall flow detected with the Doppler technique. The other controls also in-

fluence the appearance of the Doppler signal. Many of these controls have as much aesthetic value as diagnostic importance. The major principle is that one must be familiar with a given instrument.[54] It is difficult to compare studies done on one instrument with another with any degree of accuracy. The qualitative diagnosis is rarely an issue, although attempts at comparing the size of a Doppler signal can be difficult.

To enhance the frame rate, the amount of image in which the Doppler signal is interrogated is variable. Making the area for sampling Doppler flow smaller in-

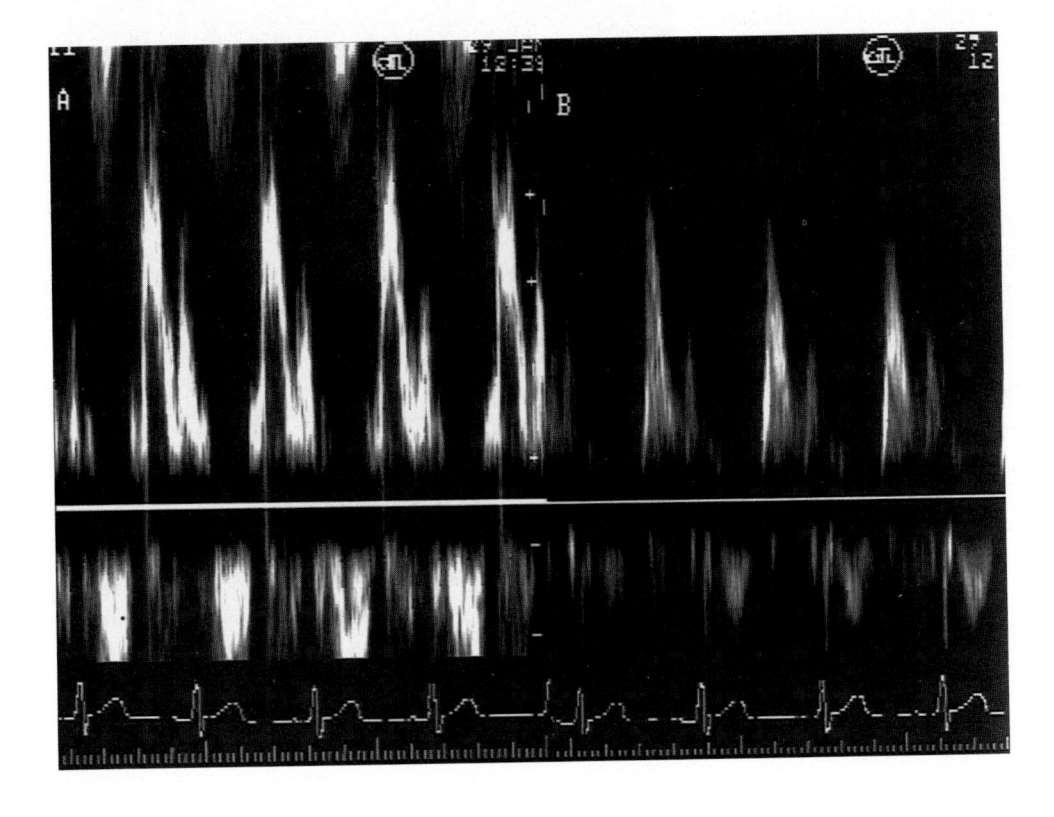

**Fig. 2–80.** Pulsed (A) and continuous wave (B) Doppler mitral flow velocities.

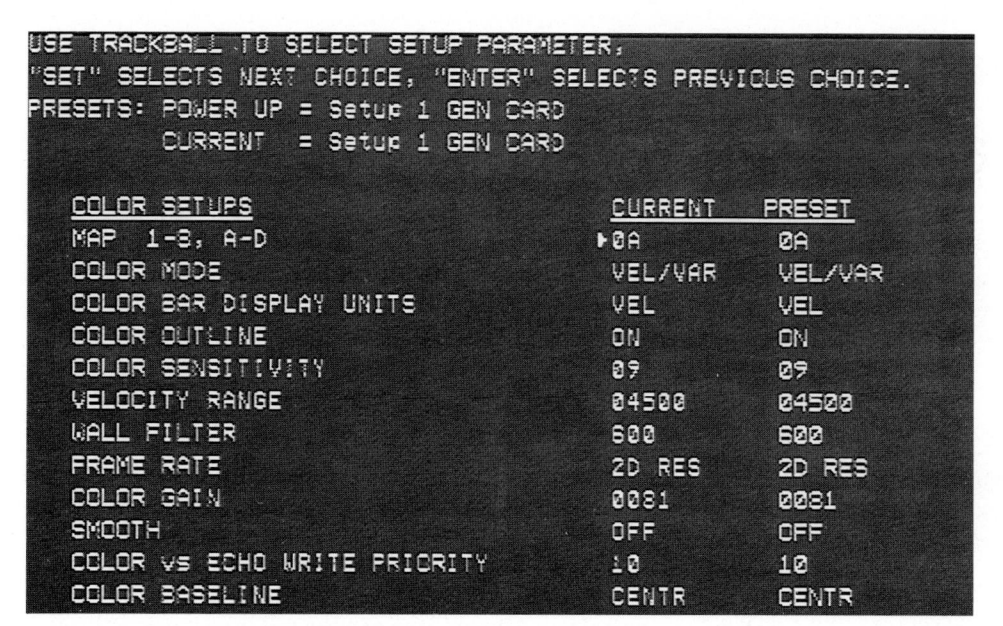

```
USE TRACKBALL TO SELECT SETUP PARAMETER;
"SET" SELECTS NEXT CHOICE, "ENTER" SELECTS PREVIOUS CHOICE.
PRESETS: POWER UP = Setup 1 GEN CARD
         CURRENT  = Setup 1 GEN CARD

COLOR SETUPS                    CURRENT   PRESET
MAP 1-3, A-D                  ▶0A         0A
COLOR MODE                     VEL/VAR    VEL/VAR
COLOR BAR DISPLAY UNITS        VEL        VEL
COLOR OUTLINE                  ON         ON
COLOR SENSITIVITY              09         09
VELOCITY RANGE                 04500      04500
WALL FILTER                    600        600
FRAME RATE                     2D RES     2D RES
COLOR GAIN                     0081       0081
SMOOTH                         OFF        OFF
COLOR vs ECHO WRITE PRIORITY   10         10
COLOR BASELINE                 CENTR      CENTR
```

**Fig. 2–81.** Listing of various options available in setting up a color Doppler examination.

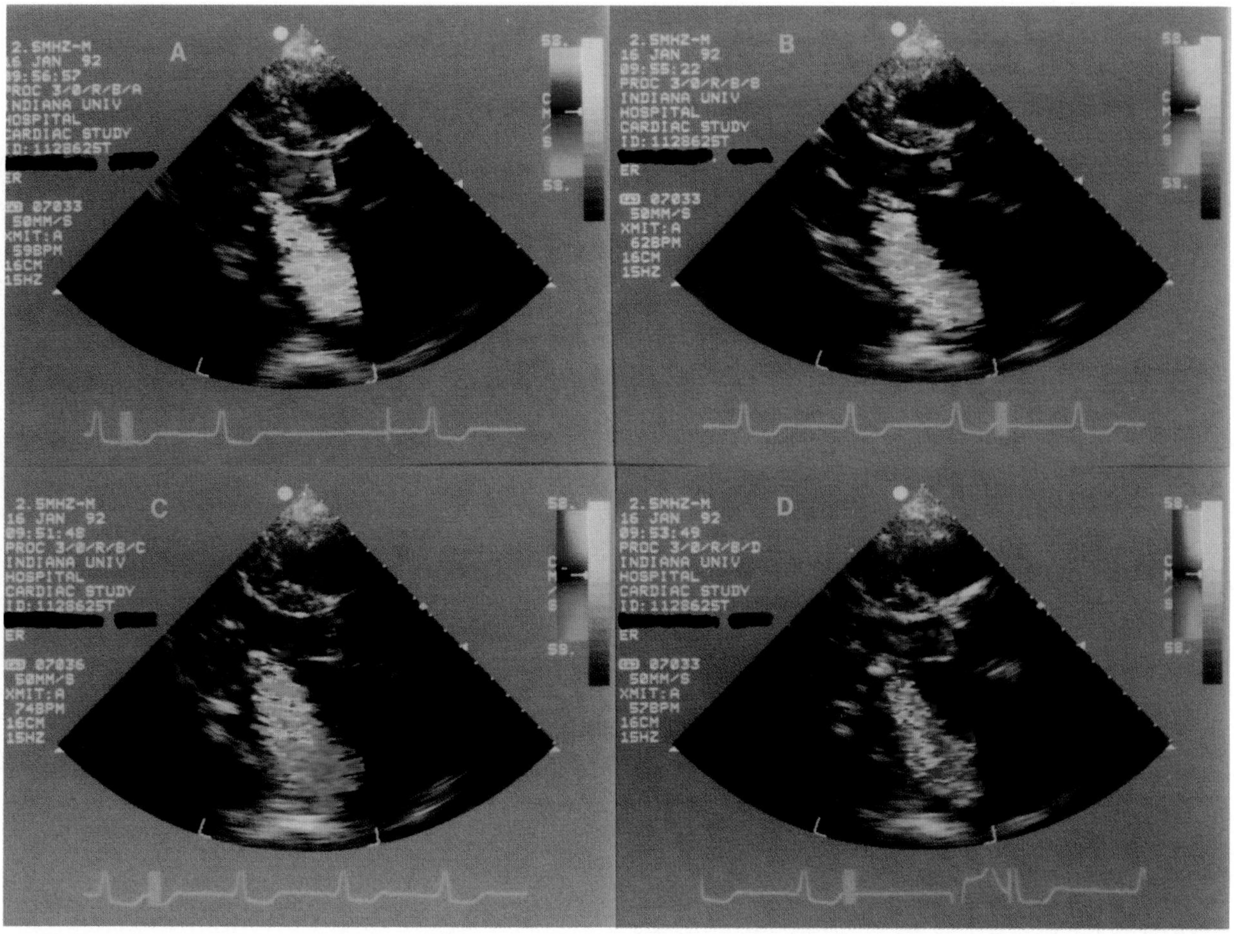

**Fig. 2–82.** Four different color maps demonstrating how turbulent mitral regurgitation can appear with different settings on the echocardiograph.

creases the frame rate. One can vary the size of the sample and limit it to the critical areas in question. To avoid being confused by what is recorded on the color Doppler examination, one should review the technical details and limitations of this type of examination as discussed in Chapter 1. In addition, one should carefully read the instruction manual before attempting a color Doppler study with a new instrument.

Figure 2-85 demonstrates the color flow Doppler pattern in the parasternal long-axis and apical four-chamber views of a normal subject. In diastole, blood flows through the mitral valve. Because the blood moves toward the transducer, it is encoded in red. During systole, the blood flows through the left ventricular outflow tract into the aorta. It is now moving away from the transducer and is seen as blue. Because the flow is more parallel to the ultrasonic beam in the apical views, the color is brighter and registers as being at higher velocity.

Figure 2-86 demonstrates an M-mode color flow examination of a normal individual. In early diastole, as the mitral valve opens, one can see red flow moving through the mitral valve. One also sees diastolic red flow in the right ventricle with flow moving through the tricuspid orifice. Some blue flow is noted in diastole above the mitral orifice as the flow turns around and heads toward the mitral valve. Figure 2-87 is another example of blood flowing in and out of a normal left ventricle from the apical four-chamber view. The left

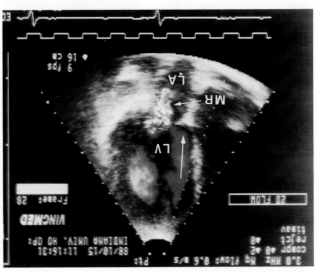

Fig. 2-83. Color flow Doppler study in a patient with mitral regurgitation. The regurgitant flow appears as a series of colors in the left atrium (LA). MR = mitral regurgitation; LV = left ventricle. (From Feigenbaum, H.: Doppler color flow imaging. In Heart Disease Update. Edited by E. Braunwald. Philadelphia, W.B. Saunders Co., 1988.)

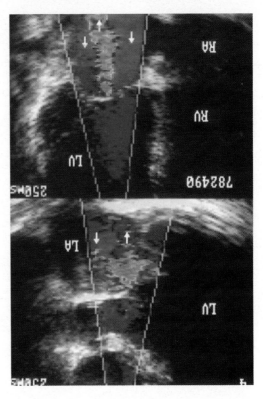

Fig. 2-84. Color flow Doppler recordings in a patient with mitral regurgitation. In the parasternal long-axis view (upper recording), the regurgitant flow appears as a greenish blue flow moving away from the transducer that then turns around and becomes red as it moves toward the transducer. In the apical four-chamber view, again a central, turbulent jet is seen moving away from the transducer. The blood then moves laterally toward the transducer.

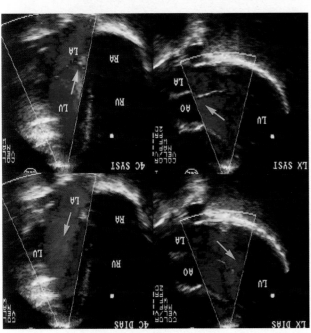

Fig. 2-85. Doppler flow imaging of a normal individual showing normal flow through the mitral orifice in red in both the long-axis (LX) and four-chamber (4C) views. In systole, the blood flowing through the left ventricular outflow tract moves away from the transducer and is inscribed in blue. Because the flow is more parallel to the beam in the four-chamber view, the velocity is a brighter shade of blue. LV = left ventricle; LA = left atrium; RV = right ventricle; RA = right atrium.

ventricular inflow is moving toward the apex and is in red. The blood moving toward the left ventricular outflow is in blue. This particular image is obtained toward the end of diastole and the beginning of systole. Because of the long time it takes to create a Doppler image, the end diastolic and early systolic flow patterns are superimposed. This is a temporal artifact. The frame rate of the study is only 9/sec and is responsible for the superimposition of these two flow patterns.

Figure 2–88 demonstrates that normal flow may exceed the Nyquist limit and will alias. In Figure 2–88B, normal flow through the mitral valve is in shades of red.

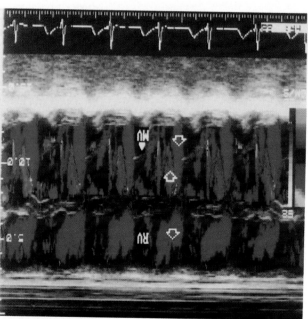

**Fig. 2–86.** M-mode color flow recording (M/Q) at the level of the mitral valve. When the valve opens, blood flows toward the transducer and is encoded in red (*up arrow*). In early diastole, the blood moves away from the transducer and is recorded in blue (*down arrow*). Tricuspid flow passing through the right ventricular inflow in diastole is shown within the right ventricle as a red-encoded Doppler signal (*up arrow*).

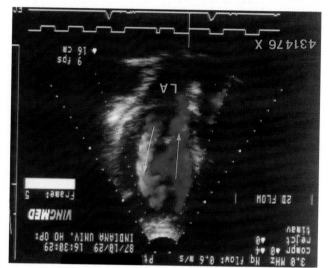

**Fig. 2–87.** Color flow Doppler showing mitral inflow and outflow in the same frame. The two flow patterns are seen simultaneously because of the time it takes to process the image and is a temporal artifact. (From Feigenbaum, H.: Doppler color flow imaging. *In* Heart Disease Update. Edited by E. Braunwald. Philadelphia, W.B. Saunders Co., 1988.)

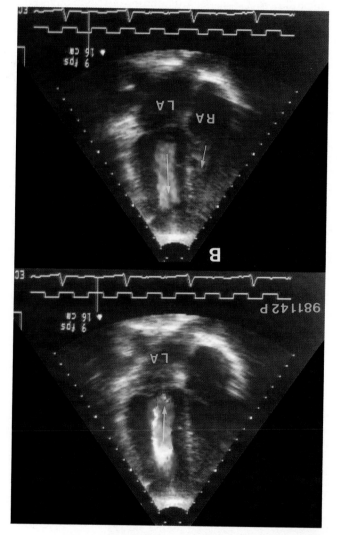

**Fig. 2–88.** Apical four-chamber Doppler flow imaging study of a normal individual during systole (A) and diastole (B). The normal outflow during systole exceeds the Nyquist limit and the color aliases. The lower velocity blood near the apex is properly encoded in blue. The velocity increases as it approaches the aorta and the color changes to white and then to shades of red. In diastole, the flow passing into the right and left ventricles does not alias and is displayed in shades of red. LA = left atrium; RA = right atrium. (From Feigenbaum, H.: Doppler color flow imaging. *In* Heart Disease Update. Edited by E. Braunwald, Philadelphia, W.B. Saunders Co., 1988.)

In systole (Fig. 2–88A), however, the flow through the left ventricular outflow tract exceeds the Nyquist limit and aliases. As a result, the flow goes from blue to red. Thus, although blood moving toward the transducer is usually in red and that moving away is blue, aliasing reverses the situation.

Doppler flow imaging is normally recorded in color; however, it is also possible to view the flow in shades of black and white. Figure 2–89 demonstrates flow into (IF) and out of (OF) the left ventricle in shades of gray. The inflow, which normally is red, is somewhat brighter than the outflow, which normally is blue. Turbulent flow would have a bright speckled appearance.

In several areas of the heart, flow is not visualized because the velocity is too low to be detected. In addition, normal flow is not always in one direction and may turn around. In Figure 2–86, one can see blue diastolic flow above the mitral valve. The flow velocity may also change depending on the angle between the ultrasonic beam and the flow. The velocity will appear to be higher when the ultrasound and the blood flow are parallel to each other. It must be remembered that the blood flow is three dimensional, and one is interrogating with a two-dimensional tomographic examination. Thus, multiple views and angles are frequently necessary to appreciate fully the moving column of blood.

The transducer placement for recording the various Doppler flow patterns is similar to that with spectral Doppler. For example, aortic flow is seen best with right parasternal or suprasternal placement of the transducer. Looking for a discrete jet of abnormal flow may require unusual transducer positioning and angulation. At times, finding the proper jet and following its path can be complicated and tedious.

## TRANSESOPHAGEAL ECHOCARDIOGRAPHY

The transesophageal echocardiographic examination is significantly different from examinations using the transthoracic approach. Using the transesophageal probe to obtain information is clearly invasive and requires a totally different level of expertise and personnel. The potential risk and discomfort to the patient is higher with this relatively invasive approach.[55-60] As a result, far greater precautions and preparations are necessary for this type of examination.[61-70] For example, buckling of the transesophageal probe has been reported.[71] The operator being bitten by the patient is another potential problem.[72]

Transesophageal echocardiography is basically a form of upper endoscopy. Physicians performing this examination must be knowledgeable with this form of intubation. It is best to begin by gaining experience from gastroenterologists in the technical details involved with inserting a probe into the esophagus and stomach.[73,74] Some of the preparation of the patient is controversial. In some laboratories, use of medication such as sedation with benzodiazepine-type drugs is routine. This medication allays apprehension and also produces some amnesia. Excessive anxiety can also be reduced with the use of meperidine. As a general rule, younger patients are more anxious than are older individuals. The use of medication seems to be more popular in the United States than in other countries.[75] Although medication may make the examination more pleasant for the patient, it also introduces some complications. For example, respiration can be affected, and it is best to use a pulse oximeter to monitor oxygenation. Use of this device is probably preferred for all patients undergoing trans-

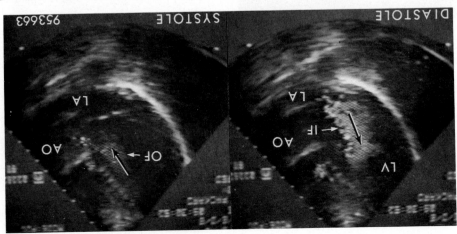

**Fig. 2–89.** Doppler flow images displayed in black and white. The normal homogeneous inflow (IF) can be seen passing from the left atrium (LA) to the left ventricle (LV). This flow is displayed in red on the color recording and is brighter in black and white than the blue-encoded outflow (OF) blood. Cross-hatching is noted in all of the flow recordings. This electronic artifact helps distinguish blood flow from tissue echoes when displayed in black and white. (From Feigenbaum, H.: Echocardiography. *In* Textbook of Internal Medicine. Edited by W.N. Kelly. Philadelphia, J.B. Lippincott Co., 1988.)

esophageal echocardiography, but it is particularly im-portant in patients who are premedicated or who are seriously ill. Furthermore, patients who receive medica-tion must be observed for a period of time after the ex-amination because of the inability to function normally for several hours.

Secretions are always a potential problem when doing endoscopy. Suction should be available. In addition, some authorities recommend using drying agents, such as glycopyrrolate. With all of these potential problems and cautions, it is preferred that trained health care per-sonnel, such as a registered nurse, be in attendance to monitor the patient's condition throughout the proce-dure. Bacterial endocarditis prophylaxis is still some-what controversial.[62,64,76] The bulk of the evidence thus far indicates that the risk of bacteremia is no greater than with other minor procedures,[66] and that prophylactic use of antibiotics is not routinely necessary.[76a] This situ-ation may be altered in patients with prosthetic valves because of the devastating effect that endocarditis has with such valves.

For esophageal intubation, the pharynx is anesthe-tized with a topical anesthetic. Cetacaine or Lidocaine spray can be used to supress the gag reflex. The patient is placed in the left lateral decubitus position with the head slightly flexed forward (Fig. 2-90). If necessary, the patient can be in other positions, but the left lateral position is the safest for managing secretions. A bite block is inserted unless the patient is edentulous.[72] The bite block is necessary to protect the expensive esopha-geal probe. The probe is lubricated with a surgical jelly. The transducer is then slowly introduced until resistance is encountered. The patient then swallows and with

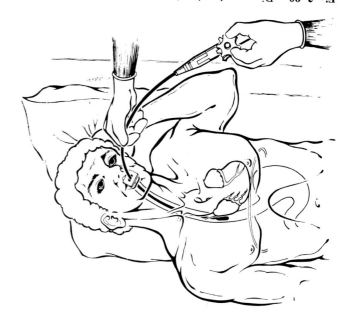

**Fig. 2-90.** Diagram showing the position of the patient during the insertion of a transesophageal echocardiographic probe.

gentle pressure, the probe is passed and advanced to a position behind the heart.

Certain patients should be excluded from considera-tion of transesophageal echocardiography. Primarily, these are individuals with pathologic conditions involv-ing the esophagus.[77] Patients should be questioned care-fully for any swallowing difficulty. An occasional patient will be totally uncooperative and the procedure may need to be aborted. Occasionally, a laryngoscope may be helpful in passing the probe.

Pediatric transesophageal echocardiography has its unique challenges.[67,68,78,78a,78b] The probe must be smaller and patients must be heavily sedated or anesthe-tized.

## Transesophageal Echocardiographic Views

Transesophageal echocardiography offers an excel-lent view of the heart because the ultrasonic beam is unobstructed by lung or chest wall. The examining tech-nique continues to evolve. With the various probes and manipulations currently available, one can record an al-most infinite number of examining planes, some of which can be confusing.[69,79-82] The following discussion of the transesophageal examination is somewhat simpli-fied. Naturally, anyone intending to perform trans-esophageal echocardiography will have to learn all of the many potential views.

Figure 2-91 demonstrates the ways in which the trans-esophageal probe can be manipulated by the operator. First of all, the transducer can be withdrawn or ad-vanced more deeply into the throat. The probe can be rotated. In addition, the knobs on the control handle give the ability to flex the tip in four different directions. Basically three positions are used for transesophageal echocardiography to examine the heart and great vessels (Fig. 2-92). The furthest or most inferior position is ac-tually within the stomach. Withdrawal of the transducer puts the probe in a mid-position behind the heart. The third or most superior transducer position is at the base of the heart. Describing the various transesophageal planes and views of the heart is complicated by the lack of unanimity of opinion as to how these views are to be displayed. The biggest controversy is whether or not the point of the sector should be at the top of the oscillo-scope[83,84] or at the bottom.[85,86] One of the arguments for placing the transesophageal sector with the point of the sector at the bottom is to keep the views comparable to the transthoracic examination of the heart. Figure 2-93 explains this approach. The transesophageal and transthoracic examinations view the heart from opposite directions. Thus, the respective recordings should re-flect this fact. When viewed in this fashion, the orienta-tion of the heart is similar for both the transthoracic and transesophageal approaches. Unfortunately, many physicians have recorded transesophageal studies with the point of the sector at the top for so long that they have become accustomed to viewing the heart in this way. Thus, many are reluctant to invert the image. This problem is still unresolved. Figure 2-92 shows two dif-

2-95 shows that one can flex the transducer superiorly and record the left ventricular outflow tract and aorta and obtain a five-chamber view. Tilting the transducer caudally moves the plane of the ultrasonic beam through the coronary sinus.

Pulling the transducer further toward the base of the heart provides a short-axis view through the aortic valve, left atrium, right atrium, and right ventricular outflow tract (Fig. 2-92, 1A, 1B). This short-axis view can then be modified to see the coronary arteries, the left atrial appendage, pulmonary veins, and superior vena cava (Fig. 2-96).

Figure 2-97 shows the longitudinal views that can be obtained from the same three transesophageal positions.

ferent ways of looking at the same view. One with the sector at the top (1A, 2A, 3A) and the same views when displayed with the sector apex at the bottom (1B, 2B, 3B).

Figure 2-92 essentially shows the horizontal or transverse transesophageal planes. With the transducer in the gastric position and the transducer tilted cephalad, one transects the left ventricle through the short-axis plane (Fig. 2-92, 2A and 2B). By altering the flexion of the probe, one can obtain serial short-axis slices as one would with a transthoracic examination (Fig. 2-94). Moving the transducer to the middle portion of the heart and tilting the transducer inferiorly provides a four-chamber view of the heart (Fig. 2-92, 3A and 3B). Figure

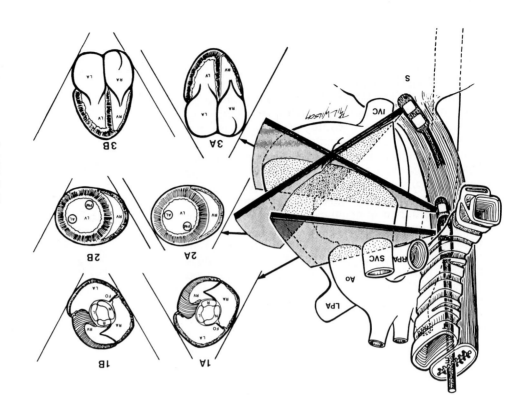

**Fig. 2-92.** Diagram demonstrating the positions of a transesophageal probe and the horizontal images that can be obtained from the transgastric (2A, 2B), the mid-esophageal (3A, 3B), and the upper esophageal (1A, 1B) positions. The echocardiographic images can be displayed with the apex of the sector up (1A, 2A, 3A) or with the apex of the sector down (1B, 2B, 3B).

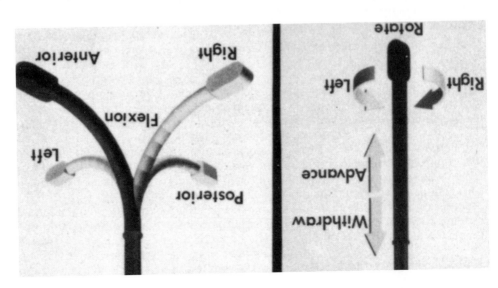

**Fig. 2-91.** Illustration showing how a transesophageal echocardiographic probe can be manipulated. The tip of the scope can be advanced, withdrawn, rotated, and flexed in four directions (anterior, posterior, left, and right). (From Seward, J.B., et al.: Biplanar transesophageal echocardiography: Anatomic correlations, image orientation, and clinical applications. Mayo Clin. Proc., 65:1193, 1990.)

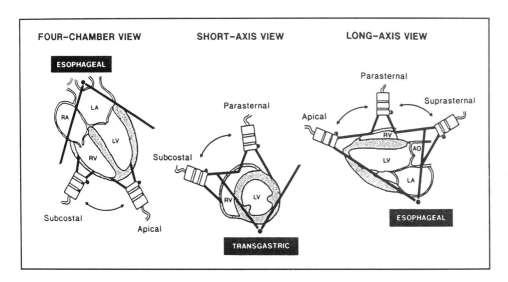

**Fig. 2–93.** Diagram showing the relationship of the esophageal and transthoracic echocardiographic examinations. The short-axis and long-axis views demonstrate the rationale for displaying the apex of the sector down to correspond with the transthoracic examinations. (From Seward, J.B., et al.: Biplanar transesophageal echocardiography: Anatomic correlations, image orientation, and clinical applications. Mayo Clin. Proc., 65:1193, 1990.)

Again, the diagram shows the heart with the sector apex at the top (1A, 2A, 3A) and with the sector apex at the bottom (1B, 2B, 3B). With the transducer in the stomach, one obtains long-axis views of the heart somewhat similar to the parasternal long-axis examination through the chest (Fig. 2–97, 3B). This particular view is the one that best justifies the sector apex down approach. With the longitudinal transducer in the middle cardiac region, a two-chamber view is obtained, demonstrating the left ventricle and left atrium. A feature of this view is that the left atrial appendage and left upper pulmonary vein are commonly visualized. The superior position of the longitudinal transducer provides a view of the left atrium, right atrium, inferior vena cava, and superior vena cava. Figure 2–98 shows how flexion and rotation of the longitudinal transducer can give traditional short-axis and long-axis planes of the heart. For example, Figure 2–99 shows how the sector apex down approach can produce long-axis and short-axis views that are fairly similar to those seen with the transthoracic echocardio-

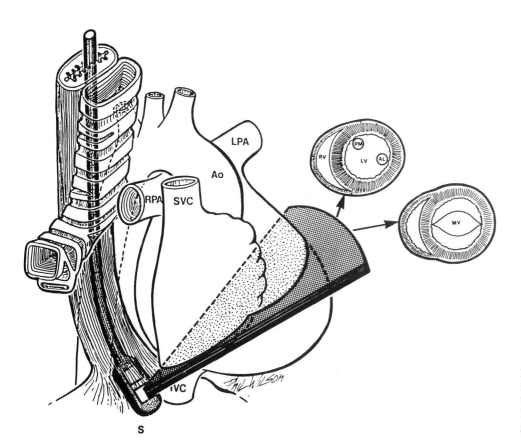

**Fig. 2–94.** Diagram illustrating two of the short-axis views that can be obtained with the longitudinal probe in the transgastric position.

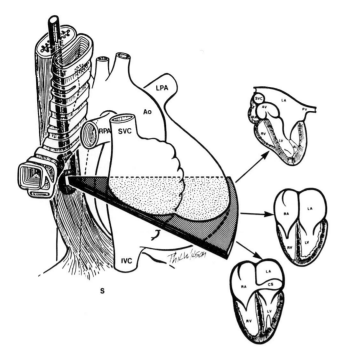

**Fig. 2–95.** Three of the echocardiographic views that can be obtained with the horizontal probe in the mid-esophageal location. LPA = left pulmonary artery; Ao = aorta; RPA = right pulmonary artery; SVC = superior vena cava; IVC = inferior vena cava; S = stomach; LA = left atrium; PV = pulmonary vein; AV = aortic valve; LV = left ventricle; RV = right ventricle; RA = right atrium; CS = coronary sinus.

graphic examination. Figure 2–100 demonstrates how one can rotate the transducer and obtain multiple tomographic views of various cardiac structures.

The most difficult part of the transesophageal echocardiographic examination is becoming oriented and familiar with the various cardiac structures viewed by this approach. There is a large number of normal variants which can mimic pathology.[86a] A variety of transesophageal recordings are demonstrated throughout this text and some of the "mimickers" will be described. Some of the more common and easily recognizable transesophageal echocardiograms are seen in the following illustrations. Figure 2–101 demonstrates the transgastric transverse view through the left ventricle in diastole and systole. This is the view that is commonly used to evaluate left ventricular function, especially in the operating room. Figure 2–102 shows a mid-esophageal level examination. The transverse and longitudinal examinations show the respective four-chamber and two-chamber views. Figure 2–103 shows how a middle level transverse examination can be modified to provide a five-chamber view with the aorta, the aortic valve, and left ventricular outflow tract.

Moving the transducer to the basal or cephalad position provides an excellent short-axis view of the aorta, left atrium, left atrial appendage, and right atrium (Fig. 2–104). This view is important for examining the left atrial appendage for possible thrombi. Modification of this examination permits visualization of the left coronary artery (Fig. 2–105). Figure 2–106 demonstrates a

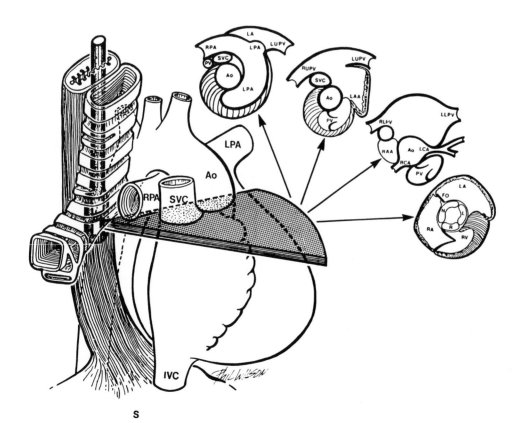

**Fig. 2–96.** Diagram demonstrating four of the short-axis views that can be obtained with the horizontal probe in the upper esophagus. LPA = left pulmonary artery; Ao = aorta; SVC = superior vena cava; RPA = right pulmonary artery; IVC = inferior vena cava; S = stomach; LA = left atrium; LUPV = left upper pulmonary vein; RUPV = right upper pulmonary vein; LAA = left atrial appendage; PV = pulmonary valve; RAA = right atrial appendage; LCA = left coronary artery; RCA = right coronary artery; FO = foramen ovale; RA = right atrium; RV = right ventricle; N = noncoronary cusp; L = left coronary cusp; R = right coronary cusp.

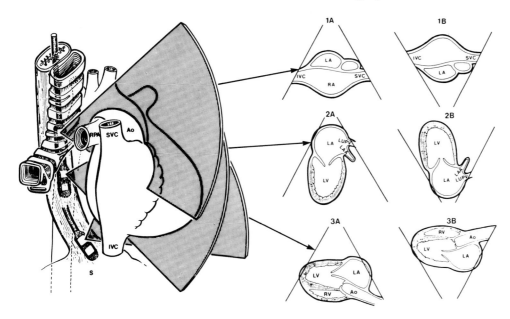

**Fig. 2–97.** Diagram illustrating the views that can be obtained with the longitudinal transducer in the gastric (3A, 3B), mid-esophageal (2A, 2B), and upper esophageal (1A, 1B) positions. RPA = right pulmonary artery; SVC = superior vena cava; Ao = aorta; IVC = inferior vena cava; LA = left atrium; RA = right atrium; LUPV = left upper pulmonary vein; LAA = left atrial appendage; LV = left ventricle; RV = right ventricle.

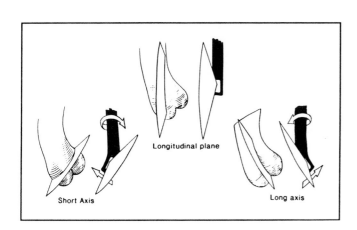

**Fig. 2–98.** Diagram demonstrating how the longitudinal plane can be manipulated to produce short-axis and long-axis views. (From Seward, J.B., et al.: Biplanar transesophageal echocardiography: Anatomic correlations, image orientation, and clinical applications. Mayo Clin. Proc., *65*:1193, 1990.)

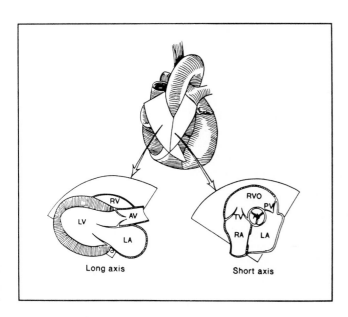

**Fig. 2–99.** Biplanar transesophageal echocardiographic long-axis and short-axis views in the longitudinal plane. Lateral fixation of the tip of the endoscope re-orients the longitudinal plane into the long-axis view. Medial flexion re-orients the plane into the short-axis view. RV = right ventricle; LV = left ventricle; AV = aortic valve; LA = left atrium; RVO = right ventricular outflow tract; TV = tricuspid valve; RA = right atrium; PV = pulmonary valve. (From Seward, J.B., et al.: Biplanar transesophageal echocardiography: Anatomic correlations, image orientation, and clinical applications. Mayo Clin. Proc., *65*:1193, 1990.)

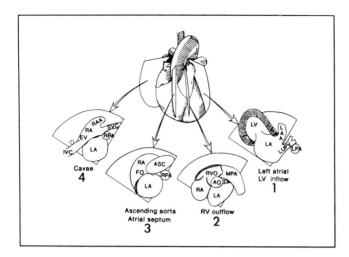

**Fig. 2–100.** Primary longitudinal views in biplanar transesophageal echocardiography. With the tip of the endoscope in the neutral long-axis orientation within the esophagus, four views are obtained by rotation of the scope from the left side to the right side of the heart. IVC = inferior vena cava; EV = eustachian valve; RA = right atrium; RAA = right atrial appendage; SVC = superior vena cava; RPA = right pulmonary artery; LA = left atrium; FO = foramen ovale; ASC = ascending aorta; AO = aorta; MPA = main pulmonary artery; LV = left ventricle; LAA = left atrial appendage; LUPV = left upper pulmonary vein; LPA = left pulmonary artery. (From Seward, J.B., et al.: Biplanar transesophageal echocardiography: Anatomic correlations, image orientation, and clinical applications. Mayo Clin. Proc., *65*:1193, 1990.)

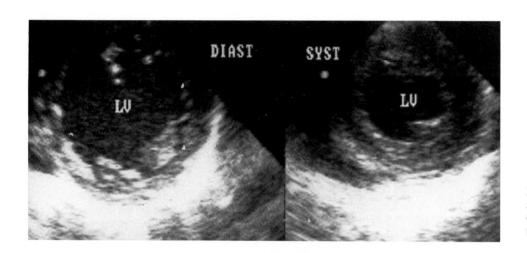

**Fig. 2–101.** Transgastric short-axis view of the left ventricle (LV) in diastole and systole using the horizontal probe.

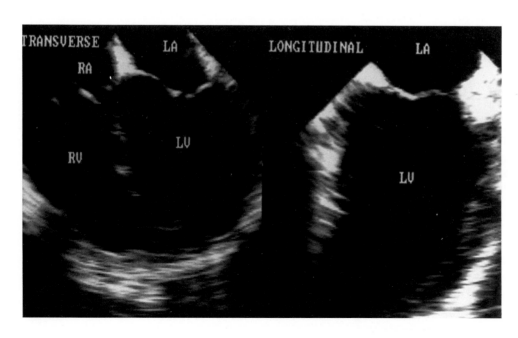

**Fig. 2–102.** Transverse and longitudinal transesophageal views of the heart with the mid-esophageal position. LA = left atrium; RA = right atrium; RV = right ventricle; LV = left ventricle.

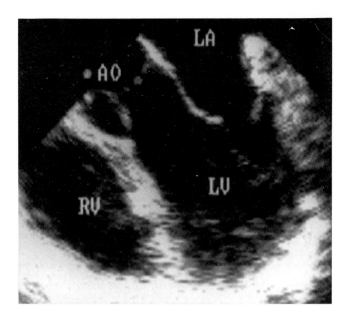

**Fig. 2–103.** Transesophageal echocardiographic five-chamber view with the transverse probe in the mid-esophageal position. AO = aorta; LA = left atrium; LV = left ventricle; RV = right ventricle.

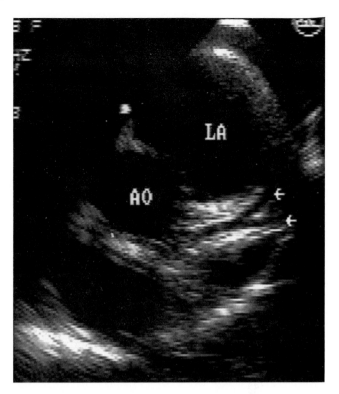

**Fig. 2–105.** Transesophageal echocardiographic study using the transverse probe demonstrating the left coronary artery (*arrows*). LA = left atrium; AO = aorta.

further modification of a short-axis transesophageal examination of the base of the heart. This study is done with an omniplane or multiplane transducer.[86b] The rotation of the transducer is indicated by the diagram on the right (*arrow*). The diagram indicates that the examination was performed at a 43° angle from the true horizontal or transverse position. A 90° angle would be equivalent to a longitudinal examination. In this particular study, the optimal short-axis view of the aorta (AO) was between the horizontal and transverse planes.

These illustrations provide examples of the more easily recognized views obtained with transesophageal echocardiography. Once one can locate and obtain these views, then experience will permit the identification of the more complicated views depicted in the diagrams.

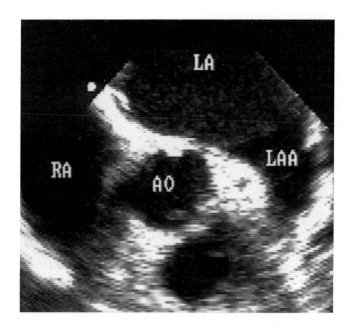

**Fig. 2–104.** Transverse esophageal echocardiogram in the upper esophageal position showing the short-axis view through the base of the heart. LA = left atrium; LAA = left atrial appendage; AO = aorta; RA = right atrium.

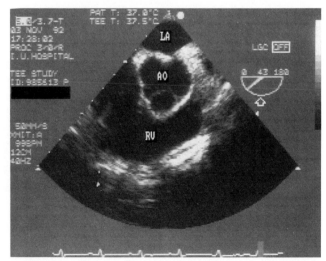

**Fig. 2–106.** Transesophageal echocardiogram obtained with a multiplane transducer. This examination of the aorta (AO) is obtained with the transducer plane 43° from the true horizontal or transverse position. The angle indicator is noted by the arrow. LA = left atrium; RV = right ventricle.

**HORIZONTAL**        **LONGITUDINAL**

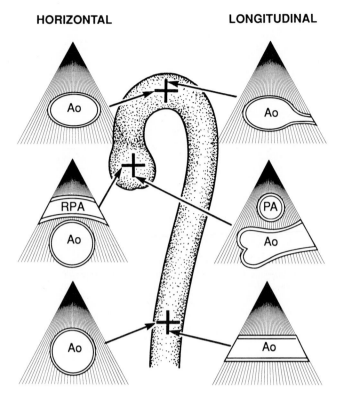

**Fig. 2–107.** Diagram demonstrating the various horizontal and longitudinal views of the aorta that can be obtained with transesophageal echocardiography. Ao = aorta; RPA = right pulmonary artery; PA = pulmonary artery.

Transesophageal echocardiography allows the clinician a unique opportunity to examine almost the entire length of the thoracic aorta,[87] especially using both horizontal and transverse transducers. As noted in Chapter 12, transesophageal echocardiography is probably the procedure of choice for detecting aortic disease, such as dissection. The ascending aorta is visualized by directing the transducer anteriorly toward the chest. The descending aorta is recorded by rotating the transducer 180° and examining structures posterior to the esophagus. The diagram in Figure 2–107 shows some of the representative two-dimensional images of the aorta at various transducer positions.

## INTRAVASCULAR ULTRASONIC EXAMINATION OF THE HEART

Great interest has been generated in using catheter-mounted ultrasonic transducers to visualize the heart from within the chambers[88] or vessels.[89] Figure 2–108 shows serial intracoronary echocardiograms in a patient with atherosclerosis. This particular ultrasonic device has a built-in artifact (*arrow*) for orientation purposes. Opposite to the artifact, the wall is thickened with an atheromatous plaque from about 9 o'clock to 5 o'clock on the circular coronary artery. More discussion about intracoronary echocardiography is provided in the chapter on coronary artery disease. This type of examination is invasive and is done in the cardiac catheterization

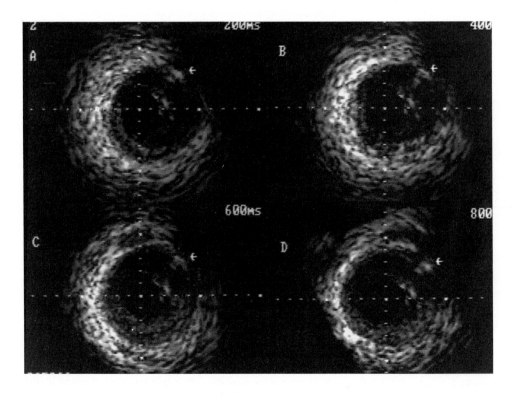

**Fig. 2–108.** Intracoronary ultra-sonic examination demonstrating several frames during a pull of the probe. A positioning artifact is noted by the arrow. Directly opposite to the arrow is an atherosclerotic plaque, which is seen as a thickening of the wall. The plaque is thickest in *C*.

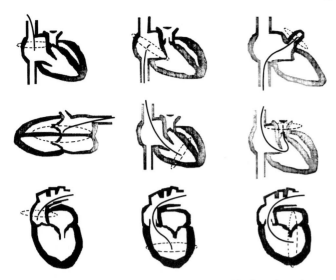

**Fig. 2–109.** Intracardiac echocardiographic imaging planes. Schematic drawing displaying the various intracardiac locations and the imaging planes from which the images can be obtained using a 12.5-MHz intracardiac catheter. (From Pandian, N.G., et al.: Real-time, intracardiac, two-dimensional echocardiography. Echocardiography, 8:407, 1991.)

laboratory. The size of the catheter is small. The examination is performed by physicians who are adept at angioplasty procedures, because much of the technique in handling angioplasty and ultrasonic catheters is similar.

Intraarterial ultrasonic catheters are 3 to 5 French. Larger catheters and lower frequency transducers can also be placed within the heart for intravascular ultrasonic images.[90–93] Figure 2–109 shows some of the positions in which a catheter can be placed for ultrasonic visualization. Figure 2–110 demonstrates an example of an intracardiac echocardiogram obtained with such a device in the left side of the heart. Again, this examination

is part of a cardiac catheterization procedure performed by physicians who are adept at cardiac catheterization. The technology is relatively new and considerable investigational efforts are underway.

## INTRAOPERATIVE ECHOCARDIOGRAPHY

In recent years, echocardiography has been playing a major role in monitoring patients during cardiac surgery. Transesophageal echocardiography is the principal technique for such ultrasonic examinations.[94–96,96a,96b] The principle advantage of the esophageal approach is that the surgeon is not hindered by the ultrasonic probe. The examination can also be performed before and after the chest is opened.

Direct recordings of the heart with an epicardial transducer is also available for the surgeon.[97,98] Figure 2–111 demonstrates a direct epicardial examination at the time of surgery. Extremely high resolution images can be recorded with these high-frequency transducers. The epicardial examination has clear advantages and disadvantages. Many views are available with the epicardial examination that cannot be duplicated with the transesophageal approach. The surgeon has control over exactly what is visualized. The epicardial examination, however, clearly interferes with the operation and obviously the study can only be done while the chest is open.

## ECHOCARDIOGRAPHIC MONITORING OF INVASIVE PROCEDURES

Echocardiography can be used to monitor a variety of invasive procedures. Echocardiography has been used for many years to follow a pericardiocentesis (see discussion in the chapter on pericardial disease). The ultra-

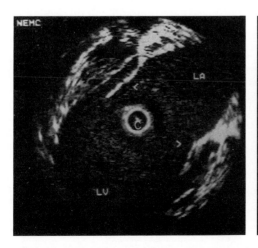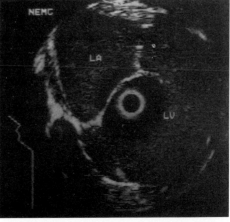

**Fig. 2–110.** Intracardiac echocardiographic images of the left side of the heart with the ultrasonic catheter (C) positioned in the left ventricular inflow region. The catheter tip has been manipulated to yield diastolic (*left*) and systolic (*right*) images of the left ventricle (LV) and left atrium (LA) in a two-chamber orientation. The diastolic opening and systolic coaptation of the mitral leaflets (*arrows*) are well seen. (From Pandian, N.G., et al.: Real-time, intracardiac, two-dimensional echocardiography. Echocardiography, 8:407, 1991.)

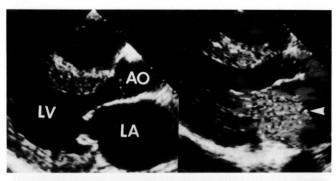

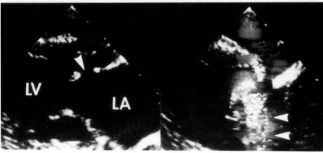

**Fig. 2–111.** Intraoperative epicardial echocardiograms of four different patients undergoing cardiac surgery. The upper left recording is of a patient with cardiac amyloidosis demonstrating thickened mitral leaflets. The upper right echogram is of a patient with severe, central mitral regurgitation. The lower left parasternal study reveals a cleft mitral valve (*arrowhead*). The right lower study shows an eccentric, posteriorly directed mitral regurgitant jet (*arrows*). (From Klein, A.L., et al.: Intraoperative epicardial echocardiography: Technique and imaging planes. Echocardiography, 7:241, 1990.)

sonic examination can also be helpful during various cardiac catheterization studies. On rare occasion, one may use echocardiography instead of fluoroscopy to monitor an invasive examination.[98a] For example, one might wish to minimize or eliminate ionizing radiation in a pregnant patient.[99] Using ultrasonic guidance of intracardiac biopsies is a fairly well-recognized technique.[100] Ultrasonic studies have also been used to assist with placement of an intraaortic balloon catheter, performing atrial balloon septostomy[100a] or doing a balloon mitral valvotomy. Investigators are also using transesophageal echocardiography to assist with catheter ablation procedures.[100b]

## DIGITAL ECHOCARDIOGRAPHY

Digital echocardiography is the recording and display of echocardiographic data in a digital form.[101] In this way, the echocardiographic recordings can be viewed and manipulated by computers. The technology provides the ability to create continuous loop recordings of cardiac cycles and to display multiple images on the same screen. Such displays are particularly useful for rapid summaries of an echocardiographic examination. These summaries are convenient for showing to refer-

ring physicians or at conferences. The ability to display multiple views simultaneously permits the direct comparison of echocardiographic studies done at different times. Another convenience associated with digital image storage is the ability to set up computer networking so that echocardiographic recordings can be viewed at computer terminals throughout an institution. These images can also be sent by way of modems to remote sites.[102] Computer-generated images are ideal for quantitation. As a result, digitally recorded images are a useful supplement to standard videotape recordings.

As digital technology accelerates, it is conceivable that it may some day obviate the need for videotape. With present day technology, however, the vast amount of information available on videotape still makes this recording medium a necessity for routine echocardiographic examinations. With a limited echocardiographic examination, such as a stress echocardiogram, the necessity for videotape may be eliminated in the near future.

Digital recording of echocardiograms requires frame grabbing capability whereby the image is converted into a digital format. Figure 2–112 demonstrates a standard echocardiograph that has a digital frame grabber mounted on the top of the instrument. This frame grabber has replaced the videotape recorder that is now in the location previously occupied by a strip chart recorder. Echographs are now commercially available that have the frame grabber built into the system so that it is not externally visible. Such frame grabbers are an integral part of the echocardiograph. Figure 2–113 shows another echocardiograph that is attached to a frame grabbing system that functions also as a review station. Such a system permits off-line analysis and quantitation as well as on-line acquisition. Figure 2–114 shows one of the major advantages of a digital echocardiographic recording system. This computer terminal resides in the coronary care unit and can display all echocardiograms at any time of the day or week at the discretion of the clinician. The convenience to the referring physician is tremendous and greatly enhances the availability, credibility, and usefulness of echocardiographic data.

How the digital images are stored can vary widely. The digital acquisition and display depend on one's priorities. Compromises are usually necessary.[101] It is impractical with current technology to digitize the entire echocardiographic recording. The amount of digital memory required for this situation is enormous and would require massive storage capability. Furthermore, the time required to retrieve such a study would be lengthy and the major feature of speed would be impaired. Sending such a massive amount of information over a telephone modem would also be impractical. Thus, one must sacrifice the amount of information recorded so that speed and convenience are not compromised. As digital technology progresses, these compromises can be modified, but it is unlikely that in the near future they will be totally eliminated.

One scheme that has been used for many years is to record the cardiac cycle in a series of eight cells or

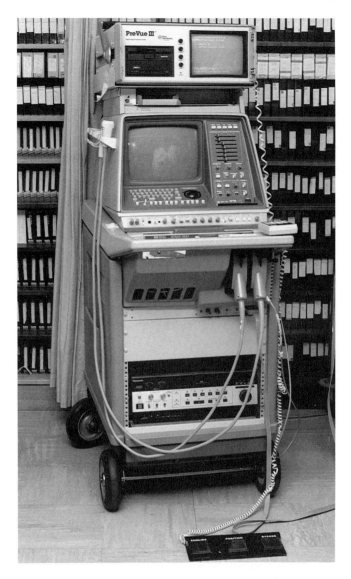

**Fig. 2–112.** Echocardiograph with a frame grabber mounted on the top.

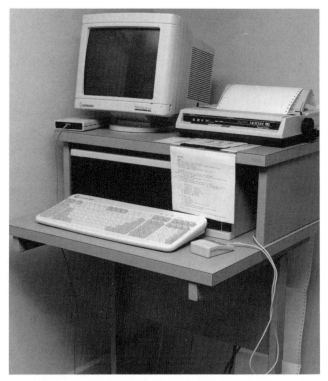

**Fig. 2–114.** Standard PC computer that is able to read digital echocardiograms and is located in the coronary care unit.

frames. The timing of the capturing is such that primarily systole is recorded. The cardiac cycle is not evenly divided into eight frames. The interval between the frames may vary from 50 to 100 msec depending on the type of examination performed. If one is looking for regional wall motion, then a 50-msec interval is the preferred technique; however, if a color Doppler study is recorded, the frame rate may not permit anything less than 100-msec intervals. An eight cell sequence with the cells or frames 50 msec apart provides a 350-msec car-

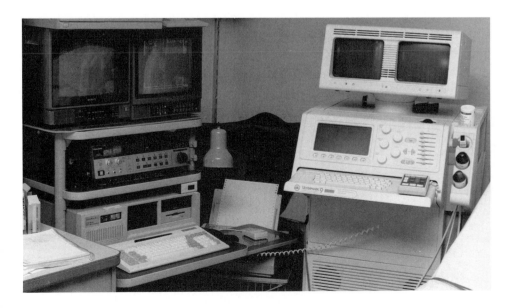

**Fig. 2–113.** A digital off-line frame grabber and analyzer attached to a standard echocardiograph.

diac cycle that is essentially systole. If one wishes to see more of diastole, then the interval can be increased to 67 or 68 msec. The playback interval has always been 100 msec. Thus, there is a slight slow motion effect of the cardiac cycle in the cine loop. This slow motion enhances the ability to analyze wall motion. Regional wall motion is also enhanced by the digital ability to look at only the first half of systole or to view the cardiac cycle in a "scan mode" so that one displays cells one through eight and then eight through one and back and forth. This type of display gives a better perception of wall thickening. All of these approaches are available with digital technology and cannot be accomplished with videotape.

The resolution can be as low as 256 × 256 pixels, which gives adequate clinical information. If one wishes slightly better quality images, the resolution can be increased. The amount of digital storage is also increased, however, and some sacrifice in speed and convenience may result. One must remember that the resolution of the raw ultrasonic two-dimensional image is no better than 256 × 256 pixels. Thus, even with this low resolution, no information is lost. The only issue is aesthetic appearance. Permanent storage is usually on floppy disks or optical disks. Hard disk storage is convenient and rapid, but it is not ideal for permanent storage. The size of all storage media is increasing dramatically.

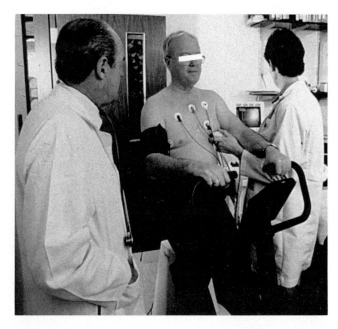

**Fig. 2–116.** Upright bicycle echocardiographic examination demonstrating how the echocardiographic probe can be placed over the cardiac apex for imaging during the examination.

## STRESS ECHOCARDIOGRAPHY

Stress testing is an indispensible part of the practice of cardiology. Many latent or known cardiac abnormalities only become manifest when provoked with some form of stress. The situation is particularly true in patients with coronary artery disease. Patients may have normal resting studies but will show wall motion abnormalities with stress-induced ischemia. Almost any form of stress can be monitored by echocardiography. One of the most common forms of stress is physical exercise. In the United States, treadmill testing is the most popular form

of exercise. Either upright[103–106] or supine[107–110] bicycle exercise is also feasible. With bicycle exercise, it is possible to perform the echocardiographic examinations during exercise. With treadmill testing, one must rely on an immediate post-exercise examination.[111–115] It is technically not feasible to obtain an adequate two-dimensional echocardiographic examination during treadmill exercise. Some investigators have used Doppler studies with treadmill exercise using the suprasternal approach.[116–119] Figure 2–115 shows a treadmill exercise laboratory in which a standard echocardiograph and an examining table are available for an immediate post-treadmill echocardiographic examination. Figure 2–116

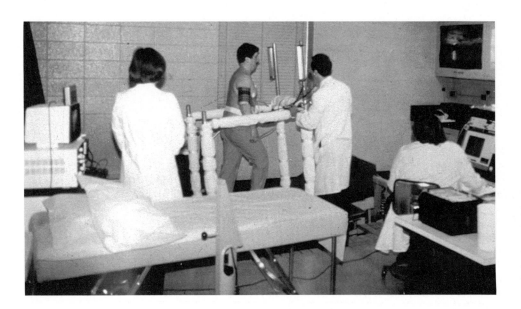

**Fig. 2–115.** Treadmill echocardiographic laboratory illustrating the position of an echocardiographic instrument and a bed for the immediate post-exercise echocardiographic examination.

demonstrates how a patient can be examined by echocardiography during an upright bicycle examination.

Other forms of stress testing include spacing,[120,121] either intracardiac or via the esophagus. In addition, pharmacologic stress testing has involved the use of either β-adrenergic stimulation, such as dobutamine,[122-124] or potent vasodilators, such as dipyridamole or adenosine.[125-128] These topics are discussed further in Chapter 8, Coronary Artery Disease.

Figure 2–117 demonstrates a two-dimensional echocardiogram before and after exercise. The systolic image after exercise exhibits the normal response to exercise, which includes a smaller left ventricular cavity, hyperdynamic left ventricular walls, and increased thickness of the walls.

The major technologic advance that has made stress echocardiography a practical examination is the introduction of digital echocardiographic recordings.[114,115,124,129,130] The digital technique permits one to eliminate the respiratory artifact that occurs with the hyperventilation that accompanies exercise. The digital approach allows one to record only cardiac cycles that are not obscured by inspiration. Furthermore, the resting and exercise images can be viewed simultaneously to facilitate direct comparisons. Heart rate indicators and timers can be displayed to assist with the interpretation (Fig. 2–118).[131]

Stress testing can also be done with other forms of heart disease.[117,132] Patients with valvular heart disease can show significant hemodynamic changes with stress. Doppler recordings are particularly important under these circumstances. One may wish to determine the effects of exercise on pulmonary artery pressure using Doppler echocardiography.

## CONTRAST ECHOCARDIOGRAPHY

The initial observation that the injection of indocyanine green dye through a cardiac catheter produces a cloud of echoes on the echocardiogram has proved to be a major development in the field.[133] The original use of this technique was to identify and verify the various cardiac structures being recorded echocardiographically.[133,134] This technique was then used for diagnostic purposes.[135-139]

Although initially investigators believed that the bubbles were produced by cavitation at the tip of the needle, the consensus is now that most of the bubbles are suspended in the liquid being injected.[140] The substances used for contrast echocardiography have included indocyanine green dye, saline, dextrose and water, the patient's own blood, carbon dioxide gas,[141] hydrogen peroxide,[142-144] sonicated ionated contrast medium and saline and, more recently, manufactured bubbles of various types. When one injects saline, one frequently agitates the liquid prior to its injection into the vascular space. This agitation, which is usually performed with

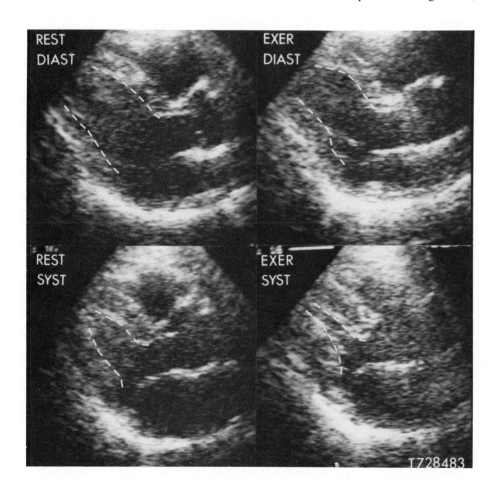

**Fig. 2–117.** Long-axis two-dimensional echocardiogram of a normal subject at rest and immediately following treadmill exercise. The end-systolic cavity is markedly reduced after exercise.

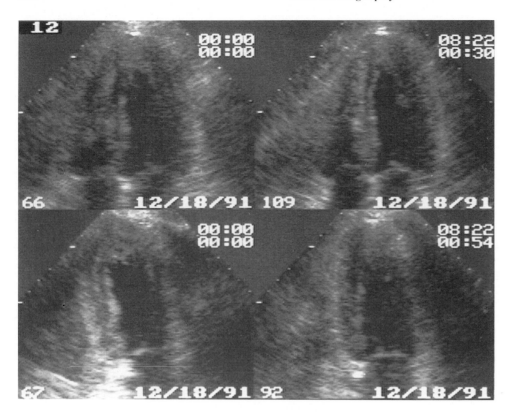

**Fig. 2–118.** Exercise echocardiogram showing the timers and heart rates superimposed on the images. Heart rates are in the lower left corner of each quadrant. The top number of the timers indicates when in exercise the examination is performed, and the lower set of numbers indicates when in the post-exercise period the examination is recorded.

two syringes connected to a stopcock, undoubtedly produces an increased number of microbubbles. In fact, the solution might even turn gray. It is important, however, to decant any visual bubbles. The possibility of producing a serious blockage of a major vessel depends on the size of the bubbles. One should not inject any visible bubbles, especially if a right-to-left shunt is evident.[145]

A considerable amount of research is being conducted in contrast echocardiography. Many new contrast agents are being studied.[146] The manufactured bubbles include sonicated albumin.[147–150] There is also a saccharide particle that apparently has an entrapped microbubble.[151–154] One or more of these manufactured contrast agents will be available for clinical use soon. The commercial microbubbles give more reproducible contrast and, it is hoped, can provide quantitative information on the number of bubbles being injected.

Most contrast agents produce bubbles that are larger than capillaries.[155] As a result, almost all the contrast-producing bubbles are filtered by the capillaries. Figure 2–119 shows an M-mode echocardiogram of the right ventricular outflow tract as a bolus of contrast passes through that area. The contrast material produces a cloud of echoes that fills the right ventricular outflow tract above the aorta. None of the bubbles appear in the left atrium or aorta because none of them pass through the pulmonary capillaries. If there is a right-to-left shunt whereby the blood can reach the left side of the heart without passing through a capillary bed, then contrast echoes are apparent on the left side of the heart (Fig. 2–120, *arrow*). As is readily apparent, this technique is extremely useful and sensitive for detecting right-to-left

shunts. This topic is discussed further in Chapter 7, Congenital Heart Disease.

The new commercial products have bubbles that are small enough to pass through the capillaries. Thus, an intravenous injection will produce contrast enhancement within the left side of the heart (Fig. 2–121).[153–157]

The contrast injections need not be made in a peripheral vein alone. Several investigators have noted the utility of using contrast injections at the time of cardiac catheterization. The injections can be used in place of contrast angiography for detecting intracardiac shunts or valvular regurgitation.[158] This technique avoids the use of both ionizing radiation and the iodinated contrast material.[159] There is also considerable investigational interest in introducing contrast-producing substances into the coronary arteries via a catheter either directly into the arteries or with a contrast injection in the root of the aorta.[160–164] Such a contrast echocardiogram produces an increase in echo intensity of the myocardium and permits an opportunity to study myocardial perfusion. Figure 2–122 shows a contrast echocardiographic study in a dog in which the injection of contrast was in the root of the aorta. Following the contrast injection (Fig. 2–122B), the myocardium (M) becomes more echogenic as the bubbles follow and identify the perfusion of blood in the myocardium.

Contrast material can also be used to enhance Doppler signals.[165–167] Figure 2–123 demonstrates a patient with a weak Doppler signal generated by mild tricuspid regurgitation. With contrast, the Doppler signal is clearer. This type of examination can be helpful because tricuspid regurgitation provides an opportunity to measure the

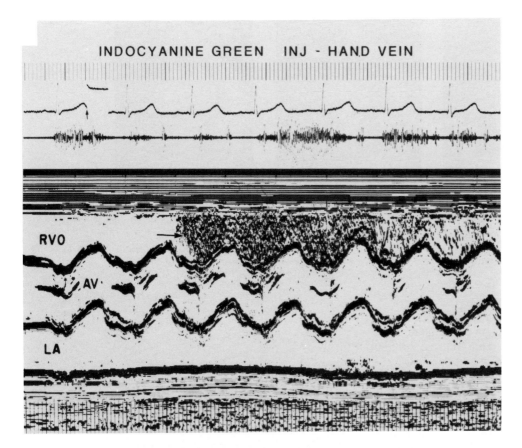

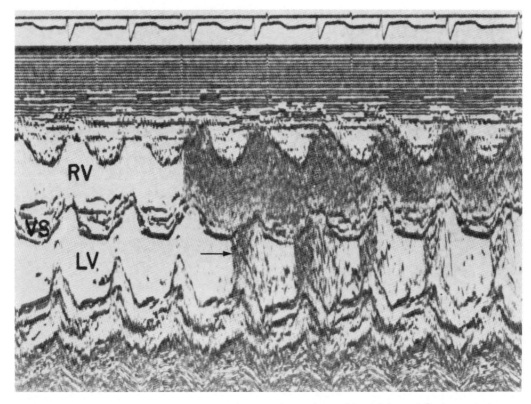

**Fig. 2–119.** A peripheral vein indocyanine green dye injection demonstrating the production of contrast echoes (*arrow*) in a patient with no evidence of an intracardiac shunt. The echoes appear in the right ventricular outflow tract (RVO) and not on the left side of the heart. AV = aortic valve; LA = left atrium. (From Seward, J.B., et al.: Peripheral venous contrast echocardiography. Am. J. Cardiol., *39*:202, 1977.)

**Fig. 2–120.** Peripheral vein contrast echocardiographic study of a patient with a right-to-left shunt at the ventricular level. Contrast echoes are seen in the left ventricle (*arrow*) above the mitral valve. RV = right ventricle; VS = ventricular septum; LV = left ventricle. (From Seward, J.B., et al.: Echocardiographic contrast studies: Initial experience. Mayo Clin. Proc., *50*: 163, 1975.) Reprinted with permission of the American College of Cardiology.

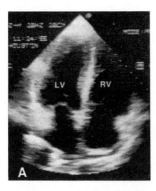
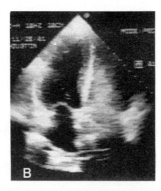
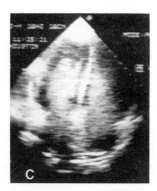

**Fig. 2–121.** Serial frames from a single intravenous injection of sonicated albumin microspheres in a patient whose heart was imaged from the apical four-chamber view. *A,* baseline image without contrast material; *B,* early image showing contrast media in the right ventricle; *C,* contrast opacification of both left and right ventricles. In these images, the left atrium (LA) and left ventricle (LV) are on the left and the right atrium (RA) and right ventricle (RV) are on the right. (From Feinstein, S.E., et al.: Safety and efficacy of a new transpulmonary ultrasound contrast agent: Initial multicenter clinical results. J. Am. Coll. Cardiol., *16*:316, 1990.)

systolic pressure within the right ventricle (see Chapter 4). Such a measurement depends on an adequate tricuspid regurgitation Doppler signal and contrast enhancement may be necessary in some individuals.

Spontaneous contrast or stagnant blood can be seen within the cardiovascular system in certain individuals.[168–170] The contrast effect is usually apparent in a patient with a large adynamic chamber with stagnant flow. Such spontaneous contrast is seen commonly within a dilated left atrium[171] or a dilated left ventricle (see Chapter 1). Some evidence suggests that the stagnant flow is a precursor to thrombi. One may also see spontaneous contrast passing through prosthetic valves

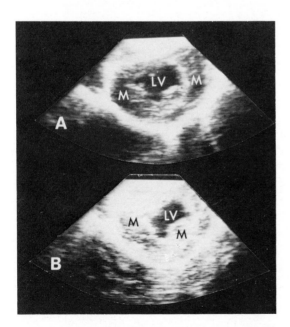

**Fig. 2–122.** Short-axis two-dimensional echocardiograms of a dog before (*A*) and after (*B*) injection of contrast echoes in the root of the aorta. The myocardium (M) becomes echogenic following injection of the contrast (*B*). LV = left ventricular cavity.

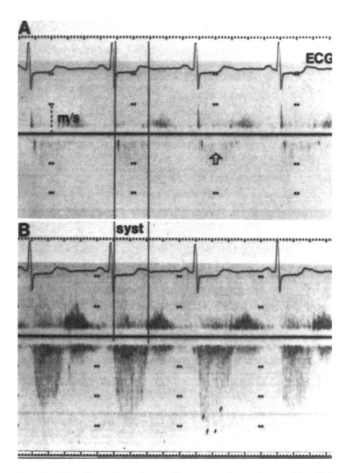

**Fig. 2–123.** Doppler echocardiograms of a patient with mild tricuspid regurgitation. The tricuspid regurgitant jet is barely seen (*A*); however, with contrast enhancement, the tricuspid jet is clearly visible (*B*). (From Torres, F., et al.: Echocardiographic contrast increases the yield for right ventricular pressure measurement by Doppler echocardiography. J. Am. Soc. Echocardiogr., *2*:423, 1989.)

(see Chapter 6). Spontaneous echoes have also been noted in the right atrium.[172]

## PRINCIPLES OF ECHOCARDIOGRAPHIC MEASUREMENTS

Because the velocity of sound in human soft tissue is known, it is possible to calibrate echocardiographs so that quantitative measurements are possible. These measurements provide a quantitative aspect to echocardiography. Many of the measurements that have been introduced into the echocardiographic literature are discussed in detail in later chapters of this book. Normal values for some of the commonly used echocardiographic measurements are listed in the appendix. Although these measurements are popular, it is important to understand some basic principles behind making echocardiographic measurements.

One may make measurements on echocardiograms in various ways. With respect to the A-mode or M-mode presentations, one should understand the concepts of "leading edges" and "trailing edges" of individual echoes. Each echo has a finite width. That edge of the echo closest to the transducer is the leading edge; the edge away from the transducer is the trailing edge (Fig. 2–124). When attempting to measure the distance between two objects, one can measure the distance between the trailing edge (TE) of the initial echo to the leading edge (LE) of the more distant echo. Such a measurement (TE-LE) is attractive because it corresponds visually to the space between the two objects. A large percentage of the echocardiographic measurements are made in this fashion. One of the problems with making measurements in this way is that the width of the individual echoes may vary from one instrument to another or may vary with the gain setting of the echocardiograph. If the instrument displays wide echoes, then the distance between the trailing edge of the first echo and the leading edge of the second echo (TE-LE) is less (Fig. 2–124B) than with an echocardiograph that displays thin echoes (Fig. 2–124A). With a system that records thick echoes, increasing the gain may aggravate the situation and make the TE-LE measurement even less (Fig. 2–124D). In those instruments that display thick echoes, the extra width displaces the trailing edge but not the leading edge. Thus, the location of the leading edge is essentially identical whether an instrument uses a thin or thick display. Therefore, measurements from leading edge to leading edge (LE-LE) are theoretically more accurate than those using the trailing edge of any echo. For this reason, the American Society of Echocardiography has recommended leading-edge-to-leading-edge M-mode measurements.[173]

The leading-edge-to-leading-edge technique for measurements is also theoretically more accurate because the leading edge of an echo actually denotes the location of a specific interface or structure in question. The location of the trailing edge is merely a function of the width of the echo as displayed on a given instrument.

Despite this recommendation and the fact that leading-edge measurements are theoretically more accurate, measurements between the trailing edge and leading edge continue to be used. The reasons are convenience and the fact that most echocardiographers use instru-

THIN ECHOES          THICK ECHOES

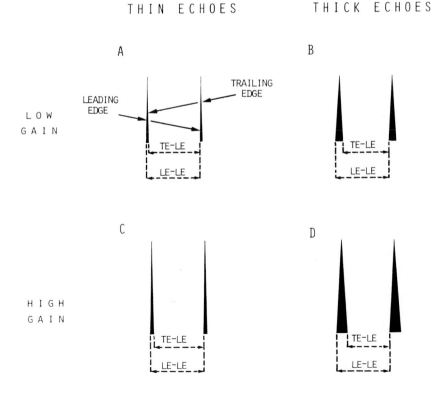

**Fig. 2–124.** Diagram demonstrating how echocardiographic measurements can differ whether one uses leading edge (LE) or trailing edge (TE) measurements. Echocardiographic measurements are commonly from leading edge to leading edge (LE-LE) or from trailing edge to leading edge (TE-LE). If the echocardiographic system has thin echoes (*A* and *C*), the gain makes little difference in either measurement. However, if the echocardiograph displays relatively thick echoes (*B* and *D*), then the trailing-edge-to-leading-edge measurement is significantly reduced with an increase in gain (*D*). The leading-edge-to-leading-edge measurement is uninfluenced by gain.

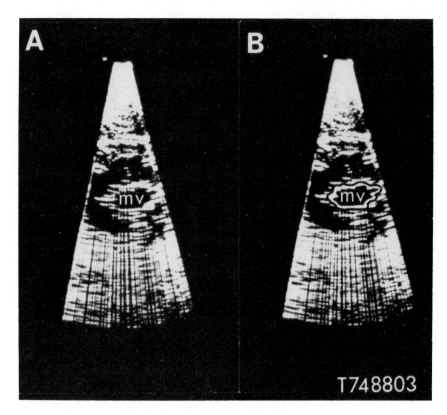

**Fig. 2–125.** Two-dimensional echocardiograms demonstrating how area measurements can be obtained from two-dimensional examinations. As noted in *B*, the measurements are usually obtained from the trailing edge of the anterior echoes, the leading edge of the posterior echoes, and the inner aspects of the lateral and medial echoes. MV = mitral valve.

ments that display thin echoes that are not as gain dependent in the axial dimension. One problem with the leading-edge-to-leading-edge standard is that finding the leading edge of the proximal echo, especially when buried among multiple echoes, is difficult. When one is using an echocardiograph that displays thin echoes, the width of the echo is not more than a millimeter. Thus, the difference between trailing-edge-to-leading-edge measurements and leading-edge-to-leading-edge measurements is no more than a millimeter or two. In adults, such a difference is of questionable significance,[174] whereas in children, in whom the measurements are small, this difference may represent a significant percentage.

With two-dimensional echocardiography, echocardiographers frequently measure the echo-free space between echoes, thus measuring between trailing edge and leading edge as well as from the right lateral border to the left lateral border of an echo (Fig. 2–125). Since leading-edge-to-leading-edge measurements are meaningless with lateral and medial echoes, the Society has adopted trailing-edge-to-leading-edge measurements for two-dimensional echocardiography.[29] This approach is also called the "black-white" interface technique (Fig. 2–125).

Any two-dimensional measurement that involves measuring area or lateral dimensions is clearly gain-dependent because lateral resolution is gain-dependent on all instruments.[175] One way of overcoming this problem is to use the minimum gain setting necessary to display all required echoes. The better focused the beam, the less of a problem one has. The error may not be significant in judging a large chamber. A millimeter or two of difference may not represent a significant problem; however, when one is measuring a small object, such as a mitral valve orifice (Fig. 2–126), an increase of a millimeter or two is significant. A basic rule is that since axial resolution is inherently better than lateral resolution, axial measurements are more accurate than lateral measurements.

Although M-mode echocardiography is not as important as it was years ago, many quantitative measurements are still made on the M-mode echocardiogram. Such measurements are taken because they have been part of the standard M-mode examination for many years and because it is convenient to make measurements on a strip-chart recording. Although computers are available for M-mode measurements, most of these can be made with simple calipers, necessitating few calculations. Unfortunately, there are many significant limitations to M-mode measurements.[176] The examination is not inherently spatially correct. Because one does not have the opportunity to examine a given individual from any interspace, the measurements are not necessarily comparable from one individual to another.

Two-dimensional echocardiography theoretically overcomes many of the limitations inherent in the M-mode measurements. The two-dimensional examination is spatially accurate, allowing one to obtain better comparative data on patients.[177] Although numerous studies have demonstrated quantitative techniques with two-dimensional echocardiography, such measurements have not been popular because of the technical inconvenience of making measurements from a recording on videotape.

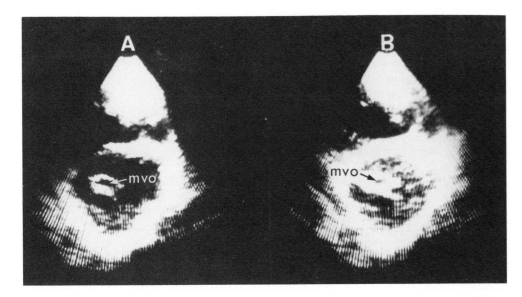

**Fig. 2–126.** Echocardiograms demonstrating how the mitral valve orifice (mvo) can be significantly influenced by gain. The orifice is virtually eliminated with a high gain setting (*B*).

The early tape recorders did not go backward, and even frame-by-frame analysis was difficult. Many of the early two-dimensional echocardiography measurements were made from hard-copy recordings, which required the use of a planimeter. Fortunately, advances in instrumentation have made the quantitation of two-dimensional echocardiograms easier and more convenient.

The biggest advance in quantitating two-dimensional echocardiograms is the availability of tape recorders that can go backward and forward both in real-time and frame-by-frame. This requirement is a major convenience for any off-line quantitative measurements. It is easier to make measurements from the videotape recordings, which can be previewed for quality, than to

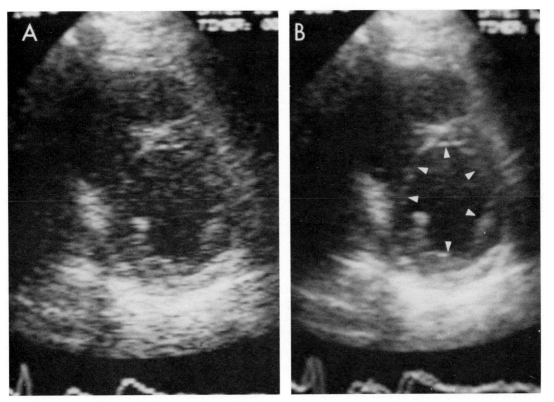

**Fig. 2–127.** Two-dimensional echocardiograms demonstrating the effect of digital averaging. The unprocessed image is in *A*. With digital averaging (*B*), the intracavity echoes are suppressed and the borders of the endocardium (*arrowheads*) are more distinct.

try to use on-line images for measurement. Although almost all instruments have on-line freeze-frame capabilities for quantitative purposes, this approach requires interrupting the examination to make measurements. New digital systems, which permit multiple images to be captured into memory in real-time with no interruption of the examination, will make on-line analysis easier.

Irrespective of whether one uses on-line or off-line analysis, it is important that any measurement be easily checked or overread. Most measurements are usually

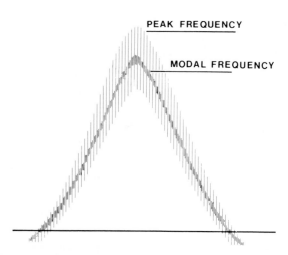

**Fig. 2–129.** Diagram of a Doppler spectral recording. The peak frequency is the highest velocity at a given time. The modal frequency is the velocity that occurs most often or is dominant. Modal frequency is identified as the frequency with the darkest spectral recording. One measures peak frequencies when interested in pressure gradients and modal frequencies when calculating flow.

made by a sonographer. The physician who makes the official interpretation must be able to check or re-do the measurements. Such overreading is difficult, if not impossible, if measurements cannot be made from videotape or from digital media.

A major problem with analyzing two-dimensional echocardiograms is that significant dropout of echo information occurs on any given frame. In real-time, the eye is integrating multiple cardiac frames, and much of the myocardium is filled in. Once the tape recorder stops and one is provided with only a single frame or field, visual integration of the multiple frames stops. With digital techniques, it is possible to overcome some of the problem with echo dropout. Digital cine-loop displays can be helpful in "filling in" myocardial dropout by viewing in continuous real time. Figure 2–127 shows a technique of digitally averaging several cardiac cycles to enhance the signal-to-noise ratio and to fill in the myocardial echoes.[178] By digitally averaging several cardiac cycles, not only are there more echoes in the area of the myocardium, but there are also fewer intracavitary echoes because many of them are random and are eliminated with averaging.

There is great interest in having the computer to identify the endocardial or epicardial border for truly automated quantitation (see Chapter 1).[179-186] This effort is being limited by the quality of the echocardiograms. Because myocardial dropout is a major problem with this approach, this effort is still investigational.

Despite the problems with M-mode dimensions, the rapid sampling rate inherent in the M-mode echocardiographic examination still makes it a potentially important quantitative examination. Several investigators have been using digitized M-mode recordings whereby the opposing anterior and posterior left ventricular walls are traced digitally for computer manipulation. One can

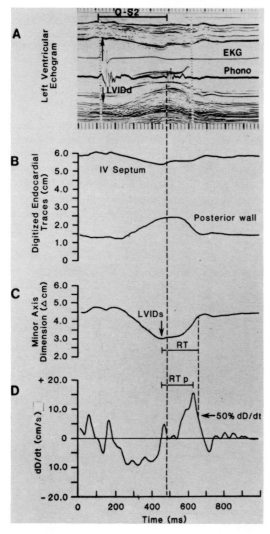

**Fig. 2–128.** Digitized M-mode echocardiogram of the left ventricle demonstrating the unprocessed M-mode recording (*A*), the digitized tracing of the interventricular septum and posterior left ventricular walls (*B*), the minor axis dimension, which is the difference between the two opposing walls (*C*), and the rate of change of the minor axis (dD/dt). LVIDd = left ventricular diastolic diameter; LVIDs = left ventricular systolic diameter; RT = relaxation time; RTp = relaxation time to peak velocity of lengthening. (From Bahler, R.C., et al.: The relation of heart rate and shortening fraction to echocardiographic indexes of left ventricular relaxation in normal subjects. J. Am. Coll. Cardiol., *2*:926, 1983.)

then analyze rapid changes in minor axis left ventricular dimensions (Fig. 2–128).[187-189]

Doppler echocardiography is also a quantitative examination. Many of the measurements are relatively simple and can be obtained using calipers on the strip-chart recording. Peak velocity or $V_{max}$ is the peak instantaneous velocity in a given cardiac cycle. Other relatively simple measurements involve time intervals. These intervals might be between various Doppler signals or between Doppler signals and events on the electrocardiogram. Such measurements, again obtained with calipers, do not require sophisticated technology. Flow measurements, however, can be more complicated. First of all, one must record the area under the Doppler curve. The area is the integral of velocity and time. A planimeter or a computer is needed for such a measurement. When measuring flow, one should measure the modal Doppler velocity. The modal velocity at any given time is the dominant frequency and is displayed as the darkest portion of the spectral display (Fig. 2–129). If the flow is purely laminar and has only one frequency, then the modal frequency and the peak frequency are identical.

Color flow imaging has unique problems with regard to quantitation.[190] Many of these problems have already been discussed in this chapter and in Chapter 1. Needless to say, measuring the area of color flow jets are gain dependent, instrument dependent, and influenced by a host of hemodynamic and anatomic limitations. These problems are addressed again in Chapter 6, Acquired Valvular Heart Disease. Despite these problems, investigators continue to measure the area of the Doppler flow jet in a variety of ways, primarily for the quantitation of valvular regurgitation. These measurements may include areas or linear dimensions.

# REFERENCES

1. Henry, W.L., et al.: Report of the American Society of Echocardiography Committee on Nomenclature and Standards in Two-dimensional Echocardiography. Circulation, *62*:212, 1980.
2. Chang, S. and Feigenbaum, H.: Subxiphoid echocardiography. JCU, *1*:14, 1973.
3. Chang, S., Feigenbaum, H., and Dillon, J.C.: Condensed M-mode echocardiographic scan of the symmetrical left ventricle. Chest, *68*:93, 1975.
4. Slovis, T.L., Clapp, S.K., and Farooki, Z.Q.: Non-invasive evaluation of the inferior vena cava. The value of sonography. Am. J. Dis. Child., *138*:277, 1984.
5. Lange, L.W., Sahn, D.J., Allen, H.D., and Goldberg, S.J.: Subxiphoid cross-sectional echocardiography in infants and children with congenital heart disease. Circulation, *59*:513, 1979.
6. Bierman, F.Z. and Williams, R.G.: Subxiphoid two-dimensional imaging of the interatrial septum in infants and neonates with congenital heart disease. Circulation, *60*: 80, 1979.
7. Goldberg, B.B.: Suprasternal ultrasonography. JAMA, *215*:245, 1971.
8. Allen, H.D., Goldberg, S.J., Sahn, D.J., Ovitt, T.W., and Goldberg, B.B.: Suprasternal notch echocardiography: Assessment of its clinical utility in pediatric cardiology. Circulation, *55*:605, 1977.
9. Light, L.H.: Transcutaneous observation of blood velocity in the ascending aorta in man. Biol. Cardiol., *26*:214, 1969.
10. D'Cruz, I.A., Jain, D.P., Hirsch, L., Levinsky, R., Cohen, H.C., and Glick, G.: Echocardiographic diagnosis of dilatation of the ascending aorta using right parasternal scanning. Radiology, *129*:465, 1978.
11. George, L., Waldman, J.D., Kirkpatrick, S.E., Turner, S.W., and Pappelbaum, S.J.: Two-dimensional echocardiographic visualization of the aortic arch by right parasternal scanning in neonates and infants. Pediatr. Cardiol., *2*:277, 1982.
12. Tei, C., Tanaka, H., Kashima, T., Yoshimura, H., Minagoe, S., and Kanehisa, T.: Real-time cross-sectional echocardiographic evaluation of the interatrial septum by right atrium-interatrial septum-left atrium direction of ultrasound beam. Circulation, *60*:539, 1979.
13. Parameswaran, R., Carr, V.F., Rao, A.V.R., and Goldberg, H.: The posterior thoracic approach in echocardiography. JCU, *7*:461, 1979.
14. Klein, A.L., Chan, K.O.L., and Walley, V.: A new paraspinal window in the echocardiographic diagnosis of descending aortic dissection. Am. Heart J., *114*:902, 1987.
15. Tajik, A.J., Seward, J.B., Hagler, D.J., Mair, D.D., and Lie, J.T.: Two-dimensional real-time ultrasonic imaging of the heart and great vessels: Technique, image orientation, structure identification, and validation. Mayo Clin. Proc., *53*:271, 1978.
16. Popp, R.L., Fowles, R., Coltart, J., and Martin, R.P.: Cardiac anatomy viewed systematically with two-dimensional echocardiography. Chest, *75*:579, 1979.
17. Keren, A., Billingham, M.E., and Popp, R.L.: Echocardiographic recognition and implications of ventricular hypertrophic trabeculations and aberrant bands. Circulation, *70*:836, 1984.
18. Okamoto, M., Nagata, S., Park, Y.D., Masuda, Y., Beppu, S., Yutani, C., Sakakibara, H., and Nimura, Y.: Visualization of the false tendon in the left ventricle with echocardiography and its clinical significance (author's translation). J. Cardiogr., *11*:265, 1981.
19. Nishimura, T., Kondo, M., Shimada, T., Shimono, Y., and Mukohyama, N.: Echocardiographic features of false tendons with special reference to phonocardiographic significance (author's translation). J. Cardiogr., *11*:253, 1981.
20. Ryssing, E., Egeblad, H., and Berning, J.: False tendons in the left ventricular outflow tract. Clinical and echocardiographic manifestations. Dan. Med. Bull., *31*:59, 1984.
21. Brenner, J.I., Baker, K., Ringel, R.E., and Berman, M.A.: Echocardiographic evidence of left ventricular bands in infants and children. J. Am. Coll. Cardiol., *3*: 1515, 1984.
22. Di Gregorio, D., Falcone, A., Mastrodicasa, M., and Vacri, A.: False chorda tendinea of the left ventricle: Possibility of diagnosis with echocardiography. G. Ital. Cardiol., *13*:311, 1983.
23. Okamoto, M., Beppu, S., Nagata, S., Park, Y.D., Masuda, Y., Sakakibara, H., and Nimura, Y.: Echocardiographic features of the eustachian valve and its clinical significance (author's translation). J. Cardiogr., *11*:271, 1981.
24. Cloez, J.L., Neimann, J.L., Chivoret, G., Danchin, N., Bruntz, J.F., Godenir, J.P., and Faivre, G.: Echocardiographic rediscovery of an anatomical structure: The Chi-

ari network. Apropos of 16 cases. Arch. Mal. Coeur, *76*: 1284, 1983.

25. Bernstein, R.F., Tei, C., Child, J.S., and Shah, P.M.: Angled interventricular septum on echocardiography: Anatomic anomaly or technical artifact? J. Am. Coll. Cardiol., *2*:297, 1983.

26. Fowles, R.E., Martin, R.P., and Popp, R.L.: Apparent asymmetric septal hypertrophy due to angled interventricular septum. Am. J. Cardiol., *46*:386, 1980.

27. Ennouri, R., Malergue, M.C., Cavailles, J., and Tricot, R.: Aorto-septal angulation: A new cause of disorder in left ventricular ejection? (A 2 dimensional echocardiographic study apropos of 56 cases.) Arch. Mal. Coeur, *77*:673, 1984.

28. Report of The American Society of Echocardiography Committee on Nomenclature and Standards: Identification of Myocardial Wall Segments. November, 1982.

29. Schiller, N.B., Shah, P.M., Crawford, M., DeMaria, A., Devereux, R., Feigenbaum, H., Gutgesell, H., Reichek, N., Sahn, D., Schnittger, I., Silverman, N., and Tajik, A.: Recommendations for Quantitation of the Left Ventricle by Two-Dimensional Echocardiography. J. Am. Soc. Echocardiogr., *5*:362, 1989.

30. Weyman, A.E., Dillon, J.C., Feigenbaum, H., and Chang, S.: Echocardiographic patterns of pulmonic valve motion in pulmonic stenosis. Am. J. Cardiol., *34*:644, 1974.

31. Sasson, Z., Hatle, L., Appleton, C.P., Jewett, M., Alderman, E.L., and Popp, R.L.: Intraventricular flow during isovolumic relaxation: Description and characterization by Doppler echocardiography. J. Am. Coll. Cardiol., *10*: 539, 1987.

32. Gindea, A.J., Slater, J., and Kronzon, I.: Doppler echocardiographic flow velocity measurements in the superior vena cava during Valsalva maneuver in normal subjects. Am. J. Cardiol., *65*:1387, 1990.

33. Appleton, C.P., Hatle, L.K., and Popp, R.L.: Superior vena cava and hepatic vein Doppler echocardiography in healthy adults. J. Am. Coll. Cardiol., 10:1032, 1987.

34. Nanda, N.C., Pinheiro, L., Sanyal, R., Jain, H., Van, T.B., and Rosenthal, S.: Transesophageal echocardiographic examination of left-sided superior vena cava and azygos and hemiazygos veins. Echocardiography, *8*:731, 1991.

35. Pinto, F.J., Wranne, B., St. Goar, F.G., Schnittger, I., and Popp, R.L.: Hepatic venous flow assessed by transesophageal echocardiography. J. Am. Coll. Cardiol., 17: 1493, 1991.

36. Reynolds, T. and Appleton, C.P.: Doppler flow velocity patterns of the superior vena cava, inferior vena cava, hepatic vein, coronary sinus, and atrial septal defect: A guide for the echocardiographer. J. Am. Soc. Echocardiogr., *4*:503, 1991.

37. Reynolds, T., Szymanski, K., Langenfeld, K., and Appleton, C.P.: Visualization of the hepatic veins: New approaches for the echocardiographer. J. Am. Soc. Echocardiogr., *4*:93, 1991.

38. Masuyama, T., Lee, J-M., Tamai, M., Tanouchi, J., Kitabatake, A., and Kamada, T.: Pulmonary venous flow velocity pattern as asessed with transthoracic pulsed Doppler echocardiography in subjects without cardiac disease. Am. J. Cardiol., *67*:1396, 1991.

39. Castello, R., Pearson, A.C., Lenzen, P., and Labovitz, A.J.: Evaluation of pulmonary venous flow by transesophageal echocardiography in subjects with a normal heart: Comparison with transthoracic echocardiography. J. Am. Coll. Cardiol., *18*:65, 1991.

40. Kuecherer, H.F., Kusumoto, F., Muhiudeen, I.A., Cahalan, M.K., and Schiller, N.B.: Pulmonary venous flow patterns by transesophageal pulsed Doppler echocardiography: Relation to parameters of left ventricular systolic and diastolic function. Am. Heart. J., *122*:1683, 1991.

41. Pinheiro, L., Nanda, N.C., Jain, H., and Sanyal, R.: Transesophageal echocardiographic imaging of the pulmonary veins. Echocardiography, *8*:741, 1991.

42. Klein, A.L. and Tajik, A.J.: Doppler assessment of pulmonary venous flow in healthy subjects and in patients with heart disease. J. Am. Soc. Echocardiogr., *4*:379, 1991.

43. Bartzokis, T., Lee, R., Yeoh, T.K., Grogin, H., and Schnittger, I.: Transesophageal echo-Doppler echocardiographic assessment of pulmonary venous flow patterns. J. Am. Soc. Echocardiogr., *4*:457, 1991.

44. Basnight, M.A., Gonzalez, M.S., Kershenovich, S.C., and Appleton, C.P.: Pulmonary venous flow velocity: Relation to hemodynamics, mitral flow velocity and left atrial volume, and ejection fraction. J. Am. Soc. Echocardiogr., *4*:547, 1991.

45. Dittrich, H.C., Blanchard, D.G., Wheeler, K.A., McCann, H.A., and Donaghey, L.B.: Influence of Doppler sample volume location on the assessment of changes in mitral inflow velocity profiles. J. Am. Soc. Echocardiogr., *3*:303, 1990.

46. Ding, Z.P., Oh, J.K., Klein, A.L., and Tajik, A.J.: Effect of sample volume location on Doppler-derived transmitral inflow velocity values. J. Am. Soc. Echocardiogr., *4*:451, 1991.

47. Miyaguchi, K., Iwase, M., Yokota, M., and Hayashi, H.: Dependency of the pulsed Doppler-derived transmitral filling profile on the sampling site. Am. Heart J., *122*:142, 1991.

48. Jaffe, W.M., Dewhurst, T.A., Otto, C.M., and Pearlman, A.S.: Influence of Doppler sample volume location on ventricular filling velocities. Am. J. Cardiol., *68*:550, 1991.

49. Gardin, J.M., Dabestani, A., Takenaka, K., Rohan, M.K., Knoll, M., Russell, D., and Henry, W.L.: Effect of imaging view and sample volume location on evaluation of mitral flow velocity by pulsed Doppler echocardiography. Am. J. Cardiol., *57*:1335, 1986.

50. Spirito, P., and Maron, B.J.: Influence of aging on Doppler echocardiographic indices of left ventricular diastolic function. Br. Heart. J., *59*:672, 1988.

51. Kuecherer, H., Ruffmann, K., and Kuebler, W.: Effect of aging on Doppler echocardiographic filling parameters in normal subjects and in patients with coronary artery disease. Clin. Cardiol., *11*:303, 1988.

52. Berman, G.O., Reichek, N., Brownson, D., and Douglas, P.S.: Effects of sample volume location, imaging view, heart rate and age on tricuspid velocimetry in normal subjects. Am. J. Cardiol., *65*:1026, 1990.

53. Baumgartner, H., Schima, H., and Kuhn, P.: Importance of technical variables for quantitative measurements by color Doppler imaging. Am. J. Cardiol., *67*:314, 1991.

54. Stewart, W.J., Cohen, G.I., and Salcedo, E.E.: Doppler color flow image size: Dependence on instrument settings. Echocardiography, *8*:319, 1991.

55. Chan, K-L., Cohen, G.I., Sochowski, R.A., and Baird, M.G.: Complications of transesophageal echocardiography in ambulatory adult patients: Analysis of 1500 consecutive examinations. J. Am. Soc. Echocardiogr., *4*: 577, 1991.

56. Marcovitz, P.A., Williamson, B.D., and Armstrong, W.F.: Toxic methemoglobinemia caused by topical anes-

thetic given before transesophageal echocardiography. J. Am. Soc. Echocardiogr., *4*:615, 1991.

57. Daniel, W.G., Erbel, R., Kasper, W., Visser, C.A., Engberding, R., Sutherland, G.R., Grube, E., Hanrath, P., Maisch, B., Dennig, K., Schartl, M., Kremer, P., Angermann, C., Iliceto, S., Curtius, J.M., and Mugge, A.: Safety of transesophageal echocardiography. A multicenter survey of 10,419 examinations. Circulation, *83*: 817, 1991.

58. Ofili, E.O., Rich, M.W., Brown, P., and Lewis, J.: Safety and usefulness of transesophageal echocardiography in persons aged greater than or equal to 70 years. Am. J. Cardiol., *66*:1279, 1990.

59. O'Shea, J.P., Southern, J.F., D'Ambra, M.N., Magro, C., Guerrero, J.L., Marshall, J.E., Vlahakes, G.V., Levine, R.A., and Weyman, A.E.: Effects of prolonged transesophageal echocardiographic imaging and probe manipulation on the esophagus—an echocardiographic-pathologic study. J. Am. Coll. Cardiol., 17:1426, 1991.

60. Geibel, A., Kasper, W., Behroz, A., Przewolka, U., Meinertz, T., and Just, H.: Risk of transesophageal echocardiography in awake patients with cardiac diseases. Am. J. Cardiol., *6*:337, 1988.

61. Fisher, E.A., Stahl, J.A., Budd, J.H., and Goldman, M.E.: Transesophageal echocardiography: Procedures and clinical application. J. Am. Coll. Cardiol., *18*:1333, 1991.

62. Steckelberg, J.M., Khandheria, B.K., Anhalt, J.P., Ballard, D.J., Seward, J.B., Click, R.L., and Wilson, W.R.: Prospective evaluation of the risk of bacteremia associated with transesophageal echocardiography. Circulation, *84*:177, 1991.

63. Pollick, C. and Taylor, D.: Assessment of left atrial appendage function by transesophageal echocardiography. Implications for the development of thrombus. Circulation, *84*:223, 1991.

64. Melendez, L.J., Chan, K-L., Cheung, P.K., Sochowski, R.A., Wong, S., and Austin, T.W.: Incidence of bacteremia in transesophageal echocardiography: A prospective study of 140 consecutive patients. J. Am. Coll. Cardiol., *18*:1650, 1991.

65. Silvey, S.V., Stoughton, T.L., Pearl, W., Collazo, W.A., and Belbel, R.J.: Rupture of the outer partition of aortic dissection during transesophageal echocardiography. Am. J. Cardiol., *68*:286, 1991.

66. Voller, H., Spielberg, C., Schroder, K., Gast, D., and Schroder, R.: Frequency of positive blood cultures during transesophageal echocardiography. Am. J. Cardiol., *68*:1538, 1991.

67. Roberson, D.A., Muhiudeen, I.A., and Silverman, N.H.: Transesophageal echocardiography in pediatrics: Technique and limitations. Echocardiography, *7*:699, 1990.

68. Ritter, S.B.: Pediatric transesophageal color flow imaging 1990: The long and short of it. Echocardiography, *7*: 713, 1990.

69. Nanda, J.C., Pinheiro, L., Sanyal, R.S., and Storey, O.: Transesophageal biplane echocardiographic imaging: Technique, planes and clinical usefulness. Echocardiography, *7*:771, 1990.

70. Seward, J.B., Khandheria, B.K., Oh, J.K., Hughes, R.W., Edwards, W.D., Nichols, B.A., Freeman, W.K., and Tajik, A.J.: Transesophageal echocardiography: Technique, anatomic correlations, implementation, and clinical applications. Mayo Clin. Proc., *63*:649, 1988.

71. Kronzon, I., Cziner, D.G., Katz, E.S., Gargiulo, A., Tunick, P.A., Freedberg, R.S., and Daniel, W.G.: Buckling of the tip of the transesophageal echocardiography

72. Lightly, G.W., Jr., Hare, C.L., and Kaplan, D.S.: Use of a mouth gag instrument to facilitate bite block insertion and prevent finger and probe bites during transesophageal echocardiography. Echocardiography, *9*:485, 1992.

73. Fleischer, D.E., and Goldstein, S.A.: Transesophageal echocardiography: What the gastroenterologist thinks the cardiologist should know about endoscopy. J. Am. Soc. Echocardiogr., *3*:428, 1990.

74. Schiller, N.B., Maurer, G., Ritter, S.B., Armstrong, W.F., Crawford, M., Spotnitz, H., Cahalan, M., Quinones, M., Meltzer, R., Feinstein, S., Konstadt, S., and Seward, J.: Transesophageal echocardiography. J. Am. Soc. Echocardiogr., *2*:354, 1989.

75. DeBelder, M.A., Leech, G., and Camm, A.J.: Transesophageal echocardiography in unsedated outpatients: Technique and patient tolerance. J. Am. Soc. Echocardiogr., *2*:375, 1989.

76. Nikutta, P., Mantey-Stiers, F., Becht, I., Hausmann, D., Mugge, A., Bohm, T., Pletschette, M., and Daniel, W.G.: Risk of bacteremia induced by transesophageal echocardiography: Analysis of 100 consecutive procedures. J. Am. Soc. Echocardiogr., *5*:168, 1992.

76a. Shyu, K-G., Hwang, J-J., Lin, S-C., Tzou, S-S., Cheng, J-J., Kuan, P., and Lien, W-P.: Prospective study of blood culture during transesophageal echocardiography. Am. Heart J., *124*:1541, 1992.

77. Freedberg, R.S., Weinreb, J., Gluck, M., and Kronzon, I.: Paraesophageal hernia may prevent cardiac imaging by transesophageal echocardiography. J. Am. Soc. Echocardiogr., *2*:202, 1989.

78. Lam, J., Neirotti, R.A., Nijveld, A., Schuller, J.L., Blom-Muilwijk, C.M., and Visser, C.A.: Transesophageal echocardiography in pediatric patients: Preliminary results. J. Am. Soc. Echocardiogr., *4*:43, 1991.

78a. Fyfe, D.A., Titter, S.B., Snider, A.R., Silverman, N.H., Stevenson, J.G., Sorensen, G., Ensing, G., Ludomirsky, A., Sahn, D.J., Murphy, D., Hagler, D., and Marx, G.R.: Guidelines for transesophageal echocardiography in children. J. Am. Soc. Echocardiogr., *5*:640–644, 1992.

78b. Scott, P.J., Blackburn, M.E., Sharton, G.A., Wilson, N., Dickinson, D.F., and Gibbs, J.L.: Transesophageal echocardiography in neonates, infants and children: Applicability and diagnostic value in everyday practice of a cardiothoracic unit. Br. Heart J., *68*:488, 1992.

79. Bansal, R.C., Shakudo, M., Shah, P.M., and Shah, P.M.: Biplane transesophageal echocardiography: Technique, image orientation, and preliminary experience in 131 patients. J. Am. Soc. Echocardiogr., *3*:348, 1990.

80. Cohen, G.I. and Chan, K-L.: Biplane transesophageal echocardiography: Clinical applications of the long-axis plane. J. Am. Soc. Echocardiogr., *4*:155, 1991.

81. Mitchell, M.M., Sutherland, G.R., Gussenhoven, E.J., Taams, M.A., and Roelandt, J.R.T.C.: Transesophageal echocardiography. J. Am. Soc. Echocardiogr., *1*:362, 1988.

82. Wang, X-F., Li, Z-A., Cheng, T.O., Deng, Y-B., Wang, J-E., and Yang, Y.: Biplane transesophageal echocardiography: An anatomic-ultrasonic-clinical correlative study. Am. Heart J., *123*:1027, 1992.

83. Richardson, S.G. and Pandian, N.G.: Echo-anatomic correlations and image display approaches in transesophageal echocardiography. Echocardiography, *8*:671, 1991.

84. Richardson, S.G., Weintraub, A.R., Schwartz, S.L., Simonetti, J., Caldeira, M.E., and Pandian, N.G.: Biplane transesophageal echocardiography utilizing transverse

and sagittal imaging planes. Echocardiography, *8*:293, 1991.

85. Seward, J.B.: Nonanatomic correlations of transesophageal echocardiography. Echocardiography, *8*:669, 1991.

86. Seward, J.B., Khandheria, B.K., Edwards, W.D., Oh, J.K., Freeman, W.K., and Tajik, A.J.: Biplanar transesophageal echocardiography: Anatomic correlations, image orientation, and clinical applications. Mayo Clin. Proc., *65*:1193, 1990.

86a. Stoddard, M.F., Liddell, N.E., Longacker, R.A., and Dawkins, P.R.: Transesophageal echocardiography: Normal variants and mimickers. Am. Heart J., *124*:1587, 1992.

86b. Pandian, N.G., Hsu, T-L., Schwartz, S.L., Weintraub, A., Cao, Q-L., Schneider, A.T., Gordon, G., England, M., and Simonetti, J.: Multiplane transesophageal echocardiography. Echocardiography *9*:649, 1992.

87. Erbel, R., Borner, N., Steller, D., Brunier, J., Thelen, M., Pfeiffer, C., Mohr-Kahaly, S., Iversen, S., Oelert, H., and Meyer, J.: Detection of aortic dissection by transoesophageal echocardiography. Br. Heart J., *58*:45, 1987

88. Seward, J.B., Khandheria, B.K., McGregor, C.G.A., Locke, T.J., and Tajik, A.J.: Transvascular and intracardiac two-dimensional echocardiography. Echocardiography, *7*:457, 1990.

89. St. Goar, F.G., Pinto, F.J., Alderman, E.L., Fitzgerald, P.J., Stadius, M.L., and Popp, R.L.: Intravascular ultrasound imaging of angiographically normal coronary arteries: An in vivo comparison with quantitative angiography. J. Am. Coll. Cardiol., *18*:952, 1991.

90. Schwartz, S.L., Pandian, N.G., Kusay, B.S., Kumar, R., Weintraub, A., Katz, S.E., and Aronovitz, M.: Real-time intracardiac two-dimensional echocardiography: An experimental study of in vivo feasibility, imaging planes, and echocardiographic anatomy. Echocardiography, *7*: 443, 1990.

91. Pandian, N.G., Kumar, R., Katz, S.E., Tutor, A., Schwartz, S.L., Weintraub, R., Gillam, L.D., McKay, R.G., Konstam, M.A., Salem, D.N., and Aronovitz, M.: Real-time, intracardiac, two-dimensional echocardiography. Echocardiography, *8*:407, 1991.

92. Pande, A., Meier, B., Fleisch, M., Kammerlander, R., Simonet, F., and Lerch, R.: Intravascular ultrasound for diagnosis of aortic dissection. Am. J. Cardiol., *67*:662, 1991.

93. Pandian, N.G., Kreis, A., Weintraub, A., Motarjeme, A., Desnoyers, M., Isner, J.M., Konstam, M., Salem, D.N., and Millen, V.: Real-time intravascular ultrasound imaging in humans. Am. J. Cardiol., *65*:1392, 1990.

94. Freeman, W.K., Schaff, H.V., Khandheria, B.K., Oh, J.K., Orszulak, T.A., Abel, M.D., Seward, J.B., and Tajik, A.J.: Intraoperative evaluation of mitral valve regurgitation and repair by transesophageal echocardiography: Incidence and significance of systolic anterior motion. J. Am. Coll. Cardiol., *20*:599, 1992.

95. Hong, Y-W., Oirhashi, K., and Oka, Y.: Intraoperative monitoring of regional wall motion abnormalities for detecting myocardial ischemia by transesophageal echocardiography. Echocardiography, *7*:323, 1990.

96. Simon, P. and Mohl, W.: Intraoperative echocardiographic assessment of global and regional myocardial function. Echocardiography, *7*:333, 1990.

96a. Eisenberg, M.J., London, M.J., Leung, J.M., Browner, W.S., Hollenberg, M., Tubau, J.F., Tateo, I.M., Schiller, N.B., and Mangano, D.T.: Monitoring for myocardial ischemia during noncardiac surgery. A technol-ogy assessment of transesophageal echocardiography and 12-lead electrocardiography. The study of perioperative ischemia research group. JAMA, *268*:210, 1992.

96b. Koolen, J.J., Visser, C.A., Reichert, S.L., Jaarsma, W.J., Kromhout, J.G., van Wezel, H.B., and Dunning, A.J.: Improved monitoring of myocardial ischemia during major vascular surgery using transesophageal echocardiography. Eur. Heart J., *13*:1028, 1992.

97. Klein, A.L., Stewart, W.C., Cosgrove, D.M., and Salcedo, E.E.: Intraoperative epicardial echocardiography: Technique and imaging planes. Echocardiography, *7*:241, 1990.

98. Isringhaus, H.: Epicardial coronary artery imaging. Echocardiography, *7*:253, 1990.

98a. Koenig, P.R., Rossi, A., and Ritter, S.B.: Bedside cardiac catheterization using transesophageal echocardiographic guidance. Echocardiography, *9*:637, 1992.

99. Stoddard, M.F., Longaker, R.A., Vuocolo, L.M., and Dawkins, P.R.: Transesophageal echocardiography in the pregnant patient. Am. Heart J., *124*:785, 1992.

100. Guttas, J.J., Brent, B.N., and Kersh, E.: Biopsy of a right atrial mass under transesophageal echocardiographic guidance. Echocardiography, *9*:129, 1992.

100a. Boutin, C., Dyck, J., Benson, L., Houde, C., and Freedom, R.M.: Balloon atrial septostomy under transesophageal echocardiographic guidance. Pediatr. Cardiol., *13*: 175, 1992.

100b. Goldman, A.P., Irwin, J.M., Glover, M.U., and Mick, W.: Transesophageal echocardiography to improve positioning of radiofrequency ablation catheters in left-sided Wolff-Parkinson-White syndrome. PACE Pacing Clin. Electrophysiol., *14*:1245, 1991.

101. Feigenbaum, H.: Digital recording, display, and storage of echocardiograms. J. Am. Soc. Echocardiogr., *1*:378, 1988.

102. Finley, J.P., Human, D.G., Nanton, M.A., Roy, D.L., Macdonald, R.G., Marr, D.R., and Chiasson, H.: Echocardiography by telephone—evaluation of pediatric heart disease at a distance. Am. J. Cardiol., *63*:1475, 1989.

103. Crawford, M.H., Amon, K.W., and Vance, W.S.: Exercise two-dimensional echocardiography: Quantitation of left ventricular performance in patients with severe angina pectoris. Am. J. Cardiol., *51*:1, 1982.

104. Visser, C.A., Van der Wieken, R.L., Kan, G., Lie, K.I., Busemann-Sokele, E., Meltzer, R.S., and Durrer, D.: Comparison of two-dimensional echocardiography with radionuclide angiography during dynamic exercise for the detection of coronary artery disease. Am. Heart J., *106*:528, 1983.

105. Ginzton, L.E., Conant, R., Brizendine, M., Lee, F., Mena, I., and Laks, M.M.: Exercise subcostal two-dimensional echocardiography: A new method of segmental wall motion analysis. Am. J. Cardiol., *53*:805, 1984.

106. Presti, C.F., Armstrong, W.F., and Feigenbaum, H.: Comparison of echocardiography at peak exercise and after bicycle exercise in evaluation of patients with known or suspected coronary artery disease. J. Am. Soc. Echocardiogr., *1*:119, 1988.

107. Wann, L.S., Faris, J.V., Childress, R.H., Dillon, J.C., Weyman, A.E., and Feigenbaum, H.: Exercise cross-sectional echocardiography in ischemic heart disease. Circulation, *60*:1300, 1979.

108. Morganroth, J., Chen, C.C., David, D., Sawin, H.S., Natio, M., Parrotto, C., and Meixell, L.: Exercise cross-sectional echocardiographic diagnosis of coronary artery disease. Am. J. Cardiol., *47*:20, 1981.

109. Takahashi, H., Koga, Y., Itaya, M., Nagata, H., Itaya,

K., Ohkita, Y., Bekki, H., Jinnouchi, J., Utsu, F., and Toshima, H.: Detection of exercise-induced left ventricular asynergy by two-dimensional echocardiography. J. Cardiogr., *11*:1193, 1981.

110. Agati, L., Arata, L., Luongo, R., Iacoboni, C., Renzi, M., Vizza, C.D., Penco, M., Fedele, F., and Dagianti, A.: Assessment of severity of coronary narrowings by quantitative exercise echocardiography and comparison with quantitative arteriography. Am. J. Cardiol., *67*: 1201, 1991.

111. Limacher, M.C., Quinones, M.A., Polner, L.R., Nelson, J.G., Wintters, Jr., W.L., and Waggoner, A.D.: Detection of coronary artery disease with exercise two-dimensional echocardiography. Circulation, *67*:1211, 1983.

112. Maurer, G. and Nanda, N.C.: Two-dimensional echocardiographic evaluation of exercise-induced left and right ventricular asynergy: Correlation with thallium scanning. Am. J. Cardiol., *48*:720, 1981.

113. Robertson, W.S., Feigenbaum, H., Armstrong, W.F., Dillon, J.C., O'Donnell, J., and McHenry, P.W.: Exercise echocardiography: A clinically practical addition in the evaluation of coronary artery disease. J. Am. Coll. Cardiol., *2*:1085, 1983.

114. Armstrong, W.F., O'Donnell, J., Dillon, J.C., McHenry, P.L., Morris, S.N., and Feigenbaum, H.: Complementary value of two-dimensional exercise echocardiography to routine treadmill exercise testing. Ann. Intern. Med., *105*:829, 1986.

115. Crouse, L.J., Harbrecht, J.J., Vacek, J.L., Rosamond, T.L., and Kramer, P.H.: Exercise echocardiography as a screening test for coronary artery disease and correlation with coronary arteriography. Am. J. Cardiol., *67*:1213, 1991.

116. Christie, J., Sheldahl, L.M., Tristani, F.E., Sagar, K.B., Ptacin, M.J., and Wann, S.: Determination of stroke volume and cardiac output during exercise: Comparison of two-dimensional and Doppler echocardiography, Fick oximetry, and thermodilution. Circulation, *76*:539, 1987.

117. Mehta, N., Boyle, G., Bennett, D., Gilmour, S., Noble, M.I.M., Mills, C.M., and Pugh, S.: Hemodynamic response to treadmill exercise in normal volunteers: An assessment by Doppler ultrasonic measurement of ascending aortic blood velocity and acceleration. Am. Heart J., *116*:1298, 1988.

118. Marx, G.R., Hicks, R.W., Allen, H.D., and Goldberg, S.J.: Noninvasive assessment of hemodynamic responses to exercise in pulmonary regurgitation after operations to correct pulmonary outflow obstruction. Am. J. Cardiol., *61*:595, 1988.

119. Ihlen, H., Endresen, K., Golf, S., and Nitter-Hauge, S.: Cardiac stroke volume during exercise measured by Doppler echocardiography: Comparison with the thermodilution technique and evaluation of reproducibility. Br. Heart J., *58*:455, 1987.

120. Pierard, L.A., Serruys, P.W., Roelandt, J., and Meltzer, R.S.: Left ventricular function at similar heart rates during tachycardia induced by exercise and atrial pacing: An echocardiographic study. Br. Heart J., *57*:154, 1987.

121. Matthews, R.V., Haskell, R.J., Ginzton, L.E., and Laks, M.M.: Usefulness of esophageal pill electrode atrial pacing with quantitative two-dimensional echocardiography for diagnosing coronary artery disease. Am. J. Cardiol., *64*:730, 1989.

122. Berthe, C., Pierard, L.A., Hiernaux, M., Trotteur, G., Lempereur, P., Carlier, J., and Kulbertus, H.E.: Predicting the extent and location of coronary artery disease in

acute myocardial infarction by echocardiography during dobutamine infusion. Am. J. Cardiol., *58*:1167, 1986.

123. Sawada, S.G., Segar, D.S., Ryan, T., Brown, S.E., Dohan, A.M., Williams, R., Fineberg, N.S., Armstrong, W.F., and Feigenbaum, H.: Echocardiographic detection of coronary artery disease during dobutamine infusion. Circulation, *83*:1605, 1991.

124. Cohen, J.L., Greene, T.O., Ottenweller, J., Bineenbaum, S.Z., Wilchfort, S.D., Kim, C.S., and Alston, J.R.: Dobutamine digital echocardiography for detecting coronary artery disease. Am. J. Cardiol., *67*:1311, 1991.

125. Bolognese, L., Sarasso, G., Aralda, D., Bondo, A.S., Rossi, L., and Rossi, P.: High dose dipyridamole echocardiography early after uncomplicated acute myocardial infarction: Correlation with exercise testing and coronary angiography. J. Am. Coll. Cardiol., *14*:357, 1989.

126. Masini, M., Picano, E., Lattanzi, F., Distante, A., and L'Abbate, A.: High dose dipyridamole-echocardiography test in women: Correlation with exercise-electrocardiography test and coronary arteriography. J. Am. Coll. Cardiol., *12*:682, 1988.

127. Picano, E., Lattanzi, F., Masini, M., Distante, A., and L'Abbate, A.: Different degrees of ischemic threshold stratified by the dipyridamole-echocardiography test. Am. J. Cardiol., *59*:71, 1987.

128. Grayburn, P.A., Popma, J.J., Pyror, S.L., Walker, B.S., Simon, T.R., and Smitherman, T.C.: Comparison of dipyridamole-Doppler echocardiography to thallium-201 imaging and quantitative coronary arteriography in the assessment of coronary artery disease. Am. J. Cardiol., *6*:1315, 1989.

129. Ryan, T., Vasey, C.G., Presti, C.F., O'Donnell, J.A., Feigenbaum, H., and Armstrong, W.F.: Exercise echocardiography: Detection of coronary artery disease in patients with normal left ventricular wall motion at rest. J. Am. Coll. Cardiol., *11*:993, 1988.

130. Cohen, J.L., Greene, T.O., Alston, J.R., Wilchfort, S.D., and Kim, C.S.: Usefulness of oral dipyridamole digital echocardiography for detecting coronary artery disease. Am. J. Cardiol., *64*:385, 1989.

131. Feigenbaum, H.: Exercise echocardiography. J. Am. Soc. Echocardiogr., *1*:161, 1988.

132. Teien, D., Wendel, H., Holm, S., and Hallberg, M.: Estimation of Doppler gradients at rest and during exercise in patients with recoarctation of the aorta. Br. Heart J., *65*:155, 1991.

133. Gramiak, R., Shah, P.M., and Kramer, D.H.: Ultrasound cardiography: Contrast studies in anatomy and function. Radiology, *92*:939, 1969.

134. Feigenbaum, H., Stone, J.M., Lee, D.A., Nasser, W.K., and Chang, S.: Identification of ultrasound echoes from the left ventricle using intracardiac injections of indocyanine green. Circulation, *41*:615, 1970.

135. Seward, J.B., Tajik, A.J., Spangler, J.G., and Ritter, D.G.: Echocardiographic contrast studies: Initial experience. Mayo Clin. Proc., *50*:163, 1975.

136. Shub, C., Tajik, A.J., Seward, J.B., and Dines, D.E.: Detecting intrapulmonary right-to-left shunt with contrast echocardiography. Mayo Clin. Proc., *51*:81, 1976.

137. Seward, J.B., Tajik, A.J., Hagler, D.J., and Ritter, D.G.: Peripheral venous contrast echocardiography. Am. J. Cardiol., *39*:202, 1977.

138. Allen, H.D., Sahn, D.J., and Goldberg, S.J.: New serial contrast technique for assessment of left-to-right shunting in patent ductus arteriosus in the neonate. Am. J. Cardiol., *41*:288, 1978.

139. Weyman, A.E., Wann, L.S., Caldwell, R.L., Hurwitz,

R.A., Dillon, J.C., and Feigenbaum, H.: Negative contrast echocardiography: A new method for detecting left-to-right shunts. Circulation, *59*:498, 1979.

140. Kort, A. and Kronzon, I.: Microbubble formation: In vitro and in vivo observation. JCU, *10*:117, 1982.

141. Meltzer, R.S., Serruys, P.W., Hugenholtz, P.G., and Roelandt, J.: Intravenous carbon dioxide as an echocardiographic contrast agent. JCU, *9*:127, 1981.

142. Gaffney, F.A., Lin, J-C., Peshock, R.M., Bush, L., and Buja, M.: Hydrogen peroxide contrast echocardiography. Am. J. Cardiol., *52*:607, 1983.

143. Wang, X., Chiaen, W., Hanjung, C., Chengfa, L., Yucken, H., and Chungte, T.: Clinical application of cardiac contrast with hydrogen peroxide. Chin. J. Phys. Med., *1*:2, 1979.

144. Winfang, W., Chiaen, W., Chengfa, L., Hanjung, C., Yucken, H., Chungte, T., and Chingkuei, K.: The application of acoustic contrast with hydrogen peroxide in the application of ultrasonophonographic cardiac anatomical structure. Natl. Med. J. Chin., *59*:321, 1979.

145. Bommer, W.J., Shah, P.M., Allen, H., Meltzer, R., and Kisslo, J.: The safety of contrast echocardiography: Report of the Committee on Contrast Echocardiography for the American Society of Echocardiography. J. Am. Coll. Cardiol., *3*:6, 1984.

146. Davis, P.L., Filly, R.A., and Goerke, J.: Echogenicity caused by stable microbubbles in a protein-lipid emulsion. JCU, *9*:249, 1981.

147. Sanders, W.E., Cheirif, J., Desir, R., Zoghbi, W.A., Hoyt, B.D., Schulz, P.E., and Quinones, M.A.: Contrast opacification of left ventricular myocardium following intravenous administration of sonicated albumin microspheres. Am. Heart J., *122*:1660, 1991.

148. Keller, M.W., Glasheen, W., and Kaul, S.: Albunex: A safe and effective commercially produced agent for myocardial contrast echocardiography. J. Am. Soc. Echocardiogr., *2*:48, 1989.

149. Feinstein, S.B., Keller, M.W., Kerber, R.E., Vandenberg, B., Hoyte, J., Kutruff, C., Bingle, J., Fraker, Jr., T.D., Chappell, R., and Welsh, A.H.: Sonicated echocardiographic contrast agents: Reproducibility studies. J. Am. Soc. Echocardiogr., *2*:125, 1989.

150. Feinstein, S.B., Cheirif, J., Ten Cate, F.J., Silverman, P.R., Heidenreich, P.A., Dick, C., Desir, R.M., Armstrong, W.F., Quinones, M.A., and Shah, P.M.: Safety and efficacy of new transpulmonary ultrasound contrast agent: Initial multicenter clinical results. J. Am. Coll. Cardiol., *16*:316, 1990.

151. Smith, M.D., Kwan, O.L., Reiser, J., and DeMaria, A.N.: Superior intensity and reproducibility of SHU-U54, a new right heart contrast agent. J. Am. Coll. Cardiol., *3*:992, 1984.

152. Rovai, D., Lombardi, M., Cini, G., Morales, M.A., Colonna, M., Bechelli, G., Marion, P., Zanolla, L., Prioli, M.A., Nicolosi, G.L., Pavan, D., Zanuttini, D., Iliceto, S., Izzi, M., Rizzon, P., and L'Abbate, A.: Echocardiographic contrast imaging of the human right heart: A multicenter study of the efficacy, safety, and reproducibility of intravenous SHU-454. JCU, *19*:523, 1991.

153. Smith, M.D., Elion, J.L., McClure, R.R., Kwan, O.L., DeMaria, A.N., Evans, J., and Fritzsch, T.H.: Left heart opacification with peripheral venous injection of a new saccharide echo contrast agent in dogs. J. Am. Coll. Cardiol., *13*:1622, 1989.

154. Berwing, K. and Schlepper, M.: Echocardiographic imaging of the left ventricle by peripheral intravenous injection of echo contrast agent. Am. Heart J., *115*:399, 1988.

155. Meltzer, R.S., Tickner, E.G., and Popp, R.L.: Clinical note. Why do the lungs clear ultrasonic contrast? Ultrasound Med. Biol., *6*:263, 1980.

156. Reid, C.L., Kawanishi, D.T., McKay, C.R., Elkayam, U., Rahimtoola, H., and Chandraratna, P.A.N.: Accuracy of evaluation of the presence and severity of aortic and mitral regurgitation by contrast 2-dimensional echocardiography. Am. J. Cardiol., *52*:519, 1983.

157. Shapiro, A.R., Reisner, S.A., Lichtenberg, G.S., and Meltzer, R.S.: Intravenous contrast echocardiography with use of sonicated albumin in humans: Systolic disappearance of left ventricular contrast after transpulmonary transmission. J. Am. Coll. Cardiol., *16*:1603, 1990.

158. Reid, C.L., Kawanishi, D.T., McKay, C.R., Elkayam, U., Rahimtoola, H., and Chandraratna, P.A.N.: Accuracy of evaluation of the presence and severity of aortic and mitral regurgitation by contrast 2-dimensional echocardiography. Am. J. Cardiol., *52*:519, 1983.

159. Elkayam, U., Kawanishi, D., Reid, C.L., Chandraratna, P.A.N., Gleicher, N., and Rahimtoola, S.H.: Contrast echocardiography to reduce ionizing radiation associated with cardiac catherization during pregnancy. Am. J. Cardiol., *52*:213, 1983.

160. Tei, C., Sakamaki, T., Shah, P.M., Meerbaum, S., Shimoura, K., Kondo, S., and Corday, E.: Myocardial contrast echocardiography: A reproducible technique of myocardial opacification for identifying regional perfusion deficits. Circulation, *67*:585, 1983.

161. Kliopera, M., Glogar, D., Mayr, H., Mohl, W., Losert, U., and Kaindl, F.: Myocardial perfusion evaluated by contrast echocardiography. A preliminary report. Chest, *82*:751, 1982.

162. Armstrong, W.F., Mueller, T.M., Kinney, E.L., Tickner, E.G., Dillon, J.C., and Feigenbaum, H.: Assessment of myocardial perfusion abnormalities with contrast-enhanced two-dimensional echocardiography. Circulation, *66*:166, 1982.

163. Jayaweera, A.R., Matthew, T.L., Sklenar, J., Spotnitz, W.D., Watson, D.D., and Kaul, S.: Method for the quantitation of myocardial perfusion during myocardial contrast two-dimensional echocardiography. J. Am. Soc. Echocardiogr., *3*:91, 1990.

164. Litchtenberg, G.S. and Meltzer, R.S.: Myocardial perfusion studies by contrast echocardiography. J. Am. Soc. Echocardiogr., *3*:170, 1990.

165. Von Bibra, H., Stempfle, H-U., Poll, A., Schlief, R., and Emslander, H.: Echo contrast agents improve flow display of color Doppler. Echocardiography, *8*:533, 1991.

166. Himelman, R.B., Stulbarg, M.S., Lee, E., Kuecherer, H.F., and Schiller, N.B.: Noninvasive evaluation of pulmonary artery systolic pressures during dynamic exercise by saline-enhanced Doppler echocardiography. Am. Heart J., *119*:685, 1990.

167. Martin, G.R., Silverman, N.H., Soifer, S.J., Lutin, W.A., and Scagnelli, S.A.: Tricuspid regurgitation in children: A pulsed Doppler, contrast echocardiographic and angiographic comparison. J. Am. Soc. Echocardiogr., *1*:257, 1988.

168. Erbel, R., Stern, H., Ehrenthal, W., Schreiner, G., Treese, N., Kramer, G., Thelen, M., Schweizer, P., and Meyer, J.: Detection of spontaneous echocardiographic contrast within the left atrium by transesophageal echocardiography: Spontaneous echocardiographic contrast. Clin. Cardiol., *9*:245, 1986.

169. Doud, D.N., Jacobs, W.R., Moran, J.F., and Scanlon, P.J.: The natural history of left ventricular spontaneous contrast. J. Am. Soc. Echocardiogr., *3*:465, 1990.

170. Beard, J.T. and Byrd, B.F.: Saline contrast enhancement of trivial Doppler tricuspid regurgitation signals for estimating pulmonary artery pressure. Am. J. Cardiol., *62*: 486, 1988.

171. Erbel, R., Stern, H., Ehrenthal, W., Schreiner, G., Treese, N., Kramer, G., Thelen, M., Schweizer, P., and Meyer, J.: Detection of spontaneous echocardiographic contrast within the left atrium by transesophageal echocardiography: Spontaneous echocardiographic contrast. Clin. Cardiol., *9*:245, 1986.

172. Iliceto, S., Papa, A., Ciociola, G., Sorino, M., Girardi, F., and Biasco, G.: Spontaneous microcavitations in the right cardiac chambers. G. Ital. Cardiol., *14*:577, 1984.

173. Sahn, D.J., DeMaria, A., Kisslo, J., and Weyman, A.: Recommendations regarding quantitation in M-mode echocardiography: Results of a survey of echocardiographic measurements. Circulation, *58*:1072, 1978.

174. Crawford, M.H., Grant, D., O'Rourke, R.A., Starling, M.R., and Grooves, B.M.: Accuracy and reproducibility of new M-mode echocardiographic recommendations for measuring left ventricular dimensions. Circulation, *61*: 137, 1980.

175. Kulas, A., Enriquea-Sarano, L., Troley, C., and Acar, J.: Value of correction by receiving gains in the determination of mitral valve surface area by two-dimensional echocardiography. Arch. Mal. Coeur, *75*:757, 1982.

176. Felner, J.M., Blumenstein, B.A., Schlant, R.C., Carter, A.D., Alimurung, B.N., Johnson, M.J., Sherman, S.W., Klicpera, M.W., Kutner, M.H., and Drucker, L.W.: Sources of variability in echocardiographic measurements. Am. J. Cardiol., *45*:995, 1980.

177. Schnittger, I., Gordon, E.P., Fitzgerald, P.J., and Popp, R.L.: Standardized intracardiac measurements of two-dimensional echocardiography. J. Am. Coll. Cardiol., *2*: 934, 1983.

178. Petrovic, O., Feigenbaum, H., Armstrong, W.F., Ryan, T., West, S.R., Green-Hess, D., Stewart, J., Mattson, J.L., and Fineberg, N.S.: Digital averaging to facilitate two-dimensional echocardiographic measurements. JCU, *14*:367, 1986.

179. Zwehl, W., Levy, R., Garcia, E., Haendchen, R.V., Childs, W., Corday, S.R., Meerbaum, S., and Corday, E.: Validation of a computerized edge detection algorithm for quantitative two-dimensional echocardiography. Circulation, *68*:1127, 1983.

180. Buda, A.J., Delp, E.J., Meyer, C.R., Jenkins, J.M., Smith, D.N., Bookstein, F.L., and Pitt, B.: Automatic computer processing of digital two-dimensional echocardiograms. Am. J. Cardiol., *52*:384, 1983.

181. Skorton, D.H., McNary, C.A., Child, J.S., Newton, F.C., and Shah, P.M.: Digital image processing of two-dimensional echocardiograms: Identification of the endocardium. Am. J. Cardiol., *48*:479, 1981.

182. Conetta, D.A., Geiser, E.A., Skorton, D.J., Pandian, N.G., Kerber, R.E., and Conti, C.R.: In vitro analysis of secondary identification techniques used in quantification of two-dimensional echocardiograms. Am. J. Cardiol., *53*:1374, 1984.

183. Collins, S.M., Skorton, D.J., Geiser, E.A., Nichols, J.A., Conetta, D.A., Pandian, N.G., and Kerber, R.E.: Computer-assisted edge detection in two-dimensional echocardiography: Comparison with anatomic data. Am. J. Cardiol., *53*:1380, 1984.

184. Geiser, E.A., Oliver, L.H., Gardin, J.M., Kerber, R.E., Parisi, A.F., Reichek, N., Werner, J.A., and Wayman, A.E.: Clinical validation of an edge detection algorithm for two-dimensional echocardiographic short-axis images. J. Am. Soc. Echocardiogr., *1*:410, 1988.

185. Perez, J.E., Waggoner, A.D., Barzilai, B., Melton, Jr., H.E., Miller, J.G., and Sobel, B.E.: On-line assessment of ventricular function by automatic boundary detection and ultrasonic backscatter imaging. J. Am. Coll. Cardiol., *19*:313, 1992.

186. Vandenberg, B.F., Rath, L.S., Stuhlmuller, P., Melton, Jr., J.E., and Skorton, D.J.: Estimation of left ventricular cavity area with an on-line, semiautomated echocardiographic edge detection system. Circulation, *86*:159, 1992.

187. St. John Sutton, M.G., Reichek, N., Kastor, J.A., and Giuliani, E.R.: Computerized M-mode echocardiographic analysis of left ventricular dysfunction in cardiac amyloid. Circulation, *66*:790, 1982.

188. Sapoznikov, D., Lewis, N., Rachmilewitz, E.A., Gotsman, M.S., and Lewis, B.S.: Left ventricular filling and emptying patterns in anemia due to beta-thalassemia. A computer-assisted echocardiographic study. Cardiology, *69*:276, 1982.

189. Bahler, R.C., Trobel, T.R., and Martin, P.: The relation of heart rate and shortening fraction to echocardiographic indexes of left ventricular relaxation in normal subjects. J. Am. Coll. Cardiol., *2*:926, 1984.

190. DeMaria, A.N. and Smith, M.D.: Quantitation of Doppler color flow recordings: An oxymoron? J. Am. Coll. Cardiol., *20*:439, 1992.

# 3

# Echocardiographic Evaluation of Cardiac Chambers

## LEFT VENTRICLE

The assessment of left ventricular function is an essential component of the evaluation of any patient with known or suspected heart disease. Thus, it is not surprising that the popularity of echocardiography rose dramatically when it was demonstrated that this noninvasive technique could be used to evaluate the status of the left ventricle. The initial echocardiographic technique for evaluating left ventricular function used M-mode measurements. Today, it is possible to use all forms of echocardiography to obtain a fairly extensive and comprehensive evaluation of the left ventricle.[1,2] Some of the measurements discussed are routinely performed on virtually all examinations, whereas many are limited to investigational purposes. Some measurements may be relatively simple and others are complex. Both qualitative and quantitative assessment of the left ventricle is possible.

### Intracavitary Dimensions, Areas, and Volumes

The observation that one could make a quantitative measurement on an M-mode echocardiogram between the interventricular septum and posterior ventricular wall was the impetus to much of the early interest in echocardiography.[3-7] Figure 3–1 illustrates how one can measure between the left side of the interventricular septum (LS) and the posterior left ventricular endocardium (EN). Measurements can be made during diastole (d) and systole (s). In Figure 3–1, the diastolic dimension is taken at the peak of the R wave and from the trailing edge of the left side of the interventricular septum (LS) to the leading edge of the posterior endocardial echo (EN). The American Society of Echocardiography (ASE) recommends that all M-mode measurements be made from leading edge to leading edge because the width of the M-mode echoes may vary from one instrument to another and at times even with gain (see Chapter 2).[8] The diagram in Figure 3–2 demonstrates the ASE recommended method for obtaining left ventricular dimensions. The measurement is made from the leading edge of the septal and endocardial echoes; thus, the septal measurement is actually taken within the substance of the septum. In addition, the ASE believes that the end of diastole is best indicated by the Q wave of the electrocardiogram rather than by the R wave. This rec-

ommendation is based on the fact that the electrocardiogram on the echocardiogram frequently is not of the highest quality and the R wave may vary. In addition, differences in the pediatric population may be significant.

Whether one uses the leading edge or trailing edge of the septal echo, and whether the measurement is made from the R wave or the Q wave, probably makes relatively little difference in adult echocardiography. As shown in Figure 3–1, there is no significant difference between a Q or an R wave diastolic measurement, and the septal echo is probably no more than a millimeter in width. In Figure 3–3, however, which shows an echocardiogram of an infant, one sees a downward motion of the posterior left ventricular wall shortly after the Q wave of the electrocardiogram. The measurement taken at the Q wave is significantly different from one taken at the R wave during the rapid downward motion of the posterior ventricular wall. Such a difference would represent a sizeable percentage of variation in this small chamber. Because the R- and Q-wave measurements are relatively minor in most adult patients, most measurements in the literature are derived from the R wave. The location for making the end-systolic measurement varies among investigators. Many authors use the peak upward motion of the posterior left ventricular endocardium as end systole. Others use the peak downward motion of the interventricular septum. One might initially assume that these two events occur simultaneously. By closer inspection, one notes that the peak downward motion of the septum occurs slightly before the maximum upward excursion of the endocardium (Fig. 3–1). A simultaneous carotid pulse tracing (Fig. 3–1) shows that the peak upward motion of the posterior endocardium usually occurs after the dicrotic notch, or the second heart sound. Thus, the peak downward motion of the interventricular septum more likely corresponds to end systole than does the posterior endocardial echo. The ASE recommends the peak downward motion of the septum as end systole; however, in many patients with abnormal septal motion, one may have to resort to peak upward motion of the posterior endocardium.

All investigators agree that left ventricular dimensions should be obtained when the ultrasonic beam is directed at the chamber between the mitral valve echoes and the papillary muscle echoes (see Fig. 3–2). Some element of the mitral valve echoes, usually chordae, is present in

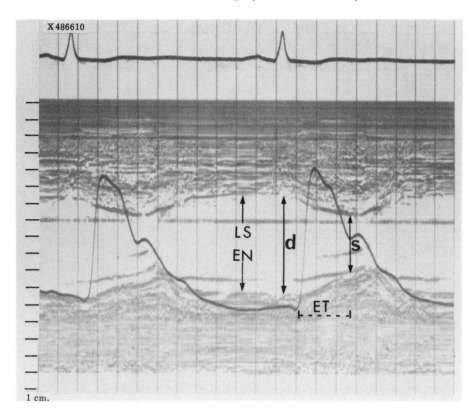

**Fig. 3–1.** Simultaneous carotid pulse tracing and left ventricular echocardiogram recorded at 100 mm/sec. The peak upward motion of the posterior left ventricular endocardium (EN) occurs after the diastolic notch on the carotid pulse. LS = left septum; d = diastolic dimension; s = systolic dimension; ET = ejection time.

such recordings. In the adult, it is unusual to record the best mitral valve echoes when making left ventricular measurements. At the mitral valve level, the posterior ventricular wall is frequently not properly seen, and one may obtain a combination of left ventricular and left atrial echoes. Whether the situation is different in pediatric echocardiography is debatable. Reasonably good mitral valve echoes are recorded in Figure 3–3 at the time left ventricular dimensions are obtained. Many pediatric echocardiographers believe that the relationship

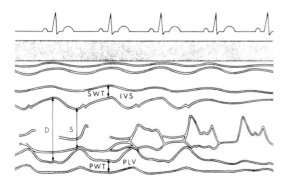

**Fig. 3–2.** Diagram of the M-mode echocardiogram demonstrating the left ventricular measurements as recommended by the American Society of Echocardiography. D = left ventricular diastolic dimension; S = left ventricular systolic dimension; SWT = septal wall thickness; IVS = interventricular septum; PWT = posterior left ventricular wall thickness; PLV = posterior left ventricular wall.

of the mitral valve to the left ventricular cavity is different in the small hearts of neonates and infants, and frequently the best and most standardized left ventricular measurements are obtained when more mitral valve echoes are present in the recording. Most M-mode measurements today are obtained with two-dimensional orientation of the ultrasonic beam. The M-mode measurements can be obtained in either the parasternal long-axis or short-axis views. The two-dimensional echocardiogram, especially in the short-axis view, helps one avoid the papillary muscles when orienting the M-mode cursor.

M-mode left ventricular cavity measurements can be used in many ways. They can be used as linear measurements to estimate the size of the left ventricle in diastole and systole. Cardiologists have become accustomed to thinking in terms of volumes. Thus, interest has been generated in converting the M-mode measurements to volumes.[4,5,7,9] The first attempt at comparing the echocardiographic measurements with angiography did demonstrate a correlation between quantitative angiography and the M-mode dimensions.[3] The correlation with left ventricular volumes was best when the echocardiographic dimensions were cubed. This reasonable relationship prompted other investigators to use the M-mode measurements for volume determinations. Their rationale was based on the following assumptions: the left ventricle could be described as a prolate ellipse (Fig. 3–4), the two short axes (D1, D2) are equal, the long axis is normally twice as long as the short axis, the echocardiographic left ventricular dimensions approximate the short axis, and the left ventricular wall contracts

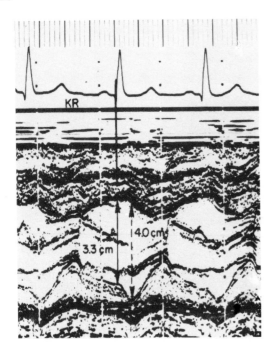

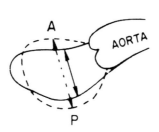

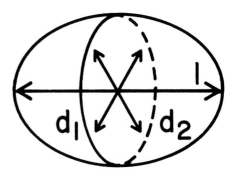

Fig. 3–3. M-mode echocardiogram of an infant demonstrating the difference in left ventricular dimensions taken at the Q wave of the electrocardiogram and after the onset of ventricular systole. A = anterior; P = posterior. (From Meyer, R.A.: Pediatric Echocardiography. Philadelphia, Lea & Febiger, 1977.)

uniformly.[4] Unfortunately, these assumptions are frequently erroneous. Measuring left ventricular volumes using a single M-mode dimension is usually unreliable and fraught with significant error.[10,11] As a result, such measurements should only be used in special situations.[9,12] Despite this caution, the ease of making M-mode measurements and converting them to volumes is so great that it is still common practice for echocardiographers to make this calculation.

Although M-mode measurements are still popular and to some extent have withstood the test of time, this type of measurement has inherent limitations.[13,14] Figure 3–5 shows one of the obvious limitations of the M-mode di-

Fig. 3–4. Prolate ellipse demonstrating the long axis (l) and the two short diameters or short axes ($d_1$ and $d_2$).

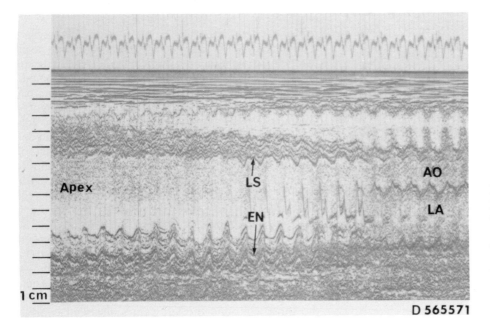

Fig. 3–5. M-mode scan of a patient with coronary artery disease. The left side of the septum (LS) moves normally at the base near the aorta (AO). Near the apex, however, septal motion is akinetic. EN = posterior left ventricular endocardium; LA = left atrium.

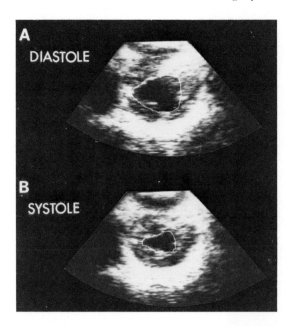

**Fig. 3–6.** Short-axis two-dimensional echocardiograms of the left ventricle in a patient with right ventricular hypertrophy and a distorted left ventricular cavity.

mensions in evaluating global left ventricular function. The patient in Figure 3–5 has coronary artery disease with regional wall motion abnormalities. The proximal septum (LS) and posterior left ventricular wall (EN) move well. The usual M-mode dimensions would be normal, although the apex is dilated and akinetic. The M-mode dimensions would not reflect this abnormality. Thus, it became apparent early that the M-mode dimensions would be limited in assessing global function in patients with regional wall motion abnormalities.

The M-mode calculations are based on the assumption that the left ventricle is essentially circular in its short-axis cross-section. Although this assumption is usually correct, in some pathologic situations, the left ventricle is not circular. Figure 3–6 shows a patient in whom the left ventricle is distorted by a hypertrophied right ventricle. An anterior-posterior dimension would not accurately reflect the cross-sectional area of this chamber.

The largest problem with the M-mode dimensions is that these measurements have been assumed to represent the minor axis of the left ventricle. The diagram in Figure 3–7 demonstrates that the M-mode dimension (*dashed line*) is rarely a true minor dimension (D). Figure 3–8 illustrates a two-dimensional echocardiogram that shows the true minor or short-axis diameter (*solid line*) versus the ultrasonic beam during an M-mode examination (*dashed line*). Not only are the measurements unequal, but also the stationary M-mode beam does not transect the same portions of the interventricular septum and the posterior left ventricular wall during diastole and systole. As the base of the heart moves toward the apex with systole, the M-mode beam transects a different portion of the walls. Figure 3–9 shows an extreme situation in a patient whose echocardiographic window is at a lower interspace than in Figure 3–8. The resultant M-

mode dimension (*dashed line*) is not even close to the minor dimension.

The fact that the M-mode measurement is not a true minor dimension is not as serious a problem as the fact that the relationship between the M-mode measurement and the minor dimension varies from patient to patient. The issue is the available echocardiographic window in a given individual. Table 3–1 shows the relationship between the minor axis and M-mode dimension in 50 consecutive adult patients. In 30% of the patients, the two measurements were within 3 mm of each other. In another 30%, the difference was between 4 and 6 mm. In 40% of the patients, the difference between the M-mode and minor dimensions was greater than 6 mm. Unfortunately, orienting the M-mode cursor with a two-dimensional scan does not overcome this problem. Knowing the location of the true minor dimension only makes the problem obvious, but it is still uncorrectable because the proper acoustic window may not be available for a true M-mode minor axis dimension. It should also be realized that M-mode measurements obtained with transesophageal echocardiography will differ from transthoracic measurements.[14a]

Two-dimensional echocardiography of course has ample possibilities for making measurements of the left ventricle. Because most cardiologists want to determine left ventricular volumes, a variety of two-dimensional echocardiographic techniques have been developed to make this calculation.[15–21,21a] A common technique is to

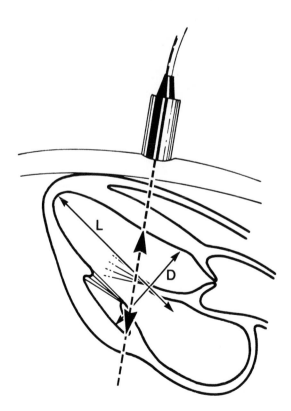

**Fig. 3–7.** Diagram showing the relationship between the direction of an M-mode ultrasonic beam through the left ventricle and the long (L) and minor (D) left ventricular dimensions.

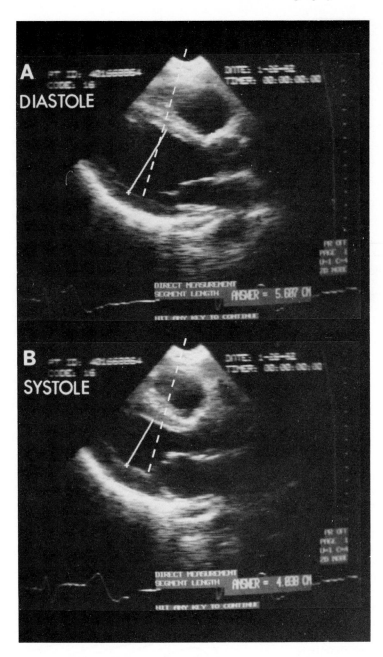

**Fig. 3–8.** Long-axis two-dimensional echocardiograms showing the relationship between the M-mode ultrasonic beam (*dashed line*) and the minor dimension of the left ventricle (*solid line*).

describe the left ventricle as a prolate ellipse (see Fig. 3–4). Two-dimensional echocardiography provides the opportunity to directly measure the two minor axes as well as the left ventricular length. An alternative technique is to measure the long axis directly and to calculate the minor axes by measuring the area of the cavity in various projections or planes. This second technique is frequently called the "area length method" for calculating the volume of a prolate ellipse. The long-axis measurements are usually obtained from apical views of the left ventricle. The minor axes can be directly measured from a short-axis examination at the level of the papillary muscles. An alternative technique is to use the area length method from the two- or four-chamber apical examination. The mathematic formula for calculating vol-

ume of a prolate ellipse is $L/2 \times D1/2 \times D2/2$ in which L is the long-axis dimension and D1 and D2 are the short-axis dimensions (see Fig. 3–4).

The principle difficulty with using the prolate ellipse model for the left ventricle is that the chamber frequently does not resemble a prolate ellipse. With any significant dilatation, the geometric model is distorted. Even a normal ventricle does not resemble a prolate ellipse in systole. As a result, may investigators have been looking for techniques to calculate volumes that do not require the assumption of a geometric model.

The technique that has proved most attractive is based on Simpson's rule. The principle for measuring volume with Simpson's rule is to divide the object into slices of known thickness. The volume of the object is then equal

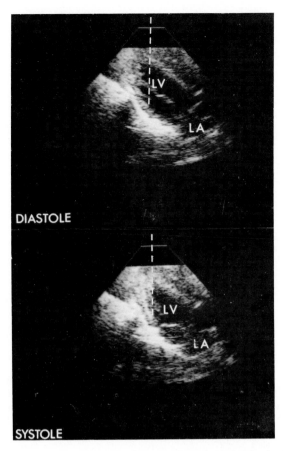

**Fig. 3–9.** Direction of the M-mode cursor through the left ventricle in a patient whose echocardiographic window is near the apex. The M-mode dimension would be much closer to the long axis than to the minor axis in this particular examination. LV = left ventricle; LA = left atrium.

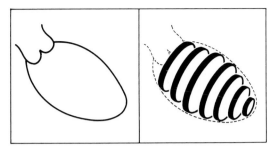

**Fig. 3–10.** Diagram demonstrating Simpson's rule. The left ventricle is expressed as a series of circular slices. (From Rogers, E.W., Feigenbaum, H., and Weyman, A.E.: Echocardiography for quantitation of cardiac chambers. *In* Progress in Cardiology. Vol. 8. Edited by P.N. Yu and J.F. Goodwin. Philadelphia, Lea & Febiger, 1979.)

shape of the left ventricle, such as with an aneurysm (Fig. 3–11), Simpson's rule permits a calculation of ventricular volume. Merely adding the volume of the individual slices provides a measure of the volume of the entire cavity.

Because two-dimensional echocardiography has the capability of obtaining multiple slices through the left ventricle, Simpson's rule should be a good method for measuring ventricular volumes. Figure 3–12A shows how one theoretically could use two-dimensional echocardiography to obtain left ventricular volumes using Simpson's rule. By moving the transducer linearly across a known width of the heart (H), one can calculate the volume. One can even do a similar examination with a sector scan technique, shown in Figure 3–12B. In this case, to calculate the width and volume of each slice,

to the sum of the volumes of the slices. One need only know the surface area and the thickness of the slice to determine the volume. If the shape of the chamber being studied is regular, only a small number of slices are required to adequately define its volume. As the shape becomes more irregular, thinner slices are needed for accurate volume quantitation. If infinitely thin slices were obtainable, one could accurately measure the volume regardless of the shape of the object. In Figure 3–10, the left ventricle is represented as a prolate ellipse and is divided into slices that are circular disks. Summing the volume of the disks provides a measurement of left ventricular volume. Even with distortion of the

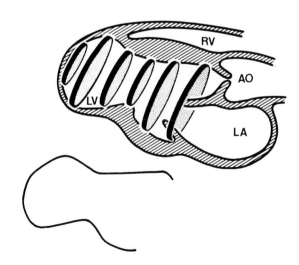

**Fig. 3–11.** Diagram demonstrating Simpson's rule. Note the series of circular slices in the case of a left ventricular aneurysm. LV = left ventricle; AO = aorta; LA = left atrium; RV = right ventricle. (From Rogers, E.W., Feigenbaum, H., and Weyman, A.E.: Echocardiography for quantitation of cardiac chambers. *In* Progress in Cardiology. Vol. 8. Edited by P.N. Yu and J.F. Goodwin. Philadelphia, Lea & Febiger, 1979.)

**Table 3–1**
M-Mode Left Ventricle Dimension Compared with 2-D Minor Diameter

| Difference (mm) | Number of Patients |
| --- | --- |
| 0–3 | 15 |
| 4–6 | 16 |
| >6 | 19 |

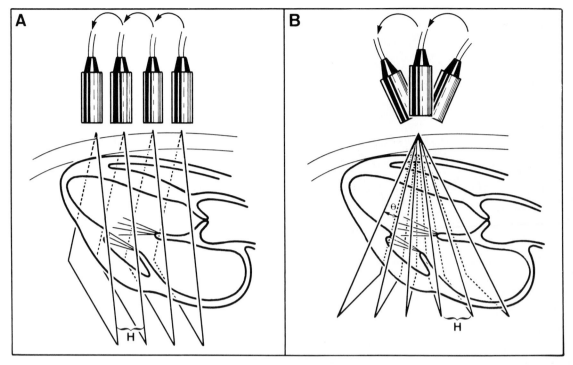

**Fig. 3–12.** Diagram of Simpson's rule. *A,* Parallel slices of the left ventricle are obtained by moving the transducer linearly across the heart. *B,* Divergent short-axis scans are obtained by angulating the transducer between scans. H = distance between echocardiographic slices. (From Rogers, E.W., Feigenbaum, H., and Weyman, A.E.: Echocardiography for quantitation of cardiac chambers. *In* Progress in Cardiology. Vol. 8. Edited by P.N. Yu and J.F. Goodwin. Philadelphia, Lea & Febiger, 1979.)

one needs to know the angle at which the transducer is directed.[22] Slices made by changing the angles of the transducer require more complicated calculations than do linear slices (Fig. 3–12*A*). Unfortunately, because of the interference of ribs, a simple examination such as that shown in Figure 3–12*A* is practical only in young infants in whom the ribs do not obstruct the examination.

Because of the limitations in obtaining multiple short-axis examinations, most investigators are using a modified approach to Simpson's rule. One approach is to use an apical two-chamber examination of the left ventricle in combination with a short-axis examination at the level of the papillary muscle. The endocardial borders of the two views are digitally traced. Then, a computer uses a modification of Simpson's rule to calculate the volumes. Each projection is divided into 20 sections along the common axis, because the two views are orthogonal to each other. As expected, the mathematics involved are somewhat complicated, but not for a computer. A more common way of using Simpson's rule is to use either or both the two-chamber and four-chamber views. The combined method of using both apical views is preferred. A recent ASE document on two-dimensional measurements recommends the modified Simpson's rule technique with the two-chamber and four-chamber views (Fig. 3–13).[23]

Other methods have been used to measure left ventricular volumes using two-dimensional echocardiography. The left ventricle can also be described as a ''bullet,'' which is a cylinder and half a prolate ellipse. The basal half of the left ventricle has a cylinder, and the apical half is a partial prolate ellipse. The volume formula is ⅚ the cross-sectional area of the cylinder times the length of the total object (V = ⅚ AL). The area would be the cross-sectional area of a short-axis left ventricular examination at the level of the papillary muscles. The long axis of the left ventricle can be measured from the apex to the mitral annulus using either an apical two-chamber or four-chamber examination. The simplicity of this approach makes it an attractive possibility for routine clinical use; however, it is limited if there is any irregularity in the shape of the left ventricle.

Another attempt at obtaining a simplified two-dimensional measurements is a technique proposed for calculating volumes from a series of minor axis dimensions.[24,25] These authors suggest making three minor-axis dimensions of the left ventricle using apical four-chamber and two-chamber views (Fig. 3–14), and two minor axis dimensions using the parasternal long-axis view (Fig. 3–15). This technique only attempts to measure ejection fraction and not the actual volumes. One can either measure the length in diastole and systole or estimate the change in length qualitatively for making the ejection fraction measurements.

The increasing use of computers for echocardiographic measurements will most likely lead to their use for calculating volumes. As a result, which formula one uses to calculate left ventricular volumes is not important. The more complicated but more accurate, modified Simpson's rule is probably the preferred technique and simplified versions are not really necessary.

## LV VOLUME

### BY METHOD OF DISCS (MODIFIED SIMPSON'S RULE)

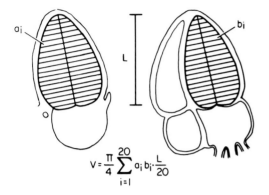

$$V = \frac{\pi}{4} \sum_{i=1}^{20} a_i \, b_i \cdot \frac{L}{20}$$

### BY SINGLE PLANE AREA LENGTH

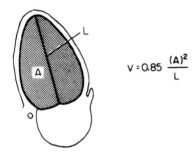

$$V = 0.85 \, \frac{(A)^2}{L}$$

**Fig. 3–13.** Diagram demonstrating how left ventricular volume can be measured using the modified Simpson's rule technique and by the single plane area length method. (From Schiller, M.B., et al.: Recommendations for quantitation of the left ventricle by two-dimensional echocardiography. J. Am. Soc. Echocardiogr., *2*:362, 1989.)

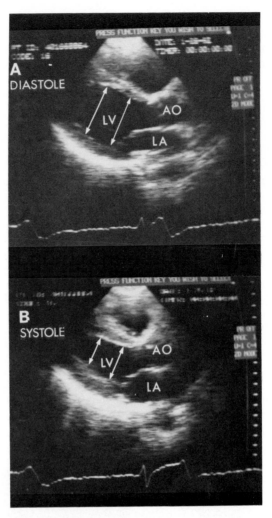

**Fig. 3–15.** Long-axis two-dimensional echocardiograms illustrating how one can obtain two minor dimensions of the left ventricle in diastole and systole. LV = left ventricle; AO = aorta; LA = left atrium.

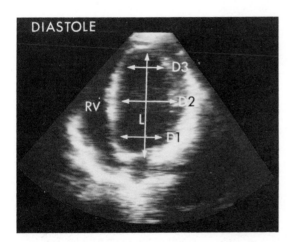

**Fig. 3–14.** Apical four-chamber, two-dimensional echocardiogram illustrating how one can utilize three minor dimensions and the length of the ventricle for calculation of ejection fraction. D1, D2, D3 = minor dimensions; L = length; RV = right ventricle.

Some investigators are using three-dimensional, spatial orientation of standard two-dimensional imaging to improve the quantitative measurements of left ventricular volumes.[25a]

Any two-dimensional technique for measuring volumes usually gives volumes that are smaller than those determined with angiography. One explanation for these differences is that echocardiography obtains tomographic views that are not necessarily the maximum dimensions. The angiographic technique relies on data from the silhouette of the angiographic dye, which visualizes the maximum distances between opposing walls. Thus, one could argue that the angiographic volumes are probably artificially too large, whereas echocardiographic volumes underestimate the true volumes. Another explanation for differences in volumes is that all of the two-dimensional echocardiographic techniques require an accurate measurement of chamber length. Unfortunately, because it is easy to foreshorten the ventricular length, the measurement may be artifactually small. In fact, when measuring left ventricular volumes, apical views are essential and one must take meticulous care to record the true apex.[26] This approach usually requires a cut out of the mattress or examining table to make certain that the transducer is over the true apex.

Another problem with two-dimensional echocardiographic calculations of left ventricular volumes is that the approach requires identification of the endocardium in the apical views. In these views, one relies on lateral resolution, and thus myocardial dropout is a frequent problem. Figure 3–16 demonstrates parasternal short-axis and apical four-chamber views from the same patient. The endocardial borders (*arrowheads*) can be appreciated in the short-axis images; however, the endocardium cannot be identified in the four-chamber views. Although echocardiographic equipment has improved over the years,[27] this lack of endocardial definition can still be a major limitation for techniques that require apical views. Investigators have tried to use color flow Doppler to identify left ventricular volume and have had some success in children.[28]

Another method for evaluating left ventricular size and function with two-dimensional echocardiography involves using spatially oriented minor axis measurements. The basis for this approach is the lengthy clinical use of M-mode measurements and the voluminous experimental data demonstrating that the left ventricle contracts through its minor axis. The principle disadvan-

tage of M-mode dimensions is that they are not consistent and rarely represent the true minor dimension. This fact became apparent with the use of two-dimensional echocardiography, an examination in which the true minor dimension could be obtained. Thus, if one wants the minor dimensions, why not use two-dimensional echocardiography?

In the parasternal long-axis view, the minor dimension of the left ventricle at the chordal level is not through the middle of the chamber. A line drawn from the posterior left ventricular wall parallel to the short axis intersects the interventricular septum close to the attachment of the aorta (Fig. 3–17). Thus, the minor dimension using the parasternal long-axis view is actually a measurement of the base of the left ventricle.[23] Figure 3–17*B* shows the systolic dimension at the base of the left ventricle. The diagram in Figure 3–18 shows that the location of the minor dimensions changes from diastole to systole because the base of the heart moves toward the apex with systole. Even though this two-dimensional fractional shortening only assesses the left ventricle at the base, this measurement has been useful in judging left ventricular function and at times is even better than using the ejection fraction.[29]

Minor axis dimensions in the long-axis view suffer from many of the same limitations as the M-mode measurements. Although one can be reasonably confident that the dimensions are consistently in the minor axis,

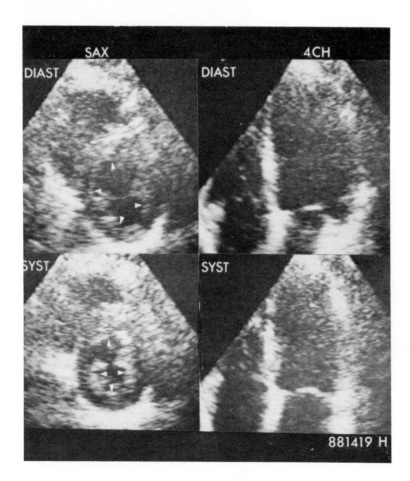

**Fig. 3–16.** Short-axis and four-chamber echocardiograms of the same patient. The endocardial echoes can be identified in the short-axis views (*arrowheads*), but are not seen in the four-chamber views.

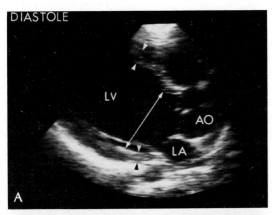

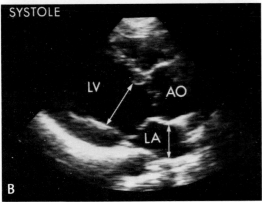

Fig. 3–17. Long-axis two-dimensional echocardiograms in diastole and systole illustrating how one can measure a minor axis dimension of the base of the left ventricle (LV), interventricular septal thickness (*upper arrowheads*), posterior left ventricular wall thickness (*lower arrowheads*), and systolic dimension of the left atrium (LA). AO = aorta.

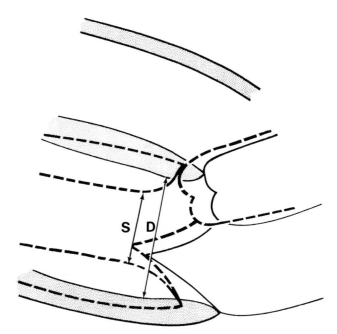

Fig. 3–18. Diagram illustrating linear dimensions of the left ventricle at the level of the base of the heart in diastole (D) and systole (S). Note how the base of the heart moves toward the apex so that the systolic measurement is more apical than is the diastolic measurement. (From Schiller, M.B., et al.: Recommendations for quantitation of the left ventricle by two-dimensional echocardiography. J. Am. Soc. Echocardiogr., 2: 362, 1989.)

the measurements only reflect the status of the base of the left ventricle and depend on only two sampling sites of the left ventricle. To overcome this problem in part, one can also measure a short-axis area at the papillary muscle level (Fig. 3–19). Because the short-axis area is at the level of the papillary muscles, the measurement is approximately in the middle portion of the left ventricular cavity and thus complements the long-axis dimensions. Not only are the two measurements from different areas of the left ventricle, but also the short-axis view includes the medial and lateral walls, which are not visualized in the long-axis examination. The short-axis area can also be combined with an apical length to provide a bullet formula measurement of the volume.

The short-axis examination also has some of the same problems as the M-mode dimensions in that it is limited by the acoustic window that is available. Because the papillary muscle level is closer to the apex than the chordal level used with M-mode dimensions, one can use the usually available lower intercostal spaces. It is easier to record the minor axis from a low interspace when examining at the papillary muscle level. Because the parasternal long-axis and short-axis views primarily use axial resolution, myocardial dropout is less of a problem than when making measurements from apical views.

## Global Systolic Function

The measurement that most cardiologists demand for global left ventricular systolic function is ejection fraction. Ejection fraction represents the percent or fraction of left ventricular diastolic volume that is ejected in systole. The measurement is made by calculating stroke volume and dividing by diastolic volume. If one uses two-dimensional echocardiography to measure volumes, then ejection fraction is a simple calculation.[30] Those who use M-mode measurements to calculate volumes can also make this determination, although its accuracy is limited. Some authors report that one can make a reasonable "eyeball" estimate of ejection fraction from the real-time two-dimensional echocardiogram without making actual measurements.[31–34]

Any systolic index or fraction can be used to assess global function. Ejection fraction uses volumes, although one can use linear dimensions to calculate fractional shortening, which is the diastolic dimensional minus the systolic dimension divided by the diastolic dimension. Fractional shortening can be calculated using M-mode or two-dimensional linear dimensions. The short-axis areas of the left ventricle provide fractional area change, which is the diastolic area minus the systolic area divided by the diastolic area. One of the advantages of fractional shortening or fractional area change is that the measurements are not squared or cubed, thus reducing the magnification of any error.

The major impetus for presenting systolic function as

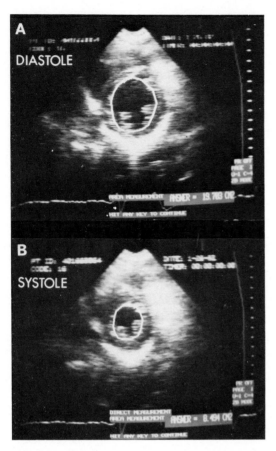

**Fig. 3–19.** Short-axis echocardiograms of the left ventricle at the level of the papillary muscles. The computer-generated circle illustrates how the cross-sectional area is obtained with exclusion of the echoes from the papillary muscles. (From Feigenbaum, H.: Echocardiography. *In* Heart Diseases, 2nd ed. Edited by E. Braunwald, Philadelphia, W.B. Saunders Co., 1984.)

"ejection fraction" is the familiarity by clinicians with this term. Furthermore, the more limited fractional shortening or fractional area change is not truly "global" if the ventricle is not contracting symmetrically to measure ejection fraction.[35] One must be aware, however, of the problems with echocardiographic calculations of volumes either with M-mode or two-dimensional techniques. Evaluating left ventricular systolic function with a combination of two-dimensional shortening and fractional area change is simpler, introduces fewer magnified potential errors, and has value even in ventricles that are not contracting symmetrically (see Chapter 8, Coronary Artery Disease). It must be remembered, however, that all systolic indices are preload and afterload dependent.[36]

M-mode measurements have been used extensively for assessing left ventricular performance. Table 3–2 lists some of these measurements. Left ventricular ejection fraction and fractional shortening are numbers 2 and 4 on this table. Circumferential shortening is a way of converting the diameter into circumference and obtaining a systolic index.[37–41] Introducing ejection time pro-

vides a measurement of mean rate of circumferential shortening (mean Vcf).[42] Some investigators also use the excursion of the interventricular septum and posterior left ventricular endocardium for assessing left ventricular function (Fig. 3–20).[43,44] One may measure the slope of the posterior ventricular wall motion ($\Delta EN/\Delta t$). Another technique is to divide the endocardial amplitude by the ejection time (see Table 3–2). This measurement can be normalized for left ventricular diastolic dimension with a formula of ENa/LVIDd × E.T. The amount and rate of left ventricular wall thickening have also been used as a marker of function.[45–48]

Doppler echocardiography can be used for determining global left ventricular systolic function. As noted in Chapter 4, the aortic Doppler velocity can be used to measure left ventricular stroke volume. The aortic velocity time integral also can give an assessment of left ventricular performance (Fig. 3–21).[49–52] The initial half of the velocity time integral, up to the peak velocity, has been used to calculate "ejection force." Some data

---

**Table 3–2**
**M-mode Echocardiographic Measurement of Left Ventricular Performance**

1. Posterior left ventricular wall velocity (cm/sec)

    a. Mean velocity $= \dfrac{Ena}{E.T.}$

    ENA = amplitude of motion of posterior left ventricular endocardium
    E.T. = ejection time

    b. Normalized velocity $= \dfrac{ENa}{LVIDd \times E.T.}$

    LVIDd = diastolic left ventricle internal dimension

2. Left ventricular ejection fraction (E.F.) (%)

    $$E.F. = \frac{LV\ diastolic\ volume - LV\ systolic\ volume}{LV\ diastolic\ volume}$$

    or

    $$E.F. = \frac{LV\ stroke\ volume}{LV\ diastolic\ volume}$$

3. Circumferential shortening of left ventricle (fraction)

    a. $\dfrac{Diastolic\ circumference - systolic\ circumference}{Diastolic\ circumference}$

    or

    $\dfrac{\pi\ LBIDd - LVIDs}{\pi\ LVIDd}$

    or

    $\dfrac{\pi\ (LVIDd - LVIDs)}{\pi\ LVIDd}$

    or

    $\dfrac{LVIDd - LVIDs}{LVIDd}$

    b. Mean rate of circumferential shortening (mean Vcf) (circumferences/sec)

    $$mean\ Vcf = \frac{LVID - LVIDs}{LVIDd \times E.T.}$$

4. Fractional shortening of left ventricle (%)

    $$\frac{LVIDd - LVIDs}{LVIDd} \times 100$$

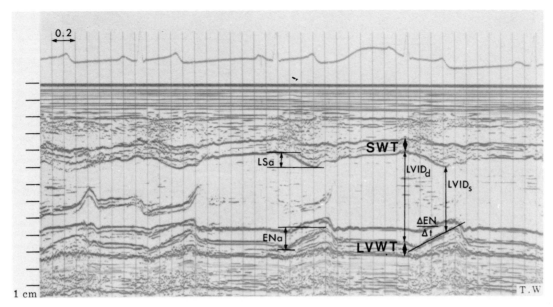

**Fig. 3–20.** M-mode echocardiogram of the left ventricle. LSa = amplitude of motion of the left side of the septum; ENa = amplitude of motion of the posterior left ventricular endocardium; SWT = septal wall thickness; LVWT = left ventricular wall thickness; LVID$_d$ = left ventricular diastolic internal dimension; LVID$_s$ = left ventricular systolic internal dimension; $\Delta$EN/$\Delta$t = rate of motion of the posterior left ventricular endocardium.

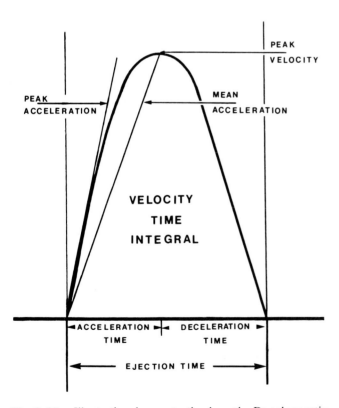

**Fig. 3–21.** Illustration demonstrating how the Doppler aortic flow can be used to obtain information concerning left ventricular systolic function. All of the measurements have been used as indicators of systolic function.

indicate that the rate or acceleration that blood leaves the left ventricle reflects the strength of left ventricular contraction. The peak acceleration is the first derivative of the aortic flow velocity, but it is difficult to measure.[53,54] An easier calculation is the slope between the onset of ejection and peak velocity, which is mean acceleration. As with almost all global assessments, these Doppler measurements are again preload and afterload dependent[55–57] and are influenced by heart rate.[58,59]

Another method of using Doppler echocardiography to assess left ventricular systolic function is to examine Doppler flow in patients who have mitral regurgitation.[60–63] The diagram in Figure 3–22 shows the relationship of a continuous wave Doppler recording of mitral regurgitation and corresponding left-sided intracardiac pressures. The rate with which the left ventricular pressure rises (dp/dt) is a measure of left ventricular contractility. The rate of rise of left ventricular pressure will be reflected by the rate that mitral regurgitant blood moves from the left ventricle into the left atrium. Figure 3–23 shows a patient with mitral regurgitation in which the rate of rise of the mitral regurgitant jet is rapid, giving a dp/dt of 1800 mm Hg/sec. Another patient with mitral regurgitation and a poor left ventricle (Fig. 3–23) has a slower rise in the mitral regurgitant velocity, giving a dp/dt of 800 mm Hg/sec. The formula in Figure 3–22 shows how to calculate the dp/dt from dv/dt. One takes two points along the slope of the mitral regurgitant flow, calculates the pressure gradient between the left ventricle and the left atrium at each point, and divides by the time between those two points. For convenience, one can make the first determination at 1 M/sec and the second at 3 M/sec. Using the modified Bernoulli equation, the 1 M/sec point is 4 mm Hg. The 3 M/sec is 36 mm Hg.

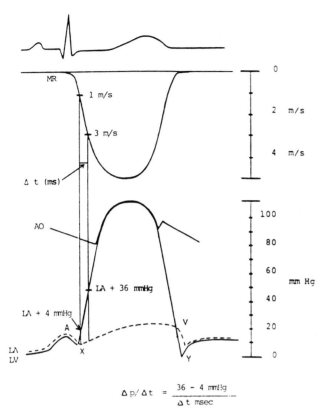

$$\Delta p / \Delta t = \frac{36 - 4 \ \text{mmHg}}{\Delta t \ \text{msec}}$$

**Fig. 3–22.** Drawing illustrating how the rate of rise of a mitral regurgitation (MR) jet can be used to determine the rate of rise of left ventricular (LV) pressure. The time required ($\Delta t$) that it takes for the mitral regurgitant velocity to go from 1 M/sec to 3 M/sec (m/s) is the same time interval that it takes for the left ventricular systolic pressure to rise from 4 to 36 mm Hg. From these data, $\Delta p / \Delta t$ can be calculated. LA = left atrium; AO, aorta. (From Pai, R.G., et al.: Doppler-derived rate of left ventricular pressure rise: Its correlation with the post-operative left ventricular function in mitral regurgitation. *Circulation, 82:*515, 1990, by permission of the American Heart Association, Inc.)

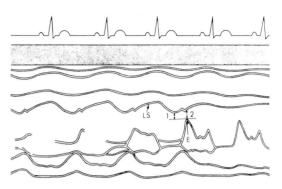

**Fig. 3–24.** Diagram of an M-mode echocardiogram demonstrating two ways of measuring the distance between the E point of the mitral valve and the left septal echo. E-point septal separation *number 1* represents the distance between the peak downward motion of the septum and the maximum upward excursion of the E point. E-point septal separation *number 2* represents the distance between the mitral valve and the septum at the time of the E point. LS = left side of the interventricular septum.

Thus, one can calculate dp/dt by dividing the difference or 32 mm Hg by dt in milliseconds.

A relatively simple echocardiographic measurement for assessing global systolic function is the mitral E-point septal separation.[64–70] This measurement is usually obtained from the M-mode echocardiogram (Fig. 3–24). Normally, the distance between the E point and the left side of the septum is less than 1 cm. Although this measurement is simple, a reasonable rationale is behind it. As the left ventricle dilates, the septum moves anteriorly. Mitral valve motion is influenced by the amount of blood flowing through the mitral valve. Thus, the excursion of the mitral valve at the E point reflects the flow through the valve. Because decreased amplitude of the mitral valve E point indicates reduced flow or stroke volume and anterior displacement of the septum indicates increased diastolic volume, it is reasonable to

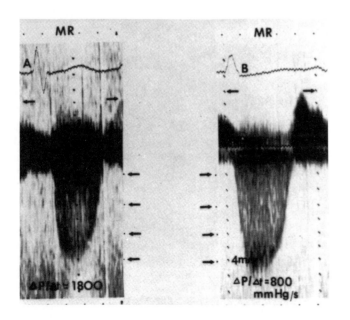

**Fig. 3–23.** Continuous wave Doppler of two patients with mitral regurgitation (MR). In patient A, the mitral regurgitant jet rises rapidly and provides a $\Delta p / \Delta t$ of 1800 mm Hg/sec. In patient B, the rise in velocity is slower and provides a calculated $\Delta p / \Delta t$ of 800 mm Hg/sec. (From Pai, R.G., et al.: Doppler-derived rate of left ventricular pressure rise: Its correlation with the post-operative left ventricular function in mitral regurgitation. *Circulation, 82:*515, 1990, by permission of the American Heart Association, Inc.)

expect an increase in the distance between the mitral valve E point and the interventricular septum with a decreased ejection fraction. There are, of course, inherent limitations. In a patient with intrinsic valve disease, such as mitral stenosis, the excursion of the mitral valve is not a reliable indicator of flow through that orifice. In patients with aortic insufficiency, mitral valve flow is not an indicator of total left ventricular stroke volume. In addition, with aortic regurgitation, the regurgitant jet may distort the excursion of the mitral valve. Furthermore, the diastolic volume may be increased by segmental dilatation or aneurysm formation that may not produce anterior displacement of the septum.

Investigators have also been using descent of the mitral annulus as an indicator of global left ventricular function.[71-74] It has been recognized for many years that the base of the heart moves whereas the apex contributes little to the ejection of blood. In an early observation, investigators used an M-mode tracing of annular motion to calculate left ventricular stroke volume.[74a,74b] The latest efforts involve the use of two-dimensional echocardiography, whereby the extent of descent of the base of the left ventricle relates to global left ventricular function (Fig. 3–25).

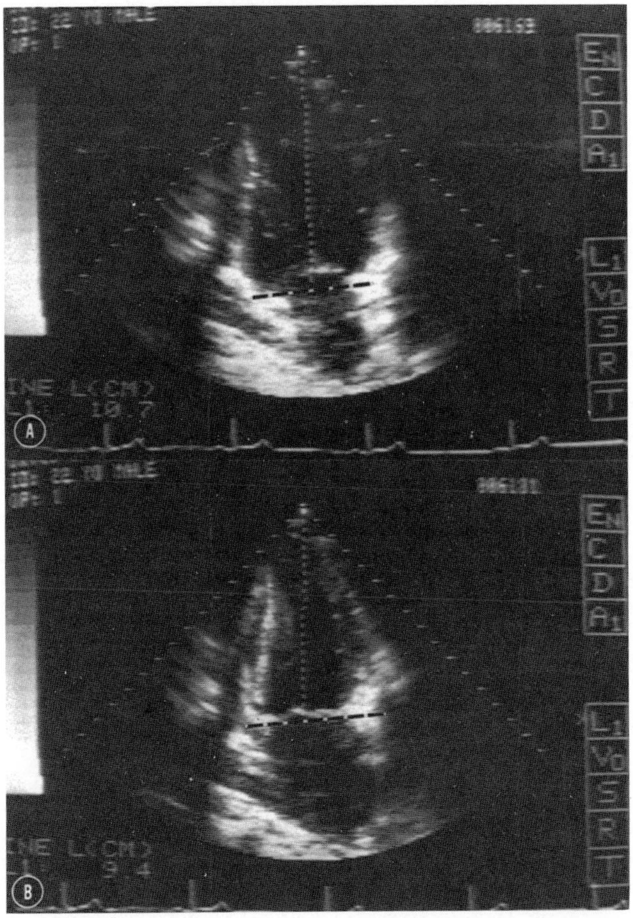

### Regional Systolic Function

One of the major advantages of two-dimensional echocardiography is that the technique provides tomographic views of the left ventricle and is ideal for assessing regional left ventricular function. This two-dimensional examination is able to visualize portions of the left ventricle that are hidden from view even with the "gold standard," contrast ventriculography. It is possible to assess regional function in many ways. The easiest and most common technique is to qualitatively analyze wall motion in real time and to indicate which segments are moving abnormally. The problem with a totally qualitative assessment is that it is subjective, and the observer frequently notices the most striking abnormalities and may overlook subtle findings.

A more systematic way to assess regional wall motion is to divide the ventricle into regions or segments. The number of segments can vary from 9 to 20 among different investigators. The original ASE document on this subject divided the left ventricle into 20 different areas. For reasons described in Chapter 2, the Society changed the recommendation and chose a 16-segment approach.[23] One of the justifications for making this change is the fact that dividing the short axis into six segments rather than eight produced a rational relationship between the three longitudinal views (long axis, two chamber, and four chamber) and the short-axis presentation (Fig. 3–26). Furthermore, one could relate the various segments to coronary artery distribution more conveniently. Figure 3–27 shows the 16 segments chosen by the Society. One can identify all 16 segments with either the longitudinal views or a series of three short-axis views. The short axis at the mitral and papillary muscle levels are divided into six segments, whereas the short axis at the apex has four divisions. This relationship works well because the four apical segments can be derived from the four-chamber and two-chamber apical views. The parasternal long-axis view does not visualize the apex and thus does not contribute. The longitudinal and short-axis examinations complement each other and give one the opportunity to look at essentially the same segments in more than one view.

The second component to using a segmental approach to analyzing regional ventricular function is to arbitrarily designate a number to indicate wall motion. Again, various investigators have used different schemes. An increasing numeric value may indicate either better or worsening wall motion. Obviously, any method is purely arbitrary. The scheme adopted by the ASE is to give a normal segment the value "one." Abnormal segments have higher numbers. A hypokinetic segment is given the value of two, akinetic is three, dyskinetic is four, and aneurysmal is five. Figure 3–28 shows a computer-generated regional evaluation of a patient using this 16-segment approach. In this example, four views were used for regional wall analysis. Each segment was as-

**Fig. 3–25.** Two-dimensional echocardiograms in diastole (*A*) and systole (*B*) showing how one can measure the excursion of the mitral annulus (*dashed line*). (From Simonson, J.S., et al.: Descent of the base of the left ventricle: An echocardiographic index of left ventricular function. J. Am. Soc. Echocardiogr., 2:27, 1989.)

## Relationship of Two-Dimensional Views And Coronary Artery Perfusion

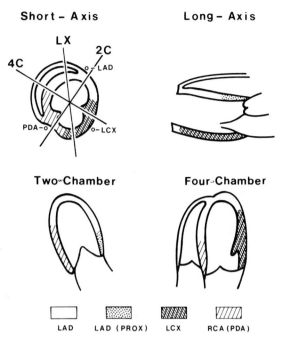

Short – Axis          Long – Axis

Two-Chamber          Four-Chamber

LAD    LAD (PROX)    LCX    RCA (PDA)

**Fig. 3–26.** Diagrams demonstrating the relationships of two-dimensional echocardiographic views and coronary artery perfusion. The long-axis, two-chamber, and four-chamber views intersect with the short-axis view. The various coronary artery perfusion beds can also be predicted reasonably well with the two-dimensional echocardiographic views.

signed a value. The patient had a fairly classic anterior myocardial infarction with an obstruction of the left anterior descending artery past the first septal perforator. Thus, all of the segments perfused by the middle and distal left anterior descending artery are akinetic (three). This particular computer program also indicates whether the segments are scarred. Akinetic with scar is given a value of six and dyskinetic with scar is given a value of seven. The designation of six and seven, however, is merely to indicate scar. For scoring purposes, akinetic with scar is still given a value of three and dyskinetic with scar is still given a value of four. The left ventricular wall motion score index is derived by totalling the scores and dividing by the number of segments scored. If a segment cannot be seen, this computer program labels it with an X. Nonscored segments are eliminated from the calculation. If a large number of segments are not seen, then the reliability of the resultant index is limited.

This particular program also calculates the percentages of normal segments and lists it as ''percent normal muscle.'' This value indicates the amount of normally contracting ventricle.

Some score index programs have a value for hyperkinesis. Hyperkinesis is a common finding with acute ischemia or with stress testing. If one uses hyperkinesis for a global score index, then the ultimate number becomes similar to ejection fraction, which is essentially

### REGIONAL WALL SEGMENTS

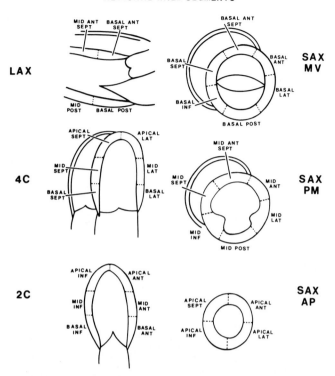

**Fig. 3–27.** Diagram demonstrating the location of the 16-segment approach to dividing the left ventricle. All 16 segments can be identified either with three longitudinal views, long-axis (LAX), four-chamber (4C), two-chamber (2C), three short-axis views at the mitral valve level (SAX MV), the papillary muscle level (SAX PM), or apical level (SAX AP).

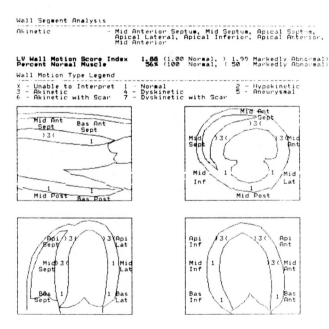

**Fig. 3–28.** Computer-generated regional wall motion report showing the 16 segments in four two-dimensional views. The diagrams identify the motion of each segment and calculate a left ventricular motion score index as well as percent normal muscle.

a summation of regional function.[75,75a] One problem in including hyperkinesis is that this number can mask a hypokinetic or akinetic area. This problem is inherent with any global measurement of a regional problem. For example, if the inferior wall is akinetic and the anterior wall is hyperkinetic, the score index may still be normal; the number would not reflect the full extent of the abnormality. A way of getting around this problem is to subdivide the score index into anterior and posterior-inferior regions. One may even divide the score index according to coronary artery distribution. Under these circumstances, one can reintroduce hyperkinesis and still appreciate the full extent of the abnormalities. Figure 3–29 illustrates a computer-generated wall motion report whereby hyperkinesis is an option and both global and regional score indices are calculated. The report also depicts the left ventricle as a ''bulls eye'' so that all 16 segments can be illustrated at once. This type of display is particularly convenient when multiple measurements are obtained with stress testing.

The score index is a qualitative evaluation. It is still better than the totally visual description because the score index forces the physician to analyze each segment. This type of evaluation is easier if the echocardiogram is recorded digitally and analyzed in a quad screen cine loop. Subtle wall motion abnormalities are easier to detect with this approach. Because of the cine loop nature of the recording, one can use a stationary marker as a reference to see whether or not a wall is moving. Figure 3–30 shows that the relationship of a circular

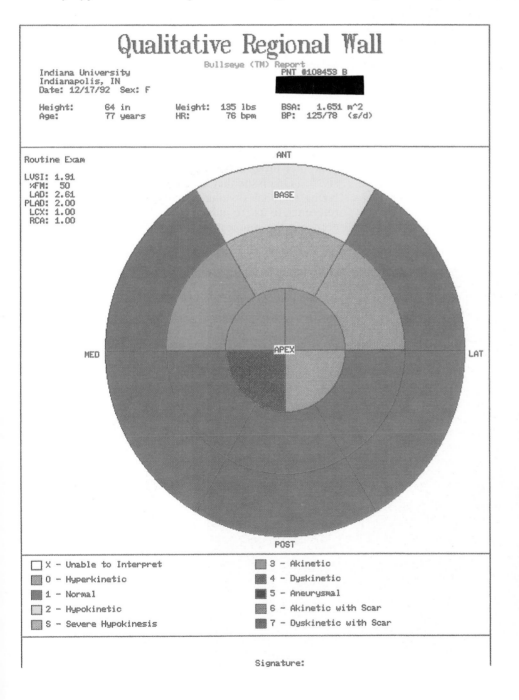

**Fig. 3–29.** Computer-generated qualitative regional wall report displaying the 16 segments of the left ventricle in a ''bull's eye'' presentation. This diagram is presented as if visualizing the left ventricle from the apex and viewing the left ventricle as three short-axis presentations. The wall motion is encoded in varying shades of color. This particular program has hyperkinesis and severe hypokinesis as options. Severe hypokinesis is given a score of 2.5, and hyperkinesis is 0. The score indices are also subdivided into coronary artery distribution indices.

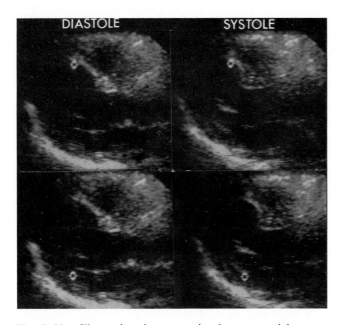

**Fig. 3–30.** Illustration demonstrating how one might use a calibrated marker to try to better quantitate the degree of wall motion. This 10-mm diameter circle shows no motion from diastole to systole of the anterior septum; however, an approximately 10-mm excursion of the posterior left ventricular wall from diastole to systole is revealed (lower echocardiograms).

marker to the akinetic distal septum is unchanged from diastole to systole. When the marker is placed at the basal portion of the normally contracting lateral wall, however, the marker is at the edge of the endocardium in diastole and in the middle of the myocardium in systole. This technique can increase the sensitivity and reliability of judging wall motion. The marker could be calibrated so that one could judge the extent of excursion. One can enlarge on this approach by colorizing the end-diastolic frame differently from systole (Fig. 3–31). Those wall segments that move well produce a rim of red. When no motion occurs, the red is absent (*arrowheads*).

The digital technique permits one to analyze wall motion frame-by-frame to evaluate not only how but also when the wall segments move. Ischemia may produce "tardokinesis" whereby wall motion is delayed. Analyzing multiple views simultaneously with a quad screen display helps confirm wall motion abnormalities by seeing them in more than one view. For all of these reasons, the qualitative regional wall score index, especially using digital recordings, is probably the most practical technique currently available for the everyday analysis of regional systolic function.

For those who wish to take the time to obtain a more quantitative analysis of regional function, a variety of computer programs are available for this type of analysis.[76,77] One issue that needs to be addressed when analyzing regional systolic function quantitatively is what reference to use to judge segmental motion. A fixed reference is the simplest, but if the heart moves during the

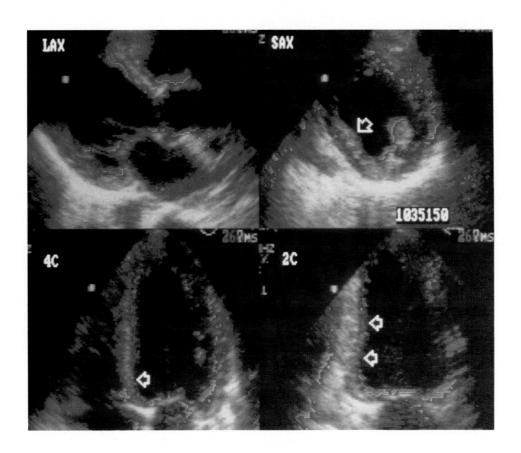

**Fig. 3–31.** Colorized digital echocardiograms showing moving wall motion in rims of red. Those areas that do not move show no red rim (*arrows*).

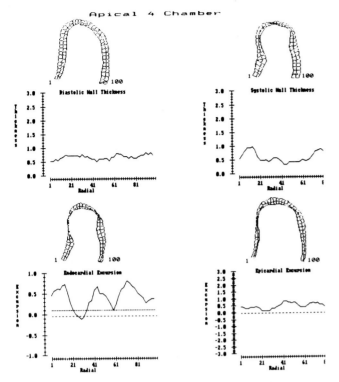

**Fig. 3–32.** Computer-generated quantitative assessment of regional wall motion. This calculation requires tracing the endocardial borders of the apical four-chamber view in diastole and systole. This program also uses tracing of the epicardial borders. With this information, it is possible to calculate and display diastolic and systolic wall thickness as well as endocardial and epicardial excursions.

cardiac cycle, error is introduced. A method of overcoming this problem calculates center of mass of the left ventricle in diastole and systole.[78,79] The centers are superimposed and segmental motion is compared to that point. The problem with this approach is that it masks or minimizes real wall motion abnormalities and probably introduces more error than just using a fixed reference system.

A popular current technique involves the centerline analysis. By tracing the diastolic and systolic endocardial outlines, the computer calculates the centerline between the two tracings and judges motion compared to that centerline. One can also enlarge on that analysis by including wall thickness, which requires tracing the epicardial echoes as well. Figure 3–32 shows a computer-generated report using the centerline analysis method. This particular program includes wall thickness. This same program also calculates regional ejection fractions and regional segment area changes (Fig. 3–33). This approach is clearly more quantitative and objective, although it requires high-quality echocardiographic recordings and is more time consuming than the qualitative technique.

Some investigators have also looked at the descent of the base of the heart from both a global and regional perspective. The global assessment using the base of the left ventricle has already been described. Figure 3–34 shows how one can use the motion of the mitral annulus to indicate whether anterior or posterior-inferior akinesis is present. If the corresponding wall is dysfunctioning, then that portion of the annulus will not move as well as that attached to normal muscle.

**Diastolic Function**

Virtually every echocardiographic technique has been used to evaluate left ventricular diastolic function. This

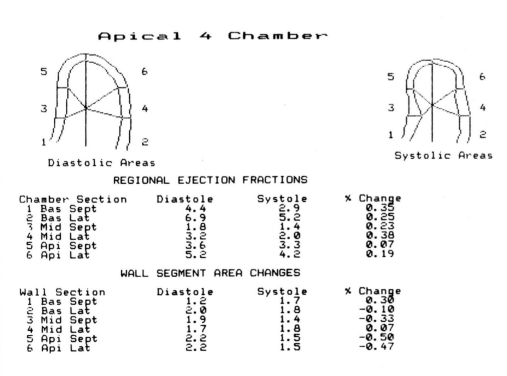

REGIONAL EJECTION FRACTIONS

| Chamber Section | Diastole | Systole | % Change |
|---|---|---|---|
| 1 Bas Sept | 4.4 | 2.9 | 0.35 |
| 2 Bas Lat | 6.9 | 5.2 | 0.25 |
| 3 Mid Sept | 1.8 | 1.4 | 0.23 |
| 4 Mid Lat | 3.2 | 2.0 | 0.38 |
| 5 Api Sept | 3.6 | 3.3 | 0.07 |
| 6 Api Lat | 5.2 | 4.2 | 0.19 |

WALL SEGMENT AREA CHANGES

| Wall Section | Diastole | Systole | % Change |
|---|---|---|---|
| 1 Bas Sept | 1.2 | 1.7 | 0.30 |
| 2 Bas Lat | 2.0 | 1.8 | -0.10 |
| 3 Mid Sept | 1.9 | 1.4 | -0.33 |
| 4 Mid Lat | 1.7 | 1.8 | 0.07 |
| 5 Api Sept | 2.2 | 1.5 | -0.50 |
| 6 Api Lat | 2.2 | 1.5 | -0.47 |

**Fig. 3–33.** Another computer-generated, quantitative, regional wall motion program. In this case, regional ejection fractions and wall segment area changes are calculated.

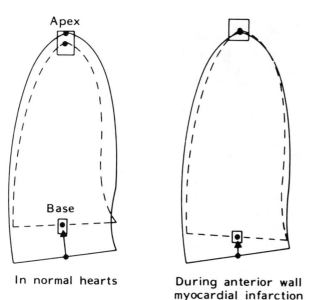

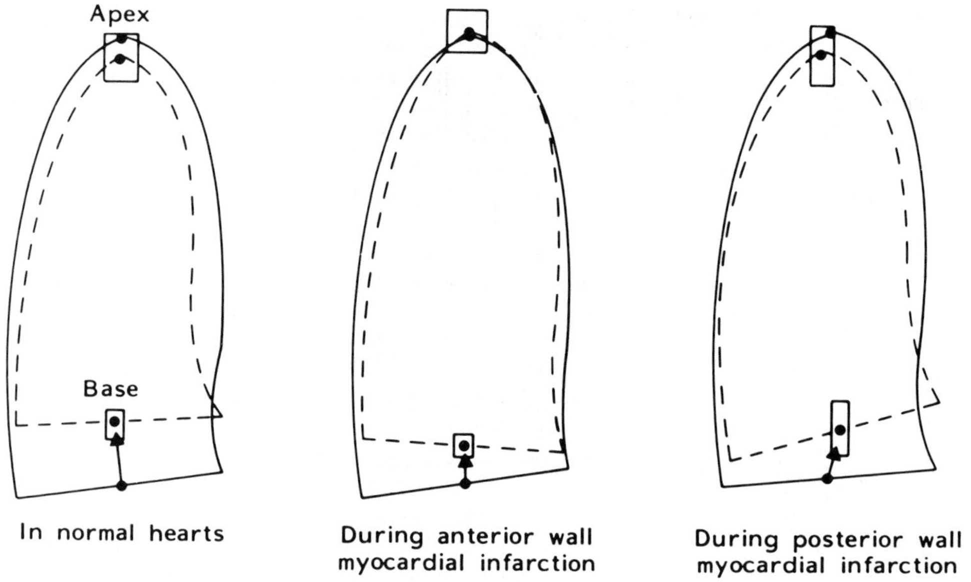

In normal hearts

During anterior wall
myocardial infarction

During posterior wall
myocardial infarction

**Fig. 3–34.** Diagram showing how excursion of the base of the heart can provide regional as well as global assessment. That portion of the mitral annulus involved with infarction does not move as well as the opposing wall without infarction. (From Assman, P.E., et al.: Two-dimensional echocardiographic analysis of the dynamic geometry of the left ventricle. The basis for an improved model of wall motion. J. Am. Soc. Echocardiogr., 6: 396, 1988.)

aspect of the left ventricle is clearly more complicated and is still unsettled.[80] Spectral Doppler is currently the technique of choice for evaluating left ventricular diastolic function.[80a,81–91] Figure 3–35 illustrates the relationship between left ventricular inflow velocities and left ventricular and atrial pressures. Figure 3–35A shows

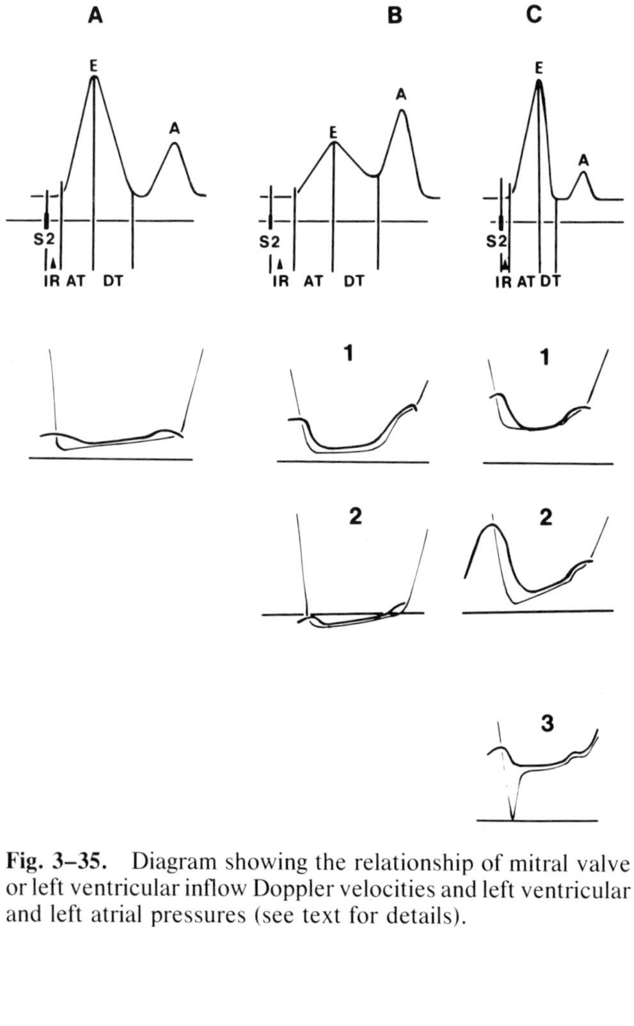

**Fig. 3–35.** Diagram showing the relationship of mitral valve or left ventricular inflow Doppler velocities and left ventricular and left atrial pressures (see text for details).

the normal situation. The early inflow of blood reaches a peak at the E point. Flow then decelerates until atrial systole, at which time the left atrial pressure rises above the left ventricular pressure and flow again passes through the mitral valve. Figure 3–36 shows an example of normal mitral flow.

Alterations in left ventricular diastolic function may reduce the height of the E wave and increase the height of the A wave (Figs. 3–35B and 3–37). This type of abnormality is usually accompanied by prolongation of the isovolumic relaxation time (IR),[91a,91b] and prolongation of the deceleration time (DT). The hemodynamic abnormalities responsible for this pattern usually are reduced left ventricular relaxation and slower fall in left ventricular pressure (Fig. 3–35B-1). This situation occurs with left ventricular hypertrophy,[92–94] myocardial ischemia, cardiomyopathy, or even normal aging. Atrial contraction occurs with an incompletely empty left atrium and blood is propelled into the left ventricle with increased velocity accounting for the heightened A wave.

This pattern of left ventricular filling can also be seen with a decrease in the filling pressure of the left ventricle (Fig. 3–35B-2). If there is dehydration or hypovolemia, or if flow into the left side of the heart is reduced because of pulmonary hypertension, the low filling pressure will also reduce early diastolic filling of the left ventricle. Systemic vasodilators could also produce a similar effect.

The other pathologic pattern that is seen with mitral flow velocities is the reverse—a tall E wave and a short A wave (Fig. 3–35C, Fig. 3–38). This pattern is accompanied by short isovolumic relaxation and deceleration times. This type of mitral flow can be produced by elevated left ventricular filling pressures (Fig. 3–35C-1), as may occur with congestive heart failure or reduced compliance. With elevated early diastolic pressures (Fig. 3–35C-2), the flow into the left ventricle is accelerated, and there may be relatively little blood to propel with atrial systole. Mitral regurgitation with a tall V wave in left atrial pressure will produce a large E-wave

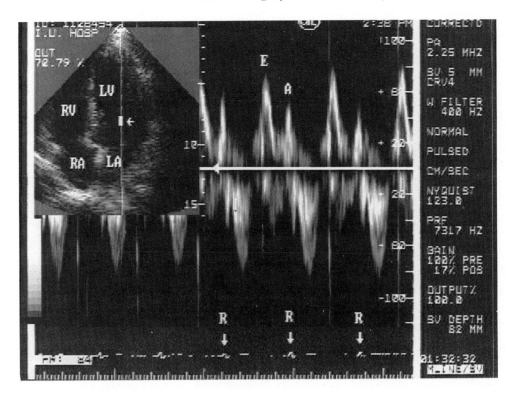

**Fig. 3–36.** Normal Doppler mitral valve flow. LV = left ventricle; RV = right ventricle; RA = right atrium; LA = left atrium.

velocity. A third pathologic situation that produces a similar pattern is restrictive or constrictive left ventricular filling (Fig. 3–35C-3). Under these circumstances, an initial rapid drop in left ventricular pressure is such so that the gradient between the left atrium and the left ventricle is high, producing accelerated flow into the left ventricle; however, the restriction or constriction causes the left ventricular pressure to rebound rapidly,

and flow into the left atrium stops abruptly. The constriction or restriction also limits atrial filling of the ventricle any further and the A wave is diminished.

In summary, basically three recognized patterns of mitral flow or left ventricular inflow have clinical significance. The first is the normal pattern in which the E wave is somewhat higher than the A wave. The second pattern is when the E wave is lower than the A wave,

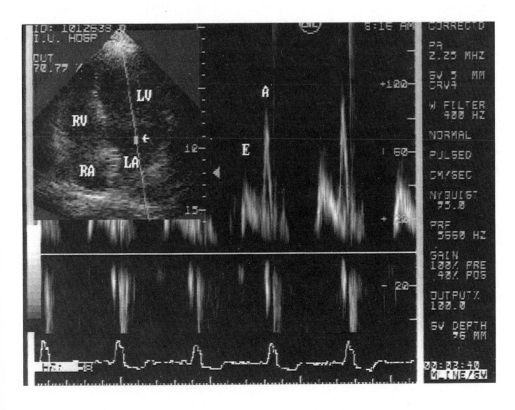

**Fig. 3–37.** Left ventricular inflow Doppler examination in a patient with abnormal left ventricular relaxation and short E wave and tall A wave. LV = left ventricle; RV = right ventricle; RA = right atrium; LA = left atrium.

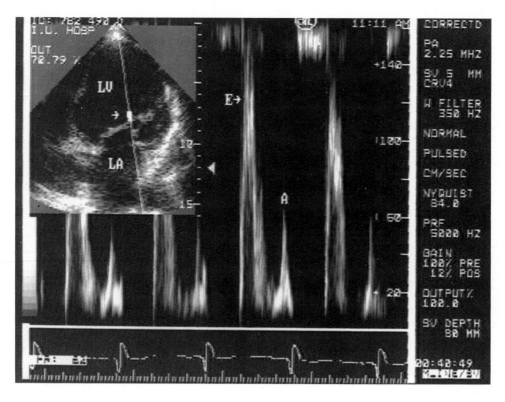

**Fig. 3–38.** Pulsed Doppler left ventricular inflow recording of a patient with reduced left ventricular compliance and a tall E wave and short A wave. LV = left ventricle; LA = left atrium.

and the third is when the E wave is taller and the A wave is reduced. In some disease states, the initial pathologic pattern is abnormal relaxation with a short E wave and a tall A wave. If mitral regurgitation or congestive heart failure raises the left ventricular filling pressure, then the pattern may reverse and the E wave will become taller and the A wave will become shorter. Thus, a transition situation can occur whereby "pseudo normalization" of the mitral flow can occur.[94a] One might find a patient with an essentially normal mitral flow pattern that is actually a transition between one type and the other.

To complicate matters even further, as already noted, normal aging produces a type 3–35B inflow.[95-101] One can usually expect patients older than age 45 or 50 years to have such a pattern. Figure 3–39 shows right ventricular and left ventricular inflow in a 28-year-old man and in a 66-year-old man. The E to A ratios across both orifices reverse with age.[102,103,103a] Heart rate,[104-107] preload[108-112] and afterload[113-116] systolic function,[117-119] and autonomic stimulation[120] or blockade[121] will have major effects on mitral flow patterns. Thus, one must include all of these factors when analyzing diastolic function using Doppler techniques.[122] In addition, as noted in Chapter 2, the location of the Doppler sample volume influences the pattern of flow recorded.[123]

Pulmonary venous flow also reflects changes in left ventricular diastolic function (Fig. 3–40).[124] With reduced early relaxation, the diastolic component decreases and the reversed A wave increases (Fig. 3–40B). When early filling is rapid (Fig. 3–40C), the pulmonary venous flow exhibits almost no systolic phase and tall diastolic and atrial components.

M-mode echocardiography has been used extensively to assess left ventricular diastolic function. An early observation was that the mitral valve E to F or diastolic slope was prolonged in patients with abnormal filling of the left ventricle. Such a situation might occur with left ventricular hypertrophy.

A useful M-mode observation involves mitral valve closure.[125,126] Normally, the mitral valve begins to close with atrial relaxation and completes closure with ventricular contraction. This closure is smooth and uninter-

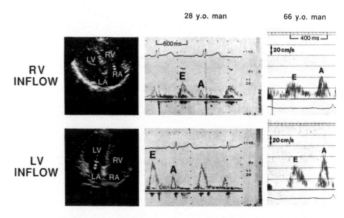

**Fig. 3–39.** Right ventricular inflow and left ventricular inflow Doppler studies of a 28-year-old man and a 66-year-old man. The E wave decreases and the A wave increases with aging. LV = left ventricle; RV = right ventricle; LA = left atrium; RA = right atrium. (From Soghbi, W.A., et al.: Doppler assessment of right ventricular filling in a normal population comparison with left ventricular filling dynamics. *Circulation,* 82:1317, 1990, by permission of the American Heart Association, Inc.)

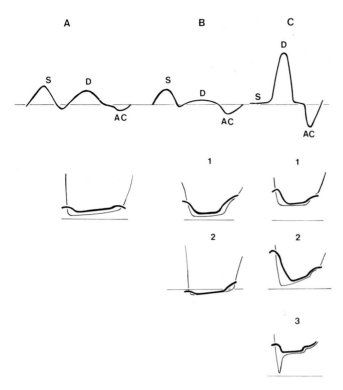

**Fig. 3–40.** Diagram demonstrating the relationship of pulmonary venous flow to left ventricular and left atrial pressure (see text for details).

rupted (Fig. 3–41*A*). In patients with abnormal ventricular performance as characterized by a tall A wave in left ventricular pressure, one commonly sees alteration in mitral closure whereby the B point is interrupted immediately before ventricular contraction (Fig. 3–41*B*). Although investigators originally thought that one could use this finding to quantitate left ventricular diastolic pressure, later studies showed that the correlation was unreliable. An index relating the A to C points as a function of the electrocardiographic PR interval was derived, but it proved not to be useful and essentially has been abandoned. The qualitative appearance of a "B bump" or notch on the mitral valve, however, still can be helpful in identifying patients who have elevated left ventricular diastolic pressure secondary to a tall A wave. Figure 3–42 shows a fairly characteristic B bump (*arrow*) in a patient with a cardiomyopathy and elevated diastolic pressures.

Other investigators have used a more complex technique for evaluating left ventricular end-diastolic function using M-mode echocardiography. The borders of the left ventricle can be traced and digitized (Fig. 3–43).[127–132] This approach provides an instantaneous left ventricular dimension, which can be analyzed for its rate of motion. A variety of indices have been developed to use this technique for assessing global diastolic function. Some investigators have studied the diastolic motion of just the posterior left ventricular wall.[133] With increasing interest in the Doppler technique, however, the digitized M-mode approach has become less popular.

The displacement of the atrioventricular plane or annulus has been used as a measure of left ventricular diastolic function.[134] With real-time left ventricular endocardial border tracking (see Chapter 1), it is possible to record the pattern of left ventricular filling.[135] This technique is under investigation as another method for evaluating left ventricular diastolic function.

Another M-mode sign that is still used commonly for identifying left ventricular diastolic pressure occurs in patients with acute aortic regurgitation. With the influx of blood into the left ventricle from the aorta, left ventricular diastolic pressure rises to the point that it exceeds left atrial pressure and the mitral valve closes before the onset of ventricular systole (Fig. 3–44). This sign is still useful for identifying hemodynamically compromised patients with acute aortic regurgitation.

## Wall Thickness, Mass, and Stress

One of the unique features of echocardiography is its ability to measure left ventricular wall thickness. Figure 3–20 shows how an M-mode echocardiogram can be used to measure the thickness of the interventricular septum (SWT) and the posterior left ventricular wall (LVWT).[136] Two-dimensional echocardiography obviously can also be used to measure wall thickness. In some ways, the two-dimensional approach is more accurate because the M-mode beam does not always cut across the walls perpendicularly. Figure 3–45 demonstrates how septal (VS) and posterior wall (PW) thickness can be measured on a two-dimensional echocardiogram. In this particular patient, the walls are thick. Also, a small echo-free space from pericardial effusion is evident behind the heart, which helps to identify the epicardial surface of the posterior left ventricular free wall.

Left ventricular hypertrophy can be indicated by

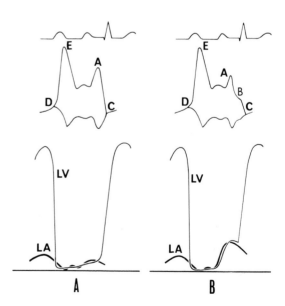

**Fig. 3–41.** Diagrams illustrating how the mitral valve echocardiogram may reflect changes in left ventricular diastolic pressure (see text for details). LV = left ventricle; LA = left atrium.

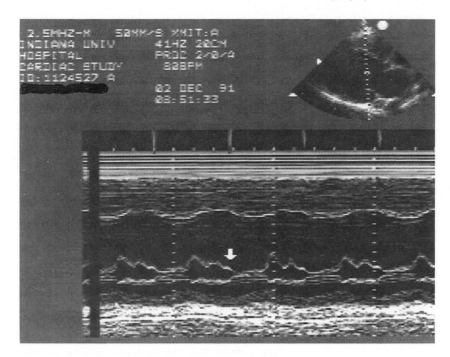

**Fig. 3–42.** M-mode mitral valve echocardiogram of a patient who exhibits incomplete closure of the mitral valve or "B" bump (*arrow*).

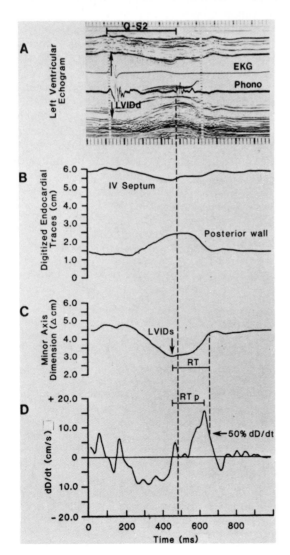

**Fig. 3–43.** Digitized M-mode echocardiogram of the left ventricle demonstrating the unprocessed M-mode recording (*A*), the digitized tracing of the interventricular septum and posterior left ventricular walls (*B*), the minor axis dimension, which is the difference between the two opposing walls (*C*), and the rate of change of the minor axis (dD/dt). LVIDd = left ventricular diastolic diameter; LVIDs = left ventricular systolic diameter; RT = relaxation time; RTp relaxation time to peak velocity of lengthening. (From Bahler, R.C., et al.: The relation of heart rate and shortening fraction to echocardiographic indexes of left ventricular relaxation in normal subjects. J. Am. Coll. Cardiol., *2*:926, 1983.)

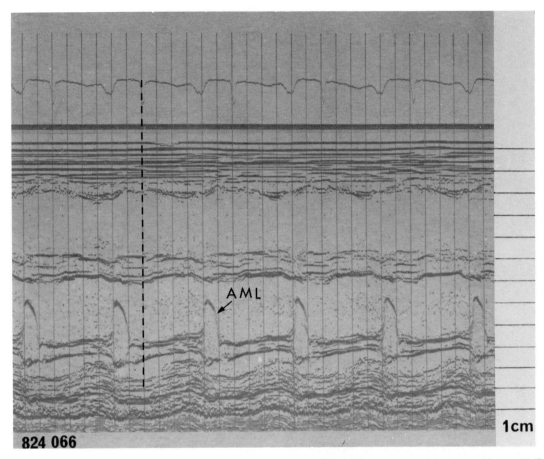

**Fig. 3–44.** M-mode recording of an anterior mitral leaflet (AML) in a patient with severe aortic regurgitation and left ventricular dysfunction. The valve closes long before the onset of ventricular systole (*dashed line*). Opening of the valve is markedly delayed and occurs following atrial systole.

merely thickened ventricular walls. A more classic description of left ventricular hypertrophy is possible by measuring left ventricular mass.[137–143,143a] This method is used by pathologists to make this assessment. The M-mode technique for measuring mass calculates the volume of the left ventricle using a dimension between the right side of the septum and the posterior left ventricular epicardium. The measurement represents the volume of the left ventricle including the walls. One then subtracts the volume of the cavity using a minor axis endocardial dimension to calculate the volume of the walls. One uses the specific gravity of cardiac muscle to convert the left ventricular wall volume into left ventricular mass.

The principle limitation of the M-mode technique is, of course, the inaccuracy of a single dimension to measure volumes. Hence, two-dimensional echocardiography has been used to measure left ventricular mass.[144–146] Area length and truncated ellipse models are used for assessing mass. Because myocardial thickness measurements require good endocardial definition, a parasternal view, such as the parasternal short-axis view, is used for this calculation. Figure 3–46 shows the technique for measuring mass that has been recommended by the ASE.[23] For both methods, the short-axis

view is obtained at the papillary muscle level. This view is usually the widest short-axis ventricular diameter. Assuming a circular cross-section, the cavity short-axis radius and the mean wall thickness can be calculated from the mean area values. As with most short-axis measurements, the papillary muscles are excluded and are considered part of the cavity. The length of the ventricular image is obtained from apical four- or two-chamber views. With the area length technique, the entire major axis is used, whereas the truncated ellipsoid approach divides the major axis into two parts at the level of the widest minor axis. The two segments are called the semimajor axis and the truncated semi-major axis.

Wall thickness and cavity dimensions can be combined with blood pressure values to produce a measure of left ventricular wall stress.[138–152] The measurement is usually obtained in systole. The calculation includes the left ventricular systolic dimension as well as the systolic thickness of the posterior left ventricular wall. The left ventricular meridian wall stress (G-CM$^2$) is usually calculated according to the following formula: systolic stress equals 0.334 (P)(d)/h [1 + (h/d)], in which P is systolic pressure, d is systolic left ventricular diameter, and h is systolic posterior wall thickness. A simplified formula for wall stress is P (R/Th), in which P is systolic

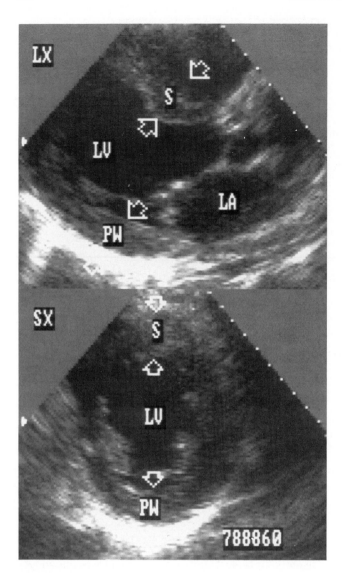

**Fig. 3–45.** Two-dimensional echocardiogram of a patient with left ventricular hypertrophy demonstrating how the ventricular septum (S) and the posterior left ventricular wall (PW) can be measured in both long-axis (LX) and short-axis (SX) views. LV = left ventricle; LA = left atrium.

pressure, R is radius of the left ventricle, and Th is left ventricular wall thickness. Circumferential wall stress equals $1.35 \, P \times [D'/2h] \times [D3/2L^2(D + h)]$, in which D is minor axis and L is long axis. There have been efforts to measure regional wall stress.[153]

The interest in calculating wall stress is stimulated by the realization that systolic ejection indices, such as ejection fraction, fractional shortening, or circumferential shortening, depend on preload and afterload. A theoretic basis exists for suggesting that stress is less dependent on loading conditions.[154] Whether an isolated resting stress measurement is a true measurement of left ventricular contractility is uncertain. Some authors believe that one should compare stress measurements obtained by changing the hemodynamics, such as altering the afterload, to assess ventricular contractility.[155] One

can then measure a slope between two stress measurements. Other investigators have also been using regional stress measurements that require determining the curvature of individual wall segments. This technique is complicated and requires high-quality echocardiograms.

## RIGHT VENTRICLE

The echocardiographic examination of the right ventricle has many limitations. This observation is not surprising when one considers the inherent difficulties in examining this chamber echocardiographically. Much of the right ventricle lies directly beneath the sternum, the chamber has an irregular shape, the walls are trabeculated, and the location of the chamber within the chest may vary significantly, depending on the position of the patient. Despite these formidable problems, echocardiography can reveal useful information concerning the status of the right ventricle. Although right ventricular measurements are admittedly crude, they are helpful in selected patients.

### Right Ventricular Dimensions, Areas, and Volumes

A qualitative assessment of the right ventricle is performed routinely with every echocardiogram. One technique is to look at the apical four-chamber view. If the right ventricular area equals or exceeds the left ventricular area, one can assume that the right ventricle is dilated.

The M-mode examination still provides the simplest right ventricular dimension for quantitation of the right ventricle.[156] Figure 3–47 shows the M-mode echocardiogram through the right ventricle demonstrating the anterior right ventricular wall (ARV) and the cavity of the

LV MASS BY AREA LENGTH (AL) AND TRUNCATED ELLIPSOID (TE)

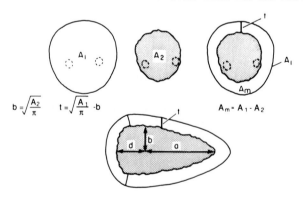

**Fig. 3–46.** Diagram demonstrating how left ventricular mass can be measured by the area length and truncated ellipsoid technique. (From Schiller, M.B., et al.: Recommendations for quantitation of the left ventricle by two-dimensional echocardiography. J. Am. Soc. Echocardiogr., *2*:362, 1989.)

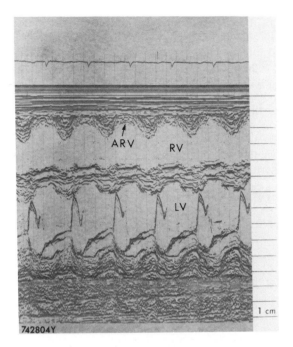

**Fig. 3–47.** M-mode echocardiogram demonstrating the anterior right ventricular wall (ARV). RV = right ventricle; LV = left ventricle.

right ventricle (RV). Figure 3–48 shows an M-mode echocardiogram with a dilated right ventricle and an increased right ventricular dimension.

Two-dimensional echocardiography provides multiple opportunities for quantitating the right ventricle.[157–165] Figures 3–49 and 3–50 show some of the numerous right ventricular measurements that can be obtained with two-dimensional echocardiography. With standardized examinations, one can use these dimensions to assess the size of the right ventricular chamber and to compare the values to a normal range. Many efforts at measuring right ventricular volumes have been made. An area length or Simpson's rule technique has been used. The right ventricle has been considered a pyramid or a crescent with the appropriate mathematic formulae.[165] One technique combined the right ventricular chamber in the four-chamber view and the right ventricular outflow tract in the subcostal view.[159] Areas and length were measured in both views. The area in one was combined with the length in the other view. A somewhat novel approach to calculating right ventricular volumes is to calculate the total volume of both chambers and then subtract the combined volume of the left ventricular cavity and the interventricular septum.[166]

Thus far, no generally accepted technique for calculating right ventricular volumes has been introduced into routine echocardiographic examinations. All of the techniques are relatively complicated. Instead of trying to measure volumes, the simpler measurements are probably all that is worthwhile for routine use at the present

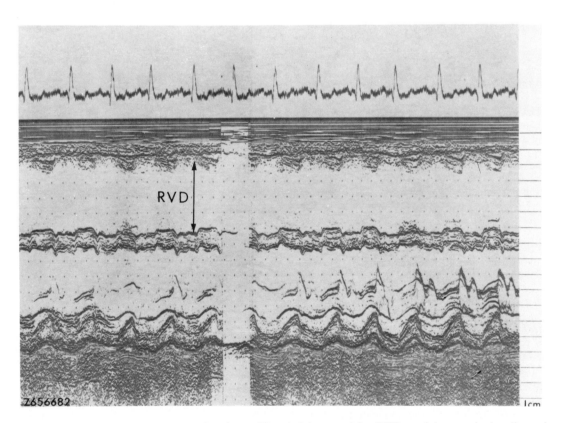

**Fig. 3–48.** M-mode echocardiogram showing a dilated right ventricle. RVD = right ventricular dimension.

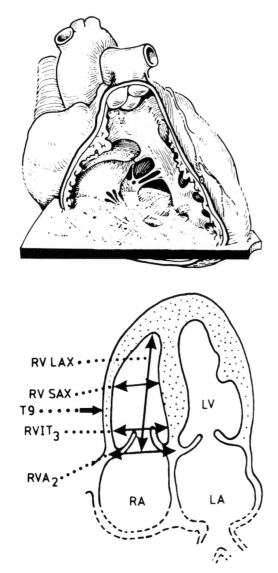

sion of the tricuspid annulus in systole recorded in the apical four-chamber view (Fig. 3–51).[168,169] The authors found this measurement to correlate well with radionuclide right ventricular ejection fraction (R = .92). Other authors enlarged on this approach by using the M-mode recording of the tricuspid annulus, which not only quantitates the excursion but also provides a temporal appreciation of the right ventricular annulus motion (Fig. 3–52). Another suggested technique for measuring right ventricular systolic function is to use contrast two-dimensional echocardiography and to apply a digital subtraction technique for measuring right ventricular ejection fraction.[170]

**Fig. 3–49.** Drawings illustrating how the right ventricle can be measured in the apical four-chamber view. RV LAX = right ventricular long axis; RV SAX = right ventricular short axis; RVIT = right ventricular inflow tract; RVA = right ventricular annulus; RA = right atrium; LV = left ventricle; LA = left atrium. (From Foal, E.R., et al.: Echocardiographic measurement of normal adult right ventricle. Br. Heart J., *56*: 36, 1986.)

time. Either the simple M-mode measurement or a single maximum two-dimensional measurement of the right ventricular cavity in the four-chamber view (see Fig. 3–49) may suffice.

### Global Systolic Function

The usual technique for measuring chamber systolic function is to take a systolic index of the dimensions or volumes of the chamber.[167] Because measurements of the right ventricle are difficult to obtain, this technique is used rarely. A simplified assessment of the right ventricular ejection fraction has been suggested as excur-

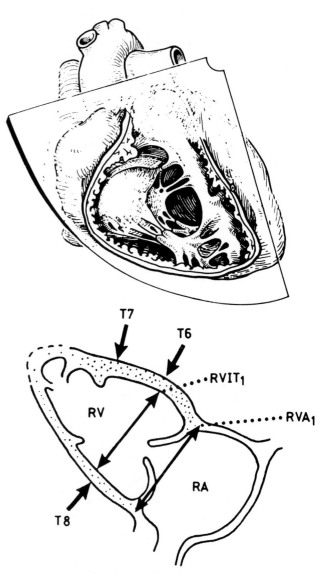

**Fig. 3–50.** Diagram demonstrating right ventricular linear dimensions that are possible with the two-dimensional right ventricular inflow view. RV = right ventricle; RA = right atrium; RVIT = right ventricular inflow tract; RVA = right ventricular annulus. (From Foal, E.R., et al.: Echocardiographic measurement of normal adult right ventricle. Br. Heart J., *56*:36, 1986.)

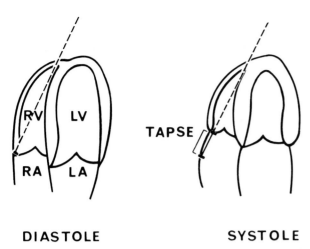

**DIASTOLE**          **SYSTOLE**

**Fig. 3–51.** Diagrams demonstrating how one can measure the systolic excursion of the plane of the tricuspid annulus. RV = right ventricle; LV = left ventricle; RA = right atrium; LA = left atrium; TAPSE = tricuspid annular plane systolic excursions.

### Echocardiographic Findings With Right Ventricular Overload

A pressure overload of the right ventricle is detected primarily by hypertrophy of the right ventricular free wall.[171–174] Occasionally, hypertrophy of the interventricular septum is a consequence of chronic right ventricular pressure overload. A pressure overload may also produce right ventricular dilatation with an increase in right ventricular echocardiographic dimensions. A characteristic finding with chronic pressure overload of the

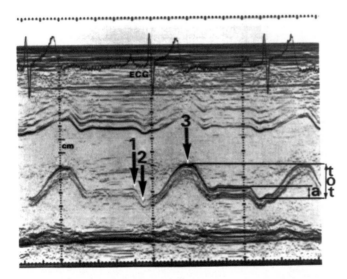

**Fig. 3–52.** M-mode echocardiogram showing the excursion of the tricuspid valve annulus at the onset of atrial systole (1), with atrial systole (2), and with right ventricular systole (3). a = amplitude of atrial motion; tot = total excursion of the annulus. (From Hammarstrom, E., et al.: Tricuspid annular motion. J. Am. Soc. Echocardiogr., *4*:133, 1991.)

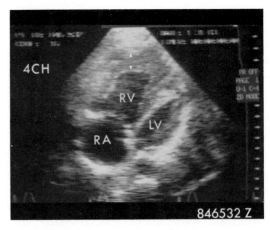

**Fig. 3–53.** Apical four-chamber view of a patient with right ventricular hypertrophy. The free wall of the right ventricle (*arrowheads*) is markedly thickened. RV = right ventricle; LV = left ventricle; RA = right atrium.

right ventricle is distortion of the interventricular septum during ventricular systole.[175–178] Figure 3–53 shows how the hypertrophied right ventricle and interventricular septum impinge on the left ventricle in the four-chamber view. The short-axis view in Figure 3–54 from the same patient shows an indentation of the interventricular septum toward the left ventricle, distorting the normally circular left ventricular cavity. Evidence suggests that the degree to which the interventricular septum is distorted in systole may be related to the systolic pressure in the right ventricle. This distortion usually produces a flattening of the septum during ventricular systole.

Right ventricular volume overload more consistently produces dilatation of the right ventricle.[156,179,180] The other finding with right ventricular volume overload is a peculiar motion of the interventricular septum.[156,181–183] The principle abnormality seen on the M-mode echocar-

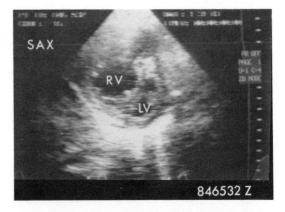

**Fig. 3–54.** Short-axis (SAX) two-dimensional echocardiogram of a patient with marked right ventricular systolic overload. The shape of the left ventricle (LV) is distorted as the septum impinges on the left ventricle. RV = right ventricle.

diogram is rapid anterior motion of the interventricular septum with the onset of ventricular systole (Fig. 3–55, *arrow*). With two-dimensional echocardiography, one can see an alteration in the shape of the interventricular septum during diastole (Fig. 3–56).[184] The increased diastolic filling of the right ventricle produces an indentation of the septum toward the left ventricle (Fig. 3–56B).[185] With ventricular systole, this indentation is rapidly corrected, and the septum moves toward the right ventricle (Fig. 3–56C).

Although M-mode echocardiography and interventricular septal motion are not used as often as in the past, the M-mode examination does provide an opportunity to see patterns of septal motion not appreciated with any other technique. Septal motion reflects relative filling of the two ventricles.[186,187] For example, a brief posterior or downward displacement of the interventricular septum normally occurs with the onset of diastole (Fig. 3–57, *arrow*). In certain conditions, such as mitral stenosis, this diastolic dip may be exaggerated (Fig. 3–58, *arrow*).[188] This exaggerated diastolic dip in mitral stenosis results from unequal filling of the two ventricles and distortion of the shape of the right ventricle.[189] The explanation for this distortion is that mitral stenosis restricts the filling of the left ventricle in early diastole, whereas the unobstructed tricuspid valve permits rapid filling of that ventricle. In early diastole, then, the right ventricle fills more rapidly and the septum bulges toward the left ventricle. It is possible that normally the more compliant right ventricle fills more rapidly than the stiffer left ventricle. This unequal rate of filling produces

the normal diastolic dip (Fig. 3–57). An alternative explanation for the diastolic dip is "twisting" of the heart at end diastole and "untwisting" with the onset of diastole.[190]

Septal motion can be extended to left ventricular volume overload as well.[191] The empiric observation is that patients with left ventricular volume overload have exaggerated septal motion (Fig. 3–59). With increased diastolic filling of the left ventricle, one expects a bulging of the septum toward the right ventricle during diastole. The increased left ventricular stroke volume would then produce exaggerated septal excursion with systole. An important technical detail to remember when evaluating septal motion is distortion of the septum occurs in the body and basal portion of the heart. Septal motion is best evaluated with an M-mode scan at the level of the tips of the mitral valve or chordae. Assessing septal motion closer to the aorta is difficult because it is influenced by aortic motion. The septum is not influenced much by the right ventricle near the apex.

Septal motion has fascinated echocardiographers since the early M-mode days. The motion of this structure provides an opportunity to study the interaction between the right and left ventricles. Some abnormalities with septal motion remain partly unexplained. For example, a characteristic paradoxic motion of the interventricular septum occurs after cardiac surgery. It has been noted for many years that after cardiac surgery involving a median sternotomy incision, septal motion usually moves toward the right ventricle instead of the left ventricle in systole. This peculiar motion is com-

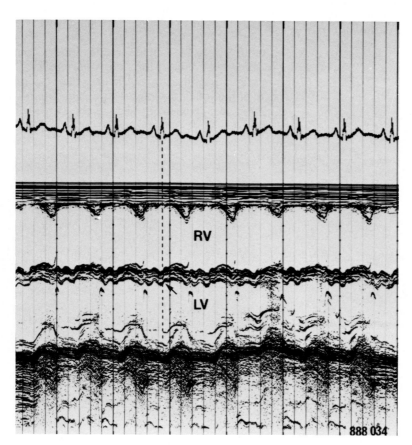

**Fig. 3–55.** M-mode echocardiogram of a patient with a right ventricular volume overload. The right ventricle (RV) is dilated. With ventricular systole (*dashed line*), there is an abrupt anterior motion of the interventricular septum (*arrow*). LV = left ventricle.

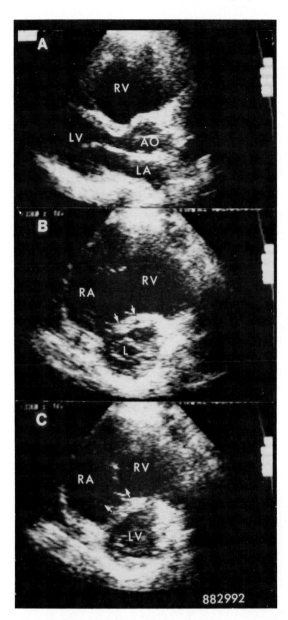

**Fig. 3–56.** Long-axis (*A*) and short-axis (*B* and *C*) two-dimensional echocardiograms of a patient with a right ventricular volume overload. The right ventricle (RV) is markedly enlarged. During diastole (*B*), the septum becomes flattened (*arrows*). With ventricular systole (*C*), the septum moves toward the right ventricle, and the left ventricle (LV) becomes more spherical. AO = aorta; LA = left atrium; RA = right atrium.

monly referred to as a post-op septum. Although there is no generally agreed on mechanism for this finding, it is thought to be a form of cardiac displacement. The abnormality occurs immediately following cardiac surgery[192] and may last indefinitely or partially return to normal after several months.

Doppler flow through the mitral orifice is also influenced by right ventricular volume or pressure overload.[185] With pressure overload, early diastolic velocity (E wave) frequently is reduced.[193] Such a situation primarily results from pulmonary hypertension and re-

duced left atrial filling pressure. The reverse situation occurs with a right ventricular volume overload. Early diastolic filling is accentuated and the atrial component is reduced.[194] Systolic overload of the right ventricle appears to produce a disproportionate distortion of the left ventricular geometry in early diastole, whereas left ventricular distortion occurs in late diastole with right ventricular volume overload. The exact mechanism for these changes in filling velocities could be a combination of hemodynamic and anatomic changes that occur with the volume overload patterns of the right ventricle.

### Diastolic Function

Much of what has been learned about left ventricular diastolic function is being applied to the right side of the heart. Velocity inflow patterns and vena cava patterns noted with different types of diastolic dysfunction of the left ventricle are being noted on the right side of the heart as well.[195,196,196a] Figure 3–60 shows right ventricular inflow velocity in a patient with a restrictive form of right ventricular dysfunction. One can note the characteristic pattern of a tall E wave and a small A wave in the tricuspid flow. The resultant hepatic vein flow shows a small systolic component and a large diastolic phase (Fig. 3–61). Figure 3–62 demonstrates the findings in a patient with impaired relaxation of the right ventricle. As with the left side of the heart, one sees an inflow velocity with a decreased E wave and a tall A wave. The hepatic vein flow demonstrates a large systolic component and a reduced diastolic phase (Fig. 3–63).

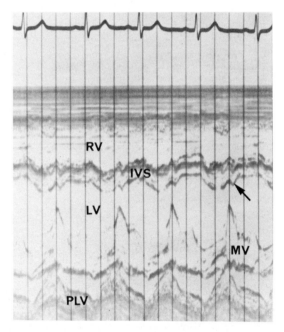

**Fig. 3–57.** Echocardiogram of a normal interventricular septum (IVS) demonstrating early diastolic dip (*arrow*). RV = right ventricle; LV = left ventricle; MV = mitral valve; PLV = posterior left ventricular wall. (From Chang, S.: Echocardiography: Techniques and Interpretation, ed 2. Philadelphia, Lea & Febiger, 1981.)

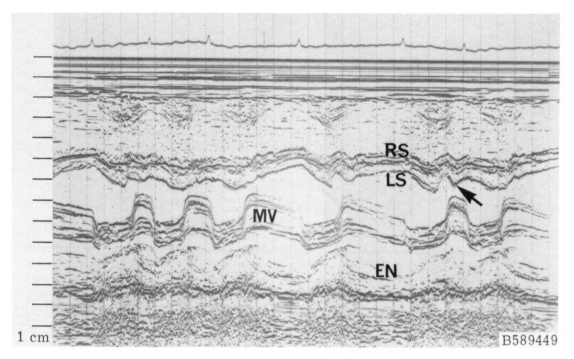

**Fig. 3–58.** M-mode echocardiogram of a patient with mitral stenosis demonstrating an exaggerated early diastolic dip (*arrow*). RS = right septum; LS = left septum; MV = mitral valve; EN = posterior left ventricular endocardium.

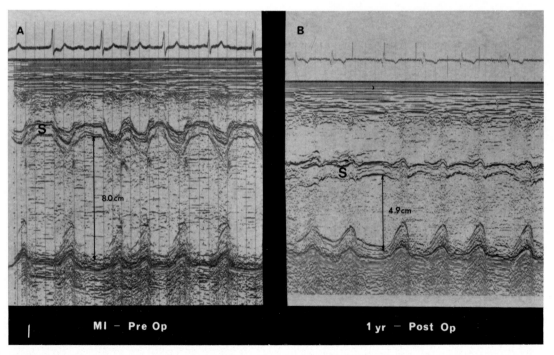

**Fig. 3–59.** Serial M-mode echocardiograms of a patient with mitral insufficiency. Before the operation, the left ventricle is dilated and the septal (S) motion is exaggerated. After the operation, the size of the left ventricle and the amplitude of septal motion are decreased markedly.

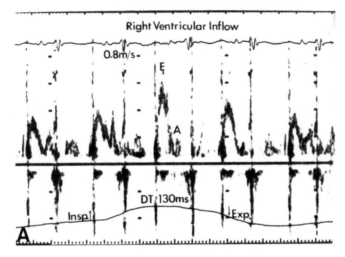

**Fig. 3–60.** Right ventricular inflow Doppler study showing a tall E wave and a short A wave during inspiration in a patient with cardiac amyloidosis. DT = deceleration time. Reprinted with permission from the American College of Cardiology. (From Klein, A.L., et al.: Comprehensive Doppler assessment of right ventricular diastolic function in cardiac amyloidosis. J. Am. Coll. Cardiol., *15*:103, 1990.)

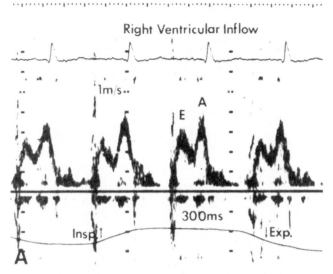

**Fig. 3–62.** Right ventricular inflow Doppler study of a patient with abnormal right ventricular relaxation showing reduced E and increased A velocities. Reprinted with permission from the American College of Cardiology. (From Klein, A.L., et al.: Comprehensive Doppler assessment of right ventricular diastolic function in cardiac amyloidosis. J. Am. Coll. Cardiol., *15*:103, 1990.)

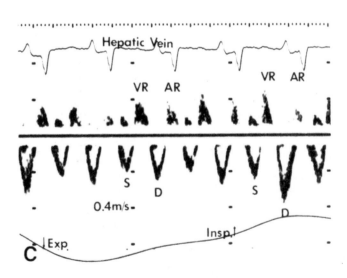

**Fig. 3–61.** Hepatic vein Doppler examination of a patient with cardiac amyloidosis demonstrating a higher diastolic velocity (D) than systolic velocity (S). VR = ventricular reverse flow; AR = atrial reverse flow. Reprinted with permission from the American College of Cardiology. (From Klein, A.L., et al.: Comprehensive Doppler assessment of right ventricular diastolic function in cardiac amyloidosis. J. Am. Coll. Cardiol., *15*:103, 1990.)

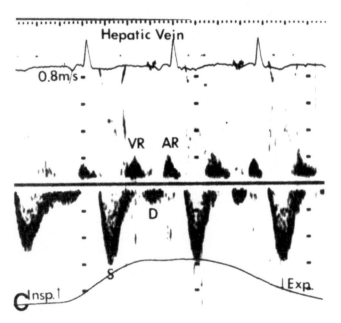

**Fig. 3–63.** Hepatic vein Doppler examination of a patient with abnormal right ventricular relaxation showing an increased systolic wave (S) and a decreased diastolic wave (D). VR = ventricular reverse flow; AR = atrial reverse flow. Reprinted with permission from the American College of Cardiology. (From Klein, A.L., et al.: Comprehensive Doppler assessment of right ventricular diastolic function in cardiac amyloidosis. J. Am. Coll. Cardiol., *15*:103, 1990.)

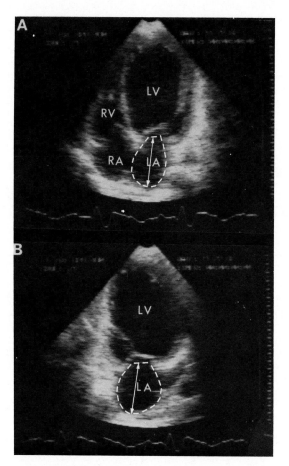

**Fig. 3–64.** Apical four-chamber (*A*) and two-chamber (*B*) two-dimensional echocardiograms demonstrating how one can measure the area (*dashed line*) and length (*arrows*) of the left atrium. LV = left ventricle; RV = right ventricle; RA = right atrium; LA = left atrium.

Abnormal tricuspid valve closure on the tricuspid valve echocardiogram similar to that seen with the mitral valve has also been observed.

## LEFT ATRIUM

The history of examining the left atrium echocardiographically parallels the history of the technologic developments in this field. M-mode echocardiography provided a relatively limited one-dimensional examination of the left atrium. Two-dimensional echocardiography widened the examination of this chamber by providing multiple tomographic planes. Areas of the left atrium, however, especially the appendage, were usually hidden from view. Transesophageal echocardiography has opened the field of view of the left atrium. Because the left atrium lies next to the esophagus, the transesophageal examination offers an opportunity to study the left atrium with a clarity not available with any other technique.

### Left Atrial Dimensions, Areas, and Volumes

Several efforts have been made to use two-dimensional echocardiography to measure left atrial volumes.[197–200] Views that have been used include the long-axis, apical four-chamber, and apical two-chamber examinations. The area, length, and minor dimensions have been measured in each of these views.[197–201] Use of a combination of two of these views is commonly suggested. A biplane, area-length formula has been proposed.[202] For example, one technique for measuring left atrial volume includes obtaining the area and length in the four- and two-chamber views (Fig. 3–64).[199–203] The formula is $V = 8, A1 \times A2 \div 3 \pi L$, in which A1 is the

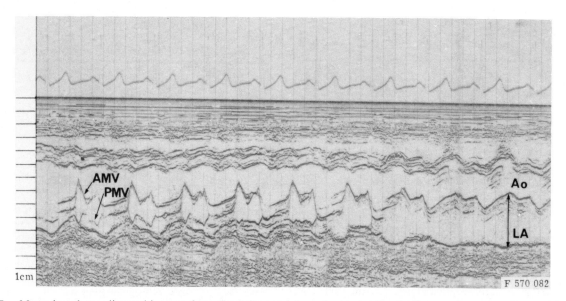

**Fig. 3–65.** M-mode echocardiographic scan from the left ventricle and mitral valve leaflets to the aorta (Ao) and left atrium (LA). The standard left atrial dimension (*arrow*) represents the distance between the atrial side of the posterior aortic wall and the anterior surface of the posterior left atrial echo at the level of the aortic valve leaflets. AMV = anterior mitral valve leaflet; PMV = posterior mitral valve leaflet. (From Chang, S.: Echocardiography Techniques and Interpretation. Philadelphia, Lea & Febiger, 1981.)

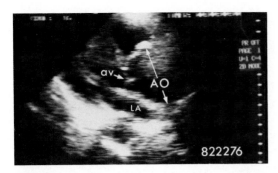

**Fig. 3–66.** Long-axis two-dimensional echocardiogram of a patient with an aortic aneurysm (AO). The left atrium (LA) is markedly distorted by the dilated aorta. av = aortic valve.

area of the four-chamber view, A2 is the area of the two-chamber view, and L is the common length in the two views. Another group of investigators uses the volume formula V = D², Lπ6, in which D is the minor axis and L is the major axis in any given view.[204] In all of the techniques, the atrial appendage and pulmonary veins are excluded from the measurements. The left atrial volume is usually obtained in systole when the chamber has its largest volume.

As is the case with right ventricular volumes, no echocardiographic technique is generally accepted as optimal for measuring left atrial volumes. The M-mode measurement between the anterior and posterior wall of the left atrium at end systole has been used for many years (Fig. 3–65).[65,205,206] Although the relationship between the measurement and the volume is not perfect, this simple dimension has provided a clinically useful estimate of left atrial size.[207] One can certainly use a similar two-dimensional echocardiographic measurement (see Fig. 3–17). Thus, one could be justified in merely measuring between the anterior and posterior left atrial walls in the parasternal long-axis view to obtain a comparable M-mode dimension that has been used for many years. As with all simple measurements, limitations are many. Although the left atrium usually dilates as a sphere, symmetric enlargement does not always occur. In addition,

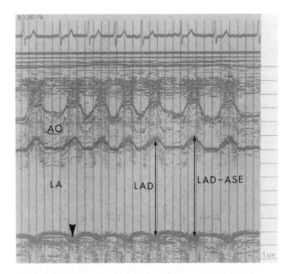

**Fig. 3–68.** M-mode echocardiogram of the aorta (AO) and left atrium (LA) in a patient with mitral regurgitation exhibiting posterior displacement of the left atrial wall in systole (*arrowhead*). LAD = left atrial dimension from trailing edge of posterior aortic wall to leading edge of posterior left atrial wall; LAD-ASE = left atrial dimension from leading edge of posterior aortic wall to leading edge of posterior left atrial wall, as recommended by the American Society of Echocardiography.

dilatation of the aorta, which is the anterior wall of the left atrium, can distort any anterior-posterior dimension (Fig. 3–66). Encroachment on the left atrium from enlarged posterior structures (Fig. 3–67) can also alter left atrial geometry. Fortunately, the qualitative two-dimensional examination readily recognizes when asymmetric dilatation or gross distortion of the left atrium occurs. Under these circumstances, one can modify any assessment of left atrial size using the simple anterior-posterior measurement.

Figure 3–68 shows how one obtains an M-mode left atrial dimension. In this tracing, the measurement is taken from the trailing edge of the echo, dividing the aorta from the left atrium to the leading edge of the echo

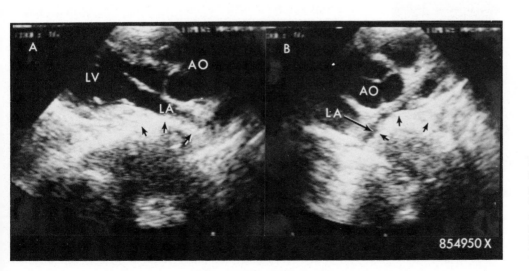

**Fig. 3–67.** Long-axis (*A*) and short-axis (*B*) echocardiograms of a patient with a posterior mediastinal mass (*arrows*). The mass greatly distorts the geometry of the left atrium (LA). AO = aorta; LV = left ventricle.

originating from the posterior left atrial wall. The measurement is taken in the vicinity of the aortic valves and is obtained at the maximum upward motion of the aortic wall, which represents end systole. According to ASE criteria, the left atrial dimension should be taken from the leading edge of the posterior aortic wall to the leading edge of the posterior left atrial wall (LAD-ASE, Fig. 3–68). This policy is in keeping with the principle that M-mode measurements are taken from leading edge to leading edge, whereas two-dimensional measurements are taken from trailing edge to leading edge.

It is not always easy to clearly identify the posterior left atrial wall to make a proper left atrial dimension. Figure 3–69 shows a parasternal long-axis view of the left atrium in which a band of fuzzy echoes is visible in the vicinity of the posterior left atrial wall. These echoes may represent stagnant blood. Angulation of the transducer will clear the fuzzy echoes so that the true left atrial border can be identified. Figure 3–70 shows another common problem with identifying the left atrial border. When the left atrium is dilated, side lobes from a strongly reflective atrioventricular groove can be seen in the dilated left atrium, making the identification of the true left atrial border confusing.

The location in the cardiac cycle from which the left atrial dimension is taken has customarily been at end systole, when the left atrium is at maximal dimension.

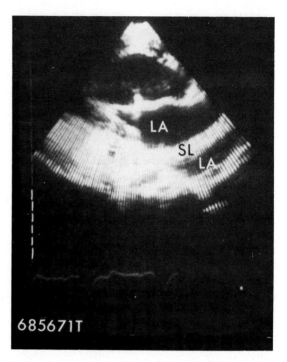

**Fig. 3–70.** Long-axis parasternal echocardiogram of a patient with a dilated left atrium (LA) showing how a side lobe artifact (SL) can appear within the echo-free cavity of the left atrium.

This technique was first used because the upward motion of the posterior aortic wall was convenient for measurement. Although other areas of the cardiac cycle have been recommended for left atrial dimensions, the end-systolic location continues to be the one most often used and is recommended by the Society.

Another way of qualitatively assessing left atrial size is to compare the left atrial dimension with the diameter of the aorta.[208] In normal subjects, the diameter of the aorta and that of the left atrium are about equal. As the left atrium dilates, this relationship changes, with the left atrial dimension becoming significantly larger than that of the aorta. Figure 3–68 demonstrates a patient with an enlarged left atrium. By any criteria, the left atrial cavity is well beyond the limits of normal. The diameter is over 6 cm, which is extremely large. Many articles in the literature correlate echocardiography and angiography for judging the size of the left atrium. The correlations between the two techniques have been good, with almost all having approximate R values of 0.9. Although the technique originally recommended correcting the dimension for body surface area, it is debatable whether the body surface area is useful when comparing one individual with another. The aorta-left atrium ratio was recommended as a better means to correct for size of the patient rather than using the body surface area. As expected, this ratio is used primarily in pediatric echocardiography. Other authors believe that merely taking the uncorrected left atrial dimension and comparing it to known normal values (see Appendix) is the best way of judging whether the chamber is dilated.

Another useful and fairly reliable sign of left atrial

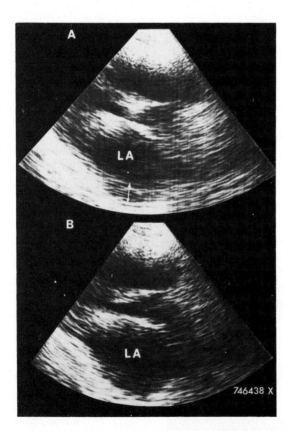

**Fig. 3–69.** Long-axis parasternal views of the left atrium (LA) demonstrating a band of faint echoes (*arrows*) along the posterior left atrial wall (*A*). These echoes can be eliminated by changes in angulation and a decrease in gain (*B*).

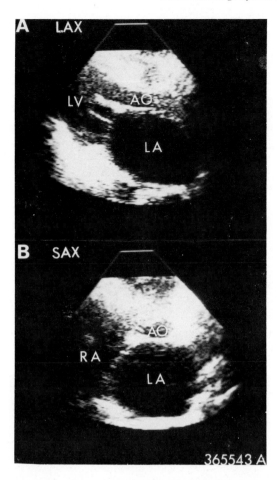

**Fig. 3–71.** Parasternal long-axis (LAX) (*A*) and short-axis (SAX) (*B*) two-dimensional echocardiograms of a patient with a dilated left atrium (LA). AO = aorta; LV = left ventricle; RA = right atrium.

dilatation is bulging of the interatrial septum toward the right atrium. This finding can be noted in any view that records the interatrial septum, such as the four-chamber or short-axis (Fig. 3–71) presentation. Figure 3–72 shows an unusual example of isolated dilatation of the left atrial appendage.[209] In this case, the anomaly is con-

genital. Partial absence of the pericardium might produce a similar echocardiographic image as the left atrial appendage herniates through the defect and is partially obstructed. Of course, transesophageal echocardiography is outstanding for detecting left atrial appendage aneurysms.[210,211]

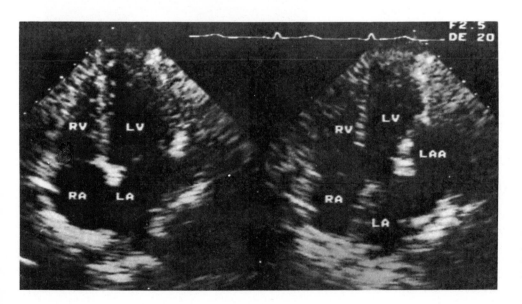

**Fig. 3–72.** Two-dimensional echocardiogram of a patient with an aneurysm of the left atrial appendage (LAA). RV = right ventricle; LV = left ventricle; RA = right atrium; LA = left atrium. (From Vargas-Barron, J., et al.: The differential diagnosis of partial absence of left pericardium and congenital left atrial aneurysm. Am. Heart J., *118*:1349, 1989.

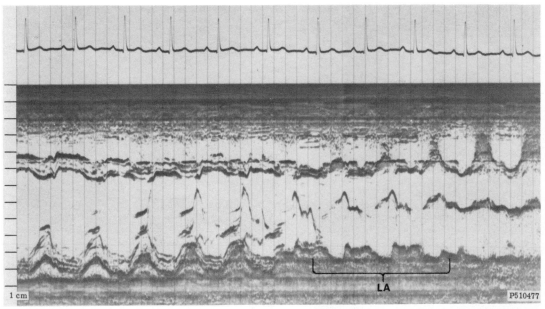

**Fig. 3–73.** M-mode scan from the left ventricle to the left atrium (LA). The best excursion of the posterior left atrial wall was seen at the junction between the posterior left ventricular wall and the left atrium.

### Left Atrial Function

Several authors have attempted to use echocardiography to assess left atrial function.[212] Initial efforts at evaluating left atrial wall motion involved the use of M-mode echocardiography.[213–215] Figure 3–73 shows an M-mode echocardiogram that displays left atrial motion at the junction between the left ventricle and the left atrium. Unfortunately, part of this motion is merely an artifact resulting from movement of the atrioventricular junction and the stationary ultrasonic beam. The beam transects the left atrium in systole and the left ventricle in diastole (Fig. 3–74).

Investigators have looked at the changes in left atrial volume by recording the motion of the posterior wall of the aorta, which is essentially the same as the anterior wall of the left atrium.[216,217] The posterior aortic wall has been used to judge both absolute and relative changes in left atrial volume.

With the advent of transesophageal echocardiography, the entire left atrium is available for examination. For example, one area of interest is the left atrial appendage, which has never been seen clearly before with echocardiography.[218,218a] In Figure 3–75, a transesophageal echocardiographic examination of the left atrial appendage shows obliteration of the appendage cavity with atrial systole. Figure 3–76 shows Doppler tracings taken from a transesophageal echocardiographic examination of the atrial appendage. One can see definite Doppler flow in the atrial appendage when the patient is in sinus rhythm (Fig. 3–76A); however, with atrial flutter (B) or fibrillation (C and D), a marked change in the flow pattern is evident within the atrial appendage.

The left atrium, especially the atrial appendage, is a common site for thrombi. A possible precursor of thrombus formation is the presence of stagnant blood or spontaneous echoes. Such echoes are best seen with trans-

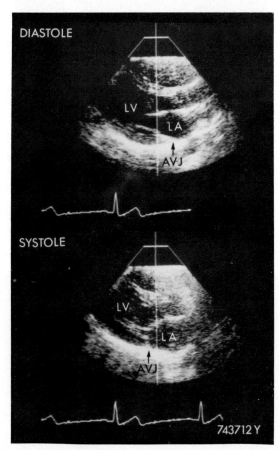

**Fig. 3–74.** Long-axis, parasternal two-dimensional echocardiograms demonstrating the mobility of the atrioventricular junction (AVJ) from diastole to systole. The M-mode ultrasonic beam (*white line*) can examine the left ventricular wall in diastole and the left atrial wall in systole without changing the direction of the transducer. LV = left ventricle; LA = left atrium.

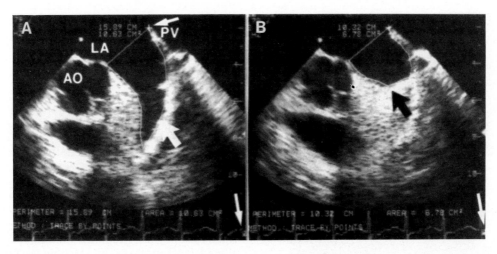

**Fig. 3–75.** Transesophageal echocardiogram showing how the cavity of the left atrial appendage (*arrow*) decreases from atrial diastole (*A*) to atrial systole (*B*). AO = aorta; LA = left atrium; PV = pulmonary vein. (From Pollick, C., et al.: Assessment of left atrial appendage function by transesophageal echocardiography: Implications for the development of thrombus. Circulation, *1*:224, 1991, by permission of the American Heart Association, Inc.)

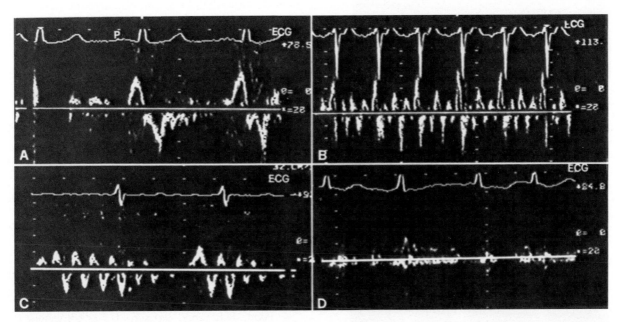

**Fig. 3–76.** Pulsed Doppler recording from the left atrial appendage using transesophageal echocardiography. With sinus rhythm (*A*), one sees fairly tall atrial velocity after the P wave of the electrocardiogram. In *B*, note atrial flutter with 2:1 block showing forward velocities after each P wave. The second P wave is within the T wave of the electrocardiogram. In *C*, the patient has flutter fibrillation and only gross oscillating velocities are noted in the left atrial appendage. With chronic atrial fibrillation (*D*), no organized flow velocity can be recorded within the left atrial appendage. (From Pozzoli, M., et al.: Left atrial appendage dysfunction: A cause of thrombosis? Evidence by transesophageal echocardiography—Doppler studies. J. Am. Soc. Echocardiogr., *5*:436, 1991.)

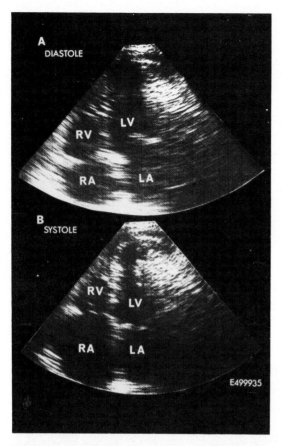

**Fig. 3–77.** Apical four-chamber views demonstrating a dramatic change in the size of the right atrium (RA) from diastole (*A*) to systole (*B*) in a patient with tricuspid stenosis and regurgitation. RV = right ventricle; LV = left ventricle; LA = left atrium.

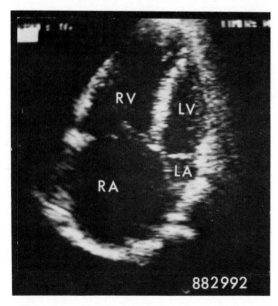

**Fig. 3–78.** Apical four-chamber echocardiogram of a patient with a dilated right ventricle (RV) and a massively dilated right atrium (RA). LV = left ventricle; LA = left atrium.

esophageal echocardiography. This topic is discussed further in Chapter 11, Cardiac Masses.

## RIGHT ATRIUM

Two-dimensional echocardiography provides several opportunities to visualize the right atrium (see Chapter 2).[219–221] Probably the most convenient examination for measuring the right atrium is the apical four-chamber view with the transthoracic examination. Figure 3–77 shows the apical four-chamber view in diastole (*A*) and in systole (*B*). The size of the right atrium, especially in comparison to the left atrium, can also be appreciated in this view. Figure 3–78 shows a massively enlarged right atrium, which impinges dramatically on a relatively small left atrium. As with a dilated left atrium, the shape of the interatrial septum helps to identify a dilated right atrium. The septum bulges toward the left atrium with right atrial dilatation, provided the left atrium also is not dilated.

Transesophageal echocardiography offers another view of the right atrium. This type of examination can provide more detail and can visualize the right atrial appendage as well as the insertions of the vena cava. Thus far, relatively little interest has been generated in quantitating right atrial volumes or function.

## REFERENCES

1. Assmann, P.E., Slager, C.J., van der Borden, S.G., Dreysse, S.T., Tijssen, J.G.P., Sutherland, G.R., and Roelandt, J.R.: Quantitative echocardiographic analysis of global and regional left ventricular function: A problem revisited. J. Am. Soc. Echocardiogr., *3*:478, 1990.
2. Kuecherer, H.F., Kee, L.L., Modin, G., Cheitlin, M.D., and Schiller, N.B.: Echocardiography in serial evaluation of left ventricular systolic and diastolic function: Importance of image acquisition, quantitation, and physiologic variability in clinical and investigational applications. J. Am. Soc. Echocardiogr., *4*:203, 1991.
3. Feigenbaum, H., et al.: Ultrasound measurements of the left ventricle: A correlative study with angiocardiography. Arch. Intern. Med., *129*:461, 1972.
4. Popp, R.L. and Harrison, D.C.: Ultrasonic cardiac echography for determining stroke volume and valvular regurgitation. Circulation, *41*:493, 1970.
5. Pombo, J.F., Troy, B.L., and Russell, R.O., Jr.: Left ventricular volumes and ejection fraction by echocardiography. Circulation, *43*:480, 1971.
6. Gibson, D.G.: Measurement of left ventricular volumes in man by echocardiography—comparison with biplane angiographs. Br. Heart J., *33*:614, 1971.
7. Teichholz, L.E., Kreulen, T., Herman, M.V., and Gorlin, R.: Problems in echocardiographic volume determinations: Echocardiographic-angiographic correlations in the presence or absence of asynergy. Am. J. Cardiol., *37*: 7, 1976.
8. Sahn, D.J., DeMaria, A., Kisslo, J., and Weyman, A.: Recommendations regarding quantitation in M-mode echocardiography: Results of a survey of echocardiographic measurements. Circulation, *58*:1072, 1978.

9. Kronik, G., Slany, J., and Mosslacher, H.: Comparative value of eight M-mode echocardiographic formulas for determining left ventricular stroke volume. A correlative study with thermodilution and left ventricular single-plane cineangiography. Circulation, *60*:1308, 1979.

10. Antani, J.A., Wayne, H.H., and Kuzman, W.J.: Ejection phase indexes by invasive and noninvasive methods: An apexcardiographic, echocardiographic, and ventriculographic correlative study. Am. J. Cardiol., *43*:239, 1979.

11. Martin, M.A.: Assessment of correction formula for echocardiographic estimation of left ventricular volume. Br. Heart J., *40*:294, 1978.

12. Bhatt, D.R., Isabel-Jones, J.B., Villoria, G.J., Naka-zawa, M., Yabek, S.M., Marks, R.A., and Jarmakani, J.M.: Accuracy of echocardiography in assessing left ventricular dimensions and volume. Circulation, *57*:699, 1978.

13. Felner, J.M., Blusmenstein, B.A., Schlant, R.C., Carter, A.D., Alimbrung, B.N., Johnson, M.J., Sherman, S.W., Klicpera, M.W., Kutner M.H., and Drucker, L.W.: Sources of variability in echocardiographic measurements. Am J. Cardiol., *45*: 995, 1980.

14. Hoenecke, H.R., Goldberg, S.J., Sahn, D.J., Allen, H.D., and Valdes-Cruz, L.M.: Effect of beam directional alterations on left ventricular shortening fraction. Am. J. Cardiol., *50*:1120, 1982.

14a. Martins, T.C., Rigby, M.L., and Redington, A.N.: Left ventricular performance in children: Transthoracic versus transesophageal measurement of M mode derived indices. Br. Heart J., *68*:485, 1992.

15. Schiller, N.B., Acquatella, H., Ports, T.A., Drew, D., Goerke, J., Ringertz, H., Silverman, N.H., Brundage, B., Botvinick, E.H., Bowell, R., Carlsson, E., and Parmley, W.W.: Left ventricular volume from paired biplane two-dimensional echocardiography. Circulation, *60*:547, 1979.

16. Wyatt, H.L., et al.: Cross-sectional echocardiography. II. Analysis of mathematical models for quantifying volume of the formalin-fixed left ventricle. Circulation, *61*: 1119, 1980.

17. Wyatt, H.L., Heng, M.K., Meerbaum, S., Hestenes, J.D., Cobo, J.M., Davidson, R.M., and Corday, E.: Cross-sectional echocardiography. I. Analysis of mathematic models for quantifying mass of the left ventricle in dogs. Circulation, *60*:1104, 1979.

18. Kan, G., Visser, C.A., Lie, K.I., and Durrer, D.: Left ventricular volumes and ejection fraction by single plane two-dimensional apex echocardiography. Eur. Heart J., *2*:339, 1981.

19. Gordon, E.P., Schnittger, I., Fitzgerald, P.J., Williams, P., and Popp, R.L.: Reproducibility of left ventricular volumes by two-dimensional echocardiography. J. Am. Coll. Cardiol., *2*:506, 1983.

20. Folland, E.D., Parisi, A.F., Moynihan, P.F., Jones, D.R., Feldman, C.L., and Tow, D.E.: Assessment of left ventricular ejection fraction and volumes by real-time, two-dimensional echocardiography. Circulation, *60*:760, 1979.

21. Starling, M.R., Crawford, M.H., Sorensen, S.G., Levi, B., Richards, K.L., and O'Rourke, R.A.: Comparative accuracy of apical biplane cross-sectional echocardiography and gated equilibrium radionuclide angiography for estimating left ventricular size and performance. Circulation, *63*:1075, 1981.

21a. Zile, M.R., Tanaka, R., Lindroth, J.R., Spinale, F., Carabello, B.A., and Mirsky, I.: Left ventricular volume determined echocardiographically by assuming a constant left ventricular epicardial long-axis/short-axis dimension ratio throughout the cardiac cycle. J. Am. Coll. Cardiol., *20*:986, 1992.

22. Zoghbi, W.A., Buckey, J.C., Massey, M.A., and Blomqvist, C.G.: Determination of left ventricular volumes with use of a new nongeometric echocardiographic method: Clinical validation and potential application. J. Am. Coll. Cardiol., *15*:610, 1990.

23. Schiller, N.B., Shah, P.M., Crawford, M., DeMaria, A., Devereux, R., Feigenbaum, H., Gutfesell, H., Reichek, N., Sahn, D., Schnittger, I., Silverman, N.H., and Tajik, A.J.: Recommendations for quantitation of the left ventricle by two-dimensional echocardiography. J. Am. Soc. Echocardiogr., *2*:358, 1989.

24. Quinones, M.A., Waggoner, A.D., Reduto, L.A., Nelson, J.G., Young, J.B., Winters, W.L., Ribeiro, L.G., and Miller, R.R.: A new, simplified and accurate method for determining ejection fraction with two-dimensional echocardiography. Circulation, *64*:744, 1981.

25. Baran, A.O., Rogal, G.J., and Nanda, N.C.: Ejection fraction determination without planimetry by two-dimensional echocardiography: A new method. J. Am. Coll. Cardiol., *1*:1471, 1983.

25a. King, D.L., Harrison, M.R., King, D.L. Jr., Gopal, A.S., Kwan, O.L., and DeMaria, A.N.: Ultrasound beam orientation during standard two-dimensional imaging: Assessment by three-dimensional echocardiography. J. Am. Soc. Echocardiogr., *5*:569, 1992.

26. Himelman, R.B., Cassidy, M.M., Landzberg, J.S., and Schiller, N.B.: Reproducibility of quantitative two-dimensional echocardiography. Am. Heart J., *115*:425, 1988.

27. Gorge, G., Erbel, R., Brennecke, R., Rupprecht, H.J., Todt, M., and Meyer, J.: High-resolution two-dimensional echocardiography improves the quantification of left ventricular function. J. Am. Soc. Echocardiogr., *5*: 125, 1992.

28. Bengur, A. R., Snider, A.R., Vermilion, R.P., and Freeland, J.C.: Left ventricular ejection fraction measured with Doppler color flow mapping techniques. Am. J. Cardiol., *68*:669, 1991.

29. Stanton, M.S., Prystowsky, E.N., Fineberg, N.S., Miles, W.M., Zipes, D.P., and Heger, J.J.: Arrhythmogenic effects of antiarrhythmic drugs: A study of 506 patients treated for ventricular tachycardia or fibrillation. J. Am. Coll. Cardiol., *14*:209, 1989.

30. Stamm, R.B., Carabello, B.A., Mayers, D.L., and Martin, R.P.: Two-dimensional echocardiographic measurement of left ventricular ejection fraction: Prospective analysis of what constitutes an adequate determination. Am. Heart J., *104*:136, 1982.

31. Rich, S., Sheikh, A., Gallastegui, J., Kondos, G.T., Mason, T., and Lam, W.: Determination of left ventricular ejection fraction by visual estimation during real-time two-dimensional echocardiography. Am. Heart J., *104*: 603, 1982.

32. Wong, M., Bruce, S., Joseph, D., and Lively, H.: Estimating left ventricular ejection fraction from two-dimensional echocardiograms: Visual and computer-processed interpretations. Echocardiography, *8*:1, 1991.

33. Mueller, X., Stauffer, J.C., Jaussi, A., Goy, J.J., and Kappenberger, L.: Subjective visual echocardiographic estimate of left ventricular ejection fraction as an alternative to conventional echocardiographic methods: Comparison with contrast angiography. Clin. Cardiol., *14*: 898, 1991.

34. Amico, A.F., Lichtenberg, G.S., Reisner, S.A., Stone,

C.K., Schwartz, R.G., and Meltzer, R.S.: Superiority of visual versus computerized echocardiographic estimation of radionuclide left ventricular ejection fraction. Am. Heart J., *118*:1259, 1989.

35. Albin, G. and Rahko, P.S.: Comparison of echocardiographic quantitation of left ventricular ejection fraction to radionuclide angiography in patients with regional wall motion abnormalities. Am. J. Cardiol., *65*:1031, 1990.

36. Lloyd, T.R. and Donnerstein, R.L.: Afterload dependence of echocardiographic left ventricular ejection force determination. Am. J. Cardiol., *67*:901, 1991.

37. Fortuin, N.J., Hood, W.P., Jr., and Craige, E.: Evaluation of left ventricular function by echocardiography. Circulation, *46*:26, 1972.

38. Benzing, G., Stockert, J., Nave, E., and Kaplan, S.: Evaluation of left ventricular performance: Circumferential fiber shortening and tension. Circulation, *49*:925, 1974.

39. Cooper, R., Karliner, J.S., O'Rourke, R.A., Peterson, K.L., and Leopold, G.R.: Ultrasound determinations of mean fiber-shortening rate in man. Am. J. Cardiol., *29*: 257, 1972.

40. Cooper, R.H., O'Rourke, R.A., Karliner, J.S., Peterson, K.L., and Leopold, G.R.: Comparison of ultrasound and cineangiographic measurements of the mean rate of circumferential shortening in man. Circulation, *46*:914, 1972.

41. Quinones, M.A., Gaasch, W.H., and Alexander, J.K.: Echocardiographic assessment of left ventricular function: With special reference to normalized velocities. Circulation, *50*:42, 1974.

42. Quinones, M.A., Gaasch, W.H., and Alexander, J.K.: Influence of acute changes in preload, afterload, contractile state, and heart rate on ejection and isovolumic indices of myocardial contractility in man. Circulation, *53*: 293, 1976.

43. Orlando, E., D'Antuono, G., Cipolla, C., et al.: Analysis of left ventricular wall motion by means of ultrasound. G. Ital. Cardiol., *2*:234, 1972.

44. Pernod, J., Terdjman, M., Kermaree, J., and Haguenauer, G.: Myocardial contraction: Study by ultrasonic echography (results in 200 normal patients). Nouv. Presse Med., *2*:2393, 1973.

45. Traill, T.A., Gibson, D.G., and Brown, D.J.: Study of left ventricular wall thickness and dimension changes using echocardiography. Br. Heart J., *40*:162, 1978.

46. Corya, B.C., Rasmussen, S., Feigenbaum, H., Knoebel, S.B., and Black, M.J.: Systolic thickening and thinning of the septum and posterior wall in patients with coronary artery disease, congestive cardiomyopathy, and atrial septal defect. Circulation, *55*:109, 1977.

47. Sasayama, S., Franklin, D., Ross, J., Kemper, W.S., and McKown, D.: Dynamic changes in left ventricular wall thickness and their use in analyzing cardiac function in the conscious dog: A study based on a modified ultrasonic technique. Am. J. Cardiol., *38*:870, 1976.

48. Feneley, M.P. and Hickie, J.B.: Validity of echocardiographic determination of left ventricular systolic wall thickening. Circulation, *70*:226, 1984.

49. Sagar, K.B., Wann, L.S., Boerboom, L.E., Kalbfleisch, J., Rhyne, T.L., and Olinger, G.N.: Comparison of peak and modal aortic blood flow velocities with invasive measures of left ventricular performance. J. Am. Soc. Echocardiogr., *1*:194, 1988.

50. Isaaz, K., Ethevenot, G., Admant, P., Brembilla, B., and Pernot, C.: A simplified normalized ejection phase index measured by Doppler echocardiography for the assessment of left ventricular performance. Am. J. Cardiol., *65*: 1246, 1990.

51. Isaaz, K., Ethevenot, G., Admant, P., Brembilla, B., Pernot, C., and Chalon, B.: A new Doppler method of assessing left ventricular ejection force in chronic congestive heart failure. Am. J. Cardiol., *64*:81, 1989.

52. Mehta, N., Bennett, D., Mannering, D., Dawkins, K., and Ward, D.E.: Usefulness of noninvasive Doppler measurement of ascending aortic blood velocity and acceleration in detecting impairment of the left ventricular functional response to exercise three weeks after acute myocardial infarction. Am. J. Cardiol., *58*:879, 1986.

53. Sabbah, H.N., Khaja, F., Brymer, J.F., McFarland, T.M., Albert, D.E., Snyder, J.E., Goldstein, S., and Stein, P.D.: Noninvasive evaluation of left ventricular performance based on peak aortic blood acceleration measured with a continuous wave Doppler velocity meter. Circulation, *74*:323, 1986.

54. Miyashita, Y., Seki, K., Takahashi, I., Takayama, K., Hara, M., Nakatsuka, T., Yoshimura, S., and Furuhata, H.: Non-invasive evaluation of cardiac function by peak aortic flow acceleration (peak dF/dt) during Exercise. Jpn. J. Med. Ultrasonics, *14*:1, 1987.

55. Bedotto, J.B., Eichhorn, E.J., and Grayburn, P.A.: Effects of left ventricular preload and afterload on ascending aortic blood velocity and acceleration in coronary artery disease. Am. J. Cardiol., *64*:856, 1989.

56. Harrison, M.R., Clifton, G.D., Berk, M.R., and DeMaria, A.N.: Effect of blood pressure and afterload on Doppler echocardiographic measurements of left ventricular systolic function in normal subjects. Am. J. Cardiol., *64*: 905, 1989.

57. Gardin, J.M.: Doppler measurements of aortic blood flow velocity and acceleration: Load-independent indexes of left ventricular performance? Am. J. Cardiol., *64*:935, 1989.

58. Harrison, M.R., Clifton, G.D., Sublett, K.L., and DeMaria, A.N.: Effect of heart rate on Doppler indexes of systolic function in humans. J. Am. Coll. Cardiol., *14*:929, 1989.

59. Wallmeyer, K., Wann, L.S., Sagar, K.B., Kalbfleisch, J., and Klopfenstein, H.S.: The influence of preload and heart rate on Doppler echocardiographic indexes of left ventricular performance: Comparison with invasive indexes in an experimental preparation. Circulation, *74*: 181, 1986.

60. Chen, C., Rodriguez, L., Guerrero, J.L., Marshall, S., Levine, R.A., Weyman, A.E., and Thomas, J.D.: Noninvasive estimation of the instantaneous first derivative of left ventricular pressure using continuous-wave Doppler echocardiography. Circulation, *83*:2101, 1991.

61. Pai, R.G., Bansal, R.C., and Shah, P.M.: Doppler-derived rate of left ventricular pressure rise. Its correlation with the postoperative left ventricular function in mitral regurgitation. Circulation, *82*:514, 1990.

62. Bargiggia, G.S., Bertucci, C., Recusani, F., Raisaro, A., DeServi, S., Valdes-Cruz, L.M., Sahn, D.J., and Tronconi, L.: A new method for estimating left ventricular dp/dt by continuous wave Doppler-echocardiography. Circulation, *80*:1287, 1989.

63. Chung, N., Nishimura, R.A., Holmes, Jr., D.R., and Tajik, A.J.: Measurement of left ventricular dp/dt by simultaneous Doppler echocardiography and cardiac catherization. J. Am. Soc. Echocardiogr., *5*:147, 1992.

64. Ahmadpour, H., Shah, A.A., Allen, J.W., Edmiston, W.A., Kim, S.J., and Haywood, L.J.: Mitral E point septal separation: A reliable index of left ventricular per-

formance in coronary artery disease. Am. Heart J., *106*: 21, 1983.

65. Engle, S.J., Disessa, T.G., Perloff, J.K., Isabel-Jones, J., Leighton, J., Gross, K., and Friedman, W.F.: Mitral valve E point to ventricular septal separation in infants and children. Am. J. Cardiol., *52*:1084, 1983.

66. Child, J.S., Krivokapick, J., and Perloff, J.K.: Effect of left ventricular size on mitral E point to ventricular septal separation in assessment of cardiac performance. Am. Heart J., *101*:797, 1981.

67. Massie, B.M., Schiller, N.B., Ratshin, R.A., and Parmley, W.W.: Mitral-septal separation: New echocardiographic index of left ventricular function. Am. J. Cardiol., *39*:1008, 1977.

68. D'Cruz, I.A., Lalmalani, G.G., Sambasivan, V., Cohen, H.C., and Glick, G.: The superiority of mitral E point-ventricular septum separation to other echocardiographic indicators of left ventricular performance. Clin. Cardiol., *2*:140, 1979.

69. Lew, W., Henning, H., Schelbert, H., and Karliner, J.S.: Assessment of mitral valve E point-septal separation as an index of left ventricular function in acute and chronic ischemic heart disease. Am. J. Cardiol., *41*:436, 1978. (Abstract)

70. Koenig, W., Gehring, J., Kollmann, G., Schinz, A., Beckmann, R., and Mathes, P.: Significance of the E point-septum distance for the evaluation of left ventricular function in coronary disease—a study using M-mode echocardiography. Z. Kardiol., *72*:649, 1983.

71. Simonson, J.S. and Schiller, N.B.: Descent of the base of the left ventricle: An echocardiographic index of left ventricular function. J. Am. Soc. Echocardiogr., *2*:25, 1989.

72. Pai, R.G., Bodenheimer, M.M., Pai, S.M., Koss, J.H., and Adamick, R.D.: Usefulness of systolic excursion of the mitral anulus as an index of left ventricular systolic function. Am. J. Cardiol., *67*:222, 1991.

73. Jones, C.J.H. and Gibson, D.G.: Functional importance of the long axis dynamics of the human left ventricle. Br. Heart J., *63*:215, 1990.

74. Keren, G., Sonnenblick, E.H., and LeJemtel, T.H.: Mitral anulus motion. Circulation, *78*:621, 1988.

74a.Zaky, A., Grabhorn, L., and Feigenbaum, H.: Movement of the mitral ring: A study of ultrasound cardiography. Cardiovasc. Res., *1*:121, 1967.

74b.Feigenbaum, H., Zaky, A., and Nasser, W.K.: Use of ultrasound to measure left ventricular stroke volume. Circulation, *35*:1092, 1967.

75. Rifkin, R.D. and Koito, H.: Comparison with radionuclide angiography of two new geometric and four nongeometric models for echocardiographic estimation of left ventricular ejection fraction using segmental wall motion scoring. Am. J. Cardiol., *65*:1485, 1990.

75a.Berning, J., Rokkedal-Nielsen, J., Launbjerg, J., Fogh, J., Mickley, H., and Andersen, P.E.: Rapid estimation of left ventricular ejection fraction in acute myocardial infarction by echocardiographic wall motion analysis. Cardiology, *80*:257, 1992.

76. Assmann, P.E., Slager, C.J., Dreysse, S.T., van der Borden, S.G., Oomen, J.A., and Roelandt, J.R.: Two-dimensional echocardiographic analysis of the dynamic geometry of the left ventricle: The basis for an improved model of wall motion. J. Am. Soc. Echocardiogr., *1*:393, 1988.

77. Guyer, D.E., Foale, R.A., Gillam, L.D., Wilkins, G.T., Guerrero, J.L., and Weyman, A.E.: An echocardiographic technique for quantifying and displaying the ex-

78. Pearlman, J.D., Hogan, R.D., Wiske, P.S., Franklin, T.D., and Weyman, A.E.: Echocardiographic definition of the left ventricular centroid. I. Analysis of methods for centroid calculation from a single tomogram. J. Am. Coll. Cardiol., *16*:986, 1990.

79. Wiske, P.S., Pearlman, J.D., Hogan, R.D., Franklin, T.D., and Weyman, A.E.: Echocardiographic definition of the left ventricular centroid. II. Determination of the optimal centroid during systole in normal and infarcted hearts. J. Am. Coll. Cardiol., *16*:993, 1990.

80. Shapiro, S.M., Bersohn, M.M., and Laks, M.M.: In search of the Holy Grail: The study of diastolic ventricular function by the use of Doppler echocardiography. J. Am. Coll. Cardiol., *17*:1517, 1991.

80a.Galderisi, M., Benjamin, E.J., Evans, J.C., D'Agostino, R.B., Fuller, D.L., Lehman, B., Wolf, P.A., and Levy, D.: Intra- and interobserver reproducibility of Doppler-assessed indexes of left ventricular diastolic function in a population-based study (the Framingham Heart Study). Am. J. Cardiol., *70*:1341, 1992.

81. Curtius, J.M., Gaebel, K., Fricke, S., Welslau, R., and Pothoff, G.: Doppler echocardiographic analysis of left ventricular diastolic blood flow. Echocardiography, *8*: 547, 1991.

82. Lin, S-L., Tak, T., Kawanishi, D.T., Rahimtoola, S.H., and Chandraratna, P.A.N.: Accuracy of Doppler ultrasound in evaluating changes of left ventricular diastolic properties. Echocardiography, *7*:515, 1990.

83. Marino, P., Destro, G., Barbieri, E., and Zardini, P.: Early left ventricular filling: An approach to its multifactorial nature using a combined hemodynamic-Doppler technique. Am. Heart J., *122*:132, 1991.

84. Thomas, J.D. and Weyman, A.E.: Echocardiographic Doppler evaluation of left ventricular diastolic function. Physics and physiology. Circulation, *84*:977, 1991.

85. Hoit, B.D., Rashwan, M., Verba, J., Pretorius, D., Sahn, D.J., and Bhargava, V.: Instantaneous transmitral flow using Doppler and M-mode echocardiography: Comparison with radionuclide ventriculography. Am. Heart J., *118*:308, 1989.

86. Nishimura, R.A., Abel, M.D., Hatle, L.K., Holmes, D.R., Housmans, P.R., Ritman, E.L., and Tajik, A.J.: Significance of Doppler indices of diastolic filling of the left ventricle: Comparison with invasive hemodynamics in a canine model. Am. Heart J., *118*:1248, 1989.

87. Myreng, Y. and Smiseth, O.A.: Assessment of left ventricular relaxation by Doppler echocardiography. Circulation, *81*:260, 1990.

88. Nishimura, R.A., Housmans, P.R., Hatle, L.K., and Tajik, A.J.: Assessment of diastolic function of the heart: Background and current applications of Doppler echocardiography. Part I. Physiologic and pathophysiologic features. Mayo Clin. Proc., *64*:71, 1989.

89. Spirito, P. and Maron, B.J.: Doppler echocardiography for assessing left ventricular diastolic function. Ann. Intern. Med., *109*:122, 1988.

90. Nishimura, R.A., Abel, M.D., Hatle, L.K., and Tajik, A.J.: Assessment of diastolic function of the heart: Background and current applications of Doppler echocardiography. Part II. Clinical studies. Mayo Clin. Proc., *64*:181, 1989.

91. Appleton, C.P., Hatle, L.K., and Popp, R.L.: Relation of transmitral flow velocity patterns to left ventricular diastolic function: New insights from a combined hemo-

dynamic and Doppler echocardiographic study. J. Am. Coll. Cardiol., *12*:426, 1988.

91a.Thomas, J.D., Flachskampf, F.A., Chen, C., Guererro, J.L., Levine, R.A., and Weyman, A.E.: Isovolumic relaxation time varies predictably with its time constant and aortic and left atrial pressures: Implications for the noninvasive evaluation of ventricular relaxation. Am. Heart J., *124*:1305, 1992.

91b.Brecker, S.J.D., Lee, C.H., and Gibson, D.G.: Relation of left ventricular isovolumic relaxation time and incoordination to transmitral Doppler filling patterns. Br. Heart J., *68*:567, 1992.

92. Buda, A.J., Li, Y., Brant, D., Kause, L.C., and Julius, S.: Changes in left ventricular diastolic filling during the development of left ventricular hypertrophy: Observations using Doppler echocardiography in a unique canine model. Am. Heart J., *121*:1759, 1991.

93. Chakko, S., Mayor, M., Allison, M.D., Kessler, K.M., Materson, B.J., and Myerburg, R.J.: Abnormal left ventricular diastolic filling in eccentric left ventricular hypertrophy of obesity. Am. J. Cardiol., *68*:95, 1991.

94. Lee, C.H., Hogan, J.C., and Gibson, D.G.: Diastolic disease in left ventricular hypertrophy: Comparison of M-mode and Doppler echocardiography for the assessment of rapid ventricular filling. Br. Heart J., *65*:194, 1991.

94a.Kono, T., Sabbah, H.N., Rosman, H., Alam, M., Stein, P.D., and Goldstein, S.: Left atrial contribution to ventricular filling during the course of evolving heart failure. Circulation, *86*:1317, 1992.

95. Legeais, S., Gaucher, S., Veyrat, C., Gourtchiglouian, C., Yafi, W.E., and Kalmanson, D.: Reference value of tricuspid flow velocity trace for assessing physiological age-variations of normal mitral traces: Value of new age-independent ratio. Cardiovasc. Imag., *2*:267, 1990.

96. Kitzman, D.W., Sheikh, K.H., Beere, P.A., Philips, J.L., and Higginbotham, M.B.: Age-related alterations of Doppler left ventricular filling indexes in normal subjects are independent of left ventricular mass, heart rate, contractility and loading conditions..J. Am. Coll. Cardiol., *18*:1243, 1991.

97. Pearson, A.C., Gudipati, C.V., and Labovitz, A.J.: Effects of aging on left ventricular structure and function. Am. Heart J., *121*:871, 1991.

98. Manning, W.J., Shannon, R.P., Santinga, J.A., Parker, J.A., Gervino, E.V., Come, P.C., and Wei, J.Y.: Reversal of changes in left ventricular diastolic filling associated with normal aging using Diltiazem. Am. J. Cardiol., *67*:894, 1991.

99. Lernfelt, B., Wikstrand, J., Svanborg, A., and Landahl, S.: Aging and left ventricular function in elderly healthy people. Am. J. Cardiol., *68*:547, 1991.

100. Vandenberg, B.F., Kieso, R.A., Fox-Eastham, K., Tomanek, R.J., and Kerber, R.E.: Effect of age on diastolic left ventricular filling at rest and during inotropic stimulation and acute systemic hypertension: Experimental studies in conscious beagles. Am. Heart J., *120*:73, 1990.

101. Spirito, P. and Maron, B.J.: Influence of aging on Doppler echocardiographic indices of left ventricular diastolic function. Br. Heart J., *59*:672, 1988.

102. Bowman, L.K., Lee, F.A., Jaffe, C.C., Mattera, J., Wackers, F.J.T., and Zaret, B.L.: Peak filling rate normalized to mitral stroke volume: A new Doppler echocardiographic filling index validated by radionuclide angiographic techniques. J. Am. Coll. Cardiol., *12*:937, 1988.

103. Courtois, M., Mechem, C.J., Barzilai, B., and Ludbrook, P.A.: Factors related to end-systolic volume are impor-tant determinants of peak early diastolic transmitral flow velocity. Circulation, *85*:1132, 1992.

103a.Stewart, R.A.H., Joshi, J., Alexander, N., Nihoyanno-poulos, P., and Oakley, C.M.: Adjustment for the influence of age and heart rate on Doppler measurements of left ventricular filling. Br. Heart J., *68*:608, 1992.

104. Appleton, C.P., Carucci, M.J., Henry, C.P., and Olajos, M.: Influence of incremental changes in heart rate on mitral flow velocity: Assessment in lightly sedated, conscious dogs. J. Am. Coll. Cardiol., *17*:227, 1991.

105. Harrison, M.R., Clifton, G.D., Pennell, A.T., DeMaria, A.N., and Cater, A.: Effect of heart rate on left ventricular diastolic transmitral flow velocity patterns assessed by Doppler echocardiography in normal subjects. Am. J. Cardiol., *67*:622, 1991.

106. Smith, S.A., Stoner, J.E., Russell, A.E., Sheppard, J.M., and Aylward, P.E.: Transmitral velocities measured by pulsed Doppler in healthy volunteers: Effects of acute changes in blood pressure and heart rate. Br. Heart J., *61*:344, 1989.

107. Danielsen, R., Nordrehaug, J.E., and Vik-mo, H.: Importance of adjusting left ventricular diastolic peak filling rate for heart rate. Am. J. Cardiol., *61*:489, 1988.

107a.Oniki, T., Hashimoto, Y., Shimizu, S., Kakuta, T., Yamima, M., and Numano, F.: Effect of increasing heart rate on Doppler indices of left ventricular performance in healthy men. Br. Heart J., *68*:425, 1992.

108. Myreng, Y., Smiseth, O.A., and Risoe, C.: Left ventricular filling at elevated diastolic pressures: Relationship between transmitral Doppler flow velocities and atrial contribution. Am. Heart J., *119*:620, 1990.

109. Suzuki, T., Sato, K., and Aoki, K.: Influence of postural change on transmitral flow velocity profile assessed by pulsed Doppler echocardiography in normal individuals and in patients with myocardial infarction. Am. Heart J., *120*:110, 1990.

110. Thomas, J.D., Choong, C.Y.P., Flachskampf, F.A., and Weyman, A.E.: Analysis of the early transmitral Doppler velocity curve: Effect of primary physiologic changes and compensatory preload adjustment. J. Am. Coll. Cardiol., *16*:644, 1990.

111. Masuyama, T., St. Goar, F.G., Alderman, E.L., and Popp, R.L.: Effects of Nitroprusside on transmitral flow velocity patterns in extreme heart failure: A combined hemodynamic and Doppler echocardiographic study of varying loading conditions. J. Am. Coll. Cardiol., *16*:1175, 1990.

112. Choong, C.Y., Herrmann, H.C., Weyman, A.E., and Fifer, M.A.: Preload dependence of Doppler-derived indexes of left ventricular diastolic function in humans. J. Am. Coll. Cardiol., *10*:800, 1987.

113. Wallmeyer, K., Wann, L.S., Sagar, K.B., Czakanski, P., Kalbfleisch, J., and Klopfenstein, H.S.: The effect of changes in afterload on Doppler echocardiographic indexes of left ventricular performance. J. Am. Soc. Echocardiogr., *1*:135, 1988.

114. Nishimura, R.A., Abel, M.D., Housmans, P.R., Warnes, C.A., and Tajik, A.J.: Mitral flow velocity curves as a function of different loading conditions: Evaluation by intraoperative transesophageal Doppler echocardiography. J. Am. Soc. Echocardiogr., *2*:79, 1989.

115. Downes, T.R., Nomeir, A-M., Stewart, K., Mumma, M., Kerensky, R., and Little, W.C.: Effect of alteration in loading conditions on both normal and abnormal patterns of left ventricular filling in healthy individuals. Am. J. Cardiol., *65*:377, 1990.

116. Wisenbaugh, T., Harlamert, E., and DeMaria, A.N.: Re-

lation of left ventricular filling dynamics to alterations in load and compliance in patients with and without pressure-overload hypertrophy. Circulation, *81*:101, 1990.

117. Himura, Y., Kumada, T., Kambayashi, M., Hayashida, W., Ishikawa, N., Nakamura, Y., and Kawai, C.: Importance of left ventricular systolic function in the assessment of left ventricular diastolic function with Doppler transmitral flow velocity recording. J. Am. Coll. Cardiol., *18*:753, 1991.

118. Miki, S., Murakami, T., Iwase, T., Tomita, T., Suzuki, Y., and Kawai, C.: Dependence of Doppler echocardiographic transmitral early peak velocity on left ventricular systolic function in coronary artery disease. Am. J. Cardiol., *67*:470, 1991.

119. Miki, S., Murakami, T., Iwase, T., Tomita, T., Nakamura, Y., and Kawai, C.: Doppler echocardiographic transmitral peak early velocity does not directly reflect hemodynamic changes in humans: Importance of normalization to mitral stroke volume. J. Am. Coll. Cardiol., *17*:1507, 1991.

120. Johannessen, K-A., Cerqueira, M., Veith, R.D., and Stratton, J.R.: Influence of sympathetic stimulation and parasympathetic withdrawal on Doppler echocardiographic left ventricular diastolic filling velocities in young normal subjects. Am. J. Cardiol., *67*:520, 1991.

121. Plotnick, G.D., Kmetzo, J.J., and Gottdiener, J.S.: Effect of autonomic blockade, postural changes and isometric exercise on Doppler indexes of diastolic left ventricular function. Am. J. Cardiol., *67*:1284, 1991.

122. Zoghbi, W.A. and Bolli, R.: The increasing complexity of assessing diastolic function from ventricular filling dynamics. J. Am. Coll. Cardiol., *17*:1237, 1991.

123. Ding, Z.P., Oh, J.K., Klein, A.L., and Tajik, A.J.: Effect of sample volume location on Doppler-derived transmitral inflow velocity values. J. Am. Soc. Echocardiogr., *4*:451, 1991.

124. Nishimura, R.A., Abel, M.D., Hatle, L.K., and Tajik, A.J.: Relation of pulmonary vein to mitral flow velocities by transesophageal Doppler echocardiography. Circulation, *81*:1488, 1990.

125. Konecke, L.L., Feigenbaum, H., Chang, S., Corya, B.C., and Fischer, J.C.: Abnormal mitral valve motion in patients with elevated left ventricular diastolic pressures. Circulation, *47*:989, 1973.

126. Lewis, J.R., Parker, J.O., and Burggraf, G.W.: Mitral valve motion and changes in left ventricular end-diastolic pressure: A correlative study of the PR-AC interval. Am. J. Cardiol., *42*:383, 1978.

127. Upton, M.T., Gibson, D.G., and Brown, D.J.: Echocardiographic assessment of abnormal left ventricular relaxation in man. Br. Heart J., *38*:1001, 1976.

128. Friedman, M.J., Sahn, D.J., Burris, H.A., Allen, H.D., and Goldberg, S.J.: Computerized echocardiographic analysis to detect abnormal systolic and diastolic left ventricular function in children with aortic stenosis. Am. J. Cardiol., *44*:478, 1979.

129. St. John Sutton, M.G., Reichek, N., Kastor, J.A., and Giuliani, E.R.: Computerized M-mode echocardiographic analysis of left ventricular dysfunction in cardiac amyloid. Circulation, *66*:790, 1982.

130. Bahler, R.C., Vrobel, T.R., and Martin, P.: The relation of heart rate and shortening fraction to echocardiographic indexes of left ventricular relaxation in normal subjects. J. Am. Coll. Cardiol., *2*:926, 1983.

131. Rhako, P.S.: Evaluation of left ventricular filling in dilated cardiomyopathy using digitized M-mode echocardiograms. Echocardiography, *8*:163, 1991.

132. Ng, K.S.K. and Gibson, D.G.: Impairment of diastolic function by shortened filling period in severe left ventricular disease. Br. Heart J., *62*:246, 1989.

133. Herve, C., Duval, A.M., Malik, J., Meguira, A., and Brun, P.: Relations between posterior wall kinetics during diastole and left ventricular filling. J. Am. Coll. Cardiol., *15*:1587, 1990.

134. Alam, M. and Hoglund, C.: Assessment by echocardiogram of left ventricular diastolic function in healthy subjects using the atrioventricular plane displacement. Am. J. Cardiol., *69*:565, 1992.

135. Perez, J.E., Waggoner, A.D., Barzilai, B., Melton, Jr., H.E., Miller, J.G., and Sobel, B.E.: On-line assessment of ventricular function by automatic boundary detection and ultrasonic backscatter imaging. J. Am. Coll. Cardiol., *19*:313, 1992.

136. Devereux, R.B., Casale, P.N., Kligfield, P., Eisenberg, R.R., Miller, D., Campo, E., and Alonso, D.R.: Performance of primary and derived M-mode echocardiographic measurements for detection of left ventricular hypertrophy in necropsied subjects and in patients with systemic hypertension, mitral regurgitation and dilated cardiomyopathy. Am. J. Cardiol., *57*:1388, 1986.

137. Devereux, R.B. and Reichek, N.: Echocardiographic determination of left ventricular mass in man. Anatomic validation of the method. Circulation, *55*:613, 1977.

138. Troy, B.L., Pombo, J., and Rackley, C.E.: Measurement of left ventricular wall thickness and mass by echocardiography. Circulation, *45*:602, 1972.

139. Devereux, R.B.: Toward a more complete understanding of left ventricular afterload. J. Am. Coll. Cardiol., *17*:122, 1991.

140. Bachenberg, T.C., Shub, C., Hauck, A.J., and Edwards, W.D.: Can anatomical left ventricular mass be estimated reliably by M-mode echocardiography? A clinicopathological study of ninety-three patients. Echocardiography, *8*:9, 1991.

141. Pearson, A.C., Pasierski, T., and Labovitz, A.J.: Left ventricular hypertrophy: Diagnosis, prognosis, and management. Am. Heart J., *121*:148, 1991.

142. Collins, H.W., Kronenberg, M.W., and Byrd, B.F.: Reproducibility of left ventricular mass measurements by two-dimensional and M-mode echocardiography. J. Am. Coll. Cardiol., *14*:672, 1989.

143. Daniels, S.R., Meyer, R.A., Liang, Y., and Bove, K.E.: Echocardiographically determined left ventricular mass index in normal children, adolescents and young adults. J. Am. Coll. Cardiol., *12*:703, 1988.

143a. Germain, P., Roul, G., Kastler, B., Mossard, J.M., Bareiss, P., and Sacrez, A.: Inter-study variability in left ventricular mass measurement. Comparison between M-mode echography and MRI. Eur. Heart J., *13*:1011, 1992.

144. Reichek, N., Helak, J., Plappert, T.A., St. John Sutton, M.G., and Weber, K.T.: Anatomic validation of left ventricular mass estimates from clinical two-dimensional echocardiography: Initial results. Circulation, *67*:348, 1983.

145. Helak, J.W. and Reichek, N.: Quantitation of human left ventricular mass and volume by two-dimensional echocardiography: In vitro anatomic validation. Circulation, *63*:1398, 1981.

146. Byrd, B.F., Finkbeiner, W., Bouchard, A., Silverman, N.H., and Schiller, N.B.: Accuracy and reproducibility of clinically acquired two-dimensional echocardiographic mass measurements. Am. Heart J., *118*:133, 1989.

147. Borow, K.M., Propper, R., Bierman, F.E., Grady, S., and Inati, A.: The left ventricular end-systolic pressure-

dimensional relation in patients with thalassemia major. A new noninvasive method for assessing contractile states. Circulation, *66*:980, 1982.

148. Reichek, N., Wilson, J., St. John Sutton, M., Plappert, T.A., Goldberg, S., and Hirshfeld, J.W.: Noninvasive determination of left ventricular end-systolic stress: Validation of the method and initial application. Circulation, *65*:99, 1982.

149. Quinones, M.A., Mokotoff, D.M., Nouri, S., Winters, W.L., and Miller, R.R.: Non-invasive quantification of left ventricular wall stress. Validation of method and application to assessment of chronic pressure overload. Am. J. Cardiol., *45*:782, 1980.

150. Roman, M.J., Devereux, R.B., and Cody, R.J.: Ability of left ventricular stress-shortening relations, end-systolic stress/volume ratio and indirect indexes to detect severe contractile failure in ischemic or idiopathic dilated cardiomyopathy. Am. J. Cardiol., *64*:1338, 1989.

151. Gardin, J.M., Matin, K., White, D., and Henry, W.L.: Effect of aging on peak systolic left ventricular wall stress in normal subjects. Am. J. Cardiol., *63*:998, 1989.

152. Douglas, P.S., Reichek, N., Plappert, T., Muhammad, A., and St. John Sutton, M.G.: Comparison of echocardiographic methods for assessment of left ventricular shortening and wall stress. J. Am. Coll. Cardiol., *9*:945, 1987.

153. Segar, D.S., Moran, M., Ryan, T., Johnson, J.K., and Johnson, M.D.: End-systolic regional wall stress-length and stress-shortening relations in an experimental model of normal, ischemic and reperfused myocardium. J. Am. Coll. Cardiol., *17*:1651, 1991.

154. Sandor, G.G.S., Popov, R., DeSouza, E., Morris, S., and Johnston, B.: Rate-corrected mean velocity of fiber shortening-stress at peak systole as a load-independent measure of contractility. Am. J. Cardiol., *69*:403, 1992.

155. Heng, M.K., Bai, J.X., and Marin, J.: Changes in left ventricular wall stress during isometric and isotonic exercise in healthy men. Am. J. Cardiol., *62*:794, 1988.

156. Popp, R.L., Wolfe, S.B., Hirata, T., and Feigenbaum, H.: Estimation of right and left ventricular size by ultrasound. A study of the echoes from the interventricular septum. Am. J. Cardiol., *24*:523, 1969.

157. Silverman, N.H. and Hudson, S.: Evaluation of right ventricular volume and ejection fraction in children by two-dimensional echocardiography. Pediatr. Cardiol., *4*: 197, 1983.

158. Levine, R.A., Gibson, T.C., Aretz, T., Gillam, L.D., Guyer, D.E., King, M.E., and Weyman, A.E.: Echocardiographic measurement of right ventricular volume. Circulation, *69*:497, 1984.

159. Starling, M.R., Crawford, M.H., Sorensen, S.G., and O'Rourke, R.A.: A new two-dimensional echocardiographic technique for evaluating right ventricular size and performance in patients with obstructive lung disease. Circulation, *66*:612, 1982.

160. Saito, A., Ueda, K., and Kalano, H.: Right ventricular volume determination by two-dimensional echocardiography. J. Cardiogr., *11*:1159, 1981.

161. Krebs, W., Erbel, R., Schweizer, P., Richter, H.A., Henn, G., Massberg, I., Meyer, J., and Effert, S.: Right ventricular volume determination by two-dimensional echocardiography and radiography of model hearts using a subtraction method. Z. Kardiol., *71*:413, 1982.

162. Aebischer, N.M. and Czegledy, F.: Determination of right ventricular volume by two-dimensional echocardiography with a crescentic model. J. Am. Soc. Echocardiogr., *2*:110, 1989.

163. Foale, R., Nihoyannopoulos, P., McKenna, W., Klienebenne, A., Nadazdin, A., Rowland, E., and Smith, G.: Echocardiographic measurement of the normal adult right ventricle. Br. Heart J., *56*:33, 1986.

164. Linker, D.T., Mortiz, W.E., and Pearlman, A.S.: A new three-dimensional echocardiographic method of right ventricular volume measurement: In vitro validation. J. Am. Coll. Cardiol., *8*:101, 1986.

165. Bommer, W., Weinert, L., Neumann, A., Neef, J., Mason, D.T., and DeMaria, A.: Determination of right atrial and right ventricular size by two-dimensional echocardiography. Circulation, *60*:91,1979.

166. Tomita, M., Masuda, H., Sumi, T., Shiraki, H., Gotoh, K., Yagi, Y., Tsukamoto, T., Terashima, Y., Miwa, Y., and Kirakawa, S.: Estimation of right ventricular volume by modified echocardiographic subtraction method. Am. Heart J., *123*:1011, 1992.

167. Mongkolsmai, D., Williams, G.A., Goodgold, H., and Labovitz, A.J.: Determination of right ventricular ejection fraction by two-dimensional echocardiographic single plane subtraction method. J. Am. Soc. Echocardiogr., *2*:119, 1989.

168. Kaul, S., Tei, C., Hopkins, J.M., and Shah, P.M.: Assessment of right ventricular function using two-dimensional echocardiography. Am. Heart J., *107*:526, 1984.

169. Hammarstrom, E., Wranne, B., Pinto, F.J., Puryear, J., and Popp, R.L.: Tricuspid annular motion. J. Am. Soc. Echocardiogr., *4*:131, 1991.

170. Wann, L.S., Stickels, K.R., Bamrah, V.S., and Gross, C.M.: Digital processing of contrast echocardiograms: A new technique for measuring right ventricular ejection fraction. Am. J. Cardiol., *53*:1164, 1984.

171. Baker, B.J., Scovil, J.A., Kane, J.J., and Murphy, M.L.: Echocardiographic detection of right ventricular hypertrophy. Am. Heart J., *105*:611, 1983.

172. Cooper, M.J., Teitel, D.F., Silverman, N.H., and Enderlein, M.: Comparison of M-mode echocardiographic measurement of right ventricular wall thickness obtained by the subcostal and parasternal approach in children. Am. J. Cardiol., *54*:835, 1984.

173. Cacho, A., Prakash, R., Sarma, R., and Kaushik, V.S.: Usefulness of two-dimensional echocardiography in diagnosing right ventricular hypertrophy. Chest, *84*:154, 1983.

174. McKenna, W.J., Kleinebenne, A., Nihoyannopoulos, P., and Foale, R.: Echocardiographic measurement of right ventricular wall thickness in hypertrophic cardiomyopathy: Relation to clinical and prognostic features. J. Am. Coll. Cardiol., *11*:351, 1988.

175. King, M.E., Braun, H., Goldblatt, A., Liberthson, R., and Weyman, A.E.: Interventricular septal configuration as a predictor of right ventricular systolic hypertension in children: A cross-sectional echocardiographic study. Circulation, *68*:68, 1983.

176. Portman, M.A., Bhat, A.M., Cohen, M.H., and Jacobstein, M.D.: Left ventricular systolic circular index: An echocardiographic measure of transseptal pressure ratio. Am. Heart J., *114*:1178, 1987.

177. Jardin, F., Dubourg, O., Gueret, P., Delorme, G., and Bourdarias, J.: Quantitative two-dimensional echocardiography in massive pulmonary embolism: Emphasis on ventricular interdependence and leftward septal displacement. J. Am. Coll. Cardiol., *10*:1201, 1987.

178. Ryan, T., Petrovic, O., Dillon, J.C., Feigenbaum, H., Conley, M.J., and Armstrong, W.F.: An echocardiographic index for separation of right ventricular volume and pressure overload. J. Am. Coll. Cardiol., *5*:918, 1985.

179. Diamond, M.A., Dillon, J.C., Haine, C.L., Chang, S., and Feigenbaum, H.: Echocardiographic features of atrial septal defect. Circulation, *43*:129, 1971.
180. Tajik, A.J., Gau, G.T., Ritter, D.G., et al.: Echocardiographic pattern of right ventricular diastolic volume overload in children. Circulation, *46*:36, 1972.
181. Kerber, R.E., Dippel, W.F., and Abboud, F.M.: Abnormal motion of the interventricular septum in right ventricular volume overload. Experimental and clinical echocardiographic studies. Circulation, *48*:86, 1973.
182. Meyer, R.A., Schwartz, D.C., Benzing, G., and Kaplan, S.: Ventricular septum in right ventricular volume overload: An echocardiographic study. Am. J. Cardiol., *30*:349, 1972.
183. Feneley, M. and Cavaghan, T.: Paradoxical and pseudo-paradoxical interventricular septal motion in patients with right ventricular volume overload. Circulation, *74*:230, 1986.
184. Weyman, A.E., Wann, L.S., Feigenbaum, H., and Dillon, J.C.: Mechanism of abnormal septal motion in patients with right ventricular volume overload: A cross-sectional echocardiographic study. Circulation, *54*:179, 1976.
185. Louie, E.K., Rich, S., Levitsky, S., and Brundage, B.H.: Doppler echocardiographic demonstration of the differential effects of right ventricular pressure and volume overload on left ventricular geometry and filling. J. Am. Coll. Cardiol., *19*:84, 1992.
186. Pearlman, A.S., Clark, C.E., Henry, W.L., Morganroth, J., Itscoitz, S.B., and Epstein, S.E.: Determinants of ventricular septal motion: Influence of relative right and left ventricular size. Circulation, *54*:83, 1986.
187. Mueller, T.N., Kerber, R.E., and Marcus, M.L.: Comparison of interventricular septal motion studied by ventriculography and echocardiography in patients with atrial septal defect. Br. Heart J., *40*:984, 1978.
188. Thompson, C.R., Kingma, I., MacDonald, R.P.R., Belenkie, I., Tyberg, J.V., and Smith, E.R.: Transseptal pressure gradient and diastolic ventricular septal motion in patients with mitral stenosis. Circulation, *76*:974, 1987.
189. Weyman, A.E., Heger, J.J., Kronik, G., Wann, L.S., Dillon, J.C., and Feigenbaum, H.: Mechanism of paradoxical early diastolic septal motion in patients with mitral stenosis: Cross-sectional echocardiographic study. Am. J. Cardiol., *40*:691, 1977.
190. McDonald, I.G., Feigenbaum, H., and Chang, S.: Analysis of left ventricular wall motion by reflected ultrasound: Application to assessment of myocardial function. Circulation, *46*:14, 1972.
191. Beppu, S., Masuda, Y., Sakakibara, H., Izumi, S., Park, Y-D., Nagata, S., Miyatake, K., and Nimura, Y.: Transient abnormal septal motion after non-surgical closure of the ductus arteriosus. Br. Heart J., *59*:706, 1988.
192. Lehmann, K.G., Lee, F.A., McKenzie, W.B., Barash, P.G., Prokop, E.K., Durkin, M.A., and Ezekowitz, M.D.: Onset of altered interventricular septal motion during cardiac surgery. Circulation, *82*:1325, 1990.
193. Dittrich, H.C., Chow, L.C., and Nicod, P.H.: Early improvement in left ventricular diastolic function after relief of chronic right ventricular pressure overload. Circulation, *80*:823, 1989.
194. Louie, E.K., Bieniarz, T., Moore, A.M., and Levitsky, S.: Reduced atrial contribution to left ventricular filling in patients with severe tricuspid regurgitation after tricuspid valvulectomy: A Doppler echocardiographic study. J. Am. Coll. Cardiol., *16*:1617, 1990.
195. Zoghbi, W.A., Habib, G.B., and Quinones, M.A.: Doppler assessment of right ventricular filling in a normal population. Circulation, *82*:1316, 1990.
196. Klein, A.L., Hatle, L.K., Burstow, D.J., Taliercio, C.P., Seward, J.B., Kyle, R.A., Bailey, K.R., Gertz, M.A., and Tajik, A.J.: Comprehensive Doppler assessment of right ventricular diastolic function in cardiac amyloidosis. J. Am. Coll. Cardiol., *15*:103, 1990.
196a. Habib, G.B. and Zoghbi, W.A.: Doppler assessment of right ventricular dynamics in systemic hypertension: Comparison with left ventricular filling. Am. Heart J., *124*:1313–1320, 1992.
197. Loperfido, F., Pennestri, F., Digaetano, A., Scabbia, E., Santarelli, P., Mongiardo, R., Schiavoni, G., Coppola, E., and Manzoli, U.: Assessment of left atrial dimensions by cross-sectional echocardiography in patients with mitral valve disease. Br. Heart J., *50*:570, 1983.
198. Schabelman, S., Schiller, N.B., Silverman, N.H., and Ports, T.A.: Left atrial volume stimulation by two-dimensional echocardiography. Cathet. Cardiovasc. Diagn., *7*:165, 1981.
199. Gehl, L.G., Mintz, G.S., Kotler, M.N., and Segal, B.L.: Left atrial volume overload in mitral regurgitation: A two-dimensional echocardiographic study. Am. J. Cardiol., *49*:33, 1982.
200. Hofstetter, R., Bartz-Bazzanella, P., Kentrup, H., and von Bernuth, G.: Determination of left atrial area and volume by cross-sectional echocardiography in healthy infants and children. Am. J. Cardiol., *68*:1073, 1991.
201. Haendchen, R.V., Povzhitkov, M., Meerbaum, S., Maurer, G., and Corday, E.: Evaluation of changes in left ventricular end-diastolic pressure by left atrial two-dimensional echocardiography. Am. Heart J., *104*:740, 1982.
202. Jones, C.J.H., Song, G.J., and Gibson, D.G.: An echocardiographic assessment of atrial mechanical behavior. Br. Heart J., *65*:31, 1991.
203. Ren, J.F., Kotler, M.N., DePace, N.L., Mintz, G.S., Kimbiris, D., Kalman, P., and Ross, J.: Two-dimensional echocardiographic determination of left atrial emptying volume: A non-invasive index in quantifying the degree of nonrheumatic mitral regurgitation. J. Am. Coll. Cardiol., *2*:729, 1983.
204. Hiraishi, S., DiSessa, T.G., Jarmakani, J.M., Nakanishi, T., Isabel-Jones, J., and Friedman, W.F.: Two-dimensional echocardiographic assessment of left atrial size in children. Am. J. Cardiol., *52*:1249, 1983.
205. Hirata, T., Wolfe, S.B., Popp, R.L., Helmen, C.H., and Feigenbaum, H.: Estimation of left atrial size using ultrasound. Am. Heart J., *78*:43, 1969.
206. TenCate, F.J., Kloster, F.E., VanDorp, W.G., Meester, G.T., and Roelandt, J.: Dimensions and volumes of left atrium and ventricle determined by single beam echocardiography. Br. Heart J., *36*:737, 1974.
207. Kronzon, I. and Mehta, S.S.: Giant left atrium. Chest, *65*:677, 1974.
208. Lester, L.A., Vitullo, D., Sodt, P., Hutcheon, N., and Arcilla, R.: An evaluation of the left atrial/aortic root ratio in children with ventricular septal defect. Circulation, *60*:364, 1979.
209. LaBarre, T.R., Stamato, N.J., Hwang, M.H., Jacobs, W.R., Stephanides, L., and Scanlon, P.J.: Left atrial appendage aneurysm with associated anomalous pulmonary venous drainage. Am. Heart J., *114*:1243, 1987.
210. Cujec, B., Bharadwaj, B., Orchard, R.C., and Lopez, J.F.: Transesophageal echocardiography in the diagnosis of left atrial appendage aneurysm. J. Am. Soc. Echocardiogr., *3*:408, 1990.

211. Comess, K.A., Labate, D.P., Winter, J.A., Hill, A.C., and Miller, D.C.: Congenital left atrial appendage aneurysm with intact pericardium: Diagnosis by transesophageal echocardiography. Am. Heart J., *120*:992, 1990.
212. Kircher, B., Abbott, J.A., Pau, S., Gould, R.G., Himelman, R.B., Higgins, C.B., Lipton, M.J., and Schiller, N.B.: Left atrial volume determination by biplane two-dimensional echocardiography: Validation by cine computed tomography. Am. Heart J., *121*:864, 1991.
213. Sasse, L.: Echocardiography of left atrial wall. JAMA, *228*:1667, 1974.
214. Yoshikawa, J., Kato, H., Owaki, T., and Tanaka, K.: Study of posterior left atrial wall motion by echocardiography and its clinical application. Jpn. Heart J., *16*:683, 1975.
215. Winsberg, F. and Goldman, H.S.: Echo patterns of cardiac posterior wall. Invest. Radiol., *4*:173, 1969.
216. Strunk, B.L., Fitzgerald, J.W., Lipton, M., Popp, R.L., and Barry, W.H.: The posterior aortic wall echocardiogram: Its relationship to left atrial volume change. Circulation, *54*:744, 1976.
217. Akgun, G. and Layton, C.: Aortic root and left atrial wall motion: An echocardiographic study. Br. Heart J., *39*:1082, 1977.
218. Pozzoli, M., Febo, O., Torbicki, A., Tramarin, R., Calsamiglia, G., Cobelli, F., Specchia, G., and Roelandt, J.R.T.C.: Left atrial appendage dysfunction: A cause of thrombosis? Evidence by transesophageal echocardiography—Doppler studies. J. Am. Soc. Echocardiogr., *4*:435, 1991.
218a.Garcia-Fernandez, M.A., Torecilla, E.G., San Roman, D., Azevedo, J., Bueno, H., Moreno, M.M., and Delcan, J.L.: Left atrial appendage Doppler flow patterns: Implications on thrombus formation. Am. Heart J., *124*:955, 1992.
219. Bommer, W., Weinert, L., Neumann, A., Neef, J., Mason, D.T., and DeMaria, A.: Determination of right atrial and right ventricular size by two-dimensional echocardiography. Circulation, *60*:91, 1979.
220. Lambertz, H., Braun, C., and Krebs, W.: Determination of the size of the right atrium using two-dimensional echocardiography. Z. Kardiol., *73*:393, 1984.
221. Iwase, M., Hurui, H., Miyaguchi, K., Hayashi, H., Yokota, M., Takeuchi, J., Ishiguro, T., and Sakuma, S.: Two-dimensional echocardiography and magnetic resonance imaging in diagnosis of idiopathic dilation of the right atrium. Am. Heart J., *120*:1231, 1990.

# 4

# Hemodynamic Information Derived from Echocardiography

The importance of echocardiography in providing hemodynamic information has increased with advances in Doppler echocardiography. Because the Doppler examination essentially records movement of red cells or blood, this technique provides a direct assessment of blood flow in the cardiovascular system. The observation that the Doppler technique can provide useful information concerning intracardiac pressure and pressure gradients has been a major stimulus to the popularity of Doppler echocardiography.

Although Doppler echocardiography is now the dominant ultrasonic technique for obtaining hemodynamic information, the other echocardiographic techniques (M-mode and two-dimensional and contrast echocardiography) also produce important data concerning pressure and flow inside the heart. The discussions in this chapter are organized to demonstrate how these various ultrasonic examinations are interrelated in providing hemodynamic information.

## ECHOCARDIOGRAPHIC DETERMINATION OF BLOOD FLOW

Doppler echocardiography is the most direct and theoretically the most accurate echocardiographic technique for assessing blood flow. The Doppler signal assesses blood velocity. Combining velocity with the cross-sectional area of the orifice or container through which the blood is flowing provides the basis for quantitating blood flow.[1-3] Figure 4–1 demonstrates the principles of using Doppler echocardiography for measuring blood flow. The Doppler signal can be converted to velocity using the standard Doppler equations (Fig. 4–2), a calculation that requires knowing the angle theta between the direction of blood flow and the ultrasonic beam. Figure 4–3 illustrates that if angle θ is 20° or less, the cosine is close to one. Under these circumstances, the angle can be ignored. An angle greater than 20° has a great effect on the calculated velocity. As the angle approaches 90°, the cosine approaches zero.

The next major determination for calculating flow is the cross-sectional area of the orifice or container through which the blood is flowing (see Fig. 4–1). This measurement is theoretically possible using any of the ultrasonic imaging techniques: M-mode, two-dimensional, or even A-mode echocardiography. For exam-

ple, if one could record the velocity of flow in the root of the aorta, one merely needs to measure the cross-sectional area of the root to obtain quantitative blood flow.

Numerous experimental and clinical studies demonstrate the feasibility of using this basic Doppler approach for measuring blood flow. Unfortunately, many limitations and technicalities remain that must be understood when one is attempting to use this type of examination. One needs to know the average velocity within the vessel in question. The velocity passing through a vessel is not necessarily uniform. As indicated in Figure 4–1, the velocity of flow in the center of a vessel (*long arrows*) is faster than that near the edges (*short arrows*). The explanation is that the friction between the red cells and the walls of the vessel reduces the velocity of those cells near the walls. Thus, the blood in the center of the vessel is moving more rapidly.

The blood flow profile is commonly described as a parabola. Ideally, one would prefer a flat or square blood profile so that one sampling velocity would indicate the average flow. Figure 4–4 illustrates how the blood profile configuration is partially a result of the size of the vessel. A large vessel has a flatter profile than a small vessel. Figure 4–5A demonstrates that the profile also varies with the length of the vessel. As flow first enters a vessel, the profile is relatively flat; with distance, however, the profile becomes more parabolic. Because it is much easier to determine the average flow velocity with a flat blood profile, it is not surprising that efforts for measuring blood flow use large orifices and flow close to the origin of vessels. Figure 4–5C shows that the shape of the vessel also influences the blood profile. If the artery curves, then wall friction varies with regard to the outside or inside of the vessel. For example, in Figure 4–5C, the velocity is higher toward the inside of a curved artery. As the artery straightens and blood leaves the curve, the blood profile is reversed, with the outside portion of the blood moving more quickly.

Despite these real differences in blood velocity, the empiric observations to date have suggested that the profile is more of a theoretic than a practical limitation. Thus far, clinicians have tended to ignore the blood profile problem, and major problems in blood flow determination have not resulted.

A more important limitation to measuring blood flow with Doppler techniques is when the caliber of the vessel

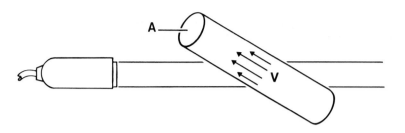
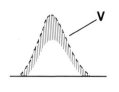

Fig. 4–1.   Principles of using Doppler echocardiography to measure blood flow.

changes, as noted in Figure 4–5*B*. If blood passes from a small cross-sectional area into a larger cross-sectional area, then the pattern of flow is altered. Laminar flow no longer exists, and it would be extremely difficult to obtain mean velocity. This situation would arise if blood were passing through a narrowed orifice or valve into a significantly larger vessel or chamber. Thus, one important prerequisite for the measurement of blood flow using Doppler echocardiography is the existence of laminar flow.

The actual measurement of flow velocity requires obtaining the area under the Doppler curve (see Fig. 4–1). Such measurement, which is the velocity time integral or flow velocity integral, can be obtained by a planimeter or, as is done more commonly, with the use of a computer. Theoretically, one should measure the modal velocity. This velocity is the dominant flow velocity at any given instant. The modal velocity is usually depicted as the most common flow velocity at any one time and is the darkest Doppler signal on the spectral display (Fig.

## DOPPLER EQUATIONS

$$f_d = f_r - f_t$$

$$f_d = 2f_t \frac{v \cdot \cos \theta}{c}$$

$$v = \frac{f_d \cdot c}{2f_t (\cos \theta)}$$

### c = velocity of sound

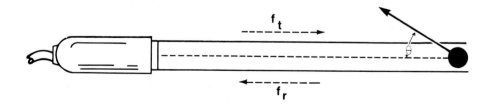

Fig. 4–2.   Doppler equations $f_d$ = Doppler frequency; $f_r$ = received frequency; $f_t$ = transmitted frequency.

**RELATIONSHIP OF ANGLE (θ) TO COSINE OF ANGLE**

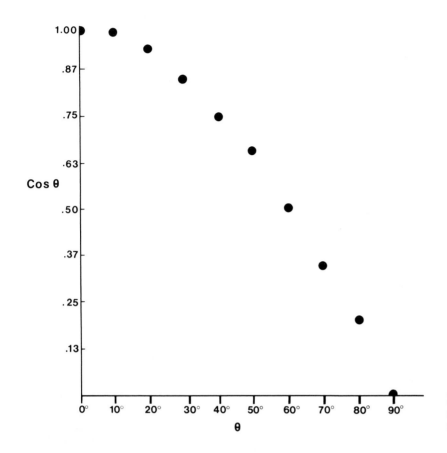

Cos θ

θ

Fig. 4–3. Relationship of an angle to the cosine of that angle.

4–6). Some data indicate that the more easily measured peak velocity envelope is just as accurate in measuring blood flow.[4]

Because the Doppler signal is velocity (distance/time), the area under the velocity-time curve is distance/time × time or distance. Thus, the velocity time integral is sometimes referred to as "stroke distance," which is

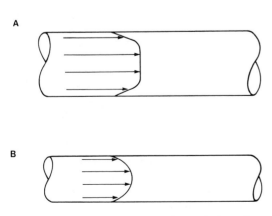

**Fig. 4–4.** Relationship of blood profile and size of a vessel. The blood flow profile is flatter when blood is flowing through a larger vessel (*A*). The profile becomes parabolic in a smaller vessel (*B*).

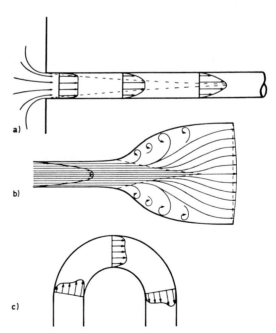

**Fig. 4–5.** The relationship of length (*a*), caliber (*b*), and shape (*c*) of a vessel and the flow profile. (From Hatle, L. and Angelsen, B.: Doppler Ultrasound in Cardiology: Physical Principles and Clinical Applications. 2nd ed. Philadelphia, Lea & Febiger, 1985.)

## PEAK FREQUENCY

## MODAL FREQUENCY

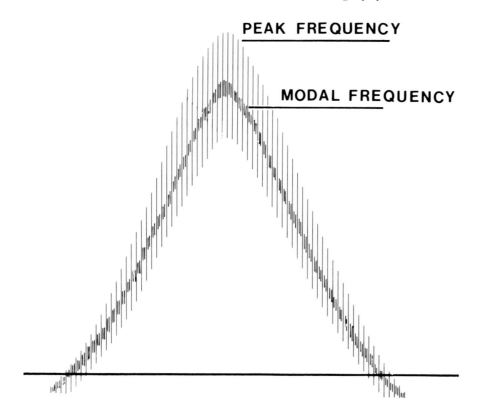

**Fig. 4–6.** Diagram indicating how the modal frequency is the darkest portion of the spectral display.

the distance traveled by the sampled volume with each heart beat.

One must remember that converting velocity to flow requires an accurate assessment of the cross-sectional area of the orifice or vessel through which the blood is flowing. To date, this determination has proved to be the weakest link in flow measurements. Thus far, cross-sectional areas using two-dimensional echocardiography have not been sufficiently accurate or reliable to provide this information. As a result, most investigators have used M-mode or two-dimensional echocardiography for obtaining a diameter of the orifice and then deriving the area. Unfortunately, by converting diameter to area, one must square the diameter or radius ($A = \pi r^2$ or $A = 0.785 d^2$). Any small error in measurement is thus squared. Because some of these diameters are obtained by using the lateral resolution of a two-dimensional system, the error can be significant, especially when squared.

Another problem that must be recognized is that the location of the cross-sectional area must be identical to where the Doppler velocity is being recorded. Because it is rarely possible to obtain high-quality M-mode or two-dimensional imaging while recording Doppler velocities, one frequently records the velocity with one examination and the diameter or cross-sectional area with a different examination. In addition, it is somewhat difficult to always know exactly where the Doppler sample is located. For example, if one records the Doppler velocity in the ascending aorta from the suprasternal notch, the location of that sample with regard to the aortic annulus is not precisely known.

Despite these limitations,[6] the use of Doppler tech-

niques combined with M-mode and two-dimensional echocardiography to provide flow measurements is progressing. The rest of this section describes the various locations within the cardiovascular system in which flow can be recorded and how these measurements are useful clinically. The other echocardiographic techniques for measuring or reflecting flow are also included in the discussions.

### Aortic Flow

Theoretically, the easiest area for flow determination with Doppler echocardiography should be within the aorta.[7,8] Because aortic flow is the blood that perfuses the systemic circulation, it should provide a measure of cardiac output.[9,10] The technique that has been most used is recording the mean velocity of blood flow in the ascending aorta using Doppler echocardiography. The diameter of the ascending aorta is then determined to provide the necessary information for calculating stroke volume or aortic flow.[11–13] The ascending aortic velocity is usually obtained with the transducer in the suprasternal notch (Fig. 4–7A). One could use either continuous or pulsed Doppler for this determination. One could also use the apical view for obtaining blood flow just past the aortic valve using the pulsed Doppler approach (Fig. 4–7C).[14,15] Initially, there was disagreement as to where the aortic diameter should be measured.[4] Several investigators measured the aorta just past the tips of the opened aortic valve.[16,17] Others emphasized the importance of the measurement being past the sinus of Valsalva (2, Fig. 4–8). Another group of investigators suggested that the most accurate measurement is at the root

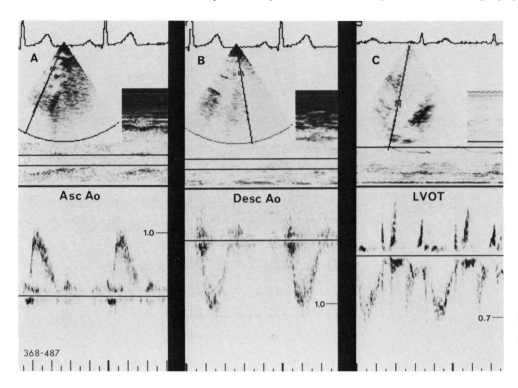

**Fig. 4–7.** *A*, Aortic flow velocity in the ascending aorta (Asc Ao); *B*, descending aorta (Desc Ao); *C*, left ventricular outflow tract (LVOT).

of the aorta (*1*, Fig. 4–8). These clinicians believe that the effective column of blood flowing into the aorta is determined by the cross-sectional area of the annulus or the aortic valve (*3*, Fig. 4–8) rather than by the diameter of the aorta.[18] This argument seems to have been generally resolved, and most aortic areas are now measured at the annulus.

Obtaining a Doppler signal from the descending aorta is technically easier using the suprasternal notch (see Fig. 4–7*B*). Some investigators have indicated that descending aortic velocity is satisfactory for measuring aortic flow.[10] There are many theoretic reasons for not using the descending aortic flow. The significant amount of blood flow that passes through the major vessels from the arch of the aorta should not be reflected by the flow

in the descending aorta. Theoretically, full aortic stroke volume should not be recorded in the descending aorta. In addition, the diameter of the descending aorta is less accurate because it is measured using lateral resolution of the two-dimensional recording.

One does not necessarily have to measure absolute flow if only directional changes are desired. One could merely follow the velocity to see whether blood flow or cardiac output is increasing or decreasing.[19–23] This approach is based on the assumption that the size of the vessel or orifice does not change as blood flow changes. This assumption may not be totally accurate because some evidence suggests that the vessel does change in size depending on the amount of blood flowing through it. This approach may also be limited by the size of the aorta.[24] In any case, reasonable data indicate that Doppler measurements are useful in following a given patient to see directional changes in blood flow.[25] The Doppler recording of the ascending aortic blood flow can also be used to evaluate left ventricular function as noted in Chapter 3. The peak velocity and the rate of acceleration may be related to the vigor with which the left ventricle is able to contract.

Simpler Doppler techniques for measuring stroke volume have been suggested but are unproven. One approach multiplies Doppler-derived ejection time and ejection rate, which is indicated by mean ejection flow velocity.[26]

Flow through the aortic orifice is also reflected by the M-mode recording of the aortic valve leaflets.[27] Figure 4–9 demonstrates an M-mode echocardiogram of a normal aortic valve. Two of the leaflets are seen in systole. With the onset of ejection of blood through the aortic valve, they separate briskly, remain parallel to each

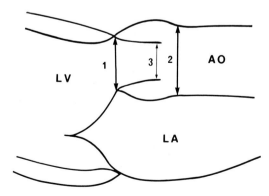

**Fig. 4–8.** Diagram demonstrating where the diameter of the aorta and aortic valve might be measured in order to calculate the cross-sectional area of the aorta for determining aortic flow. LV = left ventricle; AO = aorta; LA = left atrium.

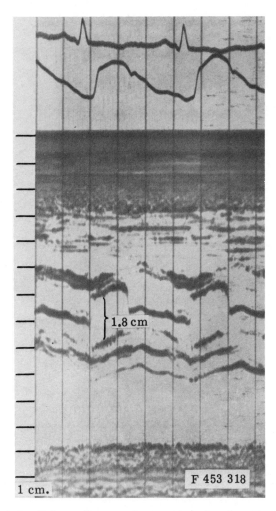

**Fig. 4–9.** Echocardiogram of a normal aortic valve. The leaflets are 1.8 cm apart during ventricular systole.

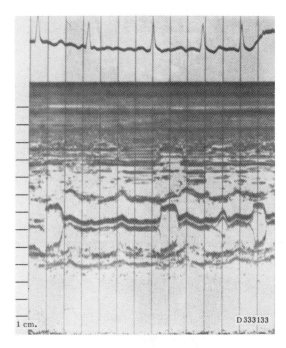

**Fig. 4–10.** Aortic valve echocardiogram of a patient with atrial fibrillation. With a short R–R interval, the separation of the leaflets in systole is either diminished or absent.

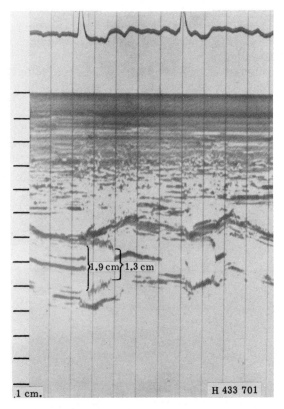

**Fig. 4–11.** Echocardiogram of the aortic valve in a patient with mitral regurgitation and decreased cardiac output. The leaflets separate normally with the onset of ventricular ejection; however, they gradually close throughout systole.

other throughout systole, and close abruptly at the end of ejection. As indicated in Figure 4–9, the separation of the leaflets is approximately 1.5 to 2 cm. Figure 4–10 demonstrates an aortic valve echocardiogram of a patient with atrial fibrillation. Aortic valve motion varies, depending on the preceding R-R interval. After the second echocardiographic QRS complex, the aortic valve does not open. This finding would certainly be compatible with the pulse deficit that commonly occurs with atrial fibrillation. The lack of aortic valve opening has even been reported in a patient with a pulmonary embolus and severe paradoxical pulse.[28] Figure 4–11 shows another pattern of aortic valve motion seen in patients with abnormal flow. The initial separation of the leaflets is greater than the separation just prior to closure of the valve. In Figure 4–9, the leaflets remain maximally opened throughout systole as blood flows through the leaflets. In Figure 4–11, the valve closes gradually during systole. This finding would suggest that the amount of blood is gradually decreasing throughout systole. It appears that the blood flow cannot be sustained at an equal rate throughout systole. This finding is usually indicative of reduced ventricular function or reduced

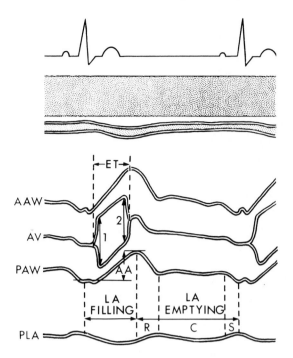

**Fig. 4–12.** Diagram of an M-mode echocardiogram of the aortic valve (AV) and left atrium (LA) demonstrating several measurements that can be made from this type of recording. Ejection time (ET) can be measured between the opening and closing points of the aortic valve. Separation of the aortic valve leaflets can be measured at the onset (*1*) and at the end (*2*) of ejection. The amplitude of motion (AA) of the posterior aortic wall (PAW) can be obtained. The posterior aortic wall motion reflects left atrial volume changes. Left atrial emptying can be divided into a rapid filling phase (R), a conduit phase (C), and a filling owing to atrial systole phase (S). AAW = anterior aortic wall; PLA = posterior left atrial wall.

stroke volume. An alternate situation exists in patients with mitral regurgitation, when the blood may be flowing back into the left atrium during the latter part of systole. Investigators have used various M-mode measurements of the aortic valve to obtain hemodynamic information. These measurements include the ejection time, the initial and final opening distances of the leaflets,[29–31] and the amplitude of motion of the aorta (Fig. 4–12).[32]

**Pulmonary Artery Flow**

Pulmonary artery flow is one of the few normal flow patterns that can be obtained with a Doppler recording from the parasternal view. The pulmonary artery is usually visualized in the short-axis, two-dimensional view with the Doppler sample placed in the pulmonary artery or right ventricular outflow tract. Figure 4–13 demonstrates a short-axis two-dimensional echocardiogram with the sample volume (*arrow*) in the right ventricular outflow tract near the pulmonary valve. The resultant pulmonary artery Doppler flow velocity is noted. One needs to determine the diameter and cross-sectional area of the pulmonary artery to convert the Doppler recording to pulmonary flow.[7,14] As noted in Figure 4–14, the frequently indistinct borders of the pulmonary artery make accurate diameter measurements difficult.[33] The Doppler sampling site may also influence the measurement.[10,34] This particular approach has been feasible in children. Investigators have used this approach to measure cardiac output in the operating room using transesophageal echocardiography.[35]

Several studies have indicated a relationship between the size of the pulmonary artery and the pulmonary blood flow.[36] Pulmonary artery size can be determined by suprasternal notch M-mode or two-dimensional ex-

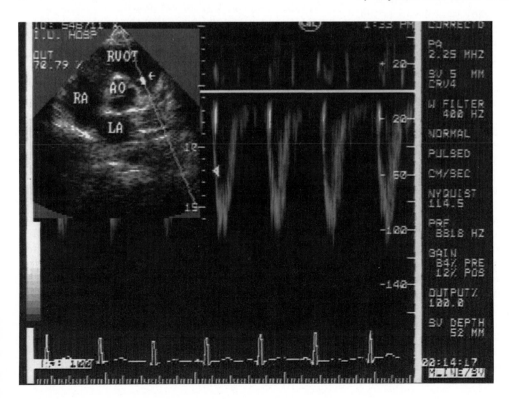

**Fig. 4–13.** Pulsed Doppler recording of pulmonary artery flow (RVOT = right ventricular outflow tract; AO = aorta; RA = right atrium; LA = left atrium).

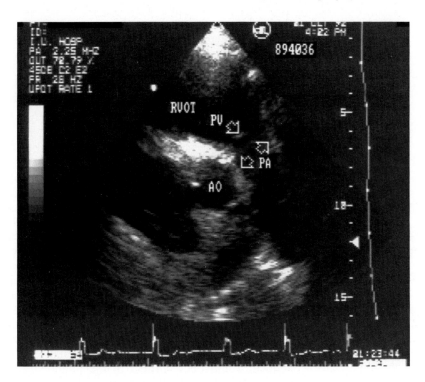

**Fig. 4–14.** Short-axis two-dimensional echocardiogram through the right ventricular outflow tract (RVOT), pulmonary valve (PV), and pulmonary artery (PA). The pulmonary artery measurement (*arrows*) frequently is difficult in the adult patient. AO = aorta.

aminations. Such a measurement is usually done to determine the blood flow in patients with congenital heart disease.

### Mitral Valve Flow

Figure 4–15 demonstrates a Doppler recording of normal flow through the mitral orifice into the left ventricular inflow tract. There are essentially two phases to the flow. The first occurs in early diastole (E) and the second after atrial systole (A). Normally, the peak velocity is greater with the early diastolic flow. Mitral flow is best recorded from the apical view. Data demonstrate that the Doppler mitral velocity can be converted to flow if one calculates the mitral valve orifice.[37–40] This complex calculation involves taking the cross-sectional area of the mitral valve orifice using a short-axis two-dimensional echocardiogram. The area is taken at peak opening, which occurs in early diastole. In addition, one uses the M-mode mitral valve recording to determine the diameter of the valve throughout diastole (Fig. 4–16).[41–43] The mean mitral diameter is then calculated. With slow heart rates, further corrections must be introduced.[41] This approach is undoubtedly too complex for routine clinical work. A somewhat simplified approach is to take the diameter of the mitral annulus as measured from the apical four-chamber view. One assumes the annulus is circular for the area measurement. This approach is the most practical and is being used by most investigators.[39,44,44a]

As noted in Chapter 3, the relative mitral flow in early and late diastole changes with the status of the left ventricle. Doppler mitral flow recordings will reflect these changes (Fig. 4–17). The M-mode mitral valve motion will also indicate alterations in left ventricular filling by a reduced E-F slope (Fig. 4–18) or reduced D-E slope (Fig. 4–19).[45–47] Figure 4–20 shows an extreme example whereby no E wave is seen except after a premature beat. This patient had pulmonary hypertension, low cardiac output, and normal left ventricular diastolic pressures.

Another empirical observation with reference to the mitral valve and blood flow is that the total amplitude of mitral motion is decreased in patients with low stroke volumes. Figure 4–21 shows two patients with differing amplitudes of mitral valve motion. The patient in Figure 4–21A had a relatively high flow through the mitral orifice, whereas the patient in Figure 4–21B had a low cardiac output and a small stroke volume.

### Left Atrial Flow

Doppler recordings within the left atrium are similar to those in the left ventricular inflow tract. Such recordings are primarily obtained to detect mitral regurgitation and not normal left atrial flow.

Investigators have been interested in changes in left atrial volume for assessing left ventricular filling. Such changes are primarily noted by the M-mode recording of the posterior aortic wall. Because the posterior left atrial wall rarely shows any significant motion, the change in left atrial volume is best reflected by the motion of its anterior wall, which is the same as that of the posterior aortic wall.

As noted in Figure 4–12, the posterior aortic wall (PAW) moves downward fairly rapidly with the onset of diastole. During mid-diastole, relatively little motion of the aortic wall occurs. After atrial systole is again a

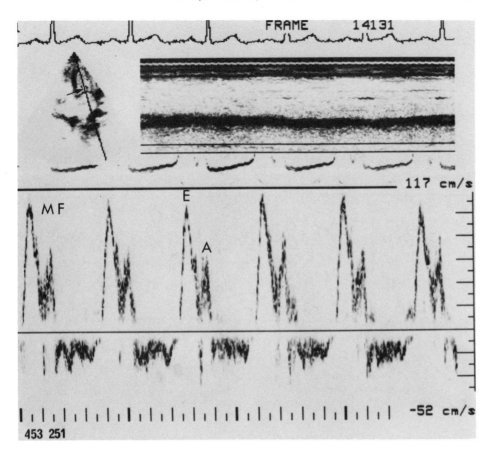

Fig. 4–15. Doppler flow velocity through a normal mitral valve orifice. MF = mitral flow; arrow = sample volume; E = early diastolic velocity; A = atrial contraction.

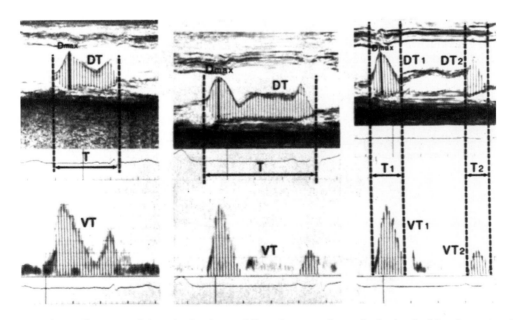

Fig. 4–16. M-mode echocardiograms of the mitral valve and Doppler recordings of mitral velocities demonstrating how mitral flow can be calculated. The diastolic distance-time area between the leaflets (DT), and the diastolic filling time (T) are indicated. The mitral Doppler spectral recording (bottom) shows the velocity-time integral (VT). The middle tracing shows the effects of bradycardia. The right tracing shows how the mid-diastolic interval, where no flow velocity is recorded, is eliminated in the calculation and one ends up with VT1 and VT2. (From Miller, W.E., et al.: Accuracy of mitral Doppler echocardiographic cardiac output determinations in adults. Am. Heart J., *119*:906, 1990.)

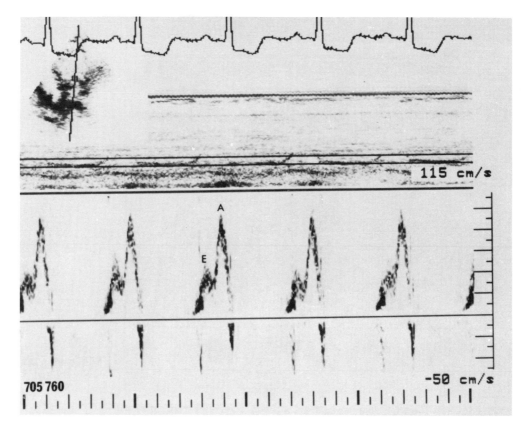

**Fig. 4–17.** Mitral valve flow pattern in a patient with reduced left ventricular relaxation. Early diastolic velocity (E) is reduced, and late velocity following atrial contraction (A) is increased.

downward displacement of the wall toward the left atrium. This pattern of wall motion can be interpreted as a sudden decrease in left atrial volume in early diastole as the mitral valve opens and blood flows from the left atrium into the left ventricle. This phase of left atrial emptying has been labeled the "rapid emptying phase"

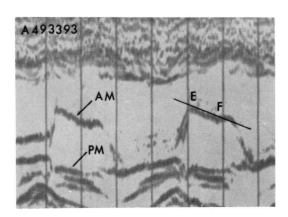

**Fig. 4–18.** Mitral valve echocardiogram of a patient with a diminished E to F slope of the anterior mitral leaflet (AM) but no evidence of mitral stenosis. Despite the diminished E to F slope, the leaflets were thin, and the posterior mitral leaflet (PM) moved normally. (From Duchak, J.M., Jr., Chang, S., and Feigenbaum, H.: The posterior mitral valve echo and the echocardiograph diagnosis of mitral stenosis. Am. J. Cardiol., 29:628, 1972.)

(R, Fig. 4–12).[48] During mid-diastole, the blood flowing from the left atrium to the left ventricle is about equal to that coming into the left atrium through the pulmonary veins. This phase has been called the "conduit phase" (C, Fig 4–12). With atrial systole, the left atrium actively contracts and produces the "systolic phase of atrial emptying" (S, Fig 4–12). During ventricular systole, the mitral valve is closed and the left atrium fills with blood coming from the pulmonary veins (LA filling). If left atrial emptying is restricted, as might occur with mitral stenosis, the rapid filling phase is decreased.[49,50] This decrease may also occur if left ventricular filling is restricted because of decreased compliance of the left ventricle.[51] One study suggests dividing the diastolic pattern of aortic wall motion into thirds to determine the ratio of emptying of the left atrium.[49] Normally, the amplitude of the first third of diastole should exceed 40% of total amplitude of left atrial emptying. A reduced left atrial emptying index could result from obstruction at the mitral orifice, either from mitral stenosis or a malfunctioning prosthetic valve,[49] or to abnormal filling of the ventricle as a result of intrinsic myocardial disease of that chamber.[51] Other studies have examined the percentage and slope of left atrial emptying with atrial systole. The investigators found that patients with a decreased left ventricular compliance had an increased percentage of left atrial emptying following atrial systole.[52]

It should be remembered that these measurements are obtained from the posterior wall of the aorta and that

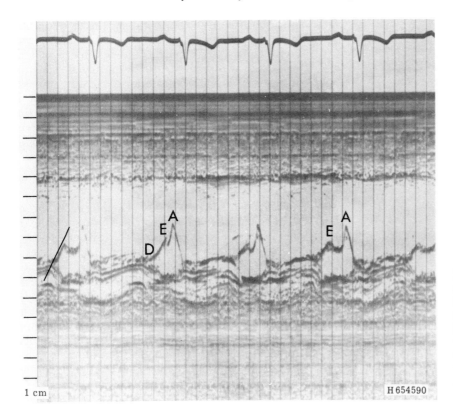

**Fig. 4–19.** Mitral valve echocardiogram of a patient with left ventricular failure, low cardiac output, and elevated left ventricular diastolic pressure. The velocity of opening of the mitral valve (D to E slope) is reduced, and the atrial component to mitral valve motion is accentuated.

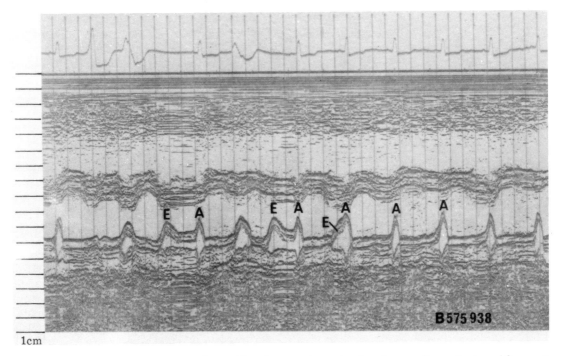

**Fig. 4–20.** Mitral valve echocardiogram of a patient with pulmonary hypertension, low cardiac output, and frequent ventricular premature beats. During sinus rhythm, the mitral valve opens only with atrial contraction.

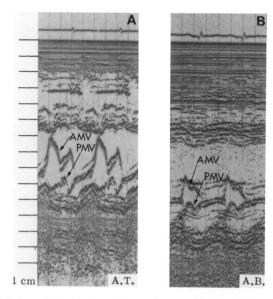

**Fig. 4–21.** Mitral valve echocardiogram of a patient with high mitral valve flow (*A*) and of a patient with low mitral valve flow (*B*). Calibrations are the same for both recordings. AMV = anterior mitral valve leaflet; PMV = posterior mitral valve leaflet.

intrinsic disease in the aorta and the ejection of blood into the aorta may also affect posterior aortic wall motion. Figure 4–16 is an echocardiogram of a patient with an aortic aneurysm. During ventricular ejection, the aorta expands and the posterior aortic wall moves downward toward the left atrium. Thus, wall motion in this patient is influenced more by blood flowing into the aorta than by blood flowing into the left atrium. The left atrial filling probably produces displacement of atrial walls not recorded on this M-mode examination.

### Tricuspid Valve Flow

Figure 4–22 demonstrates a Doppler recording of flow through the tricuspid valve. The transducer is in the apical position. The Doppler recording resembles the anterior tricuspid valve leaflet motion. One could transform the velocity to flow by determining the tricuspid valve orifice area. A technique similar to that suggested for mitral valve flow would be possible. Thus far, no investigators have attempted to make such determinations. The significance of the qualitative flow pattern should be similar to that of the variations in flow through the mitral orifice. In diseases involving alterations in right-sided hemodynamics, one should expect changes in the relationship in early to late diastolic flow.

The M-mode recording of the tricuspid valve also provides flow information across that valve orifice. Figure 4–23 demonstrates a normal tricuspid valve. Normally, only the anterior tricuspid leaflet is recorded. Distortion

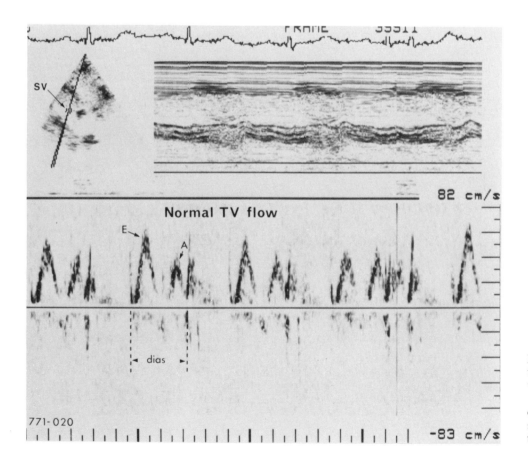

**Fig. 4–22.** Doppler flow pattern through the tricuspid valve in a normal subject. SV = sample volume; TV = tricuspid valve; E = early diastolic velocity; A = atrial contraction.

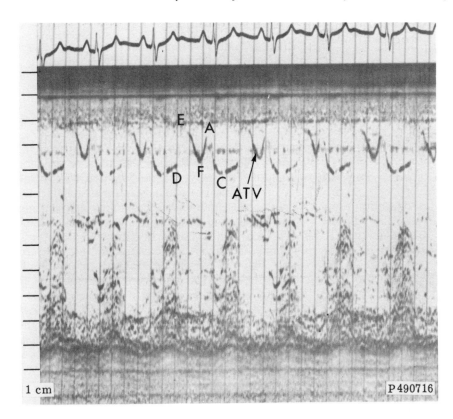

**Fig. 4–23.** Normal tricuspid valve echocardiogram. The pattern of motion of the anterior tricuspid leaflet (ATV) is essentially the same as that of the anterior mitral leaflet.

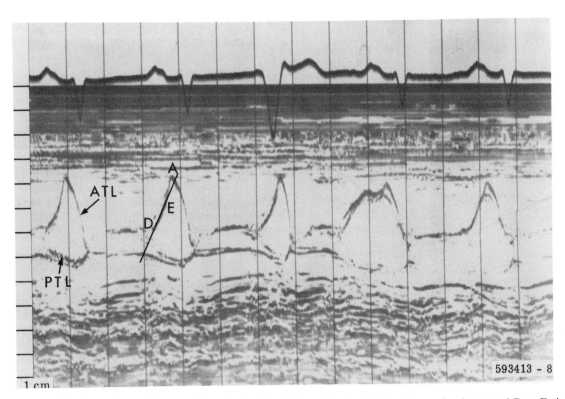

**Fig. 4–24.** Tricuspid valve echocardiogram of a patient with right ventricular dysfunction and a decreased D to E slope. ATL = anterior tricuspid valve leaflet; PTL = posterior tricuspid valve leaflet.

of the normal pattern in diastole has been noted in many disease states. Figure 4–24 shows a monophasic pattern of diastolic flow in the tricuspid valve.[53,54] This pattern is a function primarily of a reduced early diastolic flow or reduced D to E slope. Such a pattern has been noted in patients with severe right ventricular dysfunction and in patients with pulmonary hypertension, particularly acute pulmonary embolism.

### Cardiac Output

Cardiac output is the amount of blood in liters per minute flowing through the systemic circulation. Because human circulation is pulsatile, cardiac output represents stroke volume times heart rate. If no valvular insufficiency or intracardiac shunt is present, then almost any means of calculating stroke volume gives the option of calculating cardiac output. One could use aortic, mitral, pulmonary artery, or tricuspid flow for determining stroke volume and cardiac output. When valvular regurgitation or intracardiac shunts are present, then the flows that can be used for systemic cardiac output become limited. For example, with aortic regurgitation, one cannot use aortic flow for determining effective cardiac output. In such a case, the aortic flow would include the regurgitant volume in addition to the forward stroke volume. One could use mitral valve flow to determine effective forward flow provided that there is no additional mitral regurgitation. If mitral regurgitation were also present, then one might resort to pulmonary flow for measuring cardiac output, again provided there is no pulmonary regurgitation.

One can also calculate stroke volume by measuring chamber volumes. Left ventricular stroke volume can determine cardiac output provided that no aortic or mitral regurgitation is present. The use of two-dimensional echocardiography for measuring volumes was discussed in Chapter 3. Changes in left atrial volume cannot be used for calculating cardiac output because the change in left atrial volume does not necessarily indicate total stroke volume. Because there is no valve between the left atrium and the pulmonary veins, there is no assurance that with atrial contraction some of the blood does not move into the pulmonary veins. In this regard, the left atrium is more of a conduit than a propelling chamber.

Cardiac output can also be determined by the indicator dilution technique. Theoretically, contrast echocardiography offers an opportunity to use this approach for calculating cardiac output.[55] One needs a videodensitometer to sample the change in echo intensity as the contrast-producing bubbles traverse that specific area of the heart. One can obtain relative changes in flow by noting the decay or washout of the echo-producing bubbles. To obtain absolute cardiac outputs, one needs to know the number of bubbles being injected. With the development of manufactured microbubbles, whereby the number of injected bubbles is known, this approach is theoretically possible, although it is still not practical at the present time.

### Regurgitant Fraction

Regurgitant fraction is that fraction or percentage of total stroke volume that regurgitates through an incompetent valve. For example, one could determine the regurgitant fraction of aortic or mitral regurgitation if total left ventricular stroke volume and effective systemic stroke volume could be determined. The difference between the two volumes is the regurgitant volume, which when divided by the total stroke volume gives the regurgitant fraction. In the case of mitral regurgitation, one could theoretically measure total left ventricular stroke volume either by using two-dimensional echocardiographic measurements of volumes or by using mitral valve flow. The systemic stroke volume could be represented by aortic flow with either M-mode or Doppler echocardiography. For example, in nuclear cardiology, one commonly determines regurgitant fraction by comparing left ventricular stroke volume with right ventricular stroke volume. A similar approach can be used in echocardiography. One merely needs to know which stroke volume reflects the effective flow plus the regurgitant flow and which stroke volume consists only of the effective systemic flow. If one uses different Doppler flow measurements, variability in the determinations must be realized. Studies comparing aortic, mitral, tricuspid, and pulmonary flow in the same normal individuals have noted significant differences.[56]

### Shunt Ratios

In the event of a cardiac shunt, the determination of pulmonary to systemic flow ratios, or QP:QS, is the principal way of quantitating the size of the shunt.[57,58] If the resistances are normal, this shunt ratio also determines the size of the defect. Ordinarily, one would make this shunt ratio by determining the pulmonary flow and comparing it with the aortic flow.[14,59,60] This approach is being used in pediatric echocardiography with reasonable success. This approach has obvious limitations.[61] If a semilunar valve stenosis of regurgitation is present, then one must use some other stroke volume determination for either the systemic or pulmonary flow. One could resort to the mitral valve flow for the appropriate systemic or pulmonary flow in the event that the semilunar valve flow is unavailable.

### Echocardiographic Detection of Stagnant Blood

Intracardiac stagnant blood becomes echogenic and can be visualized as a cloud of echoes or spontaneous contrast on an M-mode or two-dimensional echocardiogram.[62,63] Figure 4–25 demonstrates a two-dimensional echocardiogram of a dog in which cardiac arrest has been produced. The cavity becomes echogenic in a matter of seconds (see Fig. 4–25B). If the dog is sacrificed, one finds the cavity filled with liquid blood. There is no macroscopic evidence of clot. If the heart is restarted, the echogenic blood disappears. This phenomenon has been noted in patients with dilated, hypokinetic chambers or regional wall motion abnormalities. Figure 4–26

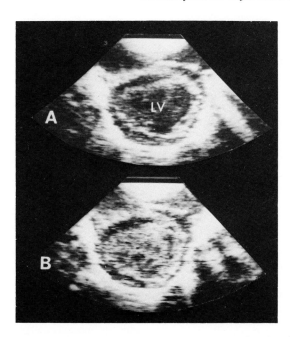

**Fig. 4–25.** Two-dimensional echocardiograms of a dog before (*A*) and after (*B*) the heart has been stopped. With cessation of flow, the cavity becomes markedly echogenic. LV = left ventricle.

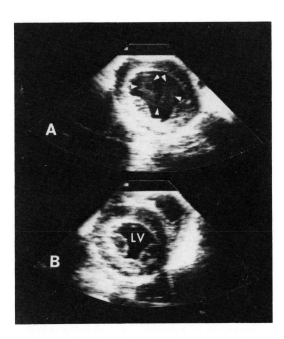

**Fig. 4–26.** Intracavitary echogenicity. In a canine experiment, regional wall akinesis is produced by coronary artery ligation. When the artery is ligated and the anterior wall fails to move (*A*), a cloud of echoes (*arrowheads*) appears in the cavity of the left ventricle next to the nonmoving anterior wall. With release of the ligature around the coronary artery (*B*), the left ventricle again contracts well, and the echoes within the left ventricular cavity disappear. LV = left ventricle.

demonstrates a canine model in which a coronary artery has been tied off and a segment of the left ventricle has become akinetic. The blood adjacent to this akinetic wall becomes echogenic (Fig. 4–26*A, arrowheads*). When the ligature around the artery is released and the wall begins to move again, this echogenic blood disappears (Fig. 4–26*B*). A similar cloud of echoes resulting from stagnant blood is commonly seen in dilated left atria, especially in patients with mitral stenosis.[63]

The mechanism for this echogenicity is unknown. This phenomenon might be a precursor to the development of a solid clot.

## MODIFIED BERNOULLI EQUATION AND INTRAVASCULAR PRESSURES

None of the echocardiographic techniques measures intravascular pressure directly. The closest echocardiography comes to obtaining direct information concerning pressure abnormalities is the use of Doppler echocardiography for determining a pressure drop or pressure gradient.[64–66] Figure 4–27 demonstrates the principle involved in using Doppler techniques for evaluating the differential in pressure across a narrowed area of the cardiovascular system. The technique is based on a modification of Bernoulli's equation. The assumptions necessary to reduce the Bernoulli equation to something that can be used clinically include eliminating the flow acceleration and viscous friction factors of the equation. The other major assumption is that the velocity distal to an obstruction is significantly greater than the velocity proximal to the obstruction so that the proximal velocity can be ignored. With these assumptions, one can convert the Bernoulli equation to $\Delta P = 4 V^2$, in which V is the peak velocity distal to an obstruction.

The modified Bernoulli equation was the development that generated the most interest in Doppler echocardiography.[65–67] The technique has proved to be extremely valuable in determining pressure gradients across obstructive valves. This application is discussed further in Chapter 6, Acquired Valvular Heart Disease. The basic principle, however, can also be used to calculate intracardiac pressures. Because valvular regurgitation is relatively common, even in essentially normal individuals, the presence of the regurgitant flow provides an opportunity to calculate intracardiac pressures. For example, Figure 4–28 demonstrates how one can use the presence of tricuspid regurgitation and the modified Bernoulli equation to calculate right ventricular systolic pressure.[68–71] In the presence of tricuspid regurgitation, a systolic pressure gradient exists between the right ventricle (P1) and the right atrium (P2). This pressure drop can be determined with the Bernoulli equation by using the peak velocity of the tricuspid regurgitant jet. If the tricuspid regurgitant signal is weak, contrast echocardiography can increase the quality of the signal and permit a more accurate measurement of the peak systolic velocity.[72–75] Color flow Doppler imaging can help to deter-

# DOPPLER ECHOCARDIOGRAPHY

## PRESSURE DROP OR GRADIENT MEASUREMENT

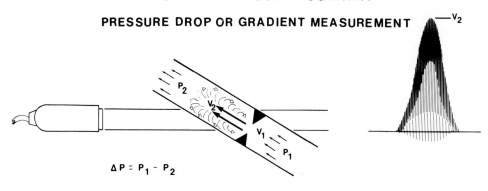

$$\Delta P = P_1 - P_2$$

### BERNOULLI EQUATION

$$P_1 - P_2 = \underbrace{\frac{1}{2}\rho\,(V_2{}^2 - V_1{}^2)}_{\substack{\text{CONVECTIVE} \\ \text{ACCELERATION}}} + \underbrace{\rho\int_1^2 \frac{\overrightarrow{DV}}{DT}\,DS}_{\substack{\text{FLOW} \\ \text{ACCELERATION}}} + \underbrace{R\overrightarrow{(V)}}_{\substack{\text{VISCOUS} \\ \text{FRICTION}}}$$

$$P_1 - P_2 = \frac{1}{2}\rho\,(V_2{}^2 - V_1{}^2)$$

$$V_1 \text{ MUCH} < V_2 \therefore \text{IGNORE } V_1$$

$$\rho = \text{MASS DENSITY OF BLOOD} = 1.06 \cdot 10^3 \text{ KG/M}^3$$

$$\therefore \Delta P = 4V_2{}^2$$

**Fig. 4–27.** Principles of using Doppler echocardiography to measure a pressure drop or gradient across an obstruction. $P_2$ = pressure distal to an obstruction; $V_2$ = blood velocity distal to an obstruction; $V_1$ = velocity proximal to an obstruction; $P_1$ = pressure proximal to an obstruction.

## ESTIMATION OF RIGHT VENTRICULAR PRESSURE

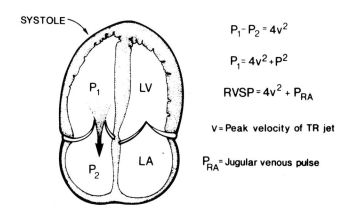

$$P_1 - P_2 = 4v^2$$

$$P_1 = 4v^2 + P^2$$

$$RVSP = 4v^2 + P_{RA}$$

v = Peak velocity of TR jet

$P_{RA}$ = Jugular venous pulse

**Fig. 4–28.** Diagram demonstrating how right ventricular systolic pressure can be measured using Doppler recording of tricuspid regurgitation. Using the modified Bernoulli equation, one can calculate the pressure gradient across the regurgitant tricuspid valve ($P_1 - P_2$). The right ventricular systolic pressure or $P_1$ is equal to four times the square of the peak velocity of the tricuspid jet (v), plus the right atrial pressure ($P_{RA}$). One way of estimating the right atrial pressure is to use the jugular venous pulse pressure.

mine the angle of the regurgitant jet for correct alignment of the ultrasonic beam.[76]

Knowing the gradient across the tricuspid valve, one needs to add the right atrial pressure to determine right ventricular systolic pressure. The right atrial pressure can be estimated clinically by judging the jugular venous pressure at the bedside. One can also give an empiric value to right atrial pressure for a simplified approach. The number given for the right atrial systolic pressure ranges from 10 to 14 mm Hg. As noted subsequently, more sophisticated approaches are available to measure right atrial mean pressure noninvasively.

Figure 4–29 diagrammatically shows how this approach can be used not only to calculate right ventricular systolic pressure from tricuspid regurgitation but also to measure pulmonary artery diastolic pressure from pulmonic regurgitation. In the setting of pulmonic regurgitation, one can measure the end-diastolic pulmonary regurgitant velocity. This measurement provides the pressure gradient between the pulmonary artery and the right ventricle at end diastole. Combining this pressure gradient with right ventricular diastolic pressure or right atrial pressure provides a measurement of pulmonary artery diastolic pressure.[77,78] Right ventricular systolic pressure can be measured by using this technique in patients with a ventricular septal defect.[79] Subtracting the pressure gradient across the defect from the systemic systolic pressure provides the systolic pressure in the right ventricle, provided no aortic stenosis is present. This approach can measure pulmonary diastolic pressure with a patent ductus arteriosus.[79a]

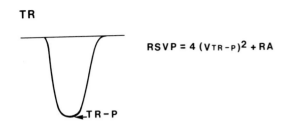

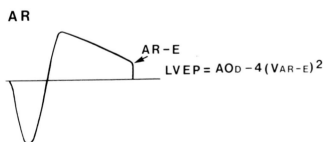

**Fig. 4–29.** Diagram demonstrating how right ventricular systolic pressure can be determined by the tricuspid regurgitation and how pulmonary artery diastolic pressure can be obtained from the pulmonary regurgitation jet (PR). The right ventricular systolic pressure (RSVP) is calculated from the peak tricuspid regurgitant velocity (TR-P) and an estimate of right atrial pressure (RA). Pulmonary artery diastolic pressure (PADP) is derived from the end-diastolic pulmonary regurgitation velocity (pr-E) and estimation of right ventricular diastolic pressure or right atrial diastolic pressure.

**Fig. 4–30.** Drawing demonstrating how left atrial pressure (LAP) and left ventricular end-diastolic pressure (LVEP) can be calculated from the peak mitral regurgitation velocity (MR-P) and the end-diastolic aortic regurgitation velocity (AR-E). Left atrial pressure is calculated using the mitral regurgitant minus the aortic systolic pressure (AO$_S$). The left ventricular end-diastolic pressure is calculated from the end-diastolic gradient across the regurgitant aortic valve minus the aortic diastolic pressure (AO$_D$).

The same basic approach can be used on the left side of the heart (Fig. 4–30).[80] With mitral regurgitation, one can convert the peak velocity of the mitral regurgitant jet into a gradient between the left ventricle and left atrium in systole. Knowing the aortic systolic pressure, which should be the same as the left ventricular systolic pressure assuming there is no aortic stenosis, one can subtract the gradient from the aortic systolic pressure to obtain the left atrial systolic pressure.[81] With aortic regurgitation, the end-diastolic velocity of the regurgitant jet provides an opportunity to calculate the left ventricular end-diastolic pressure. Subtracting the gradient from the aortic diastolic pressure gives the left ventricular diastolic pressure. Figure 4–31 is from a study that validated how the mitral regurgitant jet can produce a measurement of left atrial pressure. The gradient between the left ventricle and the left atrium is accurately reflected by the peak gradient recorded by the Doppler regurgitant jet. Figure 4–32 shows a similar study confirming the ability of Doppler imaging to use the end-

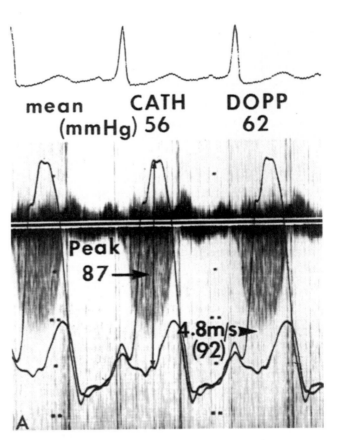

**Fig. 4–31.** Continuous wave Doppler study and simultaneous measurement of left ventricular and left atrial pressures showing the validity of using the peak mitral regurgitant jet to calculate the left atrial pressure. The catheterization calculation of peak gradient between the left ventricle and left atrium was 87 mm Hg; with the simultaneous Doppler recording, the gradient was 92 mm Hg. (From Nishimura, R.A., et al.: Determination of left-sided pressure gradients by utilizing Doppler aortic and mitral regurgitant signals: Validation by simultaneous dual catheter and Doppler studies. J. Am. Coll. Cardiol., *11*:319, 1988.)

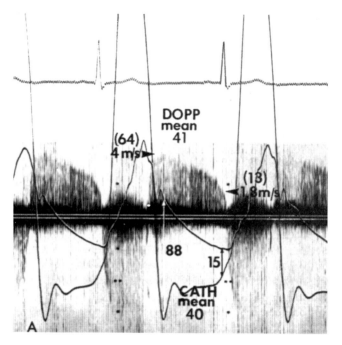

**Fig. 4–32.** Simultaneous continuous wave Doppler recording and left ventricular and aortic pressures in a patient with aortic regurgitation. The Doppler recording shows the end-diastolic gradient between the aorta and left ventricle was 13 mm Hg and the same measurement with cardiac catheterization was 15 mm Hg. (From Nishimura, R.A., et al.: Determination of left-sided pressure gradients by utilizing Doppler aortic and mitral regurgitant signs: Validation by simultaneous dual catheter and Doppler studies. J. Am. Coll. Cardiol., *11*:319, 1988.)

diastolic velocity of an aortic regurgitant jet to calculate the end-diastolic gradient between the aorta and the left ventricle.

This Doppler approach using the Bernoulli equation and valvular regurgitation is the principle technique for calculating intracardiac pressures at the present time. Other echocardiographic signs of altered intravascular pressures can also be useful.

## OTHER ECHOCARDIOGRAPHIC FINDINGS WITH ALTERED INTRAVASCULAR PRESSURE

### Elevated Left Ventricular Diastolic Pressure

Left ventricular diastolic pressure and left ventricular diastolic function are closely related phenomena. The assessment of left ventricular function during diastole was described in Chapter 3. The same echocardiographic findings with altered diastolic function will produce abnormal diastolic pressure. Figure 4–33 summarizes the relationship of mitral flow velocity and left ventricular and left atrial diastolic pressures. The diagram demonstrates how variations in mitral flow velocities in early and late diastole reflect changes in left ventricular pressure.[82,83] Normally, the E wave is taller than the A wave. With abnormal left ventricular relaxation, however, which commonly occurs with ischemic heart

disease or left ventricular hypertrophy or just aging, the E wave may be reduced. With atrial contraction, a rapid rise in left atrial pressure may occur, which produces a tall A wave. A similar mitral recording can occur coincident with lowering of the filling pressures of the left ventricle, such as in patients with vasodilatation, hypovolemia, or dehydration. Under these circumstances, the low filling pressure reduces the E-wave velocity. Atrial velocity increases with contraction of the incompletely emptied left atrium.

The third pattern of mitral flow velocity is with a tall E wave and a small A wave. This finding is indicative of high initial filling pressure in the left atrium, which could be a result of heart failure, mitral regurgitation, or constrictive restrictive physiology. In any case, the high left atrial pressure produces rapid filling of blood into the left ventricle. The filling stops relatively early in diastole, producing a short deceleration time. Atrial systole produces little additional blood flow across the mitral valve. Investigators have used the left ventricular inflow velocities to predict left ventricular end-diastolic pressure. The measurements used include the isovolumic relaxation time, atrial filling fraction, the deceleration time,

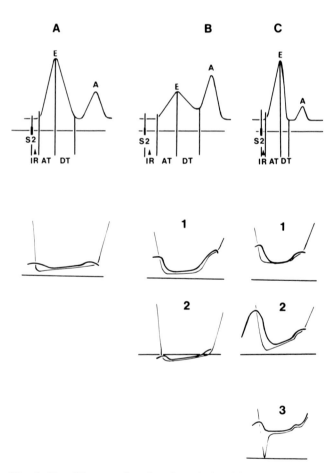

**Fig. 4–33.** Diagram showing the relationship of mitral Doppler velocities and left ventricular and left atrial pressures (see text for details). S2 = second heart sound; IR = isovolumic relaxation; AT = acceleration time; DT = deceleration time.

the E to A ratio, and the time from termination of mitral flow and the next electrocardiographic R wave.

M-mode recordings of the mitral valve also produce evidence of altered left ventricular diastolic pressure.[84,85] Figure 4–34 diagrammatically shows the relationship between mitral valve motion and left ventricular pressure in a normal subject and in a patient with an elevated left ventricular diastolic pressure secondary to an elevated atrial component.[86] This type of pressure recording is similar to that noted in Figure 4–33. In a normal individual (Fig. 4–34A), the left ventricular diastolic pressure is low initially and gradually rises during diastole. Left atrial pressure varies slightly. Corresponding mitral valve motion shows rapid opening from D to E. Closure of the mitral valve, from A to C, is smooth and of brief duration. Figure 4–34B shows the situation that may occur in a patient with an elevated left ventricular diastolic pressure as a result of a rise in pressure after atrial systole. This change in atrial pressure is followed almost immediately by a similar rise in left ventricular pressure. As a result, the two pressures cross earlier than usual, and the onset of mitral valve closure is premature. Thus, the A point occurs earlier than usual. Immediately before ventricular systole, the two pressures are nearly equal, and mitral valve closure is interrupted, as noted by a plateau or notch, between A and C. Complete closure of the mitral valve occurs at a higher left ventricular pressure and is delayed. The end result is a prolongation of the A to C interval and a "plateau," "notch," or "B bump" between the A and C points (Figs. 4–35 and 4–36). Some investigators have suggested that end-diastolic mitral regurgitation may be responsible in part for the "B bump."[87,88]

This M-mode echocardiographic sign is primarily a

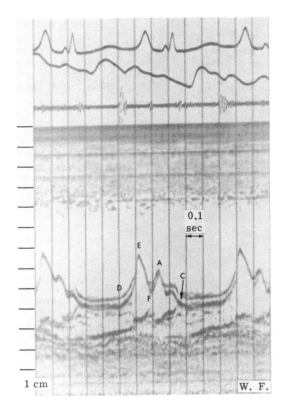

**Fig. 4–35.** Mitral valve echocardiogram of a patient with an elevated left ventricular end-diastolic pressure secondary to poor left ventricular compliance and an elevated atrial component of the left ventricular pressure. Closure of the mitral valve (A–C) is prolonged and interrupted.

qualitative identification of patients with an elevated left atrial component to their left ventricular pressure. Efforts to quantitate left ventricular diastolic pressure using this recording has not proved reliable.[89] The observation is reasonably specific but not sensitive. Usually, left ventricular end-diastolic pressure is at least 20 mm Hg before this sign appears.

A valuable M-mode finding in patients with aortic regurgitation is premature closure of the mitral valve with elevated left ventricular diastolic pressures.[90–95] Figure 4–37 shows a simultaneous mitral valve echocardiogram and left ventricular pressure in a patient with severe aortic regurgitation and atrial fibrillation. The anterior mitral leaflet shows fluttering of the valve during diastole. This phenomenon, a sign of aortic regurgitation, is discussed further in Chapter 6. Figure 4–37 shows that closure of the mitral valve (C) varies from cycle to cycle. This first cardiac cycle is relatively short, and mitral valve closure occurs immediately after the onset of electrical depolarization. Left ventricular diastolic pressure is low. The interval between the first and second cardiac complexes is much longer. In this case, closure of the valve (C) clearly precedes the onset of ventricular systole, and left ventricular diastolic pressure is considerably higher than in the preceding cardiac cycle. The next two cardiac intervals are again relatively long, and premature closure of the mitral valve again precedes the

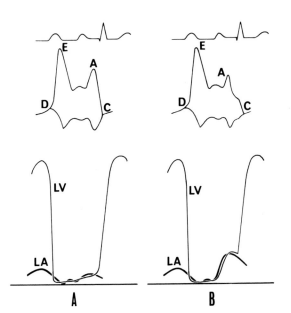

**Fig. 4–34.** Diagrams illustrating how the mitral valve echocardiogram may reflect changes in left ventricular diastolic pressure (see text for details). LV = left ventricle; LA = left atrium.

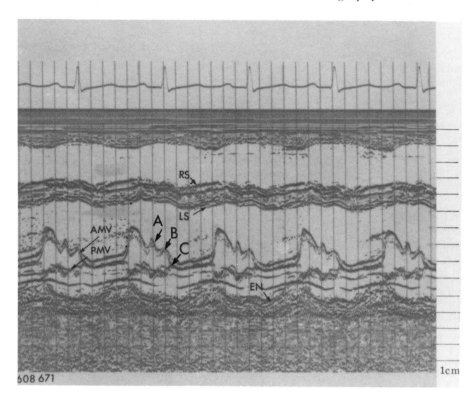

**Fig. 4–36.** Mitral valve echocardiogram of a patient with elevated left ventricular diastolic pressure. The B notch is prominent and superficially resembles an A wave. The patient has a prolonged P–R interval, and the A wave occurs earlier than usual. AMV = anterior mitral valve leaflet; PMV = posterior mitral valve leaflet; RS = right side of interventricular septum; LS = left side of interventricular septum; EN = posterior left ventricular endocardium.

onset of electrical depolarization. This finding is most striking before the last cardiac complex, at which time closure of the mitral valve is premature. This premature closure most likely occurs because the regurgitant aortic blood elevates the left ventricular diastolic pressure beyond that of the left atrial pressure. Thus, the mitral valve closes.

Figure 4–38 shows another example of a patient with severe aortic regurgitation. This time, the patient is in sinus rhythm, which is more usual. Again, the two leaflets abruptly approach each other before the onset of electrical depolarization (C'). There is actually a small amount of separation between the leaflets from C' to C. The mitral valve, however, is functionally closed at C',

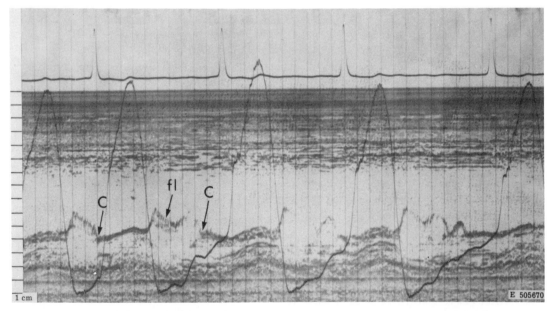

**Fig. 4–37.** Simultaneous left ventricular pressure and mitral valve echocardiogram in a patient with severe aortic regurgitation and atrial fibrillation. With a prolonged diastolic interval and a high left ventricular diastolic pressure, closure (C) on the mitral valve occurs before the onset of electrical depolarization. Fluttering (fl) of the mitral leaflet can be noted.

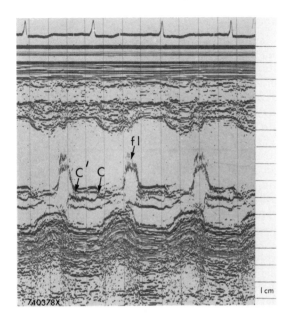

**Fig. 4–38.** Mitral valve echocardiogram of a patient with severe aortic regurgitation. The valve is almost completely closed (C') long before the onset of ventricular systole. Atrial contraction has little effect in reopening the valve. Complete closure occurs with ventricular systole (C). Note fluttering of the mitral valve (fl).

and this echocardiogram shows effective premature closure similar to that seen in Figure 4–37. Premature mitral valve closure is a clinically useful sign, because it has been shown to be a bad prognostic finding in patients with acute aortic regurgitation.

Severe aortic regurgitation and an elevated left ventricular diastolic pressure may also produce premature

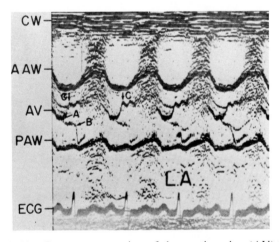

**Fig. 4–39.** Premature opening of the aortic valve (AV) in a patient with severe aortic regurgitation. The valve opens (*arrow*) before the onset of electrical depolarization (C). Additional opening of the valve occurs with ventricular ejection (B). CW = chest wall; AAW = anterior aortic wall; PAW = posterior aortic wall; LA = left atrium; ECG = electrocardiogram. (From Pietro, D.A., et al.: Premature opening of the aortic valve: An index of highly advanced aortic regurgitation. JCU, 6:170, 1978.)

opening of the aortic valve (Fig. 4–39).[96] The presumptive mechanism is that the left ventricular diastolic pressure is so high that it exceeds the aortic pressure at end diastole and the aortic valve opens.

### Left Atrial Pressure

Besides using the Doppler recording of mitral regurgitation to estimate left atrial pressure using the Bernoulli equation, several other echocardiographic techniques have been proposed for estimating left atrial pressure. The size of the left atrium has been used to predict left atrial pressure.[97] Other investigators have used time intervals to predict mean left atrial pressure.[98] A correlation between mean pulmonary capillary wedge pressure was noted with the time interval between the Q wave of the electrocardiogram and mitral valve closure divided by the interval between aortic valve closure and the mitral valve E point.[99]

The mean pulmonary capillary wedge pressure or left atrial pressure has also been estimated by pulsed Doppler recording of the mitral flow. By taking a ratio of the E to A velocities and dividing by the isovolumic relaxation time, one group of investigators found a relationship between that measurement and the pulmonary wedge pressure.[100]

It is not surprising that investigators have noted a relationship between pulmonary venous flow and left atrial pressure.[101,102] Figure 4–40 demonstrates how one can record pulmonary venous flow from both transthoracic and transesophageal echocardiography. With the transthoracic examination, one places the pulsed Doppler sample volume at the orifice of the right upper pulmonary vein. With transesophageal echocardiography, one can record pulmonary venous flow from either the upper left pulmonary vein (Fig. 4–40*A*) or the right upper pulmonary vein (Fig. 4–40*B*). The left upper pulmonary vein is recorded more easily and can be identified as being in the same tomographic plane as the left atrial appendage.

Figure 4–41 shows pulmonary venous Doppler recordings using transesophageal echocardiography in two patients with differing left atrial pressure. With a mean left atrial pressure of 9 mm Hg, a normal pulmonary venous flow pattern is noted. The diastolic component (Y) is slightly higher than the systolic component (X). In the patient with a left atrial mean pressure of 15 mm Hg, the systolic wave (X) is reduced and the diastolic component (Y) is increased. These investigators noted that the systolic fraction (i.e., the systolic velocity time integral expressed as a fraction of the total systolic and diastolic velocity integrals) correlated with the mean left atrial pressure with an R value of −0.88.[102] Other investigators have not found a good relationship between pulmonary venous flow and left atrial or pulmonary venous pressure.[103] The motion and shape of the interatrial septum also reflect left atrial pressure.[103a]

### Pulmonary Hypertension

As already discussed, the principle technique for determining pulmonary artery pressure involves the use of the tricuspid regurgitant jet and the Bernoulli equation.

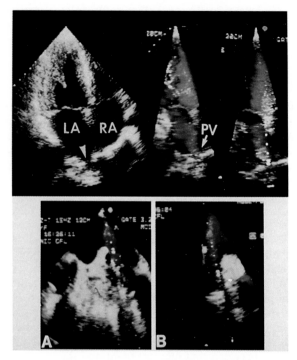

**Fig. 4-40.** Transthoracic (upper) and transesophageal (lower) echocardiograms showing the technique for recording pulmonary venous flow. The pulsed Doppler sample volume is placed distal to the orifice of the right upper pulmonary vein (upper left and upper right), and the pulmonary venous flow is depicted in orange (*arrow;* upper middle). With transesophageal echocardiography, the Doppler sample volume can be placed in the left upper pulmonary vein (*A*) or in the right upper pulmonary vein (*B*). (From Klein, A.L. and Tajik, A.J.: Doppler assessment of pulmonary venous flow in healthy subjects and in patients with heart disease. J. Am. Soc. Echocardiogr., *4*:379, 1991.)

By determining the right ventricular systolic pressure and ruling out the existence of any obstruction in the right ventricular outflow tract, one can determine the pulmonary artery systolic pressure. This technique is probably the most accurate for quantitating pulmonary artery pressure.[104]

Doppler recordings of the pulmonary artery velocity can also provide an assessment of pulmonary artery pressure and pulmonary vascular resistance.[105-111] The measurements that have been used include the pre-ejection period, which is the time interval from the onset of electrocardiographic QRS to the onset of pulmonary artery systolic flow; the acceleration time, which is the time between the onset of flow to the peak systolic flow;[112] and the ejection time, which is the interval from the onset to the cessation of flow (Fig. 4-42). The one measurement that most investigators agree is important is acceleration time. Figure 4-43 shows acceleration time in three different patients. In Figure 4-43*A*, the acceleration time is 130 msec in a patient with normal pulmonary artery pressure (2-23/11). In a patient with a pulmonary artery pressure of 65/29, the acceleration time is 100 msec (Fig. 4-43*B*). In Figure 4-43*C*, the pulmonary

artery pressure is 95/40 and the acceleration time is 65 msec. Some investigators have used the ratio of pre-ejection period and acceleration time. Others have used the ratio of acceleration time over ejection time.[107] Although the relationships have varied somewhat and one cannot predict the pulmonary artery pressure with great accuracy, some authors think that the measurement appears to be clinically useful and relates mostly to pulmonary vascular resistance.[111-113] Others have not found these measurements accurate enough for routine use.[114]

Jugular venous velocities may be altered with pulmonary hypertension. Normally, the systolic velocity exceeds that in diastole. The relationship has been noted to reverse with pulmonary hypertension.[115]

A qualitative assessment of the pulmonary artery flow is also useful in identifying pulmonary hypertension. Figure 4-44 shows a Doppler recording in a patient with severe pulmonary hypertension. Note the mid-systolic decrease in flow or notch (*arrow*).[116] This alteration in Doppler flow probably relates to reflected waves as a result of elevated pulmonary vascular resistance and systolic pressures.

The M-mode recording of the pulmonary valve also provides information concerning pulmonary artery pressure.[117-124] An absent or diminished A wave is a fairly frequent finding in pulmonary hypertension and presumably is the result of elevated pulmonary artery diastolic

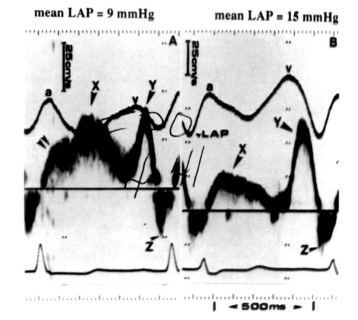

**Fig. 4-41.** Pulmonary venous Doppler recordings using transesophageal echocardiography and left atrial pressure recordings (LAP) in a patient with a mean left atrial pressure of 9 mm Hg (*A*) and another patient with mean left atrial pressure of 15 mm Hg (*B*). With the higher pressure, the systolic velocity (X) is reduced and the diastolic velocity (Y) is increased. (From Kuecher, H.F., et al.: Estimation of mean left atrial pressure from transesophageal pulsed Doppler echocardiography of pulmonary venous flow. Circulation, *82*:1127, 1990, by permission of the American Heart Association, Inc.)

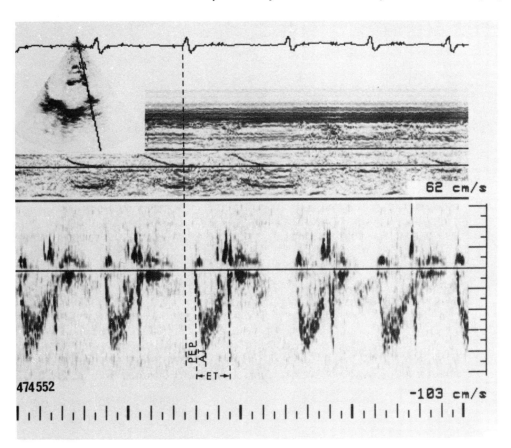

**Fig. 4–42.** Measurements of pulmonary artery flow that can be used for estimating pulmonary artery pressure. PEP = pre-ejection period; AT = acceleration time; ET = ejection time.

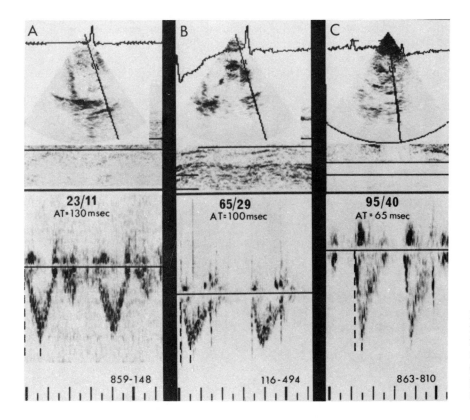

**Fig. 4–43.** Pulmonary artery flow in three patients with differing pulmonary artery pressures. The acceleration time (AT) becomes shorter as the pulmonary artery pressure rises.

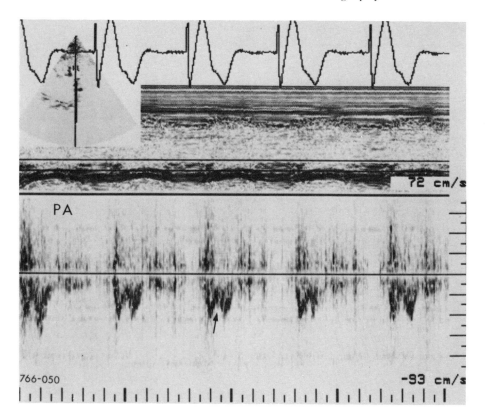

**Fig. 4–44.** Pulmonary artery flow in a patient with pulmonary hypertension and a reduction in pulmonary flow in midsystole (*arrow*). PA = pulmonary artery.

pressure (Figs. 4–45 and 4–46). In a patient with right ventricular failure, however, the A wave may reappear as the atrial component of the right ventricular diastolic component is increased (Fig. 4–47). Thus, the presence of a normal-sized A wave does not exclude pulmonary hypertension, especially when right ventricular failure is suspected. A variety of measurements of the M-mode pulmonary valve recording have been suggested, but with the decreasing reliance on M-mode echocardiography, these measurements are rarely obtained. Mid-sys-

tolic closure or notching remains a valuable qualitative sign for pulmonary hypertension.[125] Figure 4–46 demonstrates a pulmonary valve in a patient with pulmonary hypertension. A mid-systolic notch (n) is clearly visible. One can also see the lack of an A wave. A variation of the mid-systolic notch is shown in Figure 4–47. The notch is not quite as apparent because reopening of the valve in the latter half of systole is not as striking as in Figure 4–46.

The mid-systolic notch probably results from the same

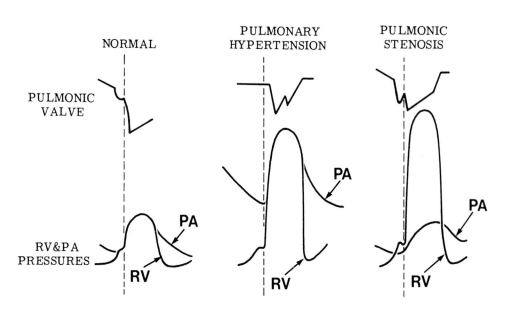

**Fig. 4–45.** Diagram demonstrating the relationship between pulmonic valve motion and pressures within the right ventricle and pulmonary artery. RV = right ventricle; PA = pulmonary artery.

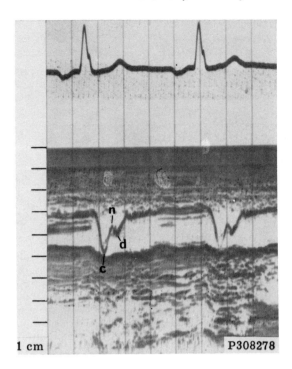

**Fig. 4–46.** Characteristic motion of the posterior pulmonary valve leaflet in a patient with pulmonary hypertension. This tracing demonstrates the absence of an A wave, negative E–F slope, and midsystolic notching (n) of the leaflet. (From Weyman, A.E., et al.: Echocardiographic patterns of pulmonic valve motion with pulmonary hypertension. Circulation, *50:* 905, 1974, by permission of the American Heart Association, Inc.)

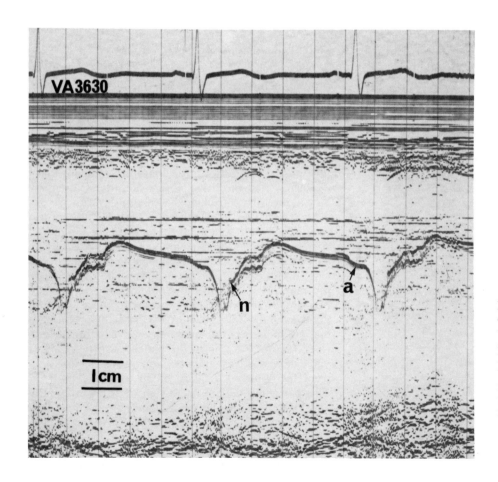

**Fig. 4–47.** Pulmonary valve echocardiogram of a patient with pulmonary hypertension and right ventricular failure. Despite the pulmonary hypertension, a small A wave (a) is still present. Midsystolic notching (n), though present, is less obvious because the valve does not reopen in late systole as much as it did in Figure 4–46.

phenomenon as the mid-systolic cessation of Doppler pulmonary artery flow. The sign is not sensitive but it appears to be fairly reliable and specific. False positives are rare.[126,127] Figure 4–48 is a pulmonary valve echogram of a patient who had a dilated pulmonary artery and normal right atrial and ventricular pressures. Despite these hemodynamics, notching (n) could be noted in the pulmonary valve. The mid-systolic closure in this patient presumably was related to eddy currents formed within the dilated pulmonary artery in systole.

Systolic time intervals derived from M-mode echocardiograms have been used to estimate pulmonary artery pressure.[128–130] The right ventricular ejection time and pre-ejection period can be measured by recording the pulmonary valve together with an electrocardiogram (Fig. 4–49). The right ventricular pre-ejection period lengthens with pulmonary hypertension. In addition, the right ventricular ejection time shortens with earlier closure of the pulmonary valve. Thus, the PEP to RVET ratio increases with pulmonary hypertension. This ratio can also be determined from the Doppler recording of the pulmonary artery flow. As a basic rule, when the interval between the tricuspid valve closure and opening barely exceeds the pulmonary ejection time, pulmonary hypertension is unlikely. When a marked difference is noted between the two intervals, significant pulmonary hypertension is indicated.

Some investigators have also noted the relationship between the size of the pulmonary artery and the pulmonary artery pressure.[131] This observation has been made

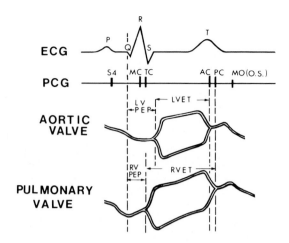

**Fig. 4–49.** Diagram of the aortic and pulmonary valve M-mode echocardiograms showing how left-sided and right-sided systolic time intervals can be measured. MC = mitral closure; TC = tricuspid closure; AC = aortic closure; PC = pulmonic closure; MO = mitral opening; PEP = pre-ejection period; LV = left ventricle; RV = right ventricle; ET = ejection time; PCG = phonocardiogram.

primarily in patients with acute pulmonary hypertension associated with pulmonary embolus.[119]

## Right Ventricular Pressure

The similarity between the tricuspid and mitral valves prompts echocardiographers to transfer their knowledge about the mitral valve to the tricuspid valve.[132,133] In patients with elevated right ventricular diastolic pressure, abnormal closure of the tricuspid valve is frequently seen, as noted in Figure 4–50. This abnormal tricuspid valve superficially resembles the mitral valve in Figure 4–35. Data in the literature indicate that the abnormal tricuspid valve closure identifies patients with elevated right ventricular diastolic pressures.

Occasionally, the right ventricular diastolic pressure may be elevated to a point that it influences pulmonary valve motion. An elevated left ventricular diastolic pressure rarely produces diastolic opening of the aortic valve (Fig. 4–39) because of the usually high aortic diastolic pressure.[134–135] Because the pulmonary artery diastolic pressure is relatively low, however, an elevated right ventricular diastolic pressure occasionally produces premature opening of the pulmonary valve before atrial systole. Figure 4–51 shows a patient whose pulmonary valve opens with a significant downward motion (*arrow*) prior to the usual location of the A dip (*dotted line*). This particular patient had a ruptured sinus of Valsalva aneurysm with blood flowing from the aorta directly into the right atrium. The sudden increase in blood and transmission of pressure from the aorta into the right atrium caused elevated right atrial and right ventricular pressures, which, as they exceeded the pulmonary artery pressure, opened the valve. After surgical correction of the aneurysm, the pulmonary valve motion returned to normal (Fig. 4–51*B*). Various other conditions produce an increase in right ventricular pressure, or right atrial

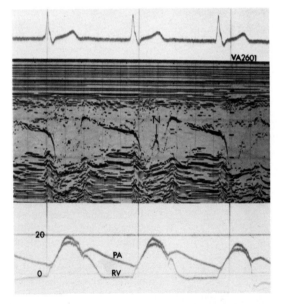

**Fig. 4–48.** Pulmonary valve echocardiogram and pulmonary artery (PA) and right ventricular (RV) pressures in a patient with a midsystolic pulmonary valve notch (N) and no pulmonary hypertension. The patient had idiopathic dilatation of the pulmonary artery and normal pulmonary artery pressure. (From Bauman, W., et al.: Mid-systolic notching of the pulmonary valve in the absence of pulmonary hypertension. Am. J. Cardiol., *43*:1049, 1979.)

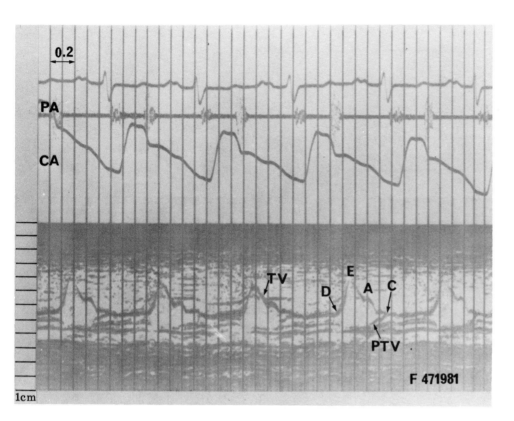

**Fig. 4–50.** Echocardiogram of the tricuspid valve in a patient with pulmonary hypertension and an elevated right ventricular diastolic pressure. Closure of the tricuspid valve (C) is delayed with a prolonged A-C interval. PA = phonocardiogram in the pulmonic area; CA = carotid pulse; TV = anterior tricuspid valve leaflet; PTV = posterior tricuspid valve leaflet. (From Chang, S.: Echocardiography: Techniques and Interpretation, ed. 2. Philadelphia, Lea & Febiger, 1981.)

pressure in diastole may produce the same phenomenon. This sign has been noted in patients with restrictive pericarditis, tricuspid regurgitation, or severe right heart failure.[134,135]

The right ventricular inflow and vena cava velocities on the right side of the heart may also be similar to that which occurs on the left side. Figures 4–52 and 4–53 show the restrictive flow patterns from the right side of the heart, which would be similar to that seen on the left side with a tall E wave and a short A wave on the ventricular inflow velocity and a small systolic and large diastolic component of the vena cava velocity.[136] Figures 4–54 and 4–55 illustrate the abnormal relaxation pattern with a reduced E wave and increased A wave across the tricuspid valve and increased systolic and decreased diastolic components in the vena cava.

Right ventricular systolic pressure has been estimated by looking at the shape of the left ventricle in the short

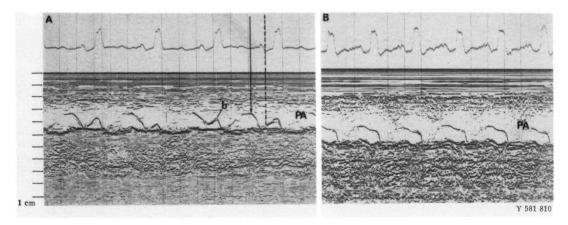

**Fig. 4–51.** *A*, Preoperative pulmonary valve echocardiogram in a patient with a sinus of Valsalva aneurysm that ruptured into the right atrium. The valve can be seen opening in early diastole (*solid arrow*) well before the onset of atrial systole. The leaflet is almost fully opened at the onset of atrial systole (*dotted line*). *B*, Following surgical closure of the fistula, the diastolic pulmonary valve opening is no longer present. (From Weyman, A.E., et al.: Premature pulmonic valve opening following sinus of Valsalva aneurysm rupture into the right atrium. Circulation, *51*:556, 1975, by permission of the American Heart Association, Inc.)

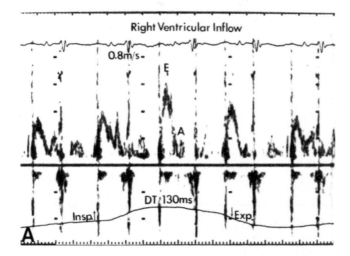

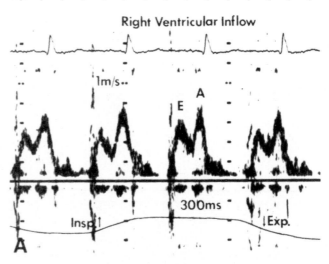

**Fig. 4–52.** Pulsed Doppler recording of right ventricular inflow in a patient with restrictive myopathy involving the right ventricle. With inspiration, the E wave is accentuated and the A wave is diminished. DT = deceleration time. (From Klein, A.L., et al.: Comprehensive Doppler assessment of right ventricular diastolic function in cardiac amyloidosis. J. Am. Coll. Cardiol., *15*:103, 1990.)

**Fig. 4–54.** Right ventricular inflow Doppler recording in a patient with abnormal right ventricular relaxation. In this patient, the E wave is reduced and the A wave is increased. (From Klein, A.L., et al.: Comprehensive Doppler assessment of right ventricular diastolic function in cardiac amyloidosis. J. Am. Coll. Cardiol., *15*:103, 1990.)

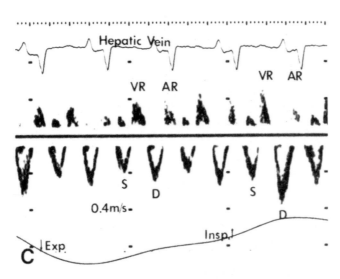

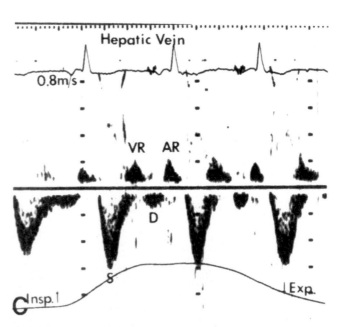

**Fig. 4–53.** Hepatic vein Doppler recording of a patient with restrictive disease of the right ventricle. The systolic velocity (S) is reduced and the diastolic velocity (D) is increased throughout the respiratory cycle. VR = ventricular reverse velocity; AR = atrial reverse velocity. (From Klein, A.L., et al.: Comprehensive Doppler assessment of right ventricular diastolic function in cardiac amyloidosis. J. Am. Coll. Cardiol., *15*:103, 1990.)

**Fig. 4–55.** Hepatic vein Doppler recording in a patient with abnormal right ventricular relaxation demonstrating accentuated systolic velocities (S) and reduced diastolic velocity (D). (From Klein, A.L., et al.: Comprehensive Doppler assessment of right ventricular function in cardiac amyloidosis. J. Am. Coll. Cardiol., *15*:103, 1990.)

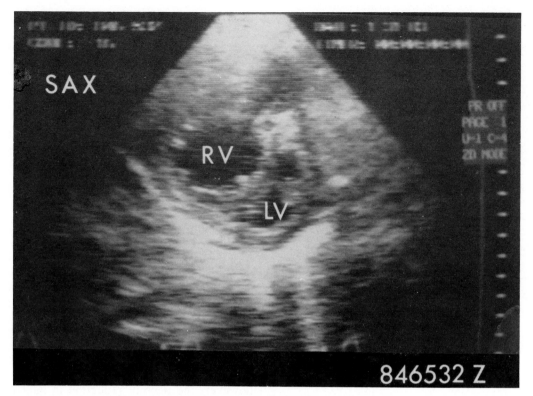

**Fig. 4–56.** Short-axis two-dimensional echocardiogram of a patient with marked increase in right ventricular systolic pressure and right ventricular hypertrophy. The interventricular septum is distorted as the right ventricle becomes more circular and the left ventricle assumes the shape of a quarter moon. RV = right ventricle; LV = left ventricle.

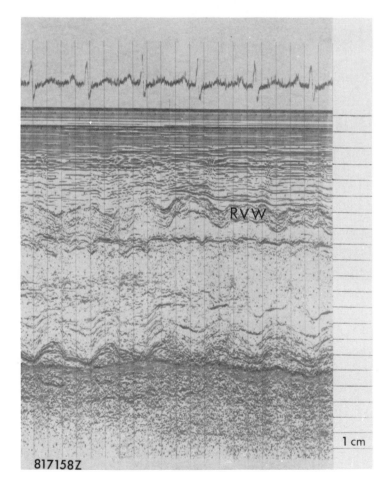

**Fig. 4–57.** M-mode echocardiogram of a thickened right ventricular free wall (RVW) in a patient with right ventricular hypertrophy.

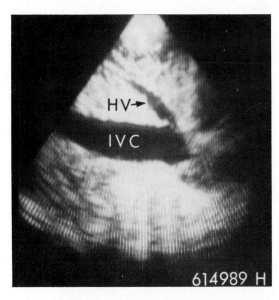

**Fig. 4–58.** Subcostal two-dimensional echocardiogram of a dilated inferior vena cava (IVC) and hepatic vein (HV) in a patient with right heart failure and elevated right atrial pressure.

axis.[137,138] Normally, the left ventricle assumes a circular configuration. If the septum is flat, or even curves toward the left ventricle (Fig. 4–56) in systole, one can be fairly certain of an increased pressure in the right ventricle.[139,140] Some investigators have even calculated left ventricular systolic circular indices.[141,142] Thickened right ventricular walls (Fig. 4–57) is another indicator of high right ventricular systolic pressure. Right ventricular dilatation commonly occurs with elevated right ventricular systolic pressure.

### Right Atrial Pressure

Elevation in right atrial pressure can best be determined by examining the inferior vena cava,[143–145] and to some extent, the hepatic veins.[146] Dilatation of these vessels is fairly specific for elevated right atrial pressures (Fig. 4–58), although the position of the patient can influence inferior vena caval size.[147] Another important finding with elevated right atrial pressure is the lack of inspiratory collapse of the inferior vena cava.[129,148] Normally, the inferior vena cava diameter decreases by 50% or more with inspiration (Fig. 4–59). Such a finding indicates a right atrial pressure of less than 10 mm Hg. If, however, the percent reduction in inferior vena caval diameter or caval index is less than 50%, a right atrial pressure of greater than 10 mm Hg is indicated. For

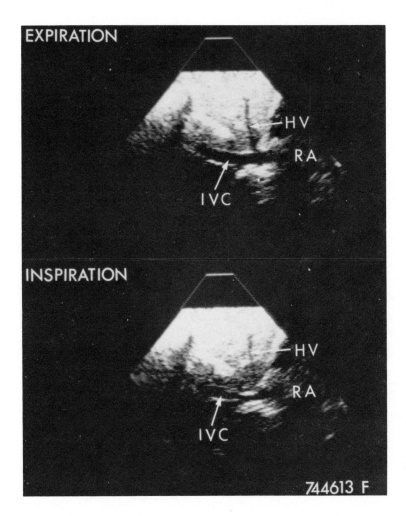

**Fig. 4–59.** Subcostal two-dimensional echocardiograms of the inferior vena cava (IVC), hepatic vein (HV), and right atrium (RA) in a normal subject. With inspiration, the caliber of the inferior vena cava and hepatic veins decreases.

those patients who cannot breathe normally, either because of pain or ventilatory status, investigators suggest having the patient "sniff" while imaging the inferior vena cava. A more complicated quantitated sonospirometry technique can be used for estimating right atrial pressure,[149] but it requires special equipment and is not used routinely. In patients receiving mechanical positive pressure ventilation, a dilated inferior vena cava does not predict right atrial pressure.[150] A small inferior vena cava, however, does exclude elevated right atrial pressures.

## REFERENCES

1. Hatle, L. and Angelsen, B.: Doppler Ultrasound in Cardiology: Physical Principles and Clinical Application. 2nd Ed. Philadelphia, Lea & Febiger, 1985.
2. Goldberg, S.J., Allen, H.D., Marx, G.R., and Flinn, C.J.: Doppler Echocardiography. Philadelphia, Lea & Febiger, 1985.
3. Thomas, J.D. and Weyman, A.E.: Seminar on *in vitro* studies of cardiac flow and their applications for clinical Doppler echocardiography—II. J. Am. Coll. Cardiol., 13:221, 1989.
4. Dubin, J., Wallerson, D.C., Cody, R.J., and Devereux, R.B.: Comparative accuracy of Doppler echocardiographic methods for clinical stroke volume determination. Am. Heart J., 120:116, 1990.
5. Moulinier, L., Venet, T., Schiller, N.B., Kurtz, T.W., Morris, R.C., and Sebastian, A.: Measurement of aortic blood flow by Doppler echocardiography: Day to day variability in normal subjects and applicability in clinical research. J. Am. Coll. Cardiol., 17:1326, 1991.
6. Meijboom, E.J., Rijsterborgh, H., Bot, H., DeBoo, J.A.J., Roelandt, J.R.T.C., and Bom, N.: Limits of reproducibility of blood flow measurements by Doppler echocardiography. Am. J. Cardiol., 59:133, 1987.
7. Goldberg, S.J., Sahn, D.J., Allen, H.D., Valldes-Cruz, L.M., Hoenecke, H., and Carnahan, Y.: Evaluation of pulmonary and systemic blood flow by two-dimensional Doppler echocardiography using fast Fourier transform spectral analysis. Am. J. Cardiol., 50:1394, 1982.
8. Nishimura, R.A., Callahan, M.J., Schaff, H.V., Ilstrup, D.M., Miller, F.A., and Tajik, A.J.: Non-invasive measurement of cardiac output by continuous-wave Doppler echocardiography: Initial experience and review of the literature. Mayo Clin. Proc., 59:484, 1984.
9. Fisher, D.C., Sahn, D.J., Friedman, M.J., Larson, D., Valdes-Cruz, L.M., Horowitz, S., Goldberg, S.J., and Allen, H.D.: The effect of variations of pulsed Doppler sampling site on calculation of cardiac output: An experimental study in open-chest dogs. Circulation, 67:370, 1983.
10. Labovitz, A.J.: The effects of sampling site on the two-dimensional echo-Doppler determination of cardiac output. Am. Heart J., 109:327, 1985.
11. Loeppky, J.A., Hoekenga, D.E., Greene, R., and Luft, U.C.: Comparison of non-invasive pulsed Doppler and Fick measurements of stroke volume in cardiac patients. Am. Heart J., 107:339, 1984.
12. Bouchard, A., Blumlein, S., Schiller, N.B., Schlitt, S., Byrd, III, B.F., Ports, T., and Chatterjee, K.: Measurement of left ventricular stroke volume using continuous wave Doppler echocardiography of the ascending aorta and M-mode echocardiography of the aortic valve. J. Am. Coll. Cardiol., 9:75, 1987.
13. Rein, A.J.J.T., Hsieh, K.S., Elixson, M., Colan, S.D., Lang, P., Sanders, S.P., and Castaneda, A.R.: Cardiac output estimates in the pediatric intensive care unit using a continuous-wave Doppler computer: Validation and limitations of the technique. Am. Heart J., 112:97, 1986.
14. Kitabatake, A., Inoue, M., Asao, M., Ito, H., Masuyama, T., Tanouchi, J., Morita, T., Hori, M., Yoshima, H., Ohnishi, K., and Abe, H.: Non-invasive evaluation of the ratio of pulmonary to systemic flow in atrial septal defect by duplex Doppler echocardiography. Circulation, 69:73, 1984.
15. Dittmann, H., Voelker, W., Karsch, K-R., and Seipel, L.: Influence of sampling site and flow area on cardiac output measurements by Doppler echocardiography. J. Am. Coll. Cardiol., 10:818, 1987.
16. Chandraratna, P.A., Nanna, M., McKay, C., Nimalasuriya, A., Swinney, R., Elkayam, U., and Rahimtoola, S.H.: Determination of cardiac output by transcutaneous continuous-wave ultrasonic Doppler computer. Am. J. Cardiol., 53:234, 1984.
17. Magnin, P.A., Stewart, J.A., Myers, S., VonRamm, O., and Kisslo, J.A.: Combined Doppler and phased-array echocardiographic estimation of cardiac output. Circulation, 63:388, 1981.
18. Ihlen, H., Amlie, J.P., Dale, J., Forfang, K., Nitter-Hauge, S., Otterstad, J.E., Simonsen, S., and Myhre, E.: Determination of cardiac output by Doppler echocardiography. Br. Heart J., 51:54, 1984.
19. Schuster, A.H. and Nanda, N.C.: Doppler echocardiographic features of mechanical alternans. Am. Heart J., 107:580, 1984.
20. Elkayam, U., Gardin, J.M., Berkley, R., Hughes, C.A., and Henry, W.L.: The use of Doppler flow velocity measurement to assess the hemodynamic response to vasodilators in patients with heart failure. Circulation, 67:377, 1983.
21. Steingart, R.M., Meller, J., Barovick, J., Patterson, R., Herman, M.V., and Teicholz, L.E.: Pulsed Doppler echocardiographic measurement of beat-to-beat changes in stroke volume in dogs. Circulation, 62:542, 1980.
22. Rose, J.S., Nanna, M., Rahimtoola, S.H., Elkayam, U., McKay, C., and Chandraratna, P.A.N.: Accuracy of determination of changes in cardiac output by transcutaneous continuous-wave Doppler computer. Am. J. Cardiol., 54:1099, 1984.
23. Maeda, M., Yokota, M., Iwase, M., Miyahara, T., Hayashi, H., and Sotobata, I.: Accuracy of cardiac output measured by continuous wave Doppler echocardiography during dynamic exercise testing in the supine position in patients with coronary artery disease. J. Am. Coll. Cardiol., 13:76, 1989.
24. Lloyd, T.R. and Shirazi, F.: Nongeometric Doppler stroke volume determination is limited by aortic size. Am. J. Cardiol., 66:883, 1990.
25. Kumar, A., Minagoe, S., Thangathurai, D., Mikhail, M., Novia, D., Vilijoen, J.F., Rahimtoola, S.H., and Chandraratna, P.A.N.: Noninvasive measurement of cardiac output during surgery using a new continuous-wave Doppler esophageal probe. Am. J. Cardiol., 64:793, 1989.
26. Spodick, D.H. and Koito, H.: Nongeometric Doppler stroke volume determination. Am. J. Cardiol., 63:883, 1989.
27. Corya, B.C., Rasmussen, S., Phillips, J.F., and Black, M.J.: Forward stroke calculated from aortic valve echograms in normal subjects and patients with mitral regurgi-

tation secondary to left ventricular dysfunction. Am. J. Cardiol., *47*:1215, 1981.

28. Winer, H., Kronzon, I., and Glassman, E.: Echocardiographic findings in severe paradoxical pulse due to pulmonary embolization. Am. J. Cardiol., *40*:808, 1977.

29. Yeh, H.C., Winsberg, F., and Mercer, E.M.: Echocardiographic aortic valve orifice dimensions: Its use in evaluating aortic stenosis and cardiac output. JCU, *1*:182, 1973.

30. Jacobs, W.R., Croke, R.P., Loeb, H.S., and Gunnar, R.M.: Echocardiographic aortic ejection area as a reflection of left ventricular stroke volume. JCU, 7:369, 1979.

31. Laniado, S., Yellin, E., Terdiman, R., Meytes, I., and Stadler, J.: Hemodynamic correlates of the normal aortic valve echogram. A study of sound, flow, and motion. Circulation, *54*:729, 1976.

32. Rasmussen, S., Corya, B.C., Lovelace, E., Black, M.J., and Phillips, J.F.: Forward stroke volume derived from aortic valve echograms. Clin. Res., 27:672A, 1979. (Abstract)

33. Lighty, G.W., Garbiulo, A., Kronzon, I., and Politzer, F.: Comparison of multiple views for the evaluation of pulmonary arterial blood flow by Doppler echocardiography. Circulation, *74*:1002, 1986.

34. Panidis, I.P., Ross, J., and Mintz, G.S.: Effect of sampling site on assessment of pulmonary artery blood flow by Doppler echocardiography. Am. J. Cardiol., *58*:1145, 1986.

35. Gorcsan, III, J., Ball, D.P., and Hattler, B.G.: Intraoperative determination of cardiac output by transesophageal continuous wave Doppler. Am. Heart J., *123*:171, 1992.

36. Kasper, W., Treese, N., Pop, T., and Meinertz, T.: Diagnosis of increased pulmonary blood flow by suprasternal M-mode echocardiography in atrial septal defect. Am. J. Cardiol., *53*:1272, 1983.

37. Fisher, D.C., Sahn, D.J., Friedman, M.J., Larson, D., Valdes-Cruz, L.M., Horowitz, S., Goldberg, S.J., and Allen, H.D.: The mitral valve orifice method for noninvasive two-dimensional echo Doppler determinations of cardiac output. Circulation, *67*:872, 1983.

38. Deleted.

39. DeZuttere, D., Touche, T., Saumon, G., Nitenberg, A., and Prasquier, R.: Doppler echocardiographic measurement of mitral flow volume: Validation of a new method in adult patients. J. Am. Coll. Cardiol., *11*:343, 1988.

40. Nicolosi, G.L., Pungercic, E., Gervesato, E., Modena, L., and Zanuttini, D.: Analysis of interobserver and intraobserver variation of interpretation of the echocardiographic and Doppler flow determination of cardiac output by the mitral orifice method. Br. Heart J., *55*:446, 1986.

41. Miller, W.E., Richards, K.L., and Crawford, M.H.: Accuracy of mitral Doppler echocardiographic cardiac output determinations in adults. Am. Heart J., *119*:620, 1990.

42. Masuyama, T., St. Goar, F.G., Alderman, E.L., and Popp, R.L.: Effects of Nitroprusside on transmitral flow velocity patterns in extreme heart failure: A combined hemodynamic and Doppler echocardiographic study of varying loading conditions. J. Am. Coll. Cardiol., *16*:1175, 1990.

43. Ascah, K.J., Stewart, W.J., Gillam, L.D., Triulzi, M.O., Newell, J.B., and Weyman, A.E.: Calculation of transmitral flow by Doppler echocardiography: A comparison of methods in a canine model. Am. Heart. J., *117*:402, 1989.

44. Meijboom, E.J., Horowitz, S., Valdes-Cruz, L.M., Larson, D.F., Bom, N., Rijsterborgh, H., Lima, C.O., and Sahn, D.J.: A simplified mitral valve method for two-dimensional echo Doppler blood flow calculation: Validation in an open-chest canine model and initial clinical studies. Am. Heart J., *113*:335, 1987.

44a. Shimamoto, H., Kito, H., Kawazoe, K., Fujita, T., and Shimamoto, Y.: Tranesophageal Doppler echocardiographic measurement of cardiac output by the mitral annulus method. Br. Heart J., *68*:510, 1992.

45. DeMaria, A., Miller, R.R., Amsterdam, E.A., Markson, W., and Mason, D.T.: Mitral valve early diastolic closing velocity on echogram: Relation to sequential diastolic flow and ventricular compliance. Am. J. Cardiol., *37*:693, 1976.

46. Quinones, M.A., Gaasch, W.H., Waisser, E., and Alexander, J.K.: Reduction in the rate of diastolic descent of the mitral valve echogram in patients with altered left ventricular diastolic pressure-volume relations. Circulation, *49*:246, 1974.

47. Vignola, P.A., Walker, H.J., Gold, H.K., and Leinbach, R.C.: Alteration of the left ventricular pressure-volume relationship in man and its effect on the mitral echocardiographic early diastolic closure slope. Circulation, *58*:586, 1977.

48. Strunk, B.L., Fitzgerald, J.W., Lipton, M., Popp, R.L., and Barry, W.H.: The posterior aortic wall echocardiogram: Its relationship to left atrial volume change. Circulation, *54*:744, 1976.

49. Strunk, B.L., London, E.J., Fitzgerald, J., Popp, R.L., and Barry, W.H.: The assessment of mitral stenosis and prosthetic mitral valve obstruction, using the posterior aortic wall echocardiogram. Circulation, *55*:885, 1977.

50. Akgun, G., and Layton, C.: Aortic root and left atrial wall motion: An echocardiographic study. Br. Heart J., *39*:1082, 1977.

51. Hall, R.J.C., Clark, S.E., and Brown, D.: Evaluation of posterior aortic wall echogram in diagnosis of mitral valve disease. Br. Heart J., *41*:522, 1979.

52. Tye, K-H., Deser, K.B., and Benchimol, A.: Relation between apexcardiographic A wave and posterior aortic wall motion. Am. J. Cardiol, *43*:24, 1979.

53. Tanimoto, M., Yamamoto, T., Makihata, S., Konishiike, A., Komasa, N., Kimura, S., Yamasaki, K., Sakuyama, K., Kawai, Y., and Iwasaki, T.: Echocardiograms of a monophasic triangular wave of the tricuspid valve. J. Cardiogr., *12*:825, 1982.

54. Iwasaki, T., Tanimoto, M., Yamamoto, T., Makihata, S., Kawai, Y., and Yorifuji, S.: Echocardiographic abnormalities of tricuspid valve motion in pulmonary embolism. Br. Heart J., *47*:454, 1982.

55. DeMaria, A.N., Bommer, W., Kwan, O.K., Riggs, K., Smith, M., and Waters, J.: In vivo correlation of thermodilution cardiac output and videodensitometric indicator-dilution curves obtained from contrast two-dimensional echocardiograms. J. Am. Coll. Cardiol., *3*:999, 1984.

56. Nicolosi, G.L., Pungercic, E., Cervesato, E., Pavan, D., Modena, L., Moro, E., Dall'Aglio, V., and Zanuttini, D.: Feasibility and variability of six methods for the echocardiographic and Doppler determination of cardiac output. Br. Heart J., *59*:299, 1988.

57. Sanders, S.P., Yeager, S., and Williams, R.G.: Measurement of systemic and pulmonary blood flow and QP/QS ratio using Doppler and two-dimensional echocardiography. Am. J. Cardiol., *51*:952, 1983.

58. Jenni, R., Ritter, M., Vieli, A., Hirzel, H.O., Schmid, E.R., Grimm, J.G., and Turina, M.: Determination of the ratio of pulmonary blood flow to systemic blood flow by derivation of amplitude weighted mean velocity from

continuous wave Doppler spectra. Br. Heart J., *61*:167, 1989.

59. Valdes-Cruz, L.M., Horowitz, S., Mesel, E., Sahn, D.J., Fisher, D.C., and Larson, D.: A pulsed Doppler echocardiographic method for calculating pulmonary and systemic blood flow in atrial level shunts: Validation studies in animals and initial human experience. Circulation, *69*:80, 1984.

60. Barron, J.V., Shan, D.J., Valdes-Cruz, L.M., Oliveira, C., Goldberg, S.J., Grenadier, E., and Allen, H.D.: Clinical utility of two-dimensional Doppler echocardiographic techniques for estimating pulmonary to systemic blood flow ratios in children with left to right shunting atrial septal defect, ventricular septal defect or patent ductus arteriosus. J. Am. Coll. Cardiol., *3*:169, 1984.

61. Okamoto, M., et al.: Noninvasive determination of the ratio of pulmonary to systemic blood flow with two-dimensional Doppler echocardiography: Efficacy and limitation. J. Cardiogr., *14*:189, 1984.

62. Machi, J., Sigel, B., Beitler, J.C., Coelho, J.C.U., and Justin, J.R.: Relation of in vivo blood flow to ultrasound echogenicity. JCU, *11*:3, 1983.

63. Garcia-Fernandez, M.A., Moreno, M., and Banuelos, F.: Two-dimensional echocardiographic identification of blood stasis in the left atrium. Am. Heart J., *109*:600, 1985.

64. Hatle, L., Brubakk, A., Tromsdal, A., and Angelsen, B.: Non-invasive assessment of pressure drop in mitral stenosis by Doppler ultrasound. Br. Heart J., *40*:131, 1978.

65. Hatle, L., Angelsen, B.A., and Tromsdal, A.: Noninvasive assessment of aortic stenosis by Doppler ultrasound. Br. Heart J., *43*:284, 1979.

66. Requarth, J.A., Goldberg, S.J., Vasko, S.D., and Allen, H.D.: In vitro verification of Doppler prediction of transvalve pressure gradient and orifice area in stenosis. Am. J. Cardiol., *53*:1369, 1984.

67. Stam, R.B., and Martin, R.P.: Quantification of pressure gradients across stenotic valves by Doppler ultrasound. J. Am. Coll. Cardiol., *2*:707, 1983.

68. Masuyama, T., Uematsu, M., Nakatani, S., Sato, H., and Kodama, K.: Doppler echocardiographic assessment of changes in pulmonary artery pressure associated with vasodilating therapy in patients with congestive heart failure. J. Am. Soc. Echocardiogr., *4*:35, 1991.

69. Beard, II, J.T., Newman, J.H., Loyd, J.E., Byrd, III, B.F.: Doppler estimation of changes in pulmonary artery pressure during hypoxic breathing. J. Am. Soc. Echocardiogr., *4*:121, 1991.

70. Stevenson, J.G.: Comparison of several noninvasive methods for estimation of pulmonary artery pressure. J. Am. Soc. Echocardiogr., *2*:157, 1989.

71. Chow, L.C., Dittrich, H.C., Hoit, B.D., Moser, K.M., and Nicod, P.H.: Doppler assessment of changes in right-sided cardiac hemodynamics after pulmonary thromboendarterectomy. Am. J. Cardiol., *61*:1092, 1988.

72. Yock, P.G., and Popp, R.L.: Non-invasive estimation of right ventricular systolic pressure by Doppler ultrasound in patients with tricuspid regurgitation. Circulation, *70*:657, 1984.

73. Torres, F., Tye, T., Gibbons, R., Puryear, J., and Popp, R.L.: Echocardiographic contrast increases the yield for right ventricular pressure measurement by Doppler echocardiography. J. Am. Soc. Echocardiogr., *2*:419, 1989.

74. Himelman, R.B., Stulbarg, M.S., Lee, E., Kuecherer, H.F., and Schiller, N.B.: Noninvasive evaluation of pulmonary artery systolic pressures during dynamic exercise by saline-enhanced Doppler echocardiography. Am. Heart J., *119*:685, 1990.

75. Himelman, R.B., Stulbarg, M., Kircher, B., Lee, E., Kee, L., Dean, N.C., Golden, J., Wolfe, C.L., and Schiller, N.B.: Noninvasive evaluation of pulmonary artery pressure during exercise by saline-enhanced Doppler echocardiography in chronic pulmonary disease. Circulation, *79*:863, 1989.

76. Hamer, H.P.M., Takens, B.L., Posma, J.L., and Lie, K.I.: Noninvasive measurement of right ventricular systolic pressure by combined color-coded and continuous-wave Doppler ultrasound. Am. J. Cardiol., *61*:668, 1988.

77. Lee, R.T., Lord, C.P., Plappert, T., and St. John Sutton, M.: Prospective Doppler echocardiographic evaluation of pulmonary artery diastolic pressure in the medical intensive care unit. Am. J. Cardiol., *64*:1366, 1989.

78. Masuyama, T., Uematsu, M., Sato, H., Nakatani, S., Nanto, S., Hirayama, A., Asada, S., Kodama, K., Kitabatake, A., and Inoue, M.: Pulmonary arterial end-diastolic pressure noninvasively estimated by continuous wave Doppler echocardiography. J. Cardiogr., *16*:669, 1986.

79. Garg, A., Shrivastava, S., Radhakrishnan, S., Dev, V., and Saxena, A.: Doppler assessment of interventricular pressure gradient across isolated ventricular septal defect. Clin. Cardiol., *13*:717, 1990.

79a. Ge, Z., Zhang, Y., Fan, D., Kang, W., Hatle, L., Duran, C.: Simultaneous measurement of pulmonary artery diastolic pressure by Doppler echocardiography and catheterization in patients with patent ductus arteriosus. Am. Heart J., *125*:263, 1993.

80. Nishimura, R.A. and Tajik, A.J.: Determination of left-sided pressure gradients by utilizing Doppler aortic and mitral regurgitant signals: Validation by simultaneous dual catheter and Doppler studies. J. Am. Coll. Cardiol., *11*:317, 1988.

81. Gorcsan, J., Snow, F.R., Paulsen, W., and Nixon, J.V.: Noninvasive estimation of left atrial pressure in patients with congestive heart failure and mitral regurgitation by Doppler echocardiography. Am. Heart J., *121*:858, 1991.

82. Myreng, Y., Smiseth, O.A., and Risoe, C.: Left ventricular filling at elevated diastolic pressures: Relationship between transmitral Doppler flow velocities and atrial contribution. Am. Heart J., *119*:620, 1990.

83. Courtois, M., Vered, Z., Barzilai, B., Ricciotti, N.A., Perez, J.E., and Ludbrook, P.A.: The transmitral pressure-flow velocity relation. Circulation, *78*:1459, 1988.

84. Konecke, L.L., Feigenbaum, H., Chang, S., Corya, B.C., and Fischer, J.C.: Abnormal mitral valve motion in patients with elevated left ventricular diastolic pressures. Circulation, *47*:989, 1973.

85. Ohte, N., Nakano, S., Mizutani, Y., Samoto, T., and Fujinami, T.: Relation of mitral valve motion to left ventricular end-diastolic pressure assessed by M-mode echocardiography. J. Cardiogr., *16*:115, 1986.

86. Ambrose, J.A., Teichholz, L.E., Meller, J., Weintraub, W., Pichard, A.D., Smith, H., Jr., Martinez, E.E., and Herman, M.V.: The influence of left ventricular late diastolic filling on the A wave of the left ventricular pressure trace. Circulation, *60*:510, 1979.

87. Ishikawa, T., Usui, T., Kashiwagi, M., Kimura, K., Yoshimura, H., Sano, T., and Nihei, T.: Contribution of end-diastolic mitral regurgitation to the B-B' step formation on M-mode echocardiography. J. Appl. Cardiol., *6*:163, 1991.

88. Otsuji, Y., Toda, H., Ishigami, T., Lee, S., Okino, H., Minagoe, S., Nakao, S., and Tanaka, H.: Mitral regurgi-

tation during B bump of the mitral valve studied Doppler echocardiography. Am. J. Cardiol., *67*:778, 1991.

89. Lewis, J.R., Parker, J.O., and Burggraf, G.W.: Mitral valve motion and changes in left ventricular end-diastolic pressure: A correlative study of the PR-AC interval. Am. J. Cardiol., *42*:383, 1978.

90. Botvinick, E.H., Schiller, N.B., Wickramasekaran, R., Klausner, S.C., and Gertz, E.: Echocardiographic demonstration of early mitral valve closure in severe aortic insufficiency: Its clinical implications. Circulation, *51*:836, 1975.

91. Pridie, R.B., Beham, R., and Oakley, C.M.: Echocardiography of the mitral valve in aortic valve disease. Br. Heart J., *33*:296, 1971.

92. Oki, T., Matsuhisa, M., Tsuyuguchi, N., Kondo, C., Matsumura, K., Niki, T., Mori, H., and Sawada, S.: Echo patterns of the anterior leaflet of the mitral valve in patients with aortic insufficiency. J. Cardiogr., *6*:307, 1976.

93. Ambrose, J.A., Meller, J., Teichholz, L.E., and Herman, M.V.: Premature closure of the mitral valve. Echocardiographic clue for the diagnosis of aortic dissection. Chest, *73*:121, 1978.

94. Fox, S., Kotler, M.N., Segal, B.L., and Parry, W.: Echocardiographic clue for the diagnosis of acute aortic valve endocarditis and its complications. Arch. Intern. Med., *137*:85, 1977.

95. Mann, T., McLaurin, L., Grossman, W., and Craige, E.: Assessing the hemodynamic severity of acute aortic regurgitation due to infective endocarditis. N. Engl. J. Med., *293*:108, 1975.

96. Pietro, D.A., Parisi, A.F., Harrington, J.J., and Askenazi, J.: Premature opening of the aortic valve: An index of highly advanced aortic regurgitation. JCU, *6*:170, 1978.

97. Haendchen, R.V., Povzhitkov, M., Meerbaum, S., Maruer, G., and Corday, E.: Evaluation of changes in left ventricular end-diastolic pressure by left atrial two-dimensional echocardiography. Am. Heart J., *104*:740, 1982.

98. Askenazi, J., Koenigsberg, D.I., Ziegler, J.H., and Lesch, M.: Echocardiographic estimates of pulmonary artery wedge pressure. N. Engl. J. Med., *305*:1566, 1981.

99. Askenazi, J., Koenigsberg, D.I., Ribner, H.S., Plucinski, D., Silverman, I.M., and Lesch, M.: Prospective study comparing different echocardiographic measurements of pulmonary capillary wedge pressure in patients with organic heart disease other than mitral stenosis. J. Am. Coll. Cardiol., *2*:919, 1983.

100. Berger, M., Bach, M., Hecht, S.R., and Van Tosh, A.: Estimation of pulmonary arterial wedge pressure by pulsed Doppler echocardiography and phonocardiography. Am. J. Cardiol., *69*:562, 1992.

101. Kuecherer, H.F., Kusumoto, F., Muhiudeen, I.A., Cahalan, M.K., and Schiller, N.B.: Pulmonary venous flow patterns by transesophageal pulsed Doppler echocardiography: Relation to parameters of left ventricular systolic and diastolic function. Am. Heart J., *122*:1683, 1991.

102. Kuecherer, H.F., Muhiudeen, I.A., Kusumoto, F.M., Lee, E., Moulinier, LE., Cahalan, M.K., and Schiller, N.B.: Estimation of mean left atrial pressure from transesophageal pulsed Doppler echocardiography of pulmonary venous flow. Circulation, *82*:1127, 1990.

103. Basnight, M.A., Gonzalez, M.S., Kershenovich, S.C., and Appleton, C.P.: Pulmonary venous flow velocity: Relation to hemodynamics, mitral flow velocity and left atrial volume, and ejection fraction. J. Am. Soc. Echocardiogr., *4*:547, 1991.

103a. Kusumoto, F.M., Muhiudeen, I.A., Kuecherer, H.F., Cahalan, M.K., Schiller, N.B.: Response of the interatrial septum to transatrial pressure gradients and its potential for predicting pulmonary capillary wedge pressure: An intraoperative study using transesophageal echocardiography in patients during mechanical ventilation. J. Am. Coll. Cardiol., *21*:721, 1993.

104. Chan, K-L., Currie, P.J., Seward, J.B., Hagler, D.J., Mair, D.D., and Tajik, A.J.: Comparison of three Doppler ultrasound methods in the prediction of pulmonary artery disease. J. Am. Coll. Cardiol., *9*:549, 1987.

105. Senecal, F., Weyman, A.E., Pyhel, H.J., Dillon, J.C., Feigenbaum, H., and Stewart, J.: Estimation of pulmonary artery pressure by pulsed Doppler echocardiography. Circulation (Suppl. III), *56*:25, 1977. (Abstract)

106. Hatle, L., Angelsen, B.A., and Tromsdal, A.: Noninvasive estimation of pulmonary artery systolic pressure with Doppler ultrasound. Br. Heart J., *45*:157, 1981.

107. Kitabatake, A., Inoue, M., Asao, M., Masuyama, T., Tanouchi, J., Morita, T., Mishima, M., Uematsu, M., Shimazu, T., Hori, M., and Abe, H.: Non-invasive evaluation of pulmonary hypertension by a pulsed Doppler technique. Circulation, *68*:302, 1983.

108. Kosturakis, D., Goldberg, S.J., Allen, H.D., and Loeber, C.: Doppler echocardiographic prediction of pulmonary arterial hypertension in congenital heart disease. Am. J. Cardiol., *53*:1110, 1984.

109. Okamoto, M., Miyatake, K., Kinoshita, N., Sakkakibara, H., and Nimura, Y.: Analysis of blood flow in pulmonary hypertension with the pulsed Doppler flowmeter combined with cross-sectional echocardiography. Br. Heart J., *51*:407, 1984.

110. Matsuda, M., Sekiguchi, T., Sugishita, Y., Kuwako, K., Iida, K., and Ito, I.: Reliability of non-invasive estimates of pulmonary hypertension by pulsed Doppler echocardiography. Br. Heart J., *56*:158, 1986.

111. Dabestani, A., Mahan, G., Gardin, J.M., Takenaka, K., Burn, C., Allfie, A., and Henry, W.L.: Evaluation of pulmonary artery pressure and resistance by pulsed Doppler echocardiography. Am. J. Cardiol., *59*:662, 1987.

112. Serwer, G.A., Cougle, A.G., Eckerd, J.M., and Armstrong, B.E.: Factors affecting use of the Doppler-determined time from flow onset to maximal pulmonary artery velocity for measurement of pulmonary artery pressure in children. Am. J. Cardiol., *58*:352, 1986.

113. Graettinger, W.F., Greene, E.R., and Voyles, W.F.: Doppler predictions of pulmonary artery pressure, flow, and resistance in adults. Am. Heart J., *113*:1426, 1987.

114. Cooper, M.J., Tyndall, M., and Silverman, N.H.: Evaluation of the responsiveness of elevated pulmonary vascular resistance in children by Doppler echocardiography. J. Am. Coll. Cardiol., *12*:470, 1988.

115. Ranganathan, N., and Sivaciyan, V.: Abnormalities in jugular venous flow velocity in pulmonary hypertension. Am. J. Cardiol., *62*:719, 1989.

116. Turkevich, D., Groves, B.M., Micco, A., Trapp, J.A., and Reeves, J.T.: Early partial systolic closure of the pulmonic valve relates to severity of pulmonary hypertension. Am. Heart J., *115*:409, 1988.

117. Nanda, N.C., Gramiak, R., Robinson, T.I., and Shah, P.M.: Echocardiographic evaluation of pulmonary hypertension. Circulation, *50*:575, 1974.

118. Weyman, A.E., Dillon, J.C., Feigenbaum, H., and Chang, S.: Echocardiographic patterns of pulmonary valve motion with pulmonary hypertension. Circulation, *50*:905, 1974.

119. Shiina, A., Yaginuma, T., Matsumoto, Y., Kawasaki,

K., Tsuchiya, M., Miyata, K., Tomita, T., Matsumoto, Y., Kawai, N., and Hosoda, S.: Echocardiographic analysis of pulmonic and aortic valve motion by simultaneous recordings of flow velocity and intravascular pressure: Genesis of mid-systolic semi-closure of the pulmonic valve in patients with pulmonary hypertension. J. Cardiogr., 7:599, 1977.

120. Lew, W., and Karliner, J.S.: Assessment of pulmonary valve echogram in normal subjects and in patients with pulmonary arterial hypertension. Br. Heart J., 42:147, 1979.

121. Marin-Garcia, J., Moller, J.H., and Mirvis, D.M.: The pulmonic valve echogram in the assessment of pulmonary hypertension in children. Pediatr. Cardiol., 4:209, 1983.

122. Haddad, K.A., Lebeau, R., and Tremblay, G.: Use of echocardiography in the diagnosis of pulmonary hypertension. Acta Cardiol., 36:21, 1981.

123. Dolara, A., Zuppiroli, A., Cecchi, F., Manetti, A., Mazzuoli, F., and Santoro, G.: Echocardiographic pitfalls in the diagnosis of pulmonary hypertension. Acta Cardiol., 36:451, 1981.

124. Lew, W. and Karliner, J.S.: Assessment of pulmonary valve echogram in normal subjects and in patients with pulmonary arterial hypertension. Br. Heart J., 42:147, 1979.

125. Tahara, M., Tanaka, H., Nakao, S., Yoshimura, H., Sakurai, S., Tei, C., and Kashima, T.: Hemodynamic determinants of pulmonary valve motion during systole in experimental pulmonary hypertension. Circulation, 64:1249, 1981.

126. Acquatella, H., Schiller, N.B., Sharpe, D.N., and Chatterjee, K.: Lack of correlation between echocardiographic pulmonary valve morphology and simultaneous pulmonary arterial pressure. Am. J. Cardiol., 43:946, 1979.

127. Bauman, W., Wann, L.S., Childress, R., Weyman, A.E., Feigenbaum, H., and Dillon, J.C.: Mid-systolic notching of the pulmonary valve in the absence of pulmonary hypertension. Am. J. Cardiol., 43:1049, 1979.

128. Hirschfeld, S., Meyer, R., Schwartz, D.C., Korfhagen, J., and Kaplan, S.: Measurement of right and left ventricular systolic time intervals by echocardiography. Circulation, 51:304, 1975.

129. Riggs, T., Hirschfeld, S., Borkat, G., Knoke, J., and Liebman, J.: Assessment of the pulmonary vascular bed by echocardiographic right ventricular systolic time intervals. Circulation, 57:939, 1978.

130. Spooner, E.W., Perry, B.L., Stern, A.M., and Sigmann, J.M.: Estimation of pulmonary/systemic resistance ratios from echocardiographic systolic time intervals in young patients with congenital or acquired heart disease. Am. J. Cardiol., 42:810, 1978.

131. Kasper, W. and Meinertz, T.: Estimation of pulmonary arterial pressure by measuring the size of the right pulmonary artery in the suprasternal echocardiogram. Klin. Wochenschr., 60:71, 1982.

132. Starling, M.R., Crawford, M.H., Walsh, R.A., and O'Rourke, R.A.: Value of the tricuspid valve echogram for estimating right ventricular end-diastolic pressure during vasodilator therapy. Am. J. Cardiol., 45:966, 1980.

133. Fujii, J., Morita, K., Watanabe, H., and Kato, K.: Tricuspid valve echograms in various right heart diseases. Cardiovasc. Sound Bull., 5:241, 1975.

134. Wann, L.S., Weyman, A.E., Dillon, J.C., and Feigenbaum, H.: Premature pulmonary valve opening. Circulation, 55:128, 1977.

135. Nishimoto, M., Tanaka, C., Oku, H., Ikuno, Y., Kawai, S., Furukawa, K., Takeuchi, K., and Shiota, K.: Presystolic pulmonary valve opening in constrictive pericarditis. J. Cardiogr., 7:55, 1977.

136. Klein, A.L., Hatle, L.K., Burstow, D.J., Taliercio, C.P., Seward, J.B., Kyle, R.A., Bailey, K.R., Gertz, M.A., and Tajik, A.J.: Comprehensive Doppler assessment of right ventricular diastolic function in cardiac amyloidosis. J. Am. Coll. Cardiol., 15:99, 1990.

137. Portman, M.A., Bhat, A.M., Cohen, M.H., and Jacobstein, M.D.: Left ventricular systolic circular index: An echocardiography measure of transseptal pressure ratio. Am. Heart J., 114:1178, 1987.

138. Dittrich, H.C., Nicod, P.H., Chow, L.C., Chappuis, F.P., Moser, K.M., and Peterson, K.L.: Early changes of right heart geometry after pulmonary thromboendarterectomy. J. Am. Coll. Cardiol., 11:937, 1988.

139. King, M.E., Braun, H., Goldblatt, A., Liberthson, R., and Weyman, A.E.: Interventricular septal configuration as a predictor of right ventricular systolic hypertension in children: A cross-section echocardiographic study. Circulation, 68:68, 1983.

140. Visner, M.S., Arentzen, C.E., O'Connor, M.J., Larson, E.V., and Anderson, R.W.: Alterations in left ventricular three-dimensional dynamic geometry and systolic function during acute right ventricular hypertension in the conscious dog. Circulation, 67:353, 1983.

141. Schreiber, T.L., Feigenbaum, H., and Weyman, A.E.: Effect of atrial septal defect repair on left ventricular geometry and degree of mitral valve prolapse. Circulation, 61:888, 1980.

142. Ryan, T., Petrovic, O., Dillon, J.C., Feigenbaum, H., Conley, M.J., and Armstrong, W.F.: An echocardiographic index for separation of right ventricular volume and pressure overload. J. Am. Cardiol., 5:918, 1985.

143. Rein, A.J., Lewis, N., Forst, L., Gotsman, M.S., and Lewis, B.S.: Echocardiography of the inferior vena cava in healthy subjects and in patients with cardiac disease. Isr. J. Med. Sci., 18:581, 1982.

144. Meltzer, R.S., McGhie, J., and Roelandt, J.: Inferior vena cava echocardiography. JCU, 10:47, 1982.

145. Gullace, G. and Savoia, M.T.: Echocardiographic assessment of the inferior vena cava wall motion for studies of right heart dynamics and function. Clin. Cardiol., 7:393, 1984.

146. Moreno, F.L.L., Hagan, A.D., Holman, J.R., Pryor, T.A., Strickland, R.D., and Castle, C.H.: Evaluation of size and dynamics of the inferior vena cava as an index of right-sided cardiac function. Am. J. Cardiol., 53:579, 1984.

147. Nakao, S., Come, P.C., McKay, R.G., and Ransil, B.J.: Effects of positional changes on inferior vena caval size and dynamics and correlations with right-sided cardiac pressure. Am. J. Cardiol., 59:125, 1987.

148. Kircher, B.J., Himelman, R.B., and Schiller, N.B.: Noninvasive estimation of right atrial pressure from the inspiratory collapse of the inferior vena cava. Am. J. Cardiol., 66:493, 1990.

149. Simonson, J.S. and Schiller, N.B.: Sonospirometry: A new method for noninvasive estimation of mean right atrial pressure based on two-dimensional echographic measurements of the inferior vena cava during measured inspiration. J. Am. Coll. Cardiol., 11:557, 1988.

150. Jue, J., Chung, W., and Schiller, N.B.: Does inferior vena cava size predict right atrial pressures in patients receiving mechanical ventilation? J. Am. Soc. Echocardiogr., 5:613, 1992.

# 5

# Echocardiographic Findings with Altered Electrical Activation

Because of its rapid sampling rate, M-mode echocardiography provides an excellent opportunity to study cardiac motion. This motion is influenced not only by anatomic and hemodynamic abnormalities, but also by changes in electrical activation. Many of the changes in motion are too subtle to be detected by angiographic or radionuclide techniques. Even real-time two-dimensional echocardiography has a relatively slow sampling rate compared with that of M-mode echocardiography. The rapid sampling rate and the use of time as one of the dimensions make M-mode echocardiography an ideal diagnostic and investigative tool for noting functional changes that occur with altered electrical activation.[1,2] Doppler echocardiography provides a real-time, beat-to-beat physiologic evaluation and is particularly valuable in assessing rhythm disturbances. Thus, the combination of M-mode and Doppler echocardiography can be helpful at times in evaluating or understanding abnormalities of electrical activation. The following discussion is not intended to be an exhaustive review of all possible relationships between the echocardiogram and electrocardiogram. It should, however, provide some principles and examples of how changes in cardiac electrical activity can influence the echocardiogram.

This knowledge should also improve our understanding of the relationship between electrical activation of the heart and cardiac function.

## ABNORMAL VENTRICULAR DEPOLARIZATION

### Bundle Branch Block

Patients with left bundle branch block serve as an excellent example of how altered electrical depolarization can influence cardiac motion. The echocardiographic findings in patients with left bundle branch block involve changes in the motion of the interventricular septum.[3–9] Figure 5–1 briefly reviews normal interventricular septal motion. Following electrical depolarization, a brief anterior motion of the interventricular septum may occur. This motion is then followed immediately by downward displacement of the septum toward the left ventricular cavity during ventricular ejection. With ventricular relaxation, the septum moves anteriorly toward the right

ventricle. Shortly after the initial mitral valve opening, or E point, a brief downward dip of the septum toward the left ventricle (*arrow*) occurs. This dip is immediately followed by resumption of the anterior motion of the interventricular septum as diastole continues. Figure 5–2 demonstrates the echocardiographic findings with left bundle branch block. Shortly after the onset of electrical depolarization (heavy vertical line at right) is a rapid downward dip of the left septum (LS) followed by a gradual anterior displacement of the interventricular septum throughout ventricular ejection. A slight downward dip of the septum corresponding to the E point of the mitral valve may occur. The principal echocardiographic feature of left bundle branch block is the downward motion of the interventricular septum with the onset of electrical depolarization (Fig. 5–2, *arrow*).

The abnormal anterior motion of the interventricular septum during ventricular ejection may be an important hemodynamic consequence of this electrical abnormality. As expected, the abnormal septal motion during ejection alters overall ventricular function. The extent to which this abnormal systolic motion occurs has been examined with two-dimensional echocardiography. Because this portion of the interventricular septum is not often recorded with the routine right anterior oblique left ventricular angiogram, the abnormal function produced by left bundle branch block pattern is not commonly recognized as an important hemodynamic factor. The left bundle branch block also appears to affect diastolic function.[10]

The abnormal septal motion during ventricular ejection is not always as striking as in Figure 5–2. Figure 5–3 demonstrates another echocardiogram of a patient with left bundle branch block. The abnormal posterior displacement of the septum with the onset of electrical depolarization is again noted (*arrows*). This downward dip, or beaking, is followed by another downward, more gradual motion of the septum toward the left ventricle. Thus, during ventricular ejection, the septum is moving toward the left ventricle rather than paradoxically as in Figure 5–2. A somewhat larger early diastolic dip is also noted in Figure 5–3. The mechanical or hemodynamic effects of the left bundle branch block would not be as adverse to overall ventricular function in the patient in Figure 5–3 as they would in the patient in Figure 5–2.

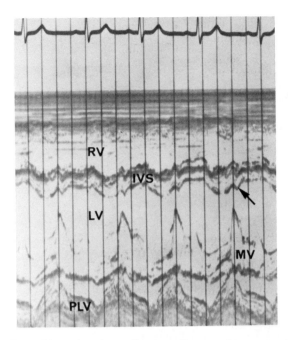

**Fig. 5–1.** M-mode echocardiogram of a normal interventricular septum (IVS). In early diastole, there is a brief diastolic downward dip (*arrow*) shortly after the opening of the mitral valve (MV). RV = right ventricle; LV = left ventricle; PLV = posterior left ventricular wall. (From Chang, S.: Echocardiography: Techniques and interpretation, ed. 2. Philadelphia, Lea & Febiger, 1981.)

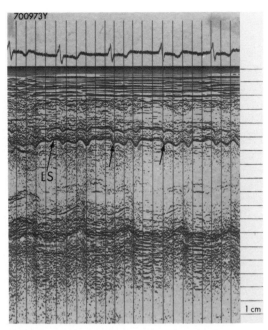

**Fig. 5–3.** M-mode echocardiogram of the interventricular septum in a patient with left bundle branch block. Note again the posterior beaking (*arrows*) following the onset of electrical depolarization. The septal motion during ventricular ejection is more normal or downward rather than anterior or paradoxic as in Figure 5–2. LS = left septum.

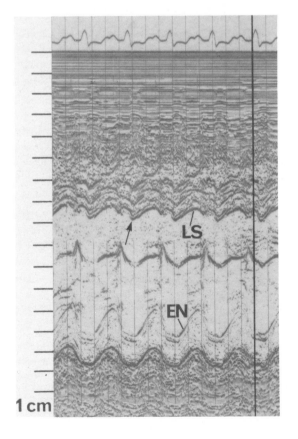

**Fig. 5–2.** M-mode echocardiogram of the left ventricle in a patient with left bundle branch block. After the onset of electrical depolarization (heavy vertical line at right) is a rapid downward displacement of the left septum (LS) followed by an upward motion during ventricular ejection. This motion produces a downward beaking (*arrow*) shortly after electrical depolarization and paradoxic septal motion during ventricular ejection. EN = posterior left ventricular endocardium. (From Dillon, J.C., et al.: Echocardiographic manifestations of left bundle branch block pattern. Circulation, *49*:876, 1974, by permission of the American Heart Association, Inc.)

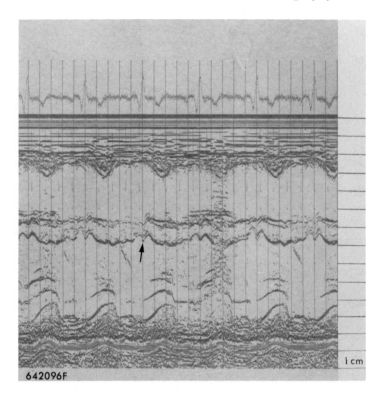

642096F

**Fig. 5–4.** M-mode echocardiogram of a patient without left bundle branch block but with an early systolic beaking (*arrow*) of the interventricular septum.

Thus, although septal motion is usually paradoxic during ventricular ejection in left bundle branch block, this situation is not always present. The early systolic downward dip, or beaking, however, immediately following electrical depolarization is a consistent and diagnostic finding in this abnormality.

According to one study, when septal motion is paradoxic during ventricular ejection with left bundle branch block, the patient usually has a more severe form of the disease with a wider QRS, a larger left ventricle, and reduced ejection fraction.[11] These individuals also frequently have left axis deviation on their electrocardiogram.[12] Thus, fairly normal septal motion during ventricular ejection may indicate that the patient has less significant clinical disease. A somewhat smaller early septal beaking (*arrow*, Fig. 5–4) can even be seen in patients who do not have left bundle branch block on the surface electrocardiogram. It is possible that this early, brief septal motion can be a variant of normal.

Few studies have attempted to delineate the mechanism of the abnormal septal motion in left bundle branch block. Most investigators assume that the abnormal contraction pattern is secondary to the altered path of depolarization.[13] Pacing the right ventricle produces both electrocardiographic and echocardiographic patterns similar to left bundle branch block.[14,14a] Figure 5–5 shows a paced beat with a pacemaker in the right ventricle. Following the paced electrical depolarization is an early systolic dip in the septum (*arrow*) identical to that seen in left bundle branch block. During ventricular ejection, the septal motion is normal and moves downward toward the left ventricle. A subsequent premature ventricular systole produces no abnormal septal motion.

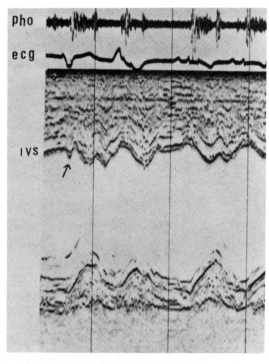

pho

ecg

IVS

**Fig. 5–5.** Left ventricular echocardiogram demonstrating the septal motion in a patient with a pacemaker in the right ventricle. The first electrocardiographic complex is a paced beat. The aberrant depolarization produces an early beaking (*arrow*) of the interventricular septum (IVS) similar to that seen with left bundle branch block. Pho = phonocardiogram. (From Zoneraich, S.O. and Rhee, J.J.: Echocardiographic evaluation of septal motion in patients with artificial pacemakers: Echocardiographic correlations. Am. Heart. J., *93*:596, 1977.)

The last two electrical complexes are normally conducted beats and septal motion is normal.[15-17] In one study of right ventricular pacing with electrocardiography and echocardiography, the authors reported that the septal motion varied depending on where the right ventricle was stimulated. If the right ventricular apex was paced, then one saw the septal beaking but not the paradoxic motion during ejection (Fig. 5–5). If the right ventricular outflow tract was paced, however, then the septal motion was similar to a left bundle branch block with paradoxic motion during ejection.[17]

In one study, a group of investigators believed that the abnormal early systolic septal motion with left bundle branch block was secondary to an early rise in pressure in the right ventricle in patients with left bundle branch block.[18] Supposedly, the abnormal depolarization produces contraction of the right ventricular chamber prior to the left ventricular chamber, thus producing an earlier rise in right ventricular pressure. This differential in pressure then produces the abnormal septal motion. The downward displacement is reversed as soon as the left ventricle begins to contract and raises the left ventricular pressure. Because this observation has not been confirmed, the exact mechanism for the septal motion with left bundle branch block still remains unproven.

No abnormal contraction pattern has been detected with right bundle branch block; however, several authors have noted a change in the intervals between closure of the mitral, tricuspid, and pulmonary valves in patients with right bundle branch block.[19.20] These authors have measured the interval between mitral valve closure (MVc) and tricuspid valve closure (TVc) and the interval between tricuspid valve closure and pulmonary valve opening (PVo). When the delay is between mitral valve closure and tricuspid valve closure (MVc − TVc), the authors believe that the bundle branch block is proximal. When the increase in interval is between TVc and pulmonary valve opening, then the block is in the distal portion of the right bundle. This relationship can also be demonstrated by the following ratio: TVc − PVo/MVc − TVc.[19] Results of another study confirmed the increase in MVc-TVc interval in patients with right bundle branch block when the injury is proximal. This particular study involved primarily the right bundle branch block, which occurs after cardiac surgery.[20]

### Wolff-Parkinson-White (WPW) Syndrome

Many articles describe the echocardiographic findings associated with Wolff-Parkinson-White (WPW) syndrome.[21-29] With so-called type B WPW syndrome, one may find an echocardiogram similar to that found in left bundle branch block. After electrical depolarization, a sharp, brief, downward or posterior dip of the interventricular septum may appear (Fig. 5–6, *arrow*).[21,23,25-29] The frequency with which this echocardiographic pattern is observed in type B WPW syndrome varies in the literature. In one study, only 4 of 22 patients demonstrated the abnormal septal motion.[23] Other series, however, had frequencies as high as 8 of 16.[28] Some authors

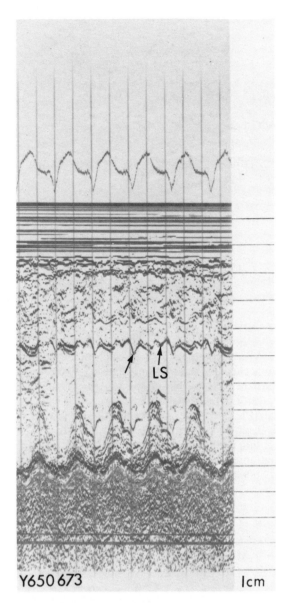

**Fig. 5–6.** Echocardiogram of the interventricular septum demonstrating an early systolic downward beaking (*arrow*) in a patient with type B Wolff-Parkinson-White syndrome. LS = left side of interventricular septum.

have noted an exaggerated diastolic dip in patients with type B WPW syndrome.[26]

In patients with type A WPW syndrome, abnormal motion of the posterior ventricular wall may be detected (Fig. 5–7).[25.28-30] The consistent finding is a brief anterior displacement of the posterior left ventricular wall following the onset of electrical depolarization (Fig. 5–7, *arrow*). The frequency with which this echocardiographic pattern occurs in patients with type A WPW syndrome again varies in the literature. One group of investigators could not find this abnormality in any of their patients,[26] whereas in another study, abnormal left ventricular posterior wall motion could be detected in all 20 patients with type A WPW syndrome.[25] It should be emphasized that the abnormal motion seen with type

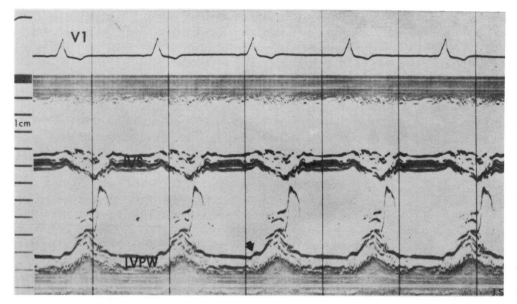

**Fig. 5–7.** Left ventricular echocardiogram in a patient with type A Wolff-Parkinson-White syndrome. Note premature contraction or anterior motion (*arrow*) in left ventricular posterior wall (LVPW) echoes. IVS = interventricular septum. (From DeMaria, A.N., et al.: Alterations in ventricular contraction pattern in the Wolff-Parkinson-White syndrome. Circulation, *53*:249, 1976, with permission of the American Heart Association, Inc.)

A WPW syndrome may be extremely subtle and thus warrants careful examination. Figure 5–8 shows an unusual patient with WPW syndrome who has an abnormal early systolic motion of both the posterior left ventricular wall (PLV) and the interventricular septum (LS). Figure 5–9 shows an M-mode echocardiogram of a patient with a left posterior accessory pathway. During atrial pacing, anterior motion of the posterior left ventricular wall is noted during diastole (*arrows*).

The fact that not all patients with WPW syndrome exhibit premature contraction patterns on the M-mode echocardiogram is not surprising. The M-mode study only samples limited areas of the heart. One should theoretically be able to identify more sites of premature activity using two-dimensional echocardiography. Unfortunately, the sampling rate is slower with the two-dimensional technique, and motion is not conveniently displayed against time on a strip chart recorder. As a result, it is more difficult to appreciate the site of premature activation with two-dimensional echocardiography. With the advent of digital echocardiography, however, it is now possible to create a continuous loop display of early systolic images. With such a display, it is easier to analyze the pattern of motion in early systole, and one can identify the wall segment that moves first in systole. This technique has already been used in the detection of sites of ventricular activation with ventricular ectopy. This same approach should be of clinical value in mapping patients with bypass tracts and WPW syndrome.

A novel approach to detect the location of accessory pathways using echocardiography involves phase imaging.[31] Using digital techniques, the investigators determined minimal and mean phased angles of various left ventricular wall segments. They then derived a histogram to determine the homogeneity of segmental contraction. The phase angle sequence was calculated to estimate the contraction sequence. The angles were displayed in color. The specific colors determined which segments moved prematurely.

Another echocardiographic technique used to help map the left ventricle during an electrophysiologic study involves the use of a transponder at the tip of a cardiac catheter.[32] The transponder emits an ultrasonic signal that is visible on an echocardiogram. In this way, the location of the catheter tip is easily identified. Such a catheter can be used in the right atrium as well.[33] Transesophageal echocardiographic monitoring is being used

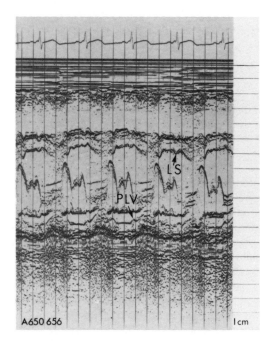

**Fig. 5–8.** Echocardiogram of the left ventricle in a patient with Wolff-Parkinson-White syndrome who shows abnormal early systolic motion of the left septum (LS) and the posterior left ventricular wall (PLV).

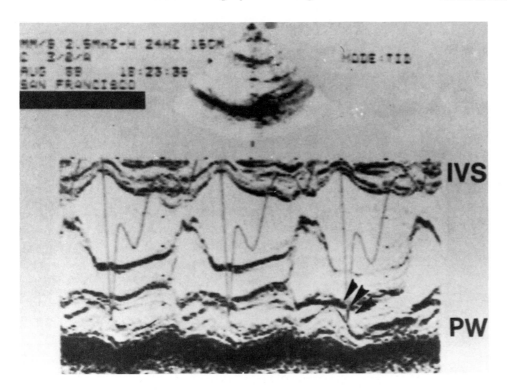

**Fig. 5–9.** M-mode echocardiogram of a patient with a left posterior accessory pathway. With atrial pacing, anterior motion of the posterior left ventricular wall occurs during diastole (*arrows*). (From Kuecher, E.R., et al.: Two-dimensional echocardiographic phase analysis: Its potential for non-invasive localization of accessory pathways in patients with Wolff-Parkinson-White syndrome. *Circulation, 85:*140, 1992, by permission of the American Heart Association.)

to improve positioning of radiofrequency ablation catheters in patients with WPW syndrome.[33a]

## ECTOPIC RHYTHM

### Ventricular Ectopy

Premature ventricular beats primarily influence the echocardiogram by the hemodynamic consequence of the premature systole. One might also expect an alteration in motion of either the interventricular septum or the posterior ventricular wall with spontaneous ventricular ectopy. Such an occurrence would result from the abnormal path of depolarization, as with left bundle branch block, WPW syndrome, or electrical pacing.

When patients with ventricular tachycardia are examined echocardiographically, one notes significant alteration in ventricular systolic function. The mechanism for hypotension in these patients is thought to be a result of the incoordinate contraction and incomplete filling.[34]

Figure 5–10 represents a common finding with a premature ventricular systole. Because the premature beat (*large arrow*) occurs before atrial depolarization, the A wave of the mitral valve is aborted in that cardiac cycle. Systolic motion of the interventricular septum (LS) and the posterior left ventricular wall (PLV) is diminished. Diastolic filling, as noted by the mitral valve, is reduced after the premature beat. The ventricular dimension between the septum and the posterior left ventricular wall increases, however, because the ventricle is inade-

quately emptied with the premature beat. With the next ventricular depolarization comes a vigorous ejection with increased motion of the septum and the posterior left ventricular endocardium. The diastolic filling after that systole shows an increased separation of the anterior and posterior mitral leaflets that is indicative of an increasing flow of blood into the ventricle.

Figure 5–11 demonstrates the hemodynamic events as reflected by the mitral valve in a patient with two consecutive premature ventricular systoles (*large arrows*). The mitral valve pattern shows abnormal hemodynamics despite the normally conducted beats. Following the first electrical depolarization, the D to E slope is reduced, and barely any E point is evident with the second diastolic interval. The first premature ventricular systole occurs when the mitral valve would ordinarily open during diastole. The premature beat prevents the opening. The second premature ectopic beat again prevents the opening of the valve until a sufficiently long interval occurs after the second premature ventricular beat. Partially because the mitral valve has been closed for such a long time (undoubtedly with increased blood volume in the left atrium), mitral valve motion following the premature beats is more normal with a brisker D to E slope, and an obvious E point.

Figure 5–12 demonstrates the hemodynamic consequences of premature ventricular beats on the aortic valve. This recording also graphically demonstrates the influence of the interval between the premature beat and the preceding normally conducted complex. Following the first premature beat (1), the aortic valve opening is clearly reduced in both amplitude and duration. Premature beat 2 occurs following two normally conducted

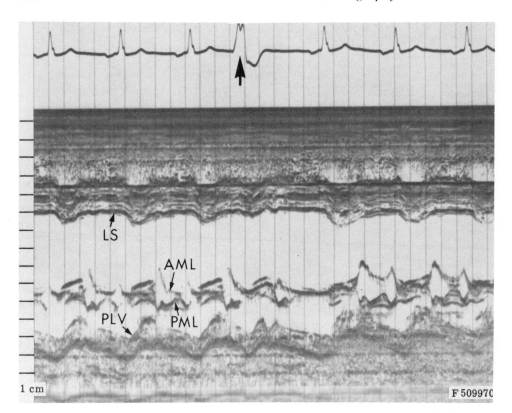

**Fig. 5–10.** M-mode echocardiogram of the left ventricle and mitral valve showing the effect of a premature ventricular systole (*large arrow*). LS = left septum; PLV = posterior left ventricular wall; PML = posterior mitral leaflet; AML = anterior mitral leaflet.

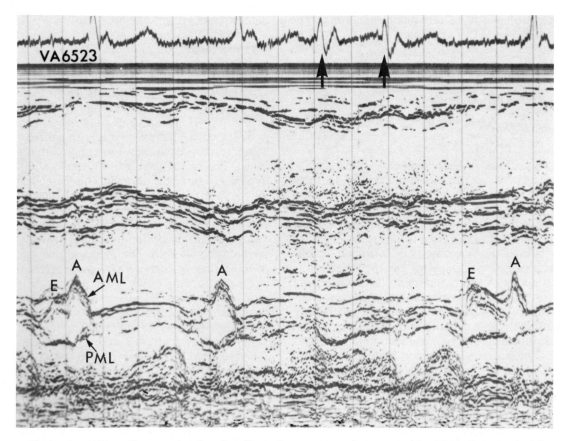

**Fig. 5–11.** Mitral valve echocardiogram showing the effect of two consecutive premature ventricular systoles (*large arrows*). The basic mitral valve motion is abnormal with a markedly decreased D to E slope and a diminished E point. No mitral opening is detected with the ventricular premature beats. Following the long pause of the second premature beat, a more normal mitral valve is recorded. AML = anterior mitral leaflet; PML = posterior mitral leaflet.

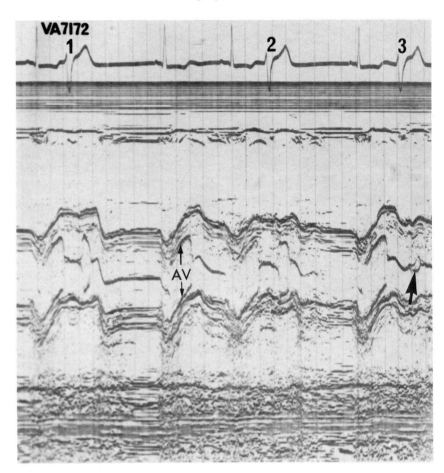

**Fig. 5–12.** Aortic valve echocardiogram showing the effect of premature ventricular systoles on aortic valve (AV) motion. Following the third premature ventricular systole (*3*), the aortic valve barely opens (*large arrow*).

beats and is slightly farther away from the preceding normal beat than is premature beat 1. The aortic valve motion following the second premature beat is clearly reduced but is more normal than that following the first premature beat. Note also a brief interval at which time both aortic leaflets are parallel to each other while open. The most interesting finding is that following premature beat 3, the aortic valve barely opens (*large arrow*). One could speculate over why the third premature beat produced such minimal blood flow into the aorta. The sequence of normal and premature beats preceding the third premature beat is undoubtedly a factor. Irrespective of the exact mechanism, however, this figure clearly demonstrates how hemodynamic consequences of ventricular premature systoles can be detected echocardiographically.

The pulmonary valve echocardiogram may also reflect the hemodynamic consequences of premature ventricular beats. Figure 5–13 is an artist's rendition of an actual electrocardiogram and echocardiogram with the proposed hemodynamic explanation for the observation as indicated by the pulmonary artery and right ventricular pressures. The interesting empiric finding is that following a single premature ventricular systole, no A wave is noted in the pulmonary valve (Fig. 5–13A). When two premature systoles occur consecutively (Fig. 5–13B), however, a prominent A wave appears on the pulmonary

valve echocardiogram. As suggested by the pulmonary valve echocardiogram in Figure 5–13A, the patient had pulmonary hypertension because no A wave was detectable on the pulmonary valve tracing. An A wave did appear, however, after the two consecutive premature systoles. The explanation for the A wave in Figure 5–13B is that the premature beats and the long diastolic interval permitted the diastolic pulmonary artery pressure to drop sufficiently so that atrial contraction could elevate the right ventricular pressure enough to open the pulmonary valve. The echocardiogram in Figure 5–13 not only represents an interesting example of the influence of premature ventricular systoles on the echocardiogram, but it also offers clinical evidence that the A wave on the pulmonary valve echocardiogram is a function of the interrelationship of the pulmonary artery and right ventricular pressures.

Premature ventricular systoles may also produce peculiar configurations of the interventricular septum. Figure 5–14 shows an example of how septal motion can be distorted by premature ventricular systoles. After normal electrical depolarization, the septal motion in this area of the heart is flat. An early diastolic dip occurs immediately prior to the full opening of the mitral valve. A second diastolic dip occurs in mid-systole; thus, this patient's septal motion is abnormal despite normal depolarization. Following a ventricular premature beat, how-

**A**

EKG

ECHO

PA

RV

**B**

EKG

ECHO

a

PA

RV

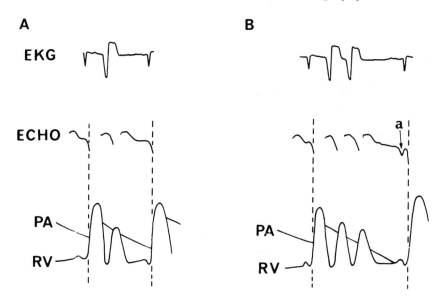

**Fig. 5–13.** Tracings demonstrating the effect of premature ventricular systoles on the pulmonary valve echocardiogram. *A,* The patient has pulmonary hypertension. No A wave is present with a single premature ventricular systole and a long diastolic pause. *B,* With two consecutive ventricular beats, however, the pulmonary artery pressure drops sufficiently so that with atrial contraction the right ventricular pressure can exceed the pulmonary artery pressure, and an A wave (a) can be recorded. PA = pulmonary artery; RV = right ventricle.

ever, there is a striking downward or posterior displacement of the interventricular septum (*arrow*). This dip is followed by anterior motion of the septum during ventricular systole. The exact explanation for this peculiar septal motion is not certain, but the motion resembles that observed in left bundle branch block (see Fig. 5–2) and may be the result of abnormal depolarization.

A more common finding with premature ventricular systoles is noted in Figure 5–15. In this patient, the septal motion following a normal beat is normal. The unu-

sual finding is that an exaggerated diastolic septal dip (*arrows*) follows the premature ventricular systoles. The diastolic dip is partially the result of the flat to absent systolic motion of the septum following ventricular ejection. Thus, the diastolic dip, which is actually not much deeper than the normal diastolic dip, is more obvious because of the flat septum during ejection. A potential misinterpretation is mistaking the diastolic dip for systolic septal motion. These brief downward displacements of the septum are clearly diastolic events. An

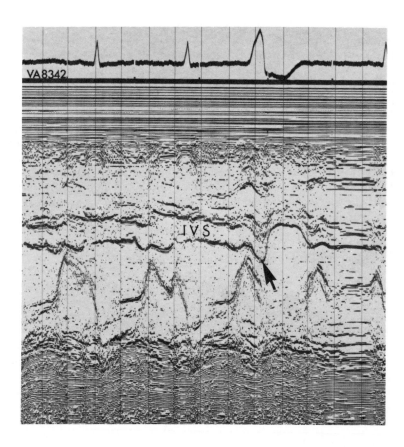

**Fig. 5–14.** M-mode echocardiogram of the interventricular septum (IVS) demonstrating a systolic downward beaking (*arrow*) of the septum and paradoxic motion during ejection with a premature ventricular systole.

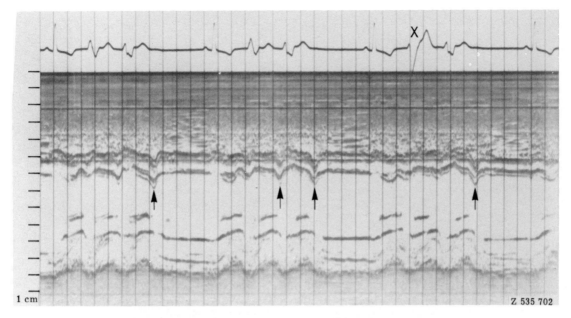

**Fig. 5–15.** M-mode examination demonstrating exaggerated diastolic septal dips (*arrows*) in a patient with premature ventricular systoles (see text for details).

unexplained feature is that a prominent diastolic dip does not occur after the premature systole that has a different pattern of depolarization (X).

With increasing interest in ablation of ventricular tachycardia, more importance is placed on identifying the site of ventricular activation. This information is usually gained by invasive electrophysiologic studies. Experimental data indicate that two-dimensional echocardiography may assist in identifying the site of ventricular activation.[35–37] Such a determination is usually obtained with multiple short-axis slices through the left ventricle. The analysis can be tedious because the recording must be examined frame by frame. With computer digitization of the two-dimensional echocardiograms, however, this application is becoming more practical.[37] Figure 5–16 demonstrates the effect of premature stimulation of the interventricular septum. At 34 msec after the stimulus artifact, one notes inward motion of the site of ventricular activation (*arrowhead,* Fig. 5–16B). At 51 msec after the electrical stimulus (Fig. 5–16B), more extensive inward motion of the septum is noted. By 136 msec after the electrical stimulus (Fig. 5–16D), the septum has returned to the control position and the rest of the ventricle may now begin to move inward. With this type of study, one can identify the portion of the left ventricle that is first activated by electrical depolarization. Transesophageal and intracardiac echocardiography can be used to help locate ablation catheters and to facilitate the procedure.

## Supraventricular Ectopy

Before discussing supraventricular ectopic rhythms, it should be apparent that sinus arrhythmia, which is a normal variant, distorts the echocardiogram. Figure 5–17 demonstrates the changes in mitral valve motion

that occur with varying R–R intervals. The principal difference is the length of the mid-diastolic filling period. It is interesting that mitral valve motion in early diastole and late diastole is unchanged by the varying diastolic intervals. The heights of the E and A points are essentially equal in all cardiac complexes. This observation helps to justify some of the formulas used for calculating mitral valve flow from the mitral valve echocardiogram (see Chapter 4).

Premature atrial systoles have similar effects on the echocardiogram as do premature ventricular systoles. Figure 5–18 demonstrates the effect of premature atrial systoles on the mitral valve echocardiogram. Despite the variation in the mitral valve motion, only three premature atrial systoles were recorded in this tracing. Three normally conducted beats occur between each atrial premature beat. The resultant A wave of the second premature atrial systole (2) is superimposed on the E point. Following ventricular systole, the mitral valve closes. The subsequent diastolic filling period shows a decreased separation of the leaflets and an indistinct E point. The next normal depolarization produces a vigorous ventricular systole, and the following mitral valve opening is brisk with an increased E wave. Because of the heart rate and possibly some left ventricular dysfunction, the subsequent A wave is superimposed on the down slope of the closing mitral valve. The following diastolic interval produces an alternating effect of the mitral valve with decreased diastolic separation, possibly as a consequence of the vigorous ventricular contraction and filling of the preceding cycle. More normal mechanical contraction and relaxation occur with the third normally conducted beat. The subsequent diastole is prematurely ended by the third premature atrial systole (3), and then the cycle is repeated. Figure 5–18 is yet another example of how echocardiography can help

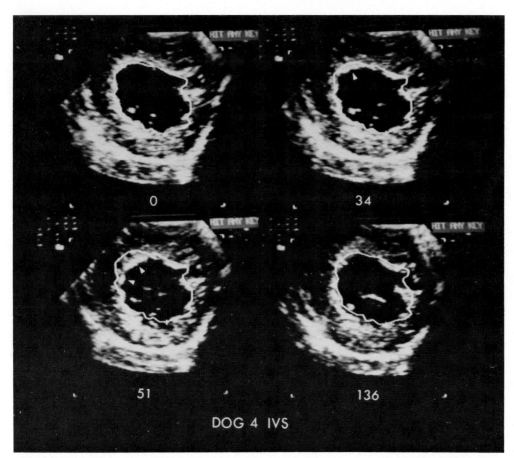

**Fig. 5–16.** Serial short-axis two-dimensional echocardiograms of a dog illustrating the effect of premature stimulation of the interventricular septum. At 34 and 51 msec after the onset of stimulation, inward motion of the interventricular septum (*arrowheads*) occurs prior to any inward motion of the rest of the myocardium.

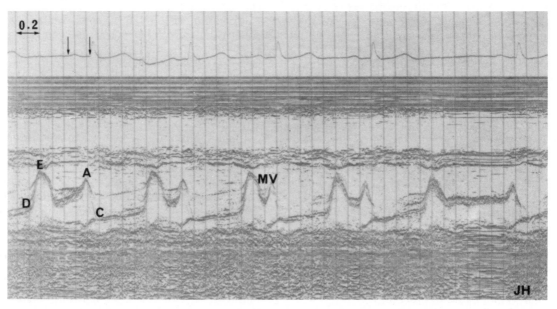

**Fig. 5–17.** Mitral valve echocardiogram demonstrating the effect of sinus arrhythmia on mitral valve (MV) motion. The principal effect of an increased R–R interval is the duration of diastasis. The heights of the E and A points are not influenced.

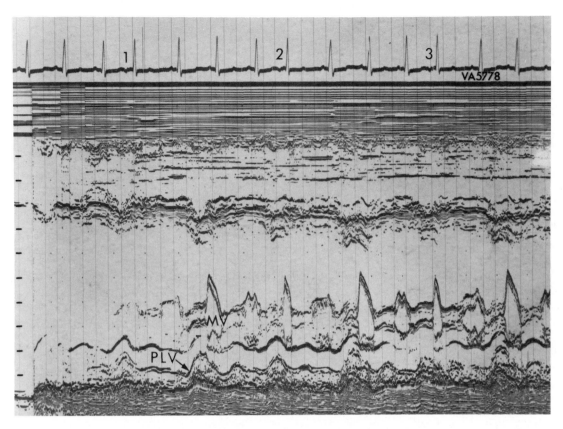

**Fig. 5–18.** The effect of atrial premature beats on an M-mode echocardiogram of the left ventricle and mitral valve (MV). PLV = posterior left ventricular wall (see text for details).

decipher the hemodynamic consequences of arrhythmias.

Figure 5–19 demonstrates the effect of a burst of supraventricular tachycardia on the left ventricle.[18] The patient has atrial fibrillation with occasional premature ventricular systole (Fig. 5–19A). During a burst of supraventricular tachycardia, which probably is only accelerated atrioventricular conduction and rapid ventricular response (Fig. 5–19B), there is a striking decrease in septal and posterior wall motion (*arrows*) and a decrease in the left ventricular diastolic dimension. The interesting clinical counterpart is that the patient became extremely short of breath during these bursts of supraventricular tachycardia and died suddenly at home 2 weeks after this echocardiogram was taken.

Most echocardiographic literature on supraventricular tachycardia relates to patients with atrial fibrillation and atrial flutter. Figure 5–20 demonstrates that patients with atrial fibrillation or atrial flutter frequently show striking oscillations of the mitral valve (*arrows*).[13] It should be noted that the posterior mitral leaflet (PML) also oscillates at the same frequency as the anterior mitral leaflet (AML) and moves in an opposite direction to that of the anterior leaflet. Thus, although organized atrial activity is not evident on this electrocardiogram, well-organized atrial contractions apparently produce sufficient blood flow to open the mitral valve with each atrial systole. Although the electrocardiogram shows

classic atrial fibrillation, one might argue that the left atrium is actually in a flutter rhythm. With electrocardiographic atrial fibrillation, one atrium may be fibrillating while the other is in flutter. Echocardiography has been used to try to determine whether the atria are in the same electrical state.[13] For example, in Figure 5–20, it is possible that the right atrium may be in atrial fibrillation and the left atrium in flutter. One may be able to establish that fact by recording the tricuspid valve and by finding no organized atrial activity sufficient to produce opening of the tricuspid valve with atrial contractions.[38–40] Dual echocardiography with recording of simultaneous mitral and tricuspid valves is one technique that has been recommended for evaluating the atria with various atrial arrhythmias.[38]

Echocardiography has a special role to play in patients with atrial fibrillation. Patients with enlarged left atria are more prone to atrial fibrillation. Some data also suggest that atrial fibrillation produces atrial enlargement.[41] Echocardiography is playing a role in managing patients before cardioversion for atrial fibrillation; for example, being certain there are no left atrial thrombi is an issue when considering cardioversion. Some investigators recommend routine transesophageal echocardiography to make certain that conversion to sinus rhythm will not dislodge an atrial thrombus. One study indicated that the Doppler examination of the fibrillating left atrium can predict whether or not cardioversion will be suc-

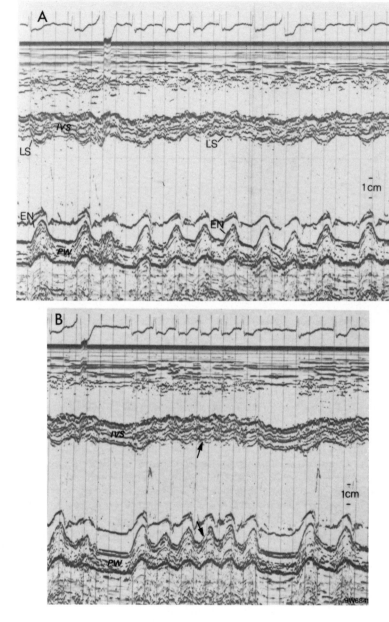

**Fig. 5–19.** The effect of a supraventricular tachycardia on the M-mode echocardiogram. The patient has atrial fibrillation with an occasional premature ventricular systole (*A*). With a burst of supraventricular tachycardia, the septal and posterior left ventricular wall motion (*arrows*) is reduced (*B*). The left ventricular diastolic dimension also decreases. LS = left septum; EN = posterior left ventricular endocardium; IVS = interventricular septum; PW = posterior wall.

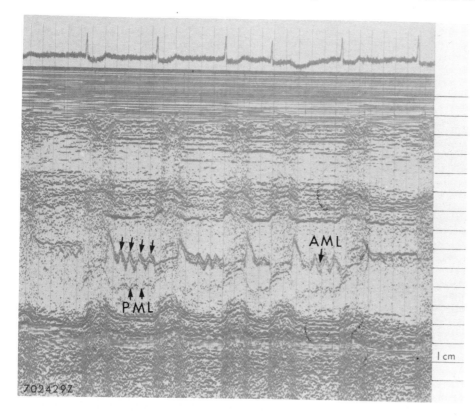

**Fig. 5–20.** The effect of atrial flutter on the mitral valve echocardiogram. With atrial systole, the anterior mitral leaflet (AML) and posterior mitral leaflet (PML) separate, indicating flow through the orifice (*arrows*).

cessful and whether it will recur.[42] A more organized Doppler signal within the left atrium indicates a better chance of longstanding success in keeping the patient in sinus rhythm. A similar judgment can be made with organized mitral valve motion on the M-mode examination.[43] After cardioversion, the atrial mechanical function can be evaluated using pulsed Doppler studies.

Occasionally, the oscillations seen on the echocardiogram may represent atrial contractions and opening of the atrioventricular valves that occur in atrial systole. Figure 5–21 shows undulating motion on the echocardiogram corresponding to the fibrillatory waves on the electrocardiogram. What distinguishes the echocardiogram in this figure from that in Figure 5–20 is that the entire heart is oscillating. Oscillations of the left septum (LS) and the posterior left ventricular wall (PLV) can also be seen, as can the obvious undulating motion of the mitral valve. In addition, the motion of the anterior mitral leaflet (AML) and the posterior mitral leaflet (PML) is in the same direction, and the leaflets do not separate following the F waves. Thus, the motion observed on the echocardiogram probably represents rocking or moving of the entire heart with the fibrillation and not necessarily propulsion of blood through the mitral valve with each atrial systole. Other echocardiographic observations noted with atrial arrhythmias are oscillations of the left atrial wall,[44,45] premature closure of the mitral valve,[46] and contractions of the right atrial wall.[47] The subcostal approach also permits recording of interatrial septal motion to help diagnose atrial flutter.[48]

Suprasternal M-mode echocardiography has also been used to identify atrial activity by noting motion of the left atrial wall.[49] Esophageal echocardiography is yet another method for detecting left atrial wall motion,[50] and has been used with endocardial mapping to localize the site of origin of atrial tachycardia.[51]

Figure 5–22 is a subcostal M-mode recording of the right atrial free wall. One notes a prominent downward motion of the right atrial echoes (A) following atrial systole (*solid line*). With atrial premature systoles (Fig. 5–23), one notes brisk posterior motion of the right atrial free wall with the premature beat (*arrow*).

Fetal echocardiography has been used to evaluate rhythm abnormalities in the fetus.[52–55] Both supraventricular and ventricular arrhythmias can be detected by noting the motion of various parts of the fetal heart.

Arrhythmias also effect Doppler recordings. Figure 5–24 shows the effect of heart rate on mitral inflow velocities. As one would predict, with increasing heart rates, diastole becomes shorter and the early and late components of diastolic filling become superimposed.[56,57] In addition, with increasing heart rate, the proportion of flow with atrial contraction increases, and when the two flows fuse, the atrial component dominates.

With the advent of transesophageal echocardiography and the ability to record flow within the left atrium with greater accuracy, the effect of atrial arrhythmias on left atrial flow can be documented. Figure 5–25 shows Doppler flow within the left atrial appendage with a variety of different atrial rhythms. Normal sinus rhythm is noted in Figure 5–25A. Flow moving toward the transducer with atrial systole can be found after each P wave. Figure 5–25B shows the flow pattern in the atrial appendage

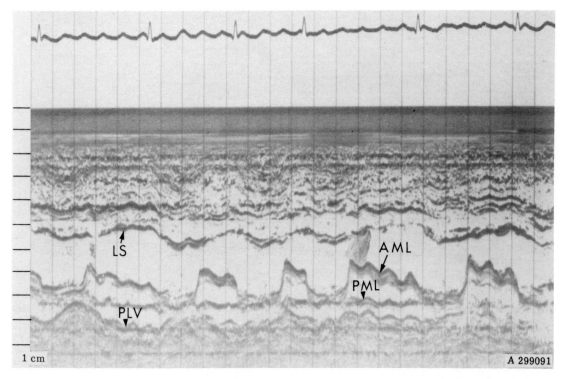

**Fig. 5–21.** M-mode echocardiogram of the left ventricle and mitral valve in a patient with atrial flutter–fibrillation. Note undulating movements of the mitral leaflets and the ventricular walls. LS = left septum; AML = anterior mitral leaflet; PML = posterior mitral leaflet; PLV = posterior left ventricular wall.

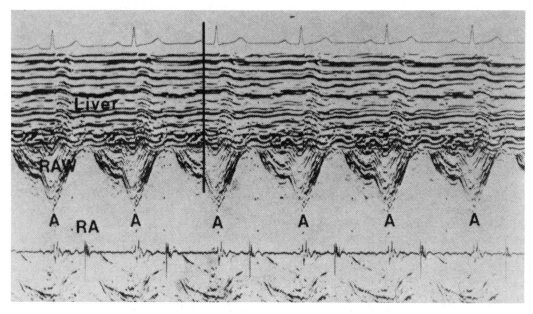

**Fig. 5–22.** Subcostal M-mode echocardiogram of the right atrial wall (RAW) demonstrating downward displacement of the right atrial echoes (A) following atrial systole (*line*). RA = right atrium. (From Drinkovic, N.: Subcostal M-mode echocardiogram of the right atrial wall and the diagnosis of cardiac arrhythmias. Am. J. Cardiol., *50*:1104, 1982.)

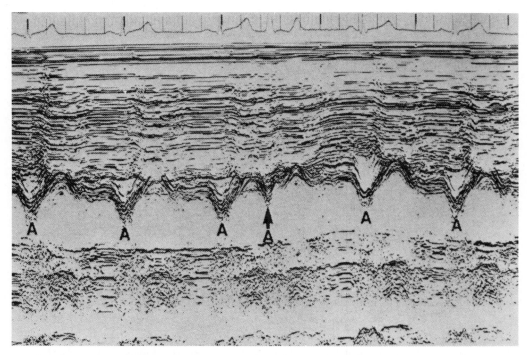

**Fig. 5–23.** Subcostal M-mode echogram of the right atrial free wall in a patient with an atrial premature systole. With the atrial premature beat (*arrow*), one records rapid downward motion of the right atrial wall. (From Drinkovic, N.: Subcostal M-mode echocardiogram of the right atrial wall and the diagnosis of cardiac arrhythmias. Am. J. Cardiol., *50*:1104, 1982.)

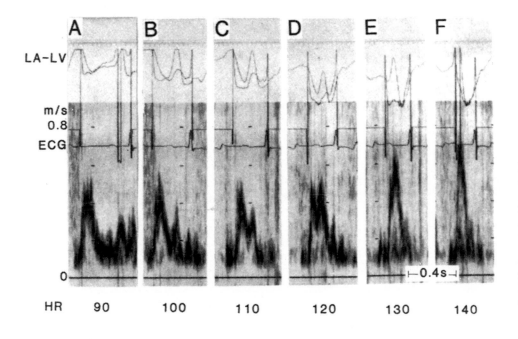

**Fig. 5–24.** Doppler echocardiogram showing the effect of increasing heart rate on mitral flow velocity. LA = left atrium; LV = left ventricle. (From Appleton, C.P., et al.: Influence of incremental changes in heart rate on mitral flow velocity: Assessment in lightly sedated, conscious dogs. J. Am. Coll. Cardiol., *17*:233, 1991.)

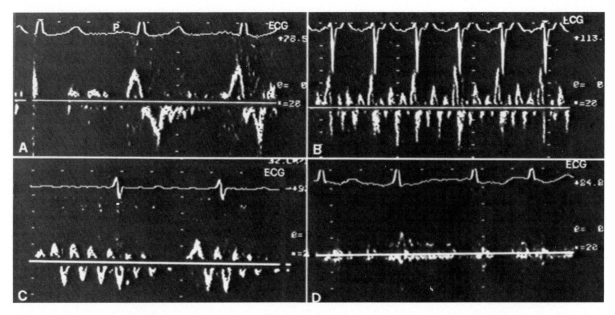

**Fig. 5–25.** Left atrial Doppler recording during transesophageal echocardiography in patients with sinus rhythm (*A*), atrial flutter (*B*), coarse atrial fibrillation (*C*), and fine atrial fibrillation (*D*). (From Pozzoli, M., et al.: Left atrial appendage dysfunction: A cause of thrombosis? Evidence by transesophageal echocardiography = Doppler studies. J. Am. Soc. Echocardiogr., *4*:436, 1991.)

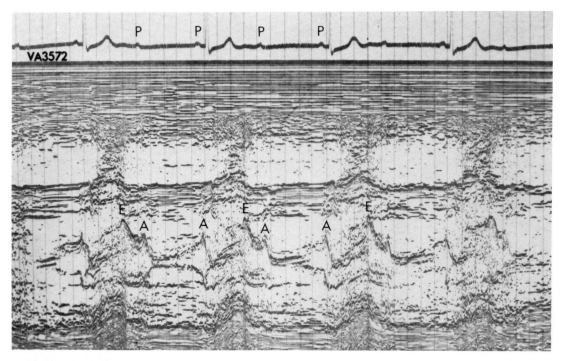

**Fig. 5–26.** Mitral valve echocardiogram in a patient with heart block and 2:1 conduction. The mitral valve A waves follow each electrocardiographic P wave.

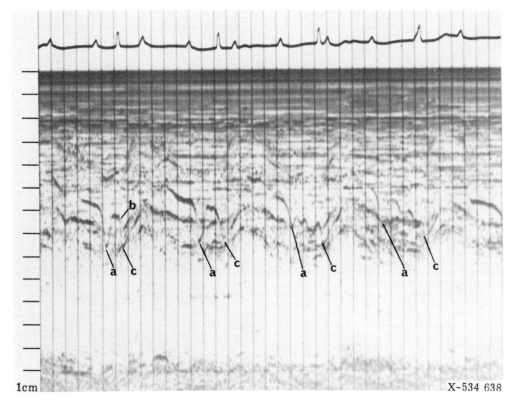

**Fig. 5–27.** The effect of complete heart block on the pulmonary valve echocardiogram. Large A waves (a) are seen corresponding with each electrocardiographic P wave. The opening of the mitral valve with ventricular systole (c) follows each ventricular depolarization. b = onset of pulmonary valve opening with ventricular systole. (From Weyman, A.E., et al.: Echocardiographic patterns of pulmonary valve motion in valvular pulmonary stenosis. Am. J. Cardiol., *34*:644, 1974.)

in a patient with atrial flutter. The multiple atrial velocities with each cardiac cycle can be noted. Figure 5–25C and D are from two patients with atrial fibrillation. The electrocardiogram shows documented flutter (F) waves on the electrocardiogram in Figure 5–25C, with corresponding well-coordinated atrial velocities within the atrial appendage. In Figure 5–25D, however, no electrocardiographic F waves are evident and there is no pulsatile atrial velocity.

## ABNORMAL ATRIOVENTRICULAR CONDUCTION

Prolonged atrioventricular conduction, or heart block, can alter the echocardiogram in a predictable manner. Echocardiographic events that depend on atrial systole follow the contractions of the atria and are not synchronous with ventricular contraction if heart block is present.[58] Figure 5–26 substantiates the fact that the mitral valve closes with atrial relaxation as well as with ventricular systole. Thus, it is not surprising to find a virtually closed mitral valve before ventricular systole in a patient with first-degree heart block and a prolonged P–R interval. In fact, heart block is one of the causes of premature mitral valve closure.

Figure 5–27 shows a pulmonary valve echocardiogram of a patient with complete heart block. Again, the consequences of atrial contraction, namely the A dips of the pulmonary valve, follow each P wave on the electrocardiogram. The C point, which represents opening of the valve following ventricular systole, remains related to ventricular depolarization. In cases in which the

atrial depolarization is not apparent on the electrocardiogram, it is sometimes possible to identify the P wave by way of echocardiographic valve motion. Thus, the echocardiogram may help in the diagnosis of arrhythmias in rare situations.

Doppler echocardiography can also show some of the hemodynamic consequences of abnormal atrioventricular conduction. Figure 5–28 shows a pulsed Doppler recording of mitral flow during first- and second-degree atrioventricular block. Left ventricular and left atrial pressures are superimposed on the recording. With a long PR interval, one can detect diastolic mitral regurgitation (dMR). With second-degree heart block, the nonconducted P wave is again followed by diastolic mitral regurgitation of even longer duration.[59] As would be expected, diastolic mitral regurgitation has also been noted with complete or third-degree heart block.[60,61]

## PACEMAKERS

The use of atrial synchronous pacemakers for patients with heart block is becoming more frequent. The variety of programmable pacemakers is increasing dramatically. Many of these more complicated pacemakers are being used to improve the hemodynamic situation. Doppler echocardiography has been suggested as a means of judging the dynamic consequences of certain forms of pacing.[62,63,63a] Using aortic flow velocity, one can note the change in left ventricular stroke volume as various types of pacing are used.[64–66]

Figure 5–29 shows left ventricular outflow recordings

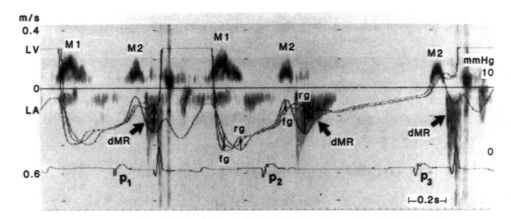

**Fig. 5–28.** Simultaneous Doppler recording of mitral flow velocity and left atrial and left ventricular pressures in a patient with heart block. After each of the P waves (P₁, P₂, P₃) is diastolic mitral regurgitation (dMR). After the nonconducted P wave (P₂), the diastolic regurgitation is longer. rg = regurgitation gradient; fg = forward gradient. (From Appleton, C.P., et al.: Diastolic mitral regurgitation with atrioventricular conduction abnormality: Relation of mitral flow velocity to transmitral pressure gradients in conscious dogs. J. Am. Coll. Cardiol., *18*:844, 1991.)

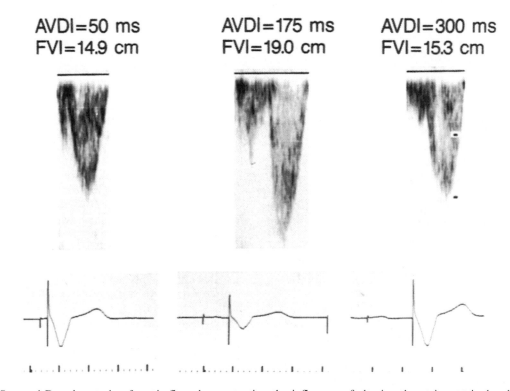

**Fig. 5–29.** Spectral Doppler study of aortic flow demonstrating the influence of altering the atrioventricular diastolic interval (AVDI) in a patient with a dual-chamber pacemaker. The optimum flow velocity integral (FVI) occurs with an AVDI of 175 msec. (From Janosik, D.L., et al.: The hemodynamic benefit of differential atrioventricular delay intervals for sensed and paced atrial events during physiologic pacing. J. Am. Coll. Cardiol., *14*:502, 1989.)

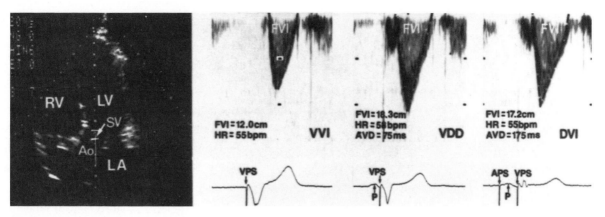

**Fig. 5–30.** Aortic Doppler velocities showing the effect of various pacemakers on Doppler flow. The flow velocity integral (FVI) is lowest with a VVI pacemaker, which stimulates only the ventricles. Atrial contractions are asynchronous. With both types of dual chamber pacemakers (VDD and DVI), whereby ventricular and atrial contractions are synchronous, aortic flow is increased. RV = right ventricle; LV = left ventricle; Ao = aorta; LA = left atrium; SV = sample volume. (From Pearson, A.C., et al.: Hemodynamic benefit of atrioventricular synchrony: Prediction from baseline Doppler-echocardiographic variables. J. Am. Coll. Cardiol., *13*:1616, 1989.)

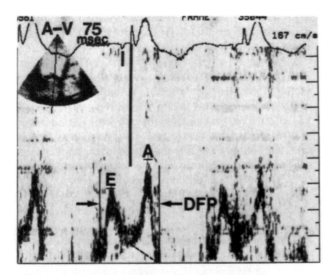

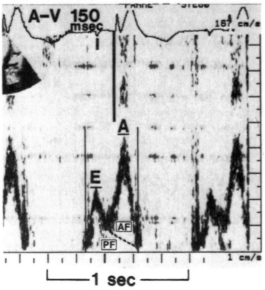

**Fig. 5–31.** Mitral flow velocities showing the effect of varying the atrioventricular pacemaker interval on left ventricular filling. Prolonging the atrioventricular (A-V) delay from 75 to 150 msec decreases the E wave and increases the A wave of the mitral flow. AF = atrial filling; PF = passive filling; DFP = diastolic filling period. (From Rokey, R., et al.: Influence of left atrial systolic emptying on left ventricular early filling dynamics by Doppler in patients with sequential atrial ventricular pacemakers. Am. J. Cardiol., *62*:969, 1988.)

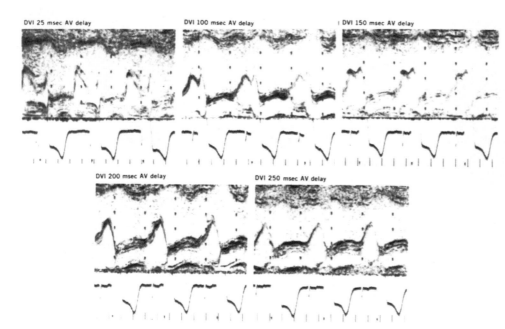

**Fig. 5–32.** Mitral valve M-mode echocardiogram showing the effect of atrioventricular (AV) delay on mitral valve motion in a patient with a dual-chamber pacemaker (DVI). (From Wish, M., et al.: M-mode echocardiograms for determination of optical left atrial timing in patients with dual chamber pacemakers. Am. J. Cardiol., *61*:319, 1988.)

with different delays with an atrioventricular (A-V) synchronous pacemaker.[67] The optimal systolic flow velocity occurs with a A-V delay interval of 175 msec compared with that of 50 or 300 msec. Doppler echocardiography can also demonstrate how the lack of an atrioventricular synchronous pacemaker eliminates atrial filling and how this deficiency effects hemodynamics.[68] Figure 5–30 illustrates the effect of various pacemakers on aortic flow. With a VVI pacemaker, which stimulates the ventricle and has no synchronization with atrial contraction, the flow velocity integral is 12.0 cm. Using two types of atrial synchronous pacemakers (VDD and DVI), the velocity flow integral is significantly increased.[69] Figure 5–31 demonstrates how the mitral flow velocity can be influenced by A-V delays of atrioventricular pacemakers.[69] Increasing the A-V delay from 75 to 150 msec produces a significant decrease in the E velocity and a modest increase in the A velocity. Figure 5–32 represents another example of how a progressive increase in the A-V delay produces a decrease in the early diastolic velocity and dependence on atrial systole for left ventricular filling.[71] Occasionally, echocardiography may identify atrial mechanical systole after implantation of a dual-chamber pacemaker, even without an electrocardiographic P wave.[72] Echocardiography provides an opportunity to study the functional and hemodynamic effects of various pacemakers.[73] In patients with a ventricular pacemaker, Doppler venous flow patterns can differentiate sinus node dysfunction from atrioventricular block.[74]

## REFERENCES

1. DeMaria, A.N., and Mason, D.T.: Echocardiographic evaluation of disturbances of cardiac rhythm and conduction. Chest, *71*:439, 1977.
2. Drinkovic, N.: Use of echocardiography in the diagnosis of cardiac arrhythmias. Pract. Cardiol., *11*:124, 1985.
3. Dillon, J.C., Chang, S., and Feigenbaum, H.: Echocardiographic manifestations of left bundle branch block. Circulation, *49*:876, 1974.
4. Abbasi, A.S., Eber, L.M., MacAlpin, R.N., and Kattus, A.A.: Paradoxical motion of the interventricular septum in left bundle branch block. Circulation, *49*:423, 1974.
5. McDonald, I.G., Feigenbaum, H., and Chang, S.: Analysis of left ventricular wall motion by reflected ultrasound: Application to assessment of myocardial function. Circulation, *46*:14, 1972.
6. McDonald, I.G.: Echocardiographic demonstration of abnormal motion of the interventricular septum in left bundle branch block. Circulation, *48*:272, 1973.
7. Burch, G.E., Giles, T.D., and Martinez, E.C.: Echocardiographic abnormalities of interventricular septum associated with absent Q syndrome. JAMA, *228*:1665, 1974.
8. Fujii, J., Watanabe, H., Watanabe, T., Takahashi, N., Ohta, A., and Kato, K.: M-mode and cross-sectional echocardiographic study of the left ventricular wall motions in complete left bundle branch block. Br. Heart J., *42*:255, 1979.
9. DeMaria, A.N., Vismara, L.A., Vera, Z., Miller, R.R., Amsterdam, E.A., and Mason, D.T.: Hemodynamic effects of cardiac arrhythmias. Angiology, *28*:427, 1977.
10. Xiao, H.B., Lee, C.H., and Gibson, D.G.: Effect of left bundle branch block on diastolic function in dilated cardiomyopathy. Br. Heart J., *66*:443, 1991.
11. Curtius, J.M., Nowitzki, G., Kohler, E., Kuhn, H., and Loogen, F.: Left bundle-branch block: Inferences from ventricular septal motion in the echocardiogram concerning left ventricular function. Z. Kardiol., *72*:635, 1983.
12. Strasberg, B., Rich, S., Lam, W., Swiryn, S., Bauernfeind, R., and Rosen, K.M.: M-mode echocardiography in left bundle branch block: Significance of frontal plane QRS axis. Am. Heart J., *104*:775, 1982.
13. Endo, N., Shimada, E., Asano, H., and Yamane, Y.: Paradoxical septal motion in left bundle branch block. J. Cardiogr., *7*:313, 1977.
14. Tsuji, Y., Matsukubo, H., Inoue, D., Furukawa, K., Wa-

tanabe, T., Tohara, M., Katsume, H., Endo, N., Matsuura, T., and Kunishige, H.: Study of ventricular wall movements in patients with left bundle branch block by echocardiography. J. Cardiogr., 8:745, 1978.

14a. Xiao, H.B., Brecker, S.J.D., Gibson, D.G.: Differing effects of right ventricular pacing and left bundle branch block on left ventricular function. Br. Heart J., 69:166, 1992.

15. Fujino, T., Ito, M., Kanaya, S., Ito, S., Fukumoto, T., Kawamura, T., Yasuda, H., Fukushima, I., Tetsuo, M., Hirata, T., and Mashiba, H.: Abnormal septal motion in the cases with various intraventricular conduction disturbances. Cardiovasc. Sound Bull., 5:77, 1975.

16. Zoneraich, S., Zoneraich, O., and Rhee, J.J.: Echocardiographic evaluation of septal motion in patients with artificial pacemakers: Vectorcardiographic correlations. Am. Heart J., 93:596, 1977.

17. Gomes, J.A.C., Damato, A.N., Akhtar, M., Dhatt, M.S., Calon, A.H., Reddy, C.P., and Moran, H.E.: Ventricular septal motion and left ventricular dimensions during abnormal ventricular activation. Am. J. Cardiol., 39:641, 1977.

18. Little, W.C., Reeves, R.C., Arciniegas, J., Katholi, R.E., and Rogers, E.W.: Mechanism of abnormal interventricular septal motion. Circulation, 65:1486, 1982.

19. Dancy, M., Leech, G., and Leatham, A.: Significance of complete right bundle-branch block when an isolated finding. An echocardiographic study. Br. Heart J., 48:217, 1982.

20. Pickott, A.S., Mehta, A.V., Casta, A., Ferrer, P.L., Wolff, G.S., Tamer, D.F., Garcia, O.L., and Gelband, H.: Echocardiographic assessment of right bundle branch injury after repair of tetralogy of Fallot. Circulation, 63:174, 1981.

21. Chandra, M.S., Kerber, R.E., Brown, D.D., and Funk, D.C.: Echocardiography in Wolff-Parkinson-White syndrome. Circulation, 53:943, 1976.

22. DeMaria, A.N., Vera, Z., Neumann, A., and Mason, D.T.: Alterations in ventricular contraction pattern in the Wolff-Parkinson-White syndrome. Circulation, 53:249, 1976.

23. Lebovitz, J.A., Mandel, W.J., Laks, M.M., Kraus, R., and Weinstein, S.: Relationship between the electrical (electrocardiographic) and mechanical (echocardiographic) events in Wolff-Parkinson-White syndrome. Chest, 71:463, 1977.

24. Gimbel, K.S.: Left ventricular wall motion in patients with the Wolff-Parkinson-White syndrome. Am. Heart J., 93:160, 1977.

25. Hishida, H., Sotobata, I., Koike, Y., Okumura, M., and Mizuno, Y.: Echocardiographic patterns of ventricular contraction in the Wolff-Parkinson-White syndrome. Circulation, 54:567, 1976.

26. Francis, G.S., Theroux, P., O'Rourke, R.A., Hagan, A.D., and Johnson, A.D.: An echocardiographic study of interventricular septal motion in the Wolff-Parkinson-White syndrome. Circulation, 54:174, 1976.

27. Chandra, M.S., Kerber, R.E., Brown, D.D., and Funk, D.C.: Echocardiography in Wolff-Parkinson-White syndrome. Circulation, 53:943, 1976.

28. Ticzon, A.R., Damato, A.N., Caracta, A.R., Russo, G., Foster, J.R., and Lau, S.H.: Interventricular septal motion during preexcitation and normal conduction in Wolff-Parkinson-White syndrome. Am. J. Cardiol., 37:840, 1976.

29. Sasse, L. and Del Puerto, H.A.: Echocardiography of ventricular septal movement in Wolff-Parkinson-White syndrome. Arch. Inst. Cardiol. Mex., 46:445, 1976.

30. Berman, N.D., Gilbert, B.W., McLaughlin, P.R., and Morch, J.E.: Mitral stenosis with posterior diastolic movement of posterior leaflet. Can. Med. Assoc. J., 112:976, 1975.

31. Kuecherer, H.F., Abbott, J.A., Botvinick, E.H., Scheinman, E.D., O'Connell, J.W., Scheinman, M.M., Foster, E., and Schiller, N.B.: Two-dimensional echocardiographic phase analysis. Circulation, 85:130, 1992.

32. Langberg, J.J., Franklin, J.O., Landzberg, J.S., Herre, J.M., Kee, L., Chin, M.C., Bharati, S., Lev, M., Himelman, R.B., Schiller, N.B., Griffin, J.C., and Scheinman, M.V.M.: The echo-transponder electrode catheter: a new method for mapping the left ventricle. J. Am. Coll. Cardiol., 12:218, 1988.

33. Landzberg, J.S., Franklin, J.O., Langberg, J.J., Herre, J.M., Scheinman, M.M., and Schiller, N.B.: The transponder system: A new method of precise catheter placement in the right atrium under echocardiographic guidance. J. Am. Coll. Cardiol., 12:753, 1988.

33a. Goldman, A.P., Irwin, J.M., Glover, M.U., and Mick, W.: Transesophageal echocardiography to improve positioning of radiofrequency ablation catheters in left-sided Wolff-Parkinson-White syndrome. PACE Pacing Clin. Electrophysiol., 14:1245, 1991.

34. Lima, J.A.C., Weiss, J.L., Guzman, P.A., Weisfeldt, M.A., Reid, P.R., and Traill, T.A.: Incomplete filling and incoordinate contraction as mechanisms of hypotension during ventricular tachycardia in man. Circulation, 68:928, 1983.

35. Machiro, I., Heckel, R.R., Nelson, R.R., Cohn, J.N., and Franciosa, J.A.: Site of premature ventricular contractions demonstrated by echocardiography. Jpn. Circ. J., 45:532, 1981.

36. Torres, M.A.R., Corday, E., Meerbaum, S., Sakamaki, T., Peter, T., and Uchiyama, T.: Characterization of left ventricular mechanical function during arrhythmias by two-dimensional echocardiography. II. Location of the site of onset of premature ventricular systoles. J. Am. Coll. Cardiol., 1:819, 1983.

37. Windle, J.R., Armstrong, W.F., Feigenbaum, H., Miles, W.M., and Prystowsky, E.N.: Determination of the earliest site of ventricular activation in Wolff-Parkinson-White syndrome: Application of digital continuous loop two-dimensional echocardiography. J. Am. Coll. Cardiol., 7:1286, 1986.

38. Fujii, J., Foster, J.R., Mills, P.G., Moos, S., and Craige, E.: Dual echocardiographic determination of atrial contraction sequence in atrial flutter and other related atrial arrhythmias. Circulation, 58:314, 1978.

39. Fujii, J., Watanabe, H., Kuboki, M., and Kato, K.: Echocardiographic study of atrial flutter. Jpn. Circ. J., 41:1393, 1977.

40. Procacci, P.M., Levites, R., Kotler, M.N., and Anderson, G.J.: Dissimilar atrial rhythm diagnosed by echocardiography. Chest, 73:429, 1978.

41. Sanfilippo, A.J., Abascal, V.M., Sheehan, M., Oertel, L.B., Harrigan, P., Hughes, R.A., and Weyman, A.E.: Atrial enlargement as a consequence of atrial fibrillation. Circulation, 82:792, 1990.

42. Dethy, M., Chassat, C., Roy, D., and Mercier, L-A.: Doppler echocardiographic predictors of recurrence of atrial fibrillation after cardioversion. Am. J. Cardiol., 62:723, 1988.

43. Manning, W.J., Leeman, D.E., Gotch, P.J., and Come, P.C.: Pulsed Doppler evaluation of atrial mechanical function after electrical cardioversion of atrial fibrillation. J. Am. Coll. Cardiol., 13:617, 1989.

44. Fujii, J., Watanabe, H., Kuboki, M., Morita, K., and Kato, K.: Echocardiograms of the left atrial wall, mitral valve, and tricuspid valve in atrial flutter. Cardiovasc. Sound Bull., 5:751, 1975.

45. Sasse, L. and Frolich, C.R.: Suprasternal notch echocardiography and atrial arrhythmias. Cardiovasc. Dis., 6:61, 1979.

46. Greenberg, M., Herman, L.S., and Cohen, M.V.: Mitral valve closure in atrial flutter. Circulation, 59:902, 1979.

47. Drinkovic, N.: Subcostal M-mode echocardiography of the right atrial wall in the diagnosis of cardiac arrhythmias. Am. J. Cardiol., 50:1104, 1982.

48. Goldbaum, T.S., Goldstein, S.A., and Lindsay, J.: Subcostal M-mode echocardiography of atrial septum for diagnosis of atrial flutter. Am. J. Cardiol., 54:1143, 1984.

49. Ruckel, A., Kasper, W., Treese, N., Henkel, B., Pop, T., and Meinertz, T.: Atrioventricular dissociation detected by suprasternal M-mode echocardiography: A clue to the diagnosis of ventricular tachycardia. Am. J. Cardiol., 54:561, 1984.

50. Nawata, T., Toma, Y., Date, T., Takahashi, T., Hiroyama, N., Tamitani, M., Maeda, T., Hesaka, K., Maeda, R., Yonezawa, F., et al.: Study of atrial contraction in sick sinus syndrome using conventional and esophageal echocardiography. J. Cardiogr., 13:981, 1983.

51. Kay, G.N., Holman, W.L., and Nanda, N.C.: Combined use of transesophageal echocardiography and endocardial mapping to localize the site of origin of ectopic atrial tachycardia. Am. J. Cardiol., 65:1284, 1990.

52. Shapiro, I., Sharf, M., and Abinader, E.G.: Prenatal diagnosis of fetal arrhythmias: A new echocardiographic technique. JCU, 12:369, 1984.

53. DeVore, G.R., Siassi, B., and Platt, L.D.: Fetal echocardiography. III. The diagnosis of cardiac arrhythmias using real-time-directed M-mode ultrasound. Am. J. Obstet. Gynecol., 146:792, 1983.

54. Allan, L.D., Anderson, R.H., Sullivan, I.D., Campbell, S., Holt, D.W., and Tynan, M.: Evaluation of fetal arrhythmias by echocardiography. Br. Heart J., 50:240, 1983.

55. Strasburger, J.F., Huhta, J.C., Carpentier, Jr., R.J., Garson, Jr., A., and McNamara, D.G.: Doppler echocardiography in the diagnosis and management of persistent fetal arrhythmias. J. Am. Coll. Cardiol., 7:1386, 1986.

56. Schaefer, S., Taylor, A.L., Lee, H.R., Niggemann, E.H., Levine, B.D., Popma, J.J., Mitchell, J.H., and Hillis, L.D.: Effect of increasing heart rate on left ventricular performance in patients with normal cardiac function. Am. J. Cardiol., 61:617, 1988.

57. Appleton, C.P., Carucci, M.J., Henry, C.P., and Olajos, M.: Influence of incremental changes in heart rate on mitral flow velocity: Assessment in lightly sedated, conscious dogs. J. Am. Coll. Cardiol., 17:233, 1991.

58. D'Cruz, I.A., Prabhu, R., Cohen, H.C., and Glick, G.: Echocardiographic features of second degree atrioventricular block. Chest, 72:459, 1977.

59. Appleton, C.P., Basnight, M.A., Gonzalez, M.S., Carucci, M.J., Henry, C.P., and Olajos, M.: Diastolic mitral regurgitation with atrioventricular conduction abnormalities: Relation of mitral flow velocity to transmitral pressure gradients in conscious dogs. J. Am. Coll. Cardiol., 18:843, 1991.

60. Clyne, C.A., Cuenoud, H.F., and Pape, L.A.: Diastolic mitral regurgitation occurring with complete atrioventricular block detected by color Doppler flow mapping. Echocardiography, 6:543, 1989.

61. Schnittger, I., Appleton, C.P., Hatle, L.K., and Popp, R.L.: Diastolic mitral and tricuspid regurgitation by Doppler echocardiography in patients with atrioventricular block: New insight into the mechanism of atrioventricular valve closure. J. Am. Coll. Cardiol., 11:83, 1988.

62. Zugibe, F.T., Jr., Nanda, N.C., Barold, S.S., and Akiyama, T.: Usefulness of Doppler echocardiography in cardiac pacing: Assessment of mitral regurgitation, peak aortic flow velocity and atrial capture. PACE, 6:1350, 1983.

63. Nanda, N.C., Bhandari, A., Barold, S.S., and Falkoff, M.: Doppler echocardiographic studies in sequential atrioventricular pacing. PACE, 6:811, 1983.

63a. Burns, C.A., Sperry, R.E., Arrowood, J.A., Wood, M.A., Nixon, J.V., Ellenbogen, K.A.: Doppler echocardiographic assessment of an impedance-based dual-chamber rate-responsive pacemaker. Am. J. Cardiol., 71:569, 1993.

64. Rosenqvist, M., Isaaz, K., Botvinick, E.H., Dae, M.W., Cockrell, J., Abbott, J.A., Schiller, N.B., and Griffin, J.C.: Relative importance of activation sequence compared to atrioventricular synchrony in left ventricular function. Am. J. Cardiol., 67:148, 1991.

65. Iwase, M., Hatano, K., Saito, F., Kato, K., Maeda, M., Miyaguchi, K., Aoki, T., Yokota, M., Hayashi, H., Saito, H., and Murase, M.: Evaluation by exercise Doppler echocardiography of maintenance of cardiac output during ventricular pacing with or without chronotropic response. Am. J. Cardiol., 63:934, 1989.

66. Lau, C-P. and Camm, A.J.: Role of left ventricular function and Doppler-derived variables in predicting hemodynamic benefits of rate-responsive pacing. Am. J. Cardiol., 62:906, 1988.

67. Janosik, D.L., Pearson, A.C., and Labovitz, A.J.: Applications of Doppler echocardiography in cardiac pacing. Echocardiography, 8:45, 1991.

68. Pearson, A.C., Janosik, D.L., Redd, R., Buckingham, T.A., Blum, R.I., and Labovitz, A.J.: Doppler echocardiographic assessment of the effect of varying atrioventricular delay and pacemaker mode on left ventricular filling. Am. Heart J., 115:611, 1988.

69. Pearson, A.C., Janosik, D.L., Redd, R.M., Buckingham, T.A., Labovitz, A.J., and Mrosek, D.: Hemodynamic benefit of atrioventricular synchrony: Prediction from baseline Doppler-echocardiographic variables. J. Am. Coll. Cardiol., 13:1613, 1989.

70. Rokey R., Quinones, M.A., Zoghbi, W.A., Kuo, L.C., and Abinader, E.G.: Influence of left atrial systolic emptying on left ventricular early filling dynamics by Doppler in patients with sequential atrioventricular pacemakers. Am. J. Cardiol., 62:968, 1988.

71. Wish, M., Gottdiener, J.S., Cohen, A.I., and Fletcher, R.D.: M-mode echocardiograms for determination of optimal left atrial timing in patients with dual chamber pacemakers. Am. J. Cardiol., 61:317, 1988.

72. Butman, S.M., Mechling, E., and Copeland, J.G.: Echocardiographic documentation of atrial mechanical systole after dual-chamber pacemaker implantation in a patient without electrically evident atrial activity. Clin. Cardiol., 10:481, 1987.

73. VonBibra, H., Wirtzfeld, A., Hall, R., Ulm, K., and Blomer, H.: Mitral valve closure and left ventricular filling time in patients with VDD pacemakers. Br. Heart J., 55:355, 1986.

74. Yamagishi, T., Maeda, T., Yamauchi, M., Yuki, K., Kohno, M., Yamada, H., Matsuzaki, M., and Kusukawa, R.: Differential diagnosis of sinus node dysfunction vs advanced atrioventricular block by analysis of venous flow patterns in patients with ventricular pacemakers. Am. Heart. J., 113:1243, 1987.

# 6

# Acquired Valvular Heart Disease

Echocardiography has become the examination of choice for evaluating valvular heart disease. No diagnostic procedure can visualize the cardiac valves as well as echocardiography. Two-dimensional echocardiography provides an excellent tomographic examination of all of the cardiac valves. M-mode echocardiography is able to record subtle motion of individual valves. The various Doppler techniques allow for an excellent hemodynamic evaluation of the valves. Stenotic and regurgitant valves are easily detected by their abnormal flow patterns. Furthermore, it is possible to quantitate the severity of stenosis using spectral Doppler and to provide at least a semiquantitative evaluation of valvular regurgitation with a combination of Doppler routines, including color flow imaging.

Transesophageal echocardiography provides a new opportunity to provide even further detailed study of the cardiac valves. Because of the enhanced resolution and unobstructed visualization, subtle details are now available for scrutiny with this ultrasonic technique. Thus, it is not surprising that the care for an increasing number of patients is being managed totally on the basis of cardiac ultrasonic evaluation.

## MITRAL VALVE DISEASE

### Mitral Stenosis

All of the echocardiographic techniques are valuable in assessing mitral stenosis. As with all echocardiographic examinations, one initially begins with the two-dimensional study for overall visualization of the mitral valve. Because the field of cardiac ultrasound began with the diagnosis of mitral stenosis, however, the topic will be discussed from a chronologic point of view. In many ways, a discussion of the echocardiographic evaluation of mitral stenosis is essentially a review of the history of cardiac ultrasound. As with all studies of history, there are lessons to be learned, because some limitations noted with early techniques are repeating themselves in later methods.

The initial clinical use of cardiac ultrasound was based on the M-mode observation that the anterior mitral leaflet closed differently with or without mitral stenosis. As demonstrated in Chapter 2, the normal early diastolic, or E to F, slope is steep (Fig. 6–1B). In patients with

mitral stenosis, this early diastolic closure occurs at a slower rate.[1,2] Thus, the mid-diastolic closing velocity of the valve or the E to F slope is markedly diminished (Fig. 6–1A). The explanation for this observation is that the E to F slope is a function of the rate of left atrial emptying or left ventricular filling.[3] In many ways, this observation is analogous to the Doppler flow patterns discussed subsequently.

Normally, the left atrium empties rapidly, so that in mid-diastole, the valve tends to close. With mitral stenosis, filling of the ventricle is slow and the valve is held open by a persistent pressure gradient between the left atrium and the left ventricle. Thus, the mitral E to F slope has been used to make the qualitative diagnosis, and several investigators used this measurement to judge the severity of the mitral stenosis.[4–8]

Figure 6–2 shows a patient before and after successful mitral commissurotomy. In the preoperative echocardiogram (Fig. 6–2A), the flat E to F slope of the anterior mitral leaflet is more rapid following the commissurotomy (Fig. 6–2B). Mitral re-stenosis has been detected by serial reductions in the E to F slope.[9–11] With further experience, however, the E to F slope proved not to be specific. Figure 6–3 shows a patient with a flat E to F slope with no evidence of mitral stenosis. This patient had aortic stenosis and regurgitation. The change in valve motion is believed to be related to decreased rate of left ventricular filling as a result of reduced left ventricular compliance.[12,13] For these and other reasons, the use of mitral E to F slope for quantitating mitral stenosis has been essentially discarded as unreliable and obsolete.

Another M-mode echocardiographic sign for the qualitative diagnosis of mitral stenosis is the pattern of motion of the posterior mitral leaflet.[12] As shown in Figure 6–1B, the normal posterior mitral leaflet is a virtual mirror image of the anterior leaflet. When the valve opens in diastole, the posterior leaflet moves downward while the anterior leaflet moves upward. Figure 6–1A illustrates the situation in the case of mitral stenosis. The most striking qualitative change is that, with early diastole, the posterior leaflet now moves upward in the same direction as the anterior leaflet.

Not all patients with mitral stenosis have anterior motion of the posterior leaflet during diastole.[14–19] Figure 6–4 shows a patient with some degree of mitral stenosis. The patient underwent a mitral commissurotomy, but

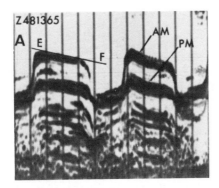

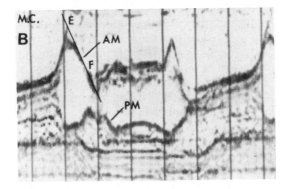

**Fig. 6–1.** Mitral valve echocardiogram of the anterior (AM) and posterior (PM) mitral valve leaflets in a patient with mitral stenosis (*A*) and in a normal subject (*B*). Note E to F slopes. (From Duchak, J.M., Chang, S., and Feigenbaum, H.: The posterior mitral valve echo and the echocardiographic diagnosis of mitral stenosis. Am. J. Cardiol., *29*:628, 1972.)

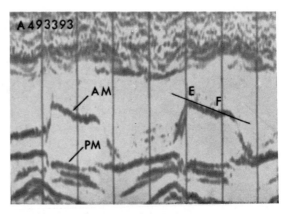

**Fig. 6–3.** Mitral valve echocardiogram of a patient with a diminished diastolic slope of the anterior mitral leaflet (AM) with no evidence of mitral stenosis. Despite the diminished E to F slope, the leaflets are thin and the posterior mitral leaflet (PM) moves normally. (From Duchak, J.M., Chang, S., and Feigenbaum, H.: The posterior mitral valve echo and the echocardiographic diagnosis of mitral stenosis. Am. J. Cardiol., *29*: 628, 1972.)

still had hemodynamically significant residual mitral stenosis. The posterior mitral leaflet clearly moves downward in diastole. The anterior motion of the anterior leaflet is certainly less than normal, and the separation between the two leaflets also is less than normal. In several studies, the number of patients with mitral stenosis who showed downward motion of the posterior leaflet varied from 10 to 17 percent.[15,16]

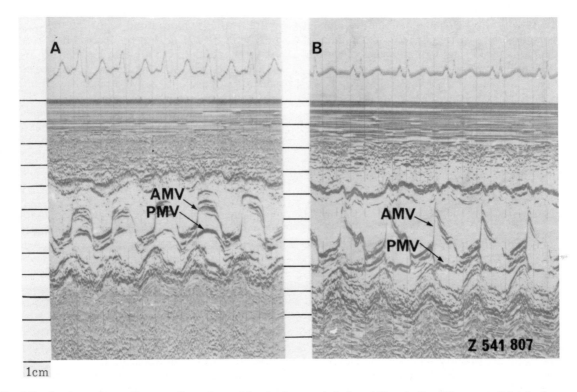

**Fig. 6–2.** Mitral valve echocardiogram of a patient with mitral stenosis before (*A*) and after (*B*) successful mitral commissurotomy. AMV = anterior mitral valve leaflet; PMV = posterior mitral valve leaflet. (From Chang, S.: Echocardiography: Techniques and Interpretation, Second Ed. Philadelphia, Lea & Febiger, 1981.)

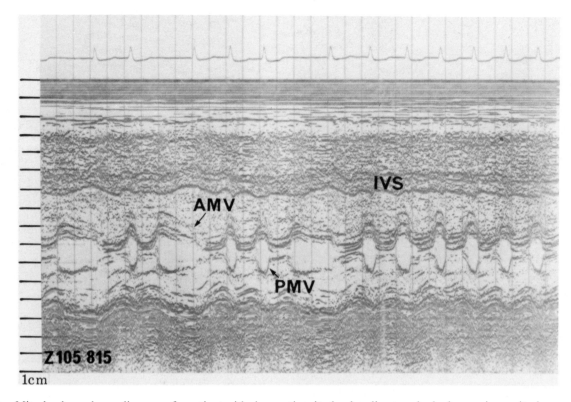

**Fig. 6–4.** Mitral valve echocardiogram of a patient with rheumatic mitral valve disease who had a previous mitral commissurotomy and some residual mitral stenosis. Despite the thickened and relatively immobile anterior mitral leaflet (AMV), the posterior mitral valve (PMV) is thinner and moves downward with diastole. IVS = interventricular septum. (From Chang, S.: Echocardiography: Techniques and Interpretation, Second Ed. Philadelphia, Lea & Febiger, 1981.)

M-mode echocardiography has been used in the past for detecting the excursion of the leaflet for valve mobility as well as for judging the degree of fibrosis and thickening. Two-dimensional echocardiography has now superseded the M-mode technique for making these judgments. In fact, M-mode echocardiography, despite its historical basis for the diagnosis and evaluation of mitral stenosis, has now been relegated to a secondary role, even in the assessment of this important valvular problem.

As with all other cardiologic abnormalities, two-dimensional echocardiography is the principle means of evaluating valvular morphology in patients with mitral stenosis. Figure 6–5 shows long-axis and short-axis two-dimensional, diastolic views of the mitral valve in a patient with mitral stenosis. The principle diagnostic feature of mitral stenosis in this view is doming of the anterior mitral leaflet in diastole. Doming indicates that the valve cannot accommodate all the blood available for delivery into the left ventricle. Thus, the body of the leaflets separates more widely than do the edges. Doming is one of the main two-dimensional features of any stenotic valve. The mitral valve may also open poorly in patients who have a low cardiac output (Fig. 6–6). If the mitral valve is intrinsically normal, however, the anterior leaflet does not dome (Fig. 6–6B).

From a historical point of view, it is interesting that one of the first applications for two-dimensional echocardiography was again the diagnosis of mitral stenosis.

The technique was used primarily to help quantitate the degree of stenosis.[20-24] Figure 6–5 demonstrates that the short-axis (SX) view gives an excellent assessment of the mitral orifice, which can be measured to provide a cross-sectional area of the stenotic orifice. This measurement is still probably the most accurate quantitation of mitral stenosis. The two-dimensional echocardiogram in Figure 6–6 is from another patient with mitral stenosis whose valve is fibrotic and immobile. The short-axis view shows a small mitral valve orifice in this patient with severe mitral stenosis. Numerous studies have demonstrated that the mitral valve area measured with two-dimensional echocardiography correlates well with the severity of mitral stenosis as determined at cardiac catheterization.[25-31]

Obvious limitations are associated with the two-dimensional measurement of mitral valve area. One potential technical error is that the measurement is influenced by any dropout of echoes. The mitral orifice in Figure 6–7 is not totally complete. The examiner must fill in some gaps where echoes are missing. Another problem is that the lateral resolution of all echocardiographic systems is less than ideal, and the echoes from the lateral and medial walls of the mitral orifice appear wider than they really are.[23] For example, in Figure 6–8, the patient has a densely calcified mitral valve, and one can barely see any remnant of a valve orifice in diastole (MVO, Fig. 6–8). Although the patient had severe mitral stenosis, one could not actually measure a valve orifice, which is

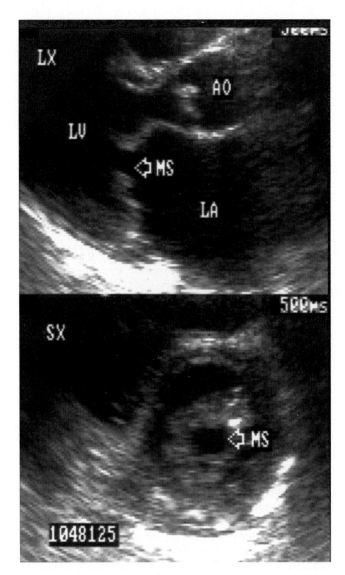

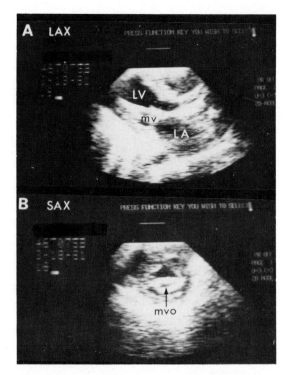

Fig. 6–6. Two-dimensional echocardiograms of a patient with severe mitral stenosis whose mitral leaflets (mv) were markedly fibrotic and immobile. The mitral valve orifice (mvo) is markedly reduced. LV = left ventricle; LA = left atrium; LAX = long axis; SAX = short axis.

Fig. 6–5. Long-axis (LX) and short-axis (SX) two-dimensional echocardiograms of a patient with mitral stenosis. The long-axis view shows typical doming of both leaflets with a diminished separation (MS) between the anterior and posterior edge. The short-axis view shows the echo-free orifice in the center of the stenotic valve (MS).

undoubtedly larger than it appears in this figure. Some two-dimensional echocardiographic systems are more gain sensitive than others.[23] Thus, the valve orifice can be influenced significantly by the gain settings (Fig. 6–9).[26] Fortunately, the echocardiogram recorded in Figure 6–9 was from an early, phased array, two-dimensional echocardiograph, which is no longer available. Most current ultrasonic instruments are not as gain sensitive as this older instrument. Furthermore, one would not ordinarily distort the image to this extent. Another technical detail that must be considered when using two-dimensional echocardiography to measure the mitral valve orifice is that, in diastole, the stenotic mitral valve assumes the shape of a funnel. If one slices the valve

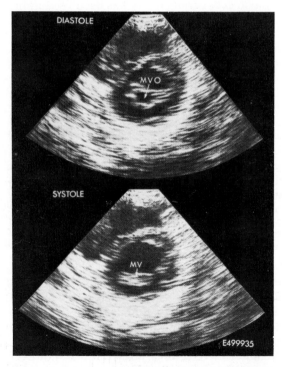

Fig. 6–7. Short-axis two-dimensional echocardiograms of a patient with mitral stenosis. Note the diastolic mitral valve orifice (MVO). In systole, the leaflets come together, and the orifice is obliterated.

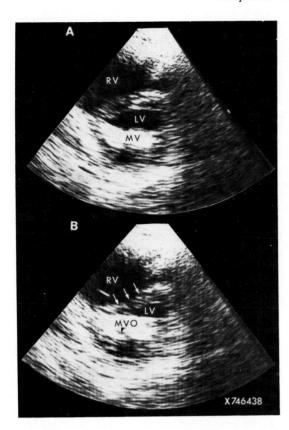

**Fig. 6–8.** Short-axis two-dimensional echocardiogram of a patient with calcific mitral stenosis. In diastole (*B*), the mitral valve orifice (MVO) is barely visible. There is also an indentation of the interventricular septum (*arrows*) toward the left ventricle in early diastole. RV = right ventricle; LV = left ventricle.

too close to the aorta, the mitral valve orifice is falsely large (Fig. 6–10).

A clinical situation whereby the two-dimensional echocardiographic technique for measuring valve area has significant limitations is in patients with a mitral commissurotomy or balloon valvuloplasty. In this situation, the valve orifice is no longer elliptic. The separation of the fractured or incised commissure may not be well visualized on the two-dimensional echocardiogram. Thus, the true orifice may be underestimated because the separation of the leaflets at the incised commissure may be excluded from the measurement. In patients with significant subvalvular fibrosis and stenosis, the valve orifice may underestimate the hemodynamic significance of the obstruction.

Despite these limitations, estimating the severity of mitral stenosis with two-dimensional echocardiography has many advantages and is still the procedure of choice for quantitating mitral stenosis. This examination comes closest to directly measuring the actual anatomic abnormality. The measurement is not influenced by accompanying mitral regurgitation. It is not surprising, therefore, that the ultrasonic measurement correlates well with the findings of the pathologist or the surgeon. Most limitations can be overcome with careful examination technique.

Doppler echocardiography offers an opportunity to assess the hemodynamic consequences of mitral stenosis.[32–40] Figure 6–11 is a pulsed Doppler echogram of mitral valve flow in a patient with mitral stenosis and sinus rhythm. One of the Doppler features of mitral stenosis is that the rate of decrease in diastolic flow after the E point is reduced. The peak velocity is also higher than normal. In this patient, the peak velocity is in excess of 150 cm/sec. Spectral broadening occurs during diastole if the sample volume is distal to the stenotic orifice. The peak velocity after atrial systole is increased as flow is forcefully transported across the narrowed valve. An increased Doppler A wave with mitral steno-

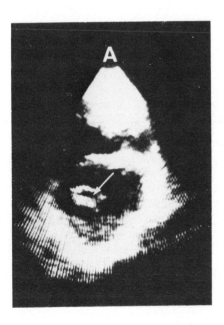
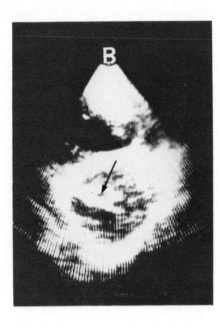

**Fig. 6–9.** Two-dimensional echocardiograms of a stenotic mitral valve with two different gain settings. Note how the apparent mitral valve orifice is much smaller with a high-gain setting (*B*).

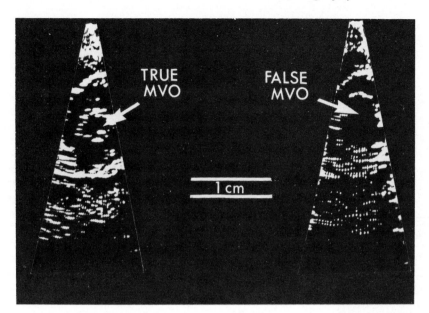

**Fig. 6–10.** Short-axis two-dimensional studies of the same patient with mitral stenosis. The true mitral valve orifice (MVO) is located at the edges of the leaflets. Note in the right-hand study how a two-dimensional slice closer to the base of the heart produces a falsely large mitral valve orifice.

sis is opposite to what one sees with mitral stenosis on the M-mode recording. With M-mode echocardiography, the A wave is reduced and usually is absent in a patient with severe mitral stenosis.[41] Some evidence shows that the Doppler A wave may also decrease with increasing severity of mitral stenosis.

Figure 6–12 shows a continuous wave Doppler recording of a patient with mitral stenosis. The configuration of the Doppler tracing is similar to the pulsed Doppler examination. Again, the A wave is accentuated. Naturally, with atrial fibrillation (Fig. 6–13), the A wave

is absent. The principle Doppler signs are reduced diastolic slope and increased velocity.

Possibly the simplest approach to using Doppler echocardiography for quantitating mitral stenosis is the concept of pressure half-time.[33,36,39,40,42] The technique is actually an adaptation of one used in the cardiac catheterization laboratory many years ago. Figure 6–14 demonstrates the principle behind this calculation. The time required for the peak gradient to be reduced to one half is quantitatively related to the degree of mitral stenosis. This approach is attractive because the calculation is

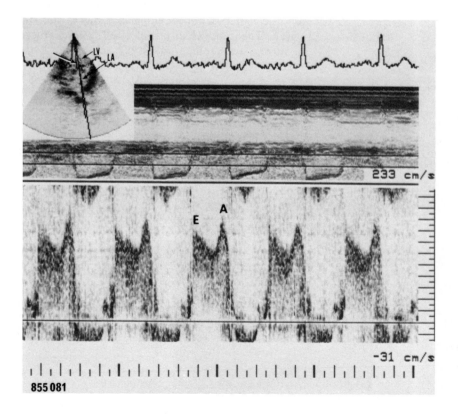

**Fig. 6–11.** Pulsed Doppler echocardiogram of mitral valve flow in a patient with mitral stenosis. Arrow = sample volume; LV = left ventricle; LA = left atrium.

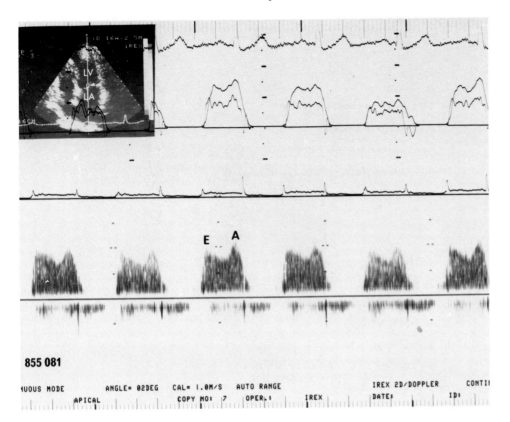

**Fig. 6–12.** Continuous wave Doppler examination of mitral flow in a patient with mitral stenosis. LV = left ventricle; LA = left atrium.

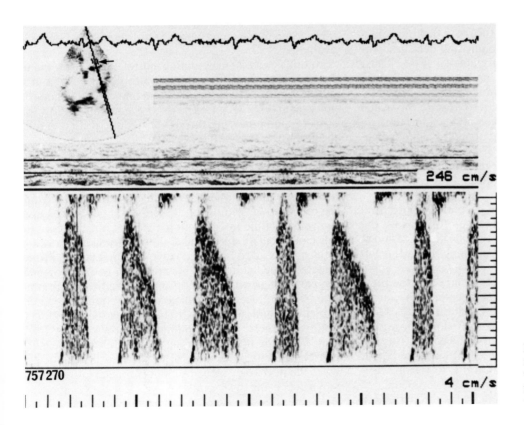

**Fig. 6–13.** Pulsed Doppler mitral valve flow in a patient with mitral stenosis and atrial fibrillation. Arrow = sample volume.

## PRESSURE HALF TIME

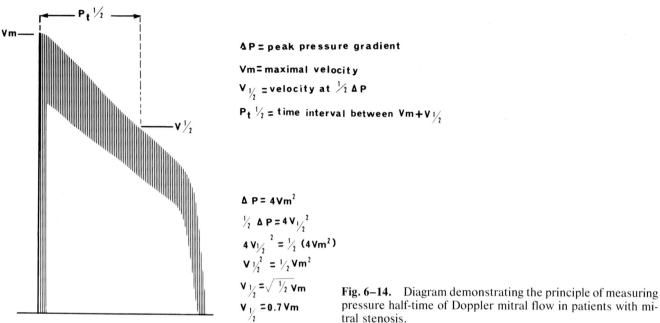

$\Delta P$ = peak pressure gradient

$V_m$ = maximal velocity

$V_{1/2}$ = velocity at $\frac{1}{2} \Delta P$

$P_{t\ 1/2}$ = time interval between $V_m + V_{1/2}$

$\Delta P = 4 V_m^2$

$\frac{1}{2} \Delta P = 4 V_{1/2}^2$

$4 V_{1/2}^2 = \frac{1}{2}(4 V_m^2)$

$V_{1/2}^2 = \frac{1}{2} V_m^2$

$V_{1/2} = \sqrt{\frac{1}{2}}\ V_m$

$V_{1/2} = 0.7 V_m$

**Fig. 6–14.** Diagram demonstrating the principle of measuring pressure half-time of Doppler mitral flow in patients with mitral stenosis.

fairly simple and can be made with a caliper or automatically by a computer with most echocardiographs or off-line analyzers.

Based on the Bernoulli equation, the pressure gradient is equal to four times the velocity squared. Therefore, the peak gradient ($\Delta P$) is four times the maximum velocity ($V_m$) squared. One-half peak gradient ($\frac{1}{2} \Delta P$) would equal four times the half peak velocity ($V_m \frac{1}{2}$) squared. After making the calculations, it turns out that the velocity ($V_m \frac{1}{2}$), which corresponds to one-half peak gradient ($\Delta P \frac{1}{2}$), is $0.7 \times$ the maximum velocity ($V_m$). Thus, multiplying the peak velocity at the E point by 0.7 gives the velocity that corresponds to the half peak pressure. The time required for the velocity to drop to this value is the pressure half-time. One then divides that time interval into an empirically derived number (220) to calculate mitral valve area (MVA = 220/pressure half-time). Figure 6–15 illustrates how the pressure half-time can be measured on a Doppler recording in a patient with severe mitral stenosis.

Another way of looking at the deceleration of mitral flow through a stenotic mitral valve is to measure the deceleration time index, which is similar to the M-mode E to F slope. This measurement is simpler than the calculation of pressure half-time.[43]

Considerable data demonstrate the fact that the pressure half-time or rate of velocity deceleration can be useful in quantitating the degree of mitral stenosis. As with the M-mode mitral valve E to F slope, however, further experience has discovered limitations to this relatively simple technique. As one might have predicted, the pressure half-time, like the mitral E to F slope, is a function of left ventricular stiffness or compliance.[44] The measurement is also influenced by the maximum

mitral gradient.[45] The presence of mitral regurgitation, which increases the maximum initial gradient, thus alters the validity of the pressure half-time.[46] Aortic regurgitation also appears to influence the pressure half-time determination.[47] And one of the principle limitations is that the pressure half-time measurement does not seem to be valid immediately after mitral balloon valvuloplasty.[45,48–50] Thus, reliance on this relatively simple measurement for quantitating mitral stenosis is being re-evaluated.[51–53]

Another way of calculating mitral valve area using Doppler techniques is to employ the continuity equation.[54] Figure 6–16 shows the principle behind the continuity equation. If one knows the amount of flow or stroke volume passing through a stenotic orifice, and if the pressure gradient across the orifice can be determined, then it is possible to calculate the area of the stenotic valve. The continuity equation basically uses the Doppler techniques of calculating a pressure gradient using the modified Bernoulli equation and measuring blood flow by knowing the cross-sectional area and the velocity time integral. In the case of mitral stenosis, one can calculate mitral valve flow by using aortic valve flow, as measured by aortic valve area and velocity time integral (see Chapter 3). This approach works provided the patient has no significant mitral or aortic regurgitation. In the presence of aortic regurgitation, one could substitute pulmonary flow by measuring the pulmonary outflow diameter and the pulmonary flow velocity integral. Knowing the flow through the orifice and measuring the velocity time integral of the mitral stenotic jet gives the necessary measurements for calculating mitral valve area using the formula: $A_2 = A_1 \times V_1/V_2$, in which $A_2$ is mitral valve area, $A_1$ is aortic valve area, $V_1$ is

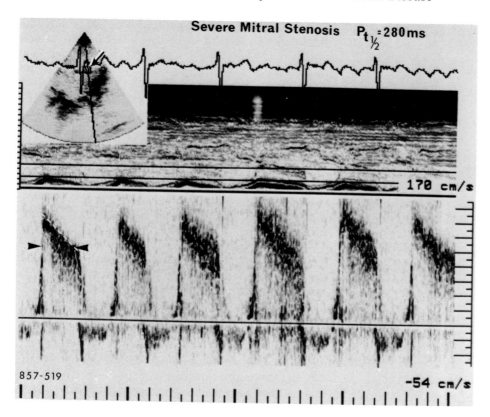

**Fig. 6–15.** Pulsed Doppler echocardiogram of mitral flow in a patient with mitral stenosis. This echocardiogram demonstrates how the pressure half time ($P_{t1/2}$) (*arrowheads*) is measured.

aortic valve velocity, and $V_2$ is mitral velocity. This approach is more complicated than using the pressure half-time; but in comparative studies, investigators find the continuity equation to be more accurate and to have fewer limitations.[45,55,56]

One could also use Doppler recordings to calculate the mitral valve area using the more standard Gorlin formula.[57] The Gorlin formula again uses pressure gradient and mitral flow. In the cardiac catheterization lab-

oratory, one measures the pressure gradient across the mitral valve directly and calculates cardiac output using an indicator dilution or Fick technique. One can make the same calculation with Doppler echocardiography by combining stroke volume using aortic or pulmonary flow and measuring the mean pressure gradient.

Pulmonary venous flow has been examined in patients with mitral stenosis. Investigators have found that mitral stenosis produces a decrease in the pulmonary venous

## DOPPLER ECHOCARDIOGRAPHY
## CONTINUITY EQUATION

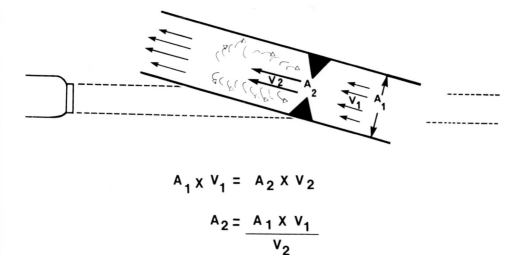

$$A_1 \times V_1 = A_2 \times V_2$$

$$A_2 = \frac{A_1 \times V_1}{V_2}$$

**Fig. 6–16.** Diagram illustrating the principle of the continuity equation in calculating a stenotic valve area. $A_1$ and $V_1$ = area and velocities proximal to the stenosis; $A_2$ and $V_2$ = area and velocities at the site of the stenosis. (From Feigenbaum, H.: Echocardiography. *In* Heart Disease, 4th ed. Edited by E. Braunwald. Philadelphia, W.B. Saunders Co., 1992.)

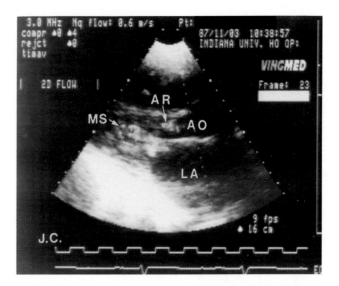

**Fig. 6–17.** Color flow Doppler study showing the turbulent jet of mitral stenosis (MS). The patient also has a color Doppler jet of aortic regurgitation (AR). AO = aorta; LA = left atrium. (From Feigenbaum, H.: Doppler color flow imaging. *In* Heart Disease Update. Edited by E. Braunwald. Philadelphia, W.B. Saunders, Co., 1988.)

diastolic flow, and flow reversal with atrial systole is accentuated.[58–60] Whether this finding adds to the understanding of mitral stenosis or the management of an individual patient is yet to be determined.

Doppler measurements in patients with mitral stenosis are sensitive to various hemodynamic conditions. Pregnancy increases the flow across the mitral valve and

enhances the gradient.[61] Exercise Doppler echocardiography can be helpful to assess changes in the pressure gradient[62–64] and flow[64a] with exertion. A unique limitation to the use of Doppler echocardiography to quantitate mitral stenosis is when the patient also has an atrial septal defect (Lutenbacher syndrome).[65] Under these circumstances, left atrial blood passes into the right atrium as well as through the mitral valve, and the Doppler gradient may be inaccurate.

Color flow imaging can assist with the qualitative diagnosis of mitral stenosis.[66] The turbulent jet going through the stenotic mitral valve can be recognized by variance or aliasing (Fig. 6–17). The location of the stenotic jet can be helpful in positioning the spectral Doppler sample for analysis.

Transesophageal echocardiography also gives an excellent view of the stenotic mitral valve. The domed leaflets are detected easily with the esophageal approach (Fig. 6–18). In addition, because the left atrium is visualized so well, one can see flow convergence using color flow Doppler on the atrial side of the stenotic mitral valve. The flow convergence is used more often with mitral regurgitation, as will be discussed, although the same phenomenon occurs with mitral stenosis. Despite the higher quality imaging with transesophageal echocardiography, transthoracic echocardiography is still the preferred technique for looking at subvalvular structures, such as fibrosed chordae.[67,68] Figure 6–19A is a transthoracic echocardiogram showing thickened subvalvular structures in a patient with mitral stenosis; however, because of shadowing, the transesophageal approach (Fig. 6–19B) did not detect subvalvular structures adequately.[69]

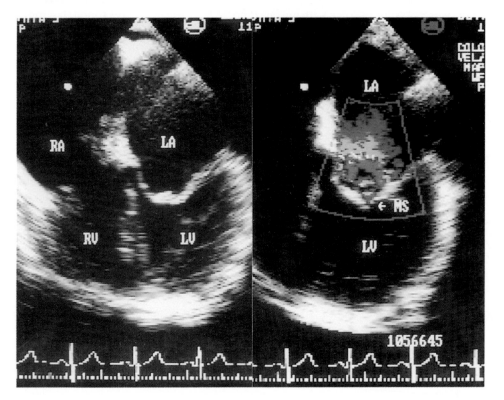

**Fig. 6–18.** Transesophageal echocardiogram of a patient with mitral stenosis. The domed mitral valve can be seen between the left atrium (LA) and left ventricle (LV). In addition, flow acceleration with multiple areas of aliasing can be seen on the left atrial side of the mitral stenotic orifice (MS). RA = right atrium; RV = right ventricle.

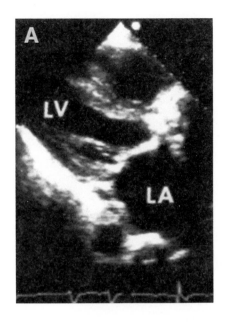

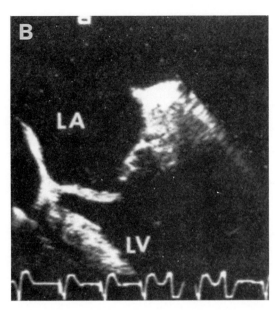

**Fig. 6–19.** Transthoracic (*A*) and transesophageal (*B*) echocardiograms of a patient with mitral stenosis and thickened chordae. The subvalvular thickening is apparent on the transthoracic examination; however, because of acoustic shadowing by the mitral valve, the subvalvular structures are not seen as easily in the transesophageal examination. (From Marwick, T.H., et al.: Assessment of the mitral valve splitability score by transthoracic and transesophageal echocardiography. Am. J. Cardiol., *68*:1107, 1991.)

The consequences of mitral stenosis, including left atrial and right ventricular dilatation (see Chapter 3), pulmonary hypertension (see Chapter 4), left atrial clots, and spontaneous contrast (see Chapter 12), are discussed in other chapters.

### Balloon Mitral Valvotomy

Balloon valvotomy has become a popular therapy for mitral stenosis. Echocardiography is playing a major role in this therapeutic option.[70] Cardiac ultrasound is important in determining whether or not balloon valvotomy should be attempted. Echocardiographic quantitation can help the physician to decide whether the stenosis is sufficiently severe to warrant balloon valvotomy. Not all valves are suitable for this procedure. One criterion for successful valvotomy is a mobile valve. One can use M-mode echocardiography to judge the mobility of the anterior leaflet (Fig. 6–20). An immobile valve is noted in Figure 6–21. Figure 6–22 shows a technique for measuring anterior leaflet mobility using two-dimensional echocardiography. This group of investigators used the height of the domed leaflet as an indicator of mobility or pliability.[71] This measurement apparently helped to predict a successful dilatation. The same group also looked at subvalvular disease, calcification, and thickening to predict the suitability for mitral valvotomy.[72] Investigators have suggested giving values of one to four for each of the parameters of mobility, thickness, calcification, and subvalvular disease and adding the numbers to create an index.[73–75] This index has been related to successful dilatations,[69] although with greater use, the predictability is not proving to be quite as reliable as originally hoped.[76,77] Nonetheless, the assessment of valve morphology with echocardiography is still used widely to evaluate the suitability of valvotomy. This index has also been used to judge the natural history of mitral stenosis.[78]

Another part of the preoperative evaluation for balloon valvotomy is using transesophageal echocardiography to explore the left atrium for any existing clots.[79–81,81a] The balloon technique requires manipulating wires and catheters throughout the left atrium and any clots could be dislodged. Many of these clots reside in the left atrial appendage and cannot be seen with transthoracic echocardiography. Clots also may be too small to be seen with the transthoracic approach. Figure 6–23 shows a transesophageal study of a patient being evaluated for balloon valvotomy. The multiple, small, left atrial clots were not seen on the routine echocardiogram. Most institutions performing trans-septal balloon valvotomy recommend routine transesophageal echocardiography prior to the procedure to rule out the presence of left atrial clots. Some institutions use transesophageal echocardiography to monitor the balloon dilatation procedure.[82–85]

Yet another use of echocardiography before a balloon valvotomy is to measure the annulus to help determine the balloon size necessary for a proper valvotomy without over inflating and producing mitral regurgitation.[86] An assessment of the interatrial septal thickness also may predict the technical ease or difficulty in carrying out the trans-septal catheterization.[87]

Echocardiography is, of course, valuable in assessing the efficacy of a balloon valvotomy.[88–90] This assessment can be done immediately after the dilatation. As mentioned earlier, using the pressure half-time immediately after a valvotomy has some limitations.[45] After 2 to 3 days, the pressure half-time accuracy improves.[49] The somewhat more complicated valve area measurements using the continuity equation[49a] or Gorlin formula are reasonably accurate provided there is no significant mitral regurgitation. The morphology of the valve, as seen using two-dimensional echocardiography, frequently changes with a successful valvotomy.[91] Figure 6–24 shows a long-axis and a four-chamber view of a patient before and after a balloon valvotomy. The

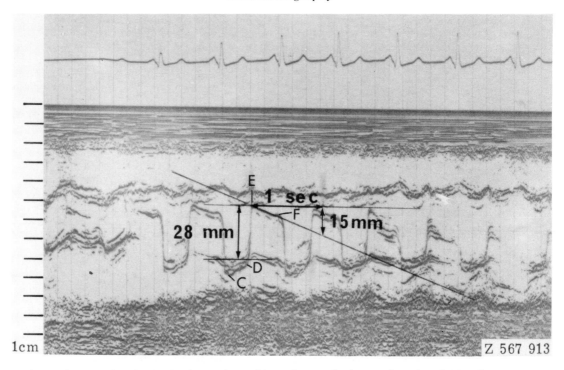

**Fig. 6–20.** Echocardiogram of a mitral valve in a patient with moderate mitral stenosis and a pliable mitral valve. Note how the diastolic closing velocity, or E to F slope, is measured and how one may measure the amplitude of opening of the mitral leaflet, or D to E amplitude. (From Chang, S.: Echocardiography: Techniques and Interpretation, Second Ed. Philadelphia, Lea & Febiger, 1981.)

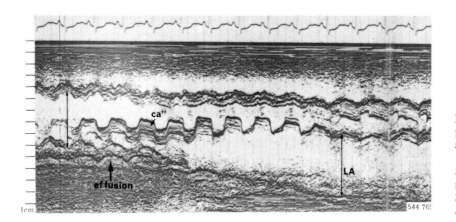

**Fig. 6–21.** M-mode scan of a patient with a calcified ($ca^{++}$) and immobile mitral valve. LA = left atrium. (From Chang, S.: Echocardiography: Techniques and Interpretation, Second Ed. Philadelphia, Lea & Febiger, 1981.)

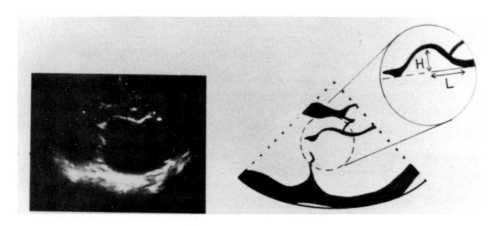

**Fig. 6–22.** A two-dimensional echocardiographic technique for measuring the pliability of the anterior leaflet of the stenotic mitral valve. H = excursion of the belly of the anterior leaflet. (From Reid, C.L., et al.: Influence of mitral valve morphology on double-balloon catheter balloon valvuloplasty in patients with mitral stenosis: Analysis of factors predicting immediate and three-month results. Circulation, *80*:518, 1989, by permission of the American Heart Association, Inc.)

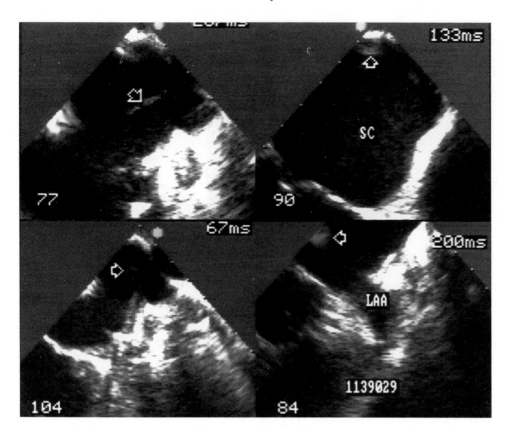

**Fig. 6–23.** Transesophageal echocardiogram of a patient being considered for a balloon mitral valvuloplasty. The examination shows multiple thrombi (*arrows*) within the left atrium. These echoes together with spontaneous contrast (SC) were not detected on the transthoracic examination. LAA = left atrial appendage.

domed, restricted orifice is clearly improved after the successful valvotomy.

Echocardiography can also assess any untoward result from the balloon valvotomy.[92,93] The detection of mitral regurgitation is an obvious application for the echocardiographic examination.[94,95] Occasionally, an

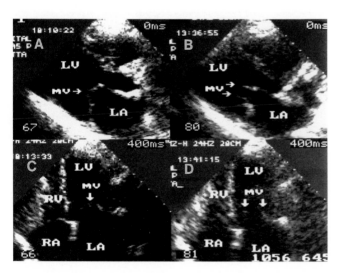

**Fig. 6–24.** Two-dimensional echocardiograms before (*A* and *C*) and after (*B* and *D*) a balloon mitral valvuloplasty. Note the significant increase in the separation of the leaflets in the long-axis (*B*) and four-chamber views (*D*) following the valvuloplasty. mv = mitral valve; LV = left ventricle; LA = left atrium; RV = right ventricle; RA = right atrium.

iatrogenic atrial septal defect will persist where the trans-septal catheter was inserted.[96–98,98a] Figure 6–25 shows a residual atrial septal defect together with mitral regurgitation in a patient who had undergone mitral balloon valvuloplasty.

## Mitral Regurgitation

Two-dimensional echocardiography and, to a lesser extent, M-mode echocardiography are the procedures of choice for visualizing mitral valve morphology in the setting of mitral regurgitation. The detection and assessment of mitral regurgitation is primarily by Doppler echocardiography.[32,34,99–106] Doppler flow imaging, or color flow Doppler, is the initial approach currently used for the diagnosis of mitral regurgitation. Figure 6–26 demonstrates a four-chamber view of a color flow Doppler study in a patient with mitral regurgitation.[107] The multicolored turbulent mitral regurgitant jet (MR) is seen easily within the left atrium (LA). Figure 6–27 illustrates another patient with mitral regurgitation. This examination is a two-chamber view. The Doppler flow study is displayed in the variance mode, and the large multicolored, somewhat greenish jet is visualized within the left atrium.

The color flow Doppler technique for detecting mitral regurgitation can use various two-dimensional views. Figure 6–28 demonstrates mitral regurgitation from the apical four-chamber and the parasternal long-axis views. The regurgitant jet is visible in both planes, although one must remember that flow is best detected when it is parallel to the ultrasonic beam. In addition, the velocity

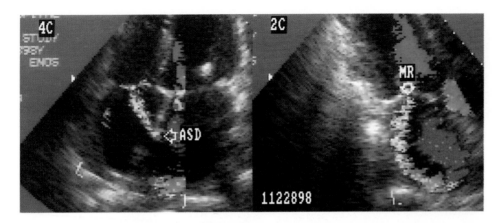

Fig. 6–25. Color flow Doppler study after a balloon mitral valvuloplasty. The patient was left with an iatrogenic atrial septal defect (ASD) and residual mitral regurgitation (MR).

that is displayed is a function of the angle between the moving red cells and the ultrasonic beam. Thus, in Figure 6–28, which is an apical four-chamber examination, the regurgitant jet aliases with areas of yellow and light green indicating turbulence or variance. In the long-axis view, however, the jet is not parallel to the ultrasonic beam and is displayed merely in shades of blue, reflecting a lower recorded velocity. The various views may give different perspectives of the three-dimensional regurgitant jet or jets. For example, Figure 6–29 shows a single mitral regurgitant jet in the long-axis view, but the four-chamber examination reveals the presence of two discrete jets.

Mitral regurgitation can be detected with color flow imaging using transesophageal echocardiography.[108–111] Figure 6–30 demonstrates a mitral regurgitant jet using the transesophageal approach. The multicolored turbulent flow is easily recognized. Figure 6–31 shows another transesophageal echocardiographic color flow study of a patient with mitral regurgitation. The eccentric jet is fairly obvious in this type of examination. As a technical note, this illustration is reproduced from videotape, and the colors are not as vivid as in the other recordings, which are obtained from a digital recording.

A major feature of color flow Doppler in assessing mitral regurgitation is the display of the regurgitant jet within the left atrium. The location and direction of the jet is readily apparent with this technique. There also is an intuitive desire to quantitate the degree of mitral regurgitation based on the size of the regurgitant jet.[112–116] Figure 6–32 shows four different patients with varying degrees of mitral regurgitation. In Figure 6–32A, the patient has a small regurgitant jet suggestive of relatively mild mitral regurgitation. In Figure 6–32D, the regurgitant jet is much larger, indicative of more severe regurgitation. In Figure 6–32B and C, the jets are intermediate in size. The most common approach for using color flow Doppler to quantitate mitral regurgitation is

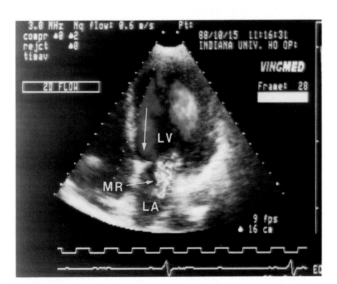

Fig. 6–26.   Color flow Doppler study of a patient with mitral regurgitation. The multicolored regurgitant jet (MR) can be seen protruding into the left atrium (LA). LV = left ventricle. (From Feigenbaum, H.: Doppler color flow imaging. *In* Heart Disease Update. Edited by E. Braunwald. Philadelphia, W.B. Saunders Co., 1988.)

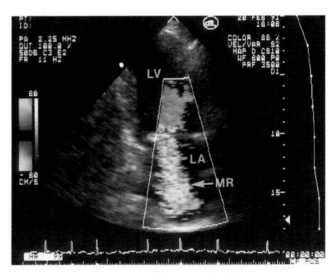

Fig. 6–27.   An apical two-chamber color flow examination of a patient with mitral regurgitation. The Doppler jet is displayed in a variance mode, which produces a multicolored, somewhat greenish jet (MR) within the left atrium (LA). LV = left ventricle.

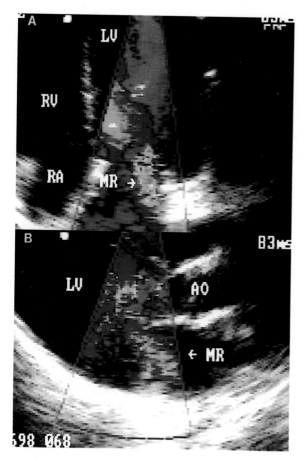

**Fig. 6–28.** Another color flow study of a patient with mitral regurgitation. With the four-chamber view (*A*), the mitral jet (MR) is parallel to the ultrasonic beam, and high velocity, aliasing, turbulent flow is displayed. The same jet seen in the parasternal long-axis view (*B*) shows only a blue, lower velocity jet (MR), because the jet is more perpendicular to the ultrasonic beam. LV = left ventricle; RV = right ventricle; RA = right atrium; AO = aorta.

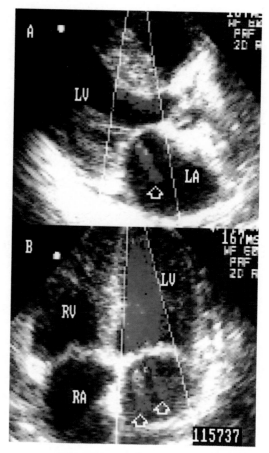

**Fig. 6–29.** Long-axis (*A*) and four-chamber (*B*) color flow imaging of a patient with mitral regurgitation. In the long-axis examination, the jet appears to be singular, whereas two jets are recorded in the four-chamber view (*arrows*). LV = left ventricle; LA = left atrium; RV = right ventricle; RA = right atrium.

to measure the area of the maximum regurgitant jet (Fig. 6–33, *arrowheads*), and to compare that value as a ratio to the area of the left atrium (Fig. 6–33, *dashed line*).[117] This measurement is relatively simple and has wide appeal. Unfortunately, this approach for quantitating mitral regurgitation has many significant limitations.[118]

Numerous instrument factors can influence the size of a Doppler flow jet.[119–122] This issue was discussed at length in Chapter 1. These factors include difference in color Doppler display from one instrument to another, gain settings, and the carrier frequency of the transducer.[123] Physiologic factors are important, such as afterload.[124] Figure 6–34 demonstrates how the size of the regurgitant jet can vary throughout systole.[125] The size of the spray or jet is different in all four images taken from the same cardiac cycle. To meet the criteria for measuring the regurgitant area, one probably should take the maximum turbulent flow area (see Fig. 6–34B). Some data suggest that measuring the turbulent mosaic pattern is more accurate than including the non-high velocity flow that surrounds the mosaic turbulent blood.

The jet is not necessarily symmetric in all planes and multiple views should be obtained to be certain that one achieves a three-dimensional appreciation of the jet size.[126]

The size of transthoracic and transesophageal regurgitant jets will differ. Because of the greater sensitivity and the unobstructed view, the regurgitant jet with transesophageal echocardiography almost always is larger (Fig. 6–35).[127–130] The difference between the transesophageal and transthoracic registration of the mitral regurgitant jet has prompted one group of investigators to indicate that when quantitating mitral regurgitation using transesophageal echocardiography, one should measure the maximum primary mosaic high flow regurgitant jet. With transthoracic echocardiography, however, one should take the entire mitral regurgitant jet, including the surrounding, lower flow spray.[127]

Figure 6–36 demonstrates one of the major clinical limitations of using the size of the color Doppler jet to quantitate mitral regurgitation. A jet flowing into the center of a chamber is able to develop to its fullest (Fig.

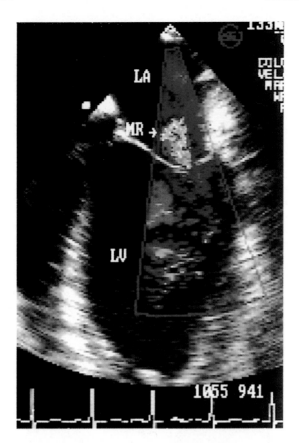

**Fig. 6–30.** Transesophageal color flow echocardiogram of a patient with mitral regurgitation. The regurgitant jet (MR) is seen as a multicolored, high-velocity aliasing display protruding into the left atrium (LA). LV = left ventricle. (From Feigenbaum, H.: Echocardiography. *In* Heart Disease, 4th ed. Edited by E. Braunwald. Philadelphia, W.B. Saunders Co., 1992.)

6–36*A*). If, however, as in Figure 6–36*B,* the jet is directed eccentrically and strikes one of the walls of the chamber, then the flow will be distorted by that wall and a totally different jet area will be recorded.[131,132] Figure 6–37 shows an eccentric mitral regurgitation jet that is initially directed toward the interatrial septum, curls around, then moves toward the left ventricle along the lateral wall of the left atrium (*reverse arrow*). Measuring the area of the turbulent multicolored jet directed toward the left ventricle would be misleading as to the severity of the mitral regurgitation.

Because of the limitations of using the area of the regurgitant jet to quantitate mitral regurgitation, investigators have been looking at other techniques for quantitation. Figure 6–38 shows the principle of flow acceleration proximal to a narrowed or regurgitant orifice.[133–140] Color flow Doppler is pulsed and the Nyquist limit is usually low; therefore, the signal aliases as the velocity accelerates toward the narrowed orifice. This aliasing produces a series of proximal multicolored rings. Each ring represents an isovelocity area (Fig. 6–39). All points equal in distance to the center of the orifice should be

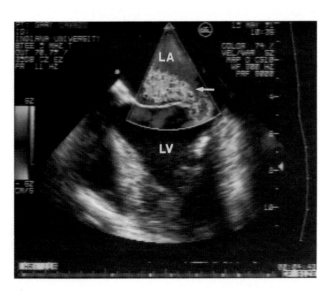

**Fig. 6–31.** Transesophageal echocardiogram of a patient with an eccentric mitral regurgitant jet (*arrow*) protruding into the left atrium (LA). LV = left ventricle. (Editor's note: Color is not quite as vivid because this image is a reproduction from a videotape rather than a direct digital recording.)

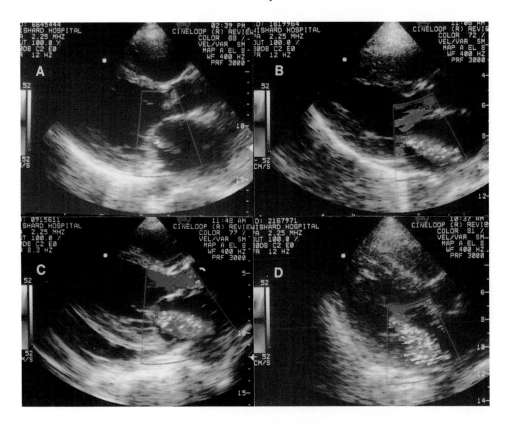

**Fig. 6–32.** Color flow Doppler examinations of four patients with varying degrees of mitral regurgitation: *A*, mild; *B* and *C*, moderate; *D*, severe. A rough relationship exists between the size of the regurgitant jet and the severity of the regurgitation.

equal in velocity (isovelocity). Using the principle of the continuity equation, the flow proximal to the orifice should equal the flow through the orifice. One can calculate the proximal flow by knowing the proximal isovelocity surface area or PISA. This calculation represents the surface of a hemisphere using the radius from the first point of aliasing or isovelocity curve to the center of the orifice (R). If one knows the surface area, it can be multiplied by the velocity that first aliases to calculate the proximal flow, which should then equal the regurgitant flow rate (FR).

Figure 6–40 shows how this principle can be used to calculate mitral regurgitation. The velocity at which an instrument aliases depends on the zero line on the instrument. In this example, if the Nyquist limit is adjusted so that the velocity aliases at 75 cm/sec, then a relatively small area of proximal convergence will be detected. If, however, the aliasing limit is changed so that it occurs at 38 cm/sec, then a larger area of convergence will be recorded. The velocity at which aliasing occurs is combined with PISA to calculate regurgitant flow. Figure 6–41 shows another patient with severe mitral regurgitation. The area of the jet entering the left atrium is relatively small, in part because it hits the lateral wall. The

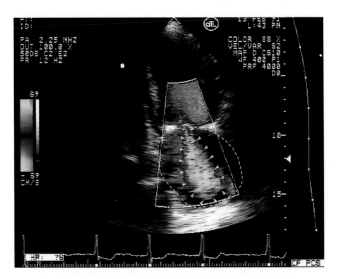

**Fig. 6–33.** Illustration demonstrating how one can attempt to quantitate the severity of mitral regurgitation using color flow Doppler. The area of the regurgitant spray (*arrowheads*) is compared as a ratio of the total area of the left atrium (*dashed line*).

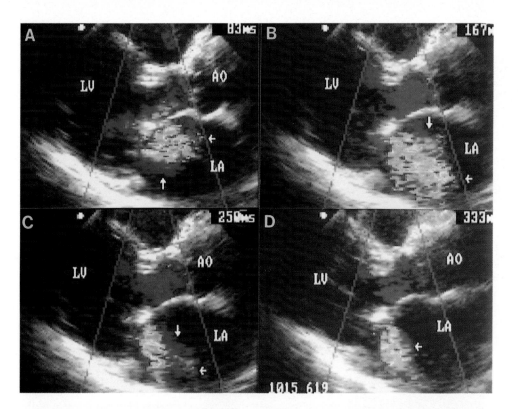

**Fig. 6–34.** Color flow echocardiograms demonstrating a mitral regurgitant jet at different times in the cardiac cycle. Although all four images were obtained during systole, the size and shape of the regurgitant jet (*arrows*) varies. LV = left ventricle; AO = aorta; LA = left atrium.

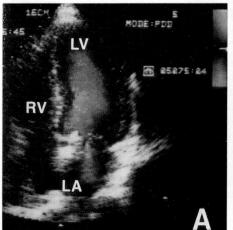
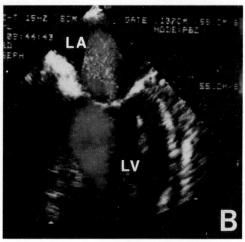

**Fig. 6–35.** Transthoracic (*A*) and transesophageal (*B*) echocardiograms of a patient with mitral regurgitation. The size of the regurgitant jet is significantly larger in the transesophageal examination than in the transthoracic study. LV = left ventricle; RV = right ventricle; LA = left atrium. (From Smith, M.D., et al.: Regurgitant jet size by transesophageal compared with transthoracic Doppler color flow imaging. Circulation, *83*: 81, 1991, by permission of the American Heart Association, Inc.)

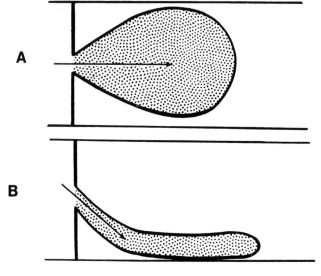

**Fig. 6–36.** Diagram illustrating how the size of the regurgitant jet is influenced by the location of the jet and the chamber into which it is flows. A jet directed into the center of the chamber will have a larger area (*A*) than one that is striking one of the walls (*B*).

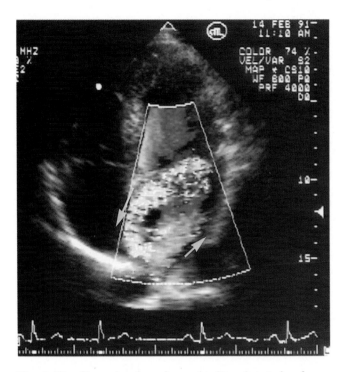

**Fig. 6–37.** Four-chamber view color Doppler study of a patient with an eccentric mitral regurgitant jet. The jet initially is directed toward the interatrial septum (*down arrow*) and then curls around and moves back toward the left ventricle (*up arrow*).

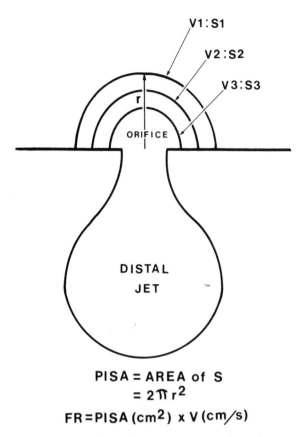

$$PISA = AREA\ of\ S$$
$$= 2\pi r^2$$
$$FR = PISA\ (cm^2) \times V\ (cm/s)$$

**Fig. 6–39** Drawing illustrating how one might calculate the regurgitant volume through an orifice based on the theory of proximal flow acceleration (see text for details). V1:S1 = initial isovelocity surface area; V2:S2 = second isovelocity surface area; V3:S3 = third isovelocity surface area; r = radius from the initial isovelocity surface area and the center of the orifice; PISA = proximal isovelocity surface area; FR = flow rate.

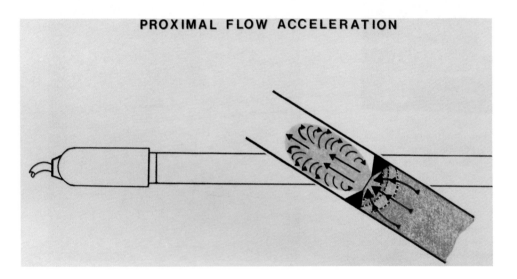

**PROXIMAL FLOW ACCELERATION**

**Fig. 6–38.** Diagram showing the principle of proximal flow acceleration. Blood flowing toward a narrow orifice accelerates. Because color flow is pulsed Doppler and aliases at a relatively low velocity, the flow increases in velocity and changes color as it approaches the orifice. This aliasing produces a series of concentric, colored rings about the narrowed orifice.

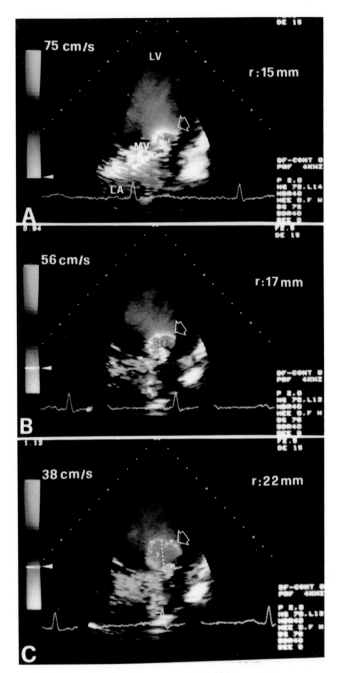

**Fig. 6-40.** Color flow Doppler studies of patients with varying degrees of mitral regurgitation show how the principle of proximal flow acceleration can be used to quantitate mitral regurgitation (see text for details). *Arrow* = initial isovelocity ring; r = radius from the initial isovelocity ring to the mitral orifice; LV = left ventricle; MV = mitral valve; LA = left atrium. (From Bargiggia, G.S., et al.: A new method for quantitation of mitral regurgitation based on color flow Doppler imaging of flow convergence proximal to regurgitant orifice. Circulation, *84*:1483, 1991, by permission of the American Heart Association, Inc.)

flow acceleration (Fig. 6-41*A, arrows*), however, is large, revealing the true severity of the regurgitation.

This technique of using flow convergence to quantitate mitral regurgitation is attractive because it does not have the same limitations as measuring regurgitant jet area. Some data suggest that the convergence technique is also more accurate.[135,138-140,140a,140b] The technique needs to be meticulous, however, to optimize the proximal convergence velocities. Further experience is needed to confirm the validity and accuracy of this approach.

Investigators are also attempting to assess the size of the regurgitant orifice by measuring the diameter of the jet at the mitral orifice (Fig. 6-41*B, arrows*).[141] Some authors are assessing regurgitant volume by measuring the orifice area and velocity to calculate flow.[142]

Color flow imaging can also be displayed as an M-mode recording. Figure 6-42 shows an M-mode color Doppler or M/Q tracing of mitral regurgitation. The blue regurgitant jet is readily visualized. The M/Q tracing provides timing of the regurgitant flow. Because the recording has no spatial orientation, it is used relatively infrequently. One application has been the study of the

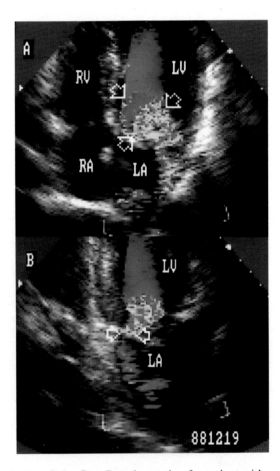

**Fig. 6-41.** Color flow Doppler study of a patient with severe mitral regurgitation. The eccentric jet entering the left atrium is relatively small. The area of the flow acceleration (*A, arrows*) is large and correctly identifies the severity of the regurgitation. *B,* Image illustrates how to measure the width of the regurgitant jet at the valve orifice (*arrows*).

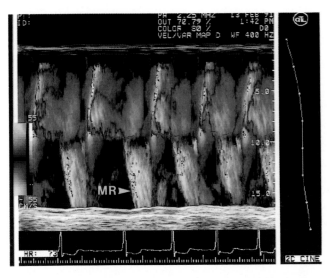

**Fig. 6–42.** M-mode color or M/Q of a patient with mitral regurgitation. The mitral regurgitant jet (MR) can be seen moving away from the transducer in systole. The initial component of the jet is high velocity and turbulent. The velocity decreases in the latter half of systole.

flow velocity profile by analyzing the timing as well as the position and velocity of mitral regurgitant flow.[143]

Spectral Doppler still plays an important role in the evaluation of patients with mitral regurgitation. Figure 6–43 is a pulsed Doppler examination with the sample volume on the atrial side of the mitral valve. The spectral recording demonstrates high-velocity, aliasing holosystolic flow. This approach is still useful for the qualitative assessment of mitral regurgitation. Occasionally, color flow Doppler may miss a regurgitant jet and pulsed spectral Doppler will make the proper diagnosis. Pulsed Doppler has been used to map the left atrium for judging the severity of mitral regurgitation (Fig. 6–44). The prin-

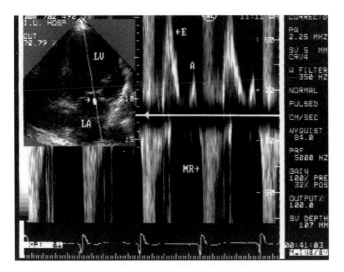

**Fig. 6–43.** Pulsed Doppler examination of patient with mitral regurgitation. The sample volume is within the left atrium (LA) and shows the high velocity, aliasing mitral regurgitant jet (MR). LV = left ventricle.

ciple is that the distance between the orifice and the furthest point that the regurgitant jet can be detected relates to the severity of regurgitation.[102,103] This approach has essentially been replaced with color flow imaging.

The pulsed Doppler technique also gives information with regard to the timing of the regurgitation. For example, in Figure 6–45, one can detect late systolic regurgitation in a patient with mitral valve prolapse. The pulsed Doppler examination also provides information about left ventricular filling. In Figure 6–46, one notes that the mitral inflow E wave is accentuated and the A wave is diminished, one of the manifestations of mitral regurgitation whereby early diastolic filling of the left ventricle is accentuated. Abnormal flow dynamics with mitral regurgitation can also be detected in pulmonary venous flow, usually recorded with transesophageal echocardiography.[144–146] Figure 6–47 shows such a recording in a patient with severe mitral regurgitation that reveals late systolic retrograde flow in the pulmonary vein and increased early diastolic flow.

Pulsed Doppler techniques can also be used to quantitate the severity of mitral regurgitation by calculating regurgitant volumes or regurgitant fractions.[147–149] As noted in Chapter 3, pulsed Doppler techniques combined with two-dimensional echocardiography can be used to calculate blood flow. There are various ways of calculating regurgitant volume or fraction by measuring flow through different orifices. For example, mitral blood flow can be combined with aortic flow to create a regurgitant fraction. Aortic flow is effective cardiac output or stroke volume. Mitral flow includes effective stroke volume plus the flow that leaks back into the left atrium. Thus, mitral flow will be greater than aortic flow. The difference between the two flows represents the regurgitant volume.

One could also calculate total left ventricular stroke volume using two-dimensional echocardiography. Subtracting aortic flow as calculated by pulsed Doppler techniques would again give regurgitant volume. These techniques require that the patient have no additional valvular disease. In the presence of aortic regurgitation, one cannot use aortic flow for determination of effective stroke volume. Under these circumstances, one might resort to pulmonary flow, provided there is no pulmonary regurgitation.

Continuous wave Doppler is also helpful in the assessment of mitral regurgitation.[150] Figure 6–48 shows a continuous wave Doppler recording of a patient with severe mitral regurgitation. The major feature is that the peak velocity occurs early in systole (*arrow*).[145] The later half of systole has a gradual decrease in velocity. This type of recording is indicative of a tall left atrial V wave, which diminishes the left atrial-left ventricular gradient during systole. The decreasing gradient results in the early peak and fall in velocity.

Some investigators have also been looking at the intensity of the continuous wave Doppler spectral recording to quantitate the severity of mitral regurgitation.[151,152] This approach is based on the theory that the number of red cells passing through the regurgitant

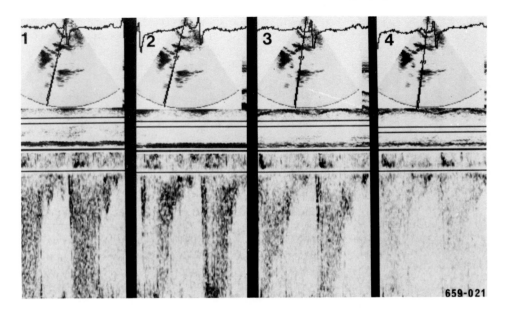

**Fig. 6–44.** Serial Doppler examinations showing mapping for mitral regurgitation with the transducer in the parasternal long-axis position.

orifice will influence the intensity of the spectral recording. Figure 6–49 shows three different Doppler recordings of mitral regurgitation in patients with varying degrees of mitral regurgitation. The intensity of the regurgitant jet is greater with more severe regurgitation. Investigators are also using contrast echocardiography to try to quantitate mitral regurgitation.[153] Injecting contrast material directly into the left ventricle permits one to analyze the washout from the left ventricle and left atrium. Analyzing the clearance of the two chambers gives a quantitative assessment as to the degree of mitral regurgitation. This approach is invasive, but some investigators hope that intravenous injection of contrast material might be able to provide a similar assessment.[153]

Several secondary signs of mitral regurgitation can be detected on M-mode and two-dimensional echocardiograms. These signs include the size of the left atrium, pulsations of the left atrial wall, the size of the left ventricle, aortic valve motion, and the pattern of motion of the interventricular septum.[154–157] Exaggerated septal motion is often seen with a volume overload of the left ventricle.[154,158] An explanation for this excessive motion has not been determined. If one wants to develop a unifying theory on septal motion, however, one can consider the septal motion in patients with left ventricular volume overload to be opposite that noted previously with right ventricular volume overload (see Chapter 3). Assuming that the septum reflects the relative filling

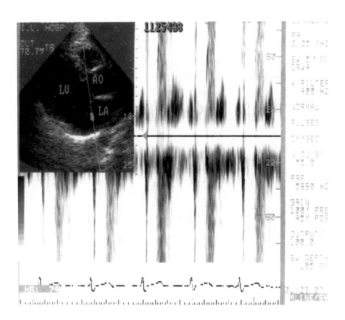

**Fig. 6–45.** Pulsed Doppler echocardiogram of a patient with late systolic mitral regurgitation. LV = left ventricle; AO = aorta; LA = left atrium.

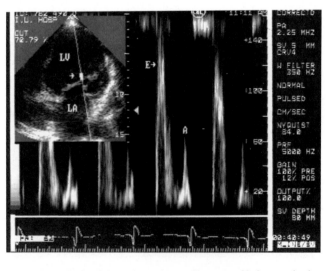

**Fig. 6–46.** Pulsed Doppler echocardiogram of left ventricular inflow of a patient with significant mitral regurgitation. The early diastolic E point is accentuated. LV = left ventricle; LA = left atrium.

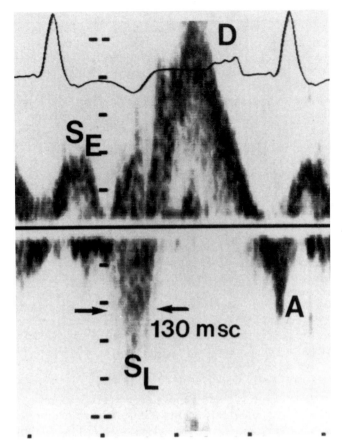

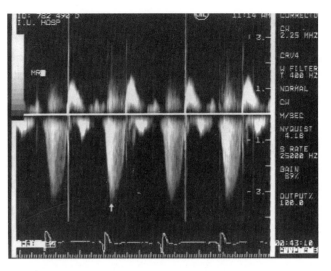

**Fig. 6–48.** Continuous wave Doppler study of a patient with severe acute mitral regurgitation. The regurgitant flow peaks early in systole (*arrow*) and then gradually decreases through the latter two thirds of systole. The shape of this curve is produced by an elevated left atrial pressure during systole (V wave), which decreases the left atrial left ventricular pressure gradient in the later half of systole.

**Fig. 6–47.** Pulmonary venous Doppler study obtained with transesophageal echocardiography of a patient with mitral regurgitation. The early systolic forward flow ($S_E$) is diminished. Late systolic flow ($S_L$) and diastolic foward flow (D) is striking. (From Castello, R., et al.: Evaluation of mitral regurgitation by Doppler echocardiography. J. Echocardiogr., *8*:706, 1991.)

patterns of the two ventricles, then it is not surprising that with the excessive inflow of blood into the left ventricle one expects increased anterior motion of the septum in early diastole. With ventricular systole, the increased left ventricular stroke volume, which exceeds that of the right ventricle, produces an increased posterior motion of the septum.

Increased septal motion is not specific for mitral regurgitation. As noted subsequently, aortic regurgitation also produces exaggerated septal motion. The exact pattern of septal motion is slightly different with mitral regurgitation and aortic insufficiency, principally in the early diastolic septal dip, which is frequently exaggerated with aortic regurgitation,[159] and may be absent with mitral regurgitation.[157] The presence of a dilated left atrium and left ventricle indicates at least moderate regurgitation, but only with chronic and not acute insufficiency.[160]

Researchers have shown considerable interest in evaluating the status of the left ventricle in patients with mitral regurgitation. Attempts have been made to identify those patients who warrant surgical replacement of

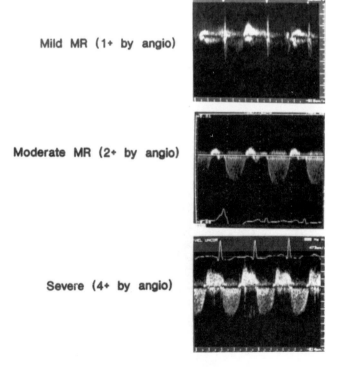

**Fig. 6–49.** Continuous wave Doppler echocardiograms of patients with different degrees of mitral regurgitation demonstrating that the intensity of the Doppler signal is related to the severity of the mitral regurgitation. (From Utsunomiya, T., et al.: Can signal intensity of the continuous wave Doppler regurgitant jet estimate the severity of mitral regurgitation? Am. Heart J., *1*:169, 1992.)

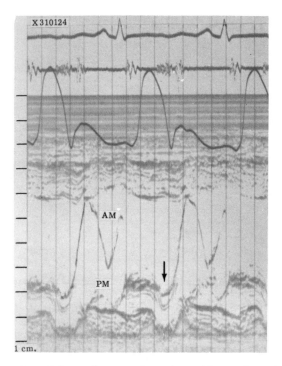

**Fig. 6–50.** Echocardiogram of a patient with a prolapsed mitral valve. Note the late systolic posterior motion of the anterior (AM) and posterior (PM) mitral valve leaflets (*arrow*). This abnormal motion corresponds with a late systolic murmur as seen on the phonocardiogram.

the mitral valve on the basis of left ventricular deterioration.[161-164] Some studies use relatively simple M-mode left ventricular dimensions.[156,157] Other authors have used more elaborate measurements of left ventricular stress (see Chapter 3).[163,164] The stress calculations may be more reliable in identifying those ventricles that will return toward normal following replacement of the mitral valve. These measurements, however, are tedious and are not being done on a routine clinical basis.

Echocardiography is particularly helpful in identifying the etiology of mitral regurgitation. Rheumatic mitral regurgitation is usually identified by finding thickening or fibrosis of the mitral valve and at least some degree of mitral stenosis. A recent study suggests that with acute rheumatic fever, the Doppler echocardiogram characteristically shows a mitral regurgitant jet that is directed toward the posterior lateral wall of the left atrium.[165] Others have also used echocardiography to assess the functional anatomy of mitral regurgitation with active rheumatic carditis.[166] Congenital mitral regurgitation, such as a cleft mitral valve, is discussed in Chapter 7, Congenital Heart Disease. Other common causes of mitral regurgitation are included in the following discussions.

**Mitral Valve Prolapse**

The diagnosis of mitral valve prolapse is probably one of the most important and most confusing applications of echocardiography. The first echocardiographic finding reported with mitral valve prolapse is demonstrated in Figure 6–50. In late ventricular systole, there is posterior displacement of the mitral valve, especially the pos-

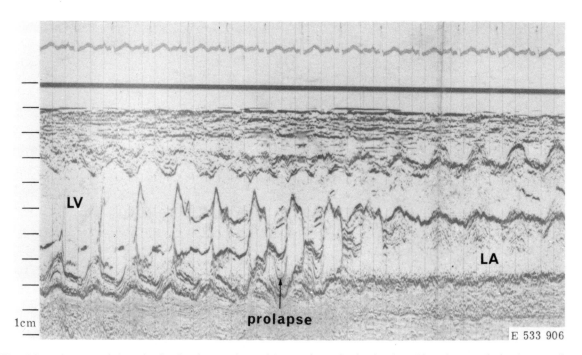

**Fig. 6–51.** M-mode scan of the mitral valve in a patient with a prolapsed mitral valve. The characteristic abnormality (*arrow*) is best seen at the junction between the left ventricle (LV) and the left atrium (LA). (From Chang, S.: Echocardiography: Techniques and Interpretation, Second Ed. Philadelphia, Lea & Febiger, 1981.)

terior leaflet toward the left atrium (*arrow*).[167,168] This posterior or downward displacement of the mitral valve in late systole corresponds with the systolic click and late systolic murmur that are clinical hallmarks of this abnormality. Figure 6–51 demonstrates an M-mode scan showing how the typical M-mode findings for mitral valve prolapse are best seen at the junction between the left ventricle and the left atrium.

The finding of late systolic prolapse, or midsystolic buckling, of the mitral valve has withstood the test of time. With rare exceptions, it has proved reliable with relatively few false positives. Figure 6–52 shows a mitral valve with posterior displacement during the latter two thirds of systole. The mitral valve motion superficially resembles that of mitral valve prolapse. This patient, however, has obvious pericardial effusion with swinging of the entire heart posteriorly during systole. Thus, the apparent mitral valve prolapse is merely a function of total cardiac motion. Although this type of echocardiogram could be misinterpreted as mitral valve prolapse, it is not a true false positive.

Most of the confusion with M-mode echocardiography with regard to mitral valve prolapse is in patients with holosystolic prolapse.[169–171] It was recognized from the beginning that under certain circumstances, the late systolic prolapse could become holosystolic. Figure 6–53A demonstrates a patient with late systolic prolapse (*arrow*). The midsystolic click and late systolic murmur can be seen on the phonocardiogram. With inhalation of amyl nitrite, the patient developed a tachycardia, and the prolapse became holosystolic (Fig. 6–53B). Many patients with mitral valve prolapse only demonstrate the

holosystolic variety (Fig. 6–54). With holosystolic prolapse, new criteria must be developed to differentiate mitral valve prolapse from a normal variant. A small degree of posterior buckling or bowing of the mitral valve in systole can occur in patients with no apparent evidence of mitral valve prolapse. One proposed criterion is that if the mitral valve leaflet extends below 3 mm of a line drawn between the C and D points, then that patient has mitral valve prolapse. This criterion, however, greatly increases the incidence of mitral valve prolapse within the general population.[172–174] One study using the more liberal criteria for mitral valve prolapse showed up to 18% of healthy young females with evidence of mitral valve prolapse.[173] Thus, some echocardiographers have been reluctant to use the 3-mm systolic bowing or hammocking of the mitral valve as the sole criterion for mitral valve prolapse.[175,176]

Another M-mode finding with mitral valve prolapse is anterior motion of the leaflets during systole.[177–179] Figure 6–55 shows a patient with classic late systolic murmur. The echocardiogram exhibits prominent early anterior systolic motion of the mitral valve. Posterior displacement of the mitral leaflets also occurs in the latter half of systole. Figure 6–56 illustrates how the M-mode recording of the prolapsing mitral leaflet may be a function of either displacement of the leaflets moving superiorly toward the left atrium (*B*) or systolic expansion of the mitral annulus (*C*). In both cases, the M-mode scan (M) would exhibit systolic posterior displacement of the posterior leaflet.[180] Annular dilatation is one of many theories with regard to the mechanism for mitral valve prolapse.[181]

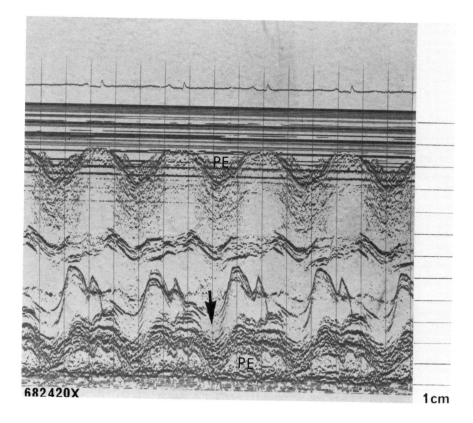

**Fig. 6–52.** M-mode echocardiogram of a patient with a large pericardial effusion (PE) with excessive cardiac motion during systole. The entire heart, including the mitral valve apparatus, moves posteriorly with systole, producing artifactual mitral valve prolapse (*arrow*).

682420X

1cm

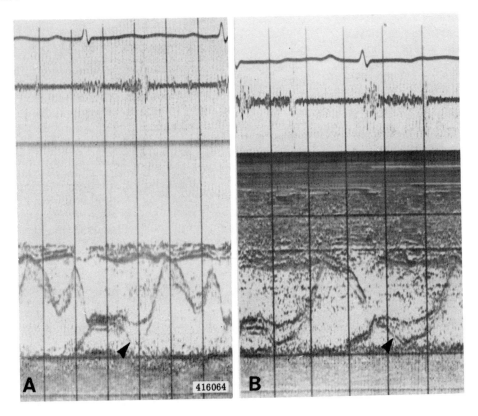

**Fig. 6–53.** Simultaneous mitral valve echocardiograms and phonocardiograms of a patient with a prolapsed mitral valve before (*A*) and after (*B*) the inhalation of amyl nitrite. With this drug, the late systolic prolapse (*arrow, A*) begins earlier, and one sees a holosystolic prolapse and a holosystolic murmur (*arrow, B*). (From Dillon, J.C., et al.: Use of echocardiography in patients with prolapsed mitral valve. Circulation, *43*:503, 1971, by permission of the American Heart Association, Inc.)

Because mitral valve prolapse is principally a displacement or bulging of the mitral leaflet into the left atrium, it would be expected that the spatial orientation inherent in two-dimensional echocardiography might be helpful in establishing this diagnosis. Figure 6–57 diagrammatically demonstrates the long-axis plane of the normal mitral valve in systole. The dotted line extends from the base of the aortic valve to the atrioventricular junction. This line is roughly parallel to the plane of the atrioventricular ring. The closed normal mitral valve does not reach this plane. Figure 6–58 diagrammatically shows how prolapsing anterior and posterior mitral leaf-

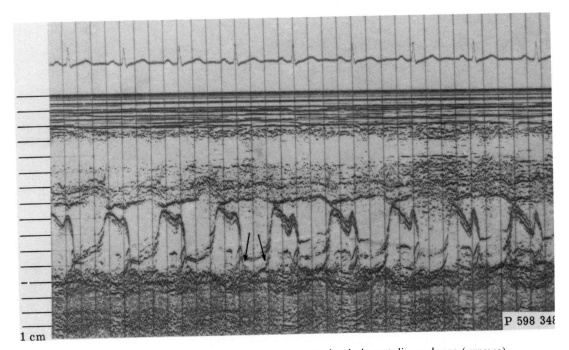

**Fig. 6–54.** Mitral valve echocardiogram demonstrating holosystolic prolapse (*arrows*).

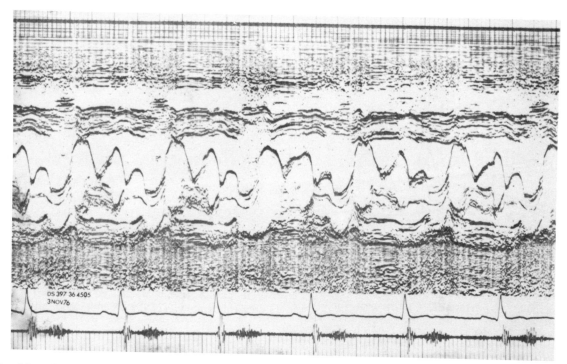

**Fig. 6–55.** M-mode echocardiogram of a patient with mitral valve prolapse. In systole there is initial anterior motion of the mitral leaflet and then posterior motion in the latter half of systole corresponding to the late systolic murmur on the phonocardiogram. (Courtesy of William Jacobs, M.D., Chicago, Illinois.)

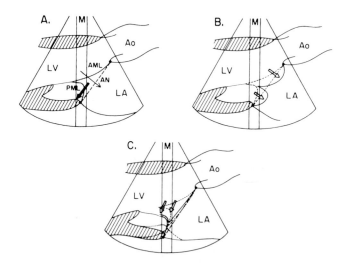

**Fig. 6–56.** Diagram showing how the M-mode ultrasonic beam (M) intersects with the posterior mitral leaflet to produce the M-mode appearance of mitral prolapse (*A*). Posterior displacement of the mitral leaflets in systole can occur with bulging of the leaflets within the left atrium (*B*) or by systolic dilatation of the mitral annulus (*C*). (Reprinted with permission from the American College of Cardiology. From Pini, R., et al.: Mitral valve dimensions and motion and familial transmission of mitral valve prolapse with and without mitral leaflet billowing. J. Am. Coll. Cardiol., *12*:1425, 1988.)

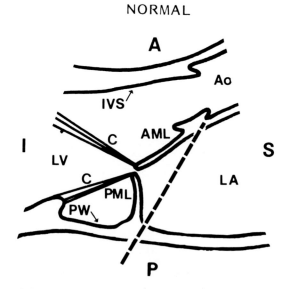

**Fig. 6–57.** Diagram demonstrating the relationship of the closed normal mitral valve to the plane of the mitral annulus (*dotted line*). A = anterior; P = posterior; I = inferior; S = superior; Ao = aorta; IVS = interventricular septum; AML = anterior mitral leaflet; C = chordae; PML = posterior mitral leaflet; PW = posterior wall; LA = left atrium; LV = left ventricle.

ANTERIOR AND POSTERIOR
LEAFLET PROLAPSE

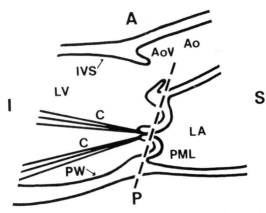

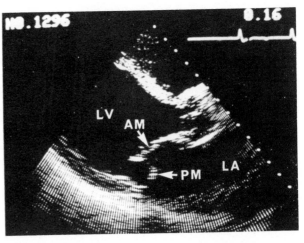

**Fig. 6–58.** Diagram showing the relationship of a prolapsed mitral valve to the plane of the mitral annulus (*dotted line*). In systole, the leaflets protrude into the left atrium and cross the plane of the annulus. A = anterior; P = posterior; I = inferior; S = superior; Ao = aorta; AoV = aorta valve; IVS = interventricular septum; LV = left ventricle; C = chordae; PW = posterior wall; PML = posterior mitral leaflet; LA = left atrium.

**Fig. 6–60.** Long-axis parasternal two-dimensional echocardiogram of a patient with prolapse of the posterior mitral leaflet (PM). AM = anterior mitral leaflet; LV = left ventricle; LA = left atrium. (From Machii, K.: Atlas of Cross-sectional Echocardiography. Tokyo, Toshiba Corporation, 1978.)

lets may bulge through this plane into the left atrium in systole. Figure 6–59 demonstrates a mitral valve echocardiogram that shows the buckling and bowing of the mitral valve (*arrows*) in a patient with mitral valve prolapse.[182] The posterior leaflet actually exhibits a sharp hairpin turn as it bends toward the left atrium. The anterior leaflet curves more gradually, producing an almost right-angle bend at the attachment of the anterior leaflet and the aorta. The posterior leaflet clearly passes through the arbitrary plane between the root of the aorta and the atrioventricular junction. The anterior leaflet is approximately parallel to this plane, well beyond the normal location for the closed mitral valve.

One may not find both leaflets to be prolapsed. Figure 6–60 shows a patient whose prolapse is limited to the posterior leaflet. The bulging of the posterior leaflet into the left atrium is obvious, whereas the anterior leaflet position is normal.

Mitral valve prolapse can also be detected in the four-chamber view.[183,184] Figure 6–61 demonstrates a four-chamber view of a patient with mitral valve prolapse. The bulging of the anterior leaflet is distinctly beyond the plane of the annulus (*dotted line*). No firm criterion has been developed as to when slight bulging beyond the plane of the annulus becomes pathologic.

Using the four-chamber rather than the long-axis view for the diagnosis of mitral valve prolapse has been popular for many years. The four-chamber view permits more

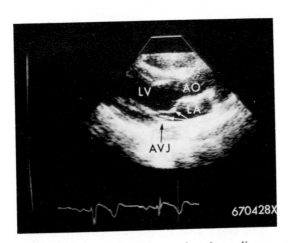

**Fig. 6–59.** Two-dimensional long-axis echocardiogram of a patient with mitral valve prolapse. Both the anterior and posterior mitral leaflets (*arrows*) curve into the left atrium (LA). The posterior leaflet makes almost a hairpin turn as it moves to the atrial side of the atrioventricular junction (AVJ). LV = left ventricle; AO = aorta.

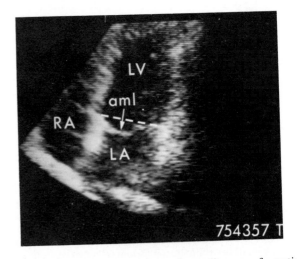

**Fig. 6–61.** Apical four-chamber echocardiogram of a patient with mitral valve prolapse demonstrating a curved anterior mitral leaflet (aml) that extends beyond the plane of the mitral annulus (*dotted line*). LV = left ventricle; LA = left atrium; RA = right atrium.

frequent visualization of the body of both leaflets because the ultrasonic beam is perpendicular to the valve in systole. In addition, the plane of the annulus is horizontal and can be readily appreciated in this view. The annular plane in the parasternal long-axis view is at an angle and its relationship to the valve leaflets is more difficult to assess. Recent findings indicate, however, that one must make the diagnosis of mitral valve prolapse in the four-chamber view with caution. It has been determined that the annulus is nonplanar and is actually shaped like a saddle.[185-188] Thus, the relationship of the leaflets to the annulus is different in the long-axis and the four-chamber views. Figure 6-62 demonstrates how a normal mitral valve could appear to be "prolapsed" when examined in the four-chamber view. This false-positive prolapse is merely a function of the shape of the

annulus, and its relationship to the leaflets in the four-chamber view. Thus, it is hazardous to make the diagnosis of mitral valve prolapse solely on the observation that leaflets bulge into the left atrium in the four-chamber view. This limitation is particularly true if both leaflets move equally. If, as noted in Figure 6-61, one leaflet prolapses more than the other, then the diagnosis is more secure.

A problem with relying solely on displacement of the mitral leaflets toward the left atrium for the diagnosis of mitral valve prolapse is that some of this displacement may be a function of body habitus and the size of the left ventricle. It is recognized that mitral valve prolapse is more common in young, thin females. For example, the incidence of prolapse is high in ballet dancers[189] and in patients with anorexia nervosa.[190] The mitral valve may bulge into the left atrium in patients with an atrial septal defect and a small left ventricle.[191,192] Even dehydration may induce echocardiographic signs of mitral valve prolapse in otherwise healthy females.[192a] In all of these cases, the leaflets may not be anatomically abnormal but may be relatively redundant for a fairly small left ventricular cavity.

Besides bowing and displacement of the valve, other two-dimensional echocardiographic criteria have been proposed to assist with the diagnosis of mitral valve prolapse. One study noted posterior displacement of the coaptation point of the two leaflets.[182,193] Figure 6-63 demonstrates a two-dimensional echocardiogram of a patient with a large anterior mitral leaflet (mv) the tip of which is close to the posterior atrioventricular groove in systole. Unfortunately, this technique has not been confirmed, and its reliability is questionable. One study revealed an abnormal contraction pattern of the interventricular septum in patients with mitral valve prolapse.[194] In the apical four-chamber view, vigorous contraction of the septum produced bending of the septum toward the left ventricle. Others have looked at left ventricular wall motion in patients with mitral valve prolapse.[195]

Although most clinicians are aware of the distortion of the mitral valve in systole, the pathologist also sees histologic changes in the valve. These changes have been referred to as "myxomatous degeneration." This term may or may not be correct since the principal histologic finding apparently is collagen degeneration within the leaflets.[196] The echocardiogram occasionally reflects the histologic changes.[197,198] Figure 6-64 demonstrates two views of a floppy, prolapsing mitral valve. The anterior leaflet is thickened and appears redundant. The short-axis view also demonstrates the thickening as well as the redundancy of the valve.

Figure 6-65 shows another example of classic mitral prolapse. Thickening of the valve, noted best during diastole, is evident, as is marked protrusion of the leaflets into the left atrium in systole.

Another possible echocardiographic sign for mitral valve prolapse is the size of the mitral valve annulus.[199] Both the size and contraction of the annulus have been noted to be abnormal in patients with mitral valve prolapse.

## SADDLE-SHAPE ANNULUS
### CONCAVE LEAFLETS
#### LONG-AXIS VIEW

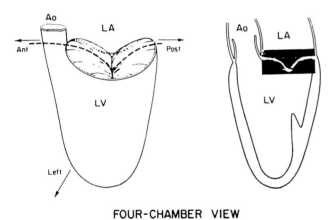

#### FOUR-CHAMBER VIEW

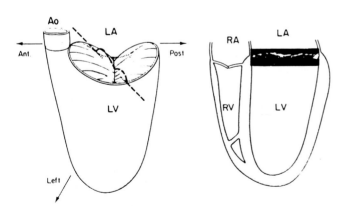

**Fig. 6-62.** Drawing demonstrating the principle of how the shape of the mitral annulus can produce apparent mitral valve prolapse in a normal individual when viewed in the four-chamber view. Because of the saddle shape of the annulus, the planar relationship of the mitral leaflets and the annulus is different in the long-axis and four-chamber views. As a result, even in the normal individual, the mitral leaflets may extend beyond the mitral annulus in the four-chamber view. (From Levine, R.A., et al.: The relationship of mitral annular shape to the diagnosis of mitral valve prolapse. Circulation, *75*:763, 1987, by permission of the American Heart Association, Inc.)

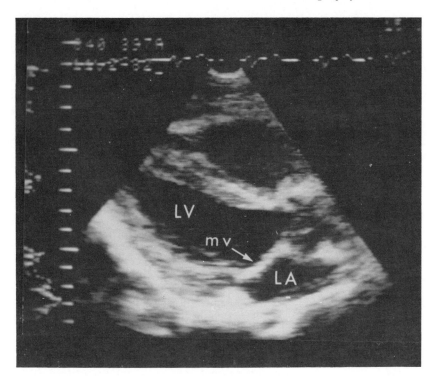

**Fig. 6–63.** Long-axis two-dimensional echocardiogram of a patient with mitral valve prolapse. The anterior mitral leaflet (mv) is large, thickened, and redundant with a coaptation point near the posterior wall. LV = left ventricle; LA = left atrium.

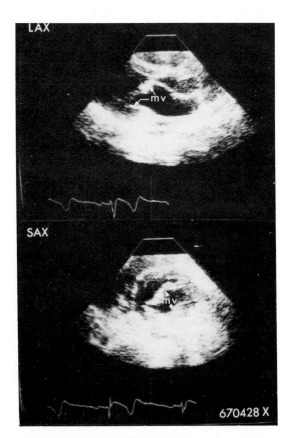

**Fig. 6–64.** Long-axis (LAX) and short-axis (SAX) two-dimensional echocardiograms of a patient with mitral valve prolapse. The leaflets are thickened and appear redundant in the short-axis view. mv = mitral valve.

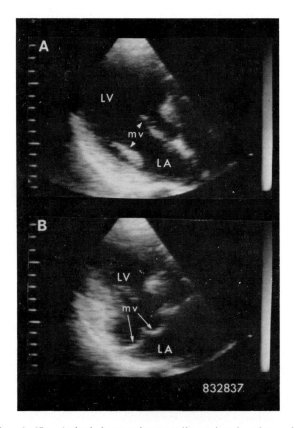

**Fig. 6–65.** Apical long-axis two-dimensional echocardiograms of a patient with marked mitral valve prolapse. The thickening of the leaflets (mv) can be observed best in diastole (A). The protrusion of the leaflets into the left atrium (LA) is striking with ventricular systole (B). LV = left ventricle.

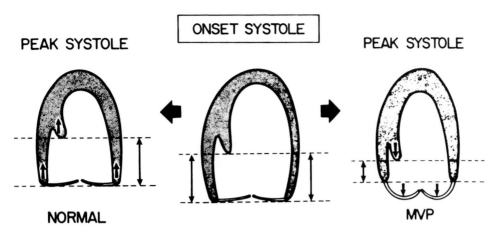

PEAK SYSTOLE      ONSET SYSTOLE      PEAK SYSTOLE

NORMAL      MVP

**Fig. 6–66.** Diagram demonstrating how the relationship of the leaflets to papillary muscles may be a mechanism for mitral valve prolapse. Normally, the papillary muscles contract toward the apex and keep the mitral leaflets aligned with the mitral annulus. With mitral prolapse (MVP), however, at peak systole, the papillary muscles fail to contract toward the apex, thus permitting the mitral leaflets to protrude toward the left atrium. (Reprinted with permission from the American College of Cardiology. From Sanfilippo, A.J., et al.: Papillary muscle traction in mitral valve prolapse: Quantitation by two-dimensional echocardiography. J. Am. Coll. Cardiol., *19*:567, 1992.)

A recent study highlighted the contribution of the papillary muscles to the mitral prolapse phenomenon.[200] Figure 6–66 demonstrates that with mitral prolapse, the relationship of the mitral annulus and the papillary muscles differs from normal. Apparently, the annulus-papillary muscle dimension is similar in both situations at end diastole. With systole, the normal annulus and papillary muscles move toward the apex. With mitral prolapse, the annulus again moves toward the apex, although the papillary muscle moves toward the base, producing a shortened dimension between the tip of the papillary muscle and the annulus. Other authors think that abnormal chordal insertion is a cause for mitral prolapse.[201]

Doppler echocardiography has also been used to assist in the diagnosis of mitral valve prolapse.[202–204] When present, mitral regurgitation is classically late systolic (see Fig. 6–45). In addition, because one leaflet prolapses more than the other, the regurgitant jet frequently is eccentric.[205]

Mitral valve prolapse has been associated with numerous complications, including rhythm disturbances, sudden death, panic attacks, systemic emboli, bacterial endocarditis, and severe mitral regurgitation. Some of these complications, such as sudden death and panic attacks, are either rare or nonexistent. The possibility of bacterial endocarditis and severe mitral regurgitation is of course a major concern and frequently requires appropriate management. Systemic emboli are extremely rare. Figure 6–67 shows an example of a patient with mitral valve prolapse who had a protruding clot at the junction between the mitral leaflet and its attachment to the septum.[206,207]

How echocardiography is to be used in patients with mitral valve prolapse is still being debated.[208–210] As indicated, the diagnostic criteria vary.[211] Some echocardiographic signs are reliable for the diagnosis of mitral prolapse. The more reliable signs include late systolic posterior bulging of the mitral leaflets on M-mode echo-

cardiography, billowing of the mitral leaflets in the parasternal long-axis view on the two-dimensional echocardiogram, and thickened, redundant, floppy mitral leaflets. Those signs that are less reliable include holosystolic prolapse on the M-mode echocardiogram and mitral valve billowing in the four-chamber, two-dimensional view. Doppler evidence of mitral regurgitation is less specific for mitral prolapse, except for the finding of late systolic mitral regurgitation and possibly an eccentric jet. Thickened leaflets appear to be associated with a poor prognosis and is more likely to progress to severe mitral regurgitation and possibly ruptured chordae.[212,213]

Naturally, esophageal echocardiography can be helpful in identifying mitral valve prolapse.[214] Figure 6–68 demonstrates an esophageal echocardiogram of mitral prolapse whereby the various mitral scallops can be seen clearly. The horizontal and longitudinal views may differ somewhat in the appearance of the prolapsing, scalloped leaflets. The esophageal approach is particularly helpful for monitoring surgical repair of the valve.

### Papillary Muscle Dysfunction

Several echocardiographic signs have been described for patients with papillary muscle dysfunction. The gold standard for this diagnosis is usually a patient with coronary artery disease or a dilated left ventricle and the presence or development of mitral regurgitation. One of the suspected mechanisms for this valvular regurgitation is dilatation of the mitral annulus. Several authors have noted two-dimensional echocardiographic evidence of mitral annulus dilatation in these patients.[215,216] Protrusion of the leaflets into the left atrium in systole, compatible with mitral valve prolapse, may also be present in patients with papillary muscle dysfunction.[215]

One of the causes of papillary muscle dysfunction is scarring of the papillary muscles secondary to myocar-

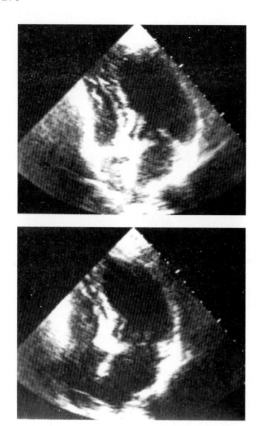

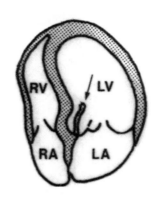

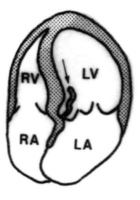

**Fig. 6–67.** Two-dimensional echocardiogram of a patient with mitral valve prolapse who demonstrates a long, filamentous thrombus (*arrows*) between the septal leaflet and the interventricular septum. (From Egeblad, H. and Hesse, B.: Mitral valve prolapse with mobile polypoid cul-de-sac thrombus and embolism to brain and lower extremity. Am. Heart J., *114*:649, 1987.)

dial infarction. With shrinkage and thinning of the papillary muscle, the chordae are pulled away from the mitral orifice. The thinning and dilatation of the muscle to which the papillary muscle is attached also contribute to shortening of the mitral valve apparatus. As a result, the leaflet or leaflets attached to the chordae and papillary muscle are prohibited from closing completely. Figure 6–69 demonstrates a scarred papillary muscle secondary to infarction in a patient with coronary artery disease. In systole, the mitral valve (mv) does not close all the way to the level of the mitral annulus (*dashed line*).[217] This observation has been confirmed by other authors.[215,218] Incomplete mitral valve closure and presumed papillary muscle dysfunction can also be seen in patients with a dilated cardiomyopathy. In these patients, the papillary muscles apparently migrate away from the annulus producing relative shortening of the valve apparatus. Complete closure of the leaflets is again prohibited.

### Flail Mitral Valve

A flail mitral valve is best detected with two-dimensional echocardiography.[219–223] Extension of part of the valve into the left atrium in systole can be readily noted with this spatially oriented examination.[219,220,222]

Figure 6–70 shows echocardiograms from a patient with a flail anterior mitral leaflet. The flail leaflet (*arrow*) is seen as a thickened valve in diastole (Fig. 6–70A). In systole, the diseased leaflet protrudes into the left atrium with the tip of the leaflet pointing toward the left atrium

(Fig. 6–70B). A short-axis view again demonstrates the flail leaflet protruding into the left atrium in systole (Fig. 6–70C). Figure 6–71 demonstrates the apical long-axis view (A) and an apical four-chamber view (B) of a patient with a flail posterior leaflet (fml). Again, the abnormal leaflet protrudes into the left atrium during systole with the tip of the leaflet pointing toward the left atrium. The direction in which the leaflet points is the principal criterion for distinguishing a flail mitral leaflet from severe mitral valve prolapse.[220,221] In one study, the authors noted that the tip of the flail leaflet may point toward the left atrium in diastole in some patients with flail mitral valve.[224]

One of the most common causes for flail mitral leaflet is ruptured chordae tendineae. In a study of 32 such patients, the authors noted three principal two-dimensional echocardiographic features.[225] Noncoaptation of the two leaflets occurred in 55% of the patients. In approximately 20% of the patients, systolic fluttering of the valve in the left atrium could be noted. Of this series of patients, 65% had diastolic chaotic motion of the leaflets seen best in the short-axis view. All three signs were specific for flail mitral leaflet. Combining the three signs provided a sensitivity of 85%.

Another less common cause of flail mitral leaflet is a ruptured papillary muscle. The ruptured papillary muscle can occasionally be visualized on two-dimensional echocardiography[226] (Fig. 6–72).

As with mitral valve prolapse, the Doppler jet is usually eccentric with flail mitral leaflet.[227] The degree of mitral regurgitation usually is more severe with a flail

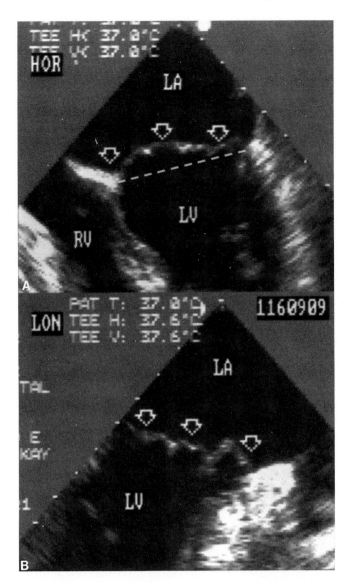

**Fig. 6–68.** Transesophageal echocardiograms of a patient with mitral valve prolapse. The horizontal examination (A) shows the billowing mitral leaflet (*arrows*) extending beyond the mitral annulus (*dashed line*) into the left atrium (LA). The longitudinal examination (B) demonstrates the multiple scallops (*arrows*) and a somewhat different appearance of the same mitral leaflet. LV = left ventricle; RV = right ventricle.

**Fig. 6–70.** Two-dimensional echocardiograms of a patient with a flail anterior mitral valve leaflet. The thickened anterior leaflet is seen best in the long-axis view in diastole (*arrow, A*). The thickened leaflet (*arrow*) protrudes into the left atrium (LA) in systole and can be seen in the parasternal long-axis view (B) and in the short-axis examination (C). LV = left ventricle; AO = aorta; RV = right ventricle.

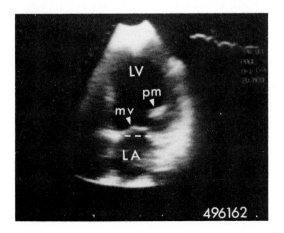

**Fig. 6–69.** Apical four-chamber two-dimensional echocardiogram of a patient with coronary artery disease, a scarred papillary muscle (pm), and papillary muscle dysfunction. With systole, the mitral valve leaflets (mv) fail to reach the level of the mitral annulus (*dashed line*). LV = left ventricle; LA = left atrium.

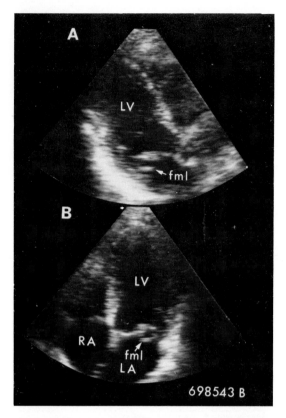

**Fig. 6–71.** Apical two-chamber and four-chamber views of a patient with a flail mitral leaflet. The flail leaflet (fml) can be seen protruding into the left atrium (LA) during ventricular systole. LV = left ventricle; RA = right atrium.

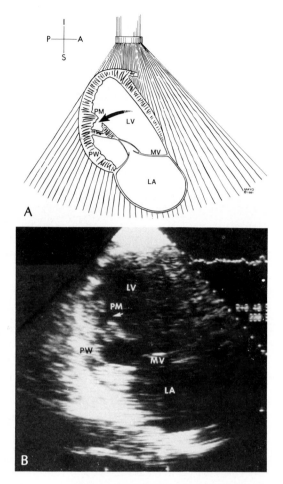

**Fig. 6–72.** Two-dimensional echocardiogram and diagram of a patient with a partial rupture of the papillary muscle (PM) following acute myocardial infarction. LV = left ventricle; PW = posterior left ventricular wall; MV = mitral valve; LA = left atrium. (From Nishimura, R.A., Shub, C., and Tajik, A.J.: Two-dimensional echocardiographic diagnosis of partial papillary muscle rupture. Br. Heart J., *48*:598, 1982.)

leaflet. The direction of the jet is opposite to the flail leaflet. For example, if the anterior leaflet is flail, the jet will be directed posteriorly.

Transesophageal echocardiography can provide spectacular views of flail mitral leaflets.[228–231] Figure 6–73 demonstrates a mitral valve with ruptured chordae protruding deeply into the left atrium in systole. The eccentric regurgitant jets that commonly accompany flail leaflets, produce striking color Doppler echocardiograms with the transesophageal approach (Fig. 6–74D). This illustration also demonstrates that a strikingly flail leaflet (Fig. 6–74B and C) may not be seen in every view of the valve (Fig. 6–74A). Transesophageal echocardiography is particularly useful in monitoring surgical repair of a flail mitral valve.[232–235] Figure 6–75 provides an example of a flail valve before and after repair.

Several M-mode echocardiographic signs of flail mitral valve have been described.[223] One pattern is indistinguishable from marked mitral valve prolapse and usually primarily involves the posterior leaflet.[236] A more common M-mode finding is coarse diastolic fluttering of the mitral leaflets.[237–240] Figure 6–76 shows a patient who had bacterial endocarditis with torn chordae and a flail mitral leaflet. The fluttering of the anterior leaflet during diastole is chaotic and coarse.

As with two-dimensional echocardiography, one of the more reliable M-mode signs of a flail mitral valve is when part of the leaflet is recorded in the left atrium.[236,238–240] Figure 6–77 shows an M-mode echocardiogram of a flail valve whereby part of the valve appears within the left atrium during ventricular systole (FML). This echocardiogram exhibits another sign of a flail valve, i.e. fine systolic fluttering of the valve.[241–243] Systolic fluttering is usually a sign of torn chordae[243] or fenestration of the valve.[241] A ruptured papillary muscle rarely produces systolic fluttering.

One investigator has described characteristic vertical striations of the Doppler signal when mitral regurgitation is the result of a flail mitral valve. The continuous wave Doppler signal has also been noted to be characteristic. Figure 6–78 shows the various types of regurgitant jets that can be recorded with continuous wave Doppler.[227] This continuous wave pattern occurs in part because of the eccentricity of the jet.

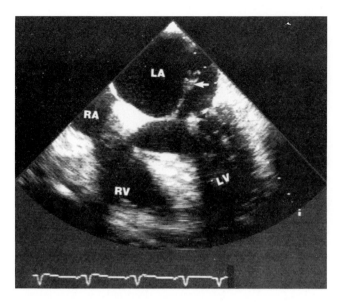

**Fig. 6–73.** Transesophageal echocardiogram of a patient with ruptured mitral chordae tendineae (*arrowhead*). The torn chordae and possible tip of the papillary muscle (*arrow*) is seen protruding deeply within the left atrium (LA). LV = left ventricle; RA = right atrium; RV = right ventricle. (From Alam, N. and Sun, I.: Superiority of transesophageal echocardiography in detecting ruptured mitral chordae tendineae. Am. Heart J., *121*:1820, 1991.)

## AORTIC VALVE DISEASE

Although isolated aortic valve disease is possibly always congenital and may be a consequence of a bicuspid aortic valve, aortic stenosis and insufficiency are progressive problems that usually affect adults. In addition, these two valvular problems are frequently secondary to rheumatic heart disease. Because rheumatic and congenital aortic valve disease may be indistinguishable echocardiographically, both aortic stenosis and aortic regurgitation are discussed in this chapter. Congenital aortic stenosis, especially in this child, is also discussed in Chapter 7, Congenital Heart Disease.

### Aortic Stenosis

Two-dimensional echocardiography provides an excellent morphologic characterization of the stenotic aortic valve.[244,245] Figure 6–79 demonstrates systolic and diastolic frames from a long-axis two-dimensional study of a normal aortic valve (av). In systole, the aortic valve appears as two thin parallel lines that lie close to the walls of the aorta (Fig. 6–79A). The echoes from the leaflets are straight and parallel to the aortic wall. During diastole, the leaflets come together. Most of the valve is parallel to the ultrasonic beam and hence is seen faintly, it at all. The point of coaptation (av) (Fig. 6–79B) is recorded as a small linear echo in the middle of the aorta.

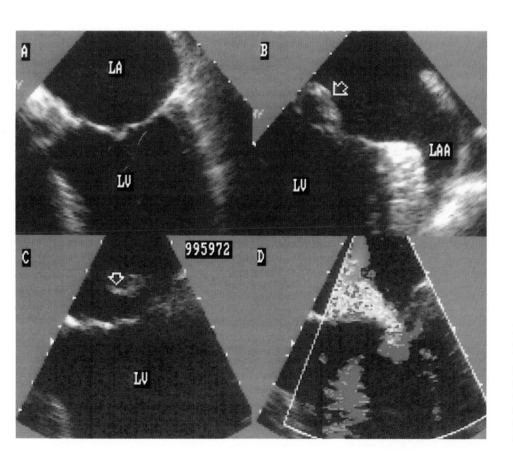

**Fig. 6–74.** Transesophageal echocardiograms of a patient with a flail mitral leaflet. The flail leaflet is readily seen in *B* and *C* (*arrows*), but is not as obvious in *A*. The eccentric color Doppler regurgitant jet is noted in *D*. LA = left atrium; LV = left ventricle.

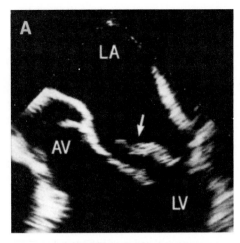 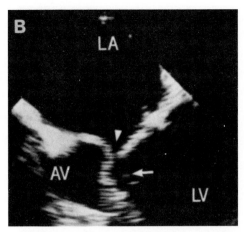

**Fig. 6–75.** Transesophageal echocardiograms obtained at the time of mitral valve repair showing the mitral leaflets before (*A*) and after (*B*) surgical correction of the valve. The lack of apposition of the leaflets (*arrow*) is obvious before repair, whereas a more normal relationship of the leaflets can be appreciated after surgery (*arrowhead*). Note also systolic anterior motion of the mitral apparatus after repair (*arrow, B*). LA = leaf atrium; AV = aortic valve; LV = left ventricle. (Reprinted with permission from the American College of Cardiology. From Freeman, W.K., et al.: Intraoperative evaluation of mitral valve regurgitation and repair by transesophageal echocardiography: Incidence and significance of systolic anterior motion. J. Am. Coll. Cardiol., *20*:599, 1992.)

With valvular aortic stenosis, the valve becomes thickened and is frequently seen in diastole (Fig. 6–80*A*). A more important sign of valvular stenosis is systolic doming (Fig. 6–80*B*). The echoes from the leaflets are no longer parallel to the aorta. The edges of the leaflets are curved toward the center of the aorta. Occasionally, only one of the aortic leaflets, usually the anterior or right coronary cusp, is visualized well in sys-

tole. If one cusp is domed (Fig. 6–81), then this finding is sufficient for the qualitative diagnosis of aortic stenosis. A semilunar valve should not be domed or curved unless the valve is unable to open widely. Doming is probably the most important two-dimensional echocardiographic finding for any form of valvular stenosis. The same type of doming is seen with mitral, pulmonic, and tricuspid stenoses.

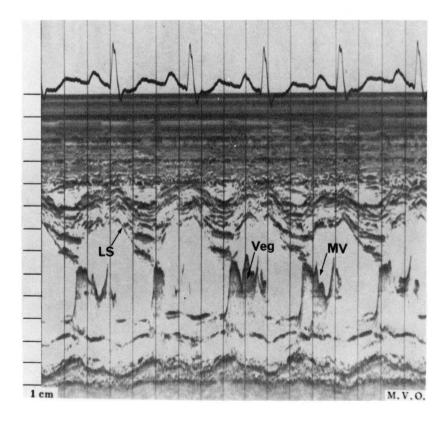

**Fig. 6–76.** Mitral valve echocardiogram of a patient with torn chordae of the anterior mitral leaflet and vegetations (Veg) secondary to bacterial endocarditis. During diastole, the anterior leaflet (MV) exhibits chaotic, coarse fluttering. LS = left side of septum.

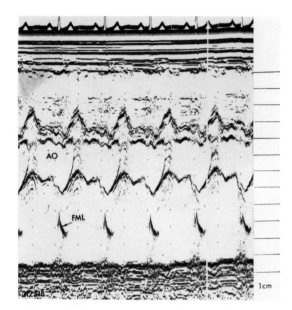

**Fig. 6–77.** M-mode echocardiogram of the aorta (AO) and left atrium of a patient with a flail mitral leaflet (FML). During systole, part of the flail mitral valve can be seen extending into the left atrial cavity.

Figure 6–82 shows a long-axis and short-axis view of a patient with valvular aortic stenosis. The domed, thickened aortic valve can be seen in the long axis. The reduced separation of the leaflets is also apparent. The short-axis view provides another way of evaluating the stenotic valve. Although efforts at quantitating aortic stenosis by measuring the cross-sectional area have been unsuccessful,[246] the short-axis view is still useful in providing a semiquantitative assessment of the aortic stenosis by looking at valve mobility.[247]

The stenotic aortic valve can be visualized with transesophageal echocardiography. Because of the higher

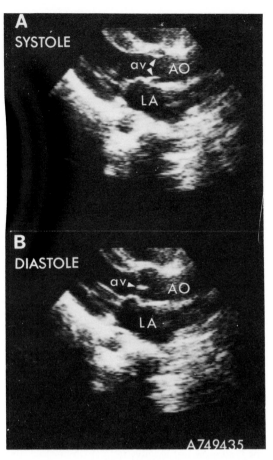

**Fig. 6–79.** Long-axis two-dimensional examination of a normal aortic valve (av). *A,* In systole, the opened aortic leaflets are parallel to each other and lie near the wall of the aorta (AO). *B,* In diastole, the point at which the leaflets coapt is seen as a bright echo within the aorta. Faint echoes from the body of the leaflets may occasionally be seen. LA = left atrium.

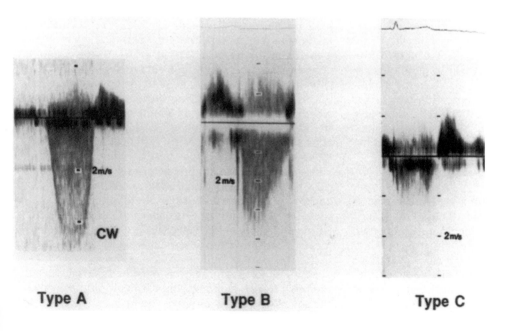

**Type A**  **Type B**  **Type C**

**Fig. 6–78.** Continuous wave Doppler examinations of patients with flail mitral leaflets. One may obtain a complete envelope of the regurgitant jet (type A). Because of the eccentric nature of the jet, however, one may detect incomplete envelopes such as type B or type C. (Reprinted with permission from the American College of Cardiology. From Pearson, A.C., et al.: Color Doppler echocardiographic evaluation of patients with a flail mitral leaflet. J. Am. Coll. Cardiol., *16*:235, 1990.)

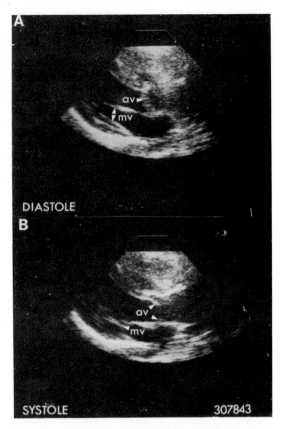

**Fig. 6–80.** Long-axis two-dimensional echocardiograms of a thickened, stenotic aortic valve (av). *A,* In diastole, the body of the thickened leaflets can be seen. *B,* In systole, doming of the aortic valve is apparent. mv = mitral valve.

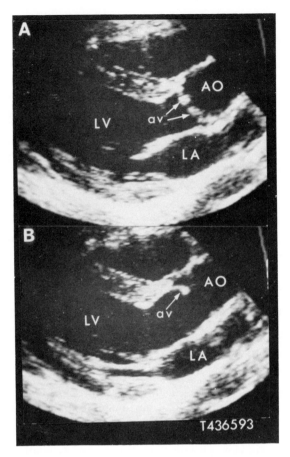

**Fig. 6–81.** Long-axis two-dimensional echocardiograms of a patient with valvular aortic stenosis. The thickened aortic leaflets (av) can easily be seen in diastole (*A*). In systole, doming of only the anterior or right coronary cusp (*B*) is visualized. LV = left ventricle; AO = aorta; LA = left atrium.

resolution inherent with this esophageal approach, investigators have revived the possibility of measuring the aortic valve area in short-axis views using the transesophageal approach.[248] Figure 6–83 demonstrates such an effort.

Figure 6–84 demonstrates long-axis views of the aortic valve in systole in a patient with calcific aortic stenosis. The two frames demonstrate that variability in aortic valve separation can occur in these often eccentrically oriented orifices. In Figure 6–84*A,* the separation is a barely visible slit (av). By changing the scanning plane, one can find a somewhat wider separation (av) (Fig. 6–84*B*). Echoes from the leaflets of the aortic valve are barely visible in the short-axis view. Frequently, the mobility or lack thereof can be appreciated in the short axis with a heavily calcified aortic valve.

The principle means of quantitating aortic stenosis is with Doppler echocardiography.[249–254] The observation that one could accurately measure a pressure gradient across the stenotic aortic valve using the modified Bernoulli equation was the development that propelled Doppler echocardiography into the prominent role that it plays today.[255–258] Valvular aortic stenosis is an important valvular problem, especially in the older population. The need to quantitate the degree of aortic stenosis is great, and Doppler techniques are playing a major role in this effort.

Figure 6–85 shows a continuous wave Doppler recording in a patient with valvular aortic stenosis. One notes a high velocity that peaks at about 4 M/sec. The velocity also peaks in mid-systole. The recording is taken with the transducer at the apex and flow is moving away from the transducer. Figure 6–86 shows another continuous wave recording from the suprasternal notch showing a high velocity jet moving toward the transducer. In this case, the flow peaks at only 2.7 L/sec, which equates to a 30-mm gradient. In addition, with this lesser degree of aortic stenosis, one can see that the peak velocity occurs in early systole. Figure 6–87 is an illustration from the study that probably confirmed the validity of using the modified Bernoulli equation to predict the pressure gradient with aortic stenosis.[259,260] As can be seen in this recording, the relationship between the aortic valve gradient measured at cardiac catheterization and the Doppler velocities is excellent. This illustration also shows how the peak velocity occurs earlier in the presence of milder disease.

Many important limitations must be realized when attempting to use Doppler echocardiography to evaluate the severity of valvular aortic stenosis.[261–263] First, the velocities involved are high, and one must use some-

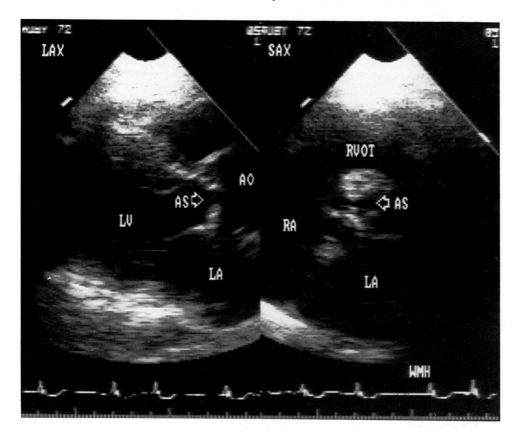

**Fig. 6–82.** Long-axis (LAX) and short-axis (SAX) views of a patient with aortic stenosis (AS). The long-axis examination shows classic doming, restricted motion, and reduced separation of the leaflets. The elliptical orifice frequently can be identified in the short-axis examination. LV = left ventricle; AO = aorta; LA = left atrium; RVOT = right ventricular outflow tract; RA = right atrium.

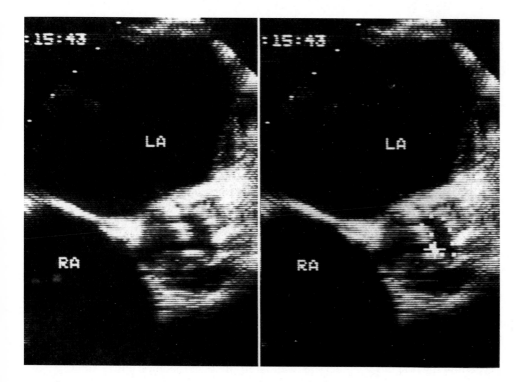

**Fig. 6–83.** Transesophageal echocardiogram showing how one might measure the aortic stenosis orifice (*dotted line*) using this type of examination. LA = left atrium; RA = right atrium. (From Stoddard, M.F., et al.: Two-dimensional transesophageal echocardiographic determination of aortic valve area in adults with aortic stenosis. Am. Heart J., *122*:1416, 1991.)

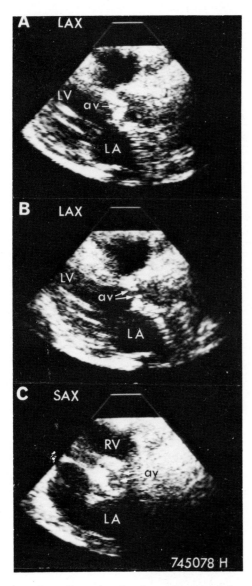

**Fig. 6–84.** Two-dimensional echocardiograms of a patient with calcific aortic stenosis. *A* and *B* are long-axis (LAX) examinations demonstrating the differences in aortic valve separation (av) that can be obtained. *C* is a short-axis (SAX) examination of the valve. LV = left ventricle; LA = left atrium; RV = right ventricle.

thing other than simple pulsed Doppler techniques. Most of the data generated thus far have been obtained with continuous wave Doppler. One can also use high pulse repetition frequency Doppler to make similar measurements.[264] One major problem is that the examiner must attempt to direct the ultrasonic beam so that it is essentially parallel to a small, high-velocity jet. Occasionally, one can use color flow imaging to help identify the direction and location of the jet to make certain that the ultrasonic beam is as parallel as possible.[265] One usually must use multiple echocardiographic windows to find the proper recording. These windows include the left parasternal, right parasternal, apical, suprasternal notch, and, especially in children, the subcostal approach.

Figure 6–88 illustrates how technique is important in obtaining the correct Doppler recording in patients with aortic stenosis. In Figure 6–88*A*, the peak velocity is approximately 2.4 M/sec. With angulation of the transducer, one finds another Doppler recording with a higher velocity jet, 3.7 M/sec. The true stenotic jet is recorded in Figure 6–88*B*. The Doppler recording in Figure 6–88*A* is probably from the larger, lower velocity parajet that surrounds the central or true jet through the stenotic orifice. A correct stenotic jet has a distinctive high velocity audible sound, and the spectral display shows a fine feathery appearance that is usually less dense than the more dominant lower frequency velocity from the parajet. One must also not confuse a mitral regurgitation jet for aortic stenosis.[266] Transpulmonary contrast administration is being suggested as a possible way to enhance a weak aortic stenosis Doppler signal.[267]

Figure 6–89 demonstrates yet another factor that must be appreciated when using Doppler echocardiography to predict pressure gradients in patients with valvular aortic stenosis. In the cardiac catheterization laboratory, it is common practice to measure the pressure gradient from the peak of the left ventricular systolic pressure to the peak pressure in the aorta. As noted in Figure 6–89, these two peak pressures do not occur at the same time, thus, the "peak-to-peak" gradient is really only a difference between two pressures and not a true instantaneous gradient. The peak instantaneous pressure gradient actually occurs before the peak aortic pressure and is larger than the peak-to-peak gradient. Thus, consistent overestimation of the peak-to-peak gradient should occur using Doppler echocardiography. The mean systolic gradients from both the Doppler and pressure recordings are both true gradients and are better for comparison purposes.[268,269]

It must also be recognized that the pressure gradient does not always reflect the severity of the aortic stenosis. In a setting of low cardiac output, the amount of blood flowing through the stenotic valve is reduced and the gradient also is reduced. Thus, the ultimate answer is not just pressure gradient but aortic valve area. In the cardiac catheterization laboratory, one uses the Gorlin formula to calculate valve area using the pressure gradient and cardiac output. One can use a similar approach with Doppler echocardiography by using a measure of cardiac output either by Doppler techniques or with invasive right heart catheterization.[270,271] Even though right heart catheterization is invasive, the determination of aortic valve area using the Doppler aortic gradient obviates the need for crossing a stenotic aortic valve with a catheter or doing a trans-septal catheterization.

A more common and simpler approach to measuring aortic valve area using Doppler echocardiography relies on the continuity equation.[272–275] The principle of the continuity equation has been described in earlier chapters as well as in the discussion of mitral stenosis. Because blood flow or stroke volume is equal to velocity times cross-sectional area, and blood flow through the left ventricular outflow tract (LVOT) must equal flow through the valve (AS), then LVOT (area) × LVOT (velocity) = AS (area) × AS (velocity) or aortic valve

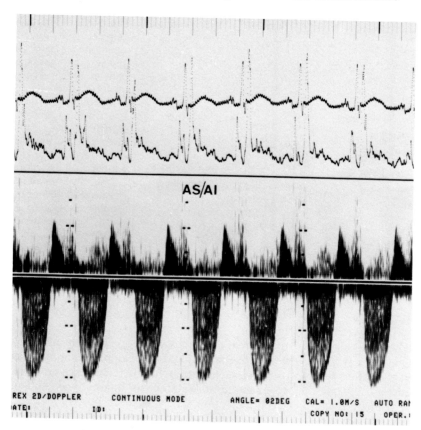

**Fig. 6–85.** Continuous wave Doppler recording of the ascending aorta in a patient with aortic stenosis (AS). The peak velocity is approximately 4 M/sec.

area = LVOT (area) × LVOT (velocity) ÷ AS (velocity). Left ventricular outflow area can be calculated from a diameter measured with two-dimensional echocardiography. Pulsed Doppler provides the means for determining LVOT velocity. Ideally, one should measure the velocity time integrals of both LVOT and AS velocities. The simpler approach of just measuring peak velocities also seems to work.[276] Occasionally, one can visualize both the low velocity outflow tract recording and the peak valvular velocity in the same recording (Fig. 6–90). One can see the somewhat darker, more dense, lower velocity envelope superimposed on the higher velocity recording.

The continuity equation calculation for aortic stenosis is the preferred echocardiographic technique for quantitating valvular stenosis. This type of calculation is particularly important when low cardiac output is suspected. It must be remembered, however, that the continuity equation calculation is different than the Gorlin formula commonly used with cardiac catheterization.[277,277a] The Gorlin formula is more sensitive to the presence of aortic regurgitation; with regurgitation, the true aortic flow cannot be calculated by the usual Fick or indicator dilution output techniques. Under these circumstances, the continuity equation is theoretically more accurate. The Gorlin formula also makes certain assumptions, including the introduction of a constant and the calculated valve area is flow dependent.[278] Thus, a discrepancy between the two measurements easily could be obtained, and the Doppler calculation may be more accurate.[279,280]

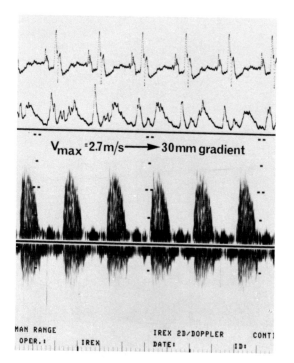

**Fig. 6–86.** Continuous wave Doppler recording in the ascending aorta in a patient with aortic stenosis and a peak velocity of 2.7 M/sec.

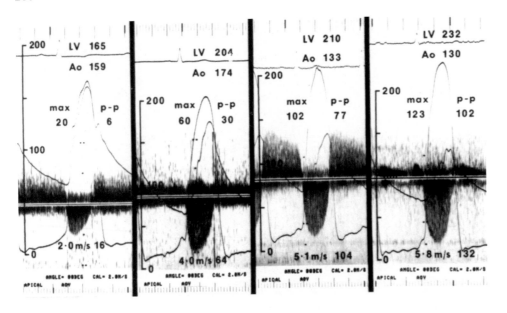

**Fig. 6–87.** Continuous wave Doppler study together with simultaneous left ventricular and aortic pressures in four patients with varying degrees of aortic stenosis. This illustration demonstrates a strong relationship between the Doppler-derived aortic gradient and the pressure differential recorded at the time of cardiac catheterization. (From Currie, P.J., et al.: Continuous wave Doppler echocardiographic assessment of severity of calcific aortic stenosis: A simultaneous Doppler-catheter correlated study in one hundred adult patients. Circulation, *71*:1162, 1985, by permission of the American Heart Association, Inc.)

M-mode echocardiography is now playing a lesser role in the assessment of aortic stenosis. One can certainly record the thickened, immobile aortic valve leaflets with the M-mode technique (Fig. 6–91). If there are any questions about the qualitative diagnosis, the M-mode examination could be helpful. For all practical purposes, however, M-mode echocardiography is redundant. Both the qualitative and quantitative evaluations are better done with two-dimensional and Doppler examinations.

Lesser echocardiographic techniques have been used to evaluate aortic stenosis qualitatively and quantitatively. Ejection time measured by Doppler recordings can be useful to judge severity.[281] The degree of left ventricular hypertrophy is another way of evaluating the

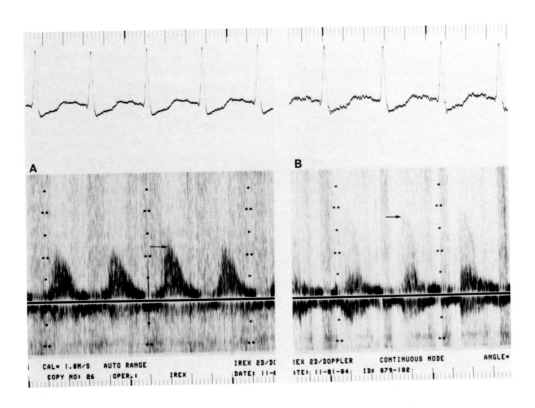

**Fig. 6–88.** Two Doppler recordings from a patient with valvular aortic stenosis. In recording A, the peak velocity is only 2.4 M/sec. In recording B, however, the peak velocity is 3.7 M/sec.

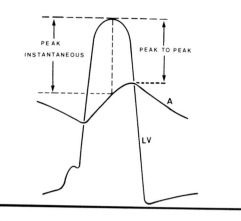

**Fig. 6–89.** Diagram of left ventricular (LV) and aortic (A) pressures in aortic stenosis. The peak instantaneous pressure difference or gradient is greater than the peak-to-peak gradient because the peak aortic pressure occurs later than the peak left ventricular pressure.

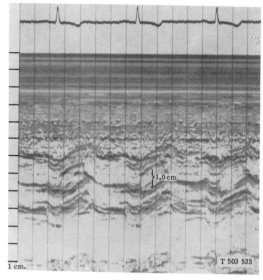

**Fig. 6–91.** Aortic valve echocardiogram of a patient with noncalcific aortic stenosis. Note multiple echoes from the valve leaflets, which separate to only 1.0 cm during systole.

long-term severity of valvular stenosis.[282–285] Before the advent of Doppler echocardiography, investigators attempted to predict left ventricular systolic pressure according to the degree of left ventricular hypertrophy. Many investigators have examined the effect of aortic stenosis on left ventricular diastolic function using Doppler imaging.[286,287]

The problem of aortic stenosis is particularly pertinent with an aging population. A systolic ejection murmur in an older patient always raises the question of possible significant aortic stenosis. Figure 6–92 illustrates a common finding in elderly patients who present with systolic

ejection murmurs and suspected valvular aortic stenosis. These individuals have distortion of the basal portion of the interventricular septum so that it impinges (*arrowhead*) on the left ventricular outflow tract.[288] This malformation is sometimes referred to as a "sigmoid septum."[289] Two-dimensional echocardiography is an excellent technique for identifying this entity. The distorted septum is easily recognized. Fortunately, these patients usually have normal valve leaflets and the differential diagnosis is relatively simple.

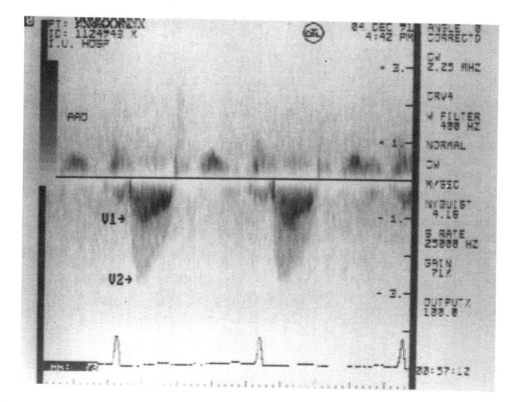

**Fig. 6–90.** Continuous wave Doppler echocardiogram showing how one can simultaneously record velocities proximal to (V1) and within (V2) a stenotic aortic valve.

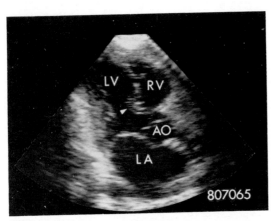

**Fig. 6–92.** Long-axis two-dimensional echocardiogram of an elderly patient who has a sigmoid septum. The base of the interventricular septum (*arrowhead*) protrudes into the left ventricular outflow tract between the left ventricle (LV) and the aorta (AO). RV = right ventricle; LA = left atrium.

### Aortic Regurgitation

Doppler echocardiography is now the principle ultrasonic technique for detecting aortic regurgitation.[290,291] Figure 6–93 illustrates a pulsed Doppler recording of a patient with aortic regurgitation. The transducer is at the apex, and the sample volume is in the left ventricular outflow tract. The Doppler recording demonstrates high-velocity turbulent flow in diastole. Because of aliasing, the direction of flow is not obvious; however, the dominant Doppler signals are above the baseline or toward the transducer.

Figure 6–94 demonstrates a continuous wave recording of a patient with both aortic regurgitation and aortic stenosis. The high-velocity diastolic flow can be seen

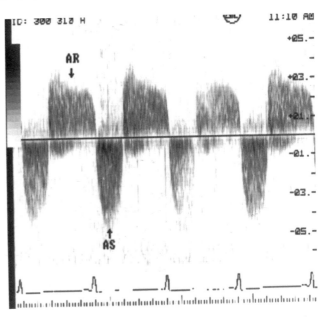

**Fig. 6–94.** Continuous wave Doppler recording of a patient with aortic stenosis and aortic regurgitation. The systolic high-velocity aortic stenosis jet (AS) and the diastolic regurgitant jet (AR) are easily recognizable.

from this apical transducer position. In Figure 6–95, a continuous wave aortic regurgitation recording is superimposed on a lower velocity mitral valve flow. The difference in timing of the two diastolic flow patterns can be readily appreciated. The aortic regurgitant flow begins slightly before normal mitral flow. Superimposition of

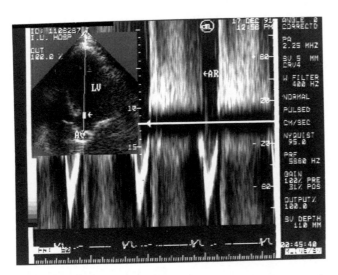

**Fig. 6–93.** Pulsed Doppler echogram of a patient with aortic regurgitation. The Doppler sample (*arrow*) is within the left ventricular outflow tract and the recording displays a high-velocity, aliasing diastolic Doppler signal (AR). LV = left ventricle; AO = aorta.

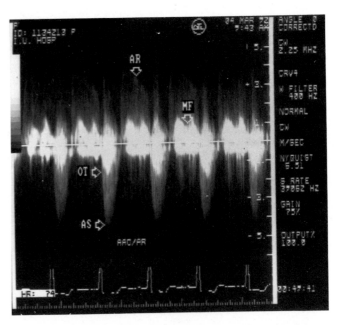

**Fig. 6–95.** Continuous wave Doppler examination of a patient with aortic stenosis and aortic regurgitation demonstrating how one can simultaneously record the Doppler signal from aortic regurgitation (AR) and mitral flow (MF), as well as the aortic stenosis (AS) and outflow tract (OT) velocities.

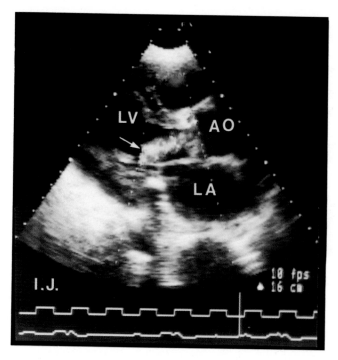

**Fig. 6–96.** Color flow Doppler examination obtained in a parasternal long-axis view demonstrating an aortic regurgitant jet (*arrow*). LV = left ventricle; AO = aorta; LA = left atrium. (From Feigenbaum, H.: Doppler color flow imaging. *In* Heart Disease Update. Edited by E. Braunwald. Philadelphia, W.B. Saunders Co., 1988.)

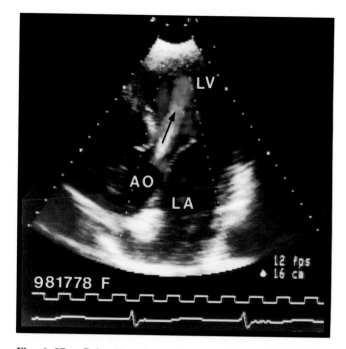

**Fig. 6–97.** Color Doppler examination in the five-chamber apical view of a patient with aortic regurgitation. The regurgitant jet (*arrow*) can be seen moving toward the transducer in shades of yellow and red. AO = aorta; LA = left atrium; LV = left ventricle.

the left ventricular outflow (OT) and aortic stenosis (AS) velocities is also seen.

Figure 6–96 shows a color Doppler recording of aortic regurgitation with the transducer in the parasternal long-axis position.[292] The turbulent blood flow passing through the aortic valve is readily appreciated. An apical five-chamber view demonstrating the high-velocity aortic regurgitant jet passing from the aorta to the left ventricle is shown in Figure 6–97. Figure 6–98 illustrates the relationship between the aortic regurgitant jet and normal mitral flow. The short-axis examination shows the cross-sectional displays of both flows. An M-mode color Doppler study of a patient with aortic regurgitation is illustrated in Figure 6–99. The turbulent regurgitant flow is displayed within the aorta as green bordered by red. The M/Q recording offers an opportunity to display the timing of the regurgitant flow. Of course, transesophageal echocardiography can detect aortic regurgitation.[293] Figure 6–100 shows a black and white recording of a transesophageal Doppler flow imaging study demonstrating an obvious aortic regurgitant jet (AR). The exact location and direction of the jet can be important. For example, an eccentric Doppler flow jet is a finding that occurs with aortic valve prolapse.[294]

All of the Doppler techniques are sensitive and reliable for the qualitative diagnosis of aortic regurgitation. Numerous efforts have been made to quantitate the degree of aortic regurgitation, however, all of them have limitations. The most obvious way is to measure the size of the regurgitant jet with color flow imaging.[295] Unfortunately, the reliability of this approach for quantitating aortic regurgitation is even worse than with mitral regurgitation.[296,297] The regurgitant aortic jet is frequently eccentric, strikes the mitral valve or interventricular septum, clashes with normal or stenotic mitral flow,[298] and is influenced by the shape of the interventricular septum and the left ventricular cavity. Thus, despite initial enthusiasm for using this criterion to quantitate aortic regurgitation, most investigators realized the many limitations. Thus, the size of the jet is only used to distinguish mild from severe regurgitation. Some investigators are attempting to use the proximal isovelocity surface area technique to quantitate aortic regurgitation.[299]

The color flow technique that probably is more reliable in judging aortic regurgitation involves measuring the width of the regurgitant jet at the orifice of the valve and comparing that diameter with the diameter of the left ventricular outflow tract (Fig. 6–101).[300,301] Figure 6–102 shows aortic jet diameters in patients with increasing degrees of aortic regurgitation. This approach also has limitations. First is the requirement of a meticulous technical examination. One must be careful to direct the ultrasonic beam through the maximum diameter of both the jet and the left ventricular outflow tract, which may not be in the same plane. In addition, data indicate that the shape of the regurgitant orifice influences the height of the color image.[302] The regurgitant orifice frequently is not perfectly round.

The rate of decline of the aortic regurgitant velocity determined with continuous wave Doppler imaging is

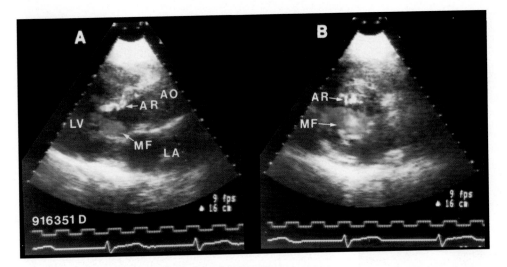

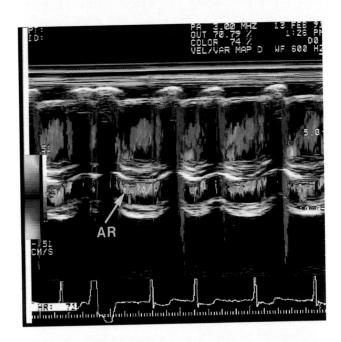

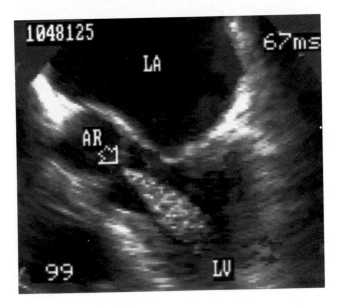

**Fig. 6–98.** Long-axis (*A*) and short-axis (*B*) color Doppler studies of a patient with aortic regurgitation. The relatively small regurgitant jet (AR) can be seen as a multicolored display in both views. The relationship of the jet to mitral inflow (MF) can be appreciated. LV = left ventricle; AO = aorta; LA = left atrium.

**Fig. 6–99.** M-mode Doppler examination of a patient with aortic regurgitation. The high-velocity turbulent aortic regurgitation (AR) can be recorded throughout diastole.

**Fig. 6–100.** Transesophageal echocardiogram demonstrating aortic regurgitant jet (AR) in this black and white Doppler flow imaging examination. LA = left atrium; LV = left ventricle.

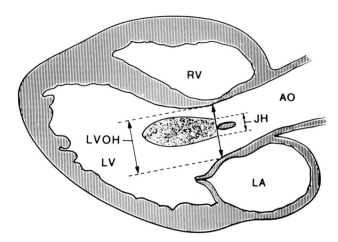

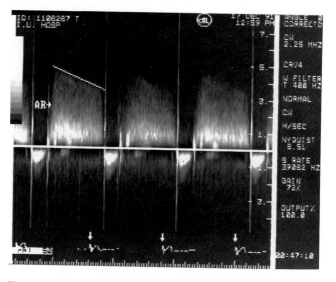

**Fig. 6–101.** Diagram illustrating how aortic regurgitation can be quantitated by measuring the jet height (JH) at the valve orifice and comparing it with the height of the left ventricular outflow tract (LVOH). RV = right ventricle; LV = left ventricle; LA = left atrium; AO = aorta. (Reprinted with permission from the American College of Cardiology. From Perry, G.J., et al.: Evaluation of aortic insufficiency by Doppler color flow mapping. J. Am. Coll. Cardiol., 9:953, 1987.)

**Fig. 6–103.** Continuous wave Doppler examination of a patient with aortic regurgitation showing how one can measure the diastolic slope (*line*) of the regurgitant signal (AR).

also used to quantitate aortic regurgitation.[303–307] Figure 6–103 demonstrates how one can measure the diastolic slope or decay of the aortic regurgitant jet. This diastolic decay can be measured as a pressure half-time, as with mitral stenosis, or as just the slope of the decay (in M/sec$^2$). Figure 6–104 demonstrates the principle behind this approach. The aortic regurgitant velocity is indica-

tive of the pressure gradient between the aorta and the left ventricle during diastole. The rapidity with which the aortic and left ventricular pressures equalize is a function of the severity of the aortic regurgitation. A larger regurgitant orifice permits a steeper fall in aortic pressure. In addition, an increasing volume of blood entering the left ventricle from the aorta produces a more rapidly rising left ventricular diastolic pressure. Thus, with severe aortic regurgitation, the gradient will de-

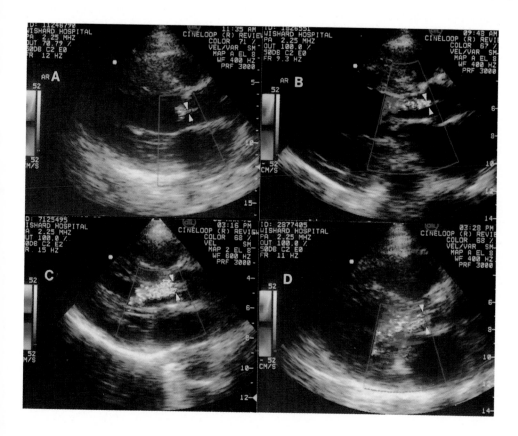

**Fig. 6–102.** Color flow Doppler studies of patients with aortic regurgitation of different severities. The width of the aortic regurgitant jet (*arrowheads*) enlarges with increasing regurgitation (*A* to *D*).

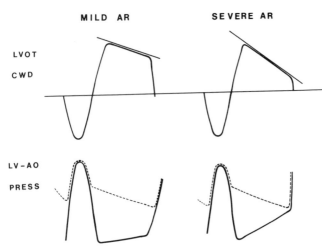

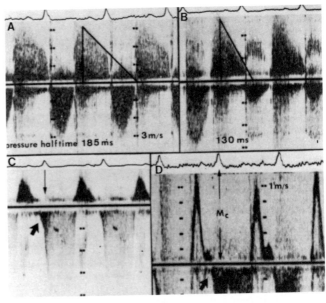

**Fig. 6–104.** Diagram illustrating the principle of how the diastolic slope of the regurgitant jet can relate to the severity of aortic regurgitation (AR). The continuous wave Doppler (CWD) signal is a function of the pressure difference between the left ventricle and the aorta (LV-AO). With relatively mild aortic regurgitation, the pressure difference gradually decreases as regurgitant blood is flowing into the left ventricle; however, with severe aortic regurgitation, the aortic pressure drops rapidly and the left ventricular pressure rises steeply as the large regurgitant volume increases the pressure. Thus, the pressure differential decreases and the slope of the diastolic regurgitant jet increases. LVOT = left ventricular outflow tract.

**Fig. 6–106.** Continuous wave Doppler recordings of a patient with progressive aortic regurgitation. The recording in *A* has a pressure half-time of 185 ms. In addition, presystolic mitral regurgitation (*large arrow*) is seen in the tracing in *C*. As the aortic regurgitation progressively worsens, the pressure half-time decreases to 130 ms and the presystolic mitral regurgitation (*arrow, D*) increases. (Reprinted with permission from the American College of Cardiology. From Oh, J.K., et al.: Characteristic Doppler echocardiographic pattern of mitral flow velocity in severe aortic regurgitation. J. Am. Coll. Cardiol., *14*:1714, 1989.)

crease rapidly and even disappear if the diastolic interval is long enough to permit equalization of aortic and left ventricular pressures. This falling gradient produces an increased slope of the regurgitant velocity. Figure 6–105 shows a deceleration rate of 13 M/sec² in a patient with severe aortic regurgitation. This slope or deceleration

rate is much greater than in Figure 6–103. In one study, a decay slope greater than 3 M/sec² was indicative of moderate to severe aortic regurgitation.[307]

Again, this technique, although useful, has limitations.[308] The rate of decline of the aortic regurgitant Doppler velocity is also a function of the systemic vascular resistance and left ventricular compliance. Increasing the systemic vascular resistance increases the rate of decline without any change in valve orifice. Reduced compliance of the left ventricle produces a more rapidly rising left ventricular pressure, which influences the diastolic slope without reflecting the severity of aortic regurgitation.[309] One group of investigators studying the use of continuous wave Doppler imaging to measure aortic regurgitation concluded that this sign is only useful to judge severe regurgitation.[310] Figure 6–106 shows another patient with severe progressive aortic regurgitation. The upper panels show the aortic diastolic regurgitant flow before and after progression. The pressure half-time decreased from 185 to 130 msec. This patient exhibited another Doppler sign of severe aortic regurgitation, late diastolic or presystolic mitral regurgitation.[311,312] With the lesser severity, one can see a mitral regurgitant jet prior to the onset of the electrocardiographic QRS (*large arrow*, lower left tracing). With more severe regurgitation (right lower tracing), one sees more impressive presystolic mitral regurgitation (*arrow*).

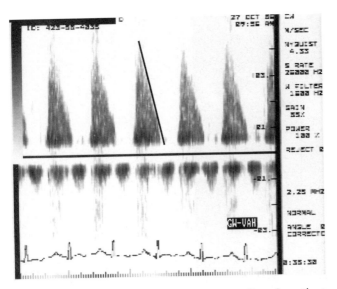

**Fig. 6–105.** Continuous wave Doppler recording of a patient with more severe regurgitation. The deceleration rate is 13 M/s².

Pulsed Doppler techniques can be used to quantitate aortic regurgitant fraction by calculating aortic flow and mitral flow and subtracting the two values to obtain aortic regurgitant volume or fraction.[313] This technique can only be done with pure aortic regurgitation. Under these circumstances, aortic flow should be greater than mitral flow and the difference should be the regurgitant volume.

Pulsed Doppler recordings of aortic flow can also be helpful in judging the presence and severity of aortic regurgitation. Figure 6–107 shows a pulsed Doppler tracing in both the ascending and descending aorta. One can see holodiastolic flow resulting from the regurgitant, reverse flow. Such a recording can also be made in any systemic artery, including the abdominal aorta with the subcostal approach.[314,315] Such regurgitant diastolic flow only occurs with moderate to severe aortic regurgitation. Figure 6–108 shows a recording of descending aortic flow in a patient with severe aortic regurgitation.

Investigational studies have been performed to measure the effective aortic regurgitant orifice. Using the continuity equation, one can make this calculation by knowing the diastolic flow velocities just above and below the regurgitant valve and the cross-sectional area of the aorta just above the valve.[316–318] There has not been great experience with this technique and the reliability and validity have yet to be determined.

All of the Doppler techniques for quantitating aortic regurgitation have some validity, but none is without limitations. The best approach is to use as many Doppler measurements as possible to improve the reliability of the examination.[319]

M-mode echocardiography plays a lesser role in the evaluation of aortic regurgitation. Figure 6–109 shows one of the earliest signs of aortic regurgitation on an M-mode echocardiogram. Fine fluttering of the anterior leaflet of the mitral valve is apparent, and, on occasion, one could even see fine fluttering of the interventricular septum.[320] This sign has become virtually obsolete with the advent of Doppler techniques.

An indirect, two-dimensional echocardiographic sign of aortic regurgitation is reverse doming of the mitral leaflet (Fig. 6–110).[112,320–323] With moderate to severe aortic regurgitation, the regurgitant jet produces diastolic indentation of the anterior mitral leaflet.

There are several useful echocardiographic signs of severe and usually acute aortic regurgitation.[324] One important sign is premature closure of the mitral valve.[325–330] Figure 6–111 shows an M-mode echocardiogram of a patient with acute severe aortic regurgitation. The mitral valve is almost completely closed (c′) long before ventricular systole. Such a sign is indicative of a high left ventricular diastolic pressure, which produces virtual closure of the mitral valve early in diastole.

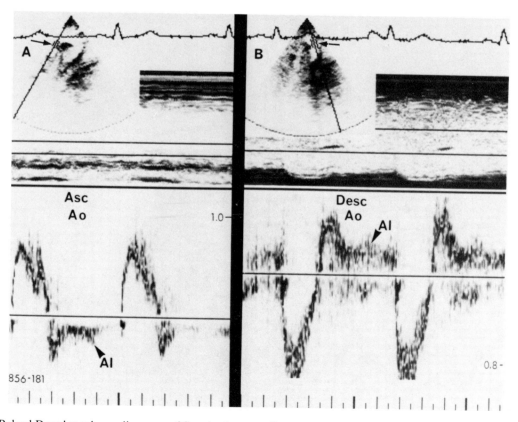

**Fig. 6–107.** Pulsed Doppler echocardiograms of flow in the ascending aorta (*A*) and in the descending aorta (*B*) of a patient with aortic regurgitation. The diastolic reverse flow from the aortic regurgitation (AI) is seen throughout diastole in both examinations. Ao = aorta; *arrows* indicate location of sample volumes.

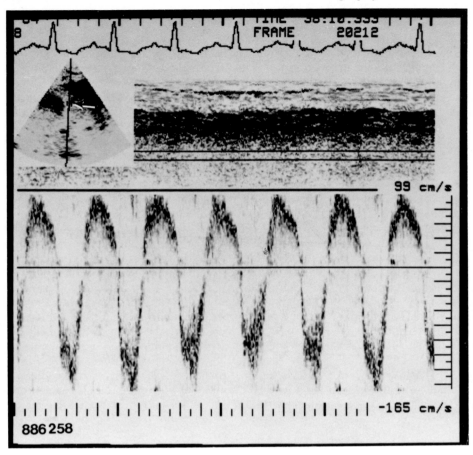

**Fig. 6–108.** Pulsed Doppler echocardiogram with the sample volume (*arrow*) in the descending aorta of a patient with severe aortic regurgitation. The retrograde diastolic flow is almost as great as the forward systolic flow.

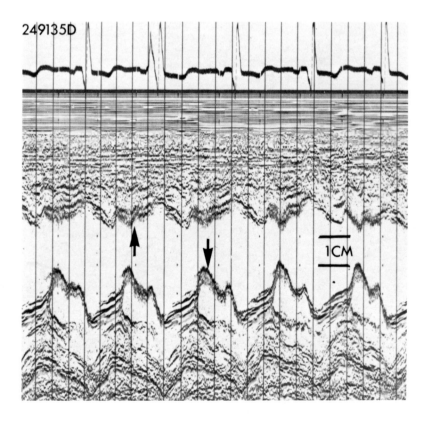

**Fig. 6–109.** M-mode echocardiogram of a patient with aortic regurgitation. Note fluttering (*arrows*) of the interventricular septum and mitral valve.

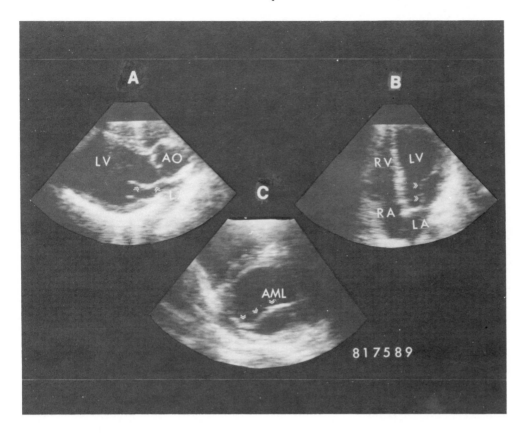

Fig. 6–110. Long-axis (*A*), four-chamber (*B*), and short-axis (*C*) two-dimensional echocardiograms of a patient with severe aortic regurgitation. During diastole, the regurgitant flow distorts the shape of the anterior mitral leaflet (*arrows*) in all three views. LV = left ventricle; AO = aorta; LA = left atrium; RV = right ventricle; RA = right atrium; AML = anterior mitral leaflet. (Reprinted with permission from the American College of Cardiology. From Robertson, W.S., et al.: Reverse doming of the anterior mitral leaflet with severe aortic regurgitation. J. Am. Coll. Cardiol., *3*: 431, 1984.)

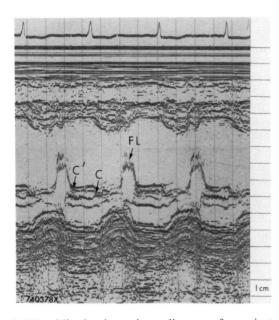

Fig. 6–111. Mitral valve echocardiogram of a patient with acute severe aortic regurgitation. The valve is almost completely closed (C′) before ventricular systole. The valve does not reopen with atrial systole and closes completely with ventricular systole (C).

Doppler recordings show the same phenomenon.[331] As noted in Figure 6–106, one may see early or late diastolic mitral regurgitation through an otherwise closed mitral valve. High left ventricular diastolic pressure associated with aortic regurgitation may produce premature opening of the aortic valve, as seen on an M-mode echocardiographic tracing (Fig. 6–112).[332–334]

Considerable research has attempted to use echocardiography to assess the left ventricle in patients with aortic regurgitation to determine the proper timing for aortic valve replacement.[335–341] Fractional shortening, diastolic and systolic dimensions, wall thickness, wall thickness-cavity dimension ratios, and left ventricular stress have all been proposed as possible echocardiographic signs for judging when intervention should occur.

The use of echocardiography to judge the timing of surgery for aortic regurgitation on the basis of the left ventricular function was stimulated by a study that indicated the following: when a left ventricular systolic dimension exceeded 55 mm or the percent fractional shortening was less than 25%, the left ventricle was decompensated and might not recover even after replacement of the valve.[335,336] Figure 6–113 is an echocardiogram of a patient with a well-compensated ventricle and severe aortic regurgitation. Figure 6–114 shows an M-mode echocardiogram of a patient with severe aortic regurgitation whose left ventricle is functioning poorly. The ventricle is dilated, and the fractional shortening is less than in Figure 6–113. Note also the lack of mitral valve opening at the E point in Figure 6–114. The

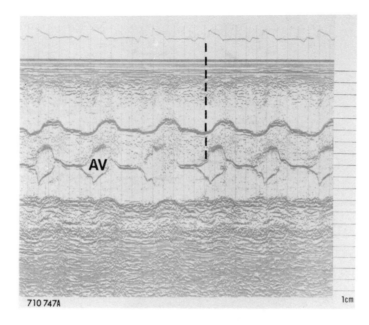

**Fig. 6–112.** M-mode echocardiogram of the aortic valve (AV) in a patient with severe aortic regurgitation and high left ventricular end-diastolic pressures. The aortic valve opens prior to the onset of ventricular systole (*dashed line*).

extreme difference between Figures 6–113 and 6–114 can be easily detected by echocardiography.

Since the original study describing the value of M-mode measurements for timing surgery for aortic regurgitation, there has been considerable controversy as to the clinical usefulness of this approach.[342–347] Later studies indicate that the criteria suggested were too rigid.[348,349] Many patients could be improperly managed by using any single measurement. The consensus is that one must use these echocardiographic measurements together with other clinical information to make the decision. Some investigators believe that adding wall thickness, possibly radius thickness ratios or stress measurements, can improve the predictive value in these patients.[350–352] These observations, however, have not withstood the test of time. Some investigators have suggested using exercise echocardiography to help make this critical assessment.[353,354,354a,354b]

Irrespective of how one obtains echocardiographic measurements of left ventricular size and function, it is certainly reasonable to use these measurements to follow individual patients with aortic regurgitation. Evidence that the ventricle is deteriorating is probably the strongest echocardiographic finding that might influence one to seriously consider aortic valve replacement.

An important role of echocardiography is to identify the etiology of aortic regurgitation.[355,356] Figure 6–115 demonstrates acute aortic regurgitation secondary to disruption of the aortic valve. This patient had bacterial endocarditis with destruction of at least one of the aortic cusps. Echoes from the aortic valve can be seen protruding into the left ventricular outflow tract in diastole. One cannot be certain whether these echoes originate from a vegetation or from valve tissue. Although the etiology of the aortic regurgitation in this particular patient was bacterial endocarditis, an almost identical echocardiogram could be displayed in patients with noninfectious disruption of the aortic valve.

Prolapsed aortic valve is being recognized with increasing frequency.[357–362] Figure 6–116 shows a two-dimensional echocardiogram of a patient with a prolapsed aortic valve. In diastole (*A*), the redundant aortic leaflets bulge into the left ventricular outflow tract.

Aortic regurgitation secondary to diseases of the aorta, such as with Marfan's syndrome or aortic dissection, is discussed in Chapter 12, Diseases of the Aorta.

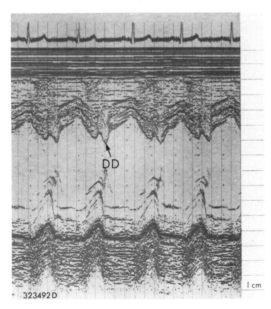

**Fig. 6–113.** Left ventricular echocardiogram of a patient with aortic regurgitation. The left ventricle is dilated, the septal and posterior walls move excessively, and there is an exaggerated diastolic dip (DD) of the interventricular septum.

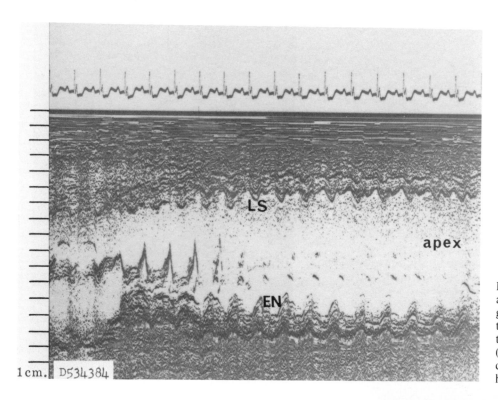

**Fig. 6–114.** M-mode scan of a patient with severe aortic regurgitation and poor left ventricular function. The left ventricle is dilated, and the septal (LS) and posterior endocardial (EN) echoes do not exhibit excessive motion.

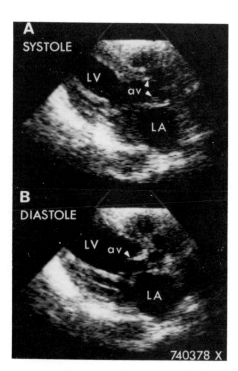

**Fig. 6–115.** Long-axis two-dimensional echocardiogram of a patient with bacterial endocarditis and a vegetation on the aortic valve. During diastole (*B*), a mass of echoes attached to the aortic valve (av) can be seen protruding into the left ventricular outflow tract. LV = left ventricle; LA = left atrium.

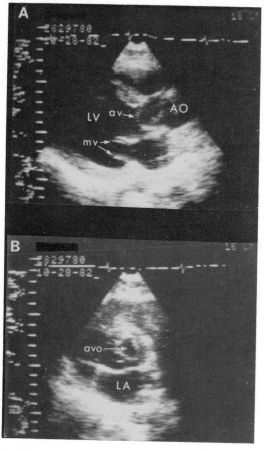

**Fig. 6–116.** Long-axis (*A*) and short-axis (*B*) two-dimensional echocardiogram of a patient with a prolapsing aortic valve (av). LV = left ventricle; AO = aorta; mv = mitral valve leaflet; LA = left atrium; avo = aortic valve orifice.

## TRICUSPID VALVE DISEASE

### Tricuspid Stenosis

Two-dimensional echocardiography is probably the most specific echocardiographic examination for tricuspid stenosis. As with all valvular stenoses, the hallmark of the diagnosis is doming of the tricuspid valve (Fig. 6–117).[363–365] The domed tricuspid valve of tricuspid stenosis can be seen in the parasternal long-axis view, as noted in Figure 6–117, or in the apical four-chamber view.[364–366] Although doming of the tricuspid valve is also visualized in the short-axis view (Fig. 6–118), this view is not as reliable as either the parasternal long-axis or apical examinations.

In addition to doming, thickening of the leaflets and restricted motion are also signs to help with the diagnosis of tricuspid stenosis.[363,364] In one study, these two-dimensional criteria for tricuspid stenosis were found to be 100% sensitive and 90% specific.[364]

The M-mode echocardiogram has also been used for the diagnosis of tricuspid stenosis.[9,367,368] Figure 6–119 shows an echocardiogram of a patient with tricuspid ste-

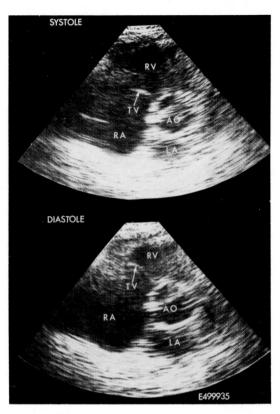

**Fig. 6–118.** Short-axis two-dimensional echocardiograms of the base of the heart and the tricuspid valve in a patient with tricuspid stenosis. Doming of the tricuspid valve (TV) is visible in diastole. RV = right ventricle; RA = right atrium; AO = aorta; LA = left atrium.

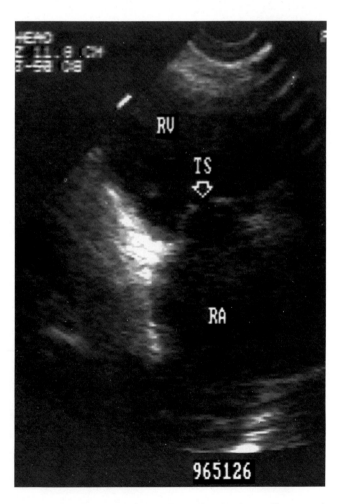

**Fig. 6–117.** Parasternal two-dimensional echocardiogram of the right ventricular inflow tract of a patient with tricuspid stenosis. The domed stenotic tricuspid valve (TS) can be seen between the right ventricle (RV) and the right atrium (RA).

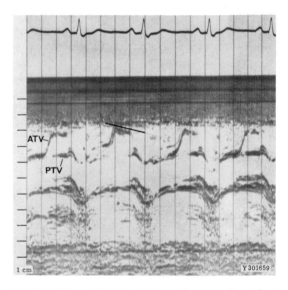

**Fig. 6–119.** Tricuspid valve echocardiogram of a patient with tricuspid stenosis. Both anterior (ATV) and posterior (PTV) tricuspid leaflets are recorded. The slope of diastolic closure is diminished, and the overall pattern is similar to that of a stenotic mitral valve.

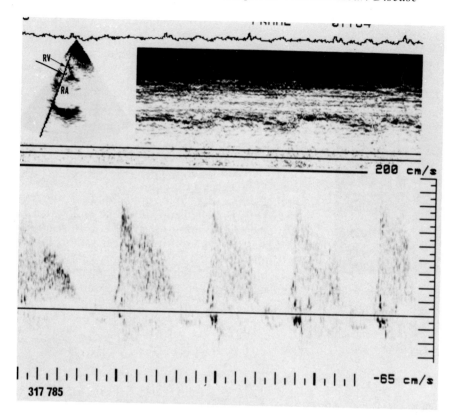

**Fig. 6–120.** Pulsed Doppler echocardiogram with a sample volume (*arrow*) in the right ventricle of a patient with tricuspid stenosis. RV = right ventricle; RA = right atrium.

nosis. The M-mode echocardiographic criteria used in the diagnosis of tricuspid stenosis are similar to those used for mitral stenosis. Again, one observes a decreased diastolic slope, thickening of the valve, and decreased separation of the leaflets. Unfortunately, these criteria have not proved to be reliable.[366] As with the mitral valve, a reduced diastolic slope is nonspecific.

Doppler echocardiography can also assist with the diagnosis of tricuspid stenosis.[369] The Doppler recording is similar to that seen with mitral stenosis. Figure 6–120 shows a pulsed Doppler echocardiogram of a patient with tricuspid stenosis. The Doppler sample is in the right ventricle, and one sees turbulent diastolic flow with a slowed reduction in velocity during diastole. The velocities are higher than normal maximal tricuspid flow. The Doppler approach offers a better opportunity for judging the severity of the stenosis. The two-dimensional technique does not permit the recording of an orifice as with mitral stenosis. Thus, two-dimensional echocardiography is more specific and sensitive for the qualitative diagnosis, whereas the Doppler examination holds the best promise for the quantitation of tricuspid stenosis.

### Tricuspid Regurgitation

As with all other forms of valvular regurgitation, Doppler echocardiography is the ultrasonic technique of choice for detection of tricuspid regurgitation. Figure 6–121 shows a pulsed Doppler recording of a patient with tricuspid regurgitation. The Doppler sample is on the right atrial side of the tricuspid valve and the turbulent systolic flow can be recorded. Figure 6–122 demon-

strates color flow Doppler studies of two patients with tricuspid regurgitation. The severity of tricuspid regurgitation is being judged primarily by the size of the regurgitant jet on the color flow image.[370–372] Figure 6–122*B* shows moderately severe tricuspid regurgitation, which fills much of the right atrium. A lesser degree of tricuspid

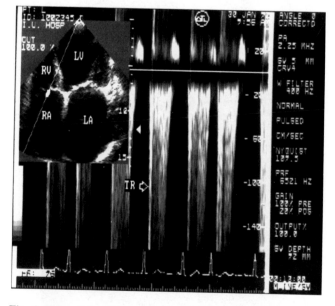

**Fig. 6–121.** Pulsed Doppler recording of a patient with tricuspid regurgitation. The sample volume is on the right atrial side of the tricuspid valve. The tricuspid regurgitation jet (TR) is noted as a high-velocity systolic recording. RV = right ventricle; LV = left ventricle; LA = left atrium; RA = right atrium.

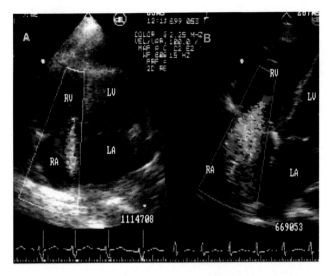

**Fig. 6–122.** Color flow Doppler recordings of a patient with relatively mild (*A*) and more severe (*B*) tricuspid regurgitation. A rough relationship exists between the size of the regurgitant jet and the severity of the regurgitation. RV = right ventricle; RA = right atrium; LV = left ventricle; LA = left atrium.

regurgitation is noted in Figure 6–122*A*. Multiple tricuspid regurgitant jets can be seen in some patients (Fig. 6–123). This illustration also demonstrates the two common two-dimensional views for detecting tricuspid regurgitation.

Continuous wave Doppler recordings of tricuspid regurgitation are used primarily to determine right ventricular systolic pressure and an estimation of pulmonary hypertension (see Chapter 4). The continuous wave Doppler recording can also give an estimate of the severity of tricuspid regurgitation. As with mitral regurgitation, the presence of a tall V wave in the right atrium produces a decrease in the gradient across the tricuspid orifice (Fig. 6–124). Thus, the shape of the tricuspid regurgitant jet can help to identify severe regurgitation. Early peaking and midsystolic deceleration of the velocity is indicative of a tall V wave in the right atrium. If the Doppler signal from the regurgitant jet is weak, it can be enhanced with an intravenous contrast injection.[373]

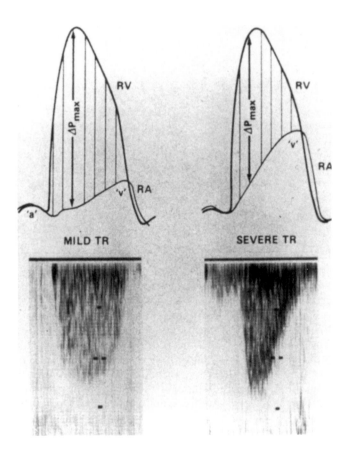

**Fig. 6–124.** Continuous wave Doppler examinations of two patients with mild and severe tricuspid regurgitation (TR). The shape of the Doppler signal is a function of the pressure gradient between the right ventricle (RV) and the right atrium (RA). With a tall V wave in the right atrium, the pressure gradient decreases through the latter half of systole, and the tricuspid regurgitant Doppler signal falls more rapidly. (From Gupta, M.K., and Sasson, Z.: The mechanisms and importance of tricuspid regurgitation and hepatic pulsations in dilated cardiomyopathy: A review. Echocardiography, *8*:195, 1991.)

**Fig. 6–123.** Parasternal (*A*) and apical four-chamber (*B*) color flow Doppler studies of a patient with tricuspid regurgitation. The regurgitant jet appears singular in *A* (*arrow*), whereas multiple jets (*arrows*) are noted in *B*.

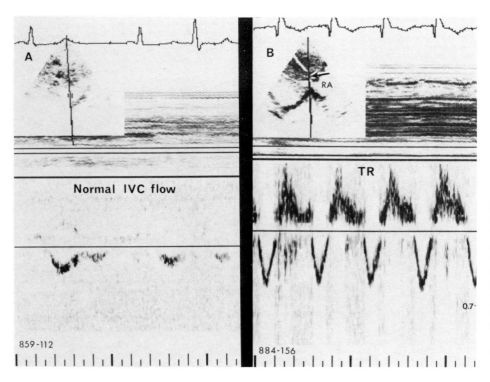

**Fig. 6–125.** Doppler echocardiograms of the inferior vena cava of a normal individual (*A*) and a patient with tricuspid regurgitation (*B*). With the sample volume (*arrow*) in the inferior vena cava or preferably the hepatic vein, one sees flow toward the transducer in systole in the presence of tricuspid regurgitation (TR). RA = right atrium; IVC = inferior vena cava.

The Doppler technique for detecting tricuspid regurgitation is proving to be extremely sensitive. In fact, many patients with no clinical evidence of tricuspid regurgitation apparently have Doppler findings of valvular insufficiency. Since there is no good gold standard, it is difficult to determine if this finding is a "false positive." It is possible that the Doppler technique is sensitive enough to detect subclinical amounts of tricuspid regurgitation. With a valve as complex as the tricuspid valve, it is not surprising that a minor degree of incompetence would be fairly common.

The Doppler technique can also be used to examine the inferior vena cava and/or the hepatic veins for the presence of tricuspid regurgitation. Figure 6–125 demonstrates both normal inferior vena cava flow and flow noted with tricuspid regurgitation. The prominent finding of tricuspid regurgitation is flow toward the transducer in systole. This abnormality is usually best seen in the hepatic vein because the flow is more parallel to the ultrasonic beam in this vessel.[374-377] Some authors have taken a ratio of forward and reverse flow to quantitate the degree of regurgitation.[375,376]

Contrast echocardiography is another technique that has been used for the diagnosis of tricuspid regurgitation.[378-383] This examination is done best by an M-mode recording of the inferior vena cava and a contrast injection in one of the arm veins.[384] With tricuspid regurgitation, one sees the appearance of contrast in the inferior vena cava during ventricular systole (Fig. 6–126).[385] This finding must be distinguished from a normal examination in which contrast can be seen following atrial systole. The necessity of distinguishing between atrial and ventricular systole is one of the reasons why the M-mode contrast study is preferable to the one done with two-dimensional echocardiography.

With the increasing use of Doppler echocardiography, the application of contrast studies for this diagnosis is decreasing.[386]

Tricuspid regurgitation is a cause for right ventricular volume overload.[243] The M-mode echocardiogram shows the typical findings of a dilated right ventricle and anterior motion of the interventricular septum during isovolumetric contraction (see Chapter 3). The two-dimensional echocardiogram also shows a dilated right ventricle with flattening of the interventricular septum during diastole.

Echocardiography, primarily two-dimensional echocardiography, offers an opportunity to identify specific causes of tricuspid regurgitation. Rheumatic tricuspid regurgitation is usually associated with an element of tricuspid stenosis. Tricuspid valve prolapse has been increasingly recognized as a cause of tricuspid regurgitation.[387-390] Figure 6–127 shows one of the earliest reports of a prolapsing tricuspid valve. A somewhat more severe form of tricuspid valve prolapse is noted in Figure 6–128. This valve had chaotic motion and wide excursions,[391] as well as late systolic posterior displacement of the leaflets (P). Tricuspid valve prolapse is primarily demonstrated with two-dimensional echocardiography (Fig. 6–129).[383,387,392,393] The four-chamber view is a common approach for this diagnosis, although the examination has been made by a subcostal approach as well.[390] Tricuspid valve prolapse almost always occurs in patients with associated mitral valve prolapse.

Incomplete closure of the tricuspid valve has been noted on two-dimensional echocardiography.[394] This finding is similar to papillary muscle dysfunction. Ruptured tricuspid valve chordae have been reported.[395,396] Diastolic fluttering of a tricuspid valve secondary to traumatic tricuspid regurgitation[395,397-399] or secondary

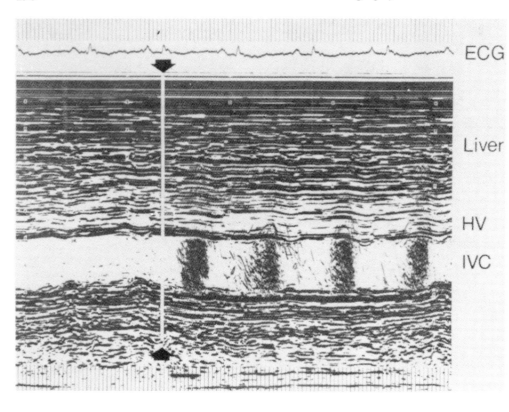

ECG

Liver

HV

IVC

**Fig. 6–126.** Contrast M-mode echocardiogram of the inferior vena cava (IVC) in a patient with tricuspid regurgitation. The contrast is seen within the inferior vena cava during ventricular systole. HV = hepatic vein. (From Wise, N.K., et al.: Contrast M-mode ultrasonography of the inferior vena cava. Circulation, *63*:1100, 1981, by permission of the American Heart Association, Inc.)

to endocarditis[398] has also been described. Figure 6–130 demonstrates a four-chamber view of a patient with tricuspid regurgitation presumably secondary to trauma many years earlier. The right ventricle and right atrium are enlarged. In addition, one sees a faint mural tricuspid leaflet that protrudes into the right atrium in systole.

Transesophageal echocardiography is proving to be useful in identifying the etiology of tricuspid regurgitation. Tricuspid valve prolapse can be detected readily with the transesophageal approach.[400] The examination is particularly helpful in identifying a flail tricuspid valve.[401] Figure 6–131 shows a transesophageal exami-

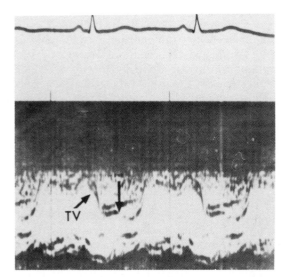

**Fig. 6–127.** Tricuspid valve echocardiogram (TV) depicting prolapse of the tricuspid valve (*arrow*). (From Chandraratna, P.A.N., et al.: Echocardiographic detection of tricuspid valve prolapse. Circulation, *51*:823, 1975, by permission of the American Heart Association, Inc.)

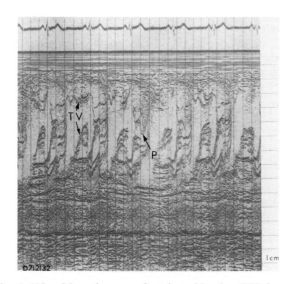

**Fig. 6–128.** M-mode scan of a tricuspid valve (TV) in a patient with tricuspid valve prolapse. The excursion and separation of the tricuspid leaflets increase, and posterior displacement of the valve (P) occurs in late systole.

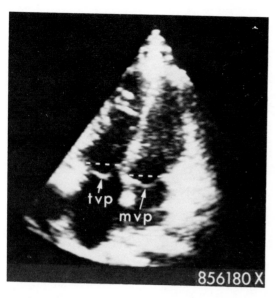

**Fig. 6–129.** Apical four-chamber two-dimensional echocardiogram of a patient with tricuspid valve prolapse (tvp) and mitral valve prolapse (mvp).

nation of a patient with a flail tricuspid valve associated with ruptured chordae (rct).

Several reports have described the echocardiographic findings with carcinoid heart disease. One of the principal clinical manifestations of this disease is tricuspid regurgitation.[402–406] Figure 6–132 demonstrates characteristic echocardiographic findings of carcinoid involvement of the tricuspid valve. The tricuspid valve leaflets

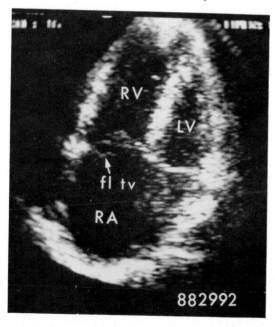

**Fig. 6–130.** Two-dimensional echocardiogram of a patient with a flail tricuspid valve leaflet. The flail leaflet (fl tv) can be seen protruding into the right atrium (RA) in systole. The right ventricle (RV) and right atrium are markedly dilated. LV = left ventricle.

are thickened and totally rigid with no change in position from diastole to systole. The leaflets produce wide open tricuspid regurgitation because there seems to be no effort toward closure of the valve during systole.

## PULMONARY VALVE DISEASE

The most common pulmonary valve problem is congenital pulmonic stenosis. Since this problem is a congenital abnormality, the topic is discussed further in the chapter on congenital heart disease. One sees an occasional acquired form of pulmonary valve disease, the most common of which is pulmonic insufficiency. This valvular regurgitation may be secondary to pulmonary hypertension, bacterial endocarditis, or iatrogenic causes secondary to a pulmonary valvotomy.

Doppler echocardiography is again the ultrasonic procedure of choice for the diagnosis of pulmonic insufficiency.[407,408] Figure 6–133 shows a pulsed echo recording with the sample volume (*arrow*) proximal to the pulmonary valve. One detects high-velocity turbulent flow in early diastole immediately after the systolic ejection of the blood into the pulmonary artery. In this patient, the pulmonary artery pressure was essentially normal. Pulmonic insufficiency frequently is a result of severe pulmonary hypertension. Figure 6–134 demonstrates a Doppler echocardiogram in a patient with pulmonic insufficiency secondary to pulmonary hypertension. Again, one sees high-velocity disturbed flow throughout diastole with the Doppler sample in the right ventricular outflow tract. The two-dimensional image is in the short-axis view. In addition, one sees the typical Doppler flow pattern of pulmonary hypertension with a short acceleration time and a decrease in flow in midsystole (*arrow*).

Figure 6-135 shows a color flow Doppler study of a patient with pulmonic regurgitation. The characteristic regurgitant turbulent jet can be seen passing from the pulmonary artery into the right ventricular outflow tract.

No one has attempted to quantitate pulmonic regurgitation with Doppler echocardiography. One must be careful not to confuse normal tricuspid flow with pulmonic insufficiency. Careful placement of the Doppler sample is necessary to avoid this confusion. As with other valvular regurgitation lesions, the Doppler technique may detect pulmonic insufficiency that is not clinically significant.

Pulmonic regurgitation is another cause for right ventricular volume overload.[409] Thus, the echocardiographic findings of a right ventricular volume overload with a dilated right ventricle and abnormal septal motion and configuration may also occur in these patients.

## PROSTHETIC VALVES

The echocardiographic evaluation of prosthetic valves has always been, and continues to be, a challenge. Many

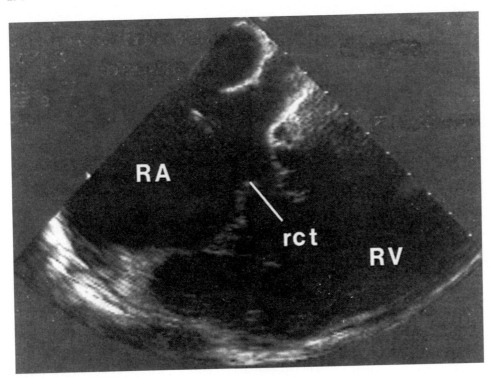

**Fig. 6–131.** Transesophageal echocardiogram of a patient with a ruptured tricuspid valve chordae (rct). The ruptured chordae can be seen displaced into the right atrium (RA). RV = right ventricle. (From Winslow, T., et al.: Transesophageal echocardiography in the diagnosis of flail tricuspid valve. Am. Heart J., *123*:1683, 1992.)

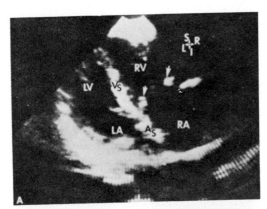

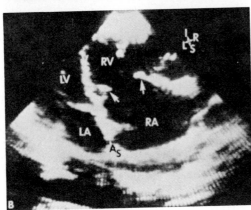

**Fig. 6–132.** Two-dimensional echocardiograms of a patient with carcinoid syndrome. The tricuspid valve leaflets (*arrows*) are markedly thickened and immobile. The valves are fixed in an open position. LV = left ventricle; VS = ventricular septum; RV = right ventricle; LA = left atrium; AS = atrial septum; RA = right atrium. (From Callahan, J.A., et al.: Echocardiographic features of carcinoid heart disease. Am. J. Cardiol., *50*:762, 1982.) S = superior; I = inferior; R = right; L = left.

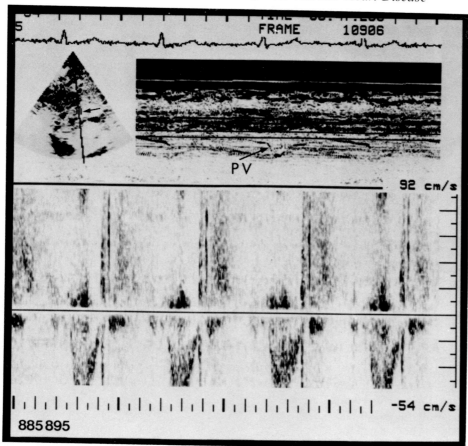

**Fig. 6–133.** Pulsed Doppler echocardiogram with the sample volume (*arrow*) in the right ventricular outflow tract of a patient with pulmonic insufficiency. High-velocity turbulent flow can be seen moving toward the transducer in diastole. PV = pulmonary valve.

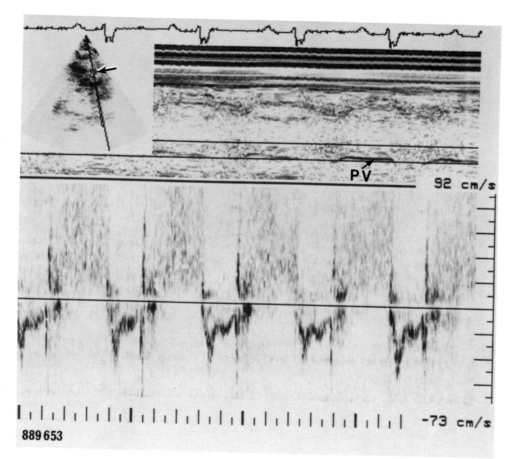

**Fig. 6–134.** Doppler echocardiogram of a patient with pulmonic insufficiency and pulmonary hypertension. The turbulent diastolic flow is seen moving toward the transducer in diastole. In systole, the pulmonary artery flow shows the characteristic pattern of pulmonary hypertension (see Chap. 4). PV = pulmonary valve. *Arrow* locates the sample volume.

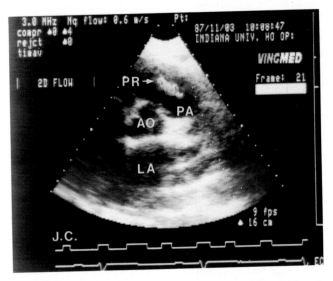

**Fig. 6–135.** Color flow Doppler study of a patient with pulmonic regurgitation (PR). PA = pulmonary artery; AO = aorta; LA = left atrium.

difficulties, technical and physiologic, arise when trying to distinguish between a normally and abnormally functioning prosthetic valve. These difficulties are based on acoustic artifacts commonly present with prosthetic valves. These artifacts include shadowing because of the highly reflective material in prosthetic valves,[410] reverberations again because of the acoustic characteristics of the valve, and the large number of echoes that occur with prosthetic valves that are difficult to distinguish from pathologic echoes, especially in the area of the sewing rings. Furthermore, the wide variety of prosthetic valves makes any type of generalization with regard to the echocardiographic evaluation difficult. Many of these problems have been overcome with the introduction of transesophageal echocardiography.[411–413,413a,413b] And even transthoracic echocardiography is highly valuable in following patients with prosthetic valves. Thus many, if not most, of the malfunctioning valves can be identified properly with echocardiographic techniques.

### Normal Function

All prosthetic valves can be imaged using two-dimensional and M-mode echocardiography. Figure 6–136 shows a characteristic two-dimensional echocardiogram of a patient with a ball-cage type prosthetic mitral valve. The echoes coming from the cage and ball are seen on the ventricular side of the mitral annulus. The curved cage can be appreciated (*vertical arrows*) within the cage. An echo from the leading edge of the ball (*horizontal arrows*) moves back and forth within the cage. The curved nature of the ball usually is not apparent. Figure 6–137 shows a characteristic porcine mitral prosthesis in the long-axis and four-chamber views. Two of the struts protruding into the left ventricle are visible and are characteristic of this type of valve. A tilting disk-type mechanical valve shows a singular echo moving up

and down on the ventricular side of mitral annulus (Fig. 6–138). The St. Jude valve, which has two semicircular leaflets, frequently shows both leaflets protruding into the left ventricle during diastole.[414] Figure 6–139 shows a St. Jude valve in the mitral position with a transthoracic (Fig. 6–139A) and transesophageal (Fig. 6–139B) examination.

The M-mode echogram still can be useful in distinguishing normal versus abnormal mechanical valves.[415] This situation is particularly true with the tilting disk or Bjork-Shiley valve and occasionally with older Starr-Edwards valves. Figure 6–140 demonstrates the normal M-mode appearance of a ball-cage mitral prosthetic valve. The normal mitral tilting disk valve is demonstrated in Figure 6–141. With a tilting disk valve, it is important to note that the opening E point is sharp (Fig. 6–141B).

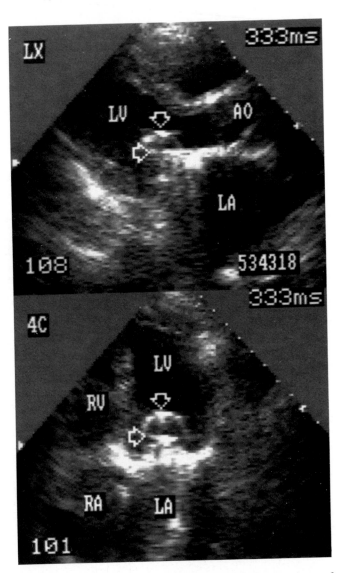

**Fig. 6–136.** Long-axis (LX) and four-chamber (4C) views of a ball-cage type prosthetic mitral valve. *Vertical arrows* = leading echoes from the cage. *Horizontal arrows* = leading echoes from the ball. LV = left ventricle; AO = aorta; LA = left atrium; RV = right ventricle; RA = right atrium.

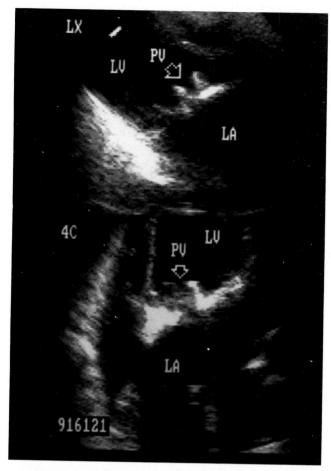

**Fig. 6–137.** Long-axis (LX) and four-chamber (4C) echocardiograms of a patient with a porcine mitral valve (PV). The characteristic struts can be seen in both views. LV = left ventricle; LA = left atrium.

All of the illustrations are of mitral prosthetic valves. It is not easy to obtain two-dimensional images of the normal prosthetic aortic valve with transthoracic echocardiography. Furthermore, such imaging does not necessarily differentiate normal from abnormally functioning valves.

Doppler echocardiography is playing the major role in assessing prosthetic valve function.[416–422] The Doppler

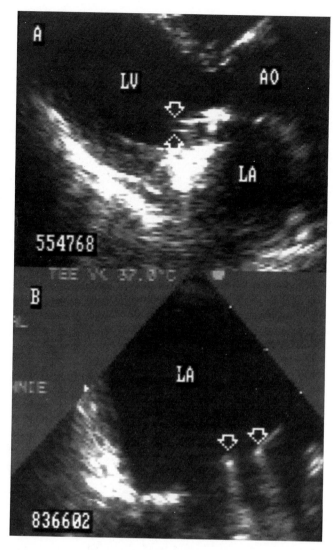

**Fig. 6–139.** Transthoracic long-axis (A) and transesophageal (B) two-dimensional echocardiograms of patients with St. Jude mitral prosthetic valves. The two leaflets (*arrows*) can be seen in diastole in both examinations. LV = left ventricle; AO = aorta; LA = left atrium.

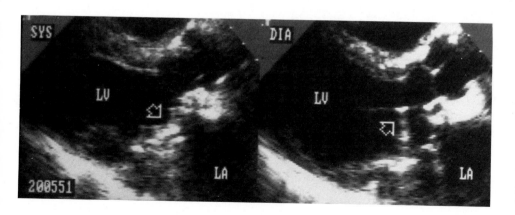

**Fig. 6–138.** Systolic (SYS) and diastolic (DIA) long-axis images of a tilting disk mitral prosthesis. The recording shows the closed and open tilting disk (*arrows*). LV = left ventricle; LA = left atrium.

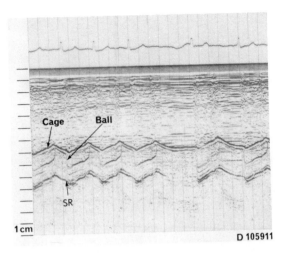

1 cm
D 105911

**Fig. 6–140.** Echocardiogram of a mitral valve-ball valve prosthesis with the transducer near the cardiac apex. The most anterior echo originates from the struts of the cage. The leading edge of the ball produces an echo resembling moderate mitral stenosis. The more posterior echo, which is parallel to the anterior cage echo, originates from the posterior portion of the cage or the sewing ring (SR). (From Schuchman, H., et al.: Intracavitary echoes in patients with mitral prosthetic valves. JCU, *3*:111, 1975.)

recordings are similar to native valve studies, except that the velocities are higher because all prosthetic valves are mildly stenotic. Figure 6–142 shows the pulsed Doppler recording of a normally functioning porcine mitral valve. The peak flow is approximately 135 cm/sec. Figure 6–143 shows another normally functioning porcine valve in a patient with atrial fibrillation.

Doppler flow of a normal Bjork-Shiley mitral prosthesis is noted in Figure 6–144. A similar recording from a St. Jude valve is illustrated in Figure 6–145.

Normal Doppler values for prosthetic valves vary widely according to the type and size of the valves.[423–425] Because all prosthetic valves are mildly stenotic, the velocity passing across the valves are flow dependent. In the appendix is listed some of the normal values obtained on a variety of prosthetic valves. The striking finding in looking at these values is the wide range of normal measurements. These measurements are primarily of value in trying to differentiate a normally functioning valve from one that is stenotic.[426] Doppler studies of prosthetic valves performed during exercise have been suggested as a way to evaluate these valves physiologically.[427–429,429a,429b]

**Stenosis**

Trying to determine prosthetic valve stenosis can be extremely difficult because of the wide range of normal velocities through these valves. Figure 6–146 shows a prosthetic aortic valve with a velocity usually out of the range of a normally functioning valve. Figure 6–147 is a pulsed Doppler examination through a porcine mitral valve that was obstructed and had an 18-mm gradient. The flow through a stenotic tricuspid porcine valve is shown in Figure 6–148. The measurements made to assess stenosis include the peak velocity, mean velocity, velocity time integral, valve area[430,431] using pressure half-time, and effective valve orifice using the continuity equation and Gorlin formula.[432,433] A simplified version of the continuity equation, effective valve orifice deter-

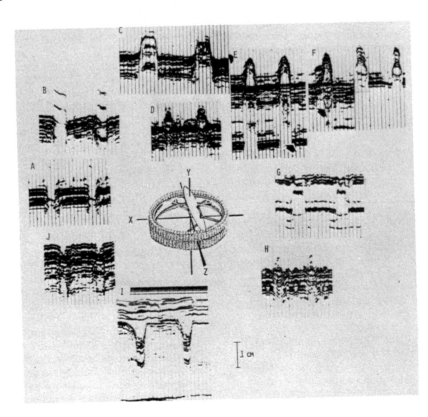

**Fig. 6–141.** Illustration demonstrating the various echocardiograms one can obtain from a Bjork-Shiley tilting disc valve. (From Douglas, J.E. and Williams, G.D.: Echocardiographic evaluation of the Bjork-Shiley prosthetic valve. Circulation, *50*:52, 1974, by permission of the American Heart Association, Inc.)

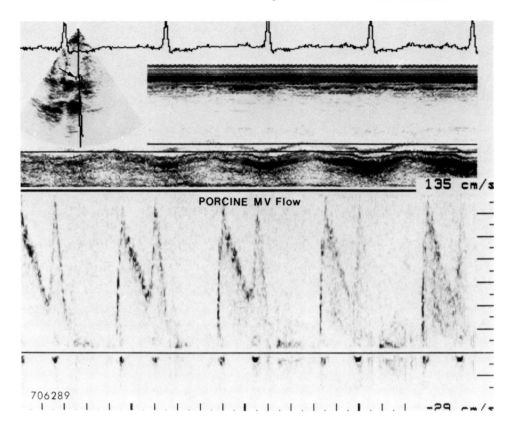

**Fig. 6–142.** Pulsed Doppler echocardiogram demonstrating flow through a normally functioning porcine mitral valve.

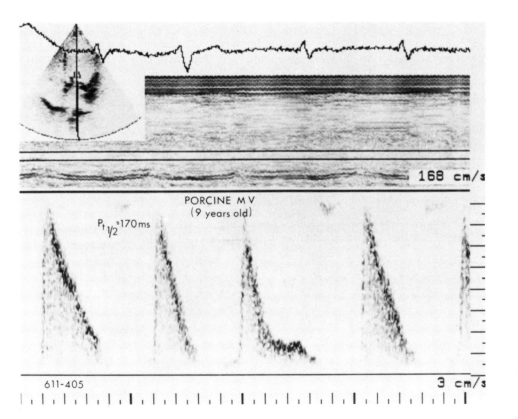

**Fig. 6–143.** Doppler flow through a normally functioning porcine mitral valve of a patient with atrial fibrillation.

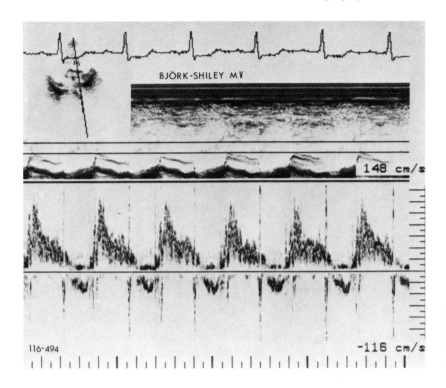

**Fig. 6–144.** Doppler flow recording of a normally functioning Bjork-Shiley mitral valve prosthesis. The sample volume is in the left ventricle.

mination would be the ratio of velocities on both sides of the valve.[434]

All efforts to calculate prosthetic valve stenosis are based on the Doppler-derived pressure gradient.[435,436] A factor that must be considered because it introduces a source of potential error is the phenomenon of "pressure recovery." This concept is based on the conserva-

tion of energy, which requires that the pressure of a fluid decreases as the velocity increases. The site of highest velocity and lowest pressure is at the narrowest point (or just downstream at the vena contracta) in a prosthetic valve. As one moves away from the prosthesis, the velocity decreases and the pressure increases. This increase in pressure represents "the pressure recov-

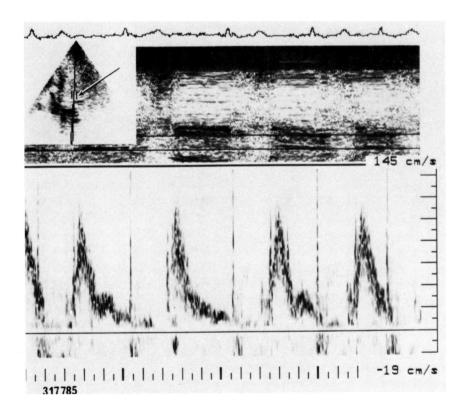

**Fig. 6–145.** Doppler flow pattern through a normally functioning St. Jude mitral valve prosthesis. *Arrow* = the Doppler sample.

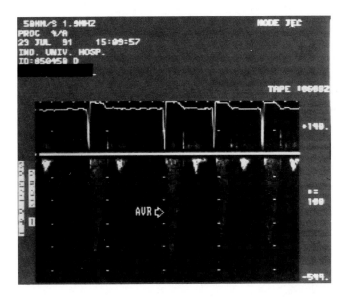

**Fig. 6–146.** Continuous wave Doppler study of a patient with a stenotic aortic valve prosthesis. The peak systolic velocity reaches 4.5 M/sec.

ery.''[437] Thus, the pressure gradient depends on where the pressure is sampled. With continuous wave Doppler imaging, the peak velocity is recorded at the site of the narrowest point of the prosthetic valve; in the catheterization laboratory, however, the pressure may be measured at varying points from the valve. Thus, the Doppler pressure gradient may be higher than that obtained invasively.[437,438] Because of the hydrodynamic flow through prosthetic valves, this pressure recovery

phenomenon is more significant than with native valves. Despite these difficulties, some data show a reasonable relationship between the continuous wave-derived Doppler gradients and those obtained at cardiac catheterization. These difficulties in calculating accurate gradients across prosthetic valves using Doppler are aggravated by small prosthetic valves.[439]

The way one would determine whether a prosthetic valve is stenotic is to obtain the various Doppler-derived estimates of valve area or gradient and compare these measurements with the expected values for that particular valve type and size. Because of the variability in normal values (see Appendix), no general, simple measurement can help separate the normally from abnormally functioning valve. One group of investigators think that one can calculate prosthetic valve area and use the number in a fashion similar to that with native valves.[440] When attempting to measure the effective valve orifice, it is probably best to measure the left ventricular outflow tract when estimating the aortic valve orifice. Sometimes, however, it is technically difficult to obtain this measurement, and it is easier to measure the diameter of the sewing ring. It should be clearly noted which diameter is used so that in follow-up studies measurements are made in the same fashion.

An approach that seems to be increasingly popular for evaluating a prosthetic valve is to take the ratio of the proximal and distal velocities. For example, with regard to the aortic prosthetic valve, one would compare the peak or velocity time integral of the left ventricular outflow tract velocity and the prosthetic valve peak or integrated velocities. This ratio is ''dimensionlessness,'' and is not as related to the type and size of the prosthetic

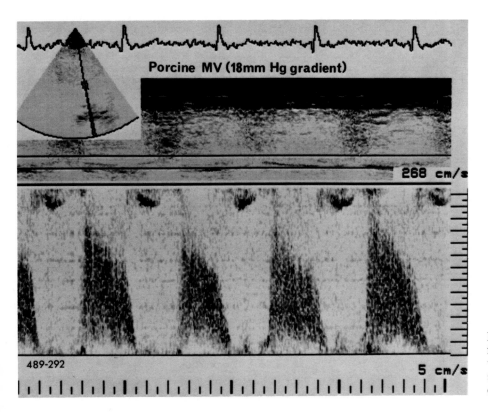

**Fig. 6–147.** Pulsed Doppler flow through a porcine mitral valve that had significant obstruction and an 18-mm gradient.

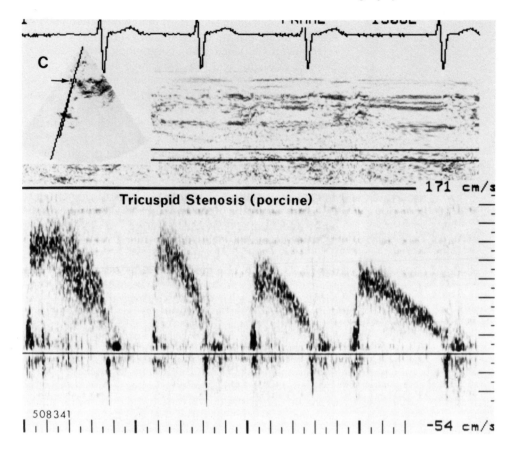

**Fig. 6–148.** Doppler flow through a stenotic porcine tricuspid valve prosthesis. The Doppler sample (*arrow*) is in the right ventricle.

valve. The ratio of left ventricular outflow tract velocity and aortic prosthesis velocity is ideal for serial studies to see whether a change has occurred, because the outflow tract size, which is the missing factor, should not change over time. Thus, for assessing aortic prosthetic valve stenosis, probably the preferred technique is either to measure the valve area by using the continuity equation[441–443] or to follow the proximal and peak velocity ratios to see whether any change is noted. This approach requires a baseline examination shortly after surgery, at which time there is confidence that the valve is functioning normally.

The mitral prosthesis can be assessed by measuring the mean gradient or by calculating a pressure half-time.[444] Pressure half-time accuracy is somewhat limited[445] and probably overestimates the true effective orifice area. If no aortic regurgitation or mitral regurgitation is present, then the continuity equation calculation of effective mitral orifice area is probably preferred. The calculation would be the left ventricular outflow tract area times the left ventricular outflow tract velocity divided by the prosthetic mitral valve velocity ($A_{PV} = A_{LVOT} \times V_{LVOT} \div V_{PV}$). In this case, one would need to use the time velocity integral for both the outflow tract and mitral valve prosthesis flows. One could not rely on a simplified peak velocity measurement. Calculations for tricuspid valves would be somewhat similar to that for mitral valves.

In summary, calculating prosthetic valve stenosis is fraught with difficulties and is not a simple procedure.[445a] One must know the type and size of the pros-

thesis in question and realize the wide range of normal velocities that can occur across these valves. Meticulous attention must be given to acquiring accurate measurements. And even despite these precautions, a given set of values is not nearly as important as following an individual and noting deterioration in effective valve orifice. Thus, it is increasingly important to obtain a baseline echocardiographic study when the valve is apparently functioning normally and using these values for comparison with future studies when the suspicion is that the valve may have become stenotic.

The difficulties in calculating effective valve orifice is not as much of a problem as would be anticipated, in part because if the valve is stenotic, the etiology for the stenosis can frequently be detected more directly. For example, if the reason for stenosis is a fibrotic, calcified, and immobile porcine mitral valve, this change in valve morphology can be detected with two-dimensional or M-mode echocardiography.[446] Furthermore, if a clot is producing obstruction, the clot can be detected.[447,447a] Figure 6–149 shows a two-dimensional echocardiogram of a patient with a Bjork-Shiley mitral valve prosthesis with a large clot obstructing inflow to the valve. Transesophageal echocardiography is more productive in detecting clots on prosthetic valves.[448–451] Figure 6–150 shows a transesophageal echocardiogram of a patient with a prosthetic mitral valve. The valve was physiologically stenotic and the explanation was a massive clot on the atrial side of the prosthesis. Visualization of the clot was far more definitive in managing the patient than was the hemodynamic measurement of valve stenosis. Occa-

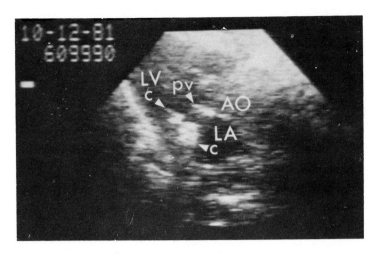

**Fig. 6–149.** Two-dimensional echocardiogram showing a large clot (c) surrounding a Bjork-Shiley mitral valve prosthesis (pv). LV = left ventricle; AO = aorta; LA = left atrium.

sionally, mobile strands of tissue that are clinically unimportant can be seen on a St. Jude valve with transesophageal echocardiography.[452]

M-mode echocardiography can still be helpful in detecting valve stenosis, especially with mechanical valves. One of the more important signs of an obstructed prosthetic mitral valve is with a tilting disk valve, such as a Bjork-Shiley prosthesis.[453–455] With obstruction to opening, the normally sharp E point is rounded (Fig. 6–151).[456] In some older ball-cage valves, ball variance was a problem whereby the ball would swell and become partially stuck in the cage.[457,458] Figure 6–152 shows an M-mode recording of such a situation whereby the excursion of the ball is restricted and does not reach the full extent of the cage. A clot effecting a ball valve can also produce intermittent obstruction to opening. Figure 6–153 shows an example of a valve that is obstructed intermittently by a thrombus in the valve.

## Regurgitation

One of the reasons echocardiography is so valuable in evaluating prosthetic valves is that one of the most common forms of malfunction is prosthetic valve regurgitation. Doppler echocardiography is extremely useful in assessing this valvular insufficiency.[459–463] Certain technical precautions are necessary when using Doppler echocardiography for prosthetic valve regurgitation. The most important of these limitations is the problem of acoustic shadowing by the highly reflective prosthetic material. Thus, it is difficult, and sometimes inaccurate, to try to detect a regurgitant velocity jet when the reflective prosthetic valve is between the transducer and the jet. For example, it is difficult to assess fully the presence or degree of mitral valvular regurgitation with the transducer at the apex. The ultrasonic beam must traverse the highly reflected valve structures before inter-

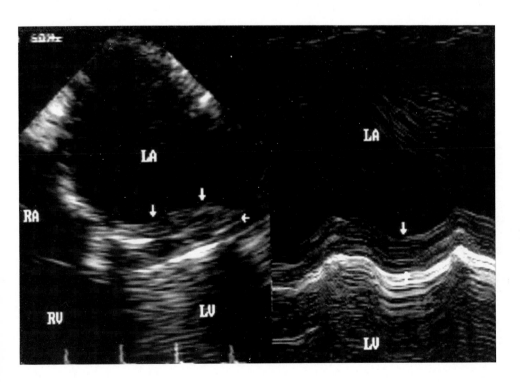

**Fig. 6–150.** Transesophageal echocardiogram of a patient with a thrombus (*arrows*) on a prosthetic mitral valve. The thrombus is on the left atrial side of the valve. LA = left atrium; LV = left ventricle; RA = right atrium; RV = right ventricle.

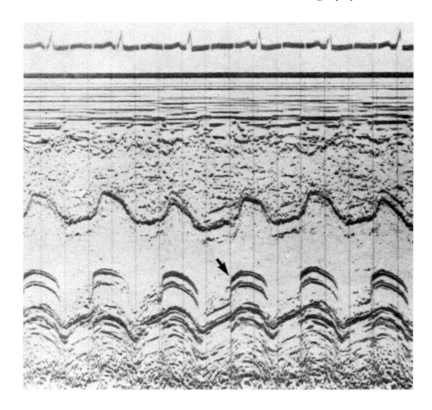

**Fig. 6–151.** Echocardiogram from a Bjork-Shiley prosthesis in the mitral position demonstrating rounding of the E point (*arrow*). Partial obstruction of the valve occurred owing to an ingrowth of fibrous tissue. (From Clements, S.D. and Perkins, J.V.: Malfunction of a Bjork-Shiley prosthetic heart valve in the mitral position producing an abnormal echocardiographic pattern. JCU, *6*:334, 1978.)

rogating the left atrium for any insufficiency. This problem is lessened if the valve is a heterograft, which is not as reflective, and if the leak if perivalvular. Figure 6–154 shows such an example of a mitral regurgitant jet in a patient with a porcine mitral valve and a perivalvular leak. One clearly can see the regurgitant jet originating in the perivalvular position. Attempting to quantitate regurgitation through prosthetic valves, however, especially in the mitral position, is extremely difficult with the transthoracic approach. Figure 6–155 demonstrates another patient with a leaking prosthetic mitral valve. One definitely can identify regurgitant flow into the left atrium (*arrows*), however, the color flow Doppler would be indicative of only moderate regurgitation. The patient, in fact, had severe regurgitation. Much of the regurgitant jet was not seen because of acoustic shadowing by the prosthetic valve.

Transesophageal echocardiography is clearly the pro-

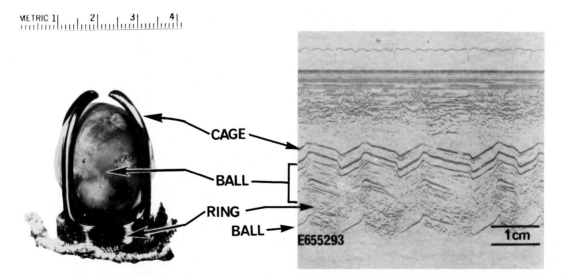

**Fig. 6–152.** Photograph and echocardiogram of a patient with ball variance. The Silastic ball swelled and became lodged within the cage. The echoes from the ball demonstrate minimal motion, and the leading edge of the ball fails to reach the leading echo from the cage. (From Wann, L.S., et al.: Ball variance in a Harken mitral prosthesis. Echocardiographic and phonocardiographic features. Chest, *72*:785, 1977.)

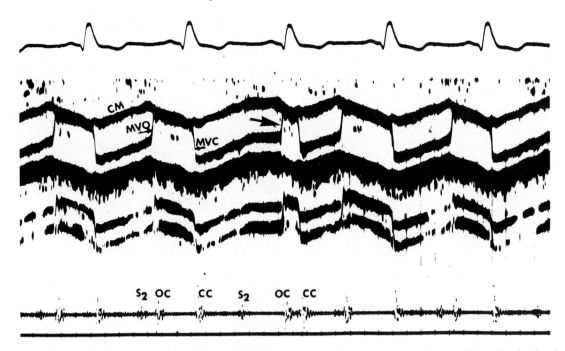

**Fig. 6–153.** Echocardiogram from a malfunctioning mitral prosthetic valve, demonstrated by a delayed mitral valve opening (MVO) in the third cardiac complex (*arrow*). CM = cage of mitral valve; MVC = mitral valve closing; S2 = second heart sound; OC = opening click; CC = closing click. (From Pfeifer, J., et al.: Malfunction of mitral ball valve prosthesis due to thrombosis. Am. J. Cardiol., *29*:95, 1972.)

cedure of choice for detecting valvular regurgitation through a mitral prosthesis.[464–469] Because the prosthesis is not between the regurgitant jet and the transducer, one obtains an unobstructed view of any regurgitant leak. In fact, the transesophageal technique is so sensitive that the normal amount of regurgitation commonly seen with prosthetic valves can also be detected.[470–473] Thus, one has to be careful about assuming that a valve is malfunctioning because of a small regurgitant leak. Figure 6–156 demonstrates a transesophageal echocardiogram of a normally functioning Medtronic Hall mitral prosthetic valve. The small central regurgitant flow is to be expected. The normal regurgitation noted with mitral St. Jude valve is illustrated in Figure

6–157. This bileaflet valve produces multiple jets. Noncentral or perivalvular leaks are always abnormal.[474] Figure 6–158 is a transesophageal echocardiogram of a patient with a porcine prosthetic mitral valve with two, noncentral regurgitant jets that definitely are abnormal.

The transthoracic approach for detecting aortic prosthesis regurgitation is easier because the apical approach easily identifies the leak. Figure 6–159 shows a gray scale Doppler imaging study of a patient with a small perivalvular leak of a prosthetic aortic valve. Figure 6–160 demonstrates a regurgitant prosthetic aortic valve using pulsed Doppler. Transesophageal echocardiography can also detect this type of leak and may give better

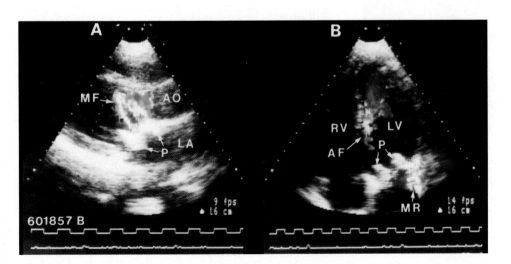

**Fig. 6–154.** Color flow Doppler examinations in diastole (*A*) and systole (*B*) of a patient with a porcine mitral valve who has a perivalvular mitral regurgitant leak (MR). P = porcine valve; AF = aortic flow; RV = right ventricle; LV = left ventricle; MF = mitral flow; AO = aorta; LA = left atrium. (From Feigenbaum, H.: Doppler color flow imaging. *In* Heart Disease Update. Edited by E. Braunwald. Philadelphia, W.B. Saunders Co., 1988.)

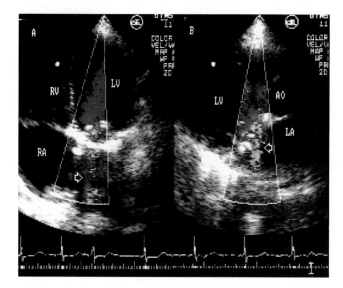

**Fig. 6–155.** Four-chamber (*A*) and long-axis (*B*) color flow Doppler studies of a severely leaking mitral porcine valve. The size of the jet (*arrows*) is limited by shadowing from the sewing ring. Thus, the degree of regurgitation artifactually appears less than it should be. RV = right ventricle; LV = left ventricle; RA = right atrium; LA = left atrium; AO = aorta.

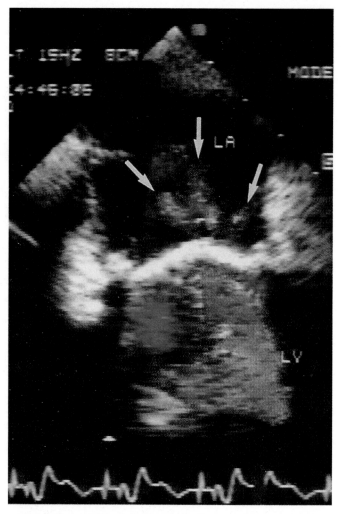

**Fig. 6–157.** Normally functioning St. Jude prosthetic mitral valve demonstrating multiple regurgitant jets (*arrows*) within the left atrium (LA) using transesophageal echocardiography. LV = left ventricle. (From Hixson, C.S., et al.: Comparison of transesophageal color flow Doppler imaging of normal mitral regurgitant jets in St. Jude Medical and Medtronic Hall cardiac protheses. J. Am. Soc. Echocardiogr., *5*:58, 1992.)

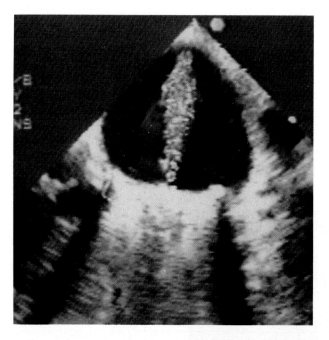

**Fig. 6–156.** Transesophageal color Doppler study of a patient with a normally functioning Medtronic Hall mitral prosthetic valve. One can see a central regurgitant jet in the left atrium in this normally functioning valve. (From Hixson, C.S., et al.: Comparison of transesophageal color flow Doppler imaging of normal mitral regurgitant jets in St. Jude Medical and Medtronic Hall cardiac protheses. J. Am. Soc. Echocardiogr., *5*: 58, 1992.)

definition as to the exact site of the regurgitation.[475,476] As a general rule, the transthoracic examination does a reasonable job with aortic prosthesis regurgitation. Transesophageal echocardiography does not provide as much information as it does in the evaluation of the mitral prosthetic valve.[466,477] In fact, if the patient also has a prosthetic mitral valve, transesophageal echocardiography may not detect aortic regurgitation because of acoustic shadowing.

Figure 6–161 shows some of the potential artifacts produced with prosthetic valves that can make the detection of regurgitation difficult. This black and white flow imaging study shows a patient with true aortic regurgitation (AR) through a native regurgitant valve. In addition, a mitral prosthesis produces a reverberation (R) that obscures part of the left atrium. A flow imaging flash (F) or ghosting resulting from a reverberation su-

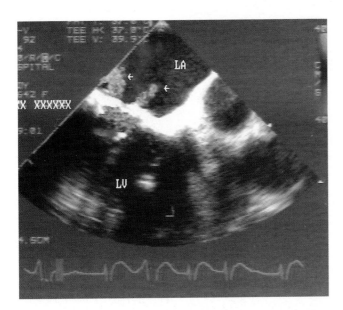

**Fig. 6–158.** Transesophageal echocardiographic examination of a patient with a porcine mitral valve and two non-central mitral regurgitant jets (*arrows*) within the left atrium (LA). LV = left ventricle.

perficially resembles a regurgitant jet. One can usually exclude this possibility because the flash is brief and does not represent any logical physiologic flow.

Other signs on the echocardiogram give evidence of prosthetic valve regurgitation. An interesting Doppler finding with a malfunctioning porcine mitral valve is a series of oscillating velocities that produce stripes on a pulsed Doppler recording (Fig. 6–162).[478] Needless to say, this coarse Doppler fluttering produces a most unu-

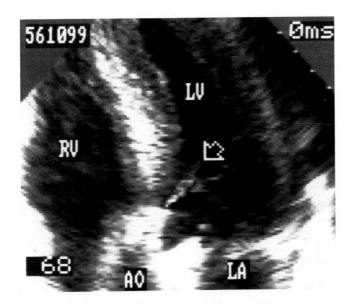

**Fig. 6–159.** Black and white Doppler flow imaging of a patient with aortic valve prosthesis and a small perivalvular aortic regurgitant jet (*arrow*). LV = left ventricle; RV = right ventricle; AO = aorta; LA = left atrium.

sual sound during the Doppler examination. This finding is highly indicative of a fractured porcine mitral valve. Flail porcine valves also are seen with two-dimensional imaging. Figure 6–163 shows such a leaflet protruding into the left atrium. The transesophageal examination would be even more spectacular in demonstrating this abnormality.

Another technique with which to evaluate prosthetic valve regurgitation, especially in the mitral position, is proximal color flow acceleration.[479,480,480a] Acoustic shadowing prevents a good assessment of valvular regurgitation within the left atrium with transthoracic echocardiography. Looking for proximal flow acceleration on the ventricular side of the prosthetic valve, however, can be useful in identifying patients with significant valvular regurgitation. This flow acceleration occurs only with significant degrees of regurgitation and can immediately identify those patients who have malfunctioning prosthetic valves, despite the inability to see regurgitation on the left atrial side of the valve.

Valvular regurgitation secondary to prosthetic valve dehiscence can be detected with two-dimensional echocardiography by noting extreme rocking of the prostheses. Disk escape from a Bjork-Shiley valve has been noted echocardiographically.[481] Dehiscence of a Carpentier mitral ring has been detected with transesophageal echocardiography.[482]

### Complications

A variety of complications can occur with prosthetic valves that require surgical revision and can be detected with echocardiography. These complications include pseudoaneurysm at the attachment of the prosthetic valve.[483–485] Also, a variety of fistulas can occur with these valves.[484] The fistulas have been noted to go from the left ventricle to a left coronary artery[486] or from the left ventricle into the right atrium. All of these complications, especially those involving the mitral protheses, can best be detected with transesophageal echocardiography. The devastating complication of infection or endocarditis is discussed in the next section, Endocarditis. Occasionally, a prosthetic valve can protrude into the interventricular septum.[487–489] This problem has also been detected with echocardiography (Fig. 6–164). Transesophageal echocardiography has identified an atrial wall aneurysm owing to an abnormal attachment of a mitral prosthesis.[489a]

There have been a few isolated reports of peculiar findings in patients with prosthetic valves. One observation is the presence of tiny echoes apparently coming through a mitral prosthetic valve.[490,491] Figure 6–165 shows an example of such a situation. The patient has a mitral Starr-Edwards valve. The transducer is at the cardiac apex. One can note rapidly moving echoes (*arrowheads*) moving from the vicinity of the mitral valve into the more anterior left ventricle during diastole. The echoes are similar to those seen with contrast echocardiography. Moving away from the ball during diastole, they turn around and move away from the transducer, possibly out the left ventricular outflow tract, during

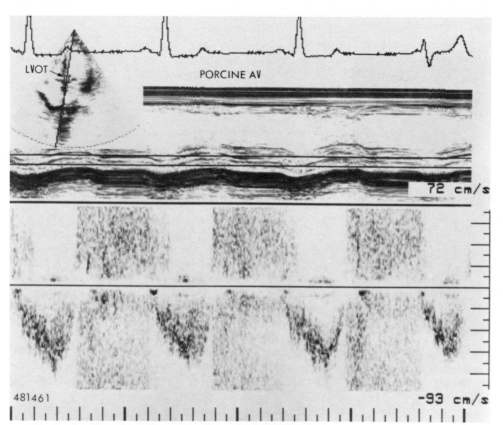

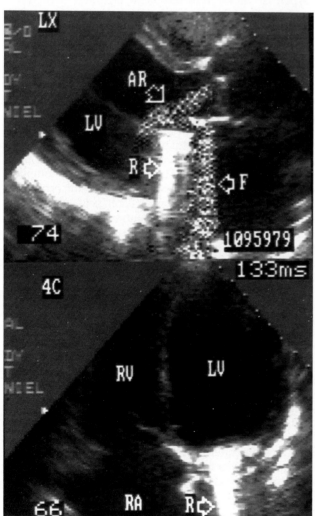

Fig. 6–160. Pulsed Doppler echocardiogram with the sample volume in the left ventricular outflow tract (LVOT) of a patient with a porcine aortic valve (AV) and marked aortic regurgitation.

Fig. 6–161. Black and white Doppler flow imaging showing some of the artifacts that can produce confusing echocardiograms in patients with prosthetic valves. The patient has true aortic regurgitation (AR). In addition, the prosthetic mitral valve produces a long reverberation (R) and a reverberation flash (F), which can simulate artifactual mitral regurgitation. LV = left ventricle; RV = right ventricle; RA = right atrium; LX = long axis; 4C = four chamber.

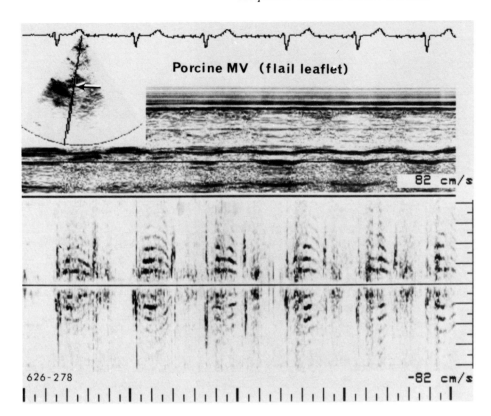

**Fig. 6–162.** Doppler echocardiogram with the sample volume (*arrow*) near a flail porcine mitral leaflet. In systole, one records bands of differing velocities possibly due to coarse fluttering of the flail leaflet.

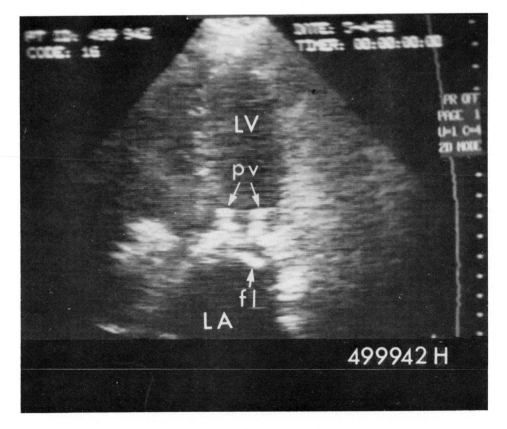

**Fig. 6–163.** Apical four-chamber view of a patient with a degenerated flail porcine mitral valve prosthesis (pv). The flail leaflet (fl) can be seen protruding into the left atrium (LA) in systole. LV = left ventricle.

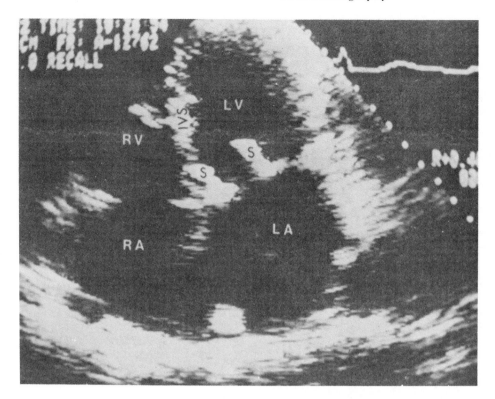

**Fig. 6–164.** Apical four-chamber echocardiogram of a patient with a prosthetic mitral prosthesis with the stents (S) protruding into the interventricular septum (IVS). LV = left ventricle; RV = right ventricle; RA = right atrium; LA = left atrium. (Reprinted with permission of the American College of Cardiology. From Solana, L.G., et al.: Two-dimensional echocardiographic assessment of complications involving the Ionescu-Shiley pericardial valve in the mitral position. J. Am. Coll. Cardiol., *3*:328, 1984.)

systole. The origin and significance of these echoes are not clear. They often occur with cloth-covered valves. Figure 6–166, however, shows similar findings in a patient with a porcine mitral valve. During systole (Fig. 6–166), the left ventricle is free of any intracavitary echoes. During diastole (Fig. 6–166), however, a shower of echoes (*arrows*) passes through the prosthetic valve (PV). Although the origin of these peculiar echoes is unknown, most patients manifesting this phenomenon have some clinical problem. These problems are not consistent, however, and all valves are not hemodynamically impaired.

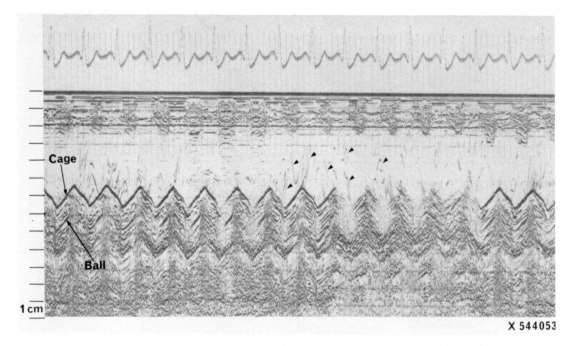

X 544053

**Fig. 6–165.** Intracavitary echoes (*arrowheads*) originating from a mitral valve prosthesis. The transducer was at the cardiac apex, the reject was low, and the gain was high in order to record these fine echoes. (From Schuchman, H., et al.: Intracavitary echoes in patients with mitral prosthetic valves. JCU, *3*:111, 1975.)

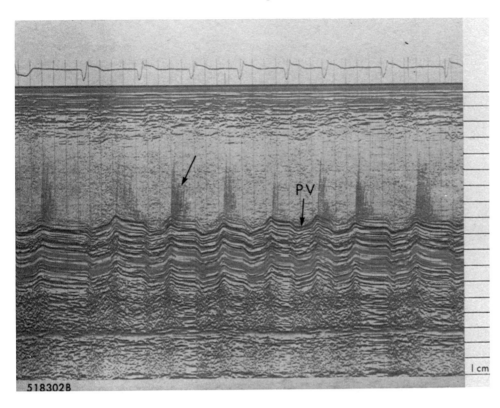

**Fig. 6–166.** M-mode echocardiogram of a porcine mitral valve (PV) in the mitral position through which a shower of echoes (*arrow*) passes in diastole.

## ENDOCARDITIS

The ability of M-mode and two-dimensional echocardiography to visualize vegetations on valves affected by endocarditis is one of the major applications of echocardiography. The echocardiographic criterion for the diagnosis of a vegetation is the finding of an echogenic mass on one of the valve leaflets. Figure 6–167 shows one of the original M-mode echocardiograms with a vegetation on a posterior mitral leaflet. The echocardiographic diagnosis consists of a mass of somewhat "shaggy" echoes on the valve leaflet.

Vegetations on the aortic valve are similar to those on the mitral valve. In some ways, the diagnosis of aortic valve vegetations is easier because multiple echoes from the aortic valve are not as common as they are in the noninfected mitral valve. Figure 6–168 is an early tracing from a patient with aortic valve vegetation. Again, one sees increased echoes from the aortic valve leaflets with no restriction of motion. The three views of this patient note the variability that one can record in a patient with an eccentrically located vegetation. The echoes from the vegetation may be seen best either in systole or in diastole depending on the direction of the ultrasonic beam. A mobile vegetation is more apparent on the M-mode echocardiogram.[396,492,493] Figure 6–169 demonstrates a vegetation on the aortic valve that is recorded as a mass of echoes within the aorta in diastole. In addition, part of the vegetation can be seen in the left ventricular outflow tract above the mitral valve. Recording these abnormal echoes within the left ventricular outflow tract is more convincing than merely finding excess echoes on the aortic valve.[494] It is not clear whether

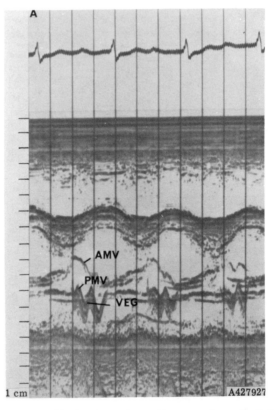

**Fig. 6–167.** Mitral valve echocardiogram of a patient with bacterial endocarditis and vegetations (VEG) on the posterior mitral valve leaflet (PMV). AMV = anterior mitral valve leaflet. (From Dillon, J.C., et al.: Echocardiographic manifestations of valvular vegetations. Am. Heart J., *86*:698, 1973.)

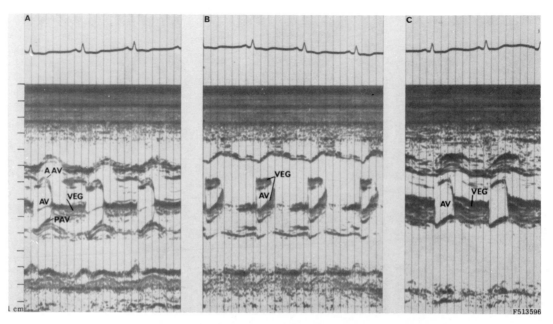

**Fig. 6–168.** Aortic valve echocardiograms of a patient with bacterial endocarditis and vegetations (VEG) on the aortic valve (AV). AAV = anterior aortic valve leaflet; PAV = posterior aortic valve leaflet. (From Dillon, J.C., et al.: Echocardiographic manifestations of valvular vegetations. Am. Heart J., *86*:698, 1973.)

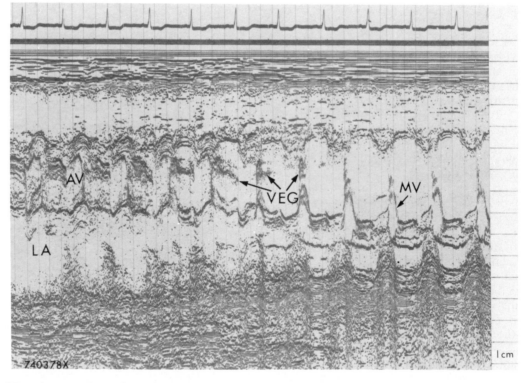

**Fig. 6–169.** M-mode scan of a patient with bacterial endocarditis and vegetations on the aortic valve (AV). During diastole, echoes from the vegetations (VEG) extend into the left ventricular outflow tract above the mitral valve (MV). LA = left atrium.

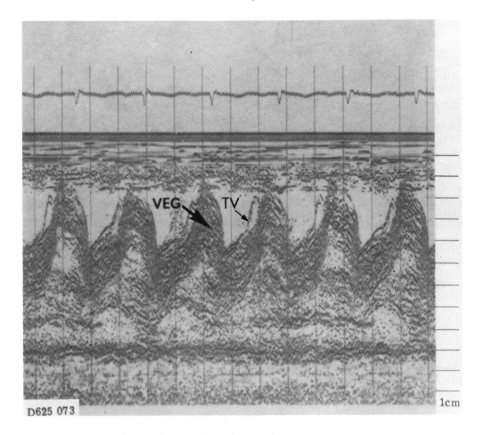

**Fig. 6–170.** M-mode echocardiogram demonstrating a massive bacterial vegetation (VEG) on the tricuspid valve (TV).

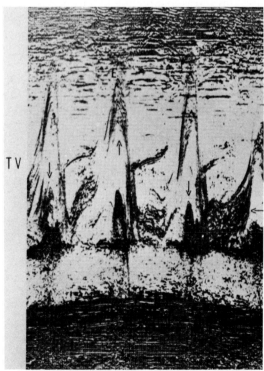

**Fig. 6–171.** Tricuspid valve echocardiogram showing multiple "shaggy" echoes (*arrows*) attached to the tricuspid valve (TV). These echoes originated from a clot that was trapped within the tricuspid valve and simulated a vegetation. (From Covarrubias, E.A., Sheikh, M.U., and Fox, L.M.: Echocardiography and pulmonary embolism. Ann. Intern. Med., *87*:720, 1977.)

the abnormal echoes originate from the vegetation or from part of a flail aortic valve.[494] Thus, the echocardiographic diagnosis would be consistent with, but not necessarily diagnostic of, a mobile vegetation on the aortic valve with or without disruption of the valve. Aortic valve vegetations may be massive.[495] One report described vegetation that produced lethal obstruction to blood flow into the aorta.[496] Vegetations large enough to obstruct the mitral valve have also been detected echocardiographically.[497,498]

Vegetations involving the tricuspid valve have been noted on the M-mode echocardiogram.[499–501] Their appearance is similar to those seen on the mitral valve. Occasionally, one might note an unusually large vegetation such as the one in Figure 6–170 involving the tricuspid valve. In this case, the mass is so large that it is difficult to distinguish from a neoplasm. It must be emphasized that finding a mass on a valve is not specific for a vegetation. In Figure 6–171, the tricuspid valve shows an echo-producing mass near the posterior tricuspid valve leaflet. These "shaggy" echoes actually originated from a clot that was trapped in the tricuspid valve. No evidence of a vegetation was found.[502]

Two-dimensional echocardiography is actually the preferred technique for detecting vegetations. The spatially oriented examination provides a better assessment of the size and motion of the abnormal masses. Figure 6–172 demonstrates a mobile vegetation on a mitral valve. This mobile mass of tissue (*arrow*), attached to a flail mitral valve, can be seen protruding into the left atrium in systole and into the left ventricular outflow tract in diastole. The real-time examination was striking

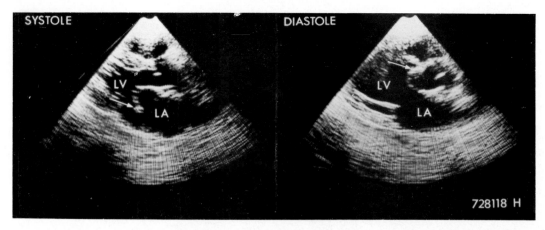

**Fig. 6–172.** Long-axis echocardiogram demonstrating a mobile vegetation (*arrows*) on the anterior mitral leaflet. In systole, the vegetation protrudes into the left atrium. In diastole, the vegetation moves into the left ventricular outflow tract. LV = left ventricle; LA = left atrium.

as this mass flopped about within the heart. Figure 6–173 demonstrates vegetations on both mitral valve leaflets.

The patient illustrated in Figure 6–174 had endocarditis involving the aortic valve. The vegetation (veg) can be seen protruding into the left ventricular outflow tract in both the long-axis and short-axis views. The larger more mobile vegetations are spectacular in the real-time two-dimensional echocardiographic examination. A tricuspid valve vegetation is illustrated in Figure 6–175. Figure 6–176 provides a two-dimensional echocardiogram of a patient who had vegetations on both the aortic valve (avv) and the mitral valve (mvv). A patient with a vegetation on the aortic, mitral, and tricuspid valves is illustrated in Figure 6–177.

One of more important complications is the presence of an abscess.[503–510] Figure 6–178 demonstrates a patient with a vegetation on the mitral leaflet with a secondary abscess involving the papillary muscle. The abscesses frequently, but not always, have an echo-free center. Figure 6–179 illustrates an important and poten-

tially devastating complication of endocarditis. This patient has developed a periannular abscess of the aortic root.[504–511] Early signs of the abscess can be seen in the upper recordings with an echo-free space (*arrows*) posterior to the aortic valve leaflets. The lower tracing shows progression of the abscess as the echo-free space becomes larger.

With the introduction of transesophageal echocardiography, this ultrasonic technique has now become, by far, the most sensitive means of detecting and evaluating

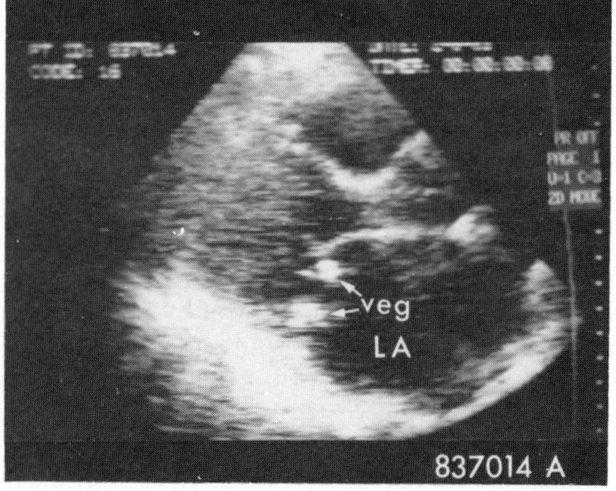

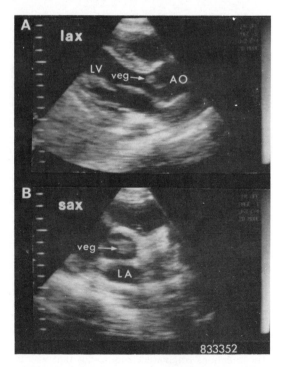

**Fig. 6–174.** Long-axis (*A*) and short-axis (*B*) two-dimensional echocardiograms of a patient with a vegetation (veg) on the aortic valve. LV = left ventricle; AO = aorta; LA = left atrium; lax = long axis; sax = short axis.

**Fig. 6–173.** Long-axis two-dimensional echocardiogram of a patient with vegetations (veg) on both mitral leaflets. LA = left atrium.

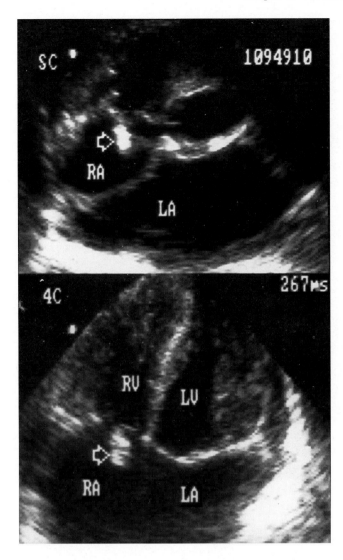

**Fig. 6–175.** Subcostal (SC) and four-chamber (4C) two-dimensional echocardiograms of a patient with a vegetation (*arrow*) on a tricuspid valve. RA = right atrium; LA = left atrium; RV = right ventricle; LV = left ventricle.

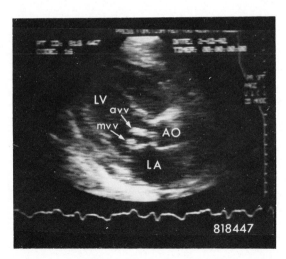

**Fig. 6–176.** Long-axis two-dimensional echocardiogram of a patient with an aortic valve vegetation (avv) and a vegetation on the anterior mitral leaflet (mvv). LV = left ventricle; AO = aorta; LA = left atrium.

vegetations on the valves.[512–517] Numerous studies have now confirmed that the transesophageal approach detects more vegetations than could be seen with the transthoracic echocardiogram. Figure 6–180 shows a patient with a small aortic valve vegetation that could not be seen with transthoracic echocardiography. Figure 6–181 demonstrates a transesophageal echocardiogram of a patient with a vegetation on the pulmonary valve.[518–520] Such vegetations are not common and may also be seen with the transthoracic examination.[521–525]

The transesophageal examination reveals more complications from endocarditis.[526–530,530a] Figure 6–182 is a transesophageal examination of a patient with an aortic root abscess. This complication is extremely important in the management of patients with bacterial endocarditis.[531,532] This abscess was difficult to identify with the standard transthoracic examination. A mitral valve abscess is illustrated in Figure 6–183. This biplane transesophageal examination demonstrates a large abscess on the left atrial side of the mitral valve in both the longitudinal (L) and transverse (T) views. This abscess (A) has

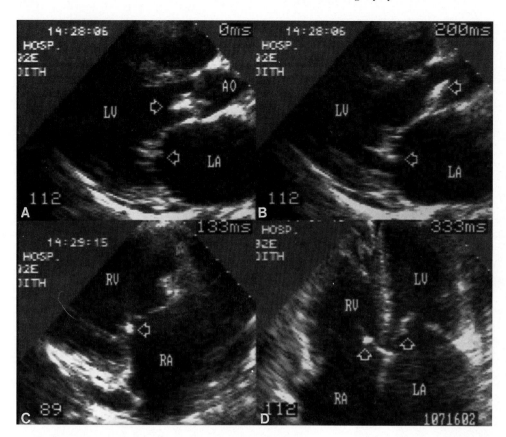

**Fig. 6–177.** Two-dimensional echocardiograms of a patient with vegetations on the mitral and aortic valves (*arrows, A* and *B*) and on the tricuspid valve (*arrows, C* and *D*). LV = left ventricle; AO = aorta; LA = left atrium; RV = right ventricle; RA = right atrium.

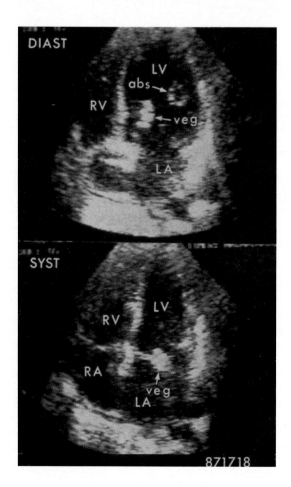

**Fig. 6–178.** Apical four-chamber echocardiograms of a patient with a vegetation (veg) on the anterior mitral leaflet and an abscess (abs) near the papillary muscle. LV = left ventricle; RV = right ventricle; LA = left atrium; RA = right atrium.

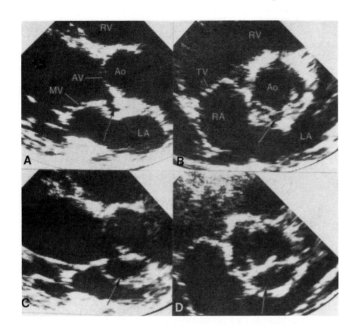

**Fig. 6–179.** Serial two-dimensional echocardiograms of a patient with a periaortic root abscess. Tracings in *A* and *B* show long-axis and short-axis views of an echo-free space (*arrows*) posterior to the aorta (AO). As the abscess grew, the echo-free space became larger (*arrows, C* and *D*). RV = right ventricle; AO = aorta; AV = aortic valve; MV = mitral valve; LA = left atrium; AO = aorta; AV = aortic valve; MV = mitral valve; TV = tricuspid valve; RA = right atrium. (From Byrd, B.F., et al.: Infective perivalvular abscess of the aortic ring: Echocardiographic features and clinical course. Am. J. Cardiol., 66:104, 1990.)

a relatively echo-free center. The color flow study shows mitral regurgitation (MR).

Figure 6–184 shows another complication of endocarditis that is best detected with transesophageal echocardiography.[533] This patient had an infection of the mitral valve that caused perforation and an aneurysm of the leaflet.[534–537] The perforation can be seen with the turbulent blood flow passing through the leaflet from the left ventricle into an aneurysm that protrudes into the left atrium.

The Eustachean valve may also become infected. Such a form of endocarditis has been noted echocardiographically.[538] Vegetations may develop on chamber walls struck by the jets of infected valves. These, too, can be detected on echocardiograms.[539–543,543a]

It is not difficult to understand why one of the major indications for transesophageal echocardiography is the detection and complete evaluation of patients with known or suspected bacterial endocarditis. The sensitivity of this semi-invasive technique is so high that it is

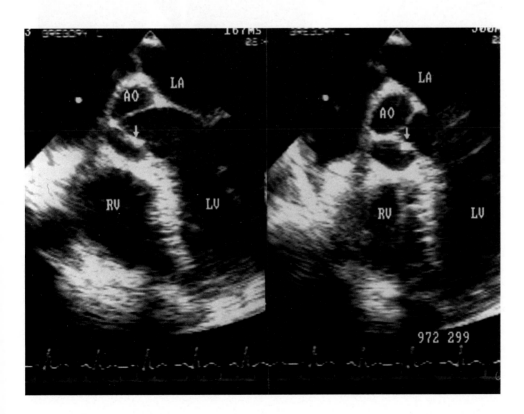

**Fig. 6–180.** Transesophageal echocardiogram of a patient with a small vegetation (*arrows*) on an aortic valve. LA = left atrium; AO = aorta; LV = left ventricle; RV = right ventricle. (From Feigenbaum, H.: Echocardiography. *In* Heart Disease, 4th ed. Edited by E. Braunwald. Philadelphia, W.B. Saunders Co., 1992.)

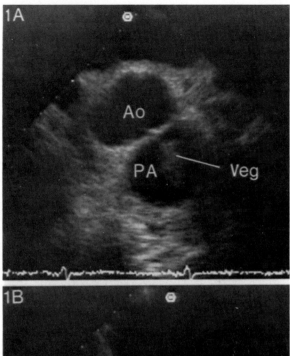

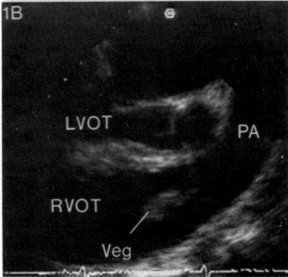

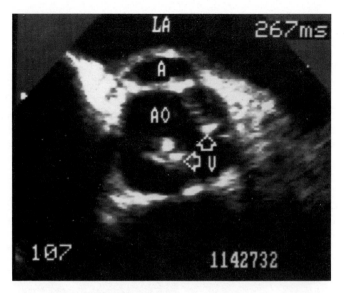

**Fig. 6–182.** Transesophageal echocardiogram of a patient with vegetations (V) on the aortic valve and a periaortic abscess (A). LA = left atrium; AO = aorta.

**Fig. 6–181.** Pulmonary valve vegetation seen with transesophageal echocardiography. The transverse examination (*A*) visualizes the vegetation (Veg) in the pulmonary artery (PA). The longitudinal study (*B*) shows the vegetation in the right ventricular outflow tract (RVOT). AO = aorta; LVOT = left ventricular outflow tract. (From Winslow, T., et al.: Pulmonary valve endocarditis: Improved diagnosis with biplane transesophageal echocardiography. J. Am. Soc. Echocardiogr., *5*:206, 1992.)

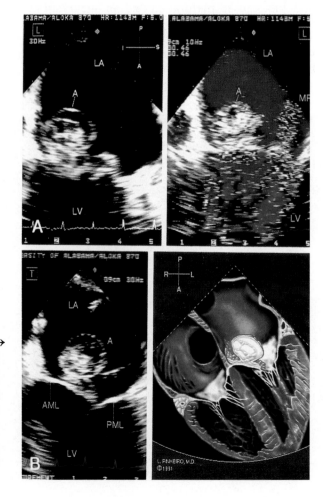

**Fig. 6–183.** Transesophageal echocardiograms of a patient with a large mitral valve abscess (A) as seen in the longitudinal (L, *A*) and transverse (T, *B*) views. The color Doppler recording shows the mitral regurgitant jet (MR); the drawing illustrates the pathology. LA = left atrium; LV = left ventricle; AML = anterior mitral leaflet; PML = posterior mitral leaflet. (From Massey, W.M.: Serial documentation of changes in mitral valve vegetation progressing to abscess rupture and fistula formation by transesophageal echocardiography. Am. Heart J., *124*:241, 1992.)

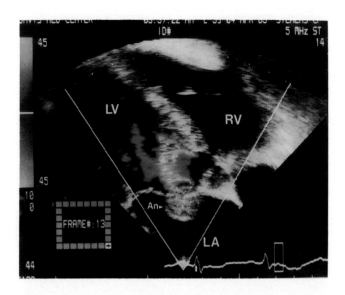

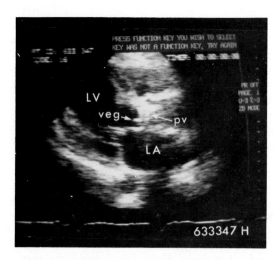

**Fig. 6–186.** Long-axis two-dimensional echocardiogram of a patient with a vegetation (veg) on an aortic prosthetic valve (pv). LV = left ventricle; LA = left atrium.

**Fig. 6–184.** Transesophageal echocardiogram of a patient with a mitral valve aneurysm (An) and perforated mitral valve secondary to mitral valve endocarditis. LV = left ventricle; RV = right ventricle; LA = left atrium. (From Behnam, R. and Bommer, W.: Fenestrated aneurysm of the mitral valve. Echocardiography, 8:525, 1991.)

coming closer to being able to exclude the possibility of endocarditis. This clinical application, however, has not been established.[543b] Some evidence shows that the intensity of the echoes on a transesophageal study may help to differentiate chronic from acute vegetation. The chronic lesions appear to be more echogenic.[544] This differentiation cannot be done with either M-mode or two-dimensional echocardiography through the chest. Making the diagnosis of endocarditis is not always suffi-

cient. One must know the full extent of the infection, whether or not other valves are involved, and whether the infection has invaded the surrounding tissues. Figure 6–185 shows some of the areas to which infection can spread.[545–547] This total assessment can best be made with the transesophageal approach.[547a]

Transesophageal echocardiography is indispensable for detecting vegetations on prosthetic valves.[548,549] It is difficult to identify vegetations on an echogenic prosthetic valve with transthoracic echocardiography. Figure 6–186 shows a vegetation on an aortic prosthetic valve. In this case, the vegetation was mobile and protruded into the left ventricular outflow tract in diastole. Unless they are mobile and protrude away from the prosthesis, it is extremely difficult to detect these vege-

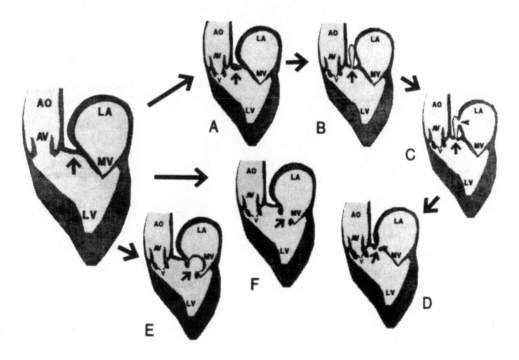

**Fig. 6–185.** Diagram showing how endocarditis can spread to produce aneurysms (B and E), perforations (D and F), and fistulae (C). (From Karalis, D.G., et al.: Transesophageal echocardiographic recognition of subaortic complications in aortic valve endocarditis. Clinical and surgical implications. Circulation, 86: 355, 1992, by permission of the American Heart Association, Inc.)

tations with transthoracic echocardiography. A transesophageal examination is more effective in detecting vegetations because of the higher resolution and because of reduced shadowing of mitral vegetations that usually are on the atrial side of the valve. Figure 6–187 shows a porcine mitral valve with a vegetation on the left atrial side of the valve. This vegetation is clearly visible. The abnormality was not seen with the transthoracic examination. Figure 6–188 shows another patient with a large vegetation on a St. Jude mitral valve. The vegetation (*arrow*) is again obvious with the transesophageal examination. Because the vegetation is on the atrial side of the valve, however, acoustic shadowing kept the transthoracic examination from clearly identifying the vegetation. Yet another example of an infected prosthetic valve is noted in Figure 6–189. This St. Jude valve is in the aortic position. The vegetation is seen protruding into the left ventricular outflow tract (*white arrow*). Even more importantly, a perivalvular abscess (*black arrowhead*) is also apparent and was not evident on the transthoracic study.

The clinical significance of finding vegetations with echocardiography is now changed with the advent of transesophageal echocardiography. The early literature

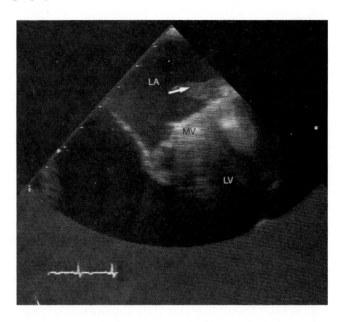

**Fig. 6–188.** Large vegetation (*arrow*) on the left atrial side of a prosthetic mitral valve (MV) as seen with transesophageal echocardiography. LA = left atrium; LV = left ventricle. (From Alam, M., et al.: Transesophageal echocardiographic evaluation of St. Jude medical and bioprosthetic valve endocarditis. Am. Heart J., *123*:237, 1992.)

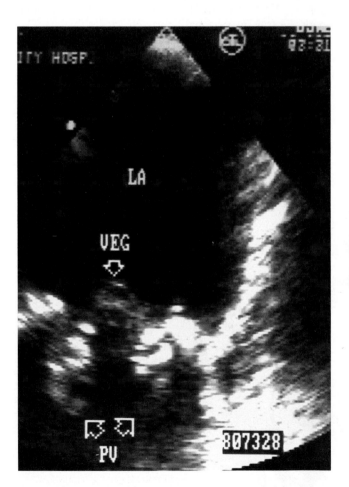

**Fig. 6–187.** Transesophageal echocardiogram of a patient with a vegetation (VEG) on a porcine mitral valve (PV). LA = left atrium.

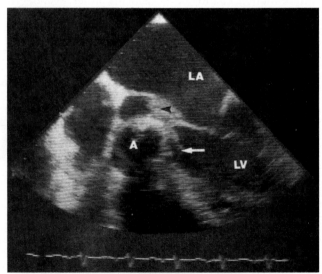

**Fig. 6–189.** Transesophageal echocardiogram showing a vegetation on the prosthetic aortic valve protruding into the left ventricular outflow tract (*arrow*). Note also a perivalvular abscess (*arrowhead*). A = prosthetic aortic valve; LA = left atrium; LV = left ventricle. (From Alam, M., et al.: Transesophageal echocardiographic evaluation of St. Jude medical and bioprosthetic valve endocarditis. Am. Heart J., *123*:237, 1992.)

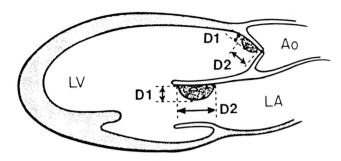

**Fig. 6–190.** Diagram demonstrating how one might measure the size of vegetations using two-dimensional echocardiography. D = diameters; LV = left ventricle; AO = aorta; LA = left atrium. (From Sanfilippo, A.J., et al.: Echocardiographic assessment of patients with infectious endocarditis: Prediction of risk complications. J. Am. Coll. Cardiol., *18*:1193, 1991.)

suggested that the echocardiographic findings indicated an advanced state of disease and that surgery was necessary.[550–555] Such an observation was based primarily on the insensitivity of the original M-mode technique. Two-dimensional echocardiography improved the sensitivity, but now with the even more sensitive transesophageal approach, merely finding a vegetation does not suggest the need for surgery.

The natural history of vegetations is being studied with echocardiography. The abnormality may have a fairly long duration. Vegetations are evident after the patient is bacteriologically cured.[556,557] Vegetations may even be larger without clinical evidence of active infection. In one study, the authors stated that the vegetation would eventually resolve, but this change may take many months.[558] Another group reported that the vege-

tation may remain stable for several years.[559] Rarely, the vegetation may increase rapidly, and when present, this finding is an ominous sign.[560] Figure 6–190 shows how one group of investigators attempts to measure the size of vegetations.[561] Vegetations may progress to form abscesses and fistulas.[562] Such progression has been observed with serial echocardiograms.[563,564] Complications and prognosis may be predicted by the size, extent, and mobility of the vegetations,[522,561,565,566] as well as the severity of regurgitation.[567]

The vegetations noted by echocardiography are not limited to bacterial infections. Many types of fungal endocarditis have been noted in the literature.[568–574] Endocarditis secondary to brucellosis[575] and gonococcus[576–578] has been reported. Noninfectious endocarditis can also be seen echocardiographically. Figure 6–191 is an M-mode echocardiogram of a patient with nonbacterial thrombotic endocarditis,[579–581,581a] and Figure 6–192 is a recording of a patient with Libman-Sacks endocarditis.[582] Libman-Sacks endocarditis has been detected with greater sensitivity using transesophageal echocardiography.[583] Löffler's endocarditis also produces changes on the echocardiogram (Fig. 6–193).[584,585] Endocarditis associated with granulomatous disease[586] and scleroderma[587] has also been described.

## CALCIFIED MITRAL ANNULUS

Numerous articles in the literature describe the echocardiographic findings in patients with a calcified mitral annulus.[588–593] The principal observation on the M-mode echocardiogram is a band of dense high-intensity

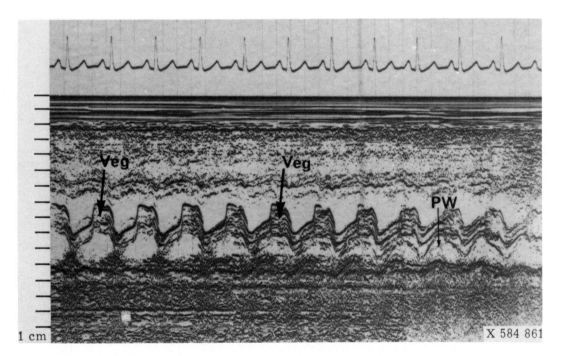

**Fig. 6–191.** Mitral valve echocardiogram of a patient with a nonbacterial thrombotic mass (Veg) involving the mitral valve. PW = posterior wall.

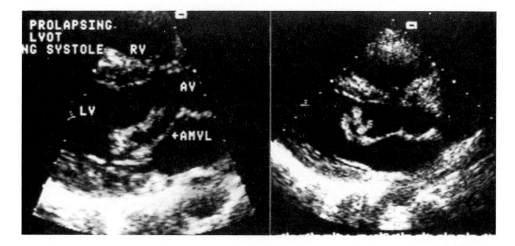

**Fig. 6–192.** Two-dimensional echocardiograms of a patient with Libman-Sacks endocarditis who exhibits large, mobile, echogenic masses on the mitral valve. LV = left ventricle; RV = right ventricle; AV = aortic valve; AMVL = anterior mitral valve leaflet. (From Applebe, A.F., et al.: Libman Sacks endocarditis mimicking intracardiac tumor. Am. J. Cardiol., *68*:817, 1991.)

echoes between the mitral valve and the posterior left ventricular wall (Fig. 6–194). This band of echoes is immediately posterior to the posterior mitral valve leaflets. Frequently, these echoes may obscure that leaflet. The echoes from the annulus may also be in direct contact with the posterior left ventricular endocardial echo and may partially obscure those echoes from acoustic shadowing (see Chapter 1). The myocardial echoes posterior to the annulus on the right side of the illustration are far weaker than those on the left side, in which the annulus echoes are absent. Figure 6–195 is a slow M-mode scan showing the extent to which the calcified annulus echoes can appear on the M-mode echocardiogram. The bright echoes (CA) can be seen extending far into the left ven-

tricular cavity and into the left atrium. Because of the highly reflective nature of the calcium, the effective beam width is wide. Thus, some apparent echoes may be artifactual. Most of the calcium appears to be posterior to the mitral valve on the left ventricular side of the atrioventricular groove. One group of investigators suggests that "calcified mitral annulus" is a misnomer.[594] The calcification is actually in the submitral region between the mitral valve and the posterior left ventricular wall and not in the annulus.

Figure 6–196 shows a two-dimensional view of a calcified mitral annulus. This patient also has pericardial effusion (pe). The calcified annulus (CA) is visible as a bright, somewhat linear echo between the mitral valve

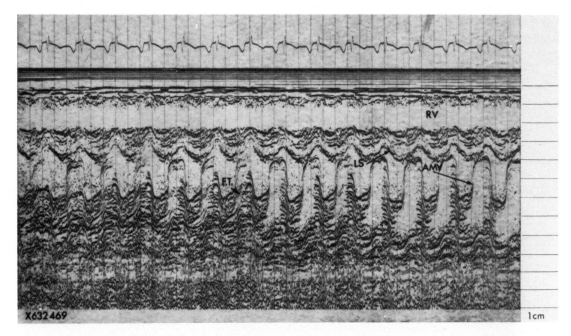

**Fig. 6–193.** M-mode echocardiogram of the mitral valve in a patient with Löffler's endocarditis. A fibrinous thrombotic mass (FT) is attached to the mitral valve and appears to be superimposed on the echoes from the left ventricular posterior wall. The left ventricular cavity is diminished. Mitral blood flow is obstructed. RV = right ventricle; AMV = anterior mitral valve leaflet; LS = left septum. (From Weyman, A.E., et al.: Loeffler's endocarditis presenting as mitral and tricuspid stenosis. Am. J. Cardiol., *40*:438, 1977.)

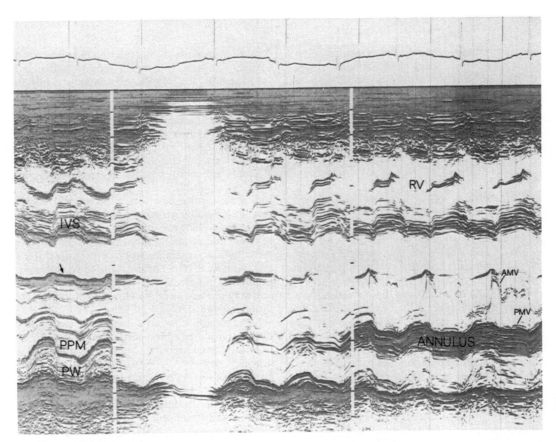

**Fig. 6–194.** M-mode echocardiogram of a patient with a calcified mitral annulus. The dense echoes from the annulus are immediately posterior to the posterior mitral valve leaflet (PMV) and partially obscure the echoes from the posterior left ventricular wall (PW). AMV = anterior mitral valve leaflet; RV = right ventricle; IVS = interventricular septum; PPM = posterior papillary muscle.

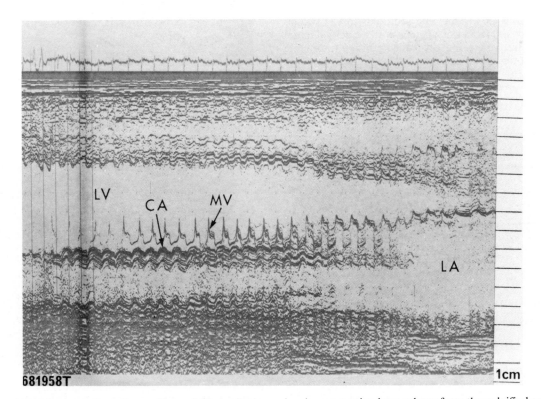

**Fig. 6–195.** M-mode scan of a patient with a calcified mitral annulus demonstrating how echoes from the calcified annulus (CA) extend from the left ventricle (LV) to the left atrium (LA). MV = mitral valve.

327

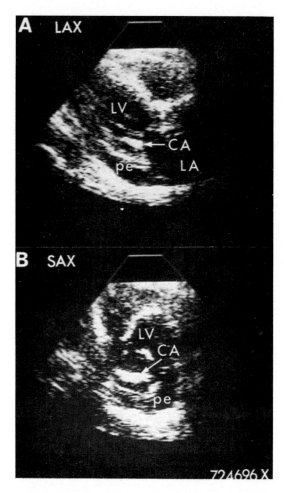

**Fig. 6–196.** Long-axis (LAX) and short-axis (SAX) two-dimensional echocardiograms of a patient with a calcified mitral annulus (CA) and a posterior pericardial effusion (pe). Note the curved nature of the calcified annulus in the short-axis view (see text for details). LV = left ventricle; LA = left atrium.

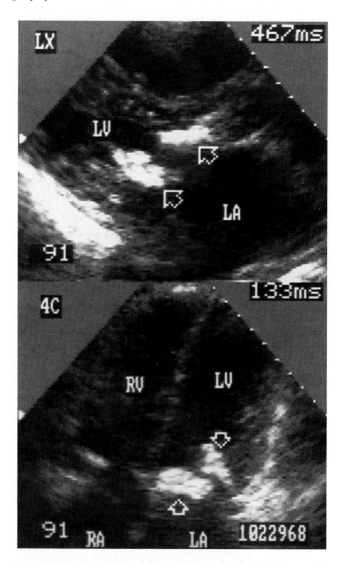

**Fig. 6–198.** Long-axis (LX) and four-chamber (4C) two-dimensional echocardiograms of a patient with extensive mitral annular calcification involving both the anterior and posterior mitral leaflets (*arrows*). LV = left ventricle; LA = left atrium; RV = right ventricle; RA = right atrium.

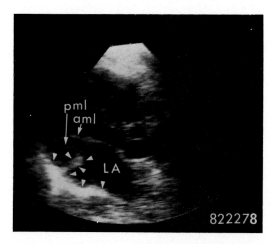

**Fig. 6–197.** Long-axis two-dimensional echocardiogram of a patient with extensive calcification of the mitral annulus and extension of the calcification into the posterior wall of the left ventricle, the left atrium, and the posterior mitral leaflet (*arrowheads*). aml = anterior mitral leaflets; pml = posterior mitral leaflets; LA = left atrium.

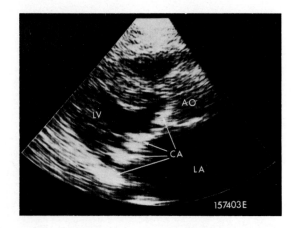

**Fig. 6–199.** Long-axis two-dimensional echocardiogram of a patient with a calcified annulus. Note extensive calcification (CA) extending from the base of the left ventricular wall through the mitral valve and into the root of the aorta (AO). LV = left ventricle; LA = left atrium.

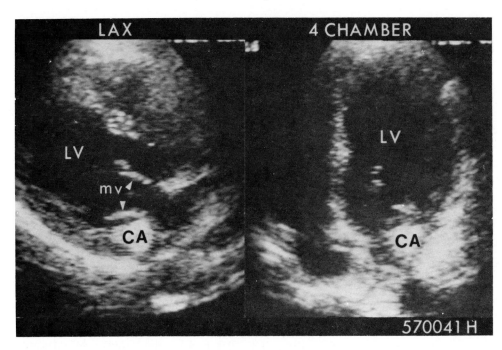

**Fig. 6–200.** Long-axis (LAX) and four-chamber two-dimensional echocardiograms of a patient with a large echo-producing caseous abscess involving the mitral annulus (CA). LV = left ventricle; mv = mitral valve leaflet.

and the posterior left ventricular wall. The long-axis view (LAX) shows the bright calcified echoes (CA) extending into the left ventricular cavity (Fig. 6–196A). The short-axis view (SAX) demonstrates the curved nature of the calcified annulus (CA, Fig. 6–196B). The echoes from the calcification obscure the posterior left ventricular endocardial echo, and it cannot be clearly identified in these recordings.

Calcification may not be limited to only the annular or submitral area. Calcification frequently extends throughout the base of the heart. It may extend into both the mitral and aortic valves.[588] Figure 6–197 shows a patient with a densely calcified annulus extending well into the left atrium. The calcium also spreads into the posterior mitral leaflet. Extension of the calcium into the valve leaflets is demonstrated in Figure 6–198. The calcific process may extend deeply into the left ventricle,[595] and can involve the aorta and aortic valve. Figure 6–199 shows a two-dimensional echocardiogram of a patient with extensive calcification involving the entire base of the heart. Calcium is seen involving the ventricular wall, the mitral valve, the root of the aorta, and even part of the aortic valve.

There are many reasons for recognizing the echocardiographic features of calcified mitral annulus. First, interpretation of the echocardiogram can be confusing. An echocardiogram, such as that in Figure 6–194, can mimic pericardial effusion in some situations.[588] The calcification may also produce echoes similar to those produced in mitral stenosis.[588,595,596] In addition, the calcification frequently obscures the posterior mitral leaflet and may prevent an adequate recording of the posterior left ventricular wall echoes.

Many conditions have been reported in association with a calcified mitral annulus. This abnormality is commonly associated with mitral regurgitation,[592,597–601] various conduction abnormalities,[598,602,603] and left ventricular outflow obstruction.[603,604] The mitral regurgita-

tion is probably due to interference with normal contraction and function of the mitral annulus. One study attempted to judge the severity of the mitral annular calcification.[605] If the diameter of the calcification was less than 5 mm on the M-mode echocardiogram, the complications secondary to the calcification were minimal. If the width of the calcification was greater than 5 mm, however, the incidence of a dilated left atrium and mitral regurgitation and conduction problems was much higher.

Occasionally, the calcification can be rapidly progressive.[606] The calcification may also be liquid and actually be a caseous abscess.[607] Figure 6–200 demonstrates a large echogenic mass in the vicinity of the mitral annulus. Because of severe mitral regurgitation, the patient had the valve replaced. At the time of surgery, the echogenic mass proved to be a liquid mass or caseous abscess. The abscess was sterile.

## REFERENCES

1. Edler, I.: Ultrasound cardiogram in mitral valve disease. Acta Chir. Scand., *111*:230, 1956.
2. Edler, I. and Gustafson, A.: Ultrasonic cardiogram in mitral stenosis. Acta Med. Scand., *159*:85, 1957.
3. Zaky, A., Nasser, W.K., and Feigenbaum, H.: Study of mitral valve action recorded by reflected ultrasound and its application in the diagnosis of mitral stenosis. Circulation, *37*:789, 1968.
4. Effert, S., Erkens, H., and Grossebrockhoff, F.: Ultrasonic echo method in cardiological diagnosis. German Med. Mth., *2*:325, 1957.
5. Gustafson, A.: Correlation between ultrasound-cardiography, haemodynamics and surgical findings in mitral stenosis. Am. J. Cardiol., *19*:32, 1967.
6. Gustafson, A.: Ultrasound cardiography in mitral stenosis. Acta Med. Scand. (Suppl.), *461*:82, 1966.
7. Joyner, C.R., Reid, J.M., and Bond, J.P.: Reflected ul-

trasound in the assessment of mitral valve disease. Circulation, *27*:506, 1963.

8. Segal, B.L., Likoff, W., and Kingsley, B.: Echocardiography: Clinical application in mitral stenosis. JAMA, *193*: 161, 1966.

9. Edler, I., Gustafson, A., Karlefors, T., and Christensson, B.: Ultrasound cardiography. Acta Med. Scand. (Suppl.), *370*:68, 1961.

10. Effert, S.: Pre- and post-operative evaluation of mitral stenosis by ultrasound. Am. J. Cardiol., *19*:59, 1967.

11. Silver, W., Rodriguez-Torres, R., and Newfelt, E.: The echocardiogram in a case of mitral stenosis before and after surgery. Am. Heart J., *78*:811, 1969.

12. Duchak, J.M., Jr., Chang, S., and Feigenbaum, H.: The posterior mitral valve echo and the echocardiographic diagnosis of mitral stenosis. Am. J. Cardiol., *29*:628, 1972.

13. Shah, P.M., Gramiak, R., and Kramer, D.H.: Ultrasound localization of left ventricular outflow obstruction in hypertrophic obstructive cardiomyopathy. Circulation, *40*: 3, 1969.

14. Hueter, D., Drew, F., McInerney, K., Flessas, A., and Ryan, T.: Analysis of diastolic motion of the posterior leaflet in mitral stenosis. Circulation (Suppl. II), *54*:99, 1976. (Abstract)

15. Levisman, J.A.: Leaflet motion in mitral stenosis. Chest, *71*:4, 1977. (Editorial)

16. Shiu, M.F., Jenkins, B.S., and Webb-Peploe, M.M.: Echocardiographic analysis of posterior mitral leaflet movement in mitral stenosis. Br. Heart J., *40*:372, 1978.

17. Glasser, S.P. and Faris, J.V.: Posterior leaflet motion in mitral stenosis. Chest, *71*:87, 1977.

18. Thomas, R.D., Mary, D.A.S., and Ionescu, M.I.: Echocardiographic pattern of posterior mitral valve leaflet movement after mitral valve repair. Br. Heart J., *41*:399, 1979.

19. Berman, N.D., Gilbert, B.W., McLaughlin, P.R., and Morch, J.E.: Mitral stenosis with posterior diastolic movement of posterior leaflet. Can. Med. Assoc. J., *112*: 976, 1975.

20. Nichol, P.M., Gilbert, B.W., and Kisslo, J.A.: Two-dimensional echocardiographic assessment of mitral stenosis. Circulation, *55*:120, 1977.

21. Wann, L.S., Weyman, A.E., Feigenbaum, H., Dillon, J.C., Johnston, K.W., and Eggleton, R.C.: Determination of mitral valve area by cross-sectional echocardiography. Ann. Intern. Med., *88*:337, 1978.

22. Henry, W.L., Griffith, J.M., Michaelis, L.L., McIntosh, C.L., Morrow, A.G., and Epstein, S.E.: Measurements of mitral orifice area in patients with mitral valve disease by real-time, two-dimensional echocardiography. Circulation, *51*:827, 1975.

23. Martin, R.P., Rakowski, H., Kleiman, J.H., Beaver, W., London, E., and Popp, R.L.: Reliability and reproducibility of two-dimensional echocardiographic measurement of the stenotic mitral valve orifice area. Am. J. Cardiol., *43*:560, 1979.

24. Kastl, D., Henry, W.L., McIntosh, C., Redwood, D.R., Griffith, J.M., Itscoitz, S.B., and Morrow, A.G.: Cross-sectional echocardiographic assessment of mitral commissurotomy: Comparison of hemodynamic and echocardiographic data. Circulation (Suppl. II), *54*:99, 1976. (Abstract)

25. Weyman, A.E., Wann, L.S., Rogers, E.W., Godley, R.W., Dillon, J.C., Feigenbaum, H., and Green, D.: Five-year experience in correlating cross-sectional echocardiographic assessment of the mitral valve area with

hemodynamic valve area determinations. Am. J. Cardiol., *43*:386, 1979. (Abstract)

26. Kulas, A., Enriquez-Sarano, L., Troley, C., and Acar, J.: Value of correction by receiving gains in the determination of mitral valve surface area by two-dimensional echocardiography. Arch. Mal. Coeur, *75*:757, 1982.

27. Schweizer, P., Bardos, P., Krebs, W., Erbel, R., Minale, C., Imm, S., Massmer, B.J., and Effert, S.: Morphometric investigations in mitral stenosis using two-dimensional echocardiography. Br. Heart J., *48*:54, 1982.

28. Glover, M.U., Warren, S.E., Vieweg, W.V.R., Ceretto, W.J., Samtoy, L.M., and Hagan, A.D.: M-mode and two-dimensional echocardiographic correlation with findings at catheterization and surgery in patients with mitral stenosis. Am. Heart J., *105*:98, 1983.

29. Jain, S.K., Pechacek, L.W., DeCastro, C.M., Garcia, E., and Hall, R.J.: Non-invasive assessment of the stenotic mitral valve orifice by two-dimensional echocardiography. Cardiovasc. Dis., *8*:29, 1981.

30. Motro, M., Schneeweiss, A., Lehrer, E., Rath, S., and Neufeld, H.N.: Correlation between cardiac catheterization and echocardiography in assessing the severity of mitral stenosis. Int. J. Cardiol., *1*:25, 1981.

31. Riggs, T.W., Lapin, G.D., Paul, M.H., Muster, A.J., Berry, T.E., Pajcic, S.E., and Berdusis, K.: Measurement of mitral valve orifice area in infants and children by two-dimensional echocardiography. J. Am. Coll. Cardiol., *1*:873, 1983.

32. Kalmanson, D., Veyrat, C., Bouchareine, F., and Degroote, A.: Non-invasive recording of mitral valve flow velocity patterns using pulsed Doppler echocardiography: Application to diagnosis and evaluation of mitral valve disease. Br. Heart J., *39*:517, 1977.

33. Hatle, L., Brubakk, A., Tromsdal, A., and Angelsen, B.: Noninvasive assessment of pressure drop in mitral stenosis by Doppler ultrasound. Br. Heart J., *40*:131, 1978.

34. Nichol, P.M., Boughner, D.R., and Persaud, J.A.: Noninvasive assessment of mitral insufficiency by transcutaneous Doppler ultrasound. Circulation, *54*:656, 1976.

35. Diebold, B., Theroux, P., Bourassa, M.G., Thuillez, C., Peronneau, P., Guermonprez, J.L., Xhaard, M., and Waters, D.D.: Non-invasive pulsed Doppler study of mitral stenosis and mitral regurgitation: Preliminary study. Br. Heart J., *42*:168, 1979.

36. Holen, J. and Simonsen, S.: Determination of pressure gradient in mitral stenosis with Doppler echocardiography. Br. Heart J., *41*:529, 1979.

37. Thuillez, C., Theroux, P., Bourassa, M.G., Blanchard, D., Peronneau, P., Guermonprez, J-L., Diebold, B., Waters, D.D., and Maurice, P.: Pulsed Doppler echocardiographic study of mitral stenosis. Circulation, *61*:381, 1980.

38. Egeblad, H., Berning, J., Saunamaki, K., Jacobsen, J.R., and Wennevold, A.: Assessment of rheumatic mitral valve disease. Value of echocardiography in patients clinically suspected of predominant stenosis. Br. Heart J., *49*:38, 1983.

39. Stamm, R.B. and Martin, R.P.: Quantification of pressure gradients across stenotic valves by Doppler ultrasound. J. Am. Coll. Cardiol., *2*:707, 1983.

40. Hatle, L. and Angelsen, B.: Doppler Ultrasound in Cardiology: Physical Principles and Clinical Applications, 2nd ed. Philadelphia, Lea & Febiger, 1985.

41. Dabestani, A., Skorton, D.J., Child, J.S., and Krivokapich, J.: Mitral valve A wave and mitral stenosis. JCU, *9*:91, 1981.

42. Geibel, A., Gornandt, L., Kasper, W., and Bubenheimer, P.: Reproducibility of Doppler echocardiographic quantification of aortic and mitral valve stenoses: Comparison between two echocardiography centers. Am. J. Cardiol., 67:1013, 1991.

43. Halbe, D., Bryg, R.J., and Labovitz, A.J.: A simplified method for calculating mitral valve area using Doppler echocardiography. Am. Heart J., 116:877, 1988.

44. Karp, K., Teien, D., Bjerle, P., and Eriksson, P.: Reassessment of valve area determinations in mitral stenosis by the pressure half-time method: Impact of left ventricular stiffness and peak diastolic pressure difference. J. Am. Coll. Cardiol., 13:594, 1989.

45. Wranne, B., Ask, P., and Loyd, D.: Analysis of different methods of assessing the stenotic mitral valve area with emphasis on the pressure gradient half-time concept. Am. J. Cardiol., 66:614, 1990.

46. Wisenbaugh, T., Berk, M., Essop, R., Middlemost, S., and Sareli, P.: Effect of mitral regurgitation and volume loading on pressure half-time before and after balloon valvotomy in mitral stenosis. Am. J. Cardiol., 67:162, 1991.

47. Flachskampf, F.A., Weyman, A.E., Gillam, L., Chun-Ming, L., Abascal, V.M., and Thomas, J.D.: Aortic regurgitation shortens Doppler pressure half-time in mitral stenosis: Clinical evidence, in vitro simulation, and theoretic analysis. J. Am. Coll. Cardiol., 16:396, 1990.

48. Nakatani, S., Nagata, S., Beppu, S., Ishikura, F., Tamai, J., Yamagishi, M., Ohmori, F., Kimura, K., Takamiya, M., and Miyatake, K.: Acute reduction of mitral valve area after percutaneous balloon mitral valvuloplasty: Assessment with Doppler continuity equation method. Am. Heart J., 121:770, 1991.

49. Chen, C., Wang, Y., Guo, B., and Lin, Y.: Reliability of the Doppler pressure half-time method for assessing effects of percutaneous mitral balloon valvuloplasty. J. Am. Coll. Cardiol., 13:1309, 1989.

49a.Derumeaux, G., Bonnemains, T., Remadi, F., Cribier, A., and Letac, B.: Non-invasive assessment of mitral stenosis before and after percutaneous balloon mitral valvotomy by Doppler continuity equation. Eur. Heart J., 13:1034, 1992.

50. Thomas, J.D., Wilkins, G.T., Choong, C.Y.P., Chir, B., Abascal, V.M., Palacios, I.G., Block, P.C., and Weyman, A.E.: Inaccuracy of mitral pressure half-time immediately after percutaneous mitral valvotomy. Circulation, 78:980, 1988.

51. Smith, M.D., Wisenbaugh, T., Grayburn, P.A., Gurley, J.C., Spain, M.G., and DeMaria, A.N.: Value and limitations of Doppler pressure half-time in quantifying mitral stenosis: A comparison with micromanometer catheter recordings. Am. Heart J., 121:480, 1991.

52. Loyd, D., Eng, D., Ask, P., and Wranne, B.: Pressure half-time does not always predict mitral valve area correctly. J. Am. Soc. Echocardiogr., 1:313, 1988.

53. Thomas, J.D. and Weyman, A.E.: Doppler mitral pressure half-time: A clinical tool in search of theoretical justification. J. Am. Coll. Cardiol., 10:923, 1987.

54. Loperfido, F., Laurenzi, F., Gimigliano, F., Pennestri, F., Biasucci, L.M., Vigna, C., DeSantis, F., Favuzzi, A., Rosse, E., and Manzoli, U.: A comparison of the assessment of mitral valve area by continuous wave Doppler and by cross-sectional echocardiography. Br. Heart J., 57:348, 1987.

55. Braverman, A.C., Thomas, J.C., and Lee, R.T.: Doppler echocardiographic estimation of mitral valve area during changing hemodynamic conditions. Am. J. Cardiol., 68:1485, 1991.

56. Nakatani, S., Masuyama, T., Kodama, K., Kitabatake, A., Fujii, K., and Kamada, T.: Value and limitations of Doppler echocardiography in the quantification of stenotic mitral valve area: Comparison of the pressure half-time and the continuity equation methods. Circulation, 77:78, 1988.

57. Fredman, C.S., Pearson, A.C., Labovitz, A.J., and Kern, M.J.: Comparison of hemodynamic pressure half-time method and Gorlin formula with Doppler and echocardiographic determinations of mitral valve area in patients with combined mitral stenosis and regurgitation. Am. Heart J., 119:121, 1990.

58. Natarajan, D., Sharma, V.P., Chandra, S., Dhar, S.K., Gaba, M., and Caroli, B.: Effects of percutaneous balloon mitral valvotomy on pulmonary venous flow in severe mitral stenosis. Am. J. Cardiol., 69:810, 1992.

59. Jolly, N., Arora, R., Mohan, J.C., and Khalilullah, M.: Pulmonary venous flow dynamics before and after balloon mitral valvuloplasty as determined by transesophageal Doppler echocardiography. Am. J. Cardiol., 70:780, 1992.

60. Keren, G., Pardes, A., Miller, H.I., Scherez, J., and Laniado, S.: Pulmonary venous flow determined by Doppler echocardiography in mitral stenosis. Am. J. Cardiol., 65:246, 1990.

61. Bryg, R.J., Gordon, P.R., Kudesia, V.S., and Bhatia, R.K.: Effect of pregnancy on pressure gradient in mitral stenosis. Am. J. Cardiol., 63:384, 1989.

62. Tunick, P.A., Freedberg, R.S., Gargiulo, A., and Kronzon, I.: Exercise Doppler echocardiography as an aid to clinical decision making in mitral valve disease. J. Am. Soc. Echocardiogr., 5:225, 1992.

63. Leavitt, J.I., Coats, M.H., and Falk, R.H.: Effects of exercise on transmitral gradient and pulmonary artery pressure in patients with mitral stenosis or a prosthetic mitral valve: A Doppler echocardiographic study. J. Am. Coll. Cardiol., 17:1520, 1991.

64. Tamai, J., Nagata, S., Akaike, M., Ishikura, F., Kimura, K., Takamiya, M., Miyatake, K., and Nimura, Y.: Improvement in mitral flow dynamics during exercise after percutaneous transvenous mitral commissurotomy. Circulation, 81:46, 1990.

64a.Dahan, M., Paillole, C., Martin, D., Gourgon, R.: Determinants of stroke volume response to exercise in patients with mitral stenosis: a Doppler echocardiographic study. J. Am. Coll. Cardiol., 21:384, 1993.

65. Vasan, R.S., Shrivastava, S., and Kumar, M.V.: Value and limitations of Doppler echocardiographic determination of mitral valve area in Lutembacher syndrome. J. Am. Coll. Cardiol., 20:1362, 1992.

66. Khandheria, B.K., Tajik, A.J., Reeder, G.S., Callahan, M.J., Nishimura, R.A., Miller, F.A., and Seward, J.B.: Doppler color flow imaging: A new technique for visualization and characterization of the blood flow jet in mitral stenosis. Mayo Clin. Proc., 61:623, 1986.

67. Zanolla, L., Marino, P., Nicolosi, G.L., Peranzoni, P.F., and Poppi, A.: Two-dimensional echocardiographic evaluation of mitral valve calcification. Sensitivity and specificity. Chest, 82:154, 1982.

68. Come, P.C. and Riley, M.F.: M-mode and cross-sectional echocardiographic recognition of fibrosis and calcification of the mitral valve chordae and left ventricular papillary muscles. Am. J. Cardiol., 49:461, 1982.

69. Marwick, T.H., Torelli, J., Obarski, T., Casale, P.N., and Stewart, W.J.: Assessment of the mitral valve split-

ability score by transthoracic and transesophageal echocardiography. Am. J. Cardiol., *68*:1106, 1991.

70. Nobuyoshi, M., Hamasaki, N., Kimura, T., Nosaka, H., Yokoi, H., Yasumoto, H., Horiuchi, H., Nakashima, H., Shindo, T., Mori, T., Miyamoto, A.T., and Inoue, K.: Indications, complications, and short-term clinical outcome of percutaneous transvenous mitral commissurotomy. Circulation, *80*:783, 1989.

71. Reid, C.L., Chandraratna, A.N., Kawanishi, D.T., Kotlewski, A., and Rahimtoola, S.H.: Influence of mitral valve morphology on double-balloon, catheter balloon valvuloplasty in patients with mitral stenosis. Circulation, *80*:515, 1989.

72. Reid, C.L., McKay, C.R., Chandraratna, P.A.N., Kawanishi, D.T., and Rahimtoola, S.H.: Mechanisms of increase in mitral valve area and influence of anatomic features in double-balloon, catheter balloon valvuloplasty in adults with rheumatic mitral stenosis: A Doppler and two-dimensional echocardiographic study. Circulation, *76*:628, 1987.

73. Abascal, V.M., Wilkins, G.T., O'Shea, J.P., Choong, C.Y., Palacios, I.F., Thomas, J.D., Rosas, E., Newell, J.B., Block, P.C., and Weyman, A.E.: Prediction of successful outcome in 130 patients undergoing percutaneous balloon mitral valvotomy. Circulation, *82*:448, 1990.

74. Wilkins, G.T., Weyman, A.E., Abascal, V.M., Block, P.C., and Palacios, I.F.: Percutaneous balloon dilatation of the mitral valve: An analysis of echocardiographic variables related to outcome and the mechanism of dilatation. Br. Heart J., *60*:299, 1988.

75. Palacios, I.F., Block, P.C., Wilkins, G.T., and Weyman, A.E.: Follow-up of patients undergoing percutaneous mitral balloon valvotomy. Circulation, *79*:573, 1989.

76. Reid, C.L., Otto, C.M., Davis, K.B., Labovitz, A., Kisslo, K.B., and McKay, C.R.: Influence of mitral valve morphology on mitral balloon commissurotomy: Immediate and six-month results from the NHLBI balloon valvuloplasty registry. Am. Heart J., *124*:657, 1992.

77. Rodriguez, L., Monterroso, V.H., Abascal, V.M., King, M.E., O'Shea, J.P., Palacios, I.F., and Weyman, A.E.: Does asymmetric mitral valve disease predict an adverse outcome after percutaneous balloon mitral valvotomy? An echocardiographic study. Am. Heart J., *123*:1678, 1992.

78. Gordon, S.P.F., Douglas, P.S., Come, P.C., and Manning, W.J.: Two-dimensional and Doppler echocardiographic determinants of the natural history of mitral valve narrowing in patients with rheumatic mitral stenosis: Implications for follow-up. J. Am. Coll. Cardiol., *19*:968, 1992.

79. Chen, W-J., Chen, M-F., Liau, C-S., Wu, C-C., and Lee, Y-T.: Safety of percutaneous transvenous balloon mitral commissurotomy in patients with mitral stenosis and thrombus in the left appendage. Am. J. Cardiol., *70*:117, 1992.

80. Manning, W.J., Reis, G.J., and Douglas, P.S.: Use of transesophageal echocardiography to detect left atrial thrombi before percutaneous balloon dilatation of the mitral valve: A prospective study. Br. Heart J., *67*:170, 1992.

81. Chan, K-L., Marquis, J-F., Ascah, C., Morton, B., and Baird, M.: Role of transesophageal echocardiography in percutaneous balloon mitral valvuloplasty. Echocardiography, *7*:115, 1990.

81a. Thomas, M.R., Monaghan, M.J., Smyth, D.W., Metcalfe, J.M., and Jewitt, D.E.: Comparative value of transthoracic and transesophageal echocardiography before

balloon dilatation of the mitral valve. Br. Heart J., *68*:493, 1992.

82. Jaarsma, W., Visser, C.A., Suttorp, M.J., Haagen, F.D.H., and Ernst, S.M.P.G.: Transesophageal echocardiography during percutaneous balloon mitral valvuloplasty. J. Am. Soc. Echocardiogr., *3*:384, 1990.

83. Kronzon, I., Tunick, P.A., Schwinger, M.E., Slater, J., and Glassman, E.: Transesophageal echocardiography during percutaneous mitral valvuloplasty. J. Am. Soc. Echocardiogr., *2*:380, 1989.

84. Ballal, R.S., Mahan, E.F., Nanda, N.C., and Dean, L.S.: Utility of transesophageal echocardiography in interatrial septal puncture during percutaneous mitral balloon commissurotomy. Am. J. Cardiol., *66*:230, 1990.

85. Vilacosta, I., Iturralde, E., San Roman, J.A., Gomez-Recio, M., Romero, C., Jimenez, J., and Martinez-Elbal, L.: Transesophageal echocardiographic monitoring of percutaneous mitral balloon valvulotomy. Am. J. Cardiol., *70*:1040, 1992.

86. Chen, C., Wang, X., Wang, Y., and Lan, Y.: Value of two-dimensional echocardiography in selecting patients and balloon sizes for percutaneous balloon mitral valvuloplasty. J. Am. Coll. Cardiol., *14*:1651, 1989.

87. Sheikh, K.H., Davidson, C.J., Skelton, T.N., Nesmith, J.W., Kisslo, K., and Bashore, T.M.: Interatrial septal thickening preventing percutaneous mitral valve balloon valvuloplasty. Am. Heart J., *117*:206, 1989.

88. Desideri, A., Vanderperren, O., Serra, A., Barraud, P., Petitclerc, R., Lesperance, J., Dyrda, I., Crepeau, J., and Bonan, R.: Long-term (9 to 33 months) echocardiographic follow-up after successful percutaneous mitral commissurotomy. Am. J. Cardiol., *69*:1602, 1992.

89. Parro, A., Helmcke, F., Mahan III, E.F., Nanda, N.C., Kandath, D., and Dean, L.S.: Value and limitations of color Doppler echocardiography in the evaluation of percutaneous balloon mitral valvuloplasty for isolated mitral stenosis. Am. J. Cardiol., *67*:1261, 1991.

90. Dev, V., Singh, L.S.K., Radhakrishnan, S., Saxena, A., and Shrivastava, S.: Doppler echocardiographic assessment of transmitral gradients and mitral valve area before and after mitral valve balloon dilatation. Clin. Cardiol., *12*:629, 1989.

91. Abascal, V.M., Wilkins, G.T., Choong, C.Y., Thomas, J.D., Palacios, I.F., Block, P.C., and Weyman, A.E.: Echocardiographic evaluation of mitral valve structure and function in patients followed for at least 6 months after percutaneous balloon mitral valvuloplasty. J. Am. Coll. Cardiol., *12*:606, 1988.

92. O'Shea, J.P., Abascal, V.M., Wilkins, G.T., Marshall, J.E., Brandi, S., Acquatella, H., Block, P.C., Palacios, I.F., and Weyman, A.E.: Unusual sequelae after percutaneous mitral valvuloplasty: A Doppler echocardiographic study. J. Am. Coll. Cardiol., *19*:186, 1992.

93. Waksmonski, C.A. and McKay, R.G.: Echocardiographic diagnosis of valve disruption following percutaneous balloon valvuloplasty. Echocardiography, *6*:277, 1989.

94. Essop, M.R., Wisenbaugh, T., Skoularigis, J., Middlemost, S., and Sareli, P.: Mitral regurgitation follow mitral balloon valvotomy. Circulation, *84*:1669, 1991.

95. Abascal, V.M., Wilkins, G.T., Ghoong, C.Y., Block, P.C., Palacios, I.F., and Weyman, A.E.: Mitral regurgitation after percutaneous balloon mitral valvuloplasty in adults: Evaluation of pulsed Doppler echocardiography. J. Am. Coll. Cardiol., *11*:257, 1988.

96. Chen, C-H., Lin, S-L., Yin, W-H., Liou, J-Y., Hsu, T-L., Ting, C-T., Chang, M-S., and Chiang, B.N.: Trans-

esophageal color Doppler flow mapping of iatrogenic left-to-right interatrial shunting after percutaneous transluminal mitral valvotomy. Echocardiography, 8:649, 1991.

97. Kronzon, I., Tunick, P.A., Goldfarb, A., Freedberg, R.S., Chinitz, L., Slater, J., Schwinger, M.E., Gindea, A.J., Glassman, E., and Danile, W.G.: Echocardiographic and hemodynamic characteristics of atrial septal defects created by percutaneous valvuloplasty. J. Am. Soc. Echocardiogr., 3:64, 1990.

98. Chen, C-H., Lin, S-L., Hsu, T-L., Chen, C-C., Wang, S-P., and Chang, M-S.: Iatrogenic Lutembacher's syndrome after percutaneous transluminal mitral valvotomy. Am. Heart J., 119:209, 1990.

98a. Thomas, M.R., Monaghan, M.J., Metcalfe, J.M., and Jewitt, D.E.: Residual atrial septal defects following balloon mitral valvuloplasty using different techniques. A transthoracic and transesophageal echocardiography study demonstrating an advantage of the Inoue balloon. Eur. Heart J., 13:496, 1992.

99. Abbasi, A.S., Allen, M.W., DeCristofaro, D., and Ungar, I.: Detection and estimation of the degree of mitral regurgitation by range-gated pulsed Doppler echocardiography. Circulation, 61:143, 1980.

100. Miyatake, K., Kinoshita, N., Nagata, S., Beppu, S., Park, Y-D., Sakakibara, H., and Nimura, Y.: Intracardiac flow pattern in mitral regurgitation studied with combined use of the ultrasonic pulsed Doppler technique and cross-sectional echocardiography. Am. J. Cardiol., 45:155, 1980.

101. Bobkov, V.V., Danilchenko, T.A., Prelatov, V.A., and Kuznetsova, L.M.: Doppler echocardiographic study of patients with mitral insufficiency. Kardiologiia, 23:79, 1983.

102. Veyrat, C., Ameur, A., Bas, S., Lessana, A., Abitbol, G., and Kalmanson, D.: Pulsed Doppler echocardiographic indices for assessing mitral regurgitation. Br. Heart J., 51:130, 1984.

103. Miyatake, K., Nimura, Y., Sakakibara, H., Kinoshita, N., Okamoto, M., Nagata, S., Kawazoe, K., and Fujita, T.: Localization and direction of mitral regurgitant flow in mitral orifice studied with combined use of ultrasonic pulsed Doppler technique and two-dimensional echocardiography. Br. Heart J., 48:449, 1982.

104. Patel, A.K., Rowe, G.G., Thomsen, J.H., Dhanani, S.P., Kosolcharoen, P., and Lyle, L.E.W.: Detection and estimation of rheumatic mitral regurgitation in the presence of mitral stenosis by pulsed Doppler echocardiography. Am. J. Cardiol., 51:986, 1983.

105. Areias, J.C., Goldberg, S.J., and de Villeneuve, V.H.: Use and limitations of time interval histogram output from echo Doppler to detect mitral regurgitation. Am. Heart J., 101:805, 1981.

106. Blanchard, D., Diebold, B., Peronneau, P., Foult, J.M., Nee, M., Guermonprez, J.L., and Maurice, P.: Non-invasive diagnosis of mitral regurgitation by Doppler echocardiography. Br. Heart J., 45:589, 1981.

107. Omoto, R., Yokote, Y., Takamoto, S., Kyo, S., Ueda, K., Asano, H., Namekawa, K., Kassai, C., Kondo, Y., and Koyano, A.: The development of real-time two-dimensional Doppler echocardiography and its clinical significance in acquired valvular diseases. With specific reference to the evaluation of valvular regurgitation. Jpn. Heart J., 25:325, 1984.

108. Jacobs, L.E., Wertheimer, J.H., Kotler, M.N., Fanning, R., Meyerowitz, C., Strauss, C.S., and Loli, A.W.: Quantification of mitral regurgitation: A comparison of

transesophageal echocardiography and contrast ventriculography. Echocardiography, 9:145, 1992.

109. Sadoshima, J., Koyanagi, S., Sugimachi, M., Hirooka, Y., and Takeshita, A.: Evaluation of the severity of mitral regurgitation by transesophageal Doppler flow echocardiography. Am. Heart J., 123:1245, 1992.

110. Kamp, O., Eijkstra, J-W., Huitink, H., Van, M.J.E., Werter, C.J.P.J., Roos, J.P., and Visser, C.A.: Transesophageal color flow Doppler mapping in the assessment of native mitral valvular regurgitation: Comparison with left ventricular angiography. J. Am. Soc. Echocardiogr., 4:598, 1991.

111. Yoshida, K., Yoshikawa, J., Yamaura, Y., Hozumi, T., Akasaka, T., and Fukaya, T.: Assessment of mitral regurgitation by biplane transesophageal color Doppler flow mapping. Circulation, 82:1121, 1990.

112. Castello, R., Lenzen, P., Aguirre, F., and Labovitz, A.J.: Quantitation of mitral regurgitation by transesophageal echocardiography with Doppler color flow mapping: Correlation with cardiac catheterization. J. Am. Coll. Cardiol., 19:1516, 1992.

113. Kurokawa, S., Takahashi, M., Sugiyama, T., Ikuri, H., Kawano, T., Tsukahara, N., Abe, W., Muramatsu, J., Kikawada, R., Nakazawa, K., and Ishii, K.: Noninvasive evaluation of the magnitude of aortic and mitral regurgitation by means of Doppler two-dimensional echocardiography. Am. Heart J., 120:638, 1990.

114. Spain, M.G., Smith, M.D., Grayburn, P.A., Harlamert, E.A., DeMaria, A.N., O'Brien, M., and Kwan, O.L.: Quantitative assessment of mitral regurgitation by Doppler color flow imaging: Angiographic and hemodynamic correlations. J. Am. Coll. Cardiol., 13:585, 1989.

115. Bolger, A.F., Eigler, N.L., Pfaff, J.M., Resser, K.J., and Maurer, G.: Computer analysis of Doppler color flow mapping images for quantitative assessment of in vitro fluid jets. J. Am. Coll. Cardiol., 12:450, 1988.

116. Veyrat, C. and Kalmanson, D.: New methodology for improved quantification of left-sided valvular lesions using color flow imaging: Evolution and update of the flow mapping procedure. Cardiovasc. Imag., 2:119, 1990.

117. Cooper, J.W., Nanda, N.C., Philpot, E.F., and Fan, P.: Evaluation of valvular regurgitation by color Doppler. J. Am. Soc. Echocardiogr., 2:56, 1989.

118. DeMaria, A.N. and Smith, M.D.: Quantitation of Doppler color flow recordings: An oxymoron? J. Am. Coll. Cardiol., 20:439, 1992.

119. Maciel, B.C., Moises, V.A., Shandas, R., Simpson, I.A., Beltran, M., Valdes-Cruz, L., and Sahn, D.J.: Effects of pressure and volume of the receiving chamber on the spatial distribution of regurgitant jets as imaged by color Doppler flow mapping. Circulation, 83:605, 1991.

120. Holen, J., Nanna, M., Lockhart, J., and Waag, R.: Doppler color flow in echocardiography: Analytical and in vitro investigations of the quantitative relationship between orifice flow and color jet dimensions. Ultrasound Med. Biol., 16:543, 1990.

121. Hoit, B.D., Jones, M., Eidbo, E.E., Elias, W., and Sahn, D.J.: Sources of variability for Doppler color flow mapping of regurgitant jets in an animal model of mitral regurgitation. J. Am. Coll. Cardiol., 13:1631, 1989.

122. Smith, M.D., Grayburn, P.A., Spain, M.G., DeMaria, A.N., Kwan, O.L., and Moffett, C.B.: Observer variability in the quantitation of Doppler color flow jet areas for mitral and aortic regurgitation. J. Am. Coll. Cardiol., 11:579, 1988.

123. Stevenson, J.G.: Two-dimensional color Doppler estimation of the severity of atrioventricular valve regurgita-

tion: Important effects of instrument gain setting, pulse repetition frequency, and carrier frequency. J. Am. Soc. Echocardiogr., *2*:1, 1989.

124. Grayburn, P.A., Pryor, S.L., Levine, B.D., Klein, M.N., Taylor, A.L., and Peters, A.: Day to day variability of Doppler color flow jets in mitral regurgitation. J. Am. Coll. Cardiol., *14*:936, 1989.

125. Smith, M.D., Kwan, O.L., Spain, M.G., and DeMaria, A.N.: Temporal variability of color Doppler jet areas in patients with mitral and aortic regurgitation. Am. Heart J., *123*:953, 1992.

126. Helmcke, F., Nanda, N.C., Hsiung, M.C., Soto, B., Adey, C.K., Goyal, R.G., and Gatewood, R.P.: Color Doppler assessment of mitral regurgitation with orthogonal planes. Circulation, *75*:175, 1987.

127. Castello, R., Lenzen, P., Aguirre, F., and Labovitz, A.: Variability in the quantitation of mitral regurgitation by Doppler color flow mapping: Comparison of transthoracic and transesophageal studies. J. Am. Coll. Cardiol., *20*:433, 1992.

128. Castello, R., Fagan, L., Lenzen, P., Pearson, A.C., and Labovitz, A.J.: Comparison of transthoracic and transesophageal echocardiography for assessment of left-sided valvular regurgitation. Am. J. Cardiol., *68*:1677, 1991.

129. Mimo, R., Sparacino, L., Nicolosi, G.L., D'Angelo, G., Dall'aglio, V., Lestuzzi, C., Pavan, D., Cervesato, E., and Zanuttini, D.: Quantification of mitral regurgitation: Comparison between transthoracic and transesophageal color Doppler flow mapping. Echocardiography, *8*:619, 1991.

130. Smith, M.D., Harrison, M.R., Pinton, R., Kandil, H., Kwan, O.L., and DeMaria, A.N.: Regurgitant jet size by transesophageal compared with transthoracic Doppler color flow imaging. Circulation, *83*:79, 1991.

131. Cape, E.G., Yoganathan, A.P., Weyman, A.E., and Levine, R.A.: Adjacent solid boundaries alter the size of regurgitant jets on Doppler color flow maps. J. Am. Coll. Cardiol., *17*:1094, 1991.

132. Chen, C., Thomas, J.D., Anconina, J., Harrigan, P., Mueller, L., Picard, M.H., Levine, R.A., and Weyman, A.E.: Impact of impinging wall jet on color Doppler quantification of mitral regurgitation. Circulation, *84*:712, 1991.

133. Shandas, R., Gharib, M., Liepmann, D., Shiota, T., and Sahn, D.J.: Experimental studies to define the geometry of the flow convergence region. Echocardiography, *9*:43, 1992.

134. Giesler, M.O. and Stauch, M.: Color Doppler determination of regurgitant flow: From proximal isovelocity surface areas to proximal velocity profiles. Echocardiography, *9*:51, 1992.

135. Bargiggia, G.S., Tronconi, L., Sahn, D.J., Recusani, F., Raisaro, A., DeServi, S., Valdes-Cruz, L.M., and Montemartini, C.: A new method for quantitation of mitral regurgitation based on color flow Doppler imaging of flow convergence proximal to regurgitant orifice. Circulation, *84*:1481, 1991.

136. Utsunomiya, T., Ogawa, T., Doshi, R., Patel, D., Quan, M., Henry, W.L., and Gardin, J.M.: Doppler color flow: "Proximal isovelocity surface area" method for estimating volume flow rate: Effects of orifice shape and machine factors. J. Am. Coll. Cardiol., *17*:1103, 1991.

137. Appleton, C.P., Hatle, L.K., Nellessen, U., Schnittger, I., and Popp, R.L.: Flow velocity acceleration in the left ventricle: A useful Doppler echocardiographic sign of he-

138. Recusani, F., Bargiggia, G.S., Yoganathan, A.P., Raisaro, A., Valdes-Cruz, L.M., Sung, H-W., Bertucci, C., Gallati, M., Moises, V.A., Simpson, I.A., Tronconi, L., and Sahn, D.J.: A new method for quantification of regurgitant flow rate using color Doppler flow imaging of the flow convergence region proximal to a discrete orifice. An in vitro study. Circulation, *83*:594, 1991.

139. Rivera, J.M., Vandervoort, P.M., Thoreau, D.H., Levine, R.A., Weyman, A.E., and Thomas, J.D.: Quantification of mitral regurgitation with the proximal flow convergence method: A clinical study. Am. Heart J., *124*:1289, 1992.

140. Bargiggia, G.S., Tronconi, L., Raisaro, A., Bertucci, C., Bramucci, E., Recusani, F., and Montemartini, C.: Color Doppler analysis of the proximal flow convergence region in patients with mitral regurgitation. Cardiovasc. Imag., *2*:137, 1990.

140a. Chen, C., Koschyk, D., Brockhoff, C., Heik, S., Hamm, C., Bleifeld, W., Kupper, W.: Noninvasive estimation of regurgitant flow rate and volume in patients with mitral regurgitation by Doppler color mapping of accelerating flow field. J. Am. Coll. Cardiol., *21*:374–383, 1993.

140b. Giesler, M., Grossmann, G., Schmidt, A., Kochs, M., Langhans, J., Stauch, M., Hombach, V.: Color Doppler echocardiographic determination of mitral regurgitant flow from the proximal velocity profile of the flow convergence region. Am. J. Cardiol., *71*:217–224, 1993.

141. Tribouilloy, C., Shen, W.F., Quere, J-P., Rey, J-L., Choquet, D., Dufosse, H., and Lesbre, J-P.: Assessment of severity of mitral regurgitation by measuring regurgitant jet width at its origin with transesophageal Doppler color flow imaging. Circulation, *85*:1248, 1992.

142. Wang, S.S., Rubenstein, J.J., Goldman, M., and Sidd, J.J.: A new Doppler-echo method to quantify regurgitant volume. J. Am. Soc. Echocardiogr., *5*:107, 1992.

143. Samstad, S.O., Rossvoll, O., Torp, H.G., Skjaerpe, T., and Hatle, L.: Cross-sectional early mitral flow-velocity profiles from color Doppler in patients with mitral valve disease. Circulation, *86*:748, 1992.

144. Kamp, O., Huitink, H., van Eenige, M.J., Visser, C.A., and Roos, J.P.: Value of pulmonary venous flow characteristics in the assessment of severity of native mitral valve regurgitation: An angiographic correlated study. J. Am. Soc. Echocardiogr., *5*:239, 1992.

145. Castello, R., Pearson, A.C., Lenzen, P., and Labovitz, A.J.: Effect of mitral regurgitation on pulmonary venous velocities derived from transesophageal echocardiography color-guided pulsed Doppler imaging. J. Am. Coll. Cardiol., *17*:1499, 1991.

146. Klein, A.L., Obarski, T.P., Stewart, W.J., Casale, P.N., Pearce, G.L., Husbands, K., Cosgrove, D.M., and Salcedo, E.E.: Transesophageal Doppler echocardiography of pulmonary venous flow: A new marker of mitral regurgitation severity. J. Am. Coll. Cardiol., *18*:518, 1991.

147. Tribouilloy, C., Shen, W.F., Slama, M.A., Dufosse, H., Choquet, D., Marek, A., and Lesbre, J.P.: Non-invasive measurement of the regurgitant fraction by pulsed Doppler echocardiography in isolated pure mitral regurgitation. Br. Heart J., *66*:290, 1991.

148. Blumlein, S., Bouchard, A., Schiller, N.B., Dae, M., Byrd, B.F., Ports, T., and Botvinick, E.H.: Quantitation of mitral regurgitation by Doppler echocardiography. Circulation, *74*:306, 1986.

149. Rokey, R., Sterling, L.L., Zoghbi, W.A., Sartori, M.P.,

Limacher, M.C., Kuo, L.C., and Quinones, M.A.: Determination of regurgitant fraction in isolated mitral or aortic regurgitation by pulsed Doppler two-dimensional echocardiography. J. Am. Coll. Cardiol., 7:1273, 1986.

150. Kisanuki, A., Tei, C., Minagoe, S., Natsugoe, K., Shibata, K., Yutsudo, T., Otsuji, Y., Abe, S., Arima, S., and Tanaka, H.: Continuous wave Doppler echocardiographic evaluations of the severity of mitral regurgitation. J. Cardiol., 19:831, 1989.

151. Utsunomiya, T., Patel, D., Doshi, R., Quan, M., and Gardin, J.M.: Can signal intensity of the continuous wave Doppler regurgitant jet estimate severity of mitral regurgitation. Am. Heart J., 123:166, 1992.

152. Jenni, R., Ritter, M., Eberli, F., Grimm, J., and Krayenbuehl, H.P.: Quantification of mitral regurgitation with amplitude-weighted mean velocity from continuous wave Doppler spectra. Circulation, 79:1294, 1989.

153. Dent, J.M., Jayaweera, A.R., Glasheen, W.P., Nolan, S.P., Spotnitz, W.D., Villanueva, F.S., and Kaul, S.: A mathematical model for the quantification of mitral regurgitation. Circulation, 86:553, 1992.

154. Fujino, T., Ito, M., Kanaya, S., Kawamura, T., Kinoshita, R., Fujino, M., Hamanaka, Y., and Mashiba, H.: Echocardiographic abnormal motion of interventricular septum in mitral insufficiency. J. Cardiogr., 6:613, 1976.

155. Ajisaka, R., Iesaka, Y., Takamoto, T., Iiizumi, T., Fujiwara, H., Taniguchi, K., and Takeuchi, J.: Echocardiographic assessment of left ventricular volume overloading in aortic insufficiency and mitral insufficiency. J. Cardiogr., 8:209, 1978.

156. Rosenblatt, A., Clark, R., Burgess, J., and Cohn, K.: Echocardiographic assessment of the level of cardiac compensation in valvular heart disease. Circulation, 54:509, 1976.

157. Fujino, T., Ito, M., Kanaya, S., Kawamura, T., Kinoshita, R., Fujino, M., Hamanaka, Y., and Mashiba, H.: Echocardiographic abnormal motion of interventricular septum in mitral insufficiency. J. Cardiogr., 6:613, 1976.

158. Levisman, J.A.: Echocardiographic diagnosis of mitral regurgitation in congestive cardiomyopathy. Am. Heart J., 93:33, 1977.

159. Sheikh, M.U., Morjaria, M., Covarrubias, E.A., Dejo, J., and Fox, L.M.: Echocardiographic demonstration of premature notching of the interventricular septal motion in aortic incompetence. Clin. Res., 26:271A, 1978. (Abstract)

160. Burwash, I.G., Blackmore, G.L., and Koilpillai, C.J.: Usefulness of left atrial and left ventricular chamber sizes as predictors of the severity of mitral regurgitation. Am. J. Cardiol., 70:774, 1992.

161. Gentile, R., Pearlman, A.S., Mastrocola, C., Rubenstein, S.S., Baratta, L., and Vitarelli, A.: The left ventricle in mitral valve insufficiency: Echocardiographic evaluation and hemodynamic correlations. G. Ital. Cardiol., 12:873, 1982.

162. Saltissi, S., Crowther, A., Byrne, C., Coltart, D.J., Jenkins, B.S., and Webb-Peploe, M.M.: Assessment of prognostic factors in patients undergoing surgery for nonrheumatic mitral regurgitation. Br. Heart J., 44:369, 1980.

163. Zile, M.R., Gaasch, W.H., Carroll, J.D., and Levine, H.J.: Chronic mitral regurgitation: Predictive value of preoperative echocardiographic indexes of left ventricular function and wall stress. J. Am. Coll. Cardiol., 3:235, 1984.

164. Carabello, B.A., Nolan, S.P., and McGuire, L.B.: Assessment of preoperative left ventricular function in patients with mitral regurgitation: Value of the end-systolic wall-stress-end-systolic volume ratio. Circulation, 64:1212, 1981.

165. Zuker, N., Goldfarb, B.L., Zalastein, E., Silber, H., Rovner, M., Goldbraich, N., and Wanderman, K.L.: A common color flow Doppler finding in the mitral regurgitation of acute rheumatic fever. Echocardiography, 8:627, 1991.

166. Marcus, R.H., Sareli, P., Pocock, W.A., Meyer, T.E., Magalhaes, M.P., Grieve, T., Antunes, M.J., and Barlow, J.B.: Functional anatomy of severe mitral regurgitation in active rheumatic carditis. Am. J. Cardiol., 63:577, 1989.

167. Dillon, J.C., Haisse, C.L., Chang, S., and Feigenbaum, H.: Use of echocardiography in patients with prolapsed mitral valve. Circulation, 43:503, 1971.

168. Kerber, R.E., Isaeff, D.M., and Hancock, E.W.: Echocardiographic patterns in patients with the syndrome of systolic click and late systolic murmur. N. Engl. J. Med., 284:691, 1971.

169. Popp, R.E., Brown, O.R., Silverman, J.F., and Harrison, D.C.: Echocardiographic abnormalities in the mitral valve prolapse syndrome. Circulation, 49:428, 1974.

170. DeMaria, A.M., King, J.F., Bogreu, H.G., Lies, J.E., and Masow, D.T.: The variable spectrum of echocardiographic manifestations of the mitral valve prolapse syndrome. Circulation, 50:33, 1974.

171. Haikal, M., Alpert, M.A., Whiting, R.B., Ahmad, M., and Kelly, D.: Sensitivity and specificity of M-mode echocardiographic signs of mitral valve prolapse. Am. J. Cardiol., 50:185, 1982.

172. Higgins, C.B., Reinke, R.T., Gosink, B.B., and Leopold, G.R.: The significance of mitral valve prolapse in middle-aged and elderly men. Am. Heart J., 91:292, 1976.

173. Markiewicz, W., Stoner, J., London, E., Hunt, S.A., and Popp, R.L.: Mitral valve prolapse in one hundred presumably healthy young females. Circulation, 53:464, 1976.

174. Darsee, J.R., Mikolich, R., Nicoloff, N.B., and Lesser, L.E.: Prevalence of mitral valve prolapse in presumably healthy young men. Circulation, 59:619, 1979.

175. Bloch, A., Vignola, P.A., Walker, H., Kaplan, A.D., Chiotellis, P.N., Lees, R.S., and Myers, G.S.: Echocardiographic spectrum of posterior systolic motion of the mitral valve in the general population. JCU, 5:243, 1977.

176. Sahn, D.J., Wood, J., Allen, H.D., Peoples, W., and Goldberg, S.J.: Echocardiographic spectrum of mitral valve motion in children with and without mitral valve prolapse: The nature of false positive diagnosis. Am. J. Cardiol., 39:422, 1977.

177. Yokota, Y., Kawanishi, H., Ohmori, K., Oda, A., Inoh, T., and Fukuzaki, H.: Studies on systolic anterior motion (SAM) pattern in idiopathic mitral valve prolapse by echocardiography. J. Cardiogr., 9:259, 1979.

178. Tharakan, J., Ahuja, G.K., Manchanda, S.C., and Khanna, A.: Mitral valve prolapse and cerebrovascular accidents in the young. Acta Neurol. Scand., 66:295, 1982.

179. Kessler, K.M., Anzola, E., Sequeira, R., Serafini, A.N., and Myerburg, R.J.: Mitral valve prolapse and systolic anterior motion: A dynamic spectrum. Am. Heart J., 105:685, 1983.

180. Pini, R., Greppi, B., Roman, M.J., Kramer-Fox, R., and Devereux, R.B.: Time-motion reconstruction of mitral leaflet motion from two-dimensional echocardiography in mitral valve prolapse. Am. J. Cardiol., 68:215, 1991.

181. Cohen, I.S., Gardner, L., Lednar, W.M., and Caceres, C.: Two-dimensional echocardiographic mitral valve pro-

lapse: Evidence for a relationship of echocardiographic morphology to clinical findings and to mitral annular size. Am. Heart J., *113*:859, 1987.

182. Gilbert, B.W., Schatz, R.A., VonRamm, O.T., Behar, V.S., and Kisslo, J.A.: Mitral valve prolapse. Two-dimensional echocardiographic and angiographic correlation. Circulation, *54*:716, 1976.

183. Morganroth, J., Jones, R.H., Chen, C.C., and Naito, M.: Two-dimensional echocardiography in mitral, aortic and tricuspid valve prolapse. The clinical problem, cardiac nuclear imaging considerations and a proposed standard for diagnosis. Am. J. Cardiol., *46*:1164, 1980.

184. Morganroth, J., Mardelli, T.J., Naito, M., and Chen, C.C.: Apical cross-sectional echocardiography. Standard for the diagnosis of idiopathic mitral valve prolapse syndrome. Chest, *79*:23, 1981.

185. Levine, R.A., Handschumacher, M.D., Sanfilippo, A.J., Hagege, A.A., Harrigan, P., Marshall, J.E., and Weyman, A.E.: Three-dimensional echocardiographic reconstruction of the mitral valve, with implications for the diagnosis of mitral valve prolapse. Circulation, *80*:589, 1989.

186. Sanfilippo, A.J., Abdollah, H., and Burggraf, G.W.: Quantitation and significance of systolic mitral leaflet displacement in mitral valve prolapse. Am. J. Cardiol., *64*: 1349, 1989.

187. Levine, R.A., Stathogiannis, E., Newell, J.B., Harrigan, P., and Weyman, A.E.: Reconsideration of echocardiographic standards for mitral valve prolapse: Lack of association between leaflet displacement isolated to the apical four-chamber view and independent echocardiographic evidence of abnormality. J. Am. Coll. Cardiol., *11*:1010, 1988.

188. Levine, R.A., Triulzi, M.O., Harrigan, P., and Weyman, A.E.: The relationship of mitral annular shape to the diagnosis of mitral valve prolapse. Circulation, *75*:756, 1987.

189. Cohen, J.L., Austin, S.M., Segal, K.R., Millman, A.E., and Kim, C.S.: Echocardiographic mitral valve prolapse in ballet dancers: A function of leanness. Am. Heart J., *113*:341, 1987.

190. Meyers, D.G., Starke, H., Pearson, P.H., and Wilken, M.K.: Mitral valve prolapse in anorexia nervosa. Ann. Intern. Med., *105*:384, 1986.

191. Ballester, M., Presbitero, P., Foale, R., Richards, A., and McDonald, L.: Prolapse of the mitral valve in secundum atrial septal defect: A functional mechanism. Eur. Heart J., *4*:472, 1983.

192. Meyer, R.A., Korfhagen, J.C., Covitz, W., and Kaplan, S.: Long-term follow-up study after closure of secundum atrial septal defect in children: An echocardiographic study. Am. J. Cardiol., *50*:143, 1982.

192a. Lax, D., Eicher, M., and Goldberg, S.J.: Mild dehydration induces echocardiographic signs of mitral valve prolapse in healthy females with prior normal cardiac findings. Am. Heart J., *124*:1533, 1992.

193. Fraker, T.D., Behar, V.S., and Kisslo, J.A.: Coaptation instead of prolapse: Refined echo descriptors for balloon mitral valve. Circulation (Suppl. II), *58*:233, 1978. (Abstract)

194. D'Cruz, I.A., Shah, S., Hirsch, L.J., and Goldberg, A.N.: Cross-sectional echocardiographic visualization of abnormal systolic motion of the left ventricle in mitral valve prolapse. Cathet. Cardiovasc. Diagn., *7*:35, 1981.

195. Doi, Y.L., Spodick, D.H., Hamashige, N., Yonezawa, Y., Sugiura, T., and Bishop, R.L.: Echocardiographic study of left ventricular wall motion in mitral valve prolapse. Am. Heart J., *108*:105, 1984.

196. Davies, M.J., Moore, B.P., and Braimbridge, M.V.: The floppy mitral valve: Study of incidence, pathology, and complications in surgical, necropsy, and forensic material. Br. Heart J., *40*:468, 1978.

197. Chun, P.K.C. and Sheehan, M.W.: Myxomatous degeneration of mitral valve M-mode and two-dimensional echocardiographic findings. Br. Heart J., *47*:404, 1982.

198. Rippe, J., Fishben, M.C., Carabello, B., Angoff, G., Sloss, L., and Collins, J.J., Jr.: Primary myxomatous degeneration of cardiac valves. Clinical, pathological, haemodynamic and echocardiographic profile. Br. Heart J., *44*:621, 1980.

199. Ormiston, J.A., Shah, P.M., Tei, C., and Wong, M.: Size and motion of the mitral valve annulus in man. II. Abnormalities in mitral valve prolapse. Circulation, *65*:713, 1982.

200. Sanfilippo, A.J., Harrigan, P., Popovic, A.D., Weyman, A.E., and Levine, R.A.: Papillary muscle traction in mitral valve prolapse: Quantitation by two-dimensional echocardiography. J. Am. Coll. Cardiol., *19*:564, 1992.

201. Virmani, R., Atkinson, J.B., Byrd, B.F., Robinowitz, M., and Forman, M.B.: Abnormal chordal insertion: A cause of mitral valve prolapse. Am. Heart J., *113*:851, 1987.

202. Shah, A.A., Quinones, M.A., Wasggoner, A.D., Barndt, R., and Miller, R.R.: Pulsed Doppler echocardiographic detection of mitral regurgitation in mitral valve prolapse: Correlation with cardiac arrhythmias. Cathet. Cardiovasc. Diagn., *8*:437, 1982.

203. Abbasi, A.S., DeCristofaro, D., Anabtawi, J., and Irwin, L.: Mitral valve prolapse: Comparative value of M-mode two-dimensional and Doppler echocardiography. J. Am. Coll. Cardiol., *2*:1219, 1983.

204. Come, P.C., Riley, M.F., Carl, L.V., and Nakao, S.: Pulsed Doppler echocardiographic evaluation of valvular regurgitation in patients with mitral valve prolapse: Comparison with normal subjects. J. Am. Coll. Cardiol., *8*: 1355, 1986.

205. Yoshida, K., Yoshikawa, J., Yamaura, Y., Hozumi, T., Shakudo, M., Akasaka, T., and Kato, H.: Value of acceleration flows and regurgitant jet direction by color Doppler flow mapping in the evaluation of mitral valve prolapse. Circulation, *81*:879, 1990.

206. Gross, C.M., Nichols, F.T., von Dohlen, T.W., and D'Cruz, I.A.: Mitral valve prolapse and stroke: Echocardiographic evidence for a missing causative link. J. Am. Soc. Echocardiogr., *2*:94, 1989.

207. Egeblad, H. and Hesse, B.: Mitral valve prolapse with mobile polypoid cul-de-sac thrombus and embolism to brain and lower extremity. Am. Heart J., *114*:648, 1987.

208. Devereux, R.B., Kramer-Fox, R., and Kligfield, P.: Mitral valve prolapse: Causes, clinical manifestations, and management. Ann. Intern. Med., *111*:305, 1989.

209. Labovitz, A.J., Pearson, A.C., McCluskey, M.T., and Williams, G.A.: Clinical significance of the echocardiographic degree of mitral valve prolapse. Am. Heart J., *115*:842, 1988.

210. Rueda, B. and Arvan, S.: The relationship between clinical and echocardiographic findings in mitral valve prolapse. Herz, *13*:277, 1988.

211. Krivokapich, J., Child, J.S., Dadourian, B.J., and Perloff, J.K.: Reassessment of echocardiographic criteria for diagnosis of mitral valve prolapse. Am. J. Cardiol., *61*: 131, 1988.

212. Okano, Y., Nagata, S., Ishikura, F., Asaoka, N., Beppu, S., Ohmori, F., Tamai, J., and Miyatake, K.: Progression of idiopathic mitral valve prolapse estimated by echocardiography. J. Cardiol., *20*:73, 1990.

213. Devereux, R.B., Kramer-Fox, R., Shear, K., Kligfield, P., Pini, R., and Savage, D.D.: Diagnosis and classification of severity of mitral valve prolapse. Methodologic, biologic, and prognostic considerations. Am. Heart J., *113*:1265, 1987.

214. Zamorano, J., Erbel, R., Mackowski, T., Alfonso, F., and Meyer, J.: Usefulness of transesophageal echocardiography for diagnosis of mitral valve prolapse. Am. J. Cardiol., *69*:419, 1992.

215. Hayakawa, M., Inoh, T., Kawanishi, H., Kaku, K., Kumaki, T., Toh, S., and Fukuzaki, H.: Two-dimensional echocardiographic findings of patients with papillary muscle dysfunction. J. Cardiogr., *12*:137, 1982.

216. Ormiston, J.A., Shah, P.M., Tei, C., and Wong, M.: Size and motion of the mitral valve annulus in man. I. A two-dimensional echocardiographic method and findings in normal subjects. Circulation, *64*:113, 1981.

217. Godley, R.W., Wann, L.S., Rogers, E.W., Feigenbaum, H., and Weyman, A.E.: Incomplete mitral leaflet closure in patients with papillary muscle dysfunction. Circulation, *63*:565, 1981.

218. Kinney, E.L. and Frangi, M.J.: Value of two-dimensional echocardiographic detection of incomplete mitral leaflet closure. Am. Heart J., *109*:87, 1985.

219. Nishimura, T., Takahashi, M., Osakada, G., Yasunaga, K., Kawai, C., Kotoura, H., Konishi, Y., and Tatsuta, N.: Two-dimensional echocardiographic findings in ruptured chordae tendineae of the mitral valve. J. Cardiogr., *8*:589, 1978.

220. Mintz, G.S., Kotler, M.N., Segal, B.L., and Parry, W.R.: Two-dimensional echocardiographic recognition of ruptured chordae tendineae. Circulation, *57*:244, 1978.

221. Ogawa, S., Mardelli, T.J., and Hubbard, F.E.: The role of cross-sectional echocardiography in the diagnosis of flail mitral leaflet. Clin. Cardiol., *1*:85, 1978.

222. Child, J.S., Skorton, D.J., Taylor, R.D., Krivokapich, J., Abbasi, A.S., Wong, M., and Shah, P.D.: M-mode and cross-sectional echocardiographic features of flail posterior mitral leaflets. Am. J. Cardiol., *44*:1383, 1979.

223. Avgeropoulou, C.C., Rahko, P.S., and Patel, A.K.: Reliability of M-mode, two-dimensional and Doppler echocardiography in diagnosing a flail mitral valve leaflet. J. Am. Soc. Echocardiogr., *1*:433, 1988.

224. Cherian, G., Tei, C., Shah, P.M., and Wong, M.: Diastolic prolapse in the flail mitral valve syndrome: A new observation providing differentiation from the mitral valve prolapse syndrome. Am. Heart J., *103*:1074, 1982.

225. Ballester, M., Foale, R., Presbitero, P., Yacoub, M., Richards, A., and McDonald, L.: Cross-sectional echocardiographic features of ruptured chordae tendineae. Eur. Heart J., *4*:795, 1983.

226. Nishimura, R.A., Schaff, H.V., Shub, C., Gersh, B.J., Edwards, W.D., and Tajik, A.J.: Papillary muscle rupture complicating acute myocardial infarction: Analysis of 17 patients. Am. J. Cardiol., *51*:373, 1983.

227. Pearson, A.C., St. Vrain, J., Mrosek, D., and Labovitz, A.J.: Color Doppler echocardiographic evaluation of patients with a flail mitral leaflet. J. Am. Coll. Cardiol., *16*:232, 1990.

228. Alam, M. and Sun, I.: Superiority of transesophageal echocardiography in detecting ruptured mitral chordae tendineae. Am. Heart J., *121*:1819, 1991.

229. Stoddard, M.F., Keedy, D.L., and Kupersmith, J.: Transesophageal echocardiographic diagnosis of papillary muscle rupture complicating acute myocardial infarction. Am. Heart J., *120*:690, 1990.

230. Sochowski, R.A., Chan, K-L., Ascah, K.J., and Bedard, P.: Comparison of accuracy of transesophageal versus transthoracic echocardiography for the detection of mitral valve prolapse with ruptured chordae tendineae (flail mitral leaflet). Am. J. Cardiol., *67*:1251, 1991.

231. Shyu, K-G., Lei, M-H., Hwang, J-J., Lin, S-C., Kuan, P., and Lien, W-P.: Morphologic characterization and quantitative assessment of mitral regurgitation with ruptured chordae tendineae by transesophageal echocardiography. Am. J. Cardiol., *70*:1152, 1992.

232. Czer, L.S.C. and Maurer, G.: Intraoperative echocardiography in mitral and tricuspid valve repair. Echocardiography, *7*:305, 1990.

233. Goldman, M.E., Guarino, T., and Mindich, B.P.: Intraoperative evaluation of valvular regurgitation: Comparison of echocardiographic techniques. Echocardiography, *7*:201, 1990.

234. Freeman, W.K., Schaff, H.V., Khandheria, B.K., Oh, J.K., Orszulak, T.A., Abel, M.D., Seward, J.B., and Tajik, A.J.: Intraoperative evaluation of mitral valve regurgitation and repair by transesophageal echocardiography: Incidence and significance of systolic anterior motion. J. Am. Coll. Cardiol., *20*:599, 1992.

235. Marwick, T.H., Stewart, W.J., Currie, P.J., and Cosgrove, D.M.: Mechanisms of failure of mitral valve repair: An echocardiographic study. Am. Heart J., *122*:149, 1991.

236. Ogawa, S., Dupler, D.A., Pauletto, F.J., Chaudry, K.R., and Drefius, L.S.: Flail mitral valve in rheumatic heart disease. Chest, *74*:88, 1978.

237. Ahmad, S., Kleiger, R.E., Connors, J., and Krone, R.: The echocardiographic diagnosis of rupture of a papillary muscle. Chest, *73*:232, 1978.

238. Matsukubo, H., Yoshioka, K., Kajita, Y., Katsuki, A., Watanabe, T., Asayama, J., Katsume, H., Kunishige, H., Endo, N., Matsuura, T., and Ijichi, H.: Echocardiographic findings of vegetation and ruptured chordae tendineae: Two cases of bacterial endocarditis. Cardiovasc. Sound Bull., *5*:717, 1975.

239. Terasawa, Y., Tsuda, K., Ohno, K., Tsugawa, K., Kawakami, A., Yoshida, T., and Takamiya, M.: Ultrasonocardiotomogram and ultrasound cardiogram of mitral regurgitation due to ruptured chordae tendineae. J. Cardiogr., *8*:349, 1978.

240. Humphries, W.C., Hammer, W.J., McDonough, M.T., Lemole, G., McCurdy, R.R., and Spann, J.F., Jr.: Echocardiographic equivalents of a flail mitral leaflet. Am. J. Cardiol., *40*:802, 1977.

241. Jamal, N., Winters, W., and Nelson, J.: Echocardiographic features of flail mitral valve leaflets: Ruptured chordae tendineae versus ruptured papillary muscle. Circulation (Suppl. II), *58*:43, 1978. (Abstract)

242. Sze, K.C., Nanda, N.C., and Gramiak, R.: Systolic flutter of the mitral valve. Am. Heart J., *96*:157, 1978.

243. Meyer, J.F., Frank, M.J., Goldberg, S., and Cheng, T.O.: Systolic mitral flutter, an echocardiographic clue to the diagnosis of ruptured chordae tendineae. Am. Heart J., *94*:3, 1977.

244. Williams, D.E., Sahn, D.J., and Friedman, W.F.: Cross-sectional echocardiographic localization of sites of left ventricular outflow tract obstruction. Am. J. Cardiol., *37*:250, 1976.

245. Weyman, A.E., Feigenbaum, H., Hurwitz, R.A., Girod, D.A., and Dillon, J.C.: Cross-sectional echocardiographic assessment of the severity of aortic stenosis in children. Circulation, *55*:773, 1977.

246. DeMaria, A.N., Bommer, J.W., Joye, J., Lee, G., Bouteller, J., and Mason, D.T.: Value and limitations of cross-sectional echocardiography of the aortic valve in

the diagnosis and quantification of valvular aortic stenosis. Circulation, *62*:304, 1980.

247. Godley, R.W., Green, D., Dillon, J.C., Rogers, E.W., Feigenbaum, H., and Weyman, A.E.: Reliability of two-dimensional echocardiography in assessing the severity of valvular aortic stenosis. Chest, *79*:657, 1981.

248. Stoddard, M.F., Arce, J., Liddell, N.E., Peters, G., Dillon, S., and Kupersmith, J.: Two-dimensional transesophageal echocardiographic determination of aortic valve area in adults with aortic stenosis. Am. Heart J., *122*:1415, 1991.

249. Otto, C.M., Nishimura, R.A., Davis, K.B., Kisslo, K.B., and Bashore, T.M.: Doppler echocardiographic findings in adults with severe symptomatic valvular aortic stenosis. Am. J. Cardiol., *68*:1477, 1991.

250. Geibel, A., Gornandt, L., Kasper, W., and Bubenheimer, P.: Reproducibility of Doppler echocardiographic quantification of aortic and mitral valve stenoses: Comparison between two echocardiography centers. Am. J. Cardiol., *67*:1013, 1991.

251. Bengur, A.R., Snider, R., Serwer, G.A., Peters, J., and Rosenthal, A.: Usefulness of the Doppler mean gradient in evaluation of children with aortic valve stenosis and comparison to gradient at catheterization. Am. J. Cardiol., *64*:756, 1989.

252. Harrison, M.R., Gurley, J.C., Smith, M.D., Grayburn, P.A., and DeMaria, A.N.: A practical application of Doppler echocardiography for the assessment of severity of aortic stenosis. Am. Heart J., *115*:622, 1988.

253. Otto, C.M. and Pearlman, A.S.: Doppler echocardiography in adults with symptomatic aortic stenosis. Arch. Intern. Med., *148*:2553, 1988.

254. Penn, I.M. and Dumesnil, J.G.: A new and simple method to measure maximal aortic valve pressure gradients by Doppler echocardiography. Am. J. Cardiol., *61*:382, 1988.

255. Hatle, L., Angelsen, B.A., and Tromsdal, A.: Noninvasive assessment of aortic stenosis by Doppler ultrasound. Br. Heart J., *43*:284, 1980.

256. Lima, C.O., Sahn, D.J., Valdes-Cruz, L.M., Allen, H.D., Goldberg, S.J., Grenadier, E., and Barron, J.V.: Prediction of the severity of left ventricular outflow tract obstruction by quantitative two-dimensional echocardiographic Doppler studies. Circulation, *68*:348, 1983.

257. Berger, M., Berdoff, R.L., Gallerstein, P.E., and Goldberg, E.: Evaluation of aortic stenosis by continuous wave Doppler ultrasound. J. Am. Coll. Cardiol., *3*:150, 1984.

258. Kosturakis, D., Allen, H.D., Goldberg, S.J., Sahn, D.J., and Valdes-Cruz, L.M.: Non-invasive quantification of stenotic semilunar valve areas by Doppler echocardiography. J. Am. Coll. Cardiol., *3*:1256, 1984.

259. Currie, P.J., Seward, J.B., Reeder, G.S., Vlietsttra, R.E., Bresnahan, D.R., Bresnahan, J.F., Smith, H.C., Hagler, D.J., and Tajik, A.J.: Continuous-wave Doppler echocardiographic assessment of severity of calcific aortic stenosis: A simultaneous Doppler-catheter correlative study in 100 adult patients. Circulation, *71*:1162, 1985.

260. Oh, J.K., Taliercio, C.P., Holmes, Jr., D.R., Reeder, G.S., Biley, K.R., Seward, J.B., and Tajik, A.J.: Prediction of the severity of aortic stenosis by Doppler aortic valve area determination: Prospective Doppler-catheterization correlation in 100 patients. J. Am. Coll. Cardiol., *11*:1227, 1988.

261. Danielsen, R., Nordrehaug, J.E., and Vik-Mo, H.: Factors affecting Doppler echocardiographic valve area assessment in aortic stenosis. Am. J. Cardiol., *63*:1107, 1989.

262. Danielsen, R., Nordrehaug, J.E., Stangeland, L., and Vik-Mo, H.: Limitations in assessing the severity of aortic stenosis by Doppler gradients. Br. Heart J., *59*:551, 1988.

263. Panidis, I.P., Mintz, G.S., and Ross, J.: Value and limitations of Doppler ultrasound in the evaluation of aortic stenosis: A statistical analysis of 70 consecutive patients. Am. Heart J., *112*:150, 1986.

264. Rothbart, R.M., Kaiser, D.L., and Gibson, R.S.: A prospective comparison of continuous wave versus high pulse repetition frequency Doppler echocardiography for quantifying transvalvular pressure gradients in adults with aortic stenosis. Am. Heart J., *114*:1155, 1987.

265. Fan, P-H., Kapur, K.K., and Nanda, N.C.: Color-guided Doppler echocardiographic assessment of aortic valve stenosis. J. Am. Coll. Cardiol., *12*:441, 1988.

266. Rifkin, R.D., Raju, P.K., and Skowronski, M.: False diagnosis of aortic stenosis due to Doppler recording of mitral regurgitation from the suprasternal notch. Echocardiography, *8*:17, 1991.

267. Nakatani, S., Imanishi, T., Terasawa, A., Beppu, S., Nagata, S., and Miyatake, K.: Clinical application of transpulmonary contrast enhanced Doppler technique in the assessment of severity of aortic stenosis. J. Am. Coll. Cardiol., *20*:973, 1992.

268. Currie, P.J., et al.: Continuous-wave Doppler echocardiographic assessment of severity of calcific aortic stenosis: A simultaneous Doppler-catheter correlative study in 100 adult patients. Circulation, *71*:1162, 1985.

269. Teien, D., Karp, K., and Eriksson, P.: Non-invasive estimation of the mean pressure difference in aortic stenosis by Doppler ultrasound. Br. Heart J., *56*:450, 1986.

270. Seitz, W.S., McIlroy, M.B., Kline, H., Operschall, J., and Kashani, I.A.: Echographic application of the Gorlin formula for assessment of aortic stenosis: Correlation with cardiac catheterization in pediatric patients. Am. Heart J., *111*:118, 1986.

271. Teirstein, P., Yeager, M., Yock, P.G., and Popp, R.L.: Doppler echocardiographic measurement of aortic valve area in aortic stenosis: A noninvasive application of the Gorlin formula. J. Am. Coll. Cardiol., *8*:1059, 1986.

272. Bengur, A.R., Snider, A.R., Meliones, J.N., and Vermilion, R.P.: Doppler evaluation of aortic valve area in children with aortic stenosis. J. Am. Coll. Cardiol., *18*:1499, 1991.

273. Taylor, R.: Evolution of the continuity equation in the Doppler echocardiographic assessment of the severity of valvular aortic stenosis. J. Am. Soc. Echocardiogr., *3*:326, 1990.

274. Otto, C.M., Pearlman, A.S., Gardner, C.L., Enomoto, D.M., Togo, T., Tsuboi, H., and Ivey, T.D.: Experimental validation of Doppler echocardiographic measurement of volume flow through the stenotic aortic valve. Circulation, *78*:435, 1988.

275. Grayburn, P.A., Smith, M.D., Harrison, M.R., Gurley, J.C., and DeMaria, A.N.: Pivotal role of aortic valve area calculation by the continuity equation for Doppler assessment of aortic stenosis in patients with combined aortic stenosis and regurgitation. Am. J. Cardiol., *61*:376, 1988.

276. Otto, C.M., Pearlman, A.S., Gardner, C.L., Kraft, C.D., and Fujioka, M.C.: Simplification of the Doppler continuity equation for calculating stenotic aortic valve area. J. Am. Soc. Echocardiogr., *1*:155, 1988.

277. Dumesnil, J.G. and Yoganathan, A.P.: Theoretical and practical differences between the Gorlin formula and the continuity equation for calculating aortic and mitral valve area. Am. J. Cardiol., *67*:1268, 1991.

277a. Wippermann, C.F., Schranz, D., Stopfkuchen, H.,

Huth, R., and Freund, M.: Evaluation of the valve area underestimation by the continuity equation. Cardiology, *80*:276–282, 1992.

278. Casale, P.N., Palacios, I.F., Abascal, V.M., Harrell, L., Davidoff, R., Weyman, A.E., and Fifer, M.A.: Effects on dobutamine on Gorlin and continuity equation valve area and valve resistance in valvular aortic stenosis. Am. J. Cardiol., *70*:1175, 1992.

279. Galan, A., Zoghbi, W.A., and Quinones, M.A.: Determination of severity of valvular aortic stenosis by Doppler echocardiography and relation of findings to clinical outcome and agreement with hemodynamic measurements determined at cardiac catheterization. Am. J. Cardiol., *67*:1007, 1991.

280. Segal, J., Lerner, D.J., Miller, C., Mitchell, R.S., Alderman, E.A., and Popp, R.L.: When should Doppler determined valve area be better than the Gorlin formula?: Variation in hydraulic constants in low flow states. J. Am. Coll. Cardiol., *9*:1294, 1987.

281. Zoghbi, W.A., Galan, A., and Quinones, M.A.: Accurate assessment of aortic stenosis severity by Doppler echocardiography independent of aortic jet velocity. Am. Heart J., *116*:855, 1988.

282. Donner, R., Black, I., Spann, J.F., and Carabello, B.A.: Improved prediction of peak left ventricular pressure by echocardiography in children with aortic stenosis. J. Am. Coll. Cardiol., *3*:349, 1984.

283. Brenner, J.I., Baker, K.R., and Berman, M.A.: Prediction of left ventricular pressure in infants with aortic stenosis. Br. Heart J., *44*:406, 1980.

284. Reichek, N. and Devereux, R.B.: Reliable estimation of peak left ventricular systolic pressure by M-mode echographic-determined end-diastolic relative wall thickness: Identification of severe valvular aortic stenosis in adult patients. Am. Heart J., *103*:202, 1982.

285. DePace, N.L., et al.: Correlation of echocardiographic wall stress and left ventricular pressure and function in aortic stenosis. Circulation, *67*:854, 1983.

286. Sheikh, K.H., Bashore, T.M., Kitzman, D.W., Davidson, C.J., Skelton, T.N., Honan, M.B., Kisslo, K.B., Higginbotham, M.B., and Kisslo, J.: Doppler left ventricular diastolic filling abnormalities in aortic stenosis and their relation to hemodynamic parameters. Am. J. Cardiol., *63*:1360, 1989.

287. Otto, C.M., Pearlman, A.S., and Amsler, L.C.: Doppler echocardiographic evaluation of left ventricular diastolic filling in isolated valvular aortic stenosis. Am. J. Cardiol., *63*:313, 1989.

288. Ennouri, R., Malergue, M.C., Cavailles, J., and Tricot, R.: Aorto-septal angulation: A new cause of disorder in left ventricular ejection? (A two-dimensional echocardiographic study apropos of 66 cases.) Arch. Mal. Coeur, *77*:673, 1984.

289. Iida, K., Sugishita, Y., Ajisaka, R., Matsumoto, R., Higuchi, Y., Tomizawa, T., Noguchi, Y., Yukisada, K., Ogawa, T., and Ito, I.: Sigmoid septum causing left ventricular outflow tract obstruction: A case report. J. Cardiogr., *16*:237, 1986.

290. Esper, R.J.: Detection of mild aortic regurgitation by range-rated pulsed Doppler echocardiography. Am. J. Cardiol., *50*:1037, 1982.

291. Ciobanu, M., Abbasi, A.S., Allen, M., Hermer, A., and Spellberg, R.: Pulsed Doppler echocardiography in the diagnosis and estimation of severity of aortic insufficiency. Am. J. Cardiol., *49*:339, 1982.

292. Cooper, J.W., Nanda, N.C., Philpot, E.F., and Fan, P.: Evaluation of valvular regurgitation by color Doppler. J. Am. Soc. Echocardiogr., *2*:56, 1989.

293. Castello, R., Fagan, L., Lenzen, J.P., Pearson, A.C., and Labovitz, A.J.: Comparison of transthoracic and transesophageal echocardiography for assessment of left-side valvular regurgitation. Am. J. Cardiol., *68*:1677, 1991.

294. Kai, H., Koyanagi, S., and Takeshita, A.: Aortic valve prolapse with aortic regurgitation assessed by Doppler color-flow echocardiography. Am. Heart J., *124*:1297, 1992.

295. Bouchard, A., Yock, P., Schiller, N.B., Blumlein, S., Botvinick, E.H., Greenburg, B., Cheitlin, M., and Massie, B.M.: Value of color Doppler estimation of regurgitant volume in patients with chronic aortic insufficiency. Am. Heart J., *117*:1099, 1989.

296. Smith, M.D., Grayburn, P.A., Spain, M.G., DeMaria, A.N., Kwan, O.L., and Moffett, C.B.: Observer variability in the quantitation of Doppler color flow jet areas for mitral and aortic regurgitation. J. Am. Coll. Cardiol., *11*: 579, 1988.

297. Reimold, S.C., Thomas, J.D., and Lee, R.T.: Relation between Doppler color flow variables and invasively determined jet variables in patients with aortic regurgitation. J. Am. Coll. Cardiol., *20*:1143, 1992.

298. Masuyama, T., Kitabatake, A., Kodama, K., Uematsu, M., Nakatani, S., and Kamada, T.: Semiquantitative evaluation of aortic regurgitation by Doppler echocardiography: Effects of associated mitral stenosis. Am. Heart J., *117*:122, 1989.

299. Nishigami, K., Yoshikawa, J., Yoshida, K., Minagoe, S., Akasaka, T., Shakudo, M., Yamaura, Y., and Matsumura, Y.: Quantification of aortic regurgitant stroke volume by Doppler color flow proximal isovelocity surface area method. Jpn. J. Med. Ultrasonics, *19*:9, 1992.

300. Reynolds, T., Abate, J., Tenney, A., and Warner, M.G.: The JH/LVOH method in the quantification of aortic regurgitation: How the cardiac sonographer may avoid an important potential pitfall. J. Am. Soc. Echocardiogr., *4*: 105, 1991.

301. Perry, G.J., Helmcke, F., Nanda, J.C., Byard, C., and Soto, B.: Evaluation of aortic insufficiency by Doppler color flow mapping. J. Am. Coll. Cardiol., *9*:952, 1987.

302. Taylor, A.L., Eichhorn, E.J., Brickner, M.E., Eberhart, R.C., and Grayburn, P.A.: Aortic valve morphology: An important in vitro determinant of proximal regurgitant jet width by Doppler color flow mapping. J. Am. Coll. Cardiol., *16*:405, 1990.

303. Slordahl, S.A., Piene, H., and Skjaerpe, T.: Pressure half-time in aortic regurgitation: Evaluation with Doppler in a cardiovascular hydromechanical simulator and in a computer model. J. Am. Soc. Echocardiogr., *3*:46, 1990.

304. Teague, S.M., Heinsimer, J.A., Anderson, J.L., Sublett, K., Olson, E.G., Voyles, W.F., and Thadani, U.: Quantification of aortic regurgitation utilizing continuous wave Doppler ultrasound. J. Am. Coll. Cardiol., *8*:592, 1986.

305. Masuyama, T., Sato, H., Nanto, S., Naka, M., Taniura, K., Hirayama, A., Kodama, K., Okamoto, K., Morita, K., Kitabatake, A., Inoue, M., and Kamada, T.: Comparison of continuous wave and pulsed Doppler method in noninvasive evaluation of aortic regurgitation. Jpn. J. Med. Ultrasonics, *13*:17, 1986.

306. Labovitz, A.J., Ferrara, R.P., Kern, M.J., Bryg, R.J., Mrosek, D.G., and Williams, G.A.: Quantitative evaluation of aortic insufficiency by continuous wave Doppler echocardiography. J. Am. Coll. Cardiol., *8*:1341, 1986.

307. Grayburn, P.A., Handshoe, R., Smith, M.D., Harrison, M.R., and DeMaria, A.N.: Quantitative assessment of the hemodynamic consequences of aortic regurgitation

by means of continuous wave Doppler recordings. J. Am. Coll. Cardiol., *10*:135, 1987.

308. Griffin, B.P., Flachskampf, F.A., Siu, S., Weyman, A.E., and Thomas, J.D.: The effects of regurgitant orifice size, chamber compliance, and systemic vascular resistance on aortic regurgitant velocity slope and pressure half-time. Am. Heart J., *122*:1049, 1991.

309. Vanoverschelde, J-L. J., Taymans-Robert, A.R., Raphael, D.A., and Cosyns, J.R.: Influence of transmitral filling dynamics on continuous-wave Doppler assessment of aortic regurgitation by half-time methods. Am. J. Cardiol., *64*:614, 1989.

310. Samstad, S.O., Hegrenaes, L., Skjaerpe, T., and Hatle, L.: Half time of the diastolic aortoventricular pressure difference by continuous wave Doppler ultrasound: A measure of the severity of aortic regurgitation? Br. Heart J., *61*:336, 1989.

311. Oh, J.K., Hatle, L.K., Sinak, L.J., Seward, J.B., and Tajik, A.J.: Characteristic Doppler echocardiographic pattern of mitral inflow velocity in severe aortic regurgitation. J. Am. Coll. Cardiol., *14*:1712, 1989.

312. Vandenbossche, J-L. and Englert, M.: Doppler color flow mapping demonstration of diastolic mitral regurgitation in severe acute aortic regurgitation. Am. Heart J., *114*:889, 1987.

313. Rokey, R., Sterling, L.L., Zoghbi, W.A., Sartori, M.P., Limacher, M.C., Kuo, L.C., and Quinones, M.A.: Determination of regurgitant fraction in isolated mitral or aortic regurgitation by pulsed Doppler two-dimensional echocardiography. J. Am. Coll. Cardiol., *7*:1273, 1986.

314. Tribouilloy, C., Avinee, P., Shen, W.F., Rey, J-L., Slama, M., and Lesbre, J-P.: End diastolic flow velocity just beneath the aortic isthmus assessed by pulsed Doppler echocardiography: A new predictor of the aortic regurgitant fraction. Br. Heart J., *65*:37, 1991.

315. Takenaka, K., Dabestani, A., Gardin, J.M., Russell, D., Clark, S., Allfie, A., and Henry, W.L.: A simple Doppler echocardiographic method for estimating severity of aortic regurgitation. Am. J. Cardiol., *57*:1340, 1986.

316. Caguioa, E.S., Reimold, S.C., Velez, S., and Lee, R.T.: Influence of aortic pressure on effective regurgitant orifice area in aortic regurgitation. Circulation, *85*:1565, 1992.

317. Yeung, A.C., Plappert, T., and St. John Sutton, M.G.: Calculation of aortic regurgitation orifice area by Doppler echocardigraphy: An application of the continuity equation. Br. Heart J., *68*:236, 1992.

318. Reimold, S.C., Ganz, P., Bittl, J.A., Thomas, M.D., Thoreau, D., Plappert, T.J., and Lee, R.T.: Effective aortic regurgitant orifice area: Description of a method based on the conservation of mass. J. Am. Coll. Cardiol., *18*:761, 1991.

319. Nishimura, R.A., Vonk, G.D., Rumberger, J.A., and Tajik, A.J.: Semiquantitation of aortic regurgitation by different Doppler echocardiographic techniques and comparison with ultrafast computed tomography. Am. Heart J., *124*:995, 1992.

320. Trappe, H-J., Daniel, W.G., Frank, G., and Lichtlen, P.R.: Comparisons between diastolic fluttering and reverse doming of anterior mitral leaflet in aortic regurgitation. Am. Heart J., *114*:1399, 1987.

321. Rowe, D.W., Pechacek, L.W., DeCastro, C.M., Garcia, E., and Hall, R.J.: Initial diastolic indentation of the mitral valve in aortic insufficiency. JCU, *10*:53, 1982.

322. Robertson, W.S., Stewart, J., Armstrong, W.F., Dillon, J.C., and Feigenbaum, H.: Reverse doming of the anterior mitral leaflet with severe aortic regurgitation. J. Am. Coll. Cardiol., *3*:431, 1984.

323. Miki, T., Yokota, Y., Nomura, H., Miki, T., Emoto, R., Kurozumi, H., Usuki, S., Chou, H., and Fukuzaki, H.: Relation between aortic regurgitant jet and reverse doming of anterior mitral leaflet in aortic regurgitation. Jpn. J. Med. Ultrasonics, *16*:25, 1989.

324. Downes, T.R., Nomeir, A-M., Hackshaw, B.T., Kellam, L.J., Watts, L.E., and Little, W.C.: Diastolic mitral regurgitation in acute but not chronic aortic regurgitation: Implications regarding the mechanism of mitral closure. Am. Heart J., *117*:1106, 1989.

325. Henzi, M., Burckhardt, D., Raeder, E.A., and Follath, F.: Echocardiography as a method for the determination of the severity of aortic insufficiency. Schweiz. Med. Wochenschr., *106*:1557, 1976.

326. Pridie, R.B., Beham, R., and Oakley, C.M.: Echocardiography of the mitral valve in aortic valve disease. Br. Heart J., *33*:296, 1971.

327. Oki, T., Matsuhisa, M., Tsuyuguchi, N., Kondo, C., Matsumura, K., Niki, T., Mori, H., and Sawada, S.: Echo patterns of the anterior leaflet of the mitral valve in patients with aortic insufficiency. J. Cardiogr., *6*:307, 1976.

328. Ambrose, J.A., Meller, J., Teichholz, L.E., and Herman, M.V.: Premature closure of the mitral valve: Echocardiographic clue for the diagnosis of aortic dissection. Chest, *73*:121, 1978.

329. Mann, T., McLaurin, L., Grossman, W., and Craige, E.: Assessing the hemodynamic severity of acute aortic regurgitation due to infective endocarditis. N. Engl. J. Med., *293*:108, 1975.

330. Fox, S., Kotler, M.N., Segal, B.L., and Parry, W.: Echocardiographic diagnosis of acute aortic valve endocarditis and its complications. Arch. Intern. Med., *137*:85, 1977.

331. Marcus, R.H., Neumann, A., Borow, K.M., and Lang, R.M.: Transmitral flow velocity in symptomatic severe arotic regurgitation: Utility of Doppler for determination of preclosure of the mitral valve. Am. Heart J., *120*:449, 1990.

332. Weaver, W.F., Wilson, C.S., Rourke, T., and Caudill, C.C.: Mid-diastolic aortic valve opening in severe acute aortic regurgitation. Circulation, *55*:145, 1977.

333. Pietro, D.A., Parisi, A.F., Harrington, J.J., and Askenazi, J.: Premature opening of the aortic valve: An index of highly advanced aortic regurgitation. JCU, *6*:170, 1978.

334. Nathan, M.P.R., Arora, R., and Rubenstein, H.: Mid-diastolic aortic valve opening in bacterial endocarditis of aortic valve. Clin. Cardiol., *5*:294, 1982.

335. Henry, W.L., Bonow, R.O., Borer, J.S., Ware, J.H., Kent, K.M., Redwood, D.R., McIntosh, C.L., Morrow, A.G., and Epstein, S.E.: Observations on the optimum time for operative intervention for aortic regurgitation. I. Evaluation of the results of aortic valve replacement in symptomatic patients. Circulation, *61*:471, 1980.

336. Henry, W.L., Bonow, R.O., Rosing, D.R., and Epstein, S.E.: Observations on the optimum time for operative intervention for aortic regurgitation. II. Serial echocardiographic evaluation of asymptomatic patients. Circulation, *61*:484, 1980.

337. Schuler, G., Peterson, K.L., Johnson, A.D., Francis, G., Ashburn, W., Dennish, G., Daily, P.O., and Ross, J.: Serial noninvasive assessment of left ventricular hypertrophy and function after surgical correction of aortic regurgitation. Am. J. Cardiol., *44*:585, 1979.

338. Borras, X., Carreras, F., Auge, J.M., and Pons-Llado, G.: Prospective validation of detection and quantitative

assessment of chronic aortic regurgitation by a combined echocardiographic and Doppler method. J. Am. Soc. Echocardiogr., *1*:422, 1988.

339. Vandenbossche, J-L., Massie, B.M., Schiller, N.B., and Karliner, J.S.: Relation of left ventricular shape to volume and mass in patients with minimally symptomatic chronic aortic regurgitation. Am. Heart J., *116*:1022, 1988.

340. Bonow, R.O., Dodd, J.T., Maron, B.J., O'Gara, P.T., White, G.G., McIntoch, C.L., Clark, R.E., and Epstein, S.E.: Long-term serial changes in left ventricular function and reversal of ventricular dilatation after valve replacement for chronic aortic regurgitation. Circulation, *78*:1108, 1988.

341. Bonow, R.O. and Epstein, S.E.: Is preoperative left ventricular function predictive of survival and functional results after aortic valve replacement for chronic aortic regurgitation? J. Am. Coll. Cardiol., *10*:713, 1987.

342. Bonow, R.O., Rosing, D.R., Kent, K.M., and Epstein, S.E.: Timing of operation for chronic arotic regurgitation. Am. J. Cardiol., *50*:325, 1982.

343. Stone, P.H., Clark, R.D., Goldschlager, N., Selzer, A., and Cohn, K.: Determinants of prognosis of patients with arotic regurgitation who undergo aortic valve replacement. J. Am. Coll. Cardiol., *3*:1118, 1984.

344. Donaldson, R.M., Florio, R., Rickards, A.F., Bennett, J.G., Yacoub, M., Ross, D.N., and Olsen, E.: Irreversible morphological changes contributing to depressed cardiac function after surgery for chronic aortic regurgitation. Br. Heart J., *48*:589, 1982.

345. Huxley, R.L., Gaffney, A., Corbett, J.R., Firth, B.G., Peshock, R., Nicod, P., Rellas, J.S., Curry, G., Lewis, S.E., and Willerson, J.T.: Early detection of left ventricular dysfunction in chronic aortic regurgitation as assessed by contrast angiography, echocardiography, and rest and exercise scintigraphy. Am. J. Cardiol., *51*:1542, 1983.

346. McDonald, I.G. and Jelinek, V.M.: Serial M-mode echocardiography in severe chronic arotic regurgitation. Circulation, *62*:1291, 1980.

347. Fioretti, P., Roelandt, J., Bos, R.J., Meltzer, R.S., Van-Hoogenhuijze, D., Serruys, P.W., Nauta, J., and Hugenholtz, P.G.: Echocardiography in chronic aortic insufficiency. Circulation, *67*:216, 1983.

348. Daniel, W.G., et al.: Chronic aortic regurgitation: Reassessment of the prognostic value of preoperative left ventricular end-systolic dimension and fractional shortening. Circulation, *71*:669, 1985.

349. Fioretti, P., et al.: Postoperative regression of left ventricular dimensions in aortic insufficiency: A long-term echocardiographic study. J. Am. Coll. Cardiol., *5*:856, 1985.

350. Gaasch, W.H., Carroll, J.D., Levine, H.J., and Criscitiello, M.G.: Chronic aortic regurgitation: Prognostic value of left ventricular end-systolic dimension and end-diastolic radius/thickness ratio. J. Am. Coll. Cardiol., *1*:775, 1983.

351. Miller, R.R.: Improtance of preoperative hypertrophy, wall stress and end-systolic dimension as echocardiographic predictors of normalization of left ventricular dilatation after valve replacement in chronic aortic insufficiency. Am. J. Cardiol., *49*:1091, 1982.

352. St. John Sutton, M.G., Plappert, T.A., Hirshfeld, J.W., and Reichek, N.: Assessment of left ventricular mechanics in patients with asymptomatic aortic regurgitation: A two-dimensional echocardiographic study. Circulation, *69*:268, 1984.

353. Paulsen, P.: Aortic regurgitation. Detection of left ventricular dysfunction by exercise echocardiography. Br. Heart J., *46*:380, 1981.

354. Gumbiner, C.H. and Gutgesell, H.P.: Response to isometric exercise in children and young adults with aortic regurgitation. Am. Heart J., *106*:540, 1983.

354a.Percy, R.F., Miller, A.B., and Conetta, D.A.: Usefulness of left ventricular wall stress at rest and after exercise for outcome prediction in asymptomatic aortic regurgitation. Am. Heart J., *125*:151, 1993.

354b.Percy, R.F., Miller, A.B., and Conetta, D.A.: Usefulness of left ventricular wall stress at rest and after exercise for outcome prediction in asymptomatic aortic regurgitation. Am. Heart J., *125*:151, 1993.

355. Imaizumi, T., Orita, Y., Koiwaya, Y., Hirata, T., and Nakamura, M.: Utility of two-dimensional echocardiography in the differential diagnosis of the etiology of aortic regurgitation. Am. Heart J., *103*:887, 1982.

356. DePace, N.L., Nestico, P.F., Kotler, M.N., Mintz, G.S., Kimbiris, D., Goel, I.P., Glazier-Laskey, E.E., and Ross, J.: Comparison of echocardiography and angiography in determining the cause of severe aortic regurgitation. Br. Heart J., *51*:36, 1984.

357. Shiu, M.F., Coltart, D.J., and Braimbridge, M.V.: Echocardiographic findings in prolapsed aortic cusp with vegetation. Br. Heart J., *41*:118, 1979.

358. El Shahawy, M., Graybeal, R., Pepine, C.J., and Conti, C.R.: Diagnosis of aortic valvular prolapse by echocardiography. Chest, *69*:411, 1976.

359. Fantini, F. and Barletta, G.: Observations of prolapse of the aortic cusps. G. Ital. Cardiol., *12*:409, 1982.

360. Mardelli, R.J., Morganroth, J., Naito, M., and Chen, C.C.: Cross-sectional echocardiographic detection of aortic valve prolapse. Am. Heart J., *100*:295, 1980.

361. Rodger, J.C. and Morley, P.: Abnormal aortic valve echoes in mitral prolapse. Echocardiographic features of floppy aortic valve. Br. Heart J., *47*:337, 1982.

362. Bullon, F.S. and Pedrero, A.C.: Prolapse of noncoronary aortic cusp with severe aortic regurgitation after a tear of the aortic root. Cardiovasc. Dis., *7*:178, 1980.

363. Guyer, D.E., Gillam, L.D., Foale, R.A., Clark, M.C., Dinsmore, R., Palacios, I., Block, P., King, M.E., and Weyman, A.E.: Comparison of the echocardiographic and hemodynamic diagnosis of rheumatic tricuspid stenosis. J. Am. Coll. Cardiol., *3*:1135, 1984.

364. Daniels, S.J., Mintz, G.S., and Kotler, M.N.: Rheumatic tricuspid valve disease: Two-dimensional echocardiographic, hemodynamic, and angiographic correlations. Am. J. Cardiol., *51*:492, 1983.

365. Nanna, M., Chandraratna, P.A., Reid, C., Nimalasuriya, A., and Rahimtoola, S.H.: Value of two-dimensional echocardiography in detecting tricuspid stenosis. Circulation, *67*:221, 1983.

366. Shimada, R., Takeshita, A., Nakamura, M., Tokunaga, K., and Hirata, T.: Diagnosis of tricuspid stenosis by M-mode and two-dimensional echocardiography. Am. J. Cardiol., *53*:164, 1984.

367. Hernandez, G., Esquivel-Avila, J.G., Villalba, R., DiSessa, T.G., and Zavala, E.: Echocardiographic evaluation of the tricuspid valve in rheumatic mitral valvulopathy. Arch. Inst. Cardiol. Mex., *53*:513, 1983.

368. Joyner, C.R., Hey, B.E., Jr., Johnson, J., and Reid, J.M.: Reflected ultrasound in the diagnosis of tricuspid stenosis. Am. J. Cardiol., *19*:66, 1967.

369. Parris, T.M., Panidis, I.P., Ross, J., and Mintz, G.S.: Doppler echocardiographic findings in rheumatic tricuspid stenosis. Am. J. Cardiol., *60*:1414, 1987.

370. Mugge, A., Danile, W.G., Herrmann, G., Simon, R., and Lichtlen, P.R.: Quantification of tricuspid regurgitant by Doppler color flow mapping after cardiac transplantation. Am. J. Cardiol., 66:884, 1990.

371. Chopra, H.K., Nanda, N.C., Fan, P., Kapur, K.K., Goyal, R., Daruwalla, D., and Pacifico, A.: Can two-dimensional echocardiography and Doppler color flow mapping identify the need for tricuspid valve repair? J. Am. Coll. Cardiol., 14:1255, 1989.

372. Fisher, E.A. and Goldman, M.E.: Simple, rapid method for quantification of tricuspid regurgitation by two-dimensional echocardiography. Am. J. Cardiol., 63:1375, 1989.

373. Waggoner, A.D., Barzilai, B., and Perez, J.E.: Saline contrast enhancement of tricuspid regurgitant jets detected by Doppler color flow imaging. Am. J. Cardiol., 65:1368, 1990.

374. Blanchard, D., Diebold, B., Guermonprez, J.L., Chitour, Z., Nee, M., Peronneau, P., Forman, J., and Maurice, P.: Doppler echocardiographic diagnosis and evaluation of tricuspid regurgitation. Arch. Mal. Coeur, 75: 1357, 1982.

375. Diebold, B., Touati, R., Blanchard, D., Colonna, G., Guermonprez, J.L., Peronneau, P., Forman, J., and Maurice, P.: Quantitative assessment of tricuspid regurgitation using pulsed Doppler echocardiography. Br. Heart J., 50:443, 1983.

376. Sakai, K., Nakamura, K., Satomi, G., Kondo, M., and Kirosawa, K.: Hepatic vein blood flow pattern measured by Doppler echocardiography as an evaluation of tricuspid valve insufficiency. J. Cardiogr., 13:33, 1983.

377. Veyrat, C., Kalmanson, D., Farjon, M., Manin, J.P., and Abitbol, G.: Non-invasive diagnosis and assessment of tricuspid regurgitation and stenosis using one and two dimensional echo-pulsed Doppler. Br. Heart J., 47:596, 1982.

378. Lieppe, W., Behar, V.S., Scallion, R., and Kisslo, J.A.: Detection of tricuspid regurgitation with two-dimensional echocardiography and peripheral vein injections. Circulation, 57:128, 1978.

379. Amano, K., Sakamoto, T., Hada, Y., Yamaguchi, T., Ishimitsu, T., and Takenake, K.: Detection of tricuspid regurgitation by contrast echocardiography. Jpn. Circ. J., 46:395, 1982.

380. Gambelli, G., Boccanelli, A., Signoretti, P., Turitto, G., DiSegni, M., and Prati, P.L.: Two-dimensional contrast echocardiography of hepatic veins in the diagnosis of tricuspid regurgitation. G. Ital. Cardiol., 11:2010, 1981.

381. Gullace, G., Savoia, M.T., Locatelli, V., Ravizza, P.F., and Ranzi, C.: Contrast echocardiography of the inferior vena cava. G. Ital. Cardiol., 11:2017, 1981.

382. Grison, D., Lassabe, G., Chemama, F., and Sacrez, A.: Two-dimensional echocardiography with contrast in tricuspid insufficiency. Cardiology, 68:75, 1981.

383. Ogawa, S., Hayashi, J., Sasaki, H., Tani, M., Akaishi, M., Mitamura, H., Sano, M., Hoshino, T., Handa, S., and Nakamura, Y.: Evaluation of combined valvular prolapse syndrome by two-dimensional echocardiography. Circulation, 65:174,1982.

384. Wise, N.K., Myers, S., Fraker, T.D., Stewart, J.A., and Kisslo, J.A.: Contrast M-mode ultrasonography of the inferior vena cava. Circulation, 63:1100, 1981.

385. Meltzer, R.S., McGhie, J., and Roelandt, J.: Inferior vena cava echocardiography. JCU, 10:47, 1982.

386. Martin, G.R., Silverman, N.H., Soifer, S.J., Lutin, W.A., and Scagnelli, S.A.: Tricuspid regurgitation in children: A pulsed Doppler, contrast echocardiographic and angiographic comparison. J. Am. Soc. Echocardiogr., 1:257, 1988.

387. Chen, C.C., Morganroth, J., Mardelli, T.J., and Naito, M.: Tricuspid regurgitation in tricuspid valve prolapse demonstrated with contrast cross-sectional echocardiography. Am. J. Cardiol., 46:983, 1980.

388. Rippe, J.M., Angoff, G., Sloss, L.J., Wynne, J., and Alpert, J.S.: Multiple floppy valves: An echocardiographic syndrome. Am. J. Med., 66:817, 1979.

389. Werner, J.A., Schiller, N.B., and Prasquier, R.: Occurrence and significance of echocardiographically demonstrated tricuspid valve prolapse. Am. Heart J., 96:180, 1978.

390. Inoue, D., Katsume, H., Watanabe, T., Matsukubo, H., Furukawa, K., Torii, Y., Sugihara, H., and Ijichi, H.: Tricuspid valve prolapse detected by subxiphoid two-dimensional echocardiography. J. Cardiogr., 9:387, 1979.

391. Bates, E.R., and Sorkin, R.P.: Echocardiographic diagnosis of flail anterior leaflet in tricuspid endocarditis. Am. Heart J., 106:161, 1983.

392. De Maria, A.N., Bommer, W., Neumann, A., Weinert, L., Barstwo, T., Kaku, R., and Mason, D.T.: Evaluation of tricuspid valve prolapse by two-dimensional echocardiography. Circulation (Suppl. II), 58:43, 1978. (Abstract)

393. Vergel, J.: Enhanced diagnosis of tricuspid valve prolapse by cross-sectional echocardiography. Am. J. Cardiol., 43:385, 1979. (Abstract)

394. Gibson, T.C., Foale, R.A., Guyer, D.E., and Weyman, A.E.: Clinical significance of incomplete tricuspid valve closure seen on two-dimensional echocardiography. J. Am. Coll. Cardiol., 4:1052, 1984.

395. Watanabe, T., Katsume, H., Matsukubo, H., Furukawa, K., and Ijichi, H.: Ruptured chordae tendineae of the tricuspid valve due to nonpenetrating trauma. Echocardiographic findings. Chest, 80:751, 1981.

396. Eckfeldt, J.H., Weir, E.K., and Chesler, E.: Echocardiographic findings in ruptured chordae tendineae of the tricuspid valve. Am. Heart J., 105:1033, 1983.

397. Kawaratani, H., Narita, M., Kurihara, T., and Usami, Y.: A case of traumatic tricuspid insufficiency. J. Cardiogr., 7:393, 1977.

398. Kessler, K.M., Foianini, J.E., Davia, J.E., Anderson, W.T., Pfuetze, K., Pinder, T., and Cheitlin, M.D.: Tricuspid insufficiency due to nonpenetrating trauma. Am. J. Cardiol., 37:442, 1976.

399. Lardouz, H., D'Allaines, C., Melanidis, J., Guerinon, J., Pornin, M., Morin, D., Ourbak, P., and Maurice, P.: Comparison of quantitative data from two-dimensional echocardiography and anatomical examination in mitral stenosis. Arch. Mal. Coeur, 77:245, 1984.

400. Liddell, N.E., Stoddard, M.F., Talley, J.D., Guinn, V.L., and Kupersmith, J.: Transesophageal echocardiographic diagnosis of isolated tricuspid valve prolapse with severe tricuspid regurgitation. Am. Heart J., 123: 230, 1992.

401. Winslow, T., Redberg, R., and Schiller, N.B.: Transesophageal echocardiography in the diagnosis of flail tricuspid valve. Am. Heart J., 123:1682, 1992.

402. Baker, B.J., McNee, V.D., Scovil, J.A., Bass, K.M., Watson, J.W., and Bissett, J.K.: Tricuspid insufficiency in carcinoid heart disease: An echocardiographic description. Am. Heart J., 101:107, 1981.

403. Forman, M.B., Byrd, B.F., Oates, J.A., and Robertson, R.M.: Two-dimensional echocardiography in the diagnosis of carcinoid heart disease. Am. Heart J., 107:492, 1984.

404. Reid, C.L., Chandraratna, P.A.N., Kawanishi, D.T., Pitha, J.V., and Rahimtoola, S.H.: Echocardiographic features of carcinoid heart disease. Am. Heart J., *107*:801, 1984.

405. Davies, M.K., Lowry, P.J., and Littler, W.A.: Cross-sectional echocardiographic features in carcinoid heart disease. A mechanism for tricuspid regurgitation in this syndrome. Br. Heart J., *51*:355, 1984.

406. Callahan, J.A., Wroblewski, E.M., Reeder, G.S., Edwards, W.D., Sewart, J.B., and Tajik, A.J.: Echocardiographic features of carcinoid heart disease. Am. J. Cardiol., *50*:762, 1982.

407. Chandraratna, P.A.N., Wilson, D., Imaizumi, T., Ritter, W.S., and Aronow, W.S.: Invasive and noninvasive assessment of pulmonic regurgitation: Clinical, angiographic, phonocardiographic, echocardiographic, and Doppler ultrasound correlation. Clin. Cardiol., *5*:360, 1982.

408. Patel, A.K., Rowe, G.G., Dhanani, S.P., Kosolcharoen, P., Lyle, L.E.W., and Thomsen, J.H.: Pulsed Doppler echocardiography in diagnosis of pulmonary regurgitation: Its value and limitations. Am. J. Cardiol., *49*:1801, 1982.

409. Takao, S., Miyatake, K., Izumi, S., Okamoto, M., Kinoshita, N., Nakagawa, H., Yamamoto, K., Sakakibara, H., and Nimura, Y.: Clinical implications of pulmonary regurgitation in healthy individuals: Detection by cross sectional pulsed Doppler echocardiography. Br. Heart J., *59*:542, 1988.

410. Sprecher, D.L., Adamick, R., Adams, D., and Kisslo, J.: In vitro color flow, pulsed and continuous wave Doppler ultrasound masking of flow by prosthetic valves. J. Am. Coll. Cardiol., *9*:1306, 1987.

411. Alam, M., Serwin, J.B., Rosman, H.S., Polanco, G.A., Sun, I., and Silverman, N.A.: Transesophageal echocardiographic features of normal and dysfunctioning bioprosthetic valves. Am. Heart J., *121*:1149, 1991.

412. Daniel, L.B., Grigg, L.E., Weisel, R.D., and Rakowski, H.: Comparison of transthoracic and transesophageal assessment of prosthetic valve dysfunction. Echocardiography, *7*:83, 1990.

413. Nellessen, U., Schnittger, I., Appleton, C.P., Masuyama, T., Bolger, A., Fischel, T.A., Tye, T., and Popp, R.L.: Transesophageal two-dimensional echocardiography and color Doppler flow velocity mapping in the evaluation of cardiac valve prostheses. Circulation, *78*:848, 1988.

413a.Alton, M.E., Pasierski, T.J., Orsinelli, D.A., Eaton, G.M., and Pearson, A.C.: Comparison of transthoracic and transesophageal echocardiography in evaluation of 47 Starr-Edwards prosthetic valves. J. Am. Coll. Cardiol., *20*:1503, 1992.

413b.Daniel, W.G., Mugge, A., Grote, J., Hausmann, D., Nikutta, P., Laas, J., Lichtlen, P.R., and Martin, R.P.: Comparison of transthoracic and transesophageal echocardiography for detection of abnormalities of prosthetic and bioprosthetic valves in the mitral and aortic positions. Am. J. Cardiol., *71*:210, 1993.

414. Panidis, I.P., Ren, J-F., Kotler, M.N., Mintz, G.S., Mundth, E.D., Goel, I.P., and Ross, J.: Clinical and echocardiographic evaluation of the St. Jude cardiac valve prosthesis: Follow-up of 126 patients. J. Am. Coll. Cardiol., *4*:454, 1984.

415. Kotler, M.N., Mintz, G.S., Panidis, I., Morganroth, J., Segal, B.L., and Ross, J.: Non-invasive evaluation of normal and abnormal prosthetic valve function. J. Am. Coll. Cardiol., *2*:151, 1983.

416. van den Brink, R.B.A., Verheul, H.A., van Capelle, F.J.L., Visser, C.A., and Dunning, A.J.: Long-term reproducibility of conventional Doppler analysis in patients with prosthetic valves. J. Am. Soc. Echocardiogr., *4*:441, 1991.

417. Pye, M., Weerasana, N., Bain, W.H., Hutton, I., and Cobbe, S.M.: Doppler echocardiographic characteristics of normal and dysfunctioning prosthetic valves in the tricuspid and mitral position. Br. Heart J., *63*:41, 1990.

418. Cooper, D.M., Stewart, W.J., Schiavone, W.A., Lombardo, H.P., Lytle, B.W., Loop, F.D., and Salcedo, E.E.: Evaluation of normal prosthetic valve function by Doppler echocardiography. Am. Heart J., *114*:576, 1987.

419. Simpson, I.A., Reece, I.J., Houston, A.B., Hutton, I., Wheatley, D.J., and Cobbe, S.M.: Non-invasive assessment by Doppler ultrasound of 155 patients with bioprosthetic valves: A comparison of the Wessex porcine, low profile Ionescu-Shiley, and Hancock pericardial prostheses. Br. Heart J., *56*:83, 1986.

420. Jaffe, W.M., Coverdale, H.A., Roche, A.H.G., Brandt, P.W.T., Ormiston, J.A., and Barratt-Boyes, B.G.: Doppler echocardiography in the assessment of the homograft aortic valve. Am. J. Cardiol., *63*:1466, 1989.

421. Kapur, K.K., Fan, P., Nanda, N.C., Yoganathan, A.P., and Goyal, R.G.: Doppler color flow mapping in the evaluation of prosthetic mitral and aortic valve function. J. Am. Coll. Cardiol., *13*:1561, 1989.

422. Melacini, P., Villanova, C., Thiene, G., Minarini, M., Fasoli, G., Bortolotti, U., Ramuscello, G., Scognamiglio, R., Ponchia, A., and Volta, S.D.: Long-term echocardiographic Doppler monitoring of Hancock bioprostheses in the mitral valve position. Am. J. Cardiol., *70*:1157, 1992.

423. Wiseth, R., Levang, O.W., Sande, E., Tangen, G., Skjaerpe, T., and Hatle, L.: Hemodynamic evaluation by Doppler echocardiography of small ($\leq 21$ mm) prostheses and bioprostheses in the aortic valve position. Am. J. Cardiol., *70*:240, 1992.

424. Heldman, D. and Gardin, J.M.: Evaluation of prosthetic valves by Doppler echocardiography. Echocardiography, *6*:63, 1989.

425. Reisner, S.A. and Meltzer, R.S.: Normal values of prosthetic valve Doppler echocardiographic parameters: A review. J. Am. Soc. Echocardiogr., *1*:201, 1988.

426. Panidis, I.P., Ross, J., and Mintz, G.S.: Normal and abnormal prosthetic valve function as assessed by Doppler echocardiography. J. Am. Coll. Cardiol., *8*:317, 1986.

427. Weiss, P., Hoffmann, A., and Burckhardt, D.: Doppler sonographic evaluation of mechanical and bioprosthetic mitral valve prostheses during exercise with a rate corrected pressure half time. Br. Heart J., *67*:466, 1992.

428. Dressler, F.A. and Labovitz, A.J.: Exercise evaluation of prosthetic heart valves by Doppler echocardiography: Comparison with catheterization studies. Echocardiography, *9*:235, 1992.

429. Reisner, S.A., Lichtenberg, G.S., Shapiro, J.R., Schwarz, K.Q., and Meltzer, R.S.: Exercise Doppler echocardiography in patients with mitral prosthetic valves. Am. Heart J., *118*:755, 1989.

429a.Wiseth, R., Levang, Q.W., Tangen, G., Rein, K.A., Skjaerpe, T., and Hatle, L.: Exercise hemodynamics in small ($-21$ mm) aortic valve prostheses assessed by Doppler echocardiography. Am. Heart J., *125*:138, 1993.

429b.Wiseth, R., Levang, O.W., Tangen, G., Rein, K.A., Skjaerpe, T., and Hatle, L.: Exercise hemodynamics in small ($-21$ mm) aortic valve prostheses assessed by Doppler echocardiography. Am. Heart J., *125*:138, 1993.

430. Dumesnil, J.G., Honos, G.N., Lemieux, M., and Beauchemin, J.: Validation and applications of mitral prosthetic valvular areas calculated by Doppler echocardiography. Am. J. Cardiol., *65*:1443, 1990.

431. Rothbart, R.M., Castriz, J.L., Harding, L.V., Russo, C.D., and Teague, S.M.: Determination of aortic valve area by two-dimensional and Doppler echocardiography in patients with normal and stenotic bioprosthetic valves. J. Am. Coll. Cardiol., *15*:817, 1990.

432. Chambers, J.B., Sprigings, D.C., Cochrane, T., Allen, J., Morris, R., Black, M.M., and Jackson, G.: Continuity equation and Gorlin formula compared with directly observed orifice area in native and prosthetic aortic valves. Br. Heart J., *67*:193, 1992.

433. Chambers, J.B., Cochrane, T., Black, M.M., and Jackson, G.: The Gorlin formula validated against directly observed orifice area in porcine mitral bioprostheses. J. Am. Coll. Cardiol., *13*:348, 1989.

434. Dumesnil, J.G., Honos, G.N., Lemieux, M., and Beauchemin, J.: Validation and applications of indexed aortic prosthetic valve areas calculated by Doppler echocardiography. J. Am. Coll. Cardiol., *16*:637, 1990.

435. Mathias, D.W., Al-Wathiqui, M.H., Sagar, K.B., and Wann, L.S.: Doppler echocardiographic assessment of prosthetic valve function: Promises and pitfalls. Echocardiography, *6*:497, 1989.

436. Chandrasekaran, K., Ross, J., Covalesky, V.A., Kresh, J.Y., and Mintz, G.S.: Two-dimensional echocardiographic visualization of turbulent intracardiac blood flow across the stenotic mitral valve. Am. Heart J., *118*:625, 1989.

437. Stewart, S.F.C., Nast, E.P., Arabia, F.A., Talbot, T.L., Proschan, M., and Clark, R.E.: Errors in pressure gradient measurement by continuous wave Doppler ultrasound: Type, size and age effects in bioprosthetic aortic valves. J. Am. Coll. Cardiol., *18*:769, 1991.

438. Rothbart, R.M., Smucker, M.L., and Gibson, R.S.: Overestimation by Doppler echocardiography of pressure gradients across Starr-Edwards prosthetic valves in the aortic position. Am. J. Cardiol., *61*:475, 1988.

439. Baumgartner, H., Khan, S., DeRobertis, M., Czer, L., and Maurer, G.: Effect of prosthetic aortic valve design on the Doppler-catheter gradient correlation: An in vitro study of normal St. Jude, Medtronic-Hall, Starr-Edward and Hancock valves. J. Am. Coll. Cardiol., *19*:324, 1992.

440. Goldrath, N., Zimes, R., and Vered, Z.: Analysis of Doppler-obtained velocity curves in functional evaluation of mechanical prosthetic valves in the mitral and aortic positions. J. Am. Soc. Echocardiogr., *1*:211, 1988.

441. Chafizadeh, E.R. and Zoghbi, W.A.: Doppler echocardiographic assessment of the St. Jude medical prosthetic valve in the aortic position using the continuity equation. Circulation, *83*:213, 1991.

442. Reimold, S.C., Yoganathan, A.P., Sung, H-W., Cohn, L.H., St. John Sutton, M.G., and Lee, R.T.: Doppler echocardiographic study or porcine bioprosthetic heart valves in the aortic valve position in patients without evidence of cardiac dysfunction. Am. J. Cardiol., *67*:611, 1991.

443. Chambers, J., Jackson, G., and Jewitt, D.: Limitations of Doppler ultrasound in the assessment of the function of prosthetic mitral valves. Br. Heart J., *63*:189, 1990.

444. Nellessen, U., Masuyama, T., Appleton, C.P., Tye, T., and Popp, R.L.: Mitral prosthesis malfunction. Circulation, *79*:330, 1989.

445. Chambers, J., McLoughlin, N., Rapson, A., and Jackson, G.: Effect of changes in heart rate on pressure half-time in normally functioning mitral valve prostheses. Br. Heart J., *60*:501, 1988.

445a. Chambers, J. and Deverall, P.: Limitations and pitfalls in the assessment of prosthetic valves with Doppler ultrasonography. J. Thorac. Cardiovasc. Surg., *204*:495, 1992.

446. Alam, M., Rosman, H.S., Polanco, G.A., Sheth, M., Garcia, R., and Serwin, J.B.: Transesophageal echocardiographic features of stenotic bioprosthetic valves in the mitral and tricuspid valve positions. Am. J. Cardiol., *68*:689, 1991.

447. Wiseth, R., Sande, E., Skaerpe, T., Gunnes, S., Levang, O.W., and Hatle, L.: Thrombotic disc impediment in a Medtronic-Hall aortic valve prosthesis diagnosed by Doppler echocardiography followed by successful reoperation. J. Am. Soc. Echocardiogr., *4*:64, 1991.

447a. Barbetseas, J., Pitsavos, C., Lalos, S., Psarros, T., and Toutouzas, P.: Partial thrombosis of a bileaflet mitral prosthetic valve: diagnosis by transesophageal echocardiography. J. Am. Soc. Echocardiogr., *6*:91, 1993.

448. Om, A., Sperry, R., and Paulsen, W.: Transesophageal echocardiography for evaluation of thrombosed mitral valve prosthesis during thrombolytic therapy. Am. Heart J., *124*:781, 1992.

449. Cassidy, J.M., Smith, M.D., Gurley, J.C., Booth, D.C., Cater, A.L., and Salley, R.K.: Detection of thrombosis of St. Jude Medical prostheses by transesophageal echocardiography. Am. Heart J., *122*:1466, 1991.

450. Dzavik, V., Cohen, G., and Chan, K.L.: Role of transesophageal echocardiography in the diagnosis and management of prosthetic valve thrombosis. J. Am. Coll. Cardiol., *18*:1829, 1991.

451. Adamick, R.D., Gleckel, L.C., and Graver, L.M.: Acute thrombosis of an aortic bioprosthetic valve: Transthoracic and transesophageal echocardiographic findings. Am. Heart J., *122*:241, 1991.

452. Stoddard, M.F., Dawkins, P.R., and Longsaker, R.A.: Mobile strands are frequently attached to the St. Jude medical mitral valve prosthesis as assessed by two-dimensional transesophageal echocardiography. Am. Heart J., *124*:671, 1992.

453. Copans, H., Lakier, J.B., Kinsley, R.H., Colsen, P.R., Fritz, V.U., and Barlow, J.B.: Thrombosed Bjork-Shiley mitral prostheses. Circulation, *61*:169, 1980.

454. Srivastava, T.N., Hussain, M., Gray, L.A., Jr., and Flowers, N.C.: Echocardiographic diagnosis of a stuck Bjork-Shiley aortic valve prosthesis. Chest, *70*:94, 1976.

455. Chandraratna, P.A.N., Lopez, J.M., Hildner, F.J., Samet, P., and Ben-Zvi, J. (with technical assistance of D. Gindlesperger): Diagnosis of Bjork-Shiley aortic valve dysfunction by echocardiography. Am. Heart J., *91*:318, 1976.

456. Clements, S.D. and Perkins, J.V.: Malfunction of a Bjork-Shiley prosthetic heart valve in the mitral position producing an abnormal echocardiographic pattern. JCU, *6*:334, 1978.

457. Pfeifer, J., Goldschlager, N., Sweatman, T., Gerbode, E., and Selzer, A.: Malfunction of mitral ball valve prosthesis due to thrombus. Am. J. Cardiol., *29*:95, 1972.

458. Wann, L.S., Pyhel, H.J., Judson, W.E., Tavel, M.E., and Feigenbaum, H.: Ball variance in a Harken mitral prosthesis: Echocardiographic and phonocardiographic features. Chest, *72*:785, 1977.

459. Chambers, J., Monaghan, M., and Jackson, G.: Colour flow Doppler mapping in the assessment of prosthetic valve regurgitation. Br. Heart J., *62*:1, 1989.

460. Faletra, F., Donatelli, F., Parmigiani, M.L., Ladelli, L., Scarpini, S., Merlini, P.A., and Pezzano, A.: Usefulness

of color flow imaging in prosthetic valve regurgitation. Cardiovasc. Imaging, *1*:52, 1989.

461. Alam, M., Rosman, H.S., McBroom, D., Graham, L., Magilligan, Jr., D.J., Khaja, F., and Stein, P.D.: Color flow Doppler evaluation of St. Jude Medical prosthetic valves. Am. J. Cardiol., *64*:1387, 1989.

462. Jones, M. and Eidbo, E.E.: Doppler color flow evaluation of prosthetic mitral valves: Experimental epicardial studies. J. Am. Coll. Cardiol., *13*:234, 1989.

463. Vandenberg, B.F., Dellsperger, K.C., Chandran, K.B., and Kerber, R.E.: Detection, localization, and quantitation of bioprosthetic mitral valve regurgitation. Circulation, *78*:529, 1988.

464. Herrera, C.J., Chaudhry, F.A., DeFrino, P.F., Mehlman, D.J., Mulhern, K.M., O'Rourke, R.A., and Zabalgoitia, M.: Value and limitations of transesophageal echocardiography in evaluating prosthetic or bioprosthetic valve dysfunction. Am. J. Cardiol., *69*:697, 1992.

465. Khandheria, B.K., Seward, J.B., Oh, J.K., Freeman, W.K., Nochols, B.A., Sinak, L.J., Miller, Jr., F.A., and Tajik, A.J.: Value and limitations of transesophageal echocardiography in assessment of mitral valve prostheses. Circulation, *83*:1956, 1991.

466. Chaudhry, F.A., Herrera, C., DeFrino, P.F., Mehlman, D.J., and Zabalgoitia, M.: Pathologic and angiographic correlations of transesophageal echocardiography in prosthetic heart valve dysfunction. Am. Heart J., *122*:1057, 1991.

467. Alam, M., Serwin, J.B., Rosman, H.S., Sheth, M., Sun, I., Silverman, N.A., and Goldstein, S.: Transesophageal color flow Doppler and echocardiographic features of normal and regurgitant St. Jude medical prostheses in the mitral valve position. Am. J. Cardiol., *66*:871, 1990.

468. Taams, M.A., Gussenhoven, E.J., Cahalan, M.K., Roelandt, J.R.T.C., van Herwerden, L.A., The, H.K., Bom, N., and deJong, N.: Transesophageal Doppler color flow imaging in the detection of native and Bjork-Shiley mitral valve regurgitation. J. Am. Coll. Cardiol., *13*:95, 1989.

469. van den Brink, R.B.A., Visser, C.A., Basart, D.C.G., Duren, D.R., de Jong, A.P., and Dunning, A.J.: Comparison of transthoracic and transesophageal color Doppler flow imaging in patients with mechanical prostheses in the mitral valve position. Am. J. Cardiol., *63*:1471, 1989.

470. Hixson, C.S., Smith, M.D., Mattson, M.D., Morris, E.J., Lenhoff, S.J., and Salley, R.K.: Comparison of transesophageal color flow Doppler imaging of normal mitral regurgitant jets in St. Jude medical and Medtronic Hall cardiac prostheses. J. Am. Soc. Echocardiogr., *5*:57, 1992.

471. Baumgartner, H., Khan, S., Derobertis, M., Czer, L., and Maurer, G.: Color Doppler regurgitant characteristics of normal mechanical mitral valve prostheses in vitro. Circulation, *85*:323, 1992.

472. Flachskampf, F.A., O'Shea, J.P., Griffin, B.P., Guerrero, L., Weyman, A.E., and Thomas, J.D.: Patterns of normal transvalvular regurgitation in mechanical valve prostheses. J. Am. Coll. Cardiol., *18*:1493, 1991.

473. Mohr-Kahaly, S., Kupferwasser, I., Erbel, R., Oelert, H., and Meyer, J.: Regurgitant flow in apparently normal valve prostheses: Improved detection and semiquantitative analysis by transesophageal two-dimensional color-coded Doppler echocardiography. J. Am. Soc. Echocardiogr., *3*:187, 1990.

474. Meloni, L., Aru, G.M., Abbruzzese, P.A., Cardu, G., Martelli, V., and Cherchi, A.: Localization of mitral periprosthetic leaks by transesophageal echocardiography. Am. J. Cardiol., *69*:276, 1992.

475. Pinto, F.J., Wranne, B., and Schnittger, I.: Transesophageal echocardiography for study of bioprostheses in the aortic valve position. Am. J. Cardiol., *69*:274, 1992.

476. Dittrich, H.C., McCann, H.A., Walsh, T.P., Blanchard, D.G., Oppenheim, G.E., Warack, T.C., Donaghey, L.B., and Wheeler, K.: Transesophageal echocardiography in the evaluation of prosthetic and native aortic valves. Am. J. Cardiol., *66*:758, 1990.

477. Karalis, D.G., Chandrasekaran, K., Ross, Jr., J.J., Micklin, A., Brown, E.M., Ren, J-F., and Mintz, G.S.: Single-plane transesophageal echocardiography for assessing function of mechanical or bioprosthetic valves in the aortic valve position. Am. J. Cardiol., *69*:1310, 1992.

478. Chambers, J.B., Monaghan, M.J., Jackson, G., and Jewitt, D.E.: Doppler echocardiographic appearance of cusp tears in tissue valve prostheses. J. Am. Coll. Cardiol., *10*:462, 1987.

479. Yoshida, K., Yoshikawa, J., Akasaka, T., Nishigami, K., and Minagoe, S.: Value of acceleration flow signals proximal to the leaking orifice in assessing the severity of prosthetic mitral vale regurgitation. J. Am. Coll. Cardiol., *19*:333, 1992.

480. Bargiggia, G.S., Tronconi, L., Raisaro, A., Recusani, F., Ragni, T., Valdes-Cruz, L.M., Sahn, D.J., and Montemartini, C.: Color Doppler diagnosis of mechanical prosthetic mitral regurgitation: Usefulness of the flow convergence region proximal to the regurgitant orifice. Am. Heart J., *120*:1137, 1990.

480a. Cohen, G.I., Davison, M.B., Klein, A.L., Salcedo, E.E., and Stewart, W.J.: A comparison of flow convergence with other transthoracic echocardiographic indexes of prosthetic mitral regurgitation. J. Am. Soc. Echocardiogr., *5*:620, 1992.

481. Vilacosta, I., San Roman, J.A., Camino, A., Castanon, J., Gil, M., De La Llana, R., Almeria, C., and Harguindey, L.S.: Disc escape after minor strut fracture in a Bjork-Shiley mitral valve prosthesis. Echocardiography, *9*:265, 1992.

482. Gindea, A.J., Schwinger, M., Freedberg, R.S., Colvin, S.B., and Kronzon, I.: Dehiscence of a Carpentier mitral ring: Diagnosis by transesophageal echocardiography. Am. Heart J., *118*:841, 1989.

483. Ascah, K.J., Patrick, E., Chilton, C., Zawalick, B., and Bedard, P.: Atypical pseudoaneurysm after mitral valve replacement: Doppler echocardiographic diagnosis. J. Am. Soc. Echocardiogr., *4*:625, 1991.

484. Comess, K.A., Baron, S.B., Cosgrove, N.A., Copeland, J.G., and Goldberg, S.J.: Doppler ultrasound diagnosis of aortic subvalvular pseudoaneurysm with left ventricular fistula. J. Am. Soc. Echocardiogr., *1*:226, 1988.

485. Sakai, K., Nakamura, K., Ishizuka, N., Nakagawa, M., and Hosoda, S.: Echocardiographic findings and clinical features of left ventricular pseudoaneurysm after mitral valve replacement. Am. Heart J., *124*:975, 1992.

486. Yee, G.W., Naasz, C., Hatle, L., Pipkin, R., and Schnittger, I.: Doppler diagnosis of left ventricle to coronary sinus fistula: An unusual complication of mitral valve replacement. J. Am. Soc. Echocardiogr., *1*:458, 1988.

487. Rosenzweig, M.S. and Nanda, N.C.: Two-dimensional echocardiographic detection of left ventricular wall impaction by mitral prosthesis. Am. Heart J., *106*:1069, 1983.

488. Solana, L.G., Pechacek, L.W., DeCastro, C.M., Klima, T., and Colley, D.A.: Two-dimensional echocardiographic assessment of complications involving the Ionescu-Shiley pericardial valve in the mitral position. J. Am. Coll. Cardiol., *3*:328, 1984.

489. Graham, S.P. and Paulsen, W.H.: Impaction of the ventricular septum by porcine mitral valves. Echocardiography, 7:523, 1990.

489a. Garcia-Fernandez, M.A., San Roman, D., Torrecilla, E., Echevarria, T., Ribeiras, R., Bueno, H., and Delcan, J.L.: Transesophageal echocardiographic detection of atrial wall aneurysm as a result of abnormal attachment of mitral prosthesis. Am. Heart J., 124:1650, 1992.

490. Schuchman, H., Feigenbaum, H., Dillon, J.C., and Chang, S.: Intracavitary echoes in patients with mitral prosthetic valves. JCU, 3:111, 1975.

491. Preis, L.K., Hess, J.P., and Austin, J.L., Craddock, G.B., McGuire, L.B., and Martin, R.P.: Left ventricular microcavitations in patients with Beall valves. Am. J. Cardiol., 45:402, 1980. (Abstract)

492. Ramirez, J., Guardiola, J., and Flowers, N.C.: Echocardiographic diagnosis of ruptured aortic valve leaflet in bacterial endocarditis. Circulation, 57:634, 1978.

493. Yoshikawa, J., Tanaka, K., Owaki, T., and Kato, H.: Cord-like aortic valve vegetation in bacterial endocarditis. Circulation, 53:911, 1976.

494. Chandraratna, P.A.N., Robinson, M.J., Byrd, C., and Pitha, J.V.: Significance of abnormal echoes in left ventricular outflow tract. Br. Heart J., 39:381, 1977.

495. Sternberg, L., Sole, M.J., Joza, P., and Scully, H.E.: Echocardiographic features of an unusual case of aortic valve endocarditis. Can. Med. Assoc. J., 115:1022, 1976.

496. Pease, H.F., Matsumoto, S., Cacchione, R.J., Richards, K.L., and Leach, J.K.: Lethal obstruction by aortic valvular vegetation: Echocardiographic studies of endocarditis without apparent aortic regurgitation. Chest, 73:658, 1978.

497. Grenadier, E., Schuger, C., Palant, A., and Ari, J.B.: Echocardiographic diagnosis of mitral obstruction in bacterial endocarditis. Am. Heart J., 106:591, 1983.

498. Neimann, J.L., Godenir, J.P., Roche, G., and Voiriot, P.: Obstructive mitral vegetations in bacterial endocarditis. Arch. Mal. Coeur, 73:1217, 1980.

499. Chandraratna, P.A.N. and Aronow, W.S.: Spectrum of echocardiographic findings in tricuspid valve endocarditis. Br. Heart J., 42:528, 1979.

500. Kisslo, J., VonRamm, O.T., Haney, R., Jones, R., Juk, S.S., and Behar, V.S.: Echocardiographic evaluation of tricuspid valve endocarditis: An M-mode and two-dimensional study. Am. J. Cardiol., 38:502, 1976.

501. Jemsek, J.G., Greenberg, S.B., Gentry, L.O., Welton, D.E., and Mattox, K.L.: Haemophilus parainfluenzae endocarditis. Two cases and review of the literature in the past decade. Am. J. Med., 66:51, 1979.

502. Covarrubias, E.A., Sheikh, M.U., and Fox, L.M.: Echocardiography and pulmonary embolism. Ann. Intern. Med., 87:720, 1977.

503. Ellis, S.G., Goldstein, J., and Popp, R.L.: Detection of endocarditis-associated perivalvular abscesses by two-dimensional echocardiography. J. Am. Coll. Cardiol., 5: 647, 1985.

504. Mardelli, T.J., Ogawa, S., Hubbard, F.E., Dreifus, L.S., and Meixell, L.L.: Cross-sectional echocardiographic detection of aortic ring abscess in bacterial endocarditis. Chest, 74:576, 1978.

505. Scanlan, J.G., Seward, J.B., and Tajik, A.J.: Valve ring abscess in infective endocarditis: Visualization with wide angle two-dimensional echocardiography. Am. J. Cardiol., 49:1794, 1982.

506. Nakamura, K., Suzuki, S., Satomi, G., Hayashi, H., and Hirosawa, K.: Detection of mitral ring abscess by two-dimensional echocardiography. Circulation, 65:816, 1982.

507. Sharma, S., Katdare, A.D., Musi, S.C., and Kinare, S.G.: M-mode echographic detection of pulmonic valve infective endocarditis. Am. Heart J., 102:131, 1981.

508. Neimann, J.L., et al.: Two-dimensional echocardiographic recognition of aortic valve ring abscess. Eur. Heart J., 5:59, 1984.

509. Agatston, A.S., Asnani, H., Ozner, M., and Kinney, E.L.: Aortic valve ring abscess: Two-dimensional echocardiographic features leading to valve replacement. Am. Heart J., 109:171, 1985.

510. Saner, H.E., Asinger, R.W., Homans, D.C., Helseth, H.K., and Elsperger, K.J.: Two-dimensional echocardiographic identification of complicated aortic root endocarditis: Implications for surgery. Am. J. Cardiol., 10:859, 1987.

511. Fisher, E.A., Estioko, M.R., Stern, E.H., and Goldman, M.E.: Left ventricular to left atrial communication secondary to a paraaortic abscess: Color flow Doppler documentation. J. Am. Coll. Cardiol., 10:222, 1987.

512. Birmingham, G.D., Rhako, P.S., and Ballantyne, F.: Improved detection of infective endocarditis with transesophageal echocardiography. Am. Heart J., 123:774, 1992.

513. Klodas, E., Edwards, W.D., and Khandheria, B.K.: Use of transesophageal echocardiography for improving detection of valvular vegetations in subacute bacterial endocarditis. J. Am. Soc. Echocardiogr., 2:386, 1989.

514. Shively, B.K., Gurule, F.T., Roldan, C.A., Leggett, J.H., and Schiller, N.B.: Diagnostic value of transesophageal compared with transthoracic echocardiography in infective endocarditis. J. Am. Coll. Cardiol., 18:391, 1991.

515. Taams, M.A., Gussenhoven, E.J., Bos, E., DeJaegere, P., Roelandt, J.R.T.C., Sutherland, G.R., and Bom, N.: Enhanced morphological diagnosis in infective endocarditis by transesophageal echocardiography. Br. Heart J., 63:109, 1990.

516. Culver, D.L., Cacchione, J., Stern, D., Shapiro, J.R., and Reisner, S.A.: Diagnosis of infective endocarditis on a Starr-Edwards prosthesis by transesophageal echocardiography. Am. Heart J., 119:972, 1990.

517. Herrera, C.J., Mehlman, D.J., Hartz, R.S., Talano, J.V., and McPherson, D.D.: Comparison of transesophageal and transthoracic echocardiograph for diagnosis of right-sided cardiac lesions. Am. J. Cardiol., 70:964, 1992.

518. Winslow, T., Foster, E., Adams, J.R., and Schiller, N.B.: Pulmonary valve endocarditis: Improved diagnosis with biplane transesophageal echocardiography. J. Am. Soc. Echocardiogr., 5:206, 1992.

519. Shapiro, S.M., Young, E., Ginzton, L.E., and Bayer, A.S.: Pulmonary valve endocarditis as an underdiagnosed disease. Role of transesophageal echocardiography. J. Am. Soc. Echocardiogr., 5:48, 1992.

520. Teskey, R.J., Chan, K-L., and Beanlands, D.S.: Diverticulum of the mitral valve complicating bacterial endocarditis: Diagnosis by transesophageal echocardiography. Am. Heart J., 118:1063, 1989.

521. Murray, N.H., Gheesman, M.G., Millar-Craig, M.: Echocardiographic demonstration of Escherichia coli endocarditis restricted to the pulmonary valve. Br. Heart J., 60:452, 1988.

522. Lewin, R.F., Sidi, Y., Hermoni, Y., Zafrir, N., Dean, H., Glazer, Y., Pinkhas, J., and Agmon, J.: Serial two-dimensional echocardiography in infective endocarditis of the pulmonic valve. Isr. J. Med. Sci., 19:53, 1983.

523. Berger, M., Wilkes, H.S., Gallerstein, P.E., Berdoff, R.L., and Goldberg, E.: M-mode and two-dimensional echocardiographic findings in pulmonic valve endocarditis. Am. Heart J., *107*:391, 1984.

524. DePace, N.L., Iskandrian, A.S., Morganroth, J., Ross, J., Mattleman, S., and Nestico, P.F.: Infective endocarditis involving a presumably normal pulmonic valve. Am. J. Cardiol., *53*:385, 1984.

525. Suwa, M., Shimizu, G., Doi, Y., Kino, M., Hirota, Y., Kubo, S., Kawamura, K., Nishimoto, T., Maeda, M., Asada, K., Sasaki, S., and Takeuchi, A.: Two-dimensional echocardiography of ruptured pulmonic valve with infective endocarditis. Am. Heart J., *107*:1027, 1984.

526. Karalis, D.G., Bansal, R.C., Hauck, A.J., Ross, Jr., J.J., Applegate, P.M., Jutzy, K.R., Mintz, G.S., and Chandrasekaran, K.: Transesophageal echocardiographic recognition of subaortic complications in aortic valve endocarditis. Circulation, *86*:353, 1992.

527. Kan, M-N., Chan, Y-T., and Lee, A. Y-S.: Comparison of transesophageal to transthoracic color Doppler echocardiography in the identification of intracardiac mycotic aneurysm in infective endocarditis. Echocardiography, *8*:643, 1991.

528. Sheppard, R.C., Chandrasekaran, K., Ross, J., and Mintz, G.S.: An acquired interatrial fistula secondary to para-aortic abscess documented by transesophageal echocardiography. J. Am. Soc. Echocardiogr., *4*:271, 1991.

529. Giannoccaro, P., Ascah, K.J., Sochowski, R.A., Chan, K-L., and Ruddy, T.D.: Spontaneous drainage of paravalvular abscess diagnosed by transesophageal echocardiography. J. Am. Soc. Echocardiogr., *4*:397, 1991.

530. Karalis, D.G., Chandrasekaran, K., Wahl, J.M., Ross, J., and Mintz, G.S.: Transesophageal echocardiographic recognition of mitral valve abnormalities associated with aortic valve endocarditis. Am. Heart J., *119*:1209, 1990.

530a.Shenoy, M.M., and Chandrasekaran, K.: Mitral and tricuspid annular endocarditis. Diagnosis by transesophageal echocardiography. Chest, *101*:1732, 1992.

531. Chow, W.H., Leung, W.H., Tai, Y.T., Lee, W.T., and Cheung, K.L.: Echocardiographic diagnosis of an aortic root abscess after Mycobacterium fortuitum prosthetic valve endocarditis. Clin. Cardiol., *14*:273, 1991.

532. Byrd, B.F., Shelton, M.E., Wilson, H., and Schillig, S.: Infective perivalvular abscess of the aortic ring: Echocardiographic features and clinical course. Am. J. Cardiol., *66*:102, 1990.

533. Nomeir, A-M., Downes, T.R., and Cordell, A.R.: Perforation of the anterior mitral leaflet caused by aortic valve endocarditis: Diagnosis by two-dimensional transesophageal echocardiography and color flow Doppler. J. Am. Soc. Echocardiogr., *5*:195, 1992.

534. Cziner, D.G., Rosenzweig, B.P., Katz, E.S., Keller, A.M., Daniel, W.G., and Kronzon, I.: Transesophageal versus transthoracic echocardiography for diagnosing mitral valve perforation. Am. J. Cardiol., *69*:1495, 1992.

535. DeLucia, F., Cunto, G.A., DeLucia, V., Parente, A., Bellizzi, G., Coppola, V., and Mottola, G.: Diagnosis of mitral valve perforation by color Doppler echocardiography. Cardiovasc. Imag., *2*:281, 1990.

536. Miyatake, K., Yamamoto, K., Park, Y-D., Izumi, S., Yamagishi, M., Sakakibara, H., and Nimura, Y.: Diagnosis of mitral valve perforation by real-time two-dimensional Doppler flow imaging technique. Am. J. Coll. Cardiol., *8*:1235, 1986.

537. Jain, S.P., Mahan, III, E.F., Nanda, N.C., Barold, S.S., and Fan, P.: Mitral valve perforation secondary to infec-

tive endocarditis: Diagnosis by Doppler color flow mapping. Echocardiography, *6*:527, 1989.

538. Vilacosta, I., San Roman, J.A.S., and Roca, V.: Eustachian valve endocarditis. Br. Heart J., *64*:340, 1990.

539. Schwinger, M.E., Tunick, P.A., Freedberg, R.S., and Kronzon, I.: Vegetations on endocardial surfaces struck by regurgitant jets: Diagnosis by transesophageal echocardiography. Am. Heart J., *119*:1212, 1990.

540. Kim, J.H., Wiseman, A., Kisslo, J., and Durack, D.T.: Echocardiographic detection and clinical significance of left atrial vegetations in active infective endocarditis. Am. J. Cardiol., *64*:950, 1989.

541. Herzog, C.A., Carson, P., Michaud, L., and Asinger, R.W.: Two-dimensional echocardiographic imaging of left ventricular mural vegetations. Am. Heart J., *115*:684, 1988.

542. Lam, D., Emilson, B., and Rapaport, E.: Four-valve endocarditis with associated right ventricular mural vegetations. Am. Heart J., *115*:189, 1988.

543. Zijlstra, F., Fioretti, P., and Roelandt, J.R.T.C.: Echocardiographic demonstration of free wall vegetative endocarditis complicated by a pulmonary embolism in a patient with ventricular septal defect. Br. Heart J., *55*:497, 1986.

543a.Shenoy, M.M., Kalakota, M., Uddin, M., and Siegel, S.: Left ventricular mural bacterial endocarditis: Diagnosis by transesophageal echocardiography. Can. J. Cardiol., *8*:57, 1992.

543b.Sochowski, R.A. and Chan, K-L.: Implication of negative results on a monoplane transesophageal echocardiographic study in patients with suspected infective endocarditis. J. Am. Coll. Cardiol., *21*:216, 1993.

544. Tak, T., Rahimtoola, S.H., Kumar, A., Gamage, N., and Chandraratna, P.A.N.: Value of digital image processing of two-dimensional echocardiograms in differentiating active from chronic vegetations of infective endocarditis. Circulation, *78*:116, 1988.

545. Trehan, N., Goldfarb, A., Gindea, A.J., and Kronzon, I.: Echocardiographic diagnosis of atrioventricular septal perforation caused by an aortic valve vegetation. J. Am. Soc. Echocardiogr., *1*:150, 1988.

546. Bansal, R.C., Graham, B.M., Jutzy, K.R., Shakudo, M., and Shah, P.M.: Left ventricular outflow tract to left atrial communication secondary to rupture of mitral-aortic intervalvular fibrosa in infective endocarditis: Diagnosis by transesophageal echocardiography and color flow imaging. J. Am. Coll. Cardiol., *15*:499, 1990.

547. Pennestri, F., Favuzzi, A., Laurenzi, F., Mazzari, M., and Loperfido, F.: Dissection of the anterior mitral leaflet causing mitral regurgitation in aortic valve endocarditis. Am. Heart J., *113*:121, 1987.

547a.Khandheria, B.K.: Suspected bacterial endocarditis: To TEE or not to TEE. J. Am. Coll. Cardiol., *21*:222, 1993.

548. Alam, M., Rosman, H.S., and Sun, I.: Transesophageal echocardiographic evaluation of St. Jude Medical and bioprosthetic valve endocarditis. Am. Heart J., *123*:236, 1992.

549. Culver, D.L., Cacchione, J., Stern, D., Shapiro, J.R., and Reisner, S.A.: Diagnosis of infective endocarditis on a Starr-Edwards prosthesis by transesophageal echocardiography. Am. Heart J., *119*:972, 1990.

550. Martin, R.P., Meltzer, R.S., Chia, B.L., Stinson, E.B., Rakowski, H., and Popp, R.L.: Clinical utility of two-dimensional echocardiography in infective endocarditis. Am. J. Cardiol., *46*:379, 1980.

551. Hickey, A.J., Wolfers, J., and Wilcken, D.E.L.: Reliability and clinical relevance of detection of vegetations by

echocardiography in bacterial endocarditis. Br. Heart J., *46*:624, 1981.

552. Wann, L.S., Dillon, J.C., Weyman, A.E., and Feigenbaum, H.: Echocardiography in bacterial endocarditis. N. Engl. J. Med., *295*:135, 1976.

553. Thompson, K.R., Nanda, N.C., and Gramiak, R.: The reliability of echocardiography in the diagnosis of infective endocarditis. Radiology, *125*:373, 1977.

554. Davis, R.S., Strom, J.A., Frishman, W., Becker, R., Matsumoto, M., LeJemtel, T.H., Sonnenblick, E.H., and Frater, R.W.M.: The demonstration of vegetations by echocardiography in bacterial endocarditis. An indication for early surgical intervention. Am. J. Med., *69*:57, 1980.

555. Come, P.C., Isaacs, R.E., and Riley, M.F.: Diagnostic accuracy of M-mode echocardiography in active infective endocarditis and prognostic implications of ultrasound-detectable vegetations. Am. Heart J., *103*:839, 1982.

556. Roudaut, R., Billes, M.A., Ginestes, J., Randazzo, W., Videau, P., Dallocchio, M., and Bricaud, H.: Outcome of echocardiographic vegetations in bacterial endocarditis during and after anti-infective therapy. Arch. Mal. Coeur, *75*:1061, 1982.

557. Sheikh, M.U., Covarrubias, E.A., Ali, N., Lee, W.R., Sheikh, N.M., and Roberts, W.C.: M-mode echocardiographic observations during and after healing of active bacterial endocarditis limited to the mitral valve. Am. Heart J., *101*:37, 1981.

558. Kavey, R.E., Frank, D.M., Byrum, C.J., Blackman, M.S., Sandheimer, H.M., and Bove, E.L.: Two-dimensional echocardiographic assessment of infective endocarditis in children. Am. J. Dis. Child., *137*:851, 1983.

559. Kisslo, J., Guadalajara, J.F., Stewart, J.A., and Stack, R.S.: Echocardiography in infective endocarditis. Herz, *8*:271, 1983.

560. Buda, A.J., MacDonald, I.L., David, T.E., and Kerwin, A.J.: Rapidly progressive vegetative endocarditis. Acta Cardiol., *37*:85, 1982.

561. Sanfilippo, A.J., Picard, M.H., Newell, J.B., Rosas, E., Davidoff, R., Thomas, J.D., and Weyman, A.E.: Echocardiographic assessment of patients with infectious endocarditis. Prediction of risk for complications. J. Am. Coll. Cardiol., *18*:1191, 1991.

562. Aragam, J.R., Keroack, M.A., and Kemper, A.J.: Doppler echocardiographic diagnosis of aortopulmonary fistula following aortic valve replacement for endocarditis. Am. Heart J., *117*:1392, 1989.

563. Massey, W.M., Samdarshi, T.E., Nanda, N.C., Sanyal, R.S., Pinheiro, L., Jain, H., and Kirklin, J.K.L.: Serial documentation of changes in a mitral valve vegetation progressing to abscess rupture and fistula formation by transesophageal echocardiography. Am. Heart J., *124*:241, 1992.

564. Tunick, P.A., Lefkow, P., and Kronzon, I.: Aorta to right atrium fistula caused by endocarditis: Diagnosis by color Doppler echocardiography. J. Am. Soc. Echocardiogr., *2*:53, 1989.

565. Rohmann, S., Erbel, R., Darius, H., Gorge, G., Markowski, T., Zotz, R., Mohr-Kahaly, S., Nixdorff, U., Drexler, M., and Meyer, J.: Prediction of rapid versus prolonged healing of infective endocarditis by monitoring vegetation size. J. Am. Soc. Echocardiogr., *4*:465, 1991.

566. Mugge, A., Daniel, W.G., Frank, G., and Lichtlen, P.R.: Echocardiography in infective endocarditis: Reassessment of prognostic implications of vegetation size determined by the transthoracic and the transesophageal approach. J. Am. Coll. Cardiol., *14*:631, 1989.

567. Jaffe, W.M., Morgan, D.E., Pearlman, A.S., and Otto, C.M.: Infective endocarditis, 1983–1988: Echocardiographic findings and factors influencing morbidity and mortality. J. Am. Coll. Cardiol., *15*:1227, 1990.

568. Arvan, S., Cagin, N., Levitt, B., and Kleid, J.J.: Echocardiographic findings in a patient with Candida endocarditis of the aortic valve. Chest, *70*:300, 1976.

569. Gomes, J.A., Calderon, J., Lajam, F., et al.: Echocardiographic detection of fungal vegetations in Candida parasilopsis endocarditis. Am. J. Med., *61*:273, 1976.

570. Pasternak, R.C., Cannom, D.S., and Cohen, L.S.: Echocardiographic diagnosis of large fungal verruca attached to mitral valve. Br. Heart J., *38*:1209, 1976.

571. Sarma, R., Prakash, R., Kaushik, V.S., Oparah, S.S., and Mandal, A.: Reliability of two-dimensional echocardiography in diagnosing fungal endocarditis. Clin. Cardiol., *6*:37, 1983.

572. Vishniavsky, N., Safar, K.B., and Markowitz, S.M.: Aspergillus fumigatus endocarditis on a normal heart valve. South. Med. J., *76*:506, 1983.

573. Stopfkuchen, H., Benzing, F., Jungst, B.K., and Meyer, W.: Echocardiographic diagnosis of Candida endocarditis of the tricuspid valve and of the right atrium in a young infant. Pediatr. Cardiol., *4*:49, 1983.

574. Sarma, R., Prakash, R., Kaushik, V.S., Oparah, S.S., and Mandal, A.: Reliability of two-dimensional echocardiography in diagnosing fungal endocarditis. Clin. Cardiol., *6*:37, 1983.

575. Heibig, J., Beall, A.C., Myers, R., Harder, E., and Feteih, N.: Brucella aortic endocarditis corrected by prosthetic valve replacement. Am. Heart J., *106*:594, 1983.

576. Rosoff, M.H., Cohen, M.V., and Jacquette, G.: Pulmonary valve gonococcal endocarditis. A forgotten disease. Br. Heart J., *50*:290, 1983.

577. Hopkins, C.B., Postic, B., and Killam, H.: Gonococcal endocarditis: Cross-sectional echocardiographic diagnosis of aortic ring abscess. JCU, *10*:279, 1982.

578. Arvan, S. and Delaverdac, C.: Early echocardiographic changes in a patient with gonococcal endocarditis. Am. Heart J., *101*:112, 1981.

579. Estevez, C.M. and Corya, B.C.: Serial echocardiographic abnormalities in nonbacterial thrombotic endocarditis of the mitral valve. Chest, *69*:801, 1976.

580. Lopez, J.A., Fishbein, M.C., and Siegel, R.J.: Echocardiographic features of nonbacterial thrombotic endocarditis. Am. J. Cardiol., *59*:478, 1987.

581. Habbab, M.A., A-Zaibag, M.A., Al-Hilali, A.M., and Al-Fagih, M.R.: Unusual presentation and echocardiographic features of surgically proven nonbacterial thrombotic endocarditis. Am. Heart J., *119*:404, 1990.

581a. Blanchard, D.G., Ross, R.S., and Dittrich, H.C.: Nonbacterial thrombotic endocarditis. Assessment by transesophageal echocardiography. Chest, *102*:954, 1992.

582. Appelbe, A.F., Olson, D., Mixon, R., Craver, J.M., and Martin, R.P.: Libman-Sacks endocarditis mimicking intracardiac tumor. Am. J. Cardiol., *68*:817, 1991.

583. Roldan, C.A., Shively, B.K., Lau, C.C., Furule, F.T., Smith, E.A., and Crawford, M.H.: Systemic Lupus Erythematosus valve disease by transesophageal echocardiography and the role of antiphospholipid antibodies. J. Am. Coll. Cardiol., *20*:1127, 1992.

584. Weyman, A.E., Rankin, R., and King, H.: Loeffler's endocarditis presenting as mitral and tricuspid stenosis. Am. J. Cardiol., *40*:438, 1977.

585. Rodger, J.C., Irvine, K.G., and Lerksi, R.A.: Echocardiography in Loeffler's endocarditis. Br. Heart J., *46*:110, 1981.

586. Fitchett, D.H. and Oakley, C.M.: Granulomatous mitral valve obstruction. Br. Heart J., *38*:112, 1976.

587. Kinney, E., Reeves, W., and Zellis, R.: The echocardiogram in scleroderma endocarditis of the mitral valve. Arch. Intern. Med., *139*:1179, 1979.

588. Dashkoff, N., Karacuschansky, M., Come, P.C., and Fortuin, N.J.: Echocardiographic features of mitral annulus calcification. Am. Heart J., *94*:585, 1977.

589. Schott, C.R., Kotler, M.N., Parry, W.R., and Segal, B.L.: Mitral annular calcification: Clinical and echocardiographic correlations. Arch. Intern. Med., *137*:1143, 1977.

590. Howard, P.F., Cabizuca, S.V., Desser, K.B., and Benchimol, A.: The echocardiographic diagnosis of calcified mitral annulus. Am. J. Med., *273*:267, 1977.

591. Curati, W.L., Petitclerc, R., and Winsberg, F.: Ultrasonic features of mitral annulus calcification: A report of 21 cases. Radiology, *122*:215, 1977.

592. Meltzer, R.S., Martin, R.P., Robbins, B.S., and Popp, R.L.: Mitral annular calcification: Clinical and echocardiographic features. Acta Cardiol., *35*:189, 1980.

593. Kronzon, I., Mitchell, J., Shapiro, J., Winer, H.E., and Newman, P.: Two-dimensional echocardiography in mitral annulus calcification. Am. J. Roentgenol., *134*:355, 1980.

594. D'Cruz, I., Panetta, F., Cohen, H., and Glick, G.: Submitral calcification or sclerosis in elderly patients: M-mode and two-dimensional echocardiography in "mitral annulus calcification." Am. J. Cardiol., *44*:31, 1979.

595. Gabor, G.E., Mohr, B.D., Goel, P.C., and Cohen, B.: Echocardiographic and clinical spectrum of mitral annular calcification. Am. J. Cardiol., *38*:836, 1976.

596. D'Cruz, I.A., Cohen, H.C., Prabhu, R., Bisla, V., and Glick, G.: Clinical manifestations of mitral annulus calcification, with emphasis on its echocardiographic features. Am. Heart J., *94*:367, 1977.

597. Ramirez, J. and Flowers, N.C.: Severe mitral stenosis secondary to massive calcification of the mitral annulus with unusual echocardiographic manifestations. Clin. Cardiol., *3*:284, 1980.

598. Nestico, R.F., DePace, N.L., Morganroth, J., Kotler, M.N., and Ross, J.: Mitral annular calcification: Clinical, pathophysiologic, and echocardiographic review. Am. Heart J., *107*:989, 1984.

599. Tominga, S., Honda, M., Yanagisawa, N., Noike, H., Nakajima, H., Yamuguchi, T., Watanabe, T., Higuchi, Y., Wada, T., and Matsuyama, S.: Mitral annular calcifications in patients with hypertrophic obstructive cardiomyopathy. An echocardiographic study. J. Cardiogr., *12*:875, 1982.

600. Lindvall, K. and Herrlin, B.: Mitral annulus calcification, systolic anterior motion of the anterior mitral leaflet and outflow obstruction in two patients without hypertrophic cardiomyopathy. An echocardiographic report. Acta Med. Scand., *209*:513, 1981.

601. Labovitz, A.J., Nelson, J.G., Windhorst, D.M., Kennedy, H.L., and Williams, G.A.: Frequency of mitral valve dysfunction from mitral annular calcium as detected by Doppler echocardiography. Am. J. Cardiol., *55*:133, 1985.

602. Takamoto, T. and Popp, R.L.: Conduction disturbances related to the site and severity of mitral annular calcification: A two-dimensional echocardiographic and electrocardiographic correlative study. Am. J. Cardiol., *51*:1644, 1983.

603. Nair, C.K., Aronow, W.S., Sketch, M.H., Mohiuddin, S.M., Pagano, T., Esterbrooks, D.J., and Hee, T.T.: Clinical and echocardiographic characteristics of patients with mitral annular calcification. Am. J. Cardiol., *51*:992, 1983.

604. Fulkerson, P.K., Beaver, B.M., Auseon, J.C., and Graber, H.L.: Calcification of the mitral annulus: Etiology, clinical associations, complications, and therapy. Am. J. Med., *66*:967, 1979.

605. Mellino, M., Salcedo, E.E., Lever, H.M., Vasudevan, G., and Kramer, J.R.: Echographic-quantified severity of mitral annulus calcification: Prognostic correlation to related hemodynamic, valvular, rhythm and conduction abnormalities. Am. Heart J., *103*:222, 1982.

606. DePace, N.L., Rohrer, A.H., Kotler, M.N., Brezin, J.H., and Parry, W.R.: Rapidly progressing, massive mitral annular calcification. Occurrence in a patient with chronic renal failure. Arch. Intern. Med., *141*:1663, 1981.

607. Kronzon, I., Winer, H.E., and Cohen, M.L.: Sterile, caseous mitral annular abscess. J. Am. Coll. Cardiol., *2*:186, 1983.

# 7

# Congenital Heart Disease

## THOMAS RYAN

"The diagnosis of congenital heart disease represents the epitome of applied clinical logic. When correct inferences are drawn from accurate observations, diagnoses are made with gratifying frequency."[1]

Joseph K. Perloff, M.D.

Congenital heart diseases are broadly defined as those cardiac anomalies that are present at birth. By their very nature, such defects have their origin in embryonic development. A number of factors are capable of adversely affecting the sequence of events that constitute cardiac morphogenesis.[2] An interaction between genetic and environmental forces probably accounts for most congenital lesions.[3] Regardless of the cause, the net result of most of these perturbations in a structural anomaly that reflects the location and timing of the causative event. Such defects may become manifest in utero, soon after birth, later in life, or not at all.

In the United States, there are currently more than 500,000 patients over the age of 21 years with congenital heart disease. Each year, approximately 25,000 infants are born with a cardiac malformation. It is now estimated that over 85% of these patients will reach adulthood, adding further to this growing population.[4,5] A variety of factors account for these observations. Improvements in the medical and surgical management of congenital heart disease have had a profound effect on survival patterns. Relatively few lesions remain inaccessible to the cardiac surgeon, and the number of postoperative patients has grown accordingly.[6] The variety and complexity of surgical options has also increased. Unfortunately, however, surgical "cure" remains an elusive goal and most patients emerge from surgery with a wide range of residua and sequelae that necessitate ongoing medical attention. We can conclude, then, that the number of adults with congenital heart lesions is growing, that these patients will continue to require specialized medical care, and that their diagnostic and functional assessment will become increasingly challenging. The number of physicians for whom a basic understanding of these diseases is mandatory must grow in parallel.[7-9]

Most congenital cardiac lesions constitute gross structural abnormalities with a spectrum of associated hemodynamic derangements. It is not surprising then that the various echocardiographic techniques are ideally suited to the study of patients with congenital heart disease. Perhaps nowhere in cardiology have these methods played a more vital role in diagnosis and management. Historically, the emergence of two-dimensional echocardiography must be viewed as a milestone in the diagnostic approach to congenital heart disease.[10,11] The tomographic nature of the technique and the unlimited number of imaging planes permit the anatomy and relationships of the cardiac structures to be defined, even in the presence of complex congenital malformations. For the noninvasive assessment of cardiac function, two-dimensional echocardiography rapidly assumed a preeminent position as the most accurate and widely applied method.[12] Later, the development of Doppler[13] and color flow imaging[14,15] contributed further to the role of ultrasound in this field. The combination of these techniques is sufficient for the diagnosis of most congenital defects and has been used effectively as a screening tool for young patients in whom congenital heart disease is suspected.[11,16] Most recently, transesophageal echocardiography has provided a novel approach to complex lesions and may be particularly beneficial to elucidate postoperative anatomy.[17-21,21a]

The echocardiographic approach to patients with congenital heart lesions differs substantially from that used to evaluate other forms of cardiac disease.[22] Imaging in children has both advantages and disadvantages compared to adults. The smaller patient size permits the use of higher frequency transducers, thereby enhancing image quality. The presence of less heavily calcified bone and the absence of hyperinflated lungs in most children increase the available acoustic windows and generally contribute to improved image quality and higher resolution. Unfortunately, the smaller patient size also creates practical problems for image acquisition. Children are more likely to be uncooperative and may have other malformations (such as a chest deformity) that complicate imaging.

Adults with congenital heart disease present an entirely different array of challenges to the echocardiographer.[7] The decision to intervene in these patients frequently hinges on the adequacy of previous interventions and the presence and severity of pulmonary vascular disease. In patients who have undergone surgery, an accurate assessment may be difficult. Those with palliative shunts or extracardiac conduits require an individualized approach and special views. When details of the clinical history are unavailable, the echocardiographer is often called on to determine which surgical procedures have been performed. The options for further intervention often depend on the echocardiographic results. As the patient with congenital heart disease ages, the superimposition of other medical conditions (such as hypertension or coronary disease) further complicates his or her evaluation and management.

Both image acquisition and interpretation can be challenging and time consuming. The diversity and complexity of congenital cardiac malformations obviate even the most basic assumptions regarding chamber orientation and great vessel relationships. These problems are magnified in the patient who has undergone a surgical procedure previously. Therefore, the initial evaluation of the patient with suspected congenital heart disease mandates a thorough and systematic echocardiographic approach, often using additional views beyond those obtained during the standard examination. Frequently, the individual responsible for interpretation of the study must be intimately involved in the performance of the examination.

This chapter focuses on the role of echocardiography in the adolescent and adult with congenital heart disease. It is not intended as an exhaustive description of all forms of congenital heart disease. Lesions that are seen more commonly in adult patients are emphasized, whereas those considered less relevant are covered only superficially. Certain conditions that are not seen in adults, such as hypoplastic left heart syndrome, are discussed briefly, primarily because their prompt recognition is so critical to proper management. Finally, the evaluation of the postoperative patient is covered in some detail.

## THE ECHOCARDIOGRAPHIC EXAMINATION: A SEGMENTAL APPROACH TO ANATOMY

The initial echocardiographic examination of the patient with suspected congenital heart disease requires a sequential and systematic approach to cardiac anatomy. Such a method is necessary to detect cardiac malpositions and to diagnose complex congenital heart disease.[23–27] The first step in this sequential approach is to determine atrial situs and to assess the venous inflow patterns to the atria. Then, atrioventricular connections are defined and ventricular morphology and position are determined. Finally, ventriculoarterial relationships are evaluated. In most cases, this approach permits the identification of even the most complex forms of congenital heart disease (Table 7–1).

**Table 7–1**
A Segmental Approach to Cardiac Situs and Malpositions

Atrial situs
  Visceral situs (and visceroatrial concordance)
  Atrial morphology (situs solitus or inversus)
  Venous inflow patterns
Ventricular localization
  Ventricular morphology (D-loop or L-loop)
  Atrioventricular concordance (AV valve morphology)
  Base-to-apex axis (levocardia or dextrocardia)
Great artery connections
  Identification of the great arteries
  Ventriculoarterial concordance or transposition
  Spatial relationship between the great arteries and ventricular septum

### Cardiac Situs

Determination of atrial situs is best accomplished by using the subcostal views.[28–30] In atrial situs solitus, the normal situation, the morphologic right atrium is to the right and the morphologic left atrium is to the left. In situs inversus, the opposite occurs, creating a mirror image effect. Atrial and visceral situs are almost always concordant. Thus, a right-sided liver and left-sided stomach are usually associated with atrial situs solitus. In the rare cases when atrial and abdominal situs are discordant, however, the likelihood of complex congenital lesions is high.[29]

Using two-dimensional echocardiography, the location and morphology of the atria can be determined. The morphologic right atrium always contains the eustachian valve, and its appendage is shorter and broader than that of the left atrium. The left atrium lacks the eustachian valve and has a more rounded shape than the right atrium. The left atrial appendage is long and thin and has a more narrow atrial junction compared to that of the right. A recent study has shown that this distinction is readily apparent using transesophageal echocardiography.[31]

Although venous inflow does not define atrial morphology, the patterns of systemic and pulmonary venous return are helpful in determining situs. This spatial relationship is best evaluated using a transverse imaging plane through the upper abdomen. Normally, the abdominal aorta lies to the left and the inferior vena cava lies to the right of the spine. Compared to the vena cava, the aorta appears larger, more rounded, and more pulsatile (Fig. 7–1). When in doubt, color flow imaging can be used to differentiate between the two vessels. Color encoding of flow is more likely in the aorta because of the higher velocity. The opposite spatial relationship is characteristic of situs inversus. By tracing the course of the inferior vena cava and hepatic veins in the subcostal long-axis view, the right atrium generally can be identified in its usual position anterior and to the right of the left atrium (Fig. 7–2). Interruption of the inferior vena cava, an uncommon anomaly often associated with polysplenia, can be detected from this view.

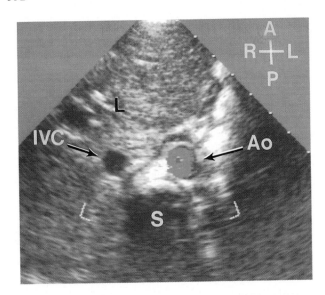

**Fig. 7–1.** Subcostal short-axis view of the subject with situs solitus. The liver (L) and inferior vena cava (IVC) are on the patient's right and the aorta (Ao) is to the patient's left. With the use of color flow imaging, flow within the aorta is detected. S = spine; A = anterior; P = posterior; R = right; L = left.

The pulmonary venous connections to the left atrium may be visualized using the four-chamber view and suprasternal window. Color Doppler imaging is particularly helpful in identifying the pulmonary veins as they enter the left atrium (Fig. 7–3). In adults, it is usually impossible to record the insertion of all four pulmonary veins using transthoracic echocardiography. With transesophageal echocardiography, however, the pulmonary venous drainage pattern can be defined more precisely. Because of the possibility of anomalous pulmonary ve-

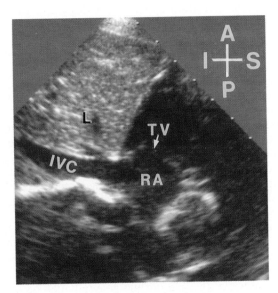

**Fig. 7–2.** Subcostal long-axis view of a normal subject. The inferior vena cava (IVC) can be seen entering the right atrium (RA). L = liver; TV = tricuspid valve; A = anterior; I = inferior; S = superior, P = posterior.

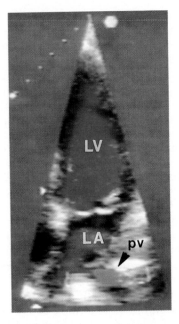

**Fig. 7–3.** Apical four-chamber view from a patient with mitral valve prolapse. Using color flow imaging, the entrance of a pulmonary vein (pv) into the left atrium (LA) is shown. LV = left ventricle.

nous drainage, the relationship between the pulmonary veins and the left atrium is not constant and their connections should not be used to define atrial morphology.

### Ventricular Morphology

Once visceroatrial situs and venous connections are established, the orientation and morphology of the ventricles should be determined. During normal embryogenesis, the straight heart tube folds to the right (a D-loop) and then pivots to occupy a position within the left side of the chest. This positioning results in the right ventricle developing anteriorly and to the right of the left ventricle. The base-to-apex axis points leftward and most of the cardiac mass lies within the left side of the chest. If the initial fold in the heart tube is leftward, an L-loop develops, with the morphologic right ventricle to the left of the morphologic left ventricle. Thus, atrioventricular discordance occurs in the presence of situs solitus and an L-loop or situs inversus and a D-loop.

Ventricular morphology is readily assessed with two-dimensional echocardiography.[32–34] Features that are useful in distinguishing the right and left ventricles are listed in Table 7–2. The presence of muscle bundles, particularly the moderator band, gives the right ventricle a trabeculated endocardial surface (Fig. 7–4). In contrast, the left ventricle is characterized by a smooth endocardial surface. This distinction is apparent using echocardiography and serves as one of the more reliable characteristics when determining ventricular morphology. The structure and position of the atrioventricular valves are additional echocardiographic features that are useful in distinguishing the right and left ventricles. If two ventricles are present, the atrioventricular valves

**Table 7–2**
Echocardiographic Characteristics of Right and
Left Ventricles

| Right Ventricle | Left Ventricle |
| --- | --- |
| Trabeculated endocardial surface | Smooth endocardial surface |
| Chordae insert into ventricular septum | Two papillary muscles |
| Infundibular muscle band | Ellipsoidal geometry |
| Moderator band | Two leaflet, mitral atrioventricular valve with relatively basal insertion |
| Triangular cavity shape | |
| Tricuspid atrioventricular valve with relatively apical insertion | |

associate with the corresponding ventricle and identification of the mitral and tricuspid valves defines the respective chambers. The tricuspid valve is more apically displaced, has three leaflets (and three papillary muscles), and has chordal insertions into the septum. The mitral valve has a more basal septal attachment and has two leaflets, which insert into two papillary muscles, but not the septum. All of these features can be assessed with echocardiography. The four-chamber view allows the echocardiographer to determine ventricular morphology and the relative positions of the atrioventricular valves. The short-axis views permit definition of the papillary muscles and chordal insertions. The relative positions of the atrioventricular valves and the presence of absence of chordal insertions into the septum are the

most helpful echocardiographic features when attempting to determine ventricular identity.

### Great Artery Connections

The final step in the segmental approach to cardiac anatomy involves identification of the great arteries and their respective connections. In the normal heart with concordant connections, the morphologic left ventricle gives rise to the aorta and the pulmonary artery serves as the outlet of the right ventricle. In the presence of normal ventricular orientation, this arrangement results in an anterior and leftward pulmonary artery and a posterior and rightward aorta with a left-sided aortic arch and descending aorta. The great arteries originate in orthogonal planes creating a "sausage and circle" appearance on short-axis imaging, which results from the rotation during development of the right ventricular outflow tract and pulmonary artery (the "sausage") around the ascending aorta (the "circle"). Discordant ventriculoarterial connections, or transposition, occur when the great arteries arise from the opposite ventricle (Fig. 7–5). Two forms of transposition exist. In D-transposition, ventricular relationship is normal, with the morphologic right ventricle to the right of the morphologic left ventricle. In L-transposition, atrioventricular discordance is present (because of formation of an L-loop during embryogenesis) so that the morphologic right ventricle lies to the left of the morphologic left ventricle. Other forms of abnormal great artery connections include double-outlet ventricle and truncus arteriosus.

Two-dimensional echocardiography permits accurate identification of the great arteries, their origins and relationship.[33,35] The short-axis view at the base of the heart is most helpful when assessing these features. In the normal heart, the pulmonary valve lies slightly anterior and to the left of the aortic valve (Fig. 7–5). The pulmonary artery then courses posteriorly and bifurcates, with the right pulmonary artery passing immediately below

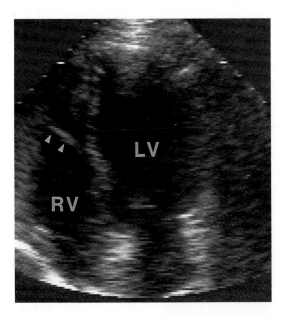

**Fig. 7–4.** Apical four-chamber view from a normal subject with a prominent moderator band (*arrowheads*), which represents a normal structure that is occasionally confused with thrombus or tumor. LV = left ventricle; RV = right ventricle.

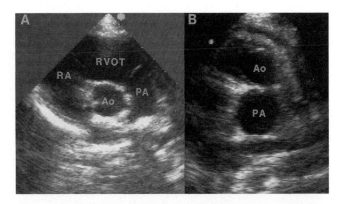

**Fig. 7–5.** Parasternal short-axis echocardiograms from a normal subject (*A*) and a patient with D-transposition of the great arteries (*B*). In the normal subject, the aorta (Ao) is posterior and the right ventricular outflow tract (RVOT) and pulmonary artery (PA) appear to wrap around the aorta. With transposition, the aorta is anterior and the two great vessels arise in parallel. RA = right atrium.

the aortic arch. These findings are best appreciated in the parasternal long- and short-axis and subcostal views. The proximal aorta is optimally recorded from the parasternal window and the suprasternal notch (Fig. 7–6). To identify the great arteries, the course of the vessel and the presence or absence of a bifurcation are the most reliable echocardiographic signs. The presence of a right aortic arch can also be detected, using a combination of suprasternal and subcostal views,[36,37] by assessing from the suprasternal short-axis view the course of the brachiocephalic vessels as they leave the arch.

A variety of complex abnormalities of cardiac situs and malpositions exist, some of which fail to adhere to the generalizations and simplifications just presented. The echocardiographic evaluation of these disorders, however, is beyond the scope of this chapter.[22,27]

## ABNORMALITIES OF RIGHT VENTRICULAR INFLOW

### Right Atrium

The right atrium can be evaluated from several echocardiographic windows. To assess right atrial size, anatomy, and venous connections, the apical and subcostal four-chamber views and the medially angulated parasternal long-axis view are most helpful. Two normal structures within the right atrium, the eustachian valve and the Chiari network, may be recorded. Recognition of these embryologic remnants is important for two reasons. First, they are useful landmarks by which to define atrial morphology. The eustachian valve is especially helpful in identifying the morphologic right atrium. Secondly, they occasionally are confused with pathologic structures, such as thrombus, vegetation, or tumor (see Chapter 11).

The eustachian valve (which functions to divert incoming inferior vena cava blood in utero) appears as a rigid elongated structure in the inferior portion of the right atrium (Fig. 7–7). It can be recorded in multiple views and sometimes is prominent. A Chiari network is a perforated, filamentous remnant of the valve to the coronary sinus. Occasionally, it is seen as a delicate, highly mobile, serpentine structure within the right atrial cavity (Figs. 7–7 and 7–8). With two-dimensional echocardiography, its undulations appear random and unrelated to valve motion.

### Right Ventricular Inflow

The right ventricular inflow tract and tricuspid valve are best visualized using the apical and subcostal four-chamber views, the short-axis view at the base, and the medially angulated parasternal long-axis view. The most important congenital pathologic entities involving the tricuspid valve are Ebstein's anomaly[38–44] and tricuspid atresia (discussed subsequently). Ebstein's anomaly consists of apical displacement of the septal and posterior (and sometimes the anterior) leaflets of the tricuspid valve into the right ventricle. Typically, the leaflets are elongated and redundant with abnormal chordal attachments. This results in "atrialization" of the basal portion of the right ventricle as the functional orifice is displaced apically relative to the anatomic annulus. Ebstein's anomaly is a spectrum of abnormalities, depending on the extent of downward displacement of the valve, the distal attachments of the leaflets, the size and function of the remaining right ventricle, the degree of tricuspid regurgitation, and the presence of right ventricular outflow tract obstruction (usually from the redundant anterior tricuspid valve leaflet).[45]

The best echocardiographic view for the evaluation of Ebstein's anomaly is the four-chamber view. The characteristic features identified in this plane are shown schematically in Figure 7–9. Of principal importance is the accurate recording of the level of insertion of the septal leaflet of the tricuspid valve relative to the annu-

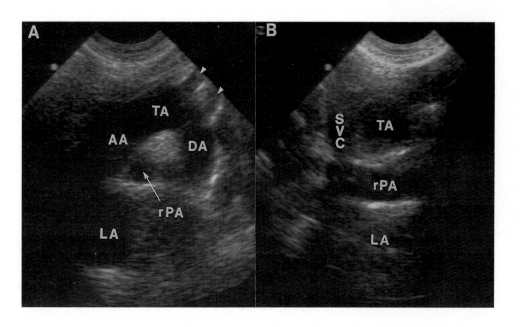

Fig. 7–6. Suprasternal long-axis (*A*) and short-axis (*B*) views from a normal subject. The right pulmonary artery (rPA) passes below the transverse aorta (TA) and above the left atrium (LA). The superior vena cava (SVC) is sometimes visualized to the right of the aortic arch. The small arrowheads indicate the left carotid and subclavian arteries. AA = ascending aorta; DA = descending aorta.

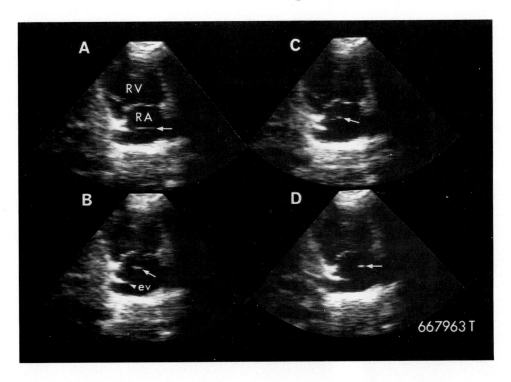

**Fig. 7–7.** Four sequential views of the right ventricular inflow tract demonstrating a Chiari network (*arrow*). In real time, random motion of the structure was evident. In *B*, the eustachian valve (ev) is also demonstrated. RA = right atrium; RV = right ventricle.

lus. Apical displacement of this insertion site is optimally assessed in this view and is the key to diagnosis (Figs. 7–10 and 7–11).[40,43,46] Because the tricuspid valve is normally positioned more apically than the mitral valve, abnormal apical displacement is relative and some investigators have suggested measuring the distance between insertion sites of the two atrioventricular valves. When normalized for body surface area, a distance of greater than 8 mm/$M^2$ is indicative of Ebstein's anomaly.[40] Other investigators have advocated a maximum displacement of more than 20 mm as the diagnostic criterion in adults.[46]

The four-chamber and medially angulated parasternal views may be used to assess the severity of Ebstein's

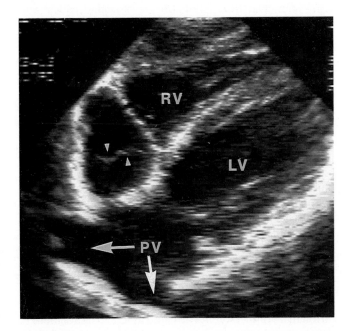

**Fig. 7–8.** Subcostal four-chamber view demonstrating a Chiari network (*arrowheads*) within the right atrium. The entrance of the superior pulmonary veins (PV) into the left atrium is also shown. LV = left ventricle; RV = right ventricle.

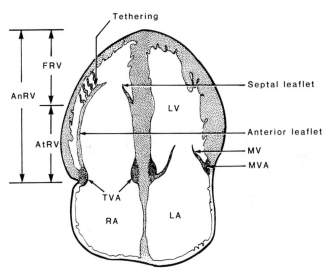

**Fig. 7–9.** Schematic of anatomic abnormalities in Ebstein's anomaly. RA = right atrium; LA = left atrium; LV = left ventricle; MV = mitral valve; MVA = mitral valve annulus; TVA = tricuspid valve annulus; AnRV = anatomic right ventricle; FRV = functional right ventricle; AtRV = atrialized right ventricle.

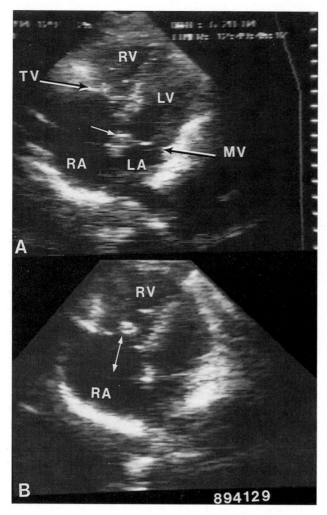

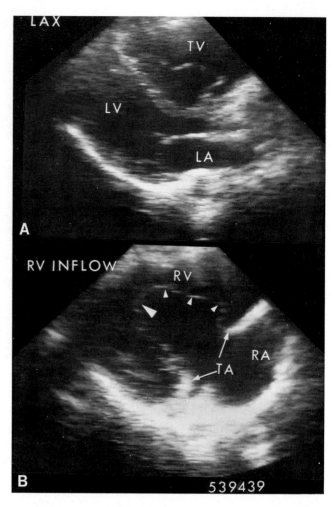

**Fig. 7–10.**   Apical four-chamber views from a patient with Ebstein's anomaly. In *A*, the apical displacement of the tricuspid valve (TV) relative to the anatomic tricuspid annulus (*white arrow*) is shown. The normal position of the mitral valve (MV) is indicated. In *B*, the extent of the displacement is identified by the double-headed arrow. This region represents the atrialized portion of the right ventricle (RV). RA = right atrium; LA = left atrium; LV = left ventricle.

**Fig. 7–11.**   Parasternal long-axis (*A*) and medially angulated right ventricular (RV) inflow (*B*) views from a patient with Ebstein's anomaly. In *A*, the elongated and redundant tricuspid leaflet (TV) is shown. In *B*, the tricuspid annulus (TA) and the displacement of the tricuspid leaflet (*small arrowheads*) are demonstrated. The large arrowhead indicates the insertion of the septal leaflet. LA = left atrium; LV = left ventricle; RA = right atrium.

anomaly and to determine surgical options.[39,47] The degree of atrialization of the ventricle, the extent of leaflet tethering, and the magnitude of deformity or dysplasia of the valve leaflets are important features with implications for surgical repair (Fig. 7–12). The extent of chordal attachments between the anterior leaflet and the anterior free wall should be assessed in multiple views. If tethering is significant, valve replacement rather than repair may be required. The degree of atrialization of the right ventricle can be expressed quantitatively in a variety of ways. The ratio of the area of the right atrium plus the "atrialized" right ventricle to the area of the "functional" right ventricle can be determined. This ratio may identify infants at risk for a poor clinical outcome.[48] If the area of the functional right ventricle is less than 35% of the total right ventricular area, overall prognosis is poor.[39] Because of the complexity of right

ventricular geometry, an accurate measure of the size of the functional right ventricle is difficult and all available views should be used.[46] Thus, most investigators conclude that the severity of Ebstein's anomaly, as assessed echocardiographically, is an important determinant of prognosis. Others, however, have not found a strong correlation between these echocardiographic features and clinical outcome.[49]

Doppler echocardiography should be used to detect tricuspid regurgitation, which is commonly seen in patients with Ebstein's anomaly. In Figure 7–13, color flow imaging demonstrated significant tricuspid regurgitation in a young patient with mild apical displacement of the tricuspid valve. A nonrestrictive atrial septal defect, commonly seen in association with Ebstein's anomaly, is also present.

After surgical repair, echocardiography plays a role

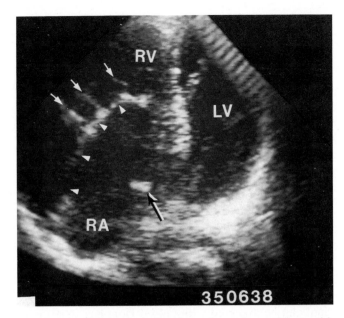

**Fig. 7–12.** Apical four-chamber view of a patient with Ebstein's anomaly. Note the pathologically elongated anterior leaflet of the tricuspid valve (*arrowheads*) and the tethering to the lateral wall (*white arrows*). The bolder arrow denotes the true tricuspid annulus. RA = right atrium; RV = right ventricle; LV = left ventricle.

in assessing the success of the procedure and the severity of residual tricuspid regurgitation.[50] An element of functional tricuspid stenosis may also be present. A redundant anterior tricuspid valve leaflet may cause functional right ventricular outflow tract obstruction, which can also be detected with Doppler. In severe cases, pulmonary atresia may be present, although it is rarely seen in adults.

Ebstein's anomaly may be associated with a variety of other abnormalities that can be detected with echocardiography, namely, atrial septal defect, mitral valve pro-

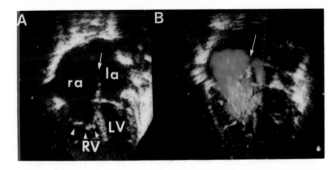

**Fig. 7–13.** Apical four-chamber view from a child with Ebstein's anomaly. *A,* Apical displacement of the tricuspid valve (*arrowheads*) is shown. A secundum atrial septal defect is indicated by the white arrow. *B,* Color flow imaging reveals significant tricuspid regurgitation and flow through the atrial septal defect. (Courtesy of Gregory J. Ensing.) la = left atrium; LV = left ventricle; ra = right atrium; RV = right ventricle.

lapse, or left ventricular dysfunction (Fig. 7–13). The etiology of the left ventricular dysfunction is not known, but its presence is associated with a poor prognosis. Some investigators speculate that abnormal septal geometry and contraction may play a role.[51]

## ABNORMALITIES OF LEFT VENTRICULAR INFLOW

### Pulmonary Veins

Obstruction to left ventricular inflow can occur at several levels (Table 7–3). Pulmonary vein stenosis may be seen as an isolated entity or in association with other congenital lesions.[52–56] In one form, discrete areas of stenosis involving one or more pulmonary veins occur at or near the junction with the left atrium. Alternatively, hypoplasia of the pulmonary veins may be present. The echocardiographic diagnosis of the discrete form of pulmonary vein stenosis is contingent on the ability to visualize the entrance of the veins into the left atrium, which is optimally recorded using the apical and subcostal four-chamber views (see Figs. 7–3 and 7–8). In younger patients, a posteriorly angulated suprasternal short-axis view (sometimes referred to as the "crab view") can also be obtained. Usually, only the right or left upper pulmonary veins are imaged. Because of the proximity of the transducer to the left atrium, transesophageal echocardiography is superior for recording the insertion of the pulmonary veins (Fig. 7–14).[56,57] In most patients, all four veins can be visualized. Echocardiography has also been used for the diagnosis of pulmonary vein obstruction from compression by an extrinsic mass.[56,57]

Even when the pulmonary veins cannot be visualized with two-dimensional echocardiography, a diagnosis of pulmonary vein stenosis may be possible using Doppler techniques. Color Doppler is useful when attempting to identify venous inflow and to detect the turbulent flow associated with stenosis. Turbulent flow in the posterior left atrium may be the initial echocardiographic abnormality and should suggest the possibility of a stenotic pulmonary vein. Then, pulsed Doppler can be used to assess the inflow pattern and determine flow veloc-

**Table 7–3**
Levels of Obstruction to Left Ventricular Inflow

Pulmonary veins
  Pulmonary vein stenosis (discrete)
  Hypoplastic pulmonary veins
  Extrinsic compression
Left atrium
  Cor triatriatum
  Supravalvular stenosing ring
Mitral valve
  Hypoplastic mitral valve
  Congenital mitral stenosis
    Parachute mitral valve
    Anomalous mitral arcade
    Double-orifice mitral valve

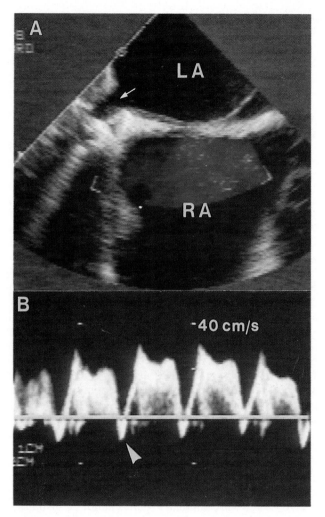

**Fig. 7–14.** In *A*, a transesophageal echocardiogram in the horizontal plane demonstrates the left atrium (LA) and right atrium (RA). The arrow indicates the entrance of the right upper pulmonary vein. In *B*, pulsed Doppler imaging at this site reveals a normal pulmonary venous flow pattern. Antegrade flow (toward the transducer) occupies most of the cardiac cycle. A brief period of flow reversal (*arrowhead*) is coincident with atrial systole.

ity.[52,53] Normally, biphasic antegrade pulmonary venous flow (during ventricular systole and early diastole) is recorded (Fig. 7–14). With stenosis, the flow velocity increases and becomes turbulent and more continuous. An example of pulmonary vein stenosis in an adult is presented in Figure 7–15. This patient had undergone repair of tetralogy of Fallot and reimplantation of an anomalous pulmonary vein 10 years prior to this study. Pulmonary vein stenosis had been unsuspected, but it was suggested on the basis of color flow imaging and then confirmed with pulsed Doppler studies. Despite these findings, visualization of the stenotic vein with two-dimensional echocardiography was not possible.

### Left Atrium

Obstruction to left ventricular filling also occurs at the atrial level, usually because of a fibrous membrane that impedes the flow of blood through the chamber. These membranes may be located in the middle of the atrium, effectively partitioning the left atrium into two chambers (a condition known as cor triatriatum) or they may occur at or near the level of the mitral annulus (a supravalvular stenosing ring). Such membranes are readily detected and localized with two-dimensional echocardiography.[58–61] Distinguishing between these two entities (and differentiating both from mitral valve stenosis) is best accomplished using the parasternal long-axis and apical four-chamber views. The membrane is visualized as a linear, echogenic structure extending from the anterosuperior to the posterolateral wall (Fig. 7–16). In most cases, the superior "chamber" receives the pulmonary veins and the inferior "chamber" is associated with the atrial appendage and mitral valve (which is usually normal). The obligatory perforation connecting the two is most often posterior and may be multiple. This communication is often difficult to record with echocardiography. Color Doppler imaging may permit localization of the opening in the membrane so that the pressure gradient can be assessed with pulsed Doppler.

Transesophageal echocardiography has also been used for the evaluation of this entity.[62,63] Figure 7–17 is an example of cor triatriatum assessed by using transesophageal echocardiography. In this patient, the diagnosis was made correctly with transthoracic echocardiography. The transesophageal echocardiogram, performed in the operating room, allowed visualization of the defect within the membrane. The insertion of all four pulmonary veins and their site of entrance relative to the membrane also were recorded, as were the degree of obstruction to left ventricular filling and the associated mitral regurgitation. Finally, the presence and severity of pulmonary hypertension were assessed.

An example of a supravalvular stenosing ring is presented in Figure 7–18. In contrast to cor triatriatum, these membranes are closer to the mitral valve and may actually adhere to the valve leaflets.[59] Distinguishing between valvular mitral stenosis and a supravalvular ring is best accomplished with two-dimensional and Doppler echocardiography. In the example presented, the membrane was not well visualized in the long-axis view, although restricted mobility of the mitral leaflets was apparent. Absence of anterior leaflet doming excludes the possibility of rheumatic mitral stenosis and the presence of the supravalvular membrane was detected from the apical window.

Using color Doppler, the identification of flow acceleration and turbulence at the level of the annulus rather than the leaflet tips is an additional clue to distinguish a supravalvular ring from mitral valve stenosis. Continuous wave Doppler can then be used to assess the severity of the obstruction. The proximity of the membrane to the valve can lead to leaflet damage, the result of high-velocity turbulent flow. Leaflet thickening and mitral regurgitation may develop as a consequence. Caution must be used when diagnosing a supravalvular stenosing ring with echocardiography. Differentiating between a thickened and calcified mitral annulus and a stenosing ring may be difficult, leading to both false-positive and false-negative results.[60] Associated anomalies are seen

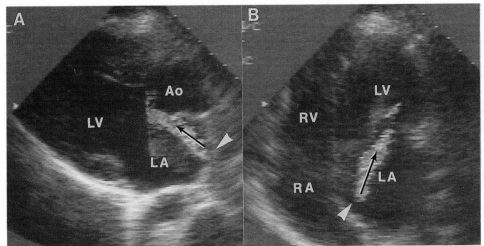

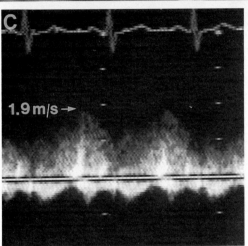

**Fig. 7–15.** Two-dimensional echocardiograms and recordings from a patient with pulmonary vein stenosis. *A* and *B* are parasternal long-axis and apical four-chamber views with color flow imaging. A turbulent jet (*double arrows*) is seen extending from the superior and medial aspect of the left atrium (LA) toward the anterior mitral valve leaflet. The jet originated from the right upper pulmonary vein and its entry into the left atrium is indicated by the large white arrowheads. In *C*, pulsed Doppler recording from the four-chamber view reveals a continuous turbulent flow pattern with a maximal velocity occurring in late diastole of 1.9 m/sec. These findings are consistent with stenosis of the right upper pulmonary vein. Ao = aorta; LV = left ventricle; RA = right atrium; RV = right ventricle.

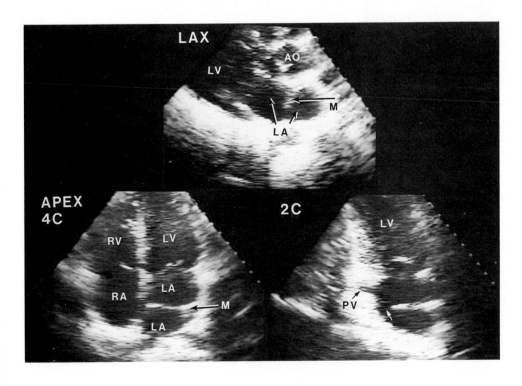

**Fig. 7–16.** Parasternal long-axis and apical views from an asymptomatic patient with cor triatriatum. A linear echo courses posterolaterally within the left atrium, dividing it into two compartments. LA = left atrium; RA = right atrium; RV = right ventricle; LV = left ventricle; Ao = aorta; M = left atrial membrane; PV = pulmonary vein.

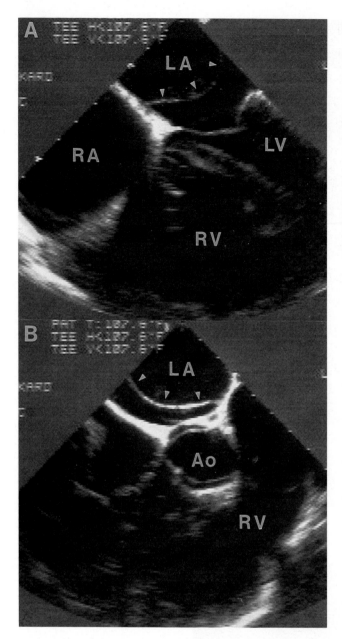

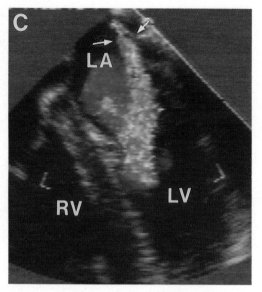

**Fig. 7–17.** A transesophageal four-chamber echocardiogram from a patient with cor triatriatum (*A*). The membrane within the left atrium (LA) is indicated by arrowheads. Note the dilated right atrium (RA) and right ventricle (RV). In the transverse plane (*B*), the membrane is clearly visualized. Color flow imaging during diastole (*C*) reveals turbulent flow through the defect in the membrane (*arrows*). LV = left ventricle; Ao = aorta.

frequently with both cor triatriatum and supravalvular stenosis. Atrial septal defect and persistent left superior vena cava are especially common and are readily detected with echocardiography. These entities may also occur in association with aortic coarctation and subaortic stenosis (Shone's complex).[64]

### Mitral Valve

Congenital mitral stenosis is less common than rheumatic mitral valve disease. Several anatomic variations exist (see Table 7–3) and all can be diagnosed accurately with echocardiography.[65–69] Because rheumatic mitral stenosis is so much more common in adults, however, the diagnosis of congenital mitral stenosis is often missed. Figure 7–19 is an example of a parachute mitral valve. In this condition, all the chordae insert into a

single, large papillary muscle (hence the term "parachute"). The parasternal short-axis view is most helpful in determining the number, size, and location of the papillary muscles. The long-axis view reveals deformity and thickening of the mitral valve, restricted leaflet excursion, and chordal thickening and fusion. Because many of these features are common to rheumatic mitral valve disease, proper diagnosis is sometimes difficult and relies on detecting the presence of a single papillary muscle.[68] The degree of stenosis is variable and is best assessed with Doppler (Fig. 7–20).[68] Because the inflow jet is often eccentric, color flow mapping is helpful for proper orientation of the Doppler beam. A supravalvular stenosing ring may coexist and its presence must be carefully sought.

Other congenital forms of mitral stenosis include anomalous mitral arcade and double-orifice mitral valve.

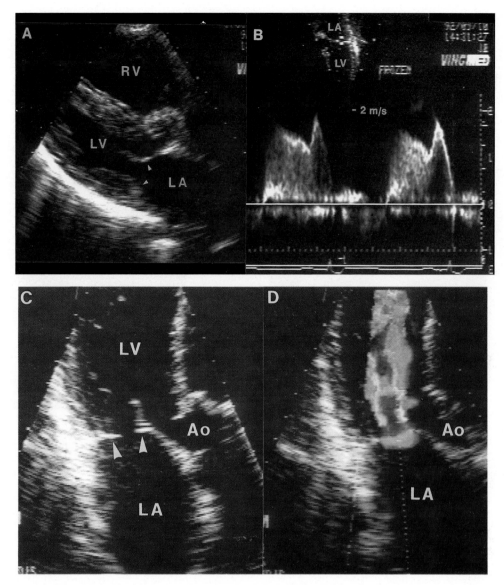

**Fig. 7–18.** A supravalvular stenosing ring is presented. In *A*, a diastolic frame demonstrates restricted opening of the mitral valve (*arrowheads*). The left atrium (LA) and right ventricle (RV) are dilated; however, the stenosing ring is not well visualized. In *B*, a Doppler recording through the mitral valve indicates significant obstruction with increased flow velocity and a prolonged pressure half-time. In *C*, an apical long-axis view demonstrates the stenosing ring (*arrowheads*). In *D*, color flow imaging in diastole reveals turbulent flow through the mitral orifice. Mitral regurgitation was also present. LV = left ventricle; Ao = aorta.

In arcade-type mitral stenosis, the chordae insert into multiple small papillary muscles. Both stenosis and regurgitation are possible. Double-orifice mitral valve occurs because of duplication of the mitral orifice with or without fusion of subvalvular chordal structures. Usually, all the chordae associated with each orifice insert into the same papillary muscle, a situation similar to parachute mitral valve. The diagnosis is made by visualization of two separate orifices in the short-axis view (Fig. 7–21). The presence and severity of stenosis are variable in this condition. Other forms of congenital mitral valve pathology, including mitral valve prolapse and cleft mitral valve, are discussed elsewhere.

## ABNORMALITIES OF RIGHT VENTRICULAR OUTFLOW

### Right Ventricle

Narrowing of the right ventricular outflow tract can occur on several different levels and obstruction may be present at multiple sites within an individual patient. Subvalvular pulmonic stenosis usually occurs at the level of the infundibulum and is less common than valvular stenosis. Infundibular pulmonic stenosis may be the result of discrete fibromuscular narrowing or hypertrophied subvalvular muscle bundles (also called double-

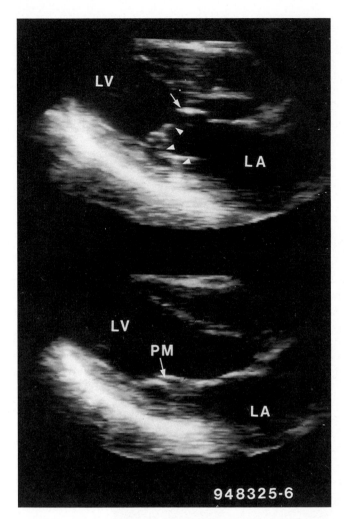

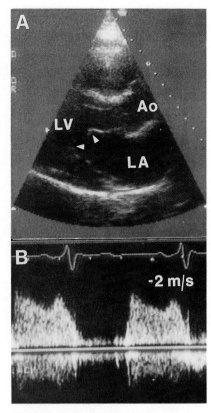

**Fig. 7–19.** Parasternal long-axis examination of a patient with a parachute mitral valve. Note the elongated posterior mitral valve leaflet (*arrowheads*) and the abnormally anteriorly located mitral orifice. LA = left atrium; LV = left ventricle; PM = papillary muscle.

**Fig. 7–20.** Parasternal long-axis view (*A*) and continuous wave Doppler recording of mitral inflow (*B*) from a child with a parachute mitral valve. The echocardiogram reveals a thickened mitral valve with restricted leaflet mobility and chordal fusion (*arrowheads*). The left atrium (LA) is dilated. Color flow imaging revealed a turbulent and anteriorly directed jet. Continuous wave Doppler demonstrates significantly increased inflow velocity and a prolonged pressure half-time consistent with mitral stenosis. In the parasternal short-axis view, a single, large posterior papillary muscle was present. Ao = aorta; LV = left ventricle.

chambered right ventricle).[70] In most cases, a ventricular septal defect is also present. Right ventricular outflow tract narrowing is occasionally secondary to stenosis at a more distal level. For example, valvular pulmonic stenosis may lead to right ventricular hypertrophy, the development of subvalvular muscle bundles, and subsequent outflow tract narrowing.

Two-dimensional echocardiography is well suited to the evaluation of the right ventricular outflow tract. The parasternal short-axis and the subcostal four-chamber views are ideal for assessing the complex geometry of this region and for determining the level and severity of stenosis.[71–73] The use of Doppler to measure the pressure gradient may be challenging, however. Orienting the ultrasound beam parallel to the outflow tract jet requires considerable effort and the use of all available windows. Furthermore, localization of the site of stenosis may be difficult if narrowing occurs at more than one level. The use of high pulse-repetition frequency (PRF)

Doppler may allow determination of the degree of stenosis at each level.[74] Typically, subvalvular stenosis is a dynamic form of obstruction with maximal velocity occurring in late systole. In children with this disorder, echocardiography plays a role in evaluating surgical options. The extent of pulmonary artery development, as determined by echocardiography, is an important factor in surgical planning, particularly in regard to tetralogy of Fallot, in which the type and timing of surgical repair is determined in part by the size of the pulmonary arteries.

A rare congenital abnormality of the right ventricle in Uhl's anomaly, or right ventricular dysplasia.[75] This condition is characterized by dysplasia of the right ventricular myocardium, the extent of which varies considerably. Functionally, the dysplastic myocardium results in a form of right ventricular cardiomyopathy with decreased contractility and a propensity for ventricular arrhythmias.[76] A spectrum of echocardiographic findings

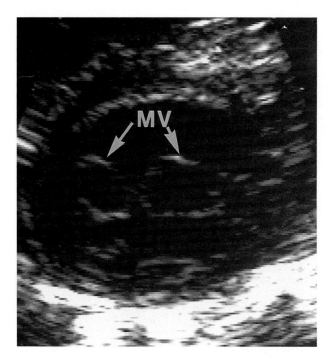

**Fig. 7–21.** Parasternal short-axis view from a patient with double-orifice mitral valve (MV). In this case, the degree of functional mitral stenosis was insignificant.

exists, depending on the extent of involvement. Thinning and hypokinesis of the free wall are characteristic. The systolic dysfunction may appear regional or, in cases of extensive dysplasia, global. Associated valvular pathology is not a feature of Uhl's dysplasia.

### Pulmonary Valve

Stenosis of the pulmonary valve is a fairly common congenital lesion that may occur in isolation or in association with other cardiac defects. The most frequently encountered form is characterized by fusion of the cusps and incompletely formed raphes resulting in a domelike structure with a narrowed orifice. Typically, the valve

annulus is normal in size. With severe stenosis, right ventricular hypertrophy may lead to variable degrees of subvalvular narrowing.

In adults, the morphology of the stenotic pulmonary valve is best visualized in the parasternal short-axis plane through the base. With two-dimensional echocardiography, the cusps appear thickened, have decreased excursion, and dome in systole (Fig. 7–22).[73,77,78] Post-stenotic pulmonary artery dilation is frequently evident, but its presence does not correlate with severity. In most cases, right ventricular size and function are normal and trabeculation of the right ventricular walls is increased. Calcification of the valve is characteristic in adults, but not children, with this disorder.

Although two-dimensional echocardiography is essential for the morphologic diagnosis of pulmonic stenosis, the technique is limited for assessing the severity of obstruction. Neither the degree of cusp thickening nor the presence of right ventricular hypertrophy provides a quantitative measure of severity. In the past, M-mode echocardiography was used to estimate the severity of the stenosis (Fig. 7–23). The depth of the a wave was found to be roughly proportional to the peak pressure gradient.[79] Currently, Doppler is the technique of choice to measure the severity of pulmonic stenosis.[71,74,80–83] Using the modified Bernoulli equation, the peak instantaneous pressure gradient can be calculated (Fig. 7–24). Several clinical studies have demonstrated an excellent correlation between Doppler and catheterization-derived pressure gradients in patients with pulmonic stenosis. In most patients, optimal alignment of the Doppler beam with the stenotic jet uses the parasternal short-axis view.[71,82] In some individuals, use of a lower interspace is necessary to better align with a superiorly directed jet. In patients with pulmonary artery dilation, anterior displacement of the valve precludes proper beam alignment from the parasternal window. In this situation, the subcostal or suprasternal approach is usually adequate. In children, particularly, the subcostal approach provides optimal beam alignment and permits detection of the maximal jet velocity.

In children with pulmonic stenosis, surgical valvot-

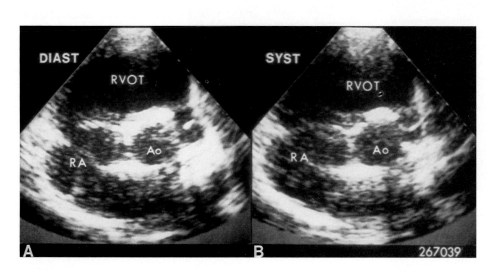

**Fig. 7–22.** Diastolic (A) and systolic (B) parasternal short-axis views through the base of the heart in a patient with severe valvular pulmonic stenosis. The right ventricle is dilated and subvalvular narrowing of the outflow tract is apparent. The pulmonic valve is thickened and immobile. Systolic doming is evident. Ao = aorta; RA = right atrium; RVOT = right ventricular outflow tract.

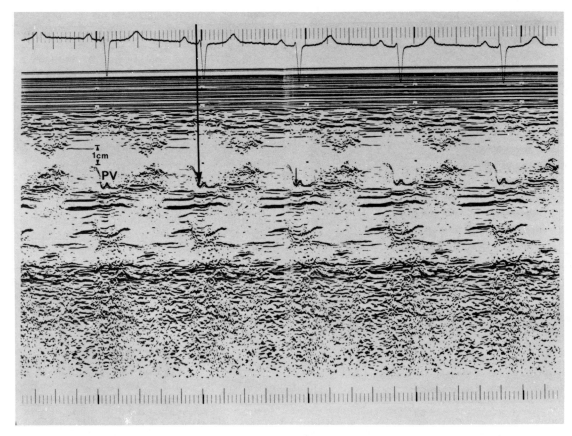

**Fig. 7–23.**   M-mode echocardiogram of the pulmonic valve (P) in a patient with valvular pulmonic stenosis. Note the increased depth of the pulmonic valve "a" wave (*arrow*).

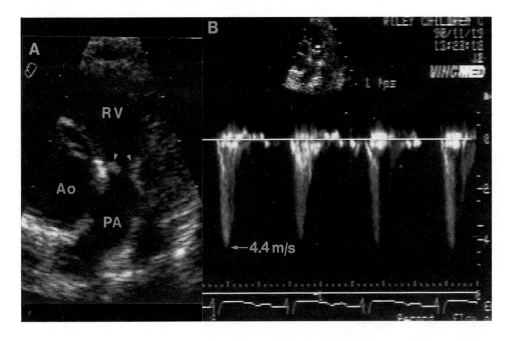

**Fig. 7–24.**   In *A*, a parasternal short-axis view of the right ventricular (RV) outflow tract in systole demonstrates a thickened, domed pulmonic valve and no evidence of infundibular stenosis. The pulmonary artery (PA) appears normal. In real time, immobility of the valve was apparent. In *B*, continuous wave Doppler through the pulmonic valve reveals a peak flow velocity of 4.4 m/sec, consistent with a maximal systolic gradient of approximately 78 mm Hg. Ao = aorta.

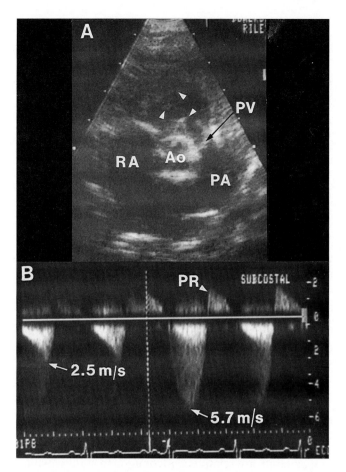

**Fig. 7–25.** Two-dimensional echocardiogram (*A*) and Doppler recording (*B*) from a patient with combined subvalvular and valvular pulmonic stenosis. From the parasternal short-axis view (*A*), right ventricular hypertrophy and infundibular narrowing are apparent (*arrowheads*). The pulmonic valve is not well visualized in this view, but thickening and immobility of the valve were apparent on real-time imaging. In *B*, from the subcostal window, Doppler demonstrates both subvalvular and valvular obstruction. On the left side is a dynamic subvalvular gradient. The maximal velocity occurs in late systole and suggests a peak gradient of approximately 25 mm Hg. On the right side, the maximal gradient at the level of the valve is 130 mm Hg. Pulmonic regurgitation (PR) is also present. Ao = aorta; RA = right atrium; PV = pulmonic valve; PA = pulmonary artery.

omy or balloon valvuloplasty is often performed to relieve the obstruction. After such interventions, Doppler echocardiography may be used for serial evaluation and to detect residual stenosis.[74,80,84–87] The magnitude of associated pulmonic insufficiency and abnormalities of right ventricular diastolic filling[88,89] can also be assessed. In patients with combined valvular and infundibular stenosis, the presence of serial obstructions may result in overestimation by continuous wave Doppler of the catheterization-derived pressure gradient.[72,90,91] This situation occurs because the method used during catheterization to determine the peak-to-peak gradient (withdrawal of a catheter across the entire length of the obstruction) actually underestimates the true maximal gradient. Pressure recovery distal to the initial stenosis

causes this underestimation. Continuous wave Doppler records the maximal gradient (wherever it occurs) and is not affected by this phenomenon. An awareness of these principles is necessary to reconcile differences between Doppler and catheterization results. Figure 7–25 is an example of combined subvalvular and valvular pulmonic stenosis. Doppler demonstrates that the most severe obstruction is valvular, whereas the subvalvular component is relatively mild.

### Pulmonary Artery

Pulmonary artery stenosis (also referred to as peripheral or supravalvular pulmonic stenosis) can occur at any level and often involves multiple sites.[92] Several morphologic forms exist, including discrete membrane-like lesions, long tubular stenoses, and tubular hypopla-

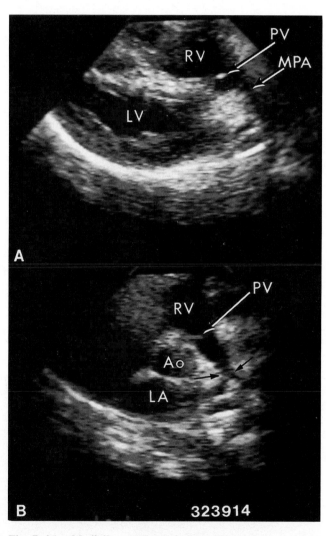

**Fig. 7–26.** Medially angulated parasternal long-axis (*A*) and short-axis (*B*) views from a patient with pulmonary artery stenosis. The pulmonic valve (PV) is mildly thickened but not stenotic. Severe narrowing occurs at the level of the distal main pulmonary artery (MPA) and the origin of the right and left branches as seen in the lower panel (*black arrows*). Ao = aorta; LA = left atrium; LV = left ventricle; RV = right ventricle.

**Table 7–4**

Classification of the Various Congenital Forms of Left
Ventricular Outflow Tract Obstruction

Subvalvular
    Discrete membranous stenosis
    Fibromuscular tunnel
    Hypertrophic obstructive cardiomyopathy
Valvular
    Unicuspid
    Bicuspid
    Dysplastic
Supravalvular
    Discrete (membranous or "hourglass")
    Aortic hypoplasia or atresia
    Interrupted aortic arch
    Coarctation of the aorta

sia. These anomalies frequently are associated with other congenital cardiac and extracardiac lesions (e.g., Williams syndrome).

The ability to detect pulmonary artery stenoses with echocardiography depends on the location of the lesions.[93,94] Proximal lesions can be visualized from the parasternal short-axis window. Figure 7–26 is an example of peripheral pulmonic stenosis involving the distal main pulmonary artery and the origin of the right and left branches. In most such cases, the diagnosis is apparent from two-dimensional echocardiographic imaging. Color Doppler should be used to demonstrate turbulence and acceleration of flow within the stenotic segment. The examiner must bear in mind, however, that a more common cause of turbulent flow within the main pulmonary artery is patent ductus arteriosus.

More peripheral stenoses may be difficult or impossible to visualize, especially in older patients. In children, the subcostal four-chamber and the suprasternal views may permit detection of distal lesions. The diagnosis should be considered in a patient with unexplained right ventricular hypertrophy, particularly in the presence of a pulsatile proximal pulmonary artery.

## ABNORMALITIES OF LEFT VENTRICULAR OUTFLOW

Congenital abnormalities of left ventricular outflow usually involve obstruction to ejection, and several important forms exist. These lesions may be categorized as subvalvular, valvular, or supravalvular (which includes coarctation of the aorta, see Table 7–4). The subvalvular forms are heterogeneous and include hypertrophic cardiomyopathy, which is discussed in Chapter 9. The most important forms are the valvular lesions, which are common causes of stenosis in children (the unicuspid or congenitally stenotic aortic valve) and in adults (the bicuspid valve). The form of supravalvular obstruction encountered most frequently in the adult patient is coarctation of the aorta. This section includes a discussion of the lesions that occur at each of these different levels in order, but the focus is on those anomalies that are most common in adults.

### Subvalvular Obstruction

Two types of subvalvular aortic stenosis are discussed here—the discrete form and the tunnel type of subaortic obstruction. Together, these lesions account for less than 20% of all cases of left ventricular outflow obstruction and both are relatively uncommon in adult patients. Discrete subaortic stenosis results from a thin, fibrous membrane or ridge that forms a crescentic barrier within the outflow tract just below the aortic valve. The membrane usually extends from the anterior septum to the anterior mitral leaflet. The degree of obstruction to flow is variable and aortic regurgitation develops in approximately 50% of patients. With two-dimensional echocardiography, these membranes are seen as a discrete linear echo in the left ventricular outflow tract perpendicular

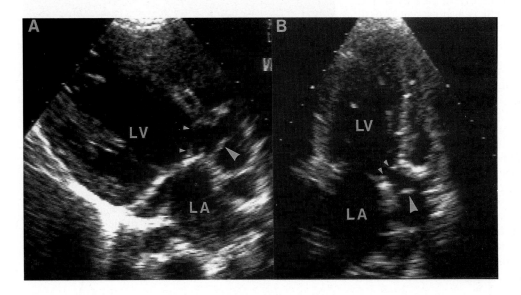

**Fig. 7–27.** Parasternal (*A*) and apical (*B*) long-axis views from a patient with discrete membranous subaortic stenosis. The aortic valve (*large arrowhead*) is thickened, but not stenotic. Immediately below the valve in the left ventricular outflow tract is a discrete membrane (*small arrowheads*). In this patient, Doppler revealed moderate left ventricular outflow tract obstruction and mild aortic regurgitation. LA = left atrium; LV = left ventricle.

to the interventricular septum (Fig. 7–27).[95–97] Because these membranes are parallel to the beam, recording these structures from the parasternal long-axis window may require the use of multiple transducer positions. In many cases, the membranes are detected more easily from the apical views (where the ultrasound beam is oriented perpendicular to the structure). In the example presented in Figure 7–27, the presence of the membrane and its location relative to the aortic valve were clearly recorded from both the parasternal and apical windows. Transesophageal echocardiography has also been used in the assessment of patients with subvalvular obstruction.[98,21a]

Historically, membranous subaortic stenosis was first diagnosed with M-mode echocardiography and the technique continues to play a role in the assessment of this entity. Figure 7–28 is an example of an M-mode echocardiographic recording from a patient with membranous subaortic stenosis, which illustrates the characteristic coarse systolic flutter of the aortic leaflets (because of turbulence and acceleration of prevalvular flow) and midsystolic partial closure of the valve (from dynamic obstruction of the outflow tract). The latter finding indicates significant subvalvular obstruction.

Doppler imaging plays an essential role in the evaluation of these patients. After the location and orientation of the jet is visualized with color flow imaging, continuous wave or high PRF Doppler can be used to estimate the peak pressure gradient across the membrane (Fig. 7–29). In the absence of aortic valve stenosis, this value correlates well with the catheterization-derived measure

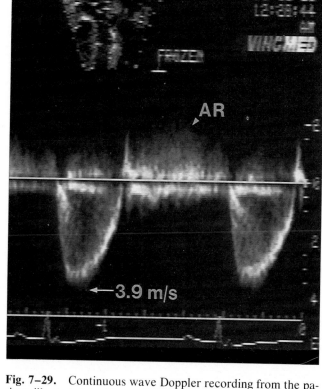

**Fig. 7–29.** Continuous wave Doppler recording from the patient illustrated in Figure 7–27. The peak systolic pressure gradient is 60 mm Hg. Aortic regurgitation (AR) is also present.

of obstruction. In the presence of multiple serial stenoses, however, Doppler may overestimate the catheterization-measured gradient, as discussed in the preceding section on pulmonic stenosis. The presence and severity of aortic regurgitation can also be assessed with Doppler techniques.

Membranous subaortic stenosis is distinguished from a subaortic fibromuscular ridge or tunnel with two-dimensional echocardiography.[99] Tunnel-type subaortic obstruction, rarely seen in adults, is characterized by diffuse thickening and narrowing of the left ventricular outflow tract with associated concentric left ventricular hypertrophy (Figs. 7–30 and 7–31).[100–102] A fibromuscular ridge may also obstruct the outflow tract. This entity is similar to discrete membranous subaortic stenosis, but the obstruction is thicker, is less discrete, and appears more muscular. These different forms of subaortic obstruction probably exist as a continuum, with a thin discrete membrane at one extreme and a diffuse tunnel at the other. Differentiating among individual cases may, therefore, be difficult and somewhat arbitrary. All of these forms of subaortic obstruction are frequently associated with ventricular septal defects.[103,104]

Occasionally, other congenital cardiac anomalies are associated with subvalvular left ventricular outflow tract obstruction, including accessory mitral valve chordae, anomalous papillary muscle insertion, and abnormal in-

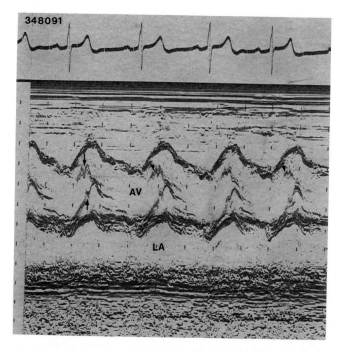

**Fig. 7–28.** Aortic valve M-mode echocardiogram in a patient with subvalvular membrane. Note the prominent midsystolic closure (*arrows*) and coarse flutter (*arrowhead*) of the aortic valve (AV). LA = left atrium.

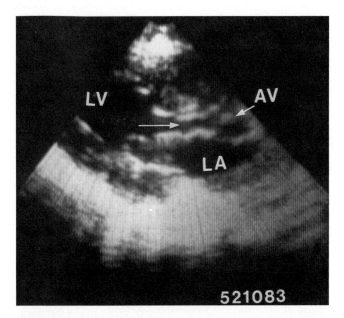

**Fig. 7–30.** Long-axis two-dimensional echocardiogram of the left ventricular outflow tract in a patient with tunnel subaortic stenosis. The subaortic narrowing (*long arrow*) is long and encompasses the entire left ventricular outflow tract. LA = left atrium; LV = left ventricle; AV = aortic valve.

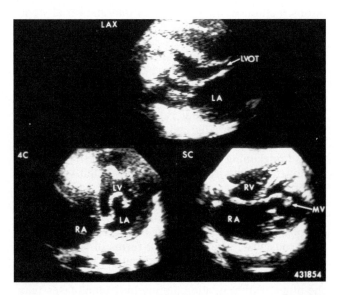

**Fig. 7–31.** Parasternal long-axis (LAX), four-chamber (4C) and subcostal (SC) views from a patient with a tunnel-type subaortic obstruction. The narrowing of the left ventricular outflow tract (LVOT) is best seen in the long-axis view. The mitral valve (MV) appears thickened and redundant. A porcine-valved left ventricular apex-to-aorta conduit is also present, but it is not visible in these frames. LA = left atrium; RA = right atrium; RV = right ventricle.

sertion of the anterior mitral leaflet. Distinguishing among these unusual causes of subvalvular aortic obstruction is readily accomplished by using two-dimensional echocardiography.

### Valvular Aortic Stenosis

Aortic stenosis may be present at birth (a congenitally stenotic aortic valve) or may develop over time in a congenitally abnormal, but not stenotic, valve.[105] In the former, the valve may be acommissural (resembling a volcano and more typical of pulmonic stenosis) or unicuspid unicommissural (with a slitlike orifice, resembling an exclamation point). A bicuspid or tricuspid valve can also be stenotic at birth, because of commissural fusion or dysplasia. Alternatively, such valves may be functionally normal at birth, but gradually become stenotic over time because of progressive fibrosis and calcification. In other cases, degeneration of the valve leads to predominant aortic regurgitation. Quadricuspid valves are rare and have a similar natural history.[106]

Bicuspid aortic valve is estimated to occur in 1 to 2% of the general population, making it the single most common congenital cardiac anomaly. As just noted, these valves often are functionally normal at birth (Fig. 7–32). Two-dimensional echocardiography plays a major role in detection of this entity (Figs. 7–33 and 7–34). Direct visualization of the aortic cusps is possible from the parasternal short-axis view through the base of the heart. During diastole, the cusps of a normal tricuspid valve are closed within the plane of the scan and the commissures form a "Y" (sometimes referred to as an inverted Mercedes Benz sign). A bicuspid valve has two cusps of nearly equal size and a single linear commissure. A raphe may or may not be present and, if present, creates the illusion of three separate cusps. By observing valve opening in systole, however, the number of distinct cusps is apparent. Confirming the presence of a bicuspid aortic valve with echocardiography requires

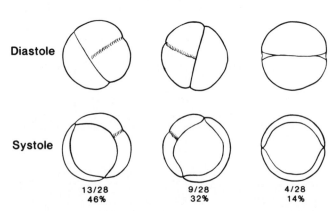

**Fig. 7–32.** Schematic of parasternal short-axis views of bicuspid aortic valves. The numbers and percentages refer to the prevalence of each orientation of valves on an anatomic basis. (From Brandenburg, R.O., et al.: Accuracy of two-dimensional echocardiographic diagnosis of congenitally bicuspid valve; Echocardiographic-anatomic correlation in 115 patients. Am. J. Cardiol., *51*:1469, 1983.)

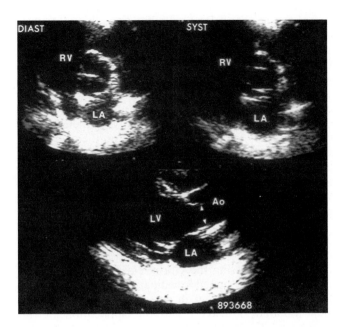

**Fig. 7–33.** Two-dimensional echocardiograms from a patient with bicuspid aortic valve. Diastolic (left) and systolic (right) parasternal short-axis views of the aortic valve demonstrate a single commissure in the horizontal plane. The parasternal long-axis view (bottom) reveals normal excursion of the cusps. No evidence of thickening or valvular stenosis is noted. Ao = aorta; LA = left atrium; LV = left ventricle; RV = right ventricle.

high-resolution images from the short-axis view for adequate visualization of valve morphology.[107–109] This assessment is relatively easy in young patients, but often presents a substantial challenge in adults and is not possible in all patients. A unicuspid valve has a single slitlike commissure and the opening is eccentric and restricted. The stenotic tricuspid valve has three cusps with variable degrees of commissural fusion. Thus, an accurate assessment of functional anatomy requires an analysis of the number of apparent cusps, the degree of cusp separation, and a recording of their mobility and excursion during systole.

Whereas the short-axis view is useful for determining the number of commissures and the degree, if any, of commissural fusion, movement of the cusps out of the imaging plane during systole precludes accurate determination of the presence and severity of stenosis. In fact, normal systolic excursion of the bodies of the cusps recorded from the short-axis view may lead to underestimation of the severity of congenital aortic stenosis. Thus, the short-axis view is useful when evaluating aortic valve anatomy, but should never be used to exclude the possibility of congenital aortic stenosis. The long-axis views have several advantages for this purpose. The thickness and excursion of the cusps can be assessed. Normally, they appear as thin, delicate structures that appear to open completely in systole and are aligned parallel to and against the aortic walls. With congenital aortic stenosis, the cusps are thickened and appear to

dome during systole, the result of restricted motion of the tips relative to the more mobile bodies of the cusps (Figs. 7–35 and 7–36). A qualitative estimate of severity is possible, based on the thickness and immobility of the cusps, the extent of leaflet tip separation in systole, the degree of left ventricular hypertrophy, and the presence of poststenotic aortic root dilation.[78,110–113] Such parameters are particularly useful in children. In adults, however, the presence of coexisting conditions that can affect these findings (e.g., hypertension) limits their value. As a result, both underestimation and overestimation of severity can occur.

Doppler imaging has had a profound impact on the noninvasive assessment of aortic stenosis.[74,114–116a] The ability to record jet velocity within the stenosis permits calculation of the peak instantaneous pressure gradient, a useful indicator of severity.[117,118] As always, proper alignment of the ultrasound beam with the jet is imperative to avoid underestimation. The apical, right parasternal, and suprasternal windows should be used to ensure that the maximal velocity is obtained. Then, through the

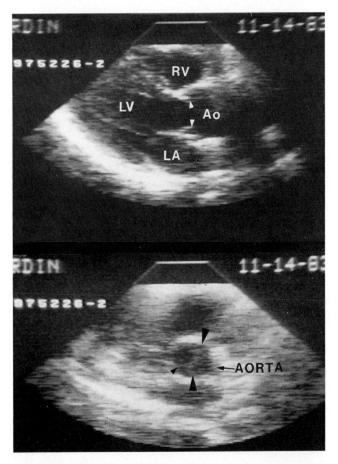

**Fig. 7–34.** Parasternal long- and short-axis views of a patient with bicuspid aortic valve. The aortic valve leaflets dome mildly in systole (*white arrowheads*). In the short-axis view, a vertically oriented commissure (*large black arrowheads*) and a smaller accessory commissure (*small black arrowhead*) are visible. LA = left atrium; LV = left ventricle; RV = right ventricle; Ao = aorta.

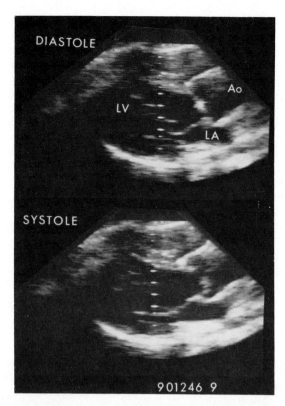

**Fig. 7–35.** Parasternal long-axis view of the aortic valve from a patient with congenital aortic stenosis. Note the systolic doming of the aortic valve leaflets as they remain tethered within the central portion of the aorta. LA = left atrium; LV = left ventricle; Ao = aorta.

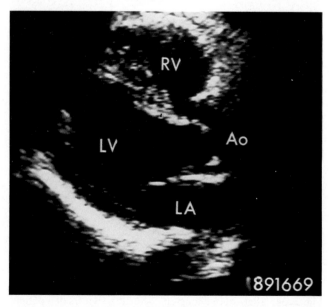

**Fig. 7–36.** Parasternal long-axis systolic frame from a patient with congenital aortic stenosis. The aortic valve cusps are thickened and dome in systole. The severity of stenosis is difficult to assess from this view alone. This patient had mild aortic stenosis. Ao = aorta; LA = left atrium; LV = left ventricle; RV = right ventricle.

use of the modified Bernoulli equation, the peak pressure gradient can be calculated. In the presence of serial stenoses, high PRF Doppler may permit localization of the site of maximal obstruction.[74] Both peak instantaneous and mean pressure gradients can be derived. The values obtained with this approach correlate well with catheterization-derived gradients. Inherent differences exist between the two methods and discrepancies should not necessarily be viewed as an error on the part of one or the other technique. In children especially, anxiety and increased activity during the examination will lead to a rise in flow velocity (both proximal and distal to the valve) and will thereby increase the measured pressure gradient.

To calculate aortic valve area, the continuity equation can be used.[119,120] In adults, correlation between valve area obtained with this technique and that obtained by catheterization using the Gorlin equation is high. Few clinical studies designed to validate the continuity equation in children have been performed. The concept is well founded, however, and the application of this method to all patients with aortic stenosis appears justified.

Clinical decision-making in children with aortic stenosis incorporates the results of the Doppler study together with other clinical information. Mean pressure gradient may be the most useful variable for this purpose. One group of investigators[121] has reported that a Doppler mean gradient greater than 27 mm Hg identifies children with a peak-to-peak gradient at catheterization of 75 mm Hg or greater, whereas a mean gradient less than 17 mm Hg correlates with a catheterization-derived peak gradient of less than 50 mm Hg. A decision regarding the need for intervention was thus possible in most of these patients. Among those with intermediate values (Doppler mean gradient of ≥17 and ≤27 mm Hg), however, the gradient alone was insufficient for clinical decision-making.

In adults with congenital aortic stenosis, an important application of the Doppler technique is to assess patients after valvotomy, primarily to detect restenosis.[85,122,123] Because these valves have been instrumented, assessing restenosis using morphologic criteria from two-dimensional echocardiography may be difficult. Doppler is an ideal technique for the serial follow-up of these patients to assess both stenosis and regurgitation (Fig. 7–37), although the orientation of the jet may be eccentric after valvotomy and proper alignment of the Doppler beam may be difficult. Here, the use of color flow imaging is helpful in identifying the jet and the position the transducer accordingly.

### Supravalvular Aortic Stenosis

The least common site for congenital aortic stenosis is in the supravalvular area.[92] Three morphologic types of supravalvular aortic stenosis have been described: (1) fibromuscular thickening producing an hourglass-shaped narrowing above the sinuses (the most common form); (2) a discrete fibrous membrane in a normal-sized aorta, usually located near the sinotubular junction; and

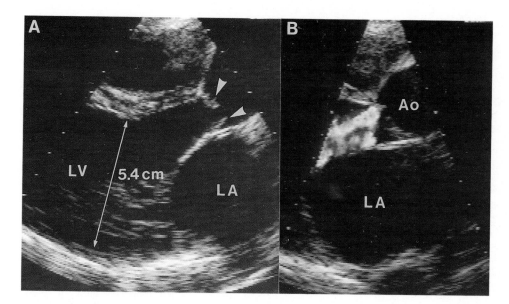

**Fig. 7–37.** Parasternal long-axis views from a patient with congenital aortic stenosis following valvotomy. In *A*, the aortic cusps are thickened and moderately immobile. Systolic doming is present. The left ventricle (LV) is dilated at 5.4 cm. The left atrium (LA) and aorta (Ao) are also dilated. In *B*, color flow imaging reveals moderate aortic regurgitation.

(3) diffuse hypoplasia of the ascending aorta, often involving the origins of the brachiocephalic arteries. Because of the presence of stenosis above the aortic valve and coronary ostia, two additional features often accompany these anomalies: (1) dilation of the coronary arteries, sometimes with ostial obstruction; and (2) thickening and fibrosis of the aortic cusps, usually with an element of aortic regurgitation. Williams syndrome includes supravalvular aortic stenosis, elfin facies, mental retardation, and, occasionally, peripheral pulmonic stenosis. Isolated supravalvular aortic stenosis with or without peripheral pulmonic stenosis may be inherited as an autosomal dominant trait.[123a]

The parasternal long-axis view or a high right parasternal view is most helpful for diagnosing supravalvular aortic stenosis.[124,125] In the normal aorta, the vessel diameter is greatest at the level of the sinuses. At the sinotubular junction, the diameter decreases slightly and approximates the size of the aortic annulus. An hourglass deformity is characterized by a segment of gradual tapering and then widening of the lumen (Fig. 7–38). The aortic walls usually appear thickened and echogenic. Aortic cusp fibrosis is often present, but poststenotic dilation of the ascending aorta is not a feature of this anomaly. A hypoplastic aorta is characterized by more diffuse and extensive narrowing with variable involvement of the branch vessels.

Assessing the severity of supravalvular aortic stenosis relies on accurate visualization, using two-dimensional echocardiography, of the magnitude and linear extent of the narrowing. Careful assessment of the aortic valve and the coronary arteries is an essential part of the evaluation of these patients. Proximal coronary artery dilation or ostial stenosis may be detected from the parasternal short-axis view. Doppler can be used to estimate the peak pressure drop across the site of aortic narrowing. In the presence of a discrete, isolated stenosis, the pressure gradient derived from Doppler is an accurate reflector of severity. As noted previously, however, if the stenoses are multiple or tubular, the correlation between Doppler and catheterization-derived gradients may be poor.[72,90,91] Doppler should also be used to determine the presence and severity of associated aortic regurgitation.

### Coarctation of the Aorta

This relatively common condition is the result of localized narrowing of the descending aorta near the origin

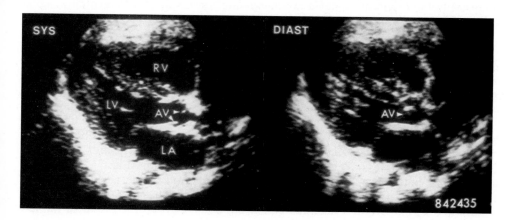

**Fig. 7–38.** Parasternal long-axis views in systole (SYS) and diastole (DIAST) from a patient with supravalvular aortic stenosis. The obstruction occurs just distal to the aortic valve (AV) and results from fibromuscular thickening producing an hourglass-shaped narrowing. The maximal systolic pressure gradient across the obstruction was 80 mm Hg. LA = left atrium; LV = left ventricle; RV = right ventricle.

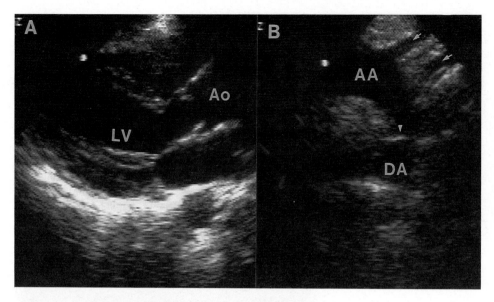

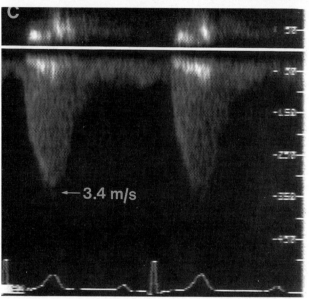

**Fig. 7–39.** In *A*, the parasternal long-axis view of a 34-year-old patient with a bicuspid aortic valve and aortic coarctation demonstrates a thickened aortic valve that domes mildly in systole. No significant aortic stenosis was present. In *B*, a suprasternal long-axis view of the aortic arch (AA) reveals a discrete, shelf-like narrowing (*arrowhead*) immediately distal to the origin of the arch vessels (*arrows*). The descending aorta (DA) beyond the coarctation is well visualized. In *C*, continuous wave Doppler of the descending aorta reveals a maximal systolic pressure gradient of 46 mm Hg. The gradient diminishes rapidly and there is little gradient during diastole. Ao = aorta; LV = left ventricle.

of the ductus arteriosus.[126] The lesion consists of a ridge-like indentation of the posterolateral wall of the aorta resulting from thickening and infolding of the aortic media. It is typically located just distal to the origin of the left subclavian artery and the specific location may be "preductal" or "postductal" depending on the position of the ridge of tissue relative to the ductus (or ligamentum) arteriosus. It is often associated with other forms of congenital heart disease, especially bicuspid aortic valve and mitral valve malformations.[64,65,127]

Echocardiographic detection of coarctation requires both an index of suspicion and careful recording of the descending aorta from the suprasternal window. In children, the evaluation of this portion of the aorta is relatively straightforward.[37] In adults, however, the assessment can be technically demanding and both false-negative and false-positive results occur. The goal is to record the arch and descending aorta in long axis from

the suprasternal notch.[128–132] False-negative results usually result from an inability to image the most distal portion of the arch (where the narrowing occurs). False-positive findings are the result of a tangential imaging plane through the vessel, creating the illusion of narrowing. The origins of the carotid and subclavian arteries serve as landmarks when localizing the juxtaductal area. The location of the left subclavian artery relative to the coarctation in an important factor in surgical management. If an area of stenosis is suspected, care should be taken to ensure proper beam alignment. If the aortic lumen can be seen beyond the narrowing, the likelihood of a false-positive result is reduced. Dilation and exaggerated pulsation of the proximal aortic arch are further evidence of significant coarctation (Fig. 7–39).

An example of coarctation of the aorta in an adult patient is shown in Figure 7–40. Note the location of a shelflike constriction just beyond the origin of the left

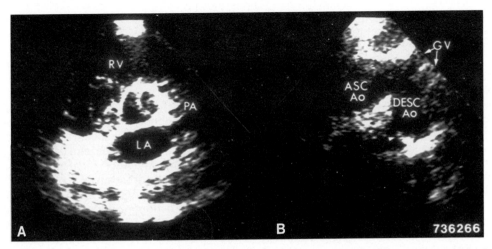

**Fig. 7–40.** Two-dimensional echocardiograms from a patient with bicuspid aortic valve and aortic coarctation. In *A*, a parasternal short-axis view through the base of the heart during diastole demonstrates a single, nearly vertical commissure consistent with a bicuspid valve. In *B*, the location of the coarctation is indicated (*arrowhead*). The descending aorta proximal to the obstruction is dilated. The location of the coarctation relative to the arch vessels (GV) is apparent. ASC Ao = ascending aorta; DESC Ao = descending aorta; LA = left atrium; RV = right ventricle; PA = pulmonary artery.

subclavian artery. Dilation of the ascending aorta is also apparent. When two-dimensional echocardiographic imaging is diagnostic of (or suspicious for) coarctation, Doppler should be performed to aid in the diagnosis and to provide an estimation of the pressure gradient.[133–140] As a first step, color Doppler can be used to detect acceleration and turbulence within the region of narrowing.[141]

The absence of Doppler evidence of acceleration and turbulence of flow should alert the examiner to the possibility of a false-positive two-dimensional echocardiographic result. Color Doppler also permits more accurate alignment of the continuous wave Doppler beam. Figure 7–41 is an example of a Doppler recording across an aortic coarctation. To estimate the peak pressure gra-

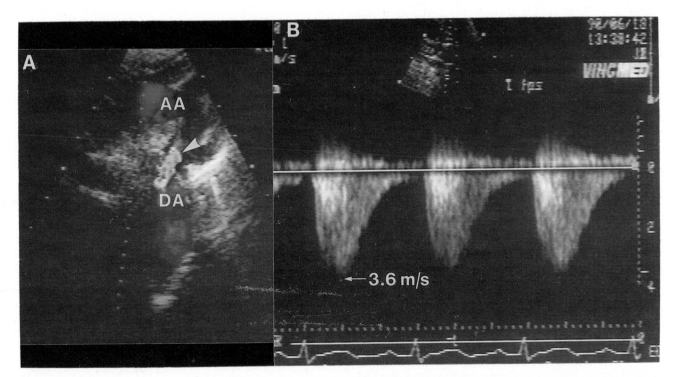

**Fig. 7–41.** In *A*, color flow imaging of the descending aorta (DA) in a patient with more severe aortic coarctation demonstrates the site of stenosis as indicated by the green turbulent flow (*arrowhead*). In *B*, continuous wave Doppler through the same area reveals a peak velocity of 3.6 m/sec consistent with a maximal gradient of 52 mm Hg. Note the persistence of the gradient well into diastole, indicating more significant obstruction. AA = aortic arch.

dient, the Bernoulli equation can be used. When this equation is applied to aortic coarctation, however, it may be inappropriate to ignore the proximal aortic flow velocity.[137] As a general rule, if this proximal velocity is less than 1 m/sec, it can be ignored and the simplified equation can be used. If it is greater than 1 m/sec, the expanded Bernoulli equation is necessary. In this way, a more accurate pressure gradient is obtained. The persistence of a high-velocity flow signal into diastole is another useful clue to the severity of the stenosis. A pressure gradient throughout the cardiac cycle indicates a more severe form of obstruction compared to a pressure gradient that is confined to systole (see Fig. 7–41). Although Doppler is sensitive for the detection of coarctation, false-negative results can occur in the presence of a patent ductus arteriosus. Left-to-right runoff of blood flow through the ductus reduces the jet velocity through the coarctation and leads to an underestimation of the pressure gradient.

Long-term follow-up after repair of aortic coarctation relies heavily on echocardiographic methods for the detection of restenosis. Estimation of the restenosis gradient by Doppler is possible and correlates well with catheterization-derived values.[142]

Aortic atresia and interrupted aortic arch are severe and uncommon forms of left ventricular outflow obstruction.[112,128,143–145] They may be diagnosed in utero or shortly after birth by using echocardiographic techniques. Interruption of the aortic arch may be thought of as an extreme form of coarctation. The length of the "missing" segment varies, as does the relative insertion sites of the arch vessels. With echocardiography, the diagnosis rests on visualization of the aortic arch as it abruptly terminates, and it is usually best seen from the suprasternal window. A patent ductus arteriosus (usually large) will also be present. When aortic arch interruption is suspected, a careful search for a right aortic arch should be undertaken to avoid confusion between these two entities.

## ABNORMALITIES OF CARDIAC SEPTATION

Defects in septation between the cardiac chambers constitute the largest single group of congenital cardiac malformations. These developmental anomalies may involve the atrial septum, the ventricular septum, or the conotruncus (the infundibulum or outlet portion of the ventricles). Within each category, specific lesions are designated on the basis of their embryologic origin and anatomic site. These anomalies often occur in association with other complex lesions; the focus of this section is on those conditions in which septation defects are the primary cardiac anomaly.

### Atrial Septal Defect

Atrial septal defects are among the most common congenital lesions encountered in adults. Because patients with an uncomplicated atrial septal defect often remain asymptomatic throughout childhood and adolescence,

the initial diagnosis of this lesion is often made in early adulthood. Because of the relative nonspecificity of both symptoms and physical findings, the diagnosis frequently is made when echocardiography is performed for unrelated reasons, revealing the unsuspected atrial septal defect.

There are four types of atrial septal defect, which correspond to abnormal development at specific stages of embryogenesis and to specific locations within the atrial septum (Fig. 7–42). The most common type is the ostrium secundum defect, located in the area of the fossa ovalis or middle of the atrial septum. In the adult population, this type comprises approximately two thirds of all cases. The ostium primum defect involves the lower (or primum) portion of the atrial septum and accounts for approximately 15% of atrial septal defects seen in adults. This type may occur alone or in association with defects in the inlet portion of the ventricular septum and atrioventricular valves (i.e., as a component of an endocardial cushion defect). The sinus venous defect is slightly less common (approximately 10% of cases) and occurs in the superior and posterior septum, near the junction of the superior vena cava. Defects in the area of the coronary sinus are rare and are not discussed.

Atrial septal defects usually are single and vary considerably in size. Direct visualization of the atrial septum with two-dimensional echocardiography is the most accurate means by which to diagnose these le-

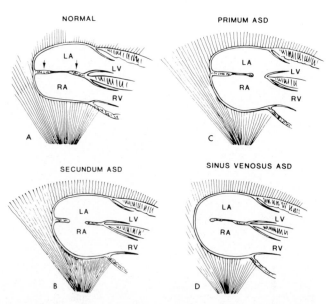

**Fig. 7–42.** Schematic of the subcostal visualization of the atrial septum in normal anatomy (*A*), secundum ASD (*B*), primum ASD (*C*), and sinus venosus ASD (*D*). In *A*, note the thicker basal and more posterior portions of the atrial septum (*arrows*) separated by the thinner valve of the foramen ovale. In the defects in *B*, *C*, and *D*, a distinct dropout of echoes is diagnostic of the ASD. LA = left atrium; RA = right atrium; RV = right ventricle; LV = left ventricle. (From Shub, O., et al.: Sensitivity of two-dimensional echocardiography and the direct visualization of atrial septal defect utilizing the subcostal approach. J. Am. Coll. Cardiol., 2:127, 1983.)

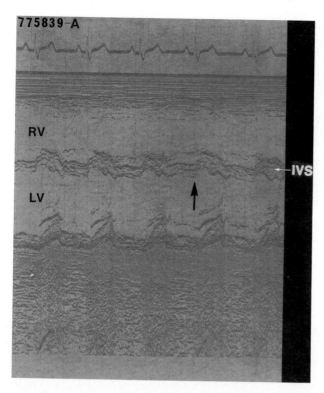

**Fig. 7–43.** M-mode echocardiogram of a patient with an uncomplicated secundum atrial septal defect. Abnormal motion of the interventricular septum (IVS) is characterized by brisk anterior motion of the septum at the onset of systole (*arrow*). RV = right ventricle; LV = left ventricle.

sions.[146–151] The presence of an atrial septal defect is often first suspected, however, on the basis of indirect echocardiographic findings.[152,153] Right ventricular dilation in an otherwise healthy young patient should always suggest this possibility. Abnormal motion of the interventricular septum is another clue to its presence.[154–158] Typically, septal motion in the presence of an atrial septal defect is characterized by brisk anterior movement in early systole or flattened motion throughout systole. These two signs are indicative of right ventricular volume overload and form the basis for the M-mode echocardiographic diagnosis of this entity (Fig. 7–43).[152,154]

Unfortunately, M-mode echocardiography does not allow direct visualization of the anatomic defect. Although the signs of right ventricular volume overload are of some diagnostic value, they are nonspecific and occur in association with other conditions, such as pulmonic and tricuspid insufficiency and anomalous pulmonary venous return.[155,158]

Two-dimensional echocardiography has several advantages compared to M-mode echocardiography for the evaluation of atrial septal defect.[150] As with M-mode echocardiography, right ventricular dilation and paradoxic septal motion can be detected. In the parasternal short-axis view, the abnormal ventricular septal geometry indicative of a right ventricular volume overload can be confirmed.[155–158] This abnormal geometry is characterized by leftward displacement (or flattening) of the septum in diastole, the result of excessive right ventricular diastolic volume. During systole, the normal transseptal pressure gradient is restored and the septum appears more rounded. Rounding of the septum in early systole causes it to be displaced anteriorly (from its abnormal posterior position in late diastole). Careful scrutiny of these events with two-dimensional echocardiography provided insight into this phenomenon and helped to explain the paradoxic motion observed on the M-mode echocardiogram.[155] Figure 7–44 is an example of left ventricular shape and septal geometry in a normal subject. Note the circular appearance of the cavity throughout the cardiac cycle with preservation of rounded septal geometry at both end diastole and end systole. In contrast, Figure 7–45 is from a patient with right ventricular volume overload as a result of an atrial septal defect. Septal flattening in diastole leads to inequality of the two minor axis dimensions (D2 > D1). During systole, however, normal circular geometry is restored (D2 = D1).

While these indirect signs of right ventricular volume overload suggest the possibility of an atrial septal defect, two-dimensional echocardiography plays a more direct diagnostic role by permitting visualization of the atrial septum.[150] To assess the presence, location, and size of an atrial septal defect, multiple echocardiographic views are required and an appreciation of the advantages and limitations of each is essential.[146,148,149] In the apical four-chamber view, the atrial septum is located in the

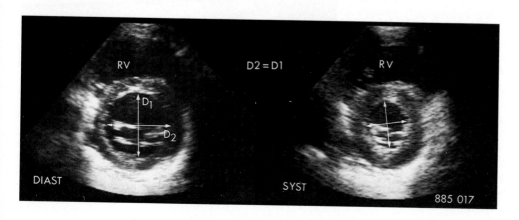

**Fig. 7–44.** Short-axis view of the left ventricle in a normal patient showing equal minor axis dimensions of the left ventricle (D1 and D2) in diastole and in systole. RV = right ventricle. (From Ryan, T., et al.: An echocardiographic index for separation of right ventricular volume and pressure overload. J. Am. Coll. Cardiol., 5:918, 1985.)

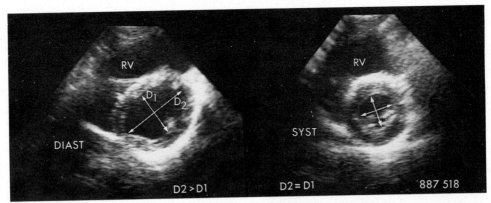

**Fig. 7–45.** Short-axis two-dimensional echocardiogram from a patient with a right ventricular volume overload showing the decreased diameter when measured perpendicular to the interventricular septum (D1). In diastole, the diameter D2 is greater than D1, and in systole they are equal. This is a pure volume overload pattern. (From Ryan, T., et al.: An echocardiographic index for separation of right ventricular volume and pressure overload. J. Am. Coll. Cardiol., 5:918, 1985.)

far field, relatively parallel to the ultrasound beam. Although the diagnosis of an ostium primum atrial septal defect can often be made with confidence from this view, detection of a secundum defect is considerably more difficult. Shadowing and echo dropout (particularly in the area of the fossa ovalis) create the potential for false-positive results. This error occasionally can be avoided if a "T-sign" is observed (Fig. 7–46). The T-sign is a bright horizontal echo that gives the edge of a true defect a more broadened appearance (forming an inverted T).[159] Such broadening is not generally present in the absence of a defect, when echo dropout creates the illusion of a secundum atrial septal defect. This sign has limited reliability and the diagnosis of an ostium secundum atrial septal defect in an adult should rarely be made solely from the apical four-chamber view.

The subcostal four-chamber view places the atrial septum perpendicular to the ultrasound beam and thereby obviates many of the limitations of the apical approach (Figs. 7–46 and 7–47).[149] From this window, the fossa ovalis is seen as a thin central region within the atrial septum. The presence and approximate size of secundum defects can be assessed accurately in well over 90% of cases. This view is also ideal when distinguishing between defects of the primum, secundum, and sinus venosus type. In fact, this is the only transthoracic view in which sinus venosus defects are consistently visualized.[151] Careful interrogation of the most superior and posterior portions of the atria is necessary to detect smaller sinus venosus defects (Fig. 7–48). By rotating the imaging plane into a subcostal sagittal view, the dimensions of the atrial septal defect can be assessed. Furthermore, the entrance of the superior vena cava and pulmonary veins frequently can be identified, thereby permitting diagnosis of anomalous pulmonary venous drainage. Finally, the subcostal views are helpful for the detection of an atrial septal aneurysm (Fig. 7–49).[160–163] These aneurysms consist of thin, billowing tissue in the area of the fossa ovalis that moves with the cardiac and respiratory cycles and usually protrudes into the right

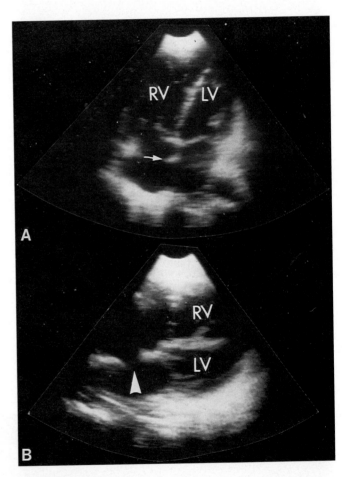

**Fig. 7–46.** Apical (*A*) and subcostal four-chamber (*B*) views in a patient with secundum atrial septal defect. In *A*, note the distinct dropout of echoes in the area of the secundum atrial septum (*arrow*). This is a characteristic "T sign." In *B*, note that the primum and most posterior (leftward) portions of the atrial septum are intact and there is a definite dropout of echoes reflecting tissue loss in the area of the secundum atrial septum (*arrowhead*). RV = right ventricle; LV = left ventricle.

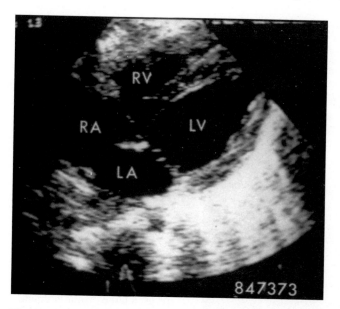

**Fig. 7–47.** Subcostal four-chamber view from a patient with a large ostium secundum atrial septal defect reveals the size and location of the defect. LA = left atrium; LV = left ventricle; RA = right atrium; RV = right ventricle.

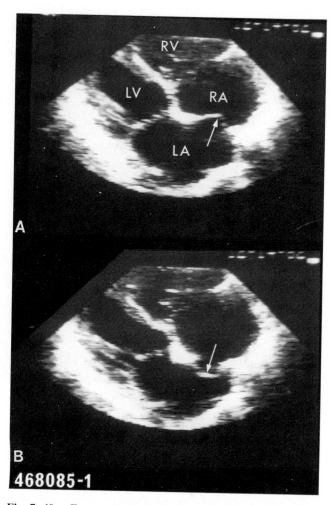

**Fig. 7–49.** Four-chamber views from a patient with an atrial septal aneurysm. In *A*, the aneurysm (*arrow*) bulges into the right atrium (RA). In *B*, the aneurysm (*arrow*) bulges into the left atrium (LA). LV = left ventricle; RV = right ventricle.

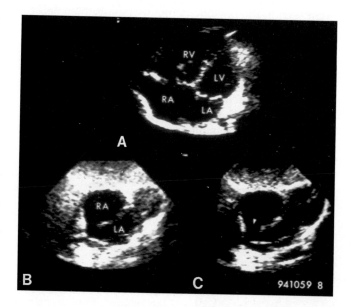

**Fig. 7–48.** In *A*, the apical four-chamber view from a patient with a sinus venosus atrial septal defect reveals a dilated right atrium (RA) and right ventricle (RV). The interatrial septum is not well visualized in this plane because of echo dropout. *B* and *C* are subcostal four-chamber views from the same patient. By tilting the transducer slightly and rotating clockwise, the defect in the superior portion of the atrial septum is recorded (*arrowhead, C*). LA = left atrium; LV = left ventricle; RA = right atrium; RV = right ventricle.

atrial cavity. In many cases, these aneurysms are an incidental finding.[164,165] They may, however, be associated with an increased risk of embolic events and thrombus may form within the concavity of the aneurysm. Some degree of patency is common and evidence of an interatrial shunt can usually be demonstrated. Detection by echocardiography is particularly important in the young patient with unexplained peripheral emboli or stroke.

Diagnosis of an ostium primum atrial septal defect is easily accomplished with two-dimensional echocardiography.[166–170] Such defects result from failure of partitioning of the atrioventricular canal and frequently involve the ventricular septum as well. Thus, an ostium primum defect may occur alone (partial artrioventricular canal) or in association with defects in the inlet ventricular septum (complete atrioventricular canal or endocardial cushion defect). Absence of tissue in the most inferior portion of the atrial septum (at the level of insertion of the septal leaflets of the atrioventricular valves) is diagnostic and serves to distinguish ostium primum from

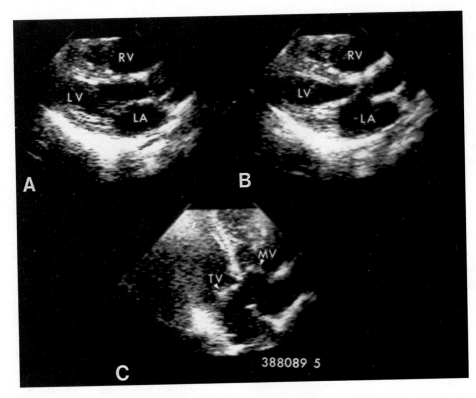

**Fig. 7–50.** Two-dimensional echocardiographic images from a patient with an ostium primum atrial septal defect are shown. The parasternal long-axis view *A* reveals abnormal insertion of the anterior mitral leaflet. With medial angulation, a portion of the anterior leaflet can be seen attached to the septum (*B*). In *C*, the apical four-chamber view demonstrates a large ostium primum atrial septal defect. The mitral (MV) and tricuspid (TV) valves are in the same plane. LA = left atrium; LV = left ventricle; RV = right ventricle.

secundum defects. This determination can be made from any of several views, although the apical four-chamber view is often best (Fig. 7–50). The presence of any atrial septal tissue above the base of the atrioventricular valves excludes the diagnosis of a primum defect. Atrioventricular canal defects are also associated with lack of separate fibrous atrioventricular valve rings. As a consequence, both atrioventricular valves lie in the same plane (rather than more apical displacement of the tricuspid valve). This finding is also readily apparent from the four-chamber view.

Once an ostium primum atrial septal defect is detected, it is essential to assess for the presence of associated abnormalities, including: (1) an inlet ventricular septal defect, (2) a cleft mitral valve, (3) the presence and severity of atrioventricular valve regurgitation, and (4) partial attachment of the septal leaflet of the mitral valve to the interventricular septum. Cleft mitral valve, often seen in the presence of an ostium primum defect, is detected more easily from the parasternal short-axis view by careful scanning at the tips of the mitral leaflets (Fig. 7–51).[169] The cleft will generally be recognized as a gap at approximately the "12 o'clock" position. Abnormal insertion of the anterior mitral valve leaflet is best appreciated from the parasternal long-axis view (Fig. 7–50). By varying the angulation of the transducer, the displaced attachment site can be visualized.

In most cases, the presence or absence of an atrial

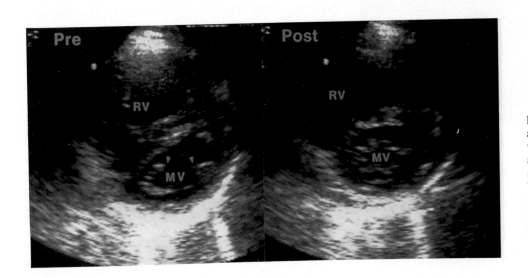

**Fig. 7–51.** Parasternal short-axis images from a patient with a cleft mitral valve (MV) are shown before (PRE) and after (POST) surgical repair. The cleft in the anterior leaflet of the valve is indicated by arrowheads. After repair, the cleft is no longer present. Note the right ventricular (RV) dilation.

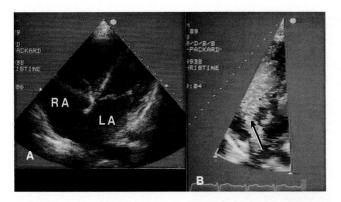

**Fig. 7–52.** Corresponding two-dimensional echocardiogram (*A*) and color flow imaging (*B*) in the apical four-chamber view from a patient with a large secundum atrial septal defect. In *A*, the right atrium (RA) and right ventricle (RV) appear dilated. The interatrial septum is not well seen although a defect would be suspected. In *B*, a turbulent jet is recorded crossing the middle of the atrial septum and extending toward the tricuspid valve into the right ventricle. In this patient, color flow imaging is diagnostic of an atrial septal defect with a large left-to-right shunt.

septal defect can be determined with confidence on the basis of transthoracic two-dimensional echocardiography.[146,149] When in doubt, contrast echocardiography and/or Doppler should be performed and will generally provide a diagnosis (Figs. 7–52 and 7–53). Contrast echocardiography is a relatively sensitive technique for detecting intracardiac shunting.[171–176] The apical four-chamber view usually is optimal because it allows simultaneous visualization of all four chambers. After injection of agitated saline (or other suitable contrast agents) into a peripheral upper extremity vein, the right side of the heart is rapidly and completely opacified. The

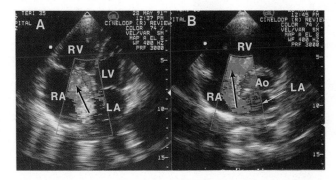

**Fig. 7–53.** The apical four-chamber (*A*) and parasternal short-axis (*B*) views from a patient with a large ostium secundum atrial septal defect are presented. In *A*, the right side of the heart is dilated. Color flow imaging demonstrates turbulent flow across the interatrial septum in a left-to-right direction (*double arrow*). The flow extends toward the tricuspid valve and right ventricle (RV). A similar flow pattern is recorded in *B*, extending into the right ventricle. The large size of the defect is suggested by the width of the color flow jet. Ao = aorta; LA = left atrium; RA = right atrium; LV = left ventricle.

demonstration of contrast echoes in the left atrium suggests right-to-left shunting at the atrial level (Fig. 7–54).[177] This phenomenon occurs both in the presence and absence of elevated pressure in the right side of the heart, even when the predominant shunt is left to right. The magnitude of this shunt, however, is often small and transient and may easily be missed. Contrast-containing blood within the left atrium also occurs in the presence of a pulmonary arteriovenous malformation.

Direct evidence of a left-to-right shunt relies on the appearance of noncontrast-containing blood within the right atrium (a so-called negative contrast effect, see Fig. 7–55).[178] Unfortunately, noncontrast-enhanced blood may enter the right atrium across an atrial septal defect, by the coronary sinus, through a left ventricle-to-right atrium communication, or from the inferior vena cava. Slow motion and frame-by-frame analysis of the echocardiogram is necessary to distinguish among these possibilities. Thus, although contrast echocardiography continues to play an important role in the assessment of patients with a suspected atrial septal defect, several limitations of the technique must be recognized. First, the method is not quantitative. Shunting is a transient phenomenon reflecting the instantaneous pressure gradient across the atrial septum (Fig. 7–56). The appearance of right-to-left shunting should not be misconstrued as evidence of pulmonary hypertension. Conversely, an apparent "negative" contrast effect with the right atrium must be analyzed carefully to avoid false-positive results. Finally, evidence of shunting at the atrial level may occur with a patent foramen ovale and does not by itself confirm the presence of an atrial septal defect.

Perhaps the most accurate technique for evaluating the integrity of the interatrial septum is transesophageal echocardiography.[179–181] The proximity and orientation of the septum relative to the esophagus permit the entire structure to be adequately visualized in virtually every patient (Figs. 7–57 and 7–58). The presence, location, and size of the defect can be determined with confidence (Fig. 7–59). The increase in sensitivity provided by this method may be particularly important for sinus venosus defects.[182] Figures 7–57 and 7–58 were recorded from a 35-year-old asymptomatic patient with a family history of congenital heart disease. Transthoracic imaging was suboptimal. Although a defect was suspected, the diagnosis could not be made with confidence. The results of the transesophageal echocardiogram, however, permitted surgical repair without the need for cardiac catheterization.

Transesophageal echocardiography has also proven valuable for the diagnosis of patent foramen ovale. Using contrast-enhanced echocardiography and/or color flow imaging, small interatrial shunts can be demonstrated (Figs. 7–60 and 7–61). At the same time, the absence of an "anatomic" atrial septal defect is confirmed with two-dimensional imaging. In these patients, contrast should be injected under basal conditions and then again during maneuvers designed to increase intrathoracic pressure, such as coughing or Valsalva.

Doppler imaging can also be used to evaluate the possibility of an atrial septal defect. By aligning the Doppler

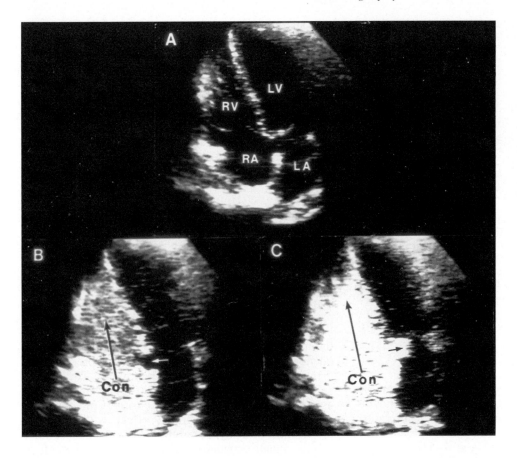

**Fig. 7–54.** Apical four-chamber views from a patient with an ostium primum atrial septal defect. In *A*, the defect is readily apparent in the inferior portion of the atrial septum. Note that the right heart does not appear significantly dilated. In *B*, following peripheral injection of agitated saline, the right atrium (RA) and right ventricle (RV) are opacified by contrast-containing blood. The white arrow indicates left-to-right shunting through the defect. In *C*, a few frames later, contrast-containing blood is seen flowing from right-to-left through the defect. LA = left atrium; LV = left ventricle; Con = contrast.

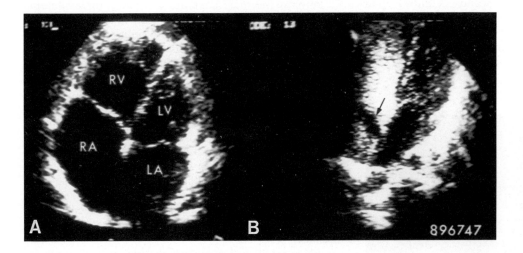

**Fig. 7–55.** *A*, an apical four-chamber view demonstrates a dilated right atrium (RA) and right ventricle (RV). There appears to be a large secundum atrial septal defect, although echo dropout in this area must be considered. In *B*, injection of agitated saline through a peripheral vein resulted in a negative contrast effect within the right atrium (*arrow*). This finding is diagnostic of left-to-right shunting through the atrial septal defect. LA = left atrium; LV = left ventricle.

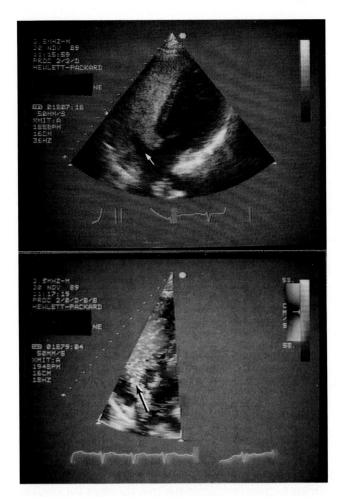

**Fig. 7–56.** Apical four-chamber views from the same patient as in Figure 7–52. The paired illustration demonstrates the similarity between contrast echocardiography (*A*) and color flow imaging (*B*). In *A*, the arrow indicates the negative contrast effect in the right atrium diagnostic of left-to-right shunting at the atrial level. In *B*, a turbulent jet in this area (*double arrow*) provides similar diagnostic information.

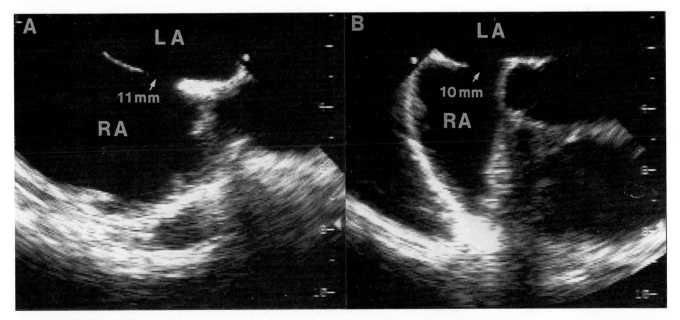

**Fig. 7–57.** Biplane transesophageal echocardiograms from a patient with a secundum atrial septal defect. In *A*, the longitudinal plane reveals the defect clearly and permits the size to be measured. In *B*, the transverse plane allows the dimension of the defect in the orthogonal plane to be determined. LA = left atrium; RA = right atrium.

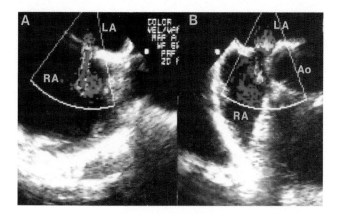

**Fig. 7–58.** Color flow images from the patient shown in Figure 7–57. Again, *A* represents the longitudinal plane and *B* the transverse plane. Color flow imaging permits the flow through the defect to be recorded. LA = left atrium; RA = right atrium; Ao = aorta.

sample volume perpendicular to the atrial septum, flow across the defect can be recorded (Fig. 7–62).[148,183,184] In adults, this study is most easily obtained by using the subcostal four-chamber view. In the usual case, pulsed Doppler will demonstrate low-velocity left-to-right flow extending from midsystole to middiastole, with a second phase of flow coincident with atrial systole. A brief period of right-to-left shunting may also be recorded in early systole. Because the pressure difference between the atria is relatively small, a high-velocity jet will not be present. The respiratory phase will also affect the flow pattern. Care must be taken to avoid confusing the low-velocity shunt flow with normal venous and atrioventricular valve flow. In patients in whom direct visualization of an atrial septal defect is not possible, color flow imaging can confirm the presence of trans-septal

flow.[183,185,186] This technique is particularly helpful when attempting to distinguish between echo dropout and a true anatomic defect.

Quantitation of the size of the shunt has been achieved with Doppler techniques.[187–191] This assessment requires determination of left and right ventricular stroke volume, which can be derived from aortic and pulmonary flow velocity profiles. In children, this method has been used to estimate the direction and magnitude of the shunt (i.e., the net shunt ratio). Correlation between Doppler and catheterization techniques for this measurement is good. In adults, however, technical problems limit the utility of this approach.

The accurate and complete evaluation of atrial septal defect provided by echocardiography has allowed many patients to undergo repair without the need for cardiac

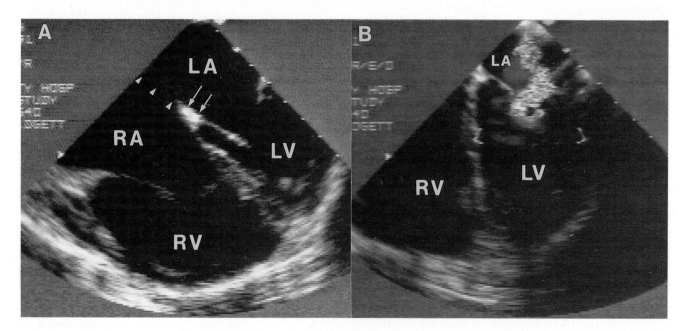

**Fig. 7–59.** Transesophageal echocardiograms recorded in the four-chamber view from a patient with a large secundum atrial septal defect. In *A*, the right side of the heart is dilated and the defect is indicated by arrowheads. The arrows indicate the presence of the septum primum, which is intact. In *B*, color flow imaging during systole reveals moderate mitral regurgitation, the result of a cleft anterior mitral leaflet. LA = left atrium; LV = left ventricle; RA = right atrium; RV = right ventricle.

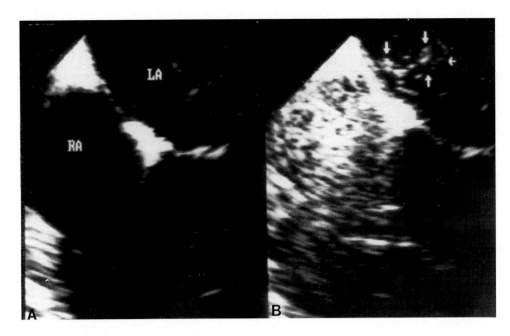

**Fig. 7–60.** Transesophageal echocardiograms from a patient with a patent foramen ovale. In *A*, the interatrial septum appears intact. The thin area in the middle portion represents the fossa ovalis. In *B*, following peripheral contrast injection, the right atrium (RA) is completely opacified. A small amount of contrast-containing blood traverses the septum and appears in the left atrium (LA) (*arrows*). This finding is diagnostic of a right-to-left shunt through a patent foramen ovale.

catheterization.[167,192–194] Although such decisions must be individualized, it is now well established that most of the necessary diagnostic information is available noninvasively. In addition to the primary diagnosis, the presence or absence of associated anomalies can be correctly determined in over 90% of patients. Most findings that are not detected preoperatively with echocardiography can be identified and repaired intraoperatively without any resultant increase in morbidity.[192] Most young patients with a secundum atrial septal defect now undergo repair without cardiac catheterization. Angiography may also be avoided in selected patients with a primum atrial septal defect if pulmonary artery pressure, papillary muscle architecture, and atrioventricular valve morphology can be adequately assessed with ultrasound.[167]

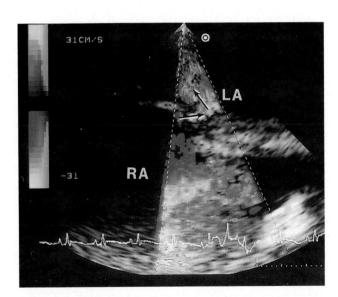

**Fig. 7–61.** Transesophageal echocardiogram in a patient with a patent foramen ovale. In two-dimensional images, the interatrial septum appeared intact. With color flow imaging, right-to-left shunting was intermittently detected through the middle portion of the septum. The flow across the septum (*double arrows*) varied with respiration. LA = left atrium; RA = right atrium.

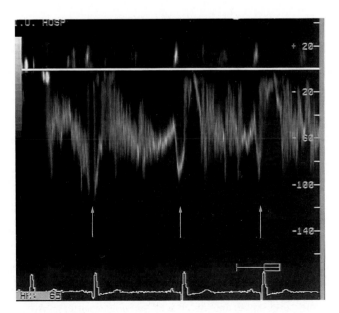

**Fig. 7–62.** Pulsed Doppler tracing from a patient with an uncomplicated secundum atrial septal defect recorded during a transesophageal echocardiographic study. From this orientation, flow below the baseline indicates left-to-right shunting through the defect. Flow persists throughout the cardiac cycle and reaches a maximal velocity of approximately 1.0 m/sec during atrial systole (*arrows*).

## Ventricular Septal Defect

This lesion is one of the most common cardiac anomalies encountered in the pediatric population.[195] It is seen considerably less often in adults, however, for several reasons. Because of the prominent murmur associated with most ventricular septal defects, detection in infancy or childhood is the rule. This discovery leads to the repair of most moderate or large defects before the patient reaches adulthood. Small ventricular septal defects may undergo spontaneous closure before adulthood. These factors are largely responsible for the relative infrequency of this lesion in the adult patient.

The interventricular septum is composed of a membranous portion and a muscular portion (Fig. 7–63). The membranous septum is small and is located directly below the aortic valve. Its right ventricular surface is adjacent to the septal leaflet of the tricuspid valve. On the left, the membranous septum forms the superior border of the left ventricular outflow tract. The remainder of the interventricular septum is composed of muscular tissue that extends out from the membranous septum in an inferior, apical, and anterior direction. Three regions are identified: the inlet septum (lying posterior to the membranous septum and between the two atrioventricular valves), the trabecular septum (extending from the membranous septum toward the cardiac apex), and the outlet or infundibular septum (extending anteriorly from the membranous septum and lying above the trabecular septum and below the great arteries). The outlet septum straddles the crista supraventricularis.

Ventricular septal defects are rarely limited to the

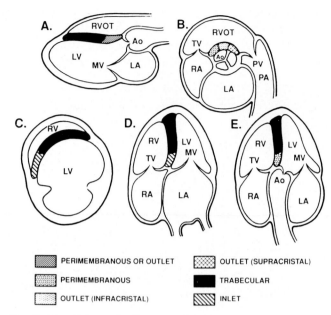

| PERIMEMBRANOUS OR OUTLET | OUTLET (SUPRACRISTAL) |
| PERIMEMBRANOUS | TRABECULAR |
| OUTLET (INFRACRISTAL) | INLET |

**Fig. 7–64.** Schematic diagram of the location of the various types of ventricular septal defect when viewed using two-dimensional echocardiography. See text for details. Ao = aorta; LA = left atrium; LV = left ventricle; RA = right atrium; RV = right ventricle; RVOT = right ventricular outflow tract; MV = mitral valve; TV = tricuspid valve; PV = pulmonic valve.

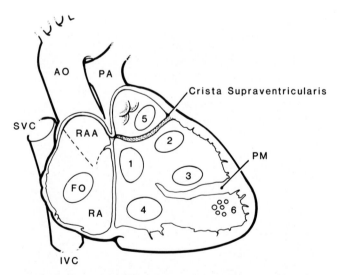

**Fig. 7–63.** Schematic of the right ventricular surface of the interventricular septum diagramming common locations of ventricular septal defects. PA = pulmonary artery; Ao = aorta; RA = right atrium; SVC = superior vena cava; IVC = inferior vena cava; RAA = right atrial appendage; FO = foramen ovale; PM = papillary muscle; region 1 = membranous interventricular septum; region 2 = outflow interventricular septum; region 3 = trabecular septum; region 4 = inflow septum; region 5 = subarterial region; region 6 = distal multiple "Swiss cheese" septal defects.

membranous septum, but more often extend into one of the three muscular regions. To describe such defects, the designation "perimembranous" is preferred to "membranous."[196] Perimembranous defects are by far the most common variety of ventricular septal defect, accounting for approximately 80% of all cases. Next most common are the trabecular ventricular septal defects, which may be multiple and vary considerably in size and location. Defects of the inlet and outlet septa are less common. Inlet ventricular septal defects occur uncommonly in isolation, but may be a component of endocardial cushion defects. Outlet ventricular septal defects, when they abut both semilunar valves, are sometimes referred to as supracristal or doubly committed subarterial defects. These anatomic distinctions have important clinical implications with regard to the chance of spontaneous closure, the surgical approach, risk of conducting system involvement, and likelihood of associated valvular dysfunction (e.g., aortic regurgitation).[197,198]

The accuracy of echocardiography for detecting a ventricular septal defect depends on its size and location. The ventricular septum is curved and therefore does not lie in only one plane. Multiple views are required to examine the entire septal region and a single imaging plane will neither interrogate the complete structure nor detect every defect (Fig. 7–64). Visualization of a ventricular septal defect in more than one imaging plane is the most direct means of diagnosis. In general, false-negative findings are more common than false-positive results. As is the case with atrial septal defects, the presence of a T-sign at the edge of the defect is helpful in distinguishing a true finding from echo dropout.[159] The size and shape of large defects can be quantitatively assessed with two-dimensional echocardiography. One study has demonstrated a high correlation between the diameter of the defect measured from multiple echocardiographic views and results obtained at autopsy.[199]

The sensitivity of two-dimensional echocardiography for diagnosis of a ventricular septal defect depends on location.[159,200-205] Sensitivity is probably highest for inlet and outlet defects (approaching 100%), slightly less for perimembranous defects (80 to 90%), and least for trabecular defects (as low as 50% in some earlier studies).[205,206] The reasons for this low detection rate are that trabecular defects can occur anywhere within a fairly large area, are sometimes small, and may be multiple. Furthermore, the ''shape'' of the defect is often complex and the orifice may be obscured in systole because of myocardial contraction. Fortunately, the addition of Doppler[207-210] and particularly color flow imaging[200,211-214] greatly enhances the accuracy for diagnosis of all varieties of ventricular septal defects.

Perimembranous defects are visible in the parasternal long and short-axis views, but generally are not seen from the four-chamber view. Slight medial angulation of the long-axis plane is required to record this area. When this adjustment is done, the membranous septum is located superior to and just below the aortic valve. From this perspective, however, distinguishing between perimembranous and outlet defects (both above and below the crista supraventricularis) may not be possible. For this purpose, the short-axis view is superior. When the scan plane is oriented just inferior to the aortic annulus, both the membranous and outlet septa are visualized. Perimembranous defects are located more medially, usually near the septal leaflet of the tricuspid valve (Figs. 7-65-7-67).

Outlet defects are more anterior and leftward (relative to the aortic annulus; Figs. 7-68 and 7-69). The short-axis view further permits classification of outlet defects as being either above or below the crista supraventricularis. Defects below the crista are to the right of midline, whereas supracristal ventricular septal defects are far leftward and adjacent to the pulmonic valve (Fig. 7-70). Supracristal defects are optimally detected from a high parasternal long-axis or parasternal short-axis view. In the long-axis plane, slight lateral angulation and rotation permit visualization of both the aortic and pulmonic valves, with the defect adjacent to both. Supracristal defects are often relatively small and may be missed, particularly if color flow imaging is not used. Once detected, a careful interrogation of the aortic valve is mandatory to exclude cusp prolapse and associated aortic regurgitation. This finding may be accompanied by sinus of Valsalva enlargement, usually involving the right sinus.

The apical four-chamber view permits visualization of

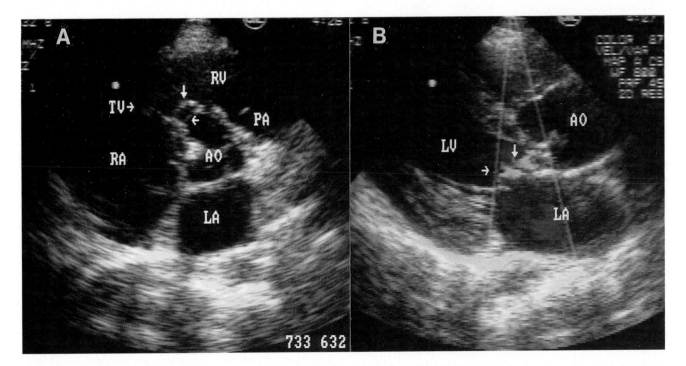

**Fig. 7-65.** An example of a perimembranous ventricular septal defect. In *A*, the parasternal short-axis view demonstrates the location of the defect below the aortic valve and adjacent to the septal leaflet of the tricuspid valve (TV) (*arrows*). The vertical arrow indicates prolapse of the right coronary cusp into the defect. In *B*, color flow imaging from the parasternal long-axis view reveals mild aortic regurgitation. In such a patient, surgical closure of the ventricular septal defect is often recommended, even when the defect is small, to prevent progression of the aortic valve disease. AO = aorta; LA = left atrium; RA = right atrium; RV = right ventricle; LV = left ventricle; PA = pulmonary artery.

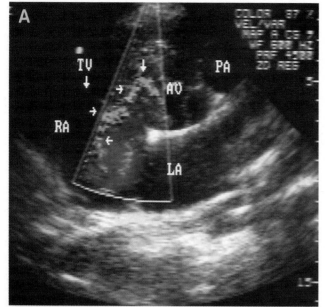

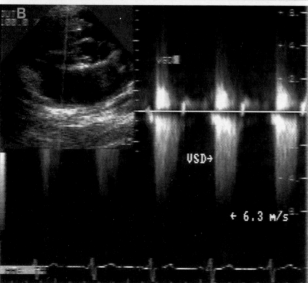

**Fig. 7–66.** In *A*, color flow imaging from the parasternal short-axis view through the base demonstrates a perimembranous ventricular septal defect. The turbulent flow through the defect (green mosaic, *arrows*) originates just below the aortic valve and extends posteriorly toward the tricuspid valve (TV) and right atrium (RA). In *B*, continuous wave Doppler in the same area demonstrates a posteriorly directed jet with a maximal systolic velocity of 6.3 m/sec consistent with a peak gradient of 160 mm Hg. LA = left atrium; PA = pulmonary artery; VSD = ventricular septal defect; Ao = aorta.

should also be used to assess the relative position of the two atrioventricular valves. In the presence of an uncomplicated inlet ventricular septal defect, the normal apical displacement of the tricuspid valve is preserved. If both valves are in the same plane, an atrioventricular canal defect is present. Because most inlet defects are large, care must be taken to avoid confusing this lesion with double-inlet left ventricle.

Malalignment between the septa can also be detected from the four-chamber view. When the atrial and ventricular septa are not aligned, it is essential that the chordal attachments of the atrioventricular valves are carefully assessed.[215–217] It is crucial to differentiate between a straddling atrioventricular valve (in which some chordae traverse the defect to insert into the opposite ventricle) and an overriding valve (which overlies the defect, but has no chordae extending through to the opposite ventricle). In the former case, the presence of chordae crossing the defect greatly complicates surgical repair (Figs. 7–72 and 7–73). Chordal attachments crossing an inlet ventricular septal defect may obscure the defect, leading to a false-negative interpretation.

Defects in the trabecular portion of the muscular septum may be difficult to record with two-dimensional echocardiography.[205] All available planes should be used to exclude the possibility of small defects in this region (Figs. 7–74 and 7–75). Trabecular defects may appear as narrow, irregular channels through the muscular septum. Thus, the orifice on one side of the septum may be displaced from the orifice on the other side, precluding visualization of the entire course in one plane. Once a trabecular defect is identified, it is essential to recognize the possibility of multiple defects and a careful search should be undertaken. Defects located in the api-

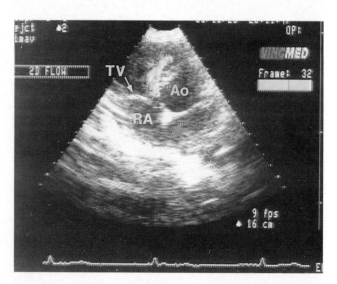

**Fig. 7–67.** Color flow mapping from the parasternal short-axis view at the base of another patient with a perimembranous ventricular septal defect demonstrates the turbulent jet originating just below the aortic valve and extending anteriorly across the base of the septal leaflet of the tricuspid valve (TV) and toward the right ventricular outflow tract. Ao = aorta; RA = right atrium.

both the inlet and trabecular ventricular septum. By tilting the scanning plane inferiorly, the inlet portion of the septum is imaged in the area between the atrioventricular valves. In infants and young children, scanning anteriorly also allows recording of the outlet portion. Although the septum is parallel to the beam in this projection, the four-chamber view is ideal for detecting inlet ventricular septal defects (Fig. 7–71). This view

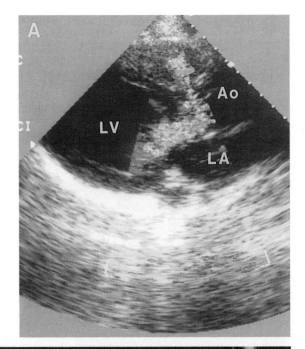

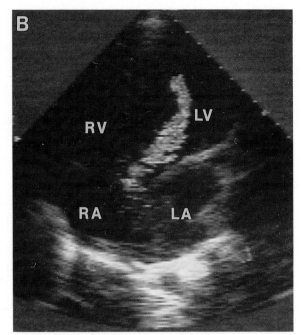

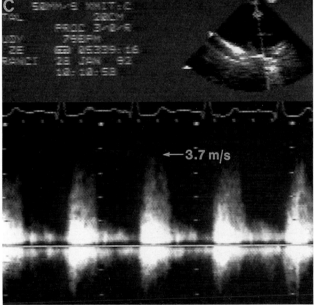

**Fig. 7–68.** An example of perimembranous outlet ventricular septal defect. In *A*, color flow mapping in the parasternal long-axis view reveals turbulent flow through the interventricular septum from left to right. Acceleration of flow within the left ventricular outflow tract is also seen in this systolic frame. In *B*, color flow imaging in the apical four-chamber view during diastole reveals severe aortic regurgitation. In *C*, continuous wave Doppler recording of the ventricular septal defect flow indicates a maximal velocity of 3.7 m/sec, indicating a peak pressure gradient of 55 mm Hg. Ao = aorta; LA = left atrium; RV = right ventricle; RA = right atrium; LV = left ventricle.

cal portion of the septum are especially likely to be multiple (so-called "Swiss cheese" defects). In such cases, detection is greatly facilitated by the simultaneous use of color Doppler imaging.[214,218]

In some instances, a ventricular septal defect is suspected, but it cannot be visualized directly with two-dimensional echocardiography. Such defects are either small or located in a part of the septum that is difficult to assess. In these situations, Doppler can enhance the sensitivity for detection. A small restrictive ventricular septal defect is recorded with Doppler as a high-velocity systolic jet crossing the septum from left to right. To detect such jets, the right ventricular septal surface is carefully and systematically interrogated using multiple views. Although any of the Doppler modes (including pulsed and continous wave) can be used for this purpose, color flow imaging is now the preferred technique. This method allows faster and more thorough scanning of the septum.[210] Small defects appear as thin jets of turbulent flow within (and on the right ventricular side of) the septum (Fig. 7–76). Larger defects are characterized by a wider jet when imaged with color Doppler (Fig. 7–77). When the location of the defect is unknown, the left parasternal, apical, and subcostal windows should be used for screening. This method is currently the most sensitive means by which to detect small ventricular

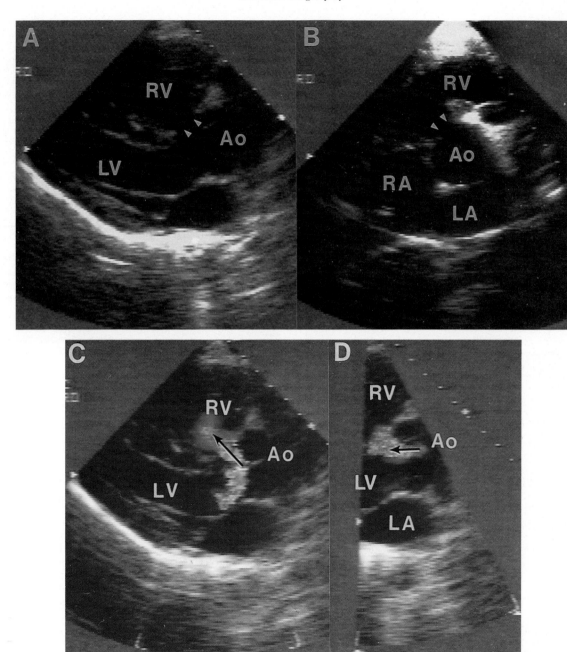

**Fig. 7–69.** In *A*, the parasternal long-axis view of a patient with a large perimembranous outlet ventricular septal defect reveals a dilated right ventricle (RV) and the defect below the aortic valve (*arrowheads*). In *B*, the parasternal short-axis view again reveals the location of the defect just below the aortic valve. In *C*, color flow imaging in the parasternal long-axis view demonstrates left-to-right shunting across the defect. In *D*, a diastolic frame from the parasternal long-axis view reveals mild aortic regurgitation, with the jet oriented toward the large defect. Ao = aorta; LA = left atrium; LV = left ventricle; RA = right atrium; RV = right ventricle.

septal defects and is the only noninvasive technique in which multiple defects can be identified reliably. With proper gain setting, false-positive results are rare.

In addition to detecting a ventricular septal defect, Doppler plays an important role in assessing the magnitude and direction of the shunt.[219] For example, with color flow imaging, a small defect is characterized by a turbulent, high-velocity jet extending from left to right

across the septum and into the right ventricular cavity. Once the jet is identified, the Doppler beam can be oriented parallel to flow to permit recording of the peak jet velocity.[220–223] With restrictive defects, the jet velocity is high, reflecting the high pressure gradient between the ventricles during systole (Fig. 7–78). With larger defects, the pressure gradient is less and, hence, the jet velocity is lower (Fig. 7–79). In the presence of a large

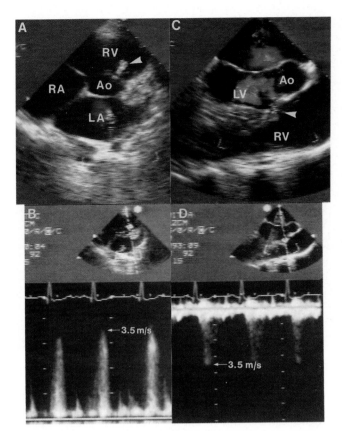

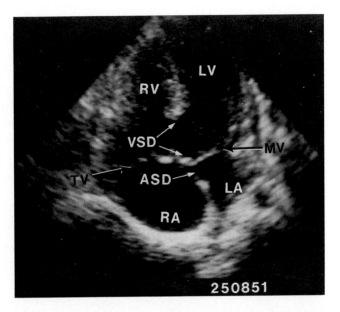

Fig. 7–71. A large inlet ventricular septal defect is demonstrated in the apical four-chamber view. An ostium primum atrial septal defect is also present. Also note that the mitral (MV) and tricuspid (TV) valves are in the same plane. These findings are diagnostic of endocardial cushion defect. LA = left atrium; LV = left ventricle; RA = right atrium; RV = right ventricle; ASD = atrial septal defect; VSD = ventricular septal defect.

Fig. 7–70. In *A*, the parasternal short-axis view at the base in a patient with a supracristal ventricular septal defect reveals the location of the defect above the crista supraventricularis and between the aortic and pulmonic valve. In *B*, continuous wave Doppler from the same view reveals a maximal systolic velocity of 3.5 m/sec. In *C*, the same patient is examined using transesophageal echocardiography in the longitudinal plane. Again, the turbulent flow throughout the defect is shown (*arrowhead*). Continuous wave Doppler from this window again demonstrates a maximal jet velocity of 3.5 m/sec, consistent with a peak pressure gradient between the left and right ventricle of 50 mm Hg. Ao = aorta; LA = left atrium; LV = left ventricle; RA = right atrium; RV = right ventricle.

ventricular septal defect and elevated right ventricular pressure, there may be relatively little flow across the defect. The flow can be assessed by using pulsed Doppler and color flow imaging and indicates the presence of Eisenmenger's physiology.

The pressure gradient between the ventricles can be estimated using the modified Bernoulli equation: gradient (mm Hg) = 4 × (peak velocity)$^2$. If the systolic blood pressure is determined by cuff recording of the upper extremity and no left ventricular outflow tract obstruction is present, the left ventricular (LV) systolic pressure can be determined. Then, right ventricular (RV) systolic pressure is calculated from the equation(s): gradient = LV (systolic) pressure − RV (systolic) pressure, or RV pressure = LV pressure − gradient, or RV pressure = cuff systolic blood pressure − [4 × (peak velocity)$^2$]. In the absence of right ventricular outflow tract obstruction, this value is equal to the

pulmonary artery systolic pressure. Thus, a noninvasive estimate of the presence and severity of pulmonary hypertension can be made. Alternatively, right ventricular systolic pressure can be calculated from the peak velocity of the tricuspid regurgitation jet using a similar equation: RV systolic pressure = right atrial pressure + [4

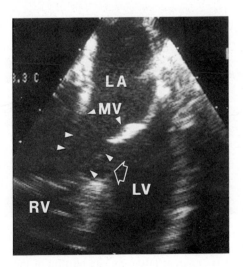

Fig. 7–72. Apical four-chamber view in a child with a large inlet ventricular septal defect (*open arrow*). The mitral valve (MV) overrides the crest of the septum and the chordae straddle the defect to insert on the right ventricular (RV) side. LA = left atrium; LV = left ventricle.

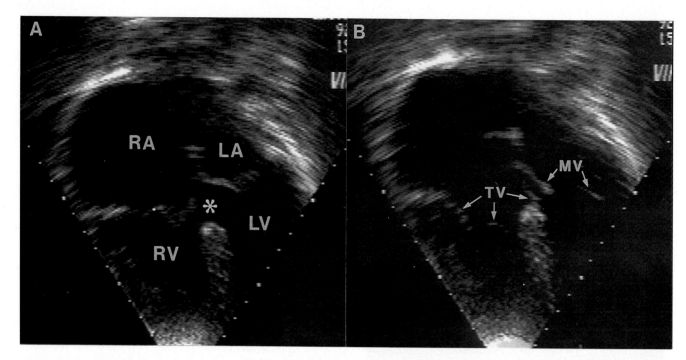

**Fig. 7–73.** Apical four-chamber views in systole (*A*) and diastole (*B*) in another patient with an inlet ventricular septal defect. The defect is seen most easily during systole (*asterisk*). The right side of the heart is dilated. There is no significant overriding of the atrioventricular valves. During diastole, a portion of the septal leaflet of the tricuspid valve (TV) appears to extend through the defect and insert into the left ventricular (LV) side. This is an example of a straddling tricuspid valve without overriding. LA = left atrium; LV = left ventricle; RA = right atrium; RV = right ventricle; MV = mitral valve.

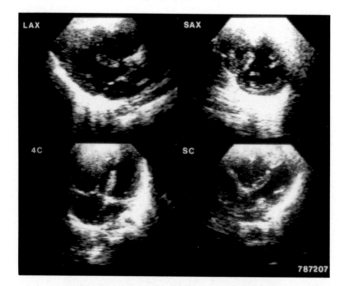

**Fig. 7–74.** A trabecular ventricular septal defect demonstrated in multiple views. In the parasternal long-axis (LAX), the defect is apparent in the middle portion of the muscular septum. In the parasternal short-axis (SAX), the defect is seen at approximately the 11 o'clock position. From the apical four-chamber (4C) view, the location of the defect appears more apical. Right atrial and ventricular dilation are apparent. From the subcostal (SC) window, the defect is again seen.

× (peak velocity)$^2$]. Using one or both of these approaches, an accurate measure of right ventricular pressure can be obtained in most patients.[223a]

A variety of associated lesions or complications occur in the setting of a ventricular septal defect, most of which are readily detected using echocardiography. Among the most common is the ventricular septal aneurysm,[224,225] a thin membrane of tissue that usually arises from the margin of the defect, sometimes by incorporation of a portion of tricuspid septal leaflet tissue (Fig. 7–80). Such aneurysms are commonly associated with perimembranous ventricular septal defects. Although aneurysms are usually patent, they may represent one mechanism for spontaneous closure of a ventricular septal defect. In one study, the presence of an aneurysm was associated with an increased likelihood of spontaneous closure.[226] The parasternal long-axis and short-axis views are most useful in detecting a ventricular septal aneurysm (Fig. 7–81). They are seen as thin, membranous pouches that bulge through the defect often with a windsock appearance. They may be highly mobile, often protruding through the defect into the right ventricle during systole. Once detected by two-dimensional echocardiography, they should be interrogated with Doppler, including color flow imaging (Fig. 7–82), which helps to determine the patency of the aneurysm. If the tricuspid valve is involved, the presence and severity of associated tricuspid regurgitation should be determined.

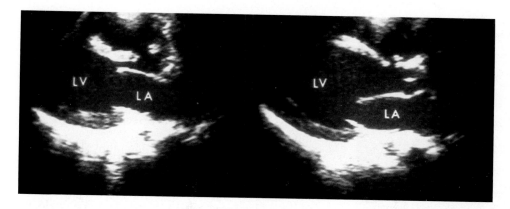

**Fig. 7–75.** Parasternal long-axis views from a patient with a large trabecular ventricular septal defect. Note that this defect is more basal than that presented in Figure 7–74. Also note that the size of the defect appears to vary considerably with the cardiac cycle. LA = left atrium; LV = left ventricle.

Another complication associated with ventricular septal defects is aortic regurgitation (see Figs. 7–65, 7–68, and 7–69), which occurs most commonly with outlet defects in which the support of the valve is undermined by an absence of myocardium below the annulus.[206] Perimembranous defects are also associated with aortic regurgitation. Prolapse of an aortic cusp through the defect occasionally is recorded. The finding of aortic regurgitation in a patient with a ventricular septal defect has important implications. Surgical closure is often recommended, even in the absence of a large shunt, to reduce the risk of progressive aortic valve dysfunction.

Echocardiography also plays a critical role in detecting endocarditis complicating a ventricular septal defect. In most cases, the vegetations tend to form on the right ventricular side of the defect, i.e., downstream from the high-velocity jet. Figure 7–83 is an example of infective

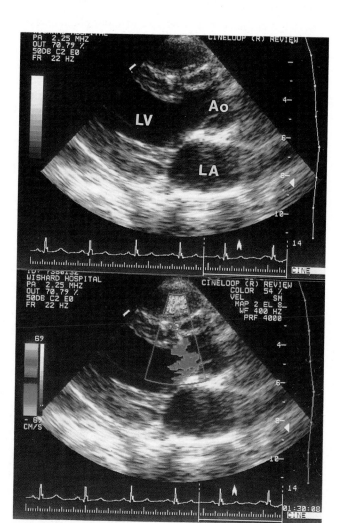

**Fig. 7–76.** Parasternal long-axis views from a patient with a small perimembranous ventricular septal defect. In *A*, the two-dimensional echocardiogram reveals no evidence of a defect. In *B*, using color flow imaging, a small defect is apparent with turbulent flow through the septum from left to right.

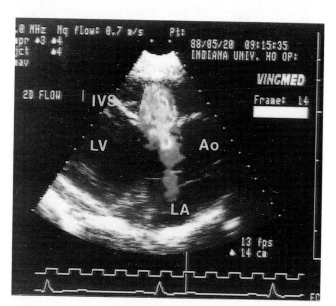

**Fig. 7–77.** Color flow imaging in the parasternal long-axis view from a patient with a large perimembranous ventricular septal defect. The width of the color flow jet indicates a larger defect than is evident in the example in Figure 7–76. Ao = aorta; LA = left atrium; LV = left ventricle; IVS = interventricular septum.

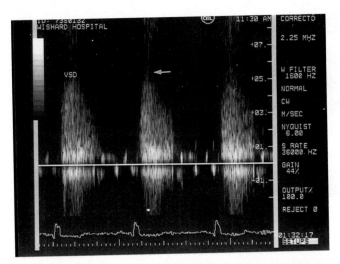

**Fig. 7-78.** Continuous wave Doppler recording from the same patient as in Figure 7-76. The recording was made from a high parasternal window. The maximal systolic flow velocity is approximately 5.5 m/sec, indicating a pressue gradient between the left and right ventricle of approximately 120 mm Hg. This finding is consistent with a small ventricular septal defect and normal right ventricular systolic pressure. VSD = ventricular septal defect.

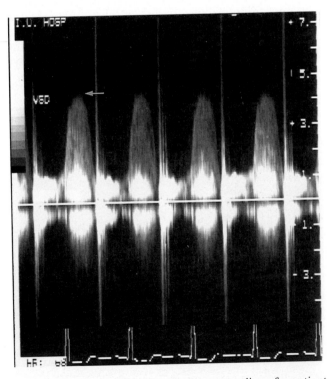

**Fig. 7-79.** Continuous wave Doppler recording of a patient with a ventricular septal defect. The maximal systolic velocity is 4.3 m/sec, indicating a peak gradient between the left and right ventricle of 74 mm Hg. In this patient, the systolic blood pressure was 140 mm Hg. Thus, the estimated right ventricular systolic pressure was elevated at 66 mm Hg.

endocarditis in a patient with a large trabecular ventricular septal defect. The vegetations are apparent on the tricuspid valve and were associated with severe tricuspid regurgitation. Another example of bacterial endocarditis complicating a ventricular septal defect is presented in Figure 7-84. Echocardiography is an excellent means by which to diagnose complications such as endocarditis and to assess for progression or regression of the infection.

After surgical repair, echocardiography can be used to determine the integrity of the ventricular septal defect patch (Fig. 7-85).[202,227,228] Color flow imaging is probably the most sensitive technique for detection of a residual shunt, which is recorded as a turbulent, high-velocity jet at the periphery of the patch (Fig. 7-86). The width of the jet has been correlated with the magnitude of the shunt and the likelihood of the need for reoperation.[227]

## Endocardial Cushion Defect

Division of the common atrioventricular canal into left and right sides occurs by fusion of the superior and inferior endocardial cushions. Failure to do so results in an atrioventricular septal defect with various combinations of ostium primum atrial septal defect, inlet ventricular septal defect, and structural abnormalities of the atrioventricular valves. Thus, an endocardial cushion defect is a spectrum of lesions including partial atrioventricular canal (implying separate atrioventricular orifices), complete atrioventricular canal (a common atrioventricular orifice), and isolated inlet ventricular septal defect.[168,229]

Two-dimensional echocardiography permits detailed assessment of virtually every morphologic feature of endocardial cushion defect.[166,168–170,230] The primum portion of the atrial septum, the inlet ventricular septum, atrioventricular valve morphology, ventriculoatrial septal malalignment, and ventricular outflow tract obstruction[231] can be accurately assessed. The four-chamber views generally yield the most diagnostic information in this entity (Figs. 7-71 and 7-87).[170] Importantly, the presence and size of the atrial and ventricular septal defects can be determined and the anatomy of the atrioventricular valves can be assessed. Because the valve leaflets move freely within the defect, accurate assessment of these features requires real-time imaging. During systole, the atrioventricular valve assumes a basal position, obscuring the primum atrial septal defect, but permitting assessment of the size of the inlet ventricular septal defect and the presence of atrioventricular valve regurgitation. As the valve opens in diastole, the atrial portion of the defect can be examined. Chordal attachments and the presence of straddling (Figs. 7-72 and 7-73) can also be determined. Although atrioventricular valve regurgitation can be detected from the four-chamber view (Fig. 7-88), the presence of a cleft anterior mitral valve leaflet is better recorded from the parasternal short-axis view (Fig. 7-89).[166,169] The short-axis view also permits visualization of both the atrial and ventricular septal defects

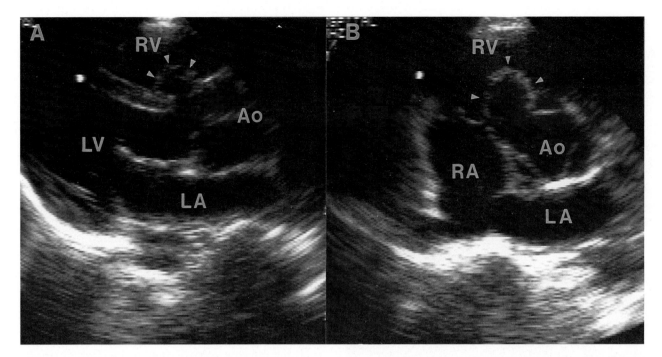

**Fig. 7–80.** Two-dimensional echocardiograms from a patient with a perimembranous ventricular septal defect. The defect has closed through the formation of a large ventricular septal aneurysm (*arrowheads*). Color flow imaging confirmed lack of blood flow through the aneurysm. On examination, this patient had no evidence of a residual septal defect, but significant aortic regurgitation was present. Ao = aorta; LA = left atrium; LV = left ventricle; RA = right atrium; RV = right ventricle.

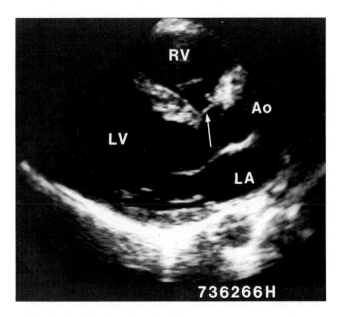

**Fig. 7–81.** Parasternal long-axis examination in an adult with a history of a spontaneously closed ventricular septal defect. In the region of the membranous ventricular septum, a fine linear echo connects the anterior aortic wall to the ventricular septum, which probably represents closure by adherence of a tricuspid leaflet to the small ventricular septal defect. LA = left atrium; LV = left ventricle; RV = right ventricle; Ao = aorta.

(Fig. 7–90). In the four-chamber view, the presence of left ventricle-to-right atrial shunting can be detected by using color flow imaging.

Because of the broad spectrum of anomalies that may occur in the setting of an endocardial cushion defect, echocardiography plays a major role in determining the feasibility of surgical repair (Fig. 7–91). Specifically, the relative size of the ventricles, the presence of septal malalignment, and the extent of the atrial and ventricular communications should be established.[169,170,232,233] The morphology of the atrioventricular valves is also critical in planning reparative surgery. Echocardiography allows the anatomy of the valves and their chordal insertions to be determined. The presence of a straddling or overriding valve and the degree of valvular regurgitation can also be assessed.[215–217,234] During surgery, the use of transesophageal echocardiography permits assessment of the adequacy of repair.[235] Most importantly, the presence and severity of residual atrioventricular valve regurgitation can be determined.

## ABNORMAL VASCULAR CONNECTIONS AND STRUCTURES

### Patent Ductus Arteriosus

The ductus arteriosus is the normal fetal vascular channel that connects the descending aorta and the main pulmonary artery, providing a conduit for blood from

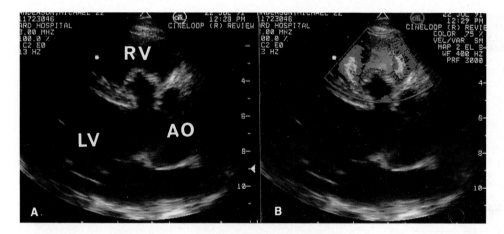

**Fig. 7–82.** *A,* Two-dimensional echocardiogram from a patient with a perimembranous ventricular septal defect and a large ventricular septal aneurysm. *B,* Color flow imaging in the parasternal long-axis view discloses left-to-right shunting at multiple sites, indicated by the turbulent mosaic flow at the edges of the aneurysm. AO = aorta; LV = left ventricle; RV = right ventricle.

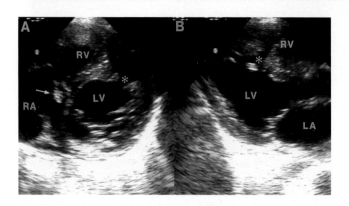

**Fig. 7–83.** In *A,* parasternal short-axis view through the midportion of the left ventricle in a patient with bacterial endocarditis complicating a trabecular ventricular septal defect reveals the defect at approximately two o'clock (*asterisk*). A large, echogenic mass is attached to the atrial side of the septal leaflet of the tricuspid valve (*arrow*). In *B,* the parasternal long-axis view again demonstrates the ventricular septal defect (*asterisk*) as a complex and irregular channel within the interventricular septum. In this patient, *Staphylococcus* was grown from multiple blood cultures. LA = left atrium; LV = left ventricle; RA = right atrium; RV = right ventricle.

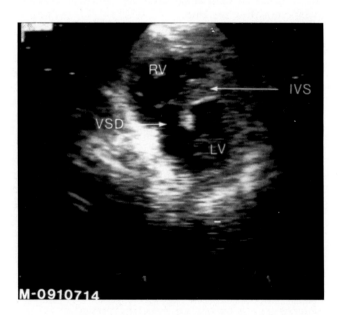

**Fig. 7–84.** Parasternal short-axis view in a patient with a large inlet ventricular septal defect (VSD). Attached to the left ventricular side of the defect is a large, echogenic, mobile mass consistent with a vegetation. IVS = interventricular septum; LV = left ventricle; RV = right ventricle.

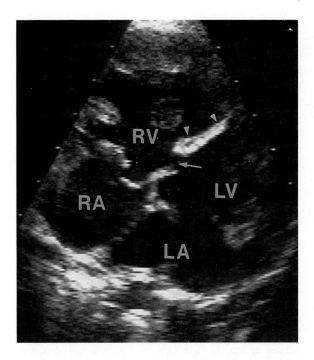

**Fig. 7–85.** Subcostal four-chamber view from a patient with D-transposition of the great arteries and a large ventricular septal defect. The patient had undergone a prior intra-atrial baffle procedure and surgical closure of the ventricular septal defect. The patch is indicated by arrowheads. The arrow depicts a gap at the superior edge of the patch caused by dehiscence of the patch. Note the hypertrophy and trabeculation within the right (systemic) ventricle (RV). The intra-atrial baffle is not well seen in this view. LA = left atrium; RA = right atrium; LV = left ventricle.

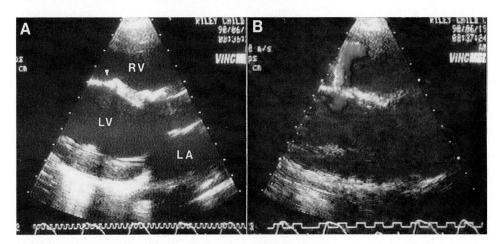

**Fig. 7–86.** Parasternal long-axis views after repair of a large trabecular ventricular septal defect. In *A*, the patch appears intact. In Panel *B*, however, color flow imaging reveals a significant residual defect with turbulent high-velocity, left-to-right shunting at the edge of the patch. LA = left atrium; LV = left ventricle; RV = right ventricle.

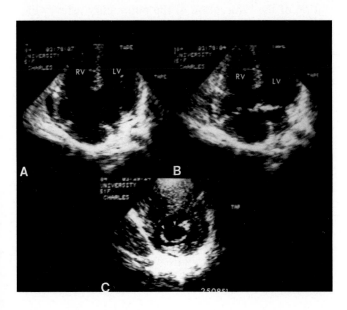

**Fig. 7–87.** Apical four-chamber views in a patient with an endocardial cushion defect during diastole (*A*) and systole (*B*). A large atrioventricular septal defect is apparent. The atrioventricular valves are at the same level and coapt within the defect. In *C*, the presence of a large cleft atrioventricular valve is indicated (*arrowheads*). LV = left ventricle; RV = right ventricle.

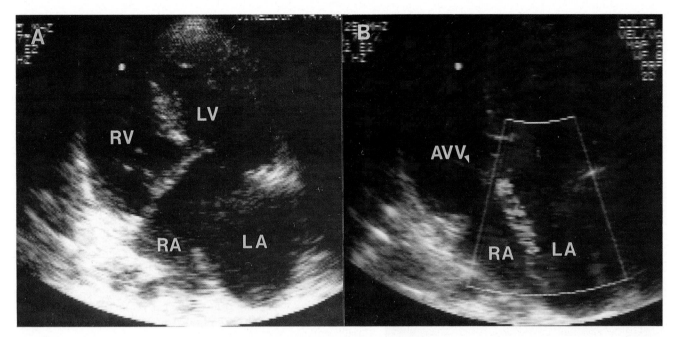

**Fig. 7–88.** Apical four-chamber views in a patient with endocardial cushion defect. In *A*, a large atrioventricular defect is apparent. A common atrioventricular valve is present. In *B*, significant atrioventricular valve regurgitation is documented with color flow imaging. LA = left atrium; LV = left ventricle; RA = right atrium; RV = right ventricle; AVV = atrioventricular valve.

the right ventricle to the thoracic aorta. Failure of the ductus to close shortly after birth is abnormal, giving rise to the term patent ductus arteriosus. This persistent patency of the ductus may be desirable or undesirable, depending on the presence of other associated anomalies. Expedient and accurate detection of this vascular channel has profound implications for the critically ill newborn.[236,237] Later in life, patent ductus arteriosus is one of the important causes of a left-to-right shunting and a volume overload of the left ventricle. The functional significance of a patent ductus arteriosus depends on the size of the channel, the pulmonary vascular resistance, and the presence and degree of left ventricular dysfunction.

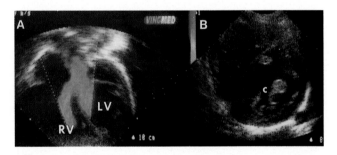

**Fig. 7–89.** In *A*, an apical four-chamber view in a patient with endocardial cushion defect. Color flow imaging demonstrates left-to-right shunting across the atrioventricular septal defect. Significant atrioventricular valve regurgitation was also present. In *B*, parasternal short-axis view at the level of the atrioventricular valve demonstrates a cleft (c) in the anterior leaflet. (Courtesy of Gregory J. Ensing.) LV = left ventricle; RV = right ventricle.

Both echocardiography and Doppler are crucial in the assessment of patients with patent ductus arteriosus. The first step in imaging a ductus is knowing where to look for it.[238,239] The pulmonary arterial end of the ductus is located to the left of the pulmonary trunk and adjacent to the left pulmonary artery. The aortic insertion is opposite to and just beyond the origin of the left subclavian artery. The aortic orifice of the channel is usually larger than the pulmonary end, giving the ductus a funnel shape. For direct visualization, the suprasternal and high parasternal short-axis views are used.[238–240] In the parasternal short-axis view, angling the imaging plane in a leftward and superior direction allows visualization of the bifurcation of the pulmonary artery (Fig. 7–92). Clockwise rotation permits recording of a greater length of the descending aorta so that the entire ductus may be visualized. From the suprasternal window, the ductus is seen as a narrow channel extending from the inferior border of the aorta to the pulmonary trunk. Unfortunately, this view has significant limitations, particularly in adults. The ductus can be recorded directly in only a few patients and care must be taken to avoid mistaking the left pulmonary artery for a large ductal channel.

Thus, the sensitivity of two-dimensional echocardiography for detecting patent ductus arteriosus is considerably higher in infants than in adults.[238,240,241] The ability of echocardiography to record a ductus depends on the width and length of the channel and the inherent difficulties in obtaining the necessary views in older patients (Fig. 7–93).[242,243] The shape and length of the ductus are variable, especially in the presence of complex congenital heart disease. In addition, the ductus is often aligned such that it is parallel to the ultrasound beam, and it is therefore subject to the limitations of lateral resolution. In adults, transesophageal echocardiography may be used to diagnose a patent ductus arteriosus when transthoracic imaging is suboptimal (Fig. 7–94).[244]

The left-to-right shunt associated with a patent ductus results in a volume overload of the left ventricle. The degree of left atrial and left ventricular dilation is a useful marker of the magnitude of shunting. In infants, the left atrium to aortic root ratio is a rough indictor of the size of the shunt. In older patients, this sign is less valuable because of the multitude of factors that can affect left atrial size. Even so, a dilated and hyperdynamic left side of the heart is an indication of volume overload and, in the absence of other causes, suggests the presence of a significant left-to-right shunt.[238,245]

Doppler echocardiography has become indispensable in the assessment of patients with patent ductus arteriosus.[237,241,243,246–250] The technique is especially helpful in confirming the presence of a small ductus when two-dimensional imaging is not diagnostic (Fig. 7–93). Early studies using Doppler for this purpose relied on the demonstration of turbulent flow in the main pulmonary artery that persisted throughout the cardiac cycle.[241] This finding is critically dependent on the presence of a left-to-right shunt and proper positioning of the Doppler sample volume. Furthermore, such a flow pattern is nonspecific and may be confused with that associated with pulmonic insufficiency, aortopulmonary window, and anomalous coronary artery arising from the pulmonary artery.

With greater experience using the various ultrasound techniques, direct recording of ductal flow became possible. Most commonly, high-velocity turbulent flow occurs continuously in a left-to-right direction, reaching a peak in late systole (Fig. 7–95).[237,249] In such cases, the peak pressure gradient can be calculated by using the modified Bernoulli equation. This method permits a quantitative estimate of pulmonary artery pressure.[251–253] If the ductus is relatively long (more than 7 mm), however, the simplified Bernoulli equation may be inaccurate. Infrequently, isolated right-to-left shunting or bidirectional shunting is noted. Bidirectional shunting always implies significantly elevated pulmonary vascular resistance.[237,249] In this situation, flow occurs from right to left in early systole and from left to right in late systole and diastole. As severity progresses, the duration and extent of right-to-left shunt flow in diastole increase.

Abnormal flow patterns can also be recorded in the descending aorta from the suprasternal notch.[254] If the sample volume is positioned in the aorta distal to the ductus, a pattern of retrograde flow in diastole may be seen. This finding is evidence of diastolic runoff of blood from the peripheral arteries into the ductus. The magnitude of this retrograde flow (i.e., the flow velocity integral) is roughly correlated with the size of the left-to-right shunt.

Color flow imaging can enhance the speed and accuracy of diagnosis.[244,255,256] In ducti too small to be detected with two-dimensional echocardiographic imag-

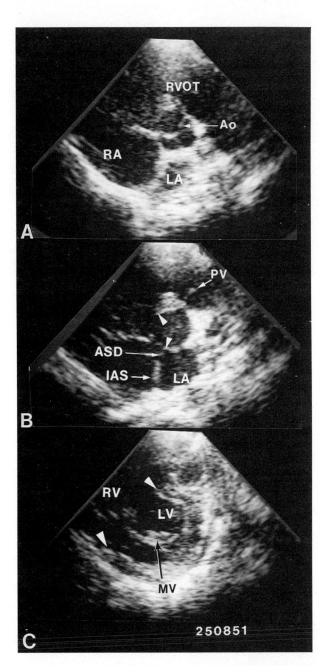

**Fig. 7–90.** Serial short-axis images from a patient with endocardial cushion defect. In *A*, the right atrium (RA) is dilated. The superior portion of the atrial septum appears intact. In *B*, a more apical plane demonstrates the atrioventricular septal defect. The atrial septal defect (ASD) involves the primum portion of the septum. In *C*, a more apical plane demonstrates the large inlet ventricular septal defect (*arrowheads*). Ao = aorta; LA = left atrium; RVOT = right ventricular outflow tract; PV = pulmonic valve; IAS = interatrial septum; MV = mitral valve; LV = left ventricle; RV = right ventricle.

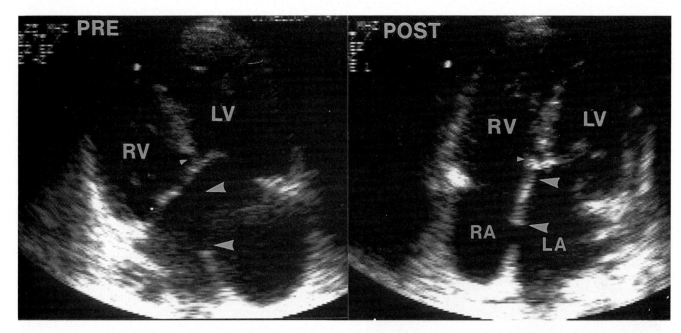

**Fig. 7–91.** Apical four-chamber views from a patient with endocardial cushion defect before (PRE) and after (POST) surgical repair. The preoperative image demonstrates a large ostium primum atrial septal defect (*large arrowheads*) and a relatively small inlet ventricular septal defect (*small arrowhead*). The postoperative image demonstrates the patch extending through the atrioventricular septal defect and supporting the atrioventricular valve. LA = left atrium; LV = left ventricle; RA = right atrium; RV = right ventricle.

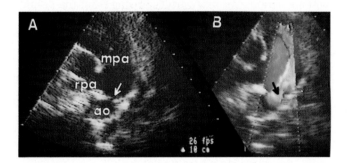

**Fig. 7–92.** Parasternal short-axis view from a patient with patent ductus arteriosus. In *A*, the two-dimensional echocardiogram demonstrates a dilated main pulmonary artery (mpa). The right pulmonary artery (rpa) and descending aorta (ao) are also seen. The site of the ductus (*arrow*) is not well visualized on two-dimensional echocardiographic imaging. In *B*, color flow mapping demonstrates turbulent high-velocity flow extending from the descending aorta into the distal main pulmonary artery. The jet flows in a proximal direction along the lateral wall of the pulmonary artery. (Courtesy of Gregory J. Ensing.)

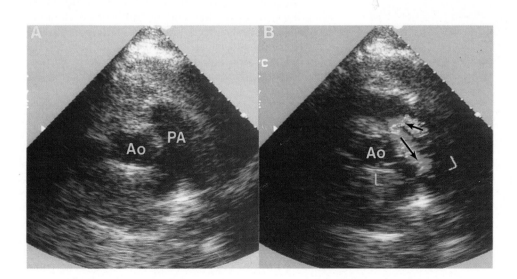

**Fig. 7–93.** Parasternal short-axis views at the base of the heart from a 68-year-old patient with patent ductus arteriosus. In *A*, the two-dimensional echocardiogram demonstrates a dilated pulmonary artery (PA). The bifurcation of a pulmonary artery is well visualized. In *B*, color flow imaging during systole reveals antegrade flow (colored blue) in the main pulmonary artery and a mosaic retrograde jet along the lateral border. This turbulent jet is the result of a patent ductus arteriosus. Ao = aorta.

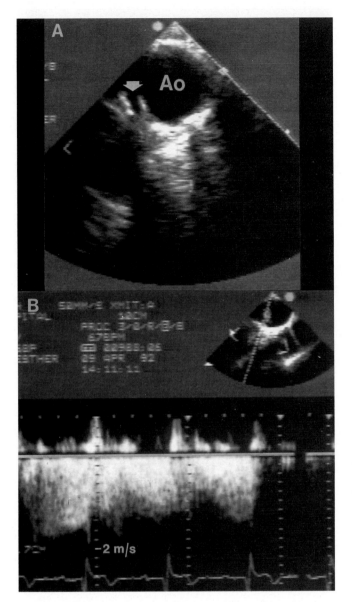

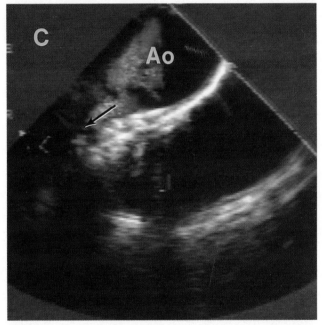

**Fig. 7–94.** Transesophageal echocardiographic images from the same patient as in Figure 7–93. In *A*, a short-axis view of the descending aorta demonstrates calcification at the origin of the ductus (*arrow*). In *B*, continuous wave Doppler recorded from the same view reveals continuous low-velocity flow from the aorta into the ductus. In *C*, color flow imaging confirms flow within this channel directed away from the descending aorta (Ao). The presence of the low-velocity flow within the ductus is primarily related to significant pulmonary hypertension and a relatively small pressure gradient between the aorta and the pulmonary artery. In addition, an inability to align the Doppler signal parallel to the ductal flow also contributes to underestimation of true velocity. Ao = aorta.

ing, a narrow jet of turbulent flow on color Doppler may be the first indication of a patent ductus arteriosus. This flow is usually best seen from the high parasternal short-axis view as a mosaic jet entering the distal pulmonary artery from the posterolateral direction (Fig. 7–96). The orientation of the jet within the pulmonary artery varies, and distinguishing it from normal pulmonary flow or pulmonic regurgitation may require slow-motion and freeze-frame analysis.

## Abnormal Systemic Venous Connections

A persistent left superior vena cava is the most common congenital anomaly involving the systemic veins. It occurs in approximately 0.5% of the general population and 3 to 10% of patients with congenital heart disease.[257] In most cases, the left superior vena cava drains into the right atrium by way of the coronary sinus (Fig. 7–97). As such, it has no physiologic consequences

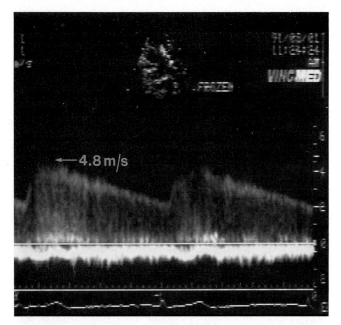

**Fig. 7–95.** Continuous wave Doppler flow within the ductus is recorded from the parasternal short-axis view. Flow above the base-line indicates flow from the aorta to the main pulmonary artery. In this young patient with normal pulmonary artery pressure, the peak velocity of the ductal flow is 4.8 m/sec, indicating a maximal gradient between the aorta and pulmonary artery of 92 mm Hg. Note that flow is continuous throughout the cardiac cycle, reaching a peak in late systole.

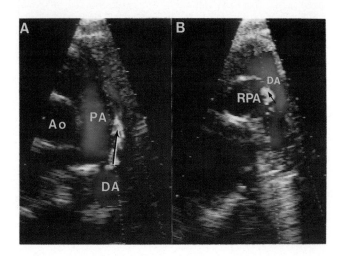

**Fig. 7–96.** Color flow images from a young patient with patent ductus arteriosus. In *A*, the angulated parasternal short-axis view at the base demonstrates the ductal flow from the descending aorta (DA) to the main pulmonary artery (PA). In *B*, a long-axis view of the descending aorta from the suprasternal notch demonstrates turbulent flow toward the right pulmonary artery (RPA). Note dilation of both the main and right pulmonary artery. Ao = aorta.

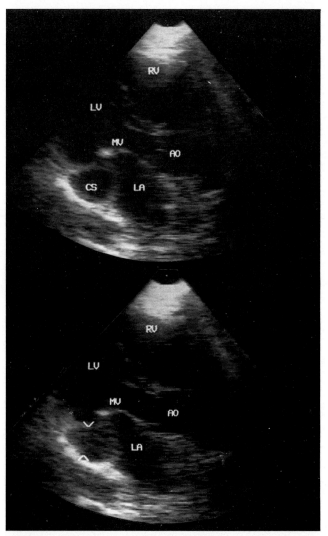

**Fig. 7–97.** Parasternal long-axis examination of a patient with a markedly dilated coronary sinus (CS) due to left superior vena cava to coronary sinus communication. The coronary sinus opacifies with contrast medium following a left arm venous injection of agitated saline. LA = left atrium; MV = mitral valve; LV = left ventricle; RV = right ventricle; Ao = aorta.

(aside from a predisposition to arrhythmias and heart block) and venous return is essentially normal. Less often, it drains into the left atrium (Fig. 7–98) or a pulmonary vein, resulting in a right-to-left shunt.[258,259] Associated lesions, especially defects of the atrial septum, are common.

Diagnosis of a persistent left superior vena cava frequently occurs after a dilated coronary sinus is detected with echocardiography.[260,261] Coronary sinus dilation is usually the result of anomalous drainage to the sinus, either from a persistent left superior vena cava or an anomalous pulmonary vein. Dilation may also occur secondary to elevated right atrial pressure. Dilation, however, usually results from some form of anomalous drainage. Occasionally, the degree of coronary sinus en-

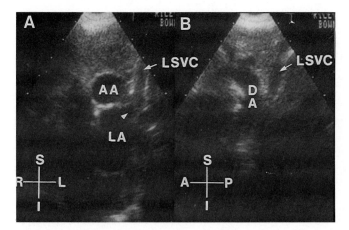

**Fig. 7–98.** The suprasternal short-axis view (*A*) of a patient with a persistent left superior vena cava (LSVC) demonstrates a vertically oriented left superior vena cava adjacent to the aortic arch (AA). In *B*, a long-axis view of the aortic arch and descending aorta (DA) again demonstrates the left superior vena cava posterior to the aorta. In this patient, the anomalous vessel (*arrow*) drained into the left atrium (LA). A = anterior; P = posterior; S = superior; I = inferior; R = right; L = left.

largement is so great that the structure is mistaken for something else, such as a pericardial effusion, pulmonary vein, or descending aorta.

The coronary sinus is best visualized in the parasternal long-axis view as a circular structure in the posterior atrioventricular groove (Figs. 7–99 and 7–100). Its location anterior to the pericardium distinguishes it from other venous and arterial structures. In the parasternal short-axis view, the coronary sinus can be recorded as a tubular, crescent-shaped structure lying within the

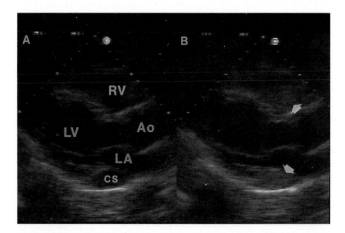

**Fig. 7–99.** Parasternal long-axis view from a patient with a dilated coronary sinus (cs). In *A*, the coronary sinus appears as an oval echo-free space behind the left atrium (LA). In *B*, opacification of both the coronary sinus and right ventricle (RV) is apparent following peripheral contrast injection into the left arm because of a persistent left superior vena cava draining into the coronary sinus. Ao = aorta; LV = left ventricle.

atrioventricular groove and communicating with the right atrium. Occasionally, a Chiari network is seen where the coronary sinus empties into the posterior right atrium. When significantly dilated, the coronary sinus occasionally is confused with the descending aorta. This distinction is readily apparent when the structure is interrogated in the long axis.

Direct visualization of a persistent left superior vena cava is easier in children than in adults. The vessel can be seen from the suprasternal window as a vertical structure to the left of the aortic arch (Fig. 7–98). This view is particularly helpful in determining if both vena cavae are present, to assess their relative size, and to detect an innominate vein. The connections between the cavae and the atria should also be examined. In adults, this determination is challenging. Doppler can be helpful in several ways. Color Doppler may be used to distinguish higher velocity arterial flow (which, at usual gain settings, appears as red or blue laminar flow in systole) from venous flow (which is often not detected with color flow imaging). Pulsed Doppler can be used to confirm venous flow, by recording low-velocity, phasic flow in a superior-to-inferior direction. More recently, transesophageal echocardiography has been used to evaluate abnormal systemic venous connections.[262,263]

Contrast-enhanced echocardiography is of great value in the differential diagnosis of a dilated coronary sinus and to assess abnormal vena caval connections (see Figs. 7–99 and 7–100).[260] If injection into the left arm results in opacification of the coronary sinus and then the right atrium, the diagnosis of a persistent left superior vena cava is likely. If the same injection leads to left atrial opacification, abnormal drainage of the vena cava (either left or common) is present. This pattern of drainage is unusual and typically is associated with other cardiac lesions. Injection into the right arm should then be performed. In the presence of a left superior vena cava (draining into either the left or right atrium), this injection should lead to the normal sequence of opacification (i.e., no opacification of the coronary sinus).

### Abnormal Pulmonary Venous Connections

Anomalous pulmonary venous return may be total or partial. Total anomalous pulmonary venous return is characterized by drainage of all four pulmonary veins into a systemic venous tributary of the right atrium or into the right atrium itself. The connections may be above or below the diaphragm and may or may not involve an element of obstruction. Some degree of interatrial admixing is mandatory and provides the only access for pulmonary venous blood to the left heart (Fig. 7–101). The degree and direction of the shunt depends on the size of the interatrial communication and the relative compliance of the two ventricles. Associated cardiac anomalies are present in more than one third of patients. Survival beyond infancy without surgical palliation or repair is unlikely, so this entity is not encountered in the adult population of patients with congenital heart disease.

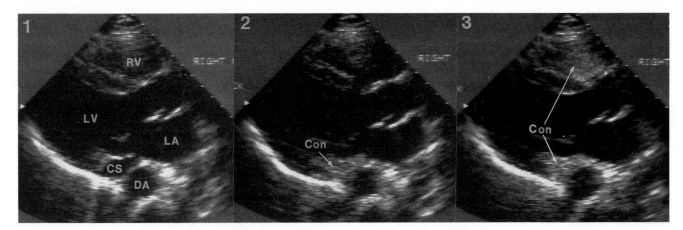

**Fig. 7–100.** Sequential frames recorded over several seconds from the parasternal long-axis view in a patient with dilated coronary sinus (CS). The relative position of the coronary sinus and descending aorta (DA) is shown. Panel *1* represents a baseline frame before peripheral injection of contrast material. Panel *2* is recorded soon after contrast injection into the right arm. The first structure to be opacified is the coronary sinus. Soon thereafter (panel *3*), the right ventricle is opacified. This sequence of events is consistent with drainage of the superior vena cava into the coronary sinus. Because opacification of the coronary sinus occurred with both right and left arm injection, this sequence is not the result of a persistent left superior vena cava. LA = left atrium; LV = left ventricle; RV = right ventricle; Con = contrast.

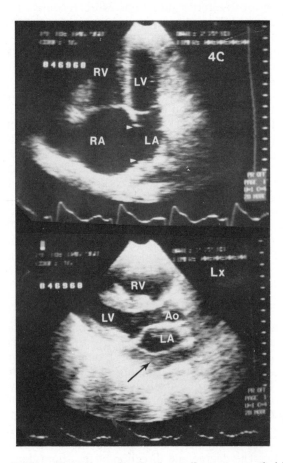

**Fig. 7–101.** Two-dimensional echocardiogram recorded in a patient with total anomalous pulmonary venous return. In the parasternal long-axis view (*B*), a linear echo is seen dividing the left atrium into a true atrium and a common posterior drainage chamber (*arrow*). In the four-chamber view (*A*), note the large atrial septal defect (*arrowheads*). RA = right atrium; LA = left atrium; RV = right ventricle; LV = left ventricle; Ao = aorta.

Partial anomalous pulmonary venous return occurs when some but not all (usually one or two) of the pulmonary veins connect to the right rather than the left atrium. The situation occurs in 10% of patients with an ostium secundum atrial septal defect and in more than 80% of patients with a sinus venosus defect. The most common anomalous connections (in decreasing order of frequency) are: (1) right upper pulmonary vein connecting to the right atrium or superior vena cava (accounting for over 90% of cases and often in association with a sinus venosus atrial septal defect), (2) left pulmonary veins connecting to an innominate vein, and (3) right pulmonary veins connecting to the inferior vena cava. The physiologic consequences of partial anomalous pulmonary venous drainage may be minor, especially if only one pulmonary vein is involved. If more of the pulmonary venous drainage is diverted to the right side of the heart, evidence of right atrial and right ventricular volume overload will be present.[264,265]

The echocardiographic diagnosis of these disorders relies on visualization of the termination of the four pulmonary veins and detection of a venous confluence with connection to the right atrium, coronary sinus, or vena cava. In total anomalous pulmonary venous return, the venous confluence may be located posterior, inferior, or superior to the left atrium (Figs. 7–102 and 7–103). The parasternal, apical, suprasternal, and subcostal views all play a role in diagnosis because the confluence may be small and difficult to image.[266–275] Imaging the pulmonary veins behind or near the left atrium does not prove that they connect to the left atrium. A careful search for the pulmonary veins entering the left atrium should be undertaken. If normal connections are not seen, a pulmonary venous confluence and abnormal connection to the right atrium should be sought. As discussed previously, a dilated coronary sinus is sometimes the initial echocardiographic abnormality detected, and

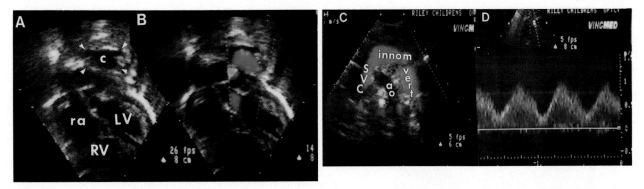

**Fig. 7–102.** In *A*, the apical four-chamber view in an infant with total anomalous pulmonary venous return reveals a structure posterior and superior to the left atrium representing the pulmonary venous confluence (c). The arrowheads indicate the entrance of the pulmonary veins. Low-velocity flow within the confluence is demonstrated in *B* using color flow imaging. In *C*, a suprasternal short-axis view reveals the presence of a vertical vein (vert), the innominate vein (innom), and the superior vena cava (SVC). Color flow imaging demonstrates red flow within the vertical vein (directed toward the transducer) and blue flow in the innominate vein and superior vena cava (directed away from the transducer). Superiorly oriented flow in the vertical vein was confirmed in *D* by using pulsed Doppler. A normal venous structure in this region would be expected to drain toward the heart, i.e., away from the transducer. (Courtesy of Gregory J. Ensing.) Ao = aorta, ra = right atrium; LV = left ventricle; RV = right ventricle.

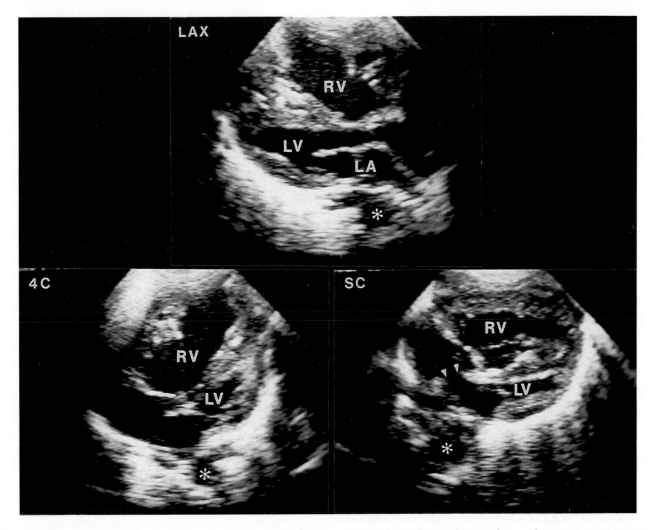

**Fig. 7–103.** Two-dimensional echocardiographic views from another patient with total anomalous pulmonary venous return. In the parasternal long-axis view (LAX), a dilated right ventricle (RV) is apparent. Posterior to the left atrium (LA) is the pulmonary venous confluence (*asterisk*). In the four-chamber view (4C), the dilated right heart is well seen. Again, the pulmonary venous confluence can be identified posterior and lateral to the left atrium. The structure is once again visualized in the subcostal (SC) image. An ostium secundum atrial septal defect is also demonstrated (*arrowheads*). LV = left ventricle.

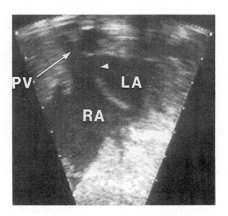

**Fig. 7–104.** A subcostal view from a patient with sinus venosus atrial septal defect. By rotating the transducer in a clockwise direction, the superior portion of the interatrial septum is clearly seen (*arrowhead*). The anomalous pulmonary vein (PV) is recorded entering the right atrium (RA). LA = left atrium.

this finding should always prompt a search for anomalous pulmonary venous drainage.[260,274] After the diagnosis is established, the interatrial communication should be characterized. Doppler is often useful in this setting to determine the direction of flow within venous channels.[276,277] The direction of venous flow may allow differentiation between a normal systemic vein and an anomalous pulmonary vein (see Fig. 7–102).

Partial anomalous pulmonary venous return may be difficult to diagnose because of the technical problems in identifying all four pulmonary venous connections to the left atrium.[278] Unless all four vessels are identified, it is impossible to completely exclude the possibility of an anomalous vein. In most cases, the possibility of anomalous pulmonary veins is considered when an atrial septal defect and/or dilation of the right side of the heart are detected (Fig. 7–104). When this situation occurs, a careful search for all four pulmonary veins should be performed. Most often, the anomaly involves the right pulmonary veins and the abnormal connection is usually near the right side of the atrial septum or the base of the superior vena cava. The suprasternal, apical four-chamber, and subcostal views should be used. Using the subcostal window, the superior portion of the interatrial septum is consistently seen. By clockwise rotation of the transducer, the entry of the right upper pulmonary vein and superior vena cava can be recorded. This view is usually the best with which to diagnose partial anomalous pulmonary venous return. Color Doppler is often helpful for identifying the pulmonary veins and their continuity (or lack thereof) with the left atrium.[278,279] More recently, transesophageal echocardiography has been used to visualize the distal pulmonary veins.[263,280] The proximity of the transducer to the left atrium makes this an ideal technique to assess pulmonary venous connections and the presence or absence of a pulmonary venous confluence. In addition, the location of the anomalous veins relative to the atrial septum and the

presence of small sinus venosus septal defects are optimally assessed with this method.

### Abnormalities of the Coronary Circulation

The most important congenital abnormalities involving the coronary circulation include anomalous origin of the coronary arteries and coronary artery fistulae. Coronary artery aneurysms, which may be congenital but more commonly are associated with Kawasaki disease, are also discussed in this section.

Anomalous origin of a coronary artery is present in approximately 1% of patients undergoing cardiac catheterization. Origin of the left circumflex artery from the right coronary sinus and origin of the right coronary artery from the left sinus are the most frequently encountered variants. These anomalies are of particular relevance when the course of the aberrant artery passes between the aorta and the pulmonary trunk. The ostia and proximal coronary arteries can be imaged with echocardiography from the parasternal short-axis view at the base. This view permits determination of the size and initial course of the arteries.[281,282] In adults, transesophageal echocardiography generally provides higher quality images of the proximal coronary arteries and anomalous vessels can be identified with a high degree of accuracy.[283–285] An inability to record the origin of the coronary artery from this view raises the possibility of an aberrant vessel.

Coronary artery anatomy may be especially important in certain forms of complex congenital heart disease, such as tetralogy of Fallot and transposition of the great arteries. In these patients, assessment of coronary artery anomalies[286–288] and vessel diameter[289] has implications for prognosis and surgical repair.

In a newborn with heart failure, origin of the left coronary artery from the pulmonary trunk should be considered.[290] These infants usually have congestive heart failure and a dilated and hypokinetic left ventricle. Distinguishing between anomalous left coronary artery and dilated cardiomyopathy as the cause of the left ventricular dysfunction is often possible by using echocardiographic techniques.[291,292] In patients with an anomalous left coronary artery, the right coronary artery is dilated and the left coronary ostium is absent from the aortic root. Wall motion abnormalities tend to be global in patients with dilated cardiomyopathy and more regional (involving the anterior wall) in patients with an anomalous left coronary artery.[293] The left coronary artery may be visualized, but does not connect with the aorta. Using a high parasternal view of the pulmonary trunk (similar to that used to evaluate a patent ductus arteriosus), the vessel can be seen arising from the posterior wall of the pulmonary trunk (Fig. 7–105).[294,295] The addition of Doppler imaging has been reported to increase the accuracy of this determination.[296,297]

Coronary artery fistula is a rare anomaly that results from the abnormal connection between a coronary artery and another vessel or chamber (either a coronary vein, pulmonary artery, or right ventricle). This connection results in a left-to-right shunt and a continuous

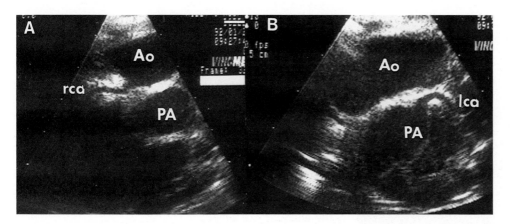

**Fig. 7–105.** An anomalous left coronary artery (lca) is illustrated. In *A*, the right coronary artery (rca) can be traced to the right coronary sinus of the aortic root (Ao). In *B*, angulation of the transducer permits recording of the left coronary artery arising from the main pulmonary artery (PA). (Courtesy of Gregory J. Ensing.)

murmur, which is often confused with patent ductus arteriosus. Two-dimensional echocardiography reveals dilation of the involved coronary artery that is uniform and often severe. In children, the course of the dilated vessel can be followed by the use of multiple imaging planes and simultaneous color flow imaging.[296,298-306] The fistula itself may be difficult to image. Color Doppler and/or contrast-enhanced echocardiography are useful when attempting to follow the path of the vessel (Figs. 7–106 and 7–107).[307] Detection of turbulent flow within the right ventricle or pulmonary artery may identify the site of fistulous connection. If the left-to-right shunt is large, chamber dilation may also be apparent.

Coronary artery aneurysms usually occur in association with Kawasaki disease.[308,309] In two-dimensional echocardiograms, these aneurysms appear as localized dilated segments, usually with a fusiform shape.[310,311] They often are multiple, may occur anywhere along the vessel, and sometimes are lined with thrombus. Detection requires the use of multiple imaging planes to record as much as possible of the distal arteries (Figs. 7–108 and 7–109). In most patients, the entire left main coronary artery and the proximal segments of the right, left circumflex, and left anterior descending arteries can be seen from the parasternal short-axis view. The parasternal long-axis view of the right ventricular outflow tract may permit recording of the more distal left anterior descending artery, whereas the apical four-chamber view can be used to assess the left circumflex and right coronary arteries. As noted previously, transesophageal echocardiography can also be used effectively to examine the coronary arteries. The diameter of the coronary artery aneurysms should be measured, because the size has prognostic implications.[312] The presence of a pericardial effusion should also be sought. Its presence increases the likelihood of coronary artery aneurysms.[313]

The coronary artery aneurysms resulting from Kawasaki disease may be associated with abnormal myocardial perfusion. Recently, stress echocardiography has been applied to these patients to induce and detect evi-

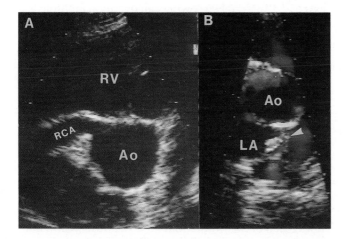

**Fig. 7–106.** Parasternal short-axis view at the base of the heart demonstrates a dilated right coronary artery (RCA) in *A*. The course of the dilated vessel could be traced to the entrance into the superior part of the left atrium (LA). In *B*, the turbulent flow at the site of entrance of the fistula is indicated by the arrowhead. Ao = aorta; RV = right ventricle.

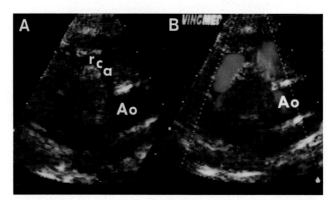

**Fig. 7–107.** In *A*, a high parasternal view at the base of the heart demonstrates a dilated right coronary artery (rca) arising from the aortic root (Ao). In *B*, color flow imaging records flow within the coronary artery. In this case, a fistulous connection between the artery and the right ventricle was demonstrated. (Courtesy of Gregory J. Ensing.)

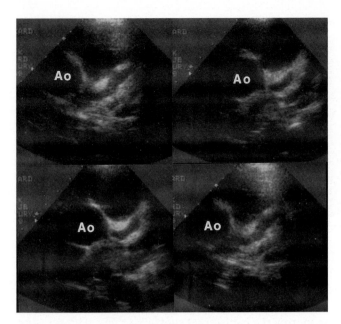

**Fig. 7–108.** Sequential images of the proximal left coronary artery are recorded from the parasternal short-axis view. Multiple, fusiform dilated segments are apparent. Such coronary artery aneurysms are seen in patients with Kawasaki disease. Ao = aorta.

dence of regional ischemia. The development of a transient wall motion abnormality during stress testing in young patients with this disorder is strong evidence of inducible ischemia (Fig. 7–110).[314] The clinical significance of this finding and its implications for management, however, are not yet known.

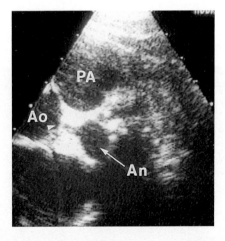

**Fig. 7–109.** Angulated parasternal short-axis view at the base from a patient with Kawasaki disease. The arrowhead indicates the ostium of the left main coronary artery. A large saccular aneurysm (An) involves the proximal left anterior descending artery (*arrow*). (Courtesy of Gregory J. Ensing.) Ao = aorta; PA = pulmonary artery.

# CONOTRUNCAL ABNORMALITIES

## Tetralogy of Fallot

Tetralogy of Fallot is one of the more common forms of cyanotic congenital heart disease and is one of the few such lesions that may escape diagnosis until later in life. This anomaly has four anatomic features: (1) anterior and rightward displacement of the aortic root, (2) ventricular septal defect, (3) right ventricular outflow tract obstruction, and (4) right ventricular hypertrophy. The echocardiographic evaluation includes de novo diagnosis of the lesion, a determination of the options for surgical intervention, and postoperative assessment of the adequacy of repair.

The critical developmental defect in Fallot's tetralogy is malalignment of the infundibular septum, resulting in a nonrestrictive (and mostly perimembranous) septal defect and overriding of the aorta.[35,315–317] Both of these fundamental anatomic features are optimally assessed using the parasternal long-axis view, which permits the viewer to determine the presence of the ventricular septal defect and the degree of aortic overriding (Fig. 7–111). Discontinuity between the infundibular septum and the anterior aortic root is readily apparent.[318–320] Proper transducer position and angulation are necessary to ensure accurate assessment of the degree of aortic overriding. This feature is variable, ranging from minimal to extreme. In the latter case, the aortic valve may appear to arise exclusively from the right ventricle and resembles double-outlet right ventricle. Most investigators follow the "50% rule" to make this distinction. If more than 50% of the aorta overlies the left ventricle, the proper designation should be tetralogy of Fallot. If more than 50% of the aorta overlies the right ventricle, double-outlet right ventricle is present.

The short-axis view allows the viewer to determine the extent and size of the septal defect.[321] More importantly, the right ventricular outflow tract can be assessed.[71,318,322,323] Narrowing can occur on multiple levels. In most cases, it is the displacement of the infundibular septum that produces the subvalvular narrowing that is characteristic of tetralogy of Fallot. In general, the greater the aortic overriding, the more severe the subpulmonic stenosis. Various combinations of infundibular hypoplasia and muscular hypertrophy may be present. Stenosis may also involve the pulmonary annulus and/or valve. Less often, the proximal pulmonary arteries are hypoplastic, resulting in supravalvular stenosis. In the most extreme situation, pulmonary atresia is present and perfusion of the lungs depends on systemic to pulmonary artery collaterals and a patent ductus arteriosus.[322,324]

Using the parasternal short-axis and subcostal coronal views, each of these potential levels of obstruction must be carefully evaluated. Color Doppler is often helpful in assessing the location of the narrowed, turbulent flow. Continuous wave Doppler is then used to determine the pressure gradient across the various levels of obstruction (Fig. 7–112).[71] Determining the size of the pulmo-

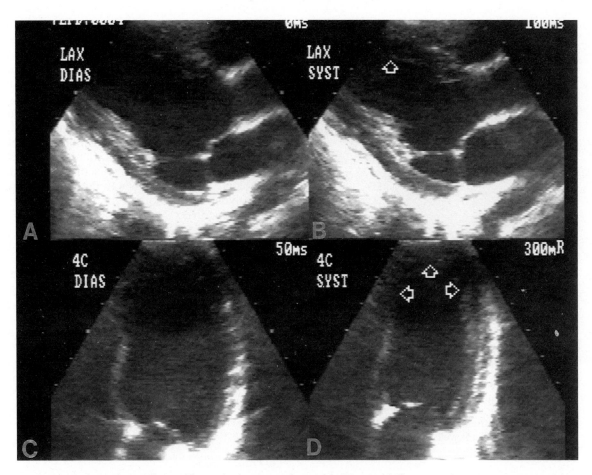

**Fig. 7–110.** An exercise echocardiographic study from a patient with Kawasaki disease and coronary artery aneurysms. Left ventricular wall motion is normal at baseline. The images were recorded immediately after treadmill exercise testing. The long-axis (*A*) and four-chamber (*C*) views at end diastole are displayed with corresponding end-systolic frames (*B* and *D*). The study demonstrates hypokinesis of the distal septum and apex (*arrows*). The deterioration in anterior and apical wall motion immediately post-exercise is strongly suggestive of inducible anterior ischemia as a result of disease of the left anterior descending artery. In this patient, multiple fusiform aneurysms were present throughout the coronary tree.

nary arteries is important in planning any surgical intervention, and it is best accomplished from the short-axis and suprasternal views. The relative sizes of the right and left pulmonary arteries can be compared. In infants, care must be taken to avoid confusing the left pulmonary artery with a patent ductus arteriosus. The diameter of the right pulmonary artery is best assessed as it passes below the aortic arch (as recorded from the suprasternal long-axis view). Coronary artery anatomy must also be examined preoperatively, and this assessment generally can be accomplished by using two-dimensional echocardiographic techniques.[286,287] A coronary artery branch crossing the right ventricular outflow tract (either an aberrant left anterior descending or conus branch) has important implications for surgical repair.

Following repair of tetralogy of Fallot, echocardiography plays a key role in assessing the surgical results.[325–327] From the parasternal long-axis view, the ventricular septal defect patch is seen as a linear structure passing obliquely from the septum to the anterior aortic root (Fig. 7–113). The oblique course is a consequence of the aortic overriding. Residual shunting may be detected with Doppler, usually at the margins of the patch. Next, right ventricular size and contractility should be assessed. These parameters have important long-term prognostic implications. Finally, the right ventricular outflow tract is interrogated. Evidence of residual stenosis may be recorded with Doppler (Fig. 7–114). The location and severity should be ascertained. In most cases, pulmonic regurgitation also is present. The magnitude varies considerably, but sometimes it is severe. The clinical implications of chronic, severe pulmonic regurgitation after repair of tetralogy of Fallot are not firmly established,[325] although close follow-up and serial assessment with echocardiography is generally recommended.

### Transposition of the Great Arteries

The term transposition is used to describe a discordant ventriculoarterial connection in which the aorta

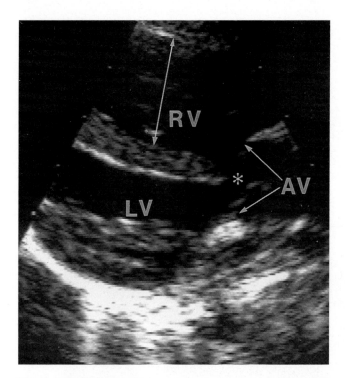

**Fig. 7–111.** Parasternal long-axis view from a patient with tetralogy of Fallot demonstrates a dilated right ventricle (RV), an overriding aorta (AV), and a subaortic ventricular septal defect (*asterisk*). Right ventricular hypertrophy, the other feature of tetralogy of Fallot, is not well illustrated in this image. LV = left ventricle.

arises from the morphologic right ventricle and the pulmonary artery arises from the left ventricle. Transposition can exist with either situs solitus or situs inversus. For simplicity, this section is a discussion of transposition in the presence of situs solitus only. The distinction between D-transposition and L-transposition is important and often is a source of confusion. In D-transposition, there is atrioventricular concordance and the morphologic right ventricle is to the right of the morphologic left ventricle. In L-transposition, there is ventricular inversion and atrioventricular discordance. Thus, the morphologic right ventricle is to the left of the morphologic left ventricle. In both cases, the great arteries arise from the "incorrect" ventricle.

With normal conotruncal development, the pulmonary artery arises anterior and to the left of the aorta. Its initial course is posterior and then it bifurcates into right and left branches. The aortic valve is more posterior and rightward and the course of the aorta is oblique with reference to the pulmonary artery. The aorta does not bifurcate, but forms an arch as it passes posteriorly and inferiorly. Thus, the outflow tracts and great arteries of the right and left sides of the heart appear to wrap around one another in a spiral fashion. Transposition results in a more parallel alignment of the great arteries. With two-dimensional echocardiography, this positioning has been described as a "double barrel" appearance rather than the normal "circle and sausage" orientation (see Fig. 7–5).[35,328,329]

### D-*Transposition*

The echocardiographic diagnosis of D-transposition requires demonstration of a right-sided right ventricle giving rise to an aorta and a left-sided left ventricle giving rise to a pulmonary artery.[330–332] In children, this ana-

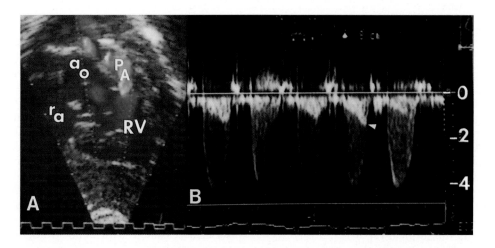

**Fig. 7–112.** Subcostal view of the right ventricular outflow tract from a patient with tetralogy of Fallot. In *A*, color flow imaging demonstrates turbulent flow within the outflow tract and pulmonary artery (PA). In *B*, continuous wave Doppler reveals a maximal velocity across the pulmonic valve of 4.0 m/sec consistent with a gradient of 64 mm Hg. In this patient, the predominant site of obstruction was valvular. The right ventricular outflow tract velocity can be seen within the Doppler signal as the darker flow peaking at approximately 1.5 m/sec in late systole (*arrowhead*). ao = aorta; ra = right atrium; RV = right ventricle.

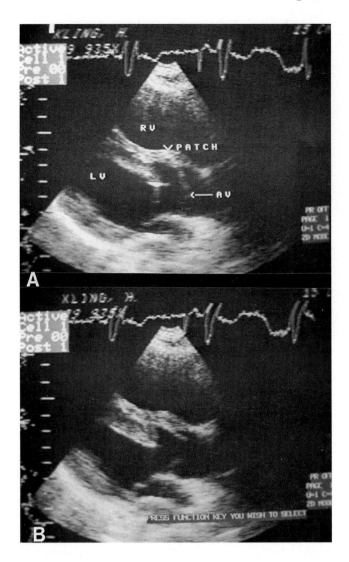

**Fig. 7–113.** Parasternal long-axis examination in diastole (*A*) and systole (*B*) from a patient after anatomic repair of tetralogy. A patch is noted in the area of the membranous ventricular septum, and there appears to be partial dehiscence at the attachment to the ventricular septum. RV = right ventricle; LV = left ventricle; AV = aortic valve.

cerned from the short-axis view at the base (Fig. 7–116).[35,328] Because the semilunar valves occupy different levels (the aortic valve being slightly more cranial), they usually are not seen in the same short-axis plane. In the long-axis view, this parallel relationship of the great arteries can often be recorded in the longitudinal plane. By demonstrating that the anterior vessel arches posteriorly and the posterior vessel bifurcates, the diagnosis of D-transposition is established. Visualization of the ostia of the coronary arteries and the brachiocephalic branch vessels also serves to identify the aorta (Fig. 7–117).

The presence of ventriculoarterial discordance alone will necessarily result in the creation of two parallel circuits and is incompatible with life. Therefore, admixture of arterial and venous blood is a prerequisite for survival and can occur at any level. An atrial septal defect, usually the secundum variety, is present in most patients. The size and direction of the interatrial shunt can be assessed with Doppler techniques. When venous admixing is inadequate, an atrial septostomy is often performed as a palliative measure. This intervention can be performed under echocardiographic guidance.[333] Echocardiography also plays a vital role in selecting candidates for this procedure and in determining its success (as judged by the size of the resulting defect).[334,335]

Approximately one third of patients with D-transposition have a ventricular septal defect (Fig. 7–118).[336] The location of these defects is variable. In most, the defect involves the outlet septum and may be associated with pulmonary artery overriding. Care must be taken to avoid confusing this condition with tetralogy of Fallot or double-outlet right ventricle.[329] In D-transposition, more than 50% of the pulmonary artery is committed to the left ventricle and there is pulmonary-mitral continuity. These features are optimally assessed from the parasternal long-axis view.

Additional associated lesions include subaortic (i.e., right ventricular outflow tract) stenosis and tricuspid (i.e., systemic atrioventricular) valve abnormalities.[52,337,338] Subpulmonic (left ventricular outflow tract) obstruction may also be present.[331,337,339] and several anatomic forms have been described. In most cases, this form of obstruction is dynamic because of systolic bowing of the septum into the left ventricle. M-mode echocardiography reveals fine fluttering of the pulmonic valve cusps, systolic anterior motion of the mitral valve, and midsystolic closure of the pulmonic valve.[340,341] When Doppler is performed, however, a significant pressure gradient is rarely detected.[342] Less commonly, fixed subpulmonic narrowing may be detected, usually resulting from a fibrous diaphragm or a fibromuscular ridge. Doppler techniques can be used to assess the pressure gradient across such stenoses.

Ventricular function and size are important parameters that should be assessed with echocardiography. The right ventricle, because it must pump against the systemic vascular resistance, becomes dilated and hypertrophied. Conversely, the left ventricle is often small and relatively thin walled.[343] The normal septal curva-

tomic structure is best evaluated from the subcostal four-chamber view, which allows all of these features of D-transposition to be displayed (Fig. 7–115). In adults, however, this assessment is technically challenging. More often, the parasternal short-axis and apical four-chamber views provide most of the diagnostic information. In the short-axis view, the aortic valve is usually anterior and to the right of the pulmonic valve and the great arteries arise in parallel. It should be emphasized that this spatial relationship between the great arteries is not essential for the diagnosis, and the aorta occasionally lies directly anterior or slightly to the left of the pulmonary valve. These arrangements are easily dis-

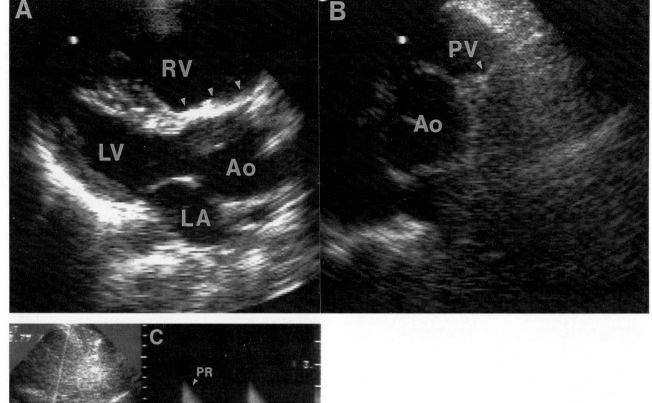

**Fig. 7-114.** A recording from a 29-year-old woman who underwent repair of tetralogy of Fallot at age 6 years. In *A*, the obliquely oriented ventricular septal defect patch is indicated by arrowheads. The right ventricle (RV) is dilated. In *B*, a short-axis view at the base provides marginal visualization of the right ventricular outflow tract and pulmonic valve (PV). In *C*, continuous wave Doppler permits detection of significant residual outflow tract obstruction with a maximal velocity of 4.7 m/sec indicating a peak systolic gradient of 88 mm Hg. Because of the technical limitations of imaging the outflow tract, the precise site of obstruction could not be determined in this tracing. The presence of pulmonic regurgitation (PR) is also demonstrated (*arrowhead*). Ao = aorta; LA = left atrium; LV = left ventricle.

ture is reversed with the right ventricle assuming a rounded configuration and the left ventricle becoming more crescent shaped. Coronary artery anomalies are present in more than one third of patients. Detection requires careful recording of the ostia and initial course of the vessels as they arise from the aortic root. An approach similar to that described in the section on tetralogy of Fallot should be used.

The evaluation of patients following surgical correction of D-transposition relies heavily on echocardiographic techniques. Two distinct surgical procedures are currently available for treatment of this condition. In the past, the most common form of palliation for D-transposition was an intra-atrial baffle (also known as a Mustard, Senning, or atrial switch) procedure. A baffle con-

nects the vena cavae to the mitral valve (and hence the pulmonary circuit) by diverting blood flow across the atrial septum while simultaneously allowing pulmonary venous blood to be routed over the baffle to the tricuspid valve (and on to the systemic circuit). Echocardiographic evaluation relies on direct visualization of the newly created systemic and pulmonary venous atria and careful assessment of right (i.e., systemic) ventricular function.[341,344–350] The presence and severity of tricuspid regurgitation should also be determined with Doppler imaging.

In the parasternal long-axis view, the baffle is seen as an oblique, linear echo within the anatomic left atrium (Fig. 7–119).[351] The pulmonary venous atrium is superior and posterior while the systemic venous atrium is

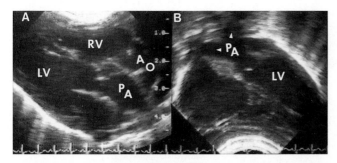

**Fig. 7–115.** Example of D-transposition of the great arteries. In *A*, the parasternal long-axis view demonstrates a normal ventricular relationship with the right ventricle (RV) anterior to the left ventricle (LV). Ventriculoarterial discordance is present with the aorta (Ao) arising from the right ventricle after the pulmonary artery (PA) arising from the left ventricle. In this view alone, the identity of the great arteries is not clear. In *B*, a modified subcostal four-chamber view demonstrates a bifurcating great artery arising from the left ventricle. This image confirms that this vessel is the pulmonary artery and secures the diagnosis of transposition. (Courtesy of Gregory J. Ensing.)

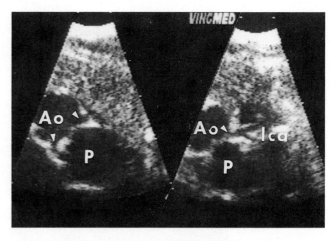

**Fig. 7–117.** Modified high parasternal views from a patient with D-transposition of the great arteries. The aorta (Ao) is anterior and rightward of the pulmonary artery (P). The ostia (*arrowheads*) and proximal course of the coronary arteries can be seen arising in the aortic root. lca = left coronary artery. (Courtesy of Gregory J. Ensing.)

in communication with the mitral valve. Medial or rightward angulation may permit visualization of the junction of the pulmonary venous atrium with the right ventricle. From the apical and subcostal four-chamber views, most regions of the baffle can be assessed. Shallow angulation of the transducer allows most of the pulmonary venous atrium to be recorded and is useful in detecting obstruction within this region (Fig. 7–120). By tilting the transducer more posteriorly, the junction between the inferior vena cava and the systemic venous atrium (an uncommon site of obstruction) is visible. Obstruction

within the superior vena caval limb of the baffle is more common, but it may be difficult to visualize, particularly in adults. The subcostal and suprasternal short-axis views can be used for this purpose.

Leaks within the baffle are best detected by using contrast echocardiography and the four-chamber view (Fig. 7–121).[351] With this technique, right-to-left baffle leaks can be diagnosed with high sensitivity.[352] Color Doppler also permits these leaks to be identified and localized. Obstruction within the superior vena caval limb of the baffle can also be detected with contrast echocardiography.[352] This approach involves imaging of the inferior vena cava during injection of contrast material into an upper extremity vein. In the absence of obstruction, contrast medium fills the systemic venous atrium from above and the inferior vena cava remains free of contrast-containing blood. With partial obstruction, normal filling of the systemic venous atrium with contrast-containing blood from above is followed by the gradual appearance of contrast material in the inferior vena cava (from collaterals). With complete obstruction, the systemic venous atrium fills with contrast medium only from below from collaterals. More recently, Doppler has been used to detect obstruction within the various limbs of the baffle (Figs. 7–122 and 7–123).[353] Obstruction within the superior vena cava can be detected from the suprasternal notch. With a normally functioning baffle, color Doppler can be used to follow the undisturbed, low-velocity flow from the vena cava to the systemic venous atrium. Pulsed Doppler can identify obstruction as continuous, turbulent flow in excess of 1 m/sec. Obstruction within the pulmonary venous atrium requires the use of Doppler techniques for detection. First, color Doppler is used to search for turbulence within the conduit. Then, pulsed Doppler can be applied to measure the increased velocity within the structure. A diastolic

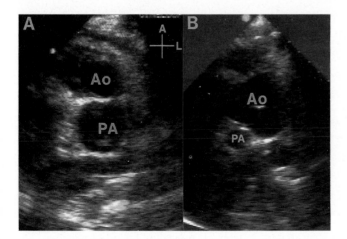

**Fig. 7–116.** Parasternal short-axis views through the base from two patients with transposition. In both cases, the great arteries arise in parallel with the aorta (Ao) in a position anterior to the pulmonary artery (PA). In *A*, the two great arteries are of roughly equal size and the aorta is directly anterior to the pulmonary artery. In *B*, the pulmonary artery is abnormally small and the aorta arises anterior and leftward.

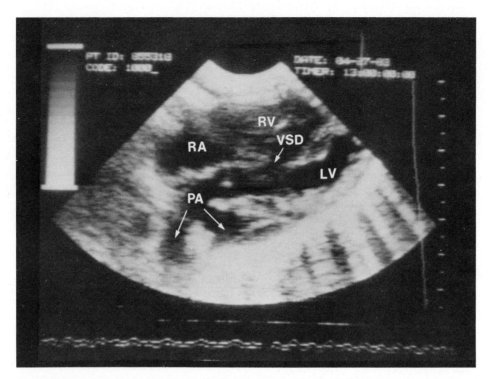

**Fig. 7–118.**   Subcostal four-chamber view of a patient with D-transposition of the great vessels and a ventricular septal defect (VSD). The great vessel arising from the left ventricle (LV) has an immediately posterior course and branches soon after the semilunar valve. This course identifies it as the pulmonary artery (PA) arising from the left ventricle. RA = right atrium; RV = right ventricle. (Courtesy of Randall L. Caldwell.)

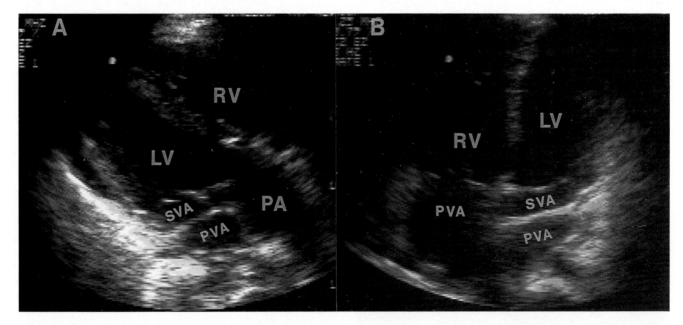

**Fig. 7–119.**   In *A*, a parasternal long-axis view from a patient following an intra-atrial baffle procedure for D-transposition. The baffle is visualized readily as a linear structure dividing the atrium to a systemic venous atrium (SVA) and a pulmonary venous atrium (PVA). In *B*, the apical four-chamber view again shows the baffle and the orientation of the atria. LV = left ventricle; RV = right ventricle.

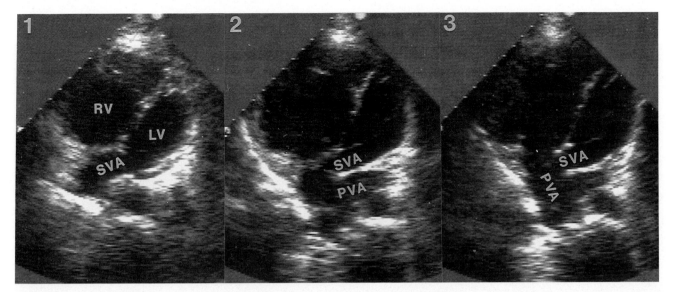

**Fig. 7–120.** A series of three modified, four-chamber views from a patient following an intra-atrial baffle procedure. By tilting the transducer at different angles, the various limbs of the baffle can be visualized. In panel *1*, the systemic venous atrium (SVA) is seen in continuity with the mitral valve and left ventricle (LV). In panel *2*, both the systemic and pulmonary venous atria (PVA) are seen. In panel *3*, by tilting the transducer to a more anterior plane, continuity between the pulmonary venous atrium and the tricuspid valve and right ventricle is demonstrated. Note the dilated right (systemic) ventricle (RV).

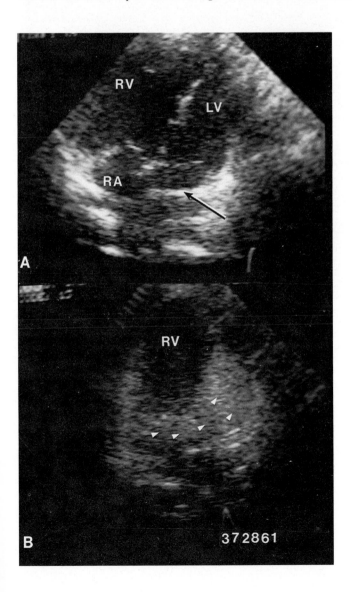

**Fig. 7–121.** Apical four-chamber view with and without contrast material in a patient with D-transposition of the great vessels following Mustard repair. The atrial baffle is noted as an echo-dense line in the region of the left atrium in *A* (*arrow*). Following peripheral venous injection of contrast material *B*, contrast flows from the region of the right atrium and then into the left ventricle (*arrowheads*). RA = right atrium; RV = right ventricle; LV = left ventricle.

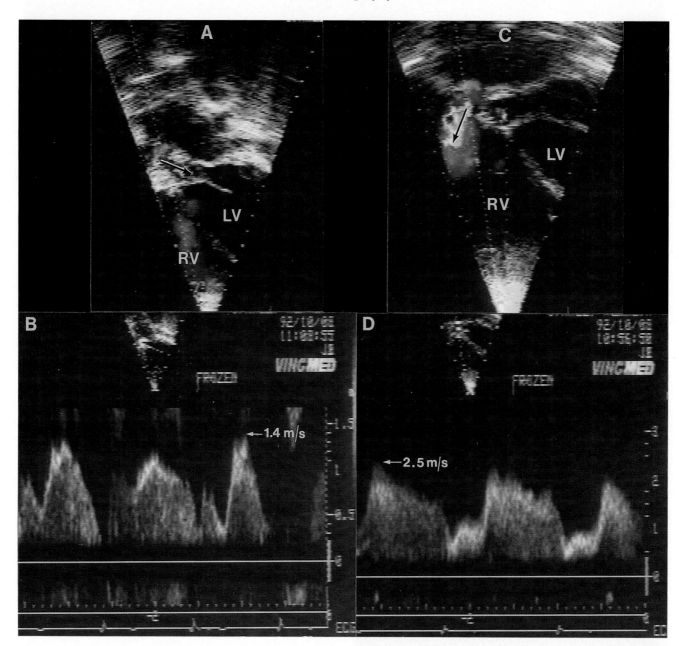

**Fig. 7–122.**  Obstruction within the various limbs of an intra-atrial baffle. In *A*, the apical four-chamber view with color flow mapping demonstrates turbulence within the systemic venous atrium as it connects to the superior vena cava (*double arrow*). In *B*, pulsed Doppler recording in this region reveals mildly elevated velocity (1.4 m/sec) consistent with a mild degree of obstruction. By tilting the transducer slightly more anteriorly, flow within the pulmonary venous atrium is recorded (*C*). Turbulence is again noted (*double arrow*). Pulsed Doppler recorded in this area consistent with significant obstruction within the pulmonary venous atrium. LV = left ventricle; RV = right ventricle.

flow velocity that is greater than 2 m/sec suggests significant obstruction. Lower velocity turbulent flow does not exclude the possibility of obstruction, however. More recently, transesophageal echocardiography has been used to more accurately assess intra-atrial baffles.[354] Use of this technique may be particularly important in adults in whom transthoracic image quality is sometimes a limitation. The detection of both obstruction and interatrial shunting is possible with this method.

The arterial switch procedure is a more recently avail-

able means of anatomic correction for D-transposition. This method has several practical and theoretic advantages over the intra-atrial baffle procedure and has now become the operation of choice in most situations. Because the technique has been in widespread use for only 10 years, experience with adult patients remains limited. The procedure involves trans-section of both great arteries and reanastomosis of the pulmonary artery to the right ventricle and the aorta to the left ventricle. Thus, the normal structure-function relationships of the ventri-

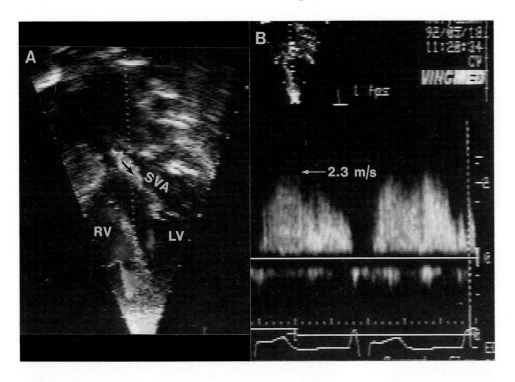

**Fig. 7–123.** In *A*, color flow imaging in a 9-year-old patient with an intra-atrial baffle demonstrates turbulence within the systemic venous atrium (SVA). In *B*, pulsed Doppler reveals significantly elevated velocity in this region, consistent with obstruction within the systemic venous atrium as it connects with the superior vena cava. LV = left ventricle; RV = right ventricle.

cles are restored. Selecting infants for this procedure depends in part on coronary artery anatomy, and echocardiography can be used for this determination. Echocardiographic evaluation after the arterial switch procedure should focus on assessment of left and right ventricular function and the detection of any newly created structural problems, either involving the ventricles, the great artery anastomoses, or the origin of the coronary arteries.[344,355–360] Both supravalvular aortic and pulmonic narrowing have been reported.[357,361] Some degree of structural distortion of the origins of the great arteries does occur commonly without significant stenosis. Therefore, Doppler must be used to determine the severity of any apparent narrowing seen with two-dimensional echocardiography. The ostia of the coronary arteries should also be visualized. This study is best performed in the parasternal short-axis view. The ability to demonstrate the proximal coronary arteries with echocardiography suggests that this technique may be helpful in detecting narrowing or kinking of the reimplanted vessels.[288]

### *L-Transposition*

In simplest terms, L-transposition can be thought of as isolated ventricular inversion in which the morphologic right ventricle is to the left of the morphologic left ventricle.[362,363] The echocardiographic diagnosis rests on demonstrating abnormal atrioventricular and ventriculoarterial connections. Determining ventricular morphology and establishing the spatial relationships of the two chambers are accomplished as described previously. The discordant connections are detected by using multiple echocardiographic windows. From the four-chamber view, the presence of ventricular inversion usually can be established (Fig. 7–124).[364–368] Apical

displacement of the left-sided tricuspid valve can also be demonstrated (Fig. 7–125). In the long-axis view, direct continuity between the pulmonary valve and anterior mitral leaflet is apparent (Fig. 7–126).

In most cases, the ventricles are oriented in a side-by-side fashion, which creates some unusual and confusing echocardiographic views.[367] For example, the parasternal long-axis plane may be vertical. In the short-axis view, the septum also appears more vertical (i.e., perpendicular to the frontal plane). The great arteries arise in parallel, with the aorta usually positioned leftward, anterior, and superior to the pulmonary valve (see Fig. 7–122). This relationship contrasts with D-transposition, in which the aortic valve is anterior and usually rightward of the pulmonic valve.

Associated anomalies are a common and important feature of L-transposition.[362,369] Structural abnormalities of the left-sided tricuspid valve occur in most patients. Apical displacement of the leaflet insertions (an Ebstein-like deformity) and tricuspid regurgitation may be detected.[370] A perimembranous ventricular septal defect is present in approximately 70% of cases. Less often, left ventricular outflow tract obstruction (valvular or subvalvular pulmonic stenosis) is present and can be assessed with Doppler. Finally, right (i.e., systemic) ventricular function may be abnormal and should be examined carefully. Gradual deterioration in function of the right side of the heart may occur over time. Echocardiography plays an important role in the detection of this problem and in the assessment of any associated tricuspid regurgitation.

### **Double-Outlet Right Ventricle**

In double-outlet right ventricle, both great arteries arise predominantly from the right ventricle. A ventricu-

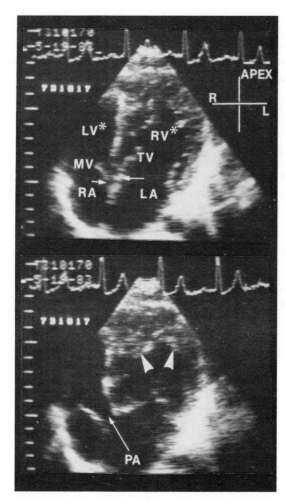

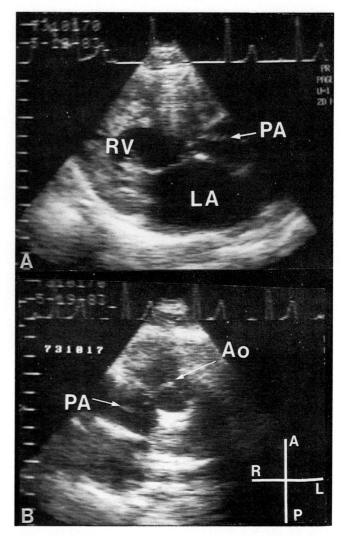

**Fig. 7–124.** Apical four-chamber views in a patient with L-transposition (corrected transposition). *A,* Note the anatomic right ventricle (RV*) in the more posterior and leftward location, and the anatomic left ventricle (LV*) in the more rightward position. The tricuspid valve (TV) insertion is more apically located than that of the mitral valve (MV). *B,* With slight anterior angulation, the first great artery visualized is more posterior and is the pulmonary artery (PA). RA = right atrium; LA = left atrium.

**Fig. 7–126.** Parasternal long-axis view (*A*) of a patient with L-transposition. The heavily trabeculated right ventricle (RV) is in communication with the left atrium (LA). The great vessel shown is the pulmonary artery, and it is not in continuity with the right ventricle. The great vessels are visualized in the short-axis view in *B*. The aorta (Ao) is anterior to and to the left of the pulmonary artery (PA).

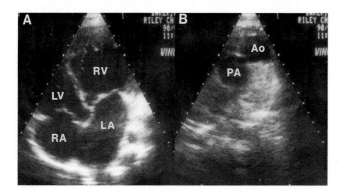

**Fig. 7–125.** Apical four-chamber (*A*) and high parasternal short-axis (*B*) views from a patient with L-transposition of the great arteries. In *A,* ventricular inversion is demonstrated. The dilated and trabeculated right ventricle (RV) receives blood from the morphologic left atrium (LA). The displaced tricuspid valve is apical to the right-sided mitral valve. In *B,* the two great arteries arise in parallel and the aorta (Ao) is anterior and to the left of the pulmonary artery (PA). RA = right atrium; LV = left ventricle.

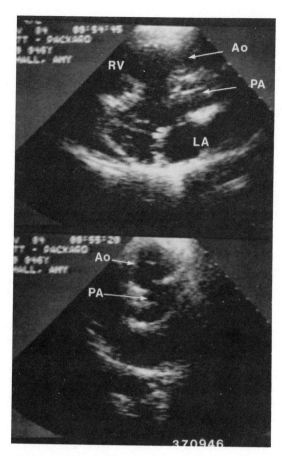

**Fig. 7–127.** Parasternal long-axis (*A*) and short-axis (*B*) views from a patient with double-outlet right ventricle. In *A*, the great arteries arise in parallel from the right ventricle (RV). Discontinuity between the anterior leaflet of the mitral valve and the posterior great vessel (PA) is apparent. In (*B*) the aorta (Ao) arises anterior to and slightly rightward of the pulmonary artery (PA). This is an example of dextromalposition. LA = left atrium; LV = left ventricle.

lar septal defect is present and is the sole outlet for the left ventricle. Partial septal overriding of the posterior great vessel may occur, but the posterior artery is primarily (more than 50%) committed to the right ventricle. In most cases, a muscular infundibulum or conus supports both great vessels, resulting in a separation (or lack of fibrous continuity) between the posterior semilunar valve and the anterior mitral leaflet. The echocardiographic evaluation of patients with double-outlet right ventricle includes an assessment of the great artery relations, determination of the size and type of ventricular septal defect, and detection of the presence of any associated lesions (especially pulmonary stenosis and atrial septal defect).[371–373]

The echocardiographic diagnosis of double-outlet right ventricle is based on the demonstration that both great arteries arise to the right of the ventricular septum (i.e., are primarily committed to the right ventricle). The origin of the great arteries in relation to the septum is best visualized from the parasternal long-axis and sub-

costal coronal views (Fig. 7–127). These views also help to determine the lack of fibrous continuity between the posterior semilunar valve and the anterior mitral valve leaflet (Fig. 7–128). This finding is not mandatory for diagnosis, however, because complete absorption of the conus below the posterior semilunar valve will allow fibrous continuity with the atrioventricular valve to be established.

Once the diagnosis is made, the great vessel relationships should be determined.[371,372] Four spatial arrangements are possible: (1) normal (pulmonary artery anterior and to the left of the aorta), (2) side-by-side (aorta to the right, but in the same transverse plane), (3) dextromalposition (aorta anterior and to the right), and (4) levomalposition (aorta anterior and to the left). This determination is made by using the parasternal short-axis and subcostal four-chamber views (Fig. 7–127). The approach is similar to that used in the assessment of transposition. A normal great vessel relationship is rare and may be confused on echocardiograms with tetralogy of Fallot. When the two vessels appear side by side in the short-axis view, determining their respective identity requires superior angulation to detect bifurcation of the pulmonary artery.

The ventricular septal defect is usually large and may be either subaortic (the most common), subpulmonic (the Taussig-Bing form), doubly committed, or noncommitted.[371–373] The defect is easily appreciated from multiple echocardiographic views. Next, the presence of pulmonary stenosis (valvular and/or subvalvular) must be determined.[372] This condition is present in approximately 50% of patients and usually is most easily detected from the parasternal long-axis view. Doppler techniques should be used to assess the pressure gra-

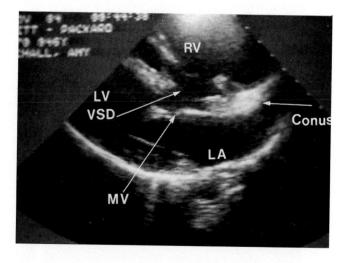

**Fig. 7–128.** Parasternal long-axis view of the same patient as in Figure 7–127. In this view, the large ventricular septal defect (VSD) is demonstrated. Discontinuity between the mitral valve (MV) and posterior great artery is again shown with the anterior mitral leaflet attached to the conus. LA = left atrium; LV = left ventricle; RV = right ventricle.

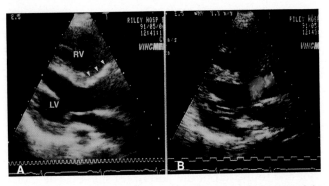

**Fig. 7–129.** A patient underwent repair of double-outlet right ventricle. In *A*, the obliquely oriented ventricular septal defect patch is indicated by arrowheads. In *B*, color flow imaging demonstrates mild aortic regurgitation. (Courtesy of Gregory J. Ensing.) LV = left ventricle; RV = right ventricle.

dient and any associated regurgitation. Other anomalies that may be detected with echocardiography include atrial septal defect, subaortic stenosis, patent ductus arteriosus, and mitral valve abnormalities.

Surgical repair of double-outlet right ventricle is complex and depends in part on the great artery relationships. Echocardiographic assessment after repair should focus on the evaluation of the ventricular septal defect patch, the presence of outflow obstruction, and the possibility of semilunar valve regurgitation (Figs. 7–129 and 7–130).

### Persistent Truncus Arteriosus

This anomaly is characterized by the presence of a single great vessel arising from the base of the heart and dividing into systemic and pulmonary arteries.[374] An outlet ventricular septal defect and a single semilunar valve are other essential features. This lesion is the result of a failure of partitioning involving the conus, truncus arteriosus, and aortic sac. The truncal valve is often large and structurally abnormal, sometimes with significant regurgitation. It is positioned directly over the ventricular septal defect and usually originates equally from the two ventricles. The origin of the pulmonary arteries from the truncus is variable and is used to classify the various types of truncus arteriosus. By far, the most common is type I, in which a short main pulmonary artery arises from the truncus before dividing into left and right branches. In type II, no main pulmonary artery is present and the left and right branches arise separately from the posterior wall of the truncus. These two forms account for over 90% of all cases.

The echocardiographic diagnosis relies on the demonstration of a single large great artery arising from the base of the heart and overriding an outlet ventricular septal defect.[375–378] In the parasternal long-axis view, the size of the great vessel and septal defect, as well as the degree of overriding, can be assessed (Fig. 7–131). The posterior truncal wall is seen in fibrous continuity with the anterior mitral leaflet. Because these features are shared by other conotruncal lesions (tetralogy of Fallot and pulmonary atresia with ventricular septal defect), the diagnosis cannot be made from the parasternal long-axis alone. The observer must evaluate the pulmonary arteries as they branch from the truncus, which is best accomplished from the parasternal short-axis view at the base (Fig. 7–132). Here, the absence of the pulmonary valve and the origin of the pulmonary arteries from the posterior truncal wall is diagnostic of this entity. Both

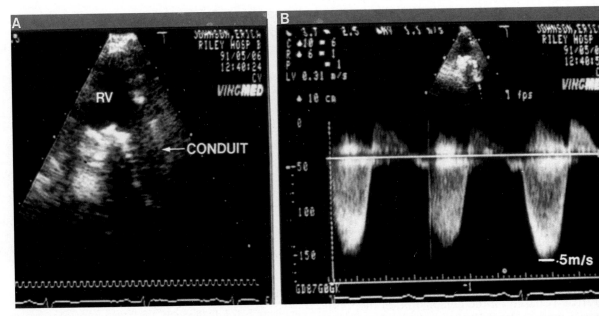

**Fig. 7–130.** Images of the same patient presented in Figure 7–129. In *A*, the proximal portion of the conduit connecting the right ventricle (RV) to the pulmonary artery is recorded. In *B*, continuous wave Doppler demonstrates severe obstruction within the conduit with a maximal velocity of 5.0 m/sec consistent with a peak systolic gradient of approximately 100 mm Hg. The obstruction was found during surgery at the level of the porcine valve in the middle portion of the conduit.

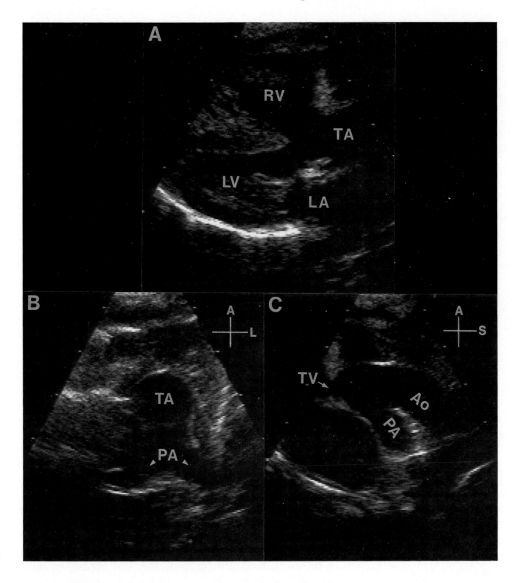

**Fig. 7–131.** In *A*, the parasternal long-axis view in a patient with truncus arteriosus reveals a large subarterial ventricular septal defect and an overriding great artery, the truncus (TA). In *B*, a high parasternal short-axis view demonstrates the origin of the pulmonary arteries (PA) from the posterior wall of the truncus. In *C*, a long-axis view at the same level again reveals the origin of the pulmonary artery from the posterior wall of the truncus. The position of the truncal valve (TV) is indicated (*arrow*). This is an example of type I truncus arteriosus. LA = left atrium; LV = left ventricle; RV = right ventricle; Ao = aortic.

pulmonary arteries must be assessed in order to exclude the possibility of unilateral absence of one artery. Classification of the anatomic type is usually possible and the number of truncal valve leaflets can often be determined. As many as six cusps may be present.[374]

The magnitude of truncal valve regurgitation and the relative sizes of the two ventricles is determined from the apical four-chamber view. From the suprasternal view, the presence of a right-sided aortic arch can be identified. Branch pulmonary artery stenosis, sometimes associated with truncus, can also be detected (Fig. 7–133). Other possible anomalies in patients with truncus arteriosus include atresia of the ductus arteriosus and anomalous origin of the coronary arteries.[379]

Aortopulmonary window is a related anomaly involving the conotruncus in which the ventricular septum is intact, two semilunar valves are present, and two great arteries arise from the base of the heart.[376,380–382] Incomplete partitioning of the truncus results in a communication between the proximal aorta and the main pulmonary artery, usually just above the semilunar valves (Fig. 7–134). The anatomic defect bears many similarities to

a ductus arteriosus and the two are sometimes confused. With echocardiography, the subcostal four-chamber view may be useful in establishing this diagnosis. The presence or absence of the proximal truncal septum distinguishes aortopulmonary window (in which it is present) from truncus arteriosus (in which it is absent). The identification of two semilunar valves clearly differentiates these entities. Finally, Doppler has proven useful in detecting aortopulmonary window and in assessing the size of the communication.

## ABNORMALITIES OF VENTRICULAR DEVELOPMENT

Anormalities of ventricular development may occur as a primary disorder, such as hypoplastic left heart syndrome, or may be secondary to other conditions, such as right ventricular hypoplasia resulting from tricuspid atresia. In either situation, hypoplasia of one or both ventricles is the primary functional anomaly.

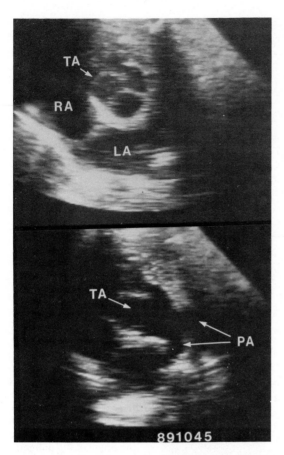

**Fig. 7–132.** Parasternal short-axis view at the base of the heart demonstrating a single large truncus type vessel (TA). With more cephalad angulation (lower panel), a branching pulmonary artery (PA) can be seen arising from the truncal vessel. LA = left atrium; RA = right atrium. (Courtesy of Randall L. Caldwell.)

### Hypoplastic Left Heart Syndrome

Hypoplasia of the left ventricle is usually associated with atresia of the aortic and mitral valves, endocardial thickening, and a small left atrium, and is properly referred to as hypoplastic left heart syndrome. The aortic diameter is reduced, but increases in size beyond the ductus arteriosus, which is dilated. The echocardiographic diagnosis is based on the presence of an abnormally small and underdeveloped left ventricle, usually in association with a dilated right ventricle (Fig. 7–135).[383-385] The ventricular septum should be carefully evaluated for the presence of a septal defect. The mitral valve, aortic valve, and aortic arch should also be assessed.[386] In the short-axis view, the relative sizes of the two ventricles can be determined. The diameter of the aortic root can be measured and is usually less than 5 mm. A dilated pulmonary artery can be seen connecting to an enlarged ductus arteriosus.

The entire aortic arch must be carefully evaluated from the parasternal and suprasternal views.[385] The dimensions of the vessel and the presence or absence of a coarctation should be determined. These features have important implications for surgical repair. The ductus

should be identified and carefully differentiated from the main pulmonary artery. In planning surgical intervention, several other anatomic features should be analyzed, right ventricular systolic function most importantly. The presence and severity of tricuspid regurgitation must also be determined. Finally, the atrial septum should be assessed for the presence of a defect.

A rare form of ventricular dysplasia, noncompaction of left ventricular myocardium, occurs because of arrested endomyocardial morphogenesis resulting in failure of trabecular "compaction" of the developing myocardium.[387,388] This condition leads to a "spongy" appearance of the myocardium, characterized by prominent ventricular trabeculations and deep intertrabecular recesses. These structural abnormalities are detectable with two-dimensional echocardiography (Fig. 7–136).

### Single Ventricle

In the simplest definition, single ventricle refers to a condition in which a single pumping chamber receives inflow from both atria (i.e., has two inlet regions and is connected to two atrioventricular valves). A second or rudimentary chamber may be present, but it has no inlet portion (hence, is not a "ventricle"). The rudimentary chamber is sometimes referred to as an outlet chamber or rudimentary pouch. Based on the morphology, location, and trabecular pattern of the pumping and rudimentary chambers, the heart is referred to as a univentricular heart of either right, left, or indeterminant ventricular type.[389,390] The most common form of single ventricle is the left ventricular type, also referred to as double-inlet left ventricle. Ventriculoarterial connections are also variable. Unfortunately, the diagnosis and classification of the univentricular heart is complex and considerable controversy exists regarding nomenclature and definitions.[391]

By using echocardiography, the type of single ventricle can be determined.[392-395] In the left ventricular type, the rudimentary chamber is anterior and superior to the pumping chamber. In the right ventricular type, it is located more posteriorly. Because the location of the rudimentary chamber varies, the echocardiographic views used to assess this structure must also vary. For the left ventricular type, the parasternal long-axis and short-axis views usually provide the best opportunities to visualize the rudimentary chamber and intervening trabecular septum. For the right ventricular type, the four-chamber view is often best. In either case, the short-axis and four-chamber views are critical to demonstrate two side-by-side inlets without an intervening inlet septum (Figs. 7–137 and 7–138). This finding secures the diagnosis and distinguishes single ventricle from other conditions in which two distinct pumping chambers are not readily apparent (Fig. 7–139), which include hypoplastic left or right heart (which has associated atrioventricular and semilunar valve hypoplasia), tricuspid atresia (characterized by a blind-ending right atrium), and a large ventricular septal defect (in which an inlet septum separates the inflow of the two atrioventricular valves). Once the rudimentary chamber is identified, the interventricular

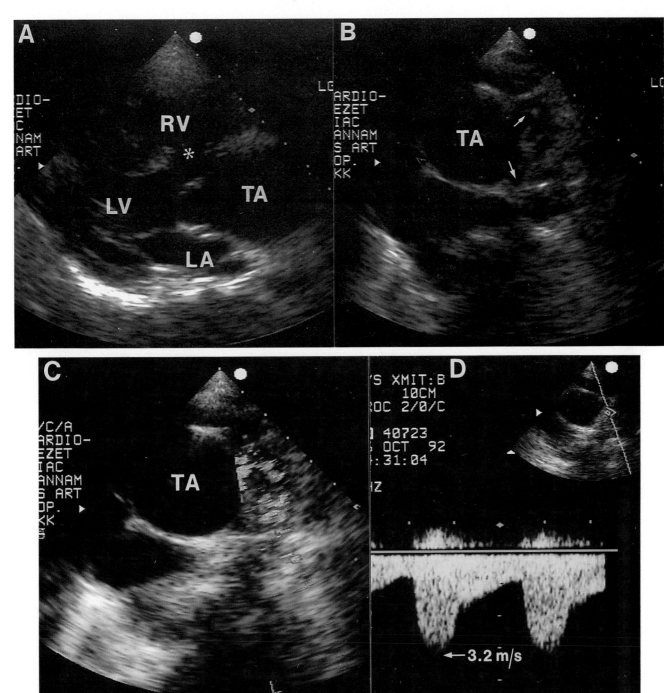

**Fig. 7–133.** An example of truncus arteriosus, type II, in a young child. In *A*, the parasternal long-axis view demonstrates the truncus arteriosus (TA) and a large ventricular septal defect (*asterisk*). In *B*, the short-axis view again demonstrates the truncus (TA). The small pulmonary arteries are barely visualized arising separately from the posterior truncal wall (*arrows*). In *C*, color flow imaging from the same view demonstrates turbulent flow within the proximal pulmonary arteries. In *D*, continuous wave Doppler reveals stenosis near their origin. The maximal velocity within the proximal pulmonary artery was 3.2 m/sec consistent with a peak systolic gradient of approximately 40 mm Hg. (Courtesy of K. Kádár, Hungarian Institute of Cardiology.) LA = left atrium; LV = left ventricle; RV = right ventricle.

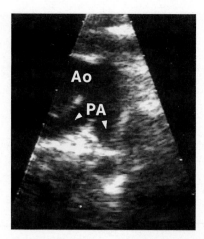

**Fig. 7–134.** A high angulated parasternal view just above the aortic valve in a patient with aortopulmonary window. The posterior wall of the aorta (Ao) communicates freely with the proximal pulmonary artery (PA). The bifurcation of the main pulmonary artery is indicated. Two separate semilunar valves were present in this patient. (Courtesy of Gregory J. Ensing.)

communication, or bulboventricular foramen, should be sought. Evidence of flow restriction through the foramen can be assessed with Doppler techniques.

Once the diagnosis of single ventricle is made, the echocardiographic evaluation should focus on two related issues that have important implications for repair.[396,397] First, the specific type of atrioventricular connections should be established.[392,393] In most cases, two separate inlet connections through two distinct atrioventricular valves are present (i.e., a double-inlet ventricle). Alternatively, in the setting of an indeterminant type of single ventricle, a single, large, common atrioventricular valve may be present (Fig. 7–140). One of the atrioventricular connections may be absent, a condition that may be difficult to distinguish from tricuspid atresia and hypoplastic left heart. Finally, the two valves themselves must be assessed carefully for the presence of straddling or overriding. As discussed previously, the insertion of the chordae relative to the trabecular septum has implications for proper classification as well as surgical repair.

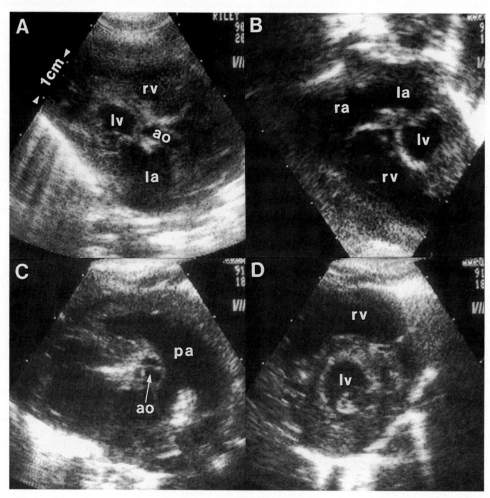

**Fig. 7–135.** Serial images from an infant with hypoplastic left heart syndrome. In *A*, the parasternal long-axis view demonstrates hypoplasia of the left ventricle (lv) and ascending aorta (ao). In *B*, the apical four-chamber view again reveals a small left ventricle with a normally developed right ventricle (rv). An atrial septal defect is also present. In *C*, the parasternal short-axis view at the base illustrates the hypoplastic aorta relative to a normal pulmonary artery (pa). In *D*, a more apical parasternal short-axis view again demonstrates left ventricular hypoplasia. ra = right atrium; la = left atrium.

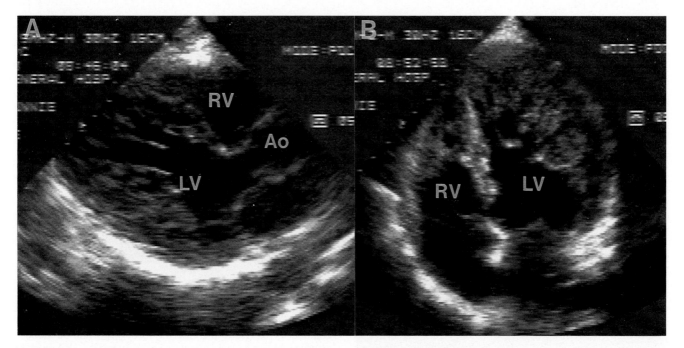

**Fig. 7–136.** Parasternal long-axis (*A*) and apical four-chamber (*B*) views from a patient with noncompaction of the ventricular myocardium. The left and right ventricular myocardium has a spongy appearance and there are prominent ventricular trabeculations and deep intertrabecular recesses. Ao = aorta; LV = left ventricle; RV = right ventricle.

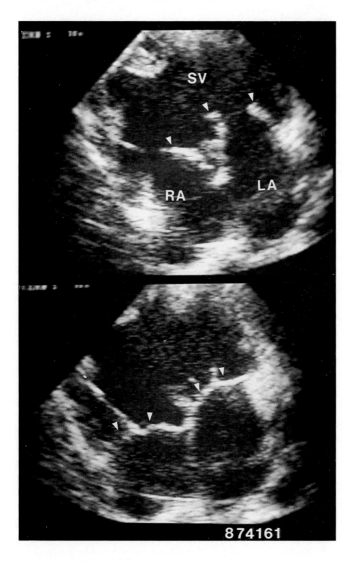

**Fig. 7–137.** Apical view of a patient with a single ventricle (SV). A single heavily trabeculated pumping chamber receives inflow from both the right atrium (RA) and left atrium (LA). Two distinct atrioventricular valves are apparent (*arrowheads*). Upper panel = diastole; lower panel = systole.

423

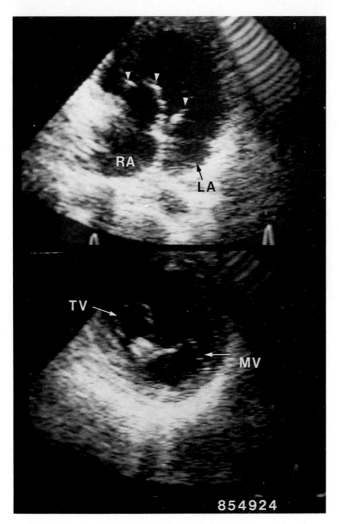

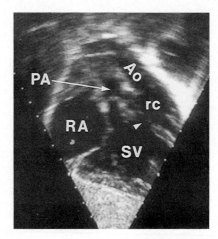

**Fig. 7–139.** Subcostal view from a patient with a single ventricle (SV). The rudimentary chamber (rc) is shown in a position anterior and to the right of the ventricle. The arrowhead indicates the bulboventricular foramen. The rudimentary chamber gives rise to the anterior aorta (Ao). The pulmonary artery (PA) can be seen arising from the ventricle. RA = right atrium.

tion. Following surgical repair, echocardiography is especially useful in assessing ventricular function and atrioventricular valve regurgitation (Fig. 7–141).

### Tricuspid Atresia

This condition is discussed here because the presence of an atretic tricuspid valve invariably leads to some degree of right ventricular hypoplasia. As a consequence, this lesion may be confused with some of the

**Fig. 7–138.** Apical and short-axis parasternal views of a patient with a left ventricular type single ventricle. Two atrioventricular valves can be seen in the four-chamber view (*arrowheads*) as well as in the short-axis view. The single pumping chamber has a smooth wall, and no ventricular septal tissue is noted. RA = right atrium; LA = left atrium; TV = tricuspid valve; MV = mitral valve.

Next, the ventriculoarterial connections should be determined.[391] Although any form of connection may occur, some are more likely than others. For example, with left ventricular type single ventricle, discordant ventriculoarterial connections are common, usually with the aorta arising from the rudimentary (anterior) chamber and the pulmonary artery from the (posterior) ventricle. Although this relationship is not properly referred to as "transposition," it bears many of the typical echocardiographic features. With the right ventricular type single ventricle, the most common connections are double outlet from the ventricle or single outlet with pulmonary atresia. Regardless of the type of outlet connection, the possibility of outflow tract obstruction from either the ventricle or rudimentary chamber should be considered. Doppler is often of value in making this determina-

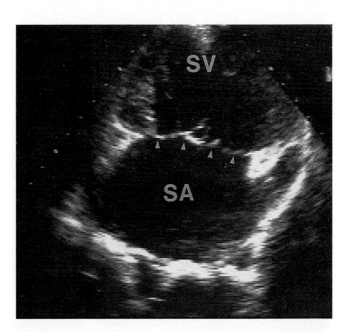

**Fig. 7–140.** An apical view in a patient reveals a single ventricle (SV) and a single atrium (SA). A large, single, common atrioventricular valve is indicated (*arrowheads*).

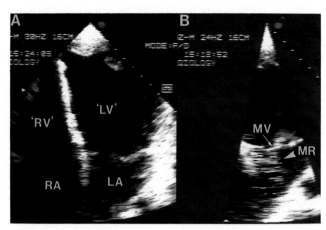

Fig. 7–141. *A*, Apical view from a patient with single ventricle after a septation procedure. The single ventricle is divided by a prosthetic patch into a ''right'' and ''left'' ventricle. The large patch is seen easily as a linear echogenic structure dividing the ventricle. In *B*, color flow imaging demonstrates mild mitral regurgitation (MR). LA = left atrium; RA = right atrium; MV = mitral valve.

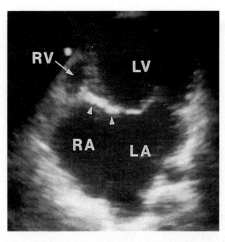

Fig. 7–143. Apical four-chamber view of a patient with tricuspid atresia. The atretic tricuspid annulus is indicated by arrowheads. A large atrial septal defect is present. The hypoplastic right ventricle (RV) is seen. RA = right atrium; LA = left atrium; LV = left ventricle.

other disorders included in this section.[398] Tricuspid atresia is characterized by an imperforate tricuspid valve, hypoplasia of the morphologic right ventricle, an interatrial communication, and a normally developed left ventricle and mitral valve.[399,400] In contrast to single ventricle, the hypoplastic chamber has an inlet portion (although it is atretic), and therefore it is properly called a ventricle. The interatrial communication is most often a patent foramen ovale and is therefore restrictive. A larger secundum defect is present in approximately 25% of patients. The clinically important variable features of tricuspid atresia include the ventriculoarterial communication (concordant or transposed), the presence and size of a ventricular septal defect, and the presence and magnitude of obstruction to pulmonary blood flow.

The echocardiographic diagnosis of tricuspid atresia is made from the four-chamber view in which the imper-forate tricuspid valve is visualized directly (Fig. 7–142).[401] The presence of severe valvular hypoplasia (rather than atresia) is established by detecting remnants of the tricuspid valve apparatus. In either case, the inlet is imperforate. When the atresia is caused by a membrane, considerable motion in the area of the annulus may be seen on two-dimensional echocardiographic images. Doppler is useful for confirming the absence of flow through the inlet.[402] The size and function of the hypoplastic right ventricle can be determined (Fig. 7–143) and the presence of mitral regurgitation can also be assessed (Fig. 7–144). The parasternal long-axis view is used to examine the septum for defects and to help determine the great artery relationships. Because any form of great artery connections is possible, the exact position of the posterior great vessel relative to the septum must also be noted.[379] By scanning superiorly, the presence or absence of transposition can usually be determined. In the short-axis view, the right ventricular

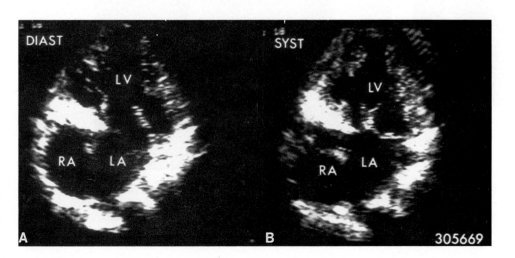

Fig. 7–142. Apical four-chamber views in diastole (*A*) and systole (*B*) of a patient with tricuspid valve atresia. A dense linear echo is present in the area of the tricuspid annulus indicating complete atresia of the valve structure. The mitral valve appears thickened and redundant. A large atrial septal defect is present. The right ventricle is hypoplastic and not seen well in these images. LA = left atrium; LV = left ventricle; RA = right atrium.

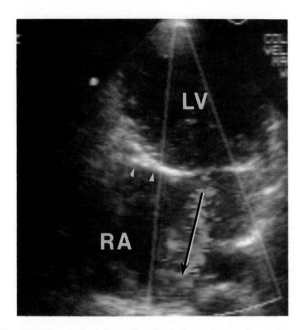

**Fig. 7–144.** Apical four-chamber view of a patient with tricuspid atresia (*arrowheads*). Color flow imaging during systole demonstrates severe mitral regurgitation (*double arrow*). LV = left ventricle; RA = right atrium.

outflow tract and pulmonary valve can be evaluated for the presence of outflow obstruction. Confirming the diagnosis of pulmonary artery atresia, however, requires the use of multiple imaging planes.[403] The subcostal views may be helpful in assessing the size of the interatrial communication. Dilation of the right atrium and bowing of the septum into the left atrium suggests a small, restrictive communication. From the suprasternal notch, the size and continuity of the pulmonary arteries can be assessed.

## ECHOCARDIOGRAPHIC EVALUATION DURING AND AFTER SURGERY

Echocardiography is extremely useful for clinical decision-making in patients undergoing palliative or reparative surgical procedures. Intraoperative echocardiography, both epicardial and transesophageal, permits additional diagnoses to be made and allows the adequacy of repair to be determined before completion of the operation.[404–409] Subsequently, echocardiography compares favorably to cardiac catheterization for the detection of postoperative residua.[410] Valvular lesions, conduit dysfunction, residual shunting, and pulmonary pressure can be accurately assessed in postoperative patients without the need for invasive procedures.

### Systemic Artery to Pulmonary Artery Shunts

Over the years, a variety of shunts have been devised to increase pulmonary artery flow by a systemic artery to pulmonary artery anastomosis. Fortunately, the most common shunt in use today, the Blalock-Taussig shunt,

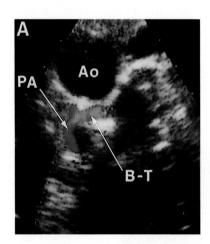
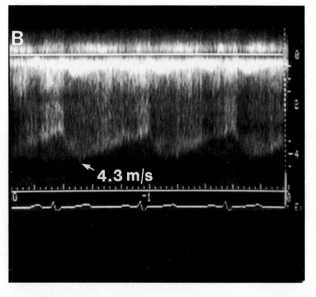

**Fig. 7–145.** In *A*, a suprasternal short-axis view with color flow imaging demonstrates a left Blalock-Taussig shunt (B-T). The junction between the shunt and the left subclavian artery is not seen in this frame. The distal anastomosis between the shunt and the pulmonary artery (PA) is indicated. In *B*, continuous wave Doppler demonstrates high-velocity continuous flow through the shunt with a maximal velocity in late systole of 4.3 m/sec indicating a gradient between the subclavian artery and pulmonary artery of approximately 74 mm Hg. Ao = aorta.

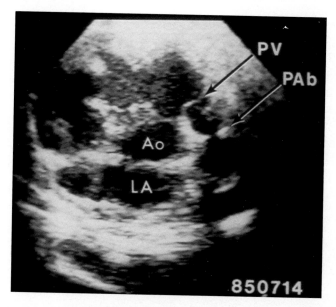

**Fig. 7–146.** Parasternal short-axis view at the base of the heart in a child with a large ventricular septal defect. A pulmonary artery band (PAb) is just distal to the pulmonic valve (PV). Ao = aorta; LA = left atrium.

is also the one that is easiest to image. This shunt is a vascular connection between the subclavian artery and a branch pulmonary artery. Thus, it may be long and can be created on either the right or left side. A direct anastomosis is commonly performed (a native shunt) or a prosthetic conduit (either Dacron or Goretex) may be used. In several situations, one might wish to evaluate a Blalock-Taussig shunt. Demonstrating the presence of such a shunt and its patency is of obvious clinical importance. Dysfunction because of stenosis can also be assessed. Finally, by determining the gradient across the conduit, the pulmonary artery pressure can be estimated.

Blalock-Taussig shunts are best viewed from the suprasternal notch or a high parasternal window.[411,412] A right-sided shunt may be seen in the suprasternal short-axis view. As the right pulmonary artery passes below the aortic arch, the insertion of the conduit can often be recorded. A left-sided shunt may be more difficult to record (Fig. 7–145). From the suprasternal notch, the scan plane is tilted far to the left to include the left pulmonary artery. The shunt may be recorded entering from the left. When the shunt cannot be observed directly, Doppler and color flow imaging are often helpful for identification. The patency of a shunt and the presence of kinking or stenosis (usually at the distal insertion site) can also be determined with Doppler. If a nonimaging probe is used, however, care must be taken to avoid mistaking the Blalock-Taussig shunt for a patent ductus arteriosus.[412]

The pressure gradient across the shunt can be measured by using the modified Bernoulli equation, and this value can be used to estimate the pulmonary pressure, both in systole and diastole. The peripheral systolic and diastolic pressures are determined from the sphygmomanometer and the pressure gradient is subtracted from these values to derive the pulmonary pressures. Doppler can underestimate the gradient of a narrow, tubular conduit (because of significant viscous friction in the vessel) leading to an overestimation of pulmonary artery pressure. The amount of shunt flow can also be estimated from the Doppler tracing.[254] Low-velocity retrograde diastolic flow in the descending aorta indicates antegrade flow through the shunt. The magnitude of the shunt flow is suggested by the size of this flow signal. The ratio of the descending aorta retrograde flow velocity integral to the forward flow velocity integral correlates with the magnitude of the left-to-right shunt.

### Pulmonary Artery Bands

A pulmonary artery band can be recorded as a linear echogenic structure positioned transversely across the main pulmonary artery (usually in its middle portion). They are best evaluated from the parasternal short-axis and subcostal views (Fig. 7–146).[413] A band can become displaced and its abnormal position can often be detected with two-dimensional echocardiography. The degree of stenosis created by these structures cannot be judged reliably with echocardiography alone, although poststenotic dilation is suggestive of significant narrowing. Doppler should be used to estimate the pressure gradient across a band (Fig. 7–147). The correlation between the Doppler estimate and the catheterization-measured gradient is high. Furthermore, in the presence of a nonrestrictive ventricular septal defect, when right and left ventricular systolic pressures are approximately equal, the pulmonary artery systolic pressure can be estimated as the brachial systolic pressure minus the gradient across the band (provided there is no left ventricular outflow tract obstruction). In patients who have had a pulmonary artery band removed, the echocardiographic

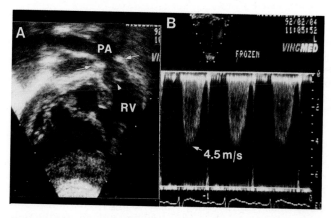

**Fig. 7–147.** A pulmonary artery band is shown. In *A*, a subcostal view demonstrates the right ventricle (RV), outflow tract, and pulmonary artery (PA). The arrows indicate the location of the pulmonary artery band immediately distal to the valve (*arrowhead*). In *B*, continuous wave Doppler recording through the band reveals a maximal velocity of 4.5 m/sec consistent with a peak systolic gradient of approximately 80 mm Hg.

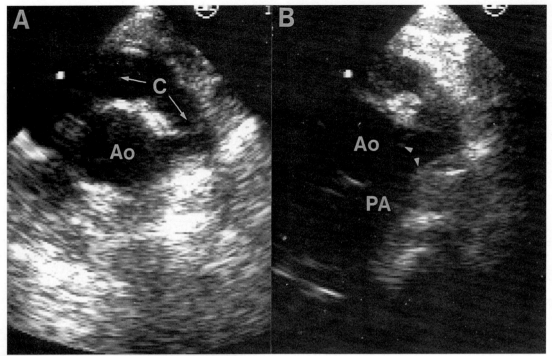

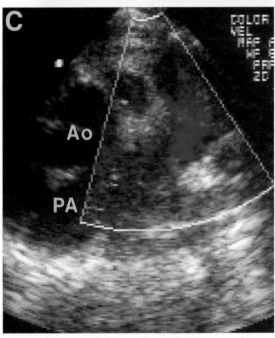

**Fig. 7–148.** In *A*, a short-axis view at the base of the heart in a patient with tricuspid atresia demonstrates a Fontan conduit passing anterior and left of the aorta (Ao). In *B*, angulation of the scan plane permits demonstration of the distal anastomosis of the conduit into the pulmonary artery (PA) (*arrowheads*). In *C*, color flow imaging in the same plane demonstrates flow within the conduit without significant turbulence, which suggests the absence of significant obstruction within the conduit.

findings may be confusing. Residual narrowing and scar tissue at the site of the banding makes it difficult to determine if the band is still in place. No echocardiographic signs alone can reliably make this distinction.

### The Fontan Procedure

For lesions such as single ventricle and tricuspid atresia, in which abnormal right ventricular structure or function prevents adequate pulmonary blood flow, the Fontan procedure is frequently used for effective palliation.[396,414] The Fontan anastomosis is a connection be-

tween the systemic atrium and the pulmonary circuit that is designed to increase pulmonary blood flow. The Fontan circuit can be created in a variety of ways. In many cases, a direct anastomosis using pericardial tissue is placed between the right atrial appendage and the pulmonary artery. In other situations, a valved or nonvalved conduit is used. Intra-atrial conduits, connecting the inferior vena cava to the pulmonary artery, are also placed.

Visualization of the Fontan anastomosis is often challenging.[415] Optimal evaluation is facilitated by knowledge of the specific type of connection that was created

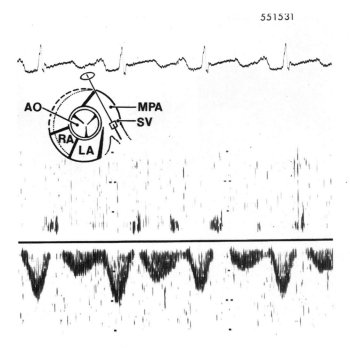

551531

**Fig. 7–149.** Pulsed Doppler interrogation of flow in the main pulmonary artery (MPA) in a patient after a Fontan procedure. The sample volume (SV) is placed in the pulmonary artery prior to its bifurcation. There is biphasic flow away from the transducer occurring in late systole and augmented by atrial contraction. LA = left atrium; RA = right atrium; AO = aorta.

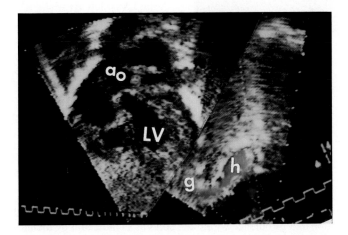

**Fig. 7–150.** A composite image from a patient with a left ventricular apex-to-descending aorta conduit. The conduit is seen arising from the left ventricular (LV) apex and consisted of a Dacron segment (g) and a valved homograft (h). Nonturbulent flow within the conduit is apparent with color flow imaging, recorded from the subcostal window. The valve within the homograft is not seen in these images. (Courtesy of Gregory J. Ensing.) ao = aorta.

surgically. The course of most of these connections is retrosternal, further complicating their echocardiographic detection. High parasternal and subcostal views are usually most effective (Fig. 7–148). Once the connection is visualized, Doppler plays an important role in assessing the flow pattern and in determining the presence of dysfunction.[416–419] Normal pulmonary artery flow after a Fontan procedure is biphasic, with one peak in late systole and a larger peak in late diastole during atrial contraction (Fig. 7–149).[416,418,419] Augmentation of flow velocity is normally seen during inspiration. Abnormal systemic ventricular function is suggested by reduced or absent late diastolic flow and diminished respiratory variation in the flow pattern. More recently, transesophageal echocardiography has been used to assess the Fontan connection.[420–422]

### Left Ventricular Apex to Descending Aorta Conduits

Complex left ventricular outflow tract obstruction is sometimes repaired by placing a prosthetic conduit between the cardiac apex and the descending aorta. In most cases, a valve (either mechanical or bioprosthetic) is positioned in the middle of these conduits. Visualization of these structures with echocardiography is challenging and requires the use of multiple views.[423,424] The prosthetic material used in the walls of the conduit is highly echogenic, a property that is useful for the initial identification of these structures. Sometimes the walls have a beaded appearance on echocardiography, the result of the ribbed surface of the synthetic material. Calcification within the conduit walls may also be detected and is not necessarily indicative of stenosis. The proximal portion of the conduit can often be seen from a modified apical window. The distal insertion, usually but not always above the diaphragm, is best recorded from the subcostal views. The middle portion containing the prosthesis may be difficult to see. In such cases, color Doppler can help to visualize the flow through the conduit (Fig. 7–150). Also, by recording turbulence within the conduit, obstruction or valvular regurgitation may be demonstrated. Pulsed and continuous wave Doppler should also be used whenever stenosis is suspected, although, proper alignment of the beam may be difficult.

### Right Ventricle to Pulmonary Artery Conduits

Both valved and nonvalved conduits have been used to shunt blood from the right ventricle to the pulmonary artery (e.g., in cases of pulmonary atresia or severe tetralogy of Fallot). The echocardiographic evaluation of these structures requires an approach similar to that just described for left ventricle to aorta conduits.[423,424] The conduits are best recorded from the high parasternal or subcostal windows (Fig. 7–151). Conduit obstruction can occur at the proximal or distal insertion site (usually because of problems in surgical positioning), at the valve (from primary tissue degeneration), or diffusely (the result of development of a neointimal peel). Turbulence on color flow imaging may provide the initial evidence of conduit stenosis (Fig. 7–152). Regurgitation, diagnosed by using Doppler, is present in many of these

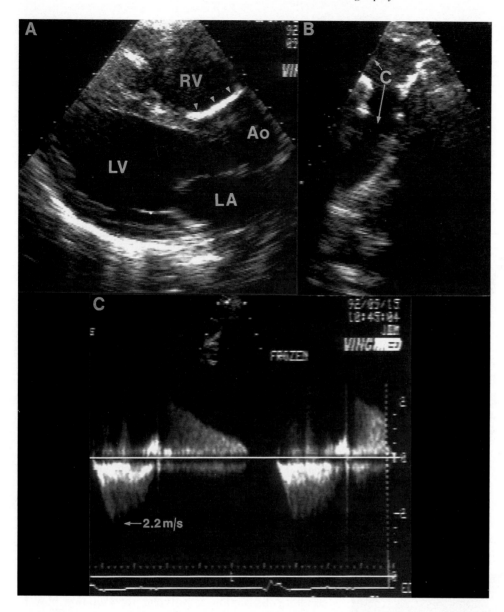

**Fig. 7–151.** In *A*, the parasternal long-axis view in a patient following repair of double-outlet right ventricle demonstrates the ventricular septal defect patch (*arrowheads*). In *B*, a high parasternal view allows visualization of the right ventricle-to-pulmonary artery conduit (C). The conduit appears patent and no valve within the structure is recorded. In *C*, Doppler imaging through the conduit demonstrates increased flow velocity during systole (2.2 m/sec) and conduit regurgitation during diastole, which suggests a maximal systolic gradient within the conduit of approximately 20 mm Hg. Ao = aorta; LV = left ventricle; RV = right ventricle; LA = left atrium.

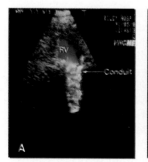
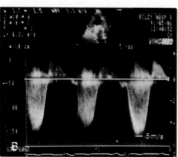

**Fig. 7–152.** An example of a right ventricle-to-pulmonary artery conduit. In *A*, color flow imaging demonstrates acceleration and turbulence within the conduit as indicated by the mosaic blood flow pattern. In *B*, continuous wave Doppler demonstrates severe obstruction. The maximal flow velocity was 5.0 m/sec, suggesting a peak pressure gradient within the conduit of approximately 100 mm Hg. RV = right ventricle.

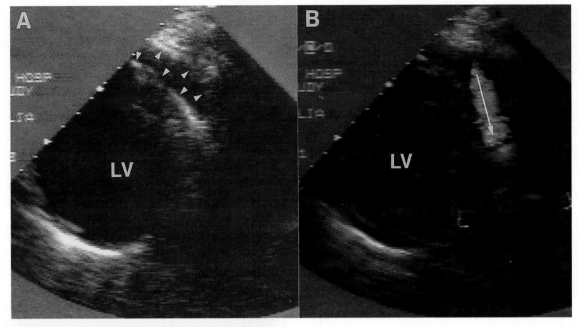

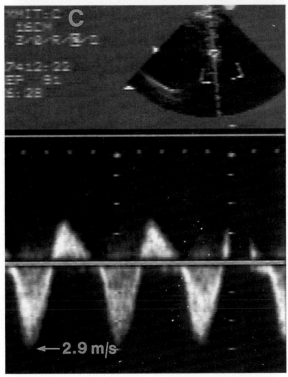

**Fig. 7–153.** In *A*, a patient with D-transposition, ventricular septal defect, and pulmonic stenosis following a Rastelli repair, the right ventricle-to-pulmonary artery conduit (*arrowheads*) is anterior and lateral to the left ventricle (LV). In *B*, color flow imaging confirms flow within the conduit in a posterior direction. In *C*, continuous wave Doppler demonstrates moderate obstruction within the conduit with a maximal systolic pressure gradient of approximately 34 mm Hg. Conduit regurgitation is also demonstrated.

valved conduits (Fig. 7–153). In one study, Doppler images revealed nearly two thirds of newly implanted valved conduits had mild regurgitation.[424]

## FETAL ECHOCARDIOGRAPHY

Examination of the fetal heart in utero is a productive and rapidly growing discipline.[425–433] Fetal echocardiography has provided a valuable new means to better understand intrauterine growth and development of the heart and great vessels. The prenatal diagnosis of structural heart disease and the physiologic evaluation of fetal arrhythmias are perhaps the most important new insights provided by this technique. The long-term effects of ultrasound energy on the developing fetus, however, are unknown. This fact may be particularly important when the higher energy levels associated with Doppler techniques are used. To date, no detrimental effects in humans have been demonstrated. Still, it is advisable

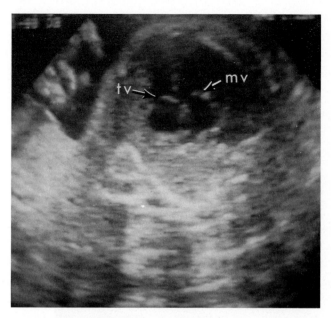

**Fig. 7–154.** Apical four-chamber view of a fetal heart recorded at approximately 30 weeks gestation reveals the mitral (mv) and tricuspid (tv) valves.

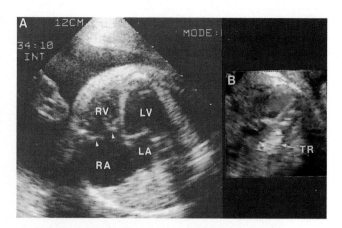

**Fig. 7–156.** A fetal echocardiogram of a patient with tricuspid valve dysplasia. In *A*, the apical four-chamber view reveals the abnormal tricuspid valve (*arrowheads*). In *B*, color flow imaging demonstrates turbulent flow through the tricuspid valve and significant tricuspid regurgitation (TR). (Courtesy of K. Kádár, Hungarian Institute of Cardiology.) LA = left atrium; LV = left ventricle; RA = right atrium; RV = right ventricle.

to avoid excess exposure of the fetus by keeping the examination time as short as possible and using the lowest possible power setting.

There are several potential indications for performing fetal echocardiography.[434] Evaluation of the heart in the setting of retarded fetal growth or fetal distress is often recommended.[431] Whenever extracardiac anomalies are detected during fetal ultrasound examination, cardiac assessment may be beneficial. The presence of chromosomal abnormalities detected with amniocentesis is strongly correlated with congenital heart disease and is another accepted indication for fetal echocardiography. The test should also be performed as part of the assessment of fetal arrhythmias.[435,436] Finally, whenever congenital heart disease is suspected for other reasons, such as maternal exposure to teratogenic substances or a pa-

rental history of previous children with congenital lesions, the examination should be considered.

The performance of a fetal echocardiogram requires experience and a systematic approach.[426] Guidelines for training have been formulated and only qualified individuals should perform this highly specialized examination. A brief description of the examination is presented here for interest only. The first step is to determine the position and orientation of the fetus within the uterus. Within the thorax, the heart, because of its motion, is usually the easiest and most recognizable structure to examine. The four-chamber view is most important and should be recorded first (Fig. 7–154). For orientation, the left atrium is identified by the presence of the septum primum and the pulmonary veins. Cardiac situs can be determined by identifying the systemic veins and the position of the atria relative to the liver and spleen. Next, the atrioventricular valves are identified, with the tricuspid valve slightly more apical than the mitral valve.[437,438] The outlet portions of the heart are than evaluated (Fig. 7–155).[110,439–441] Cardiac measurements can be made and compared to normal values that have been defined for all gestational ages.[442–445] Doppler techniques can be used to visualize blood flow through the heart, great vessels, and umbilical vessels.[432,433] Assessment of fetal arrhythmias is best accomplished by using a combination of M-mode and Doppler recordings.[435,436] When these arrhythmias are present, a careful search for structural heart disease is mandatory.[38]

Using this approach, a wealth of diagnostic information is available (Fig. 7–156). The structures in these images are small, however, and random movements of the fetus make for a challenging and time-consuming examination. For all these reasons, limitations exist and smaller defects are easily overlooked. Despite these fac-

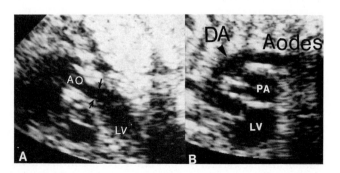

**Fig. 7–155.** The left ventricular (LV) outflow tract (*arrows*) and aorta (AO) in a normal fetus. In *A*, the ascending aorta is recorded. In *B*, the entire aortic arch, descending aorta (Ao des) and right pulmonary artery (PA) are visualized. The ductus arteriosus (DA) is indicated. (Courtesy of K. Kádár, Hungarian Institute of Cardiology.)

tors, fetal echocardiography has provided clinicians with earlier diagnosis of heart disease and a better understanding of fetal hemodynamics.

## REFERENCES

1. Perloff, J.K.: The clincial recognition of congenital heart disease. 3rd Ed. Philadelphia, W.B. Saunders Co., 1987.
2. Pyeritz, R.E. and Murphy, E.A.: Genetics and congenital heart disease: Perspectives and prospects. J. Am. Coll. Cardiol., *13*:1458, 1989.
3. Nora, J.J. and Nora, A.H.: The evolution of specific genetic and environmental counseling in congenital heart disease. Circulation, *57*:205, 1978.
4. McNamara, D.G.: The adult with congenital heart disease. Curr. Probl. Cardiol., *14*:63, 1989.
5. Perloff, J.K.: Congenital heart disease in adults: A new cardiovascular subspecialty. Circulation, *84*:1881, 1991.
6. Laks, H. and Pearl, J.M.: The surgeon's responsibility: Operation and reoperation: The UCLA experience. J. Am. Coll. Cardiol., *18*:327, 1991.
7. Celermajer, D.S. and Deanfield, J.E.: Adults with congenital heart disease. Br. Med. J., *303*:1413, 1991.
8. Perloff, J.K.: The UCLA adult congenital heart disease program. Am. J. Cardiol., *57*:1190, 1986.
9. Perloff, J.K.: Medical center experiences: Great Britain, Canada, and the United States. J. Am. Coll. Cardiol., *18*:311, 1991.
10. Child, J.S.: Echo-Doppler and color-flow imaging in congenital heart disease. Cardiol. Clin., *8*:289, 1990.
11. Rice, M.J., Seward, J.B., Hagler, D.J., Mair, D.D., Feldt, R.H., Puga, F.J., Danielson, G.K., Edwards, W.D., and Tajik, A.J.: Impact of 2-dimensional echocardiography on the management of distressed newborns in whom cardiac disease is suspected. Am. Heart. J., *51*: 228, 1983.
12. Gutgesell, H.P.: Echocardiographic assessment of cardiac function in infants and children. J. Am. Cardiol., *5*: 95S, 1985.
13. Reeder, G.S., Currie, P.J., Hagler, D.J., Tajik, A.J., and Seward, J.B.: Use of Doppler techniques (continuous-wave, pulsed-wave, and color flow imaging) in the noninvasive hemodynamic assessment of congenital heart disease. Mayo Clin. Proc., *61*:725, 1986.
14. Gnanapragasam, J.P., Houston, A.B., Doig, W.B., Fraser, R., Lilley, S., Murtagh, E., and Olafsson, G.: Influence of colour Doppler echocardiography on the ultrasonic assessment of congenital heart disease: A prospective study. Br. Heart J., *66*:238, 1991.
15. Ritter, S.B.: Two-dimensional Doppler color flow mapping in congenital heart disease. Clin. Cardiol., *9*:591, 1986.
16. Leung, M.P., Mok, C.K., Lau, K.C., Lo, R., and Yeung, C.Y.: The role of cross-sectional echocardiography and pulsed Doppler ultrasound in the management of neonates in whom congenital heart disease is suspected. Br. Heart J., *56*:73, 1986.
17. Ritter, S.B.: Transesophageal real-time echocardiography in infants and children with congenital heart disease. J. Am. Coll. Cardiol., *18*:569, 1991.
18. Weintraub, R., Shiota, T., Elkadi, T., Golebiovski, P., Zhang, J., Rothman, A., Ritter, S.B., and Sahn, D.J.: Transesophageal echocardiography in infants and chil-

dren with congenital heart disease. Circulation, *86*:711, 1992.
19. Stümper, O.: Transoesophageal echocardiography: A new diagnostic method in paediatric cardiology. Arch. Dis. Child., *66*:1175, 1991.
20. Feltes, T.F.: Advances in transesophageal echocardiography: Impact of a changing technology on children with congenital heart disease. J. Am. Coll. Cardiol., *18*:1515, 1991.
21. Stümper, O.F.W., Elzenga, N.J., Hess, J., and Sutherland, G.R.: Transesophageal echocardiography in children with congenital heart disease: An initial experience. J. Am. Coll. Cardiol., *16*:433, 1990.
21a. Hoffman, P., Stümper, O., Rydelwska-Sadowska, W., and Sutherland, G.R.: Transgastric imaging: A valuable addition to the assessment of congenital heart disease by transverse plane transesophageal echocardiography. J. Am. Soc. Echo., *6*:35, 1993.
22. Snider, A.R. and Serwer, G.A.: Echocardiography in Pediatric Heart Disease. St. Louis, Mosby-Year Book, 1990.
23. Van Praagh, R.: Diagnosis of complex congenital heart disease: Morphologic-anatomic method and terminology. Cardiovasc. Intervent. Radiol., *7*:115, 1984.
24. Van Praagh, R.: Terminology of congenital heart disease: Glossary and commentary. Circulation, *56*:139, 1977.
25. Stanger, P., Rudolph, A.M., and Edwards, J.E.: Cardiac malpositions: An overview based on study of sixty-five necropsy specimens. Circulation, *56*:159, 1977.
26. Tynan, M.G., Becker, A.E. and Macartney, F.J.: Nomenclature and classification of congenital heart disease. Br. Heart J., *41*:544, 1979.
27. Silverman, N.H.: Pediatric Echocardiography. Baltimore, Williams & Wilkins, 1993.
28. Silverman, N.H.: An ultrasonic approach to the diagnosis of cardiac situs, connections, and malpositions. Cardiol. Clin., *1*:473, 1983.
29. Sapire, D.W., Ho, S.Y., Anderson, R.H., and Rigby, M.L.: Diagnosis and significance of atrial isomerism. Am. J. Cardiol., *58*:342, 1986.
30. Huhta, J.C., Smallhorn, J.F., and Macartney, F.J.: Two-dimensional echocardiographic diagnosis of situs. Br. Heart J., *48*:97, 1982.
31. Stümper, O.F.W., Sreeram, N., Elzenga, N.J., and Sutherland, G.R.: Diagnosis of atrial situs by transesophageal echocardiography. J. Am. Coll. Cardiol., *16*:442, 1990.
32. Foale, R., Stefanini, L., Rickards, A., and Somerville, J.: Left and right ventricular morphology in complex congenital heart disease defined by two dimensional echocardiography. Am. J. Cardiol., *49*:93, 1982.
33. de la Cruz, M.V., Berrazueta, J.R., and Arteaga, M.: Rules for diagnosis of arterioventricular discordances and spatial identification of ventricles. Crossed great arteries and transposition of the great arteries. Br. Heart J., *38*:341, 1976.
34. Pasquini, L., Sanders, S.P., Parness, I., Colan, S., Keane, J.F., Mayer, J.E., Kratz, C., Foran, R.B., Marino, B., Van Praagh, S., and Van Praagh, R.: Echocardiographic and anatomic findings in atrioventricular discordance with ventriculoarterial concordance. Am. J. Cardiol., *62*:1256, 1988.
35. Henry, W.L., Maron, B.J., and Griffith, J.M.: Cross-sectional echocardiography in the diagnosis of congenital heart disease: Identification of the relation of the ventricles and great arteries. Circulation, *56*:267, 1977.
36. Celano, V., Pieroni, D.R., Gengell, R.L., and Roland,

J.-M.A.: Two-dimensional echocardiographic recognition of the right aortic arch. Am. J. Cardiol., *51*:1507, 1983.

37. Huhta, J.G., Gutgesell, H.P., Latson, L.A. and Huffines, F.D.: Two-dimensional echocardiographic assessment of the aorta in infants and children with congenital heart disease. Circulation, *70*:417, 1984.

38. Roberson, D.A. and Silverman, N.H.: Ebstein's anomaly: Echocardiographic and clinical features in the fetus and neonate. J. Am. Coll. Cardiol., *14*:1300, 1989.

39. Shiina, A., Seward, J.B., Tajik, A.J., Hagler, D.J., and Danielson, G.K.: Two-dimensional echocardiographic-surgical correlation in Ebstein's anomaly: Preoperative determination of patients requiring tricuspid valve plication vs. replacement. Circulation, *68*:534, 1983.

40. Shiina, A., Seward, J.B., Edwards, W.D., Hagler, D.J., and Tajik, A.J.: Two-dimensional echocardiographic spectrum of Ebstein's anomaly: Detailed anatomic assessment. J. Am. Coll. Cardiol., *3*:356, 1984.

41. Ports, T.A., Silverman, N.H., and Schiller, N.B.: Two-dimensional echocardiographic assessment of Ebstein anomaly. Circulation, *58*:336, 1978.

42. Farooki, Z.Q., Henry, J.C., and Green, E.W.: Echocardiographic spectrum of Ebstein anomaly of the tricuspid valve. Circulation, *53*:63, 1976.

43. Gussenhoven, W.J., Spitaels, S.E.C., Bom, N., and Ligtvoet, C.M.: Echocardiographic criteria for Ebstein's anomaly of tricuspid valve. Br. Heart J., *43*:31, 1980.

44. Jacob, J.L.B., Da Silveira, L.C., and Braile, D.M.: Echocardiographic and angiographic diagnosis of Ebstein's anomaly of mitral valve. Br. Heart J., *66*:379, 1991.

45. Lang, D., Oberhoffer, R., Cook, A., Sharland, G., Allan, L., Fagg, N., and Anderson, R.H.: Pathologic spectrum of malformations of the tricuspid valve in prenatal and neonatal life. J. Am. Coll. Cardiol., *17*:1161, 1991.

46. Gussenhoven, E.J., Stewart, P.A., Becker, A.E., Essed, C.E., Ligtvoet, K.M., and Devilleneuve, V.H.: "Offsetting" of the septal tricuspid leaflet in normal hearts and in hearts with Ebstein's anomaly. Am. J. Cardiol., *54*:172, 1984.

47. Mair, D.D.: Ebstein's anomaly: Natural history and management (editorial comment). J. Am. Coll. Cardiol., *19*:1047, 1992.

48. Celermajer, D.S., Cullen, S., Sullivan, I.D., Spiegelhalter, D.J., Wyse, R.K.H., and Deanfield, J.E.: Outcome of neonates with Ebstein's anomaly. J. Am. Coll. Cardiol., *19*:1041, 1992.

49. Nihoyannopoulos, P., McKenna, W.J., Smith, G., and Foale, R.: Echocardiographic assessment of the right ventricle in Ebstein's anomaly: Relation to clinical outcome. J. Am. Coll. Cardiol., *8*:627, 1986.

50. Quaegebeur, J.M., Sreeram, N., Fraser, A.G., Bogers, A.J.J.C., Stümper, O.F.W., Hess, J., Bos, E., and Sutherland, G.R.: Surgery for Ebstein's anomaly: The clinical and echocardiographic evaluation of a new technique. J. Am. Coll. Cardiol., *17*:722, 1991.

51. Benson, L.N., Child, J.S., Schwaiger, M., Perloff, J.K., and Schelbert, H.R.: Left ventricular geometry and function in adults with Ebstein's anomaly of the tricuspid valve. Circulation, *75*:353, 1987.

52. Vick III, G.W., Murphy, D.J., Ludomirsky, A., Morrow, W.R., Morriss, M.J.H., Danford, D.A., and Huhta, J.C.: Pulmonary venous and systemic ventricular inflow obstruction in patients with congenital heart disease: Detection by combined two-dimensional and Doppler echocardiography. J. Am. Coll. Cardiol., *9*:580, 1987.

53. Smallhorn, J.F., Freedom, R.M., and Olley, P.M.: Pulsed Doppler echocardiographic assessment of extraparenchymal pulmonary vein flow. J. Am. Coll. Cardiol., *9*:573, 1987.

54. Starc, T.J., Bierman, F.Z., Bowman, F.O., Steeg, C.N., Wang, N.K., and Krongrad, E.: Pulmonary venous obstruction and atrioventricular canal anomalies: Role of cor triatriatum and double outlet right atrium. J. Am. Coll. Cardiol., *9*:830, 1987.

55. Smallhorn, J.F., Pauperio, H., Benson, L., Freedom, R.M., and Rowe, R.D.: Pulsed Doppler assessment of pulmonary vein obstruction. Am. Heart J., *110*:483, 1985.

56. Samdarshi, T.E., Morrow, W.R., Helmcke, F.R., Nanda, N.C., Bargeron, L.M., and Pacifico, A.D.: Assessment of pulmonary vein stenosis by transesophageal echocardiography. Am. Heart J., *122*:1403, 1991.

57. Gaither, N.S., Hull, R.W., Wortham, D.C., Yost, W.J., and Jelinek, J.: Pulmonary venous obstruction: Utility of transesophageal echocardiography. Am. Heart J., *121*:203, 1991.

58. Lengyel, M., Arvay, A., and Biro, V.: Two-dimensional echocardiographic diagnosis of cor triatriatum. Am. J. Cardiol., *59*:484, 1987.

59. Sullivan, I.D., Robinson, P.J., DeLeval, M., and Graham, T.P.: Membranous supravalvular mitral stenosis: A treatable form of congenital heart disease. J. Am. Coll. Cardiol., *8*:159, 1986.

60. Jacobstein, M.D. and Hirschfeld, S.S.: Concealed left atrial membrane: Pitfalls in the diagnosis of cor triatriatum and supravalvar mitral ring. Am. J. Cardiol., *49*:780, 1982.

61. Ostman-Smith, Silverman, N.H., Oldershaw, P., Lincoln, C., and Shinebourne, E.A.: Cor triatriatum sinistrum. Diagnostic features on cross-sectional echocardiography. Br. Heart J., *51*:211, 1984.

62. Ludomirsky, A., Erickson, C., Vick, G.W., and Cooley, D.A.: Transesophageal color flow Doppler evaluation of cor triatriatum in an adult. Am. Heart J., *120*:451, 1990.

63. Schluter, M., Langstein, B.A., Thier, W., Schmiegel, W.H., Krabber, H.J., Kalmar, P., and Hanrath, P.: Transesophageal two-dimensional echocardiography in the diagnosis of cor triatriatum in the adult. J. Am. Coll. Cardiol., *2*:1011, 1983.

64. Shone, J.D., Sellers, R.D., Anderson, R.L., Adams, P., Lillehei, C.W., and Edwards, J.E.: The developmental complex of parachute mitral valve, supravalvular ring of the left atrium, subaortic stenosis, and coarctation of aorta. Am. J. Cardiol., *11*:714, 1973.

65. Celano, V., Pieroni, D.R., Morera, J.A., Roland, J.M.A., and Gengell, R.L.: Two-dimensional echocardiographic examination of mitral valve abnormalities associated with coarctation of the aorta. Circulation, *69*:924, 1984.

66. Gutgesell, N.P., Cheatham, J., Latson, L.A., Nihill, M.R., and Mullins, C.E.: Atrioventricular valve abnormalities in infancy: Two-dimensional echocardiographic and angiocardiographic comparison. J. Am. Coll. Cardiol., *2*:531, 1983.

67. Smallhorn, J., Tommasini, G., Deanfield, J., Douglas, J., Gibson, D., and Macartney, F.: Congenital mitral stenosis. Anatomic and functional assessment by echocardiography. Br. Heart J., *45*:527, 1981.

68. Grenadier, E., Sahn, D.J., Valdez-Cruz, L.M., Allen, H.D., Lima, C.O., and Goldberg, S.J.: Two-dimensional echo Doppler study of cogenital disorders of the mitral valve. Am. Heart J., *107*:319, 1984.

69. Riggs, T.W., Lapin, G.D., and Paul, M.H.: Measurement of mitral valve orifice area in infants and children by two-dimensional echocardiography. J. Am. Coll. Cardiol., *1*: 873, 1983.

70. Rowland, T.W., Rosenthal, A., and Castenada, A.R.: Doubled chamber right ventricle: Experience with 17 cases. Am. Heart J., *89*:445, 1975.

71. Johnson, G.L., Kwan, O.L., Handshoe, S., Noonan, J.A., and DeMaria, A.N.: Accuracy of combined two-dimensional echocardiography and continuous wave Doppler recordings in the estimation of pressure gradient in right ventricular outlet obstruction. J. Am. Coll. Cardiol., *3*:1013, 1984.

72. Houston, A.B., Simpson, I.A., Sheldon, C.D., Doig, W.B., and Coleman, E.N.: Doppler ultrasound in the estimation of the severity of pulmonary infundibular stenosis in infants and children. Br. Heart J., *55*:381, 1986.

73. Silove, E.D., DeGiovanni, J.V., Shiu, M.F., and Yi, M.M.: Diagnosis of right ventricular outflow obstruction in infants by cross-sectional echocardiography. Br. Heart J., *50*:416, 1983.

74. Snider, A.R., Stevenson, J.G., French, J.W., Rocchini, A.P., Dick, M., Rosenthal, A., Crowley, D.C., Beekman, R.H., and Peters, J.: Comparison of high pulse repetition frequency and continuous wave Doppler echocardiography for velocity measurement and gradient prediction in children with valvular and congenital heart disease. J. Am. Coll. Cardiol., *7*:873, 1986.

75. Marcus, F.I., Fontaine, G.H., Guiraudon, G., Frank, R., Laurenceau, J.L., Malergue, C., and Grosgogeat, Y.: Right ventricular dysplasia: A report of 24 adult cases. Circulation, *65*:384, 1982.

76. Manyari, D.E., Klein, G.J., Gulamhusein, S., Boughner, D., Guiraudon, G.M., Wyse, G., Mitchell, L.B., and Kostuk, W.J.: Arrhythmogenic right ventricular dysplasia: A generalized cardiomyopathy? Circulation, *68*:251, 1983.

77. Weyman, A.E., Hurwitz, R.A., Girod, D.A., Dillon, J.C., Feigenbaum, H., and Green, D.: Cross-sectional echocardiographic visualization of the stenotic pulmonary valve. Circulation, *56*:796, 1977.

78. Richards, K.L.: Assessment of aortic and pulmonic stenosis by echocardiography. Circulation, *84* [Suppl I]:I-182, 1991.

79. Weyman, A.E., Dillon, J.C., Feigenbaum, H., and Chang, S.: Echocardiographic pattern of pulmonic valve motion in pulmonic stenosis. Am. J. Cardiol., *34*:644, 1974.

80. Lim, M.K., Houston, A.B., Doig, W.B., Lilley, S., and Murtagh, E.P.: Variability of the Doppler gradient in pulmonary valve stenosis before and after balloon dilatation. Br. Heart J., *62*:212, 1989.

81. Lima, C.O., Sahn, D.J., Valdes-Cruz, L.M., Goldberg, S.J., Barron, J.V., Allen, H.D., and Grenadier, E.: Noninvasive prediction of transvalvular pressure gradient in patients with pulmonary stenosis by quantitative two-dimensional echocardiographic Doppler studies. Circulation, *67*:866, 1983.

82. Frantz, E.G. and Silverman, N.H.: Doppler utrasound evaluation of valvular pulmonary stenosis from multiple transducer positions in children requiring pulmonary valvuloplasty. Am. J. Cardiol., *61*:844, 1988.

83. Okamoto, M., Miyatake, K., Kinoshita, N., Matsuhisa, M., Nakasone, I., Nagata, S., Sakakibara, H., and Nimura, Y.: Blood flow analysis with pulsed echo Doppler cardiography in valvular pulmonary stenosis. J. Cardiogr., *11*:1291, 1981.

84. Marantaz, P.M., Huhta, J.C., Mullins, C.E., Murphy, D.J., Nihill, M.R., Ludomirsky, A., and Yoon, G.Y.: Results of balloon valvuloplasty in typical and dysplastic pulmonary valve stenosis: Doppler echocardiographic follow-up. J. Am. Coll. Cardiol., *12*:476, 1988.

85. Walls, J.T., Lababidi, A., Curtis, J.J., and Silver, D.: Assessment of percutaneous balloon pulmonary and aortic valvuloplasty. J. Thorac. Cardiovasc. Surg., *88*:352, 1984.

86. Kveselis, D.A., Rocchini, A.P., Snider, R., Rosenthal, A., Crowley, D.C., and Dick, M.: Results of balloon valvuloplasty in the treatment of congenital valvular pulmonary stenosis in children. Am. J. Cardiol., *56*:527, 1985.

87. Musewe, N.N., Robertson, M.A., Benson, L.N., Smallhorn, J.F., Burrows, P.E., Freedom, R.M., Moes, C.A.F., and Rowe, R.D.: The dysplastic pulmonary valve: Echocardiographic features and results of balloon dilatation. Br. Heart J., *47*:364, 1987.

88. Vermilion, R.P., Snider, A.R., Bengur, A.R., and Meliones, J.N.: Long-term assessment of right ventricular diastolic filling in patients with pulmonic valve stenosis successfully treated in childhood. Am. J. Cardiol., *68*: 648, 1991.

89. Vermilion, R.P., Snider, A.R., Meliones, J.N., Peters, J., and Merida-Asmus, L.: Pulsed Doppler evaluation of right ventricular diastolic filling in children with pulmonary valve stenosis before and after balloon valvuloplasty. *Am. J. Cardiol., 66*:79, 1990.

90. Goldberg, S.J.: The principles of pressure drop in long segment stenosis. Herz, *11*:291, 1986.

91. Simpson, I.A., Valdes-Cruz, L.M., Yoganathan, A.P., Sung, H.W., Jimoh, A., and Sahn, D.J.: Spatial velocity distribution and acceleration in serial subvalve tunnel and valvular obstructions; An in vitro study using Doppler color flow mapping. J. Am. Coll. Cardiol., *13*:241, 1989.

92. Wren, C., Oslizlok, P., and Bull, C.: Natural history of supravalvular aortic stenosis and pulmonary artery stenosis. J. Am. Coll. Cardiol., *15*:1625, 1991.

93. Swan, J.W., Chambers, J.B., Monaghan, M.J., and Jackson, G.: Echocardiographic appearance of pulmonary artery stenosis. Br. Heart J., *63*:175, 1990.

94. Tinker, D.D., Nanca, N.C., Harris, P., and Manning, J.A.: Two-dimensional echocardiographic identification of pulmonary artery branch stenosis. Am. J. Cardiol., *50*:814, 1982.

95. Motro, M., Schneeweiss, A., Shem-Tov, A., Vered, A., Hegesh, J., Neufeld, H.N., and Rath, S.: Two-dimensional echocardiography in discrete subaortic stenosis. Am. J. Cardiol., *53*:896, 1984.

96. Krueger, S.K., French, J.W., Forker, A.D., Caudill, C.C., and Popp, R.L.: Echocardiography in discrete subaortic stenosis. Am. J. Cardiol., *59*:506, 1979.

97. Wilcox, W.D., Seward, J.B., Hagler, D.J., Mair, D.D., and Tajik, A.J.: Discrete subaortic stenosis. Two-dimensional echocardiographic features with angiographic and surgical correlation. Mayo Clin. Proc., *55*:425, 1980.

98. Gnanapragasam, J.P., Houston, A.B., Doig, W.B., Jamieson, M.P.G., and Pollock, J.C.S.: Transesophageal echocardiographic assessment of fixed subaortic obstruction in children. Br. Heart J., *66*:281, 1991.

99. Choi, J.Y. and Sullivan, I.D.: Fixed subaortic stenosis: Anatomical spectrum and nature of progression. Br. Heart J., *65*:280, 1991.

100. Sreeram, N., Franks, R., and Walsh, K.: Aortic-ventricular tunnel in a neonate: Diagnosis and management based on cross sectional and colour Doppler ultrasonography. Br. Heart J., *65*:161, 1991.

101. Sreeram, N., Franks, R., Arnold, R., and Walsh, K.: Aortico-left ventricular tunnel: Long-term outcome after surgical repair. J. Am. Coll. Cardiol., *17*:950, 1991.

102. Wu, J.R., Huang, T.Y., Chen, Y.F., Lin, Y.T., and Roan, H.R.: Aortico-left ventricular tunnel: Two-dimensional echocardiographic and angiocardiographic features. Am. Heart J., *117*:697, 1989.

103. Zielinsky, P., Rossi, M., Haertel, J.C., Vitola, D., Lucchese, F.A., and Rodrigues, R.: Subaortic fibrous ridge and ventricular septal defect: Role of septal malalignment. Circulation, *75*:1124, 1987.

104. Chung, K.J., Fulton, D.R., Kreidberg, M.B., Payne, D.D., and Cleveland, R.J.: Combined discrete subaortic stenosis and ventricular septal defect in infants and children. Am. J. Cardiol., *53*:1429, 1984.

105. Borow, K.M.: Congenital aortic stenosis in the adult. J. Cardiovasc. Med., *8*:1163, 1983.

106. Barbosa, M.M. and Motta, M.S.: Quadricuspid aortic valve and aortic regurgitation diagnosed by Doppler echocardiography: Report of two cases and review of the literature. J. Am. Soc. Echocardiogr., *4*:69, 1991.

107. Radford, D.J., Blood, K.R., and Izukawa, T.: Echocardiographic assessment of bicuspid aortic valves: Angiographic and pathological correlates. Circulation, *53*:80, 1976.

108. Brandenburg, J., Tajik, A.J., Edwards, W.D., Reeder, G.S., Shub, C., and Seward, J.B.: Accuracy of 2-dimensional echocardiographic diagnosis of congenitally bicuspid aortic valve: Echocardiographic-anatomic correlation in 115 patients. Am. J. Cardiol., *51*:1469, 1983.

109. Zema, J.J. and Caccavano, M.: Two-dimensional echocardiographic assessment of aortic valve morphology: Feasibility of bicuspid valve detection. Br. Heart J., *48*:428, 1982.

110. Huhta, J.C., Carpenter, R.J., Moise, K.J., Deter, R.L., Ott, D.A., and McNamara, D.G.: Prenatal diagnosis and postnatal management of critical aortic stenosis. Circulation, *75*:573, 1987.

111. Weyman, A.E., Feigenbaum, H., Hurwitz, R.A., Girod, D.A., Dillon, J.C., and Chang, S.: Cross-sectional echocardiographic assessment of the severity of aortic stenosis in children. Circulation, *55*:773, 1977.

112. Riggs, T.W., Berry, T.E., Aziz, K.U., and Paul, M.H.: Two-dimensional echocardiographic features of interruption of the aortic arch. Am. J. Cardiol., *50*:1385, 1982.

113. Huhta, J.C., Latson, L.A., Gutgesell, H.P., Cooley, D.A., and Kearney, D.J.: Echocardiography in the diagnosis and management of symptomatic aortic valve stenosis in infants. Circulation, *70*:438, 1984.

114. Kosturakis, D., Allen, H.D., Goldberg, S.J., Sahn, D.J., and Valdes-Cruz, L.M.: Noninvasive quantification of stenotic semilunar valve areas by Doppler echocardiography. J. Am. Coll. Cardiol., *3*:1256, 1984.

115. DeKnecht, S., Hopman, J.C.W., Daniels, O., Stoelinga, G.B.A., Reneman, R.S., and Hoeks, A.P.G.: Assessment of the orifice diameter by a multigated pulsed Doppler system in children with congenital semilunar valve stenosis. Br. Heart J., *62*:50, 1989.

116. Seitz, W.S., McIlroy, M.B., Kline, H., Operschall, J., and Kashani, I.A.: Echocardiographic application of the Gorlin formula for assessment of aortic stenosis: Correlation with cardiac catheterization in pediatric patients. Am. Heart J., *111*:1118, 1986.

116a. Nishimura, R.A., Pieroni, D.R., Bierman, F.Z., Colan, S.D., Kaufman, S., Sanders, S.P., Seward, J.B., Tajik, A.J., Wiggins, J.W., and Zahka, K.G.: Second natural history study of congenital heart defects. Aortic stenosis: Echocardiography. Circulation, *87 [suppl I]*:I-66, 1993.

117. Hatle, L.: Noninvasive assessment and differentiation of left ventricular outflow obstruction with Doppler ultrasound. Circulation, *64*:381, 1981.

118. Stevenson, J.G. and Kawabori, I.: Noninvasive determination of pressure gradients in children: Two methods employing pulsed Doppler echocardiography. J. Am. Coll. Cardiol., *3*:179, 1984.

119. Skjaerpe, T., Hegrenaes, L., and Hatle, L.: Noninvasive estimation of valve area in patients with aortic stenosis by Doppler ultrasound and two-dimensional echocardiography. Circulation, *72*:810, 1985.

120. Otto, C.M., Pearlman, A.S., Comess, K.A., Reamer, R.P., Janko, C.L., and Huntsman, L.L.: Determination of stenotic aortic valve area in adults using Doppler echocardiography. J. Am. Coll. Cardiol., *7*:509, 1986.

121. Bengur, A.R., Snider, A.R., Serwer, G.A., Dick, M., Peters, J., Reynolds, P., and Rosenthal, A.: Usefulness of the Doppler mean gradient in the evaluation of children with aortic valve stenosis and comparison to gradient at catheterization. Am. J. Cardiol., *64*:756, 1989.

122. Shaddy, R.E., Boucek, M.M., Sturtevant, J.E., Ruttenberg, H.D., and Orsmond, G.S.: Gradient reduction, aortic valve regurgitation and prolapse after balloon aortic valvuloplasty in 32 consecutive patients with congenital aortic stenosis. J. Am. Coll. Cardiol., *16*:451, 1990.

123. Labadidi, Z., Wu, J., and Walls, J.T.: Percutaneous balloon aortic valvuloplasty: Results in 23 patients. Am. J. Cardiol., *53*:194, 1984.

123a. Ensing, G.J., Schmidt, M.A., Hagler, D.J., Michels, V.V., Carter, G.A., and Feldt, R.H.: Spectrum of findings in a family with nonsyndromic autosomal dominant supravalvular aortic stenosis: A Doppler echocardiography study. J. Am. Coll. Cardiol., *13*:413, 1989.

124. Vogt, J., Rupprath, G., Grimm, T., and Beuren, A.J.: Qualitative and quantitative evaluation of supravalvular aortic stenosis by cross-sectional echocardiography. A report of 80 patients. Pediatr. Cardiol., *3*:13, 1982.

125. Weyman, A.E., Caldwell, R.L., Hurwitz, R.A., Girod, D.A., Dillon, J.C., Geigenbaum, H., and Green, D.: Cross-sectional echocardiographic characterization of aortic obstruction. 1. Supravalvular aortic stenosis and aortic hypoplasia. Circulation, *57*:491, 1978.

126. Cohen, M., Fuster, V., Steele, P.M., Driscoll, D., and McGoon, D.C.: Coarctation of the aorta: Long-term follow-up and prediction of outcome after surgical correction. Circulation, *80*:840, 1989.

127. Cassidy, S.C., Van Hare, G.F., and Silverman, N.H.: The probability of detecting a subaortic ridge in children with ventricular septal defect or coarctation of the aorta. Am. J. Cardiol., *66*:505, 1990.

128. Nihoyannopoulos, P., Karas, S., Sapsford, R.N., Hallidie-Smith, K., and Foale, R.: Accuracy of two-dimensional echocardiography in the diagnosis of aortic arch obstruction. J. Am. Coll. Cardiol., *10*:1072, 1987.

129. Morrow, W.R., Huhta, J.C., Murphy, D.J., and McNamara, D.G.: Quantitative morphology of the aortic arch in neonatal coarctation. J. Am. Coll. Cardiol., *8*:616, 1986.

130. Duncan, W.J., Ninomiya, K., Cook, D.H., and Rowe, R.D.: Noninvasive diagnosis of neonatal coarctation and associated anomalies using two-dimensional echocardiography. Am. Heart J., *106*:63, 1983.

131. Weyman, A.E., Caldwell, R.L., Hurwitz, R.A., Girod, D.A., Dillon, J.C., Feigenbaum, H., and Green, G.: Cross-sectional echocardiographic detection of aortic ob-

struction. 2. Coarctation of the aorta. Circulation, *57*: 498, 1978.

132. Smallhorn, J.F., Huhta, J.C., Adams, P.A., and Anderson, R.H.: Cross-sectional echocardiographic assessment of coarctation in the sick neonate and infant. Br. Heart J., *50*:349, 1983.

133. van Son, J.A.M., Skotniki, S.H., van Asten, W.N., Daniels, O., van Lier, H.J., and Lacquet, L.K.: Quantitative assessment of coarctation in infancy by Doppler spectral analysis. Am. J. Cardiol., *62*:1282, 1989.

134. George, B., DiSessa, T.G., Williams, R., Friedman, W.F., and Laks, H.: Coarctation repair without cardiac catheterization in infants. Am. Heart J.,*114*:1421, 1987.

135. Carvalho, J.S., Redington, A.N., Shinebourne, E.A., Rigby, M.L., and Gibson, D.: Continuous wave Doppler echocardiography and coarctation of the aorta: Gradients and flow patterns in the assessment of severity. Br. Heart J., *64*:133, 1990.

136. Rao, P.S. and Carey, P.: Doppler ultrasound in the prediction of pressure gradients across aortic coarctation. Am. Heart J., *118*:299, 1989.

137. Marx, G.R. and Allen, H.D.: Accuracy and pitfalls of Doppler evaluation of the pressure gradient in aortic coarctation. J. Am. Coll. Cardiol., *7*:1379, 1986.

138. Houston, A.B., Simpson, I.A., Pollock, J.C.S., Jamieson, M.P.G., Doig, W.B., and Coleman, E.N.: Doppler ultrasound in the assessment of severity of coarctation of the aorta and interruption of the aortic arch. Br. Heart J., *57*:38, 1987.

139. Shaddy, R.E., Snider, A.R., Silverman, N.H., and Lutin, W.: Pulsed Doppler findings in patients with coarctation of the aorta. Circulation, *73*:82, 1986.

140. Sanders, S.P., MacPherson, D., and Yeager, S.B.: Temporal flow velocity profile in the descending aorta in coarctation. J. Am. Coll. Cardiol., *7*:603, 1986.

141. Simpson, I.A., Sahn, D.J., Valdes-Cruz, L.M., Chung, K.J., Sherman, F.S., and Swensson, R.E.: Color Doppler flow mapping in patients with coarctation of the aorta: New observations and improved evaluation with color flow diameter and proximal acceleration as predictors of severity. Circulation, *77*:736, 1988.

142. Syamasundar, R. and Carey, P.: Doppler ultrasound in the prediction of pressure gradients across aortic coarctation. Am. Heart J., *118*:299, 1989.

143. Marino, B., Sanders, S.P., Parness, I.A., and Colan, S.D.: Echocardiographic identification of aortic atresia with ventricular septal defect, normal left ventricle and mitral valve. Am. Heart J., *113*:1521, 1987.

144. Nihoyannopoulos, P., Karas, S., Sapsford, R.N., Hallidie-Smith, K., and Foale, R.: Accuracy of two-dimensional echocardiography in the diagnosis of aortic arch obstruction. J. Am. Coll. Cardiol., *10*:1072, 1987.

145. Smallhorn, J.F., Anderson, R.H., and Macartney, F.J.: Cross-sectional echocardiographic recognition of interruption of aortic arch between left carotid and subclavian arteries. Br. Heart J., *48*:229, 1982.

146. Mehta, R.H., Helmcke, F., Nanda, N.C., Pinheiro, L., Samdarshi, T.E., and Shah, V.K.: Uses and limitations of transthoracic echocardiography in the assessment of atrial septal defect in the adult. Am. J. Cardiol., *67*:288, 1991.

147. Forfar, J.C. and Godman, M.J.: Functional and anatomical correlates in atrial septal defect: An echocardiographic analysis. Br. Heart J., *54*:193, 1985.

148. Shub, C., Tajik, J., and Seward, J.B.: Clinically "silent" atrial septal defect: Diagnosis by two-dimensional and Doppler echocardiography. Am. Heart J., *110*:665, 1985.

149. Shub, C., Dimopoulos, I.N., Seward, J.B., Callahan, J.A., Tancredi, R.G., Schattenberg, T.T., Reeder, G.S., Hagler, D.J., and Tajik, A.J.: Sensitivity of two-dimensional echocardiography in the direct visualization of atrial septal defects utilizing the subcostal approach: Experience with 154 patients. J. Am. Coll. Cardiol., *2*:127, 1983.

150. Dillon, J.C., Weyman, A.E., Feigenbaum, H., Eggleton, R.C., and Johnston, K.: Cross-sectional echocardiographic examination of the interatrial septum. Circulation, *55*:115, 1977.

151. Nasser, F.N., Tajik, A.J., Seward, J.B., and Hagler, D.J.: Diagnosis of sinus venosus atrial septal defect by two-dimensional echocardiography. Mayo Clin. Proc., *56*:568, 1981.

152. Diamond, M.A., Dillon, J.C., Haine, C.L., Chang, S., and Feigenbaum, H.: Echocardiographic features of atrial septal defect. Circulation, *43*:129, 1971.

153. Radtke, W.E., Tajik, A.J., Gau, G.T., Schattenberg, T.T., Giuliani, E.R., and Tancredi, R.G.: Atrial septal defect: Echocardiographic observations. Studies in 120 patients. Ann. Intern. Med., *82*:246, 1976.

154. Tajik, A.J., Gau, G.T., Ritter, D.G., and Schattenberg, T.T.: Echocardiographic pattern of right ventricular diastolic volume overload in children. Circulation, *46*:36, 1972.

155. Weyman, A.E., Wann, S., Feigenbaum, H., and Dillon, J.C.: Mechanism of abnormal septal motion in patients with right ventricular volume overload. A cross-sectional echocardiographic study. Circulation, *54*:179, 1976.

156. Shimada, R., Takeshita, A., and Nakamura, M.: Noninvasive assessment of right ventricular systolic pressure in atrial septal defect: Analysis of the end-systolic configuration of the ventricular septum by two-dimensional echocardiography. Am. J. Cardiol., *53*:1117, 1984.

157. King, M.E., Braun, H., Goldblatt, A., Liberthson, R., and Weyman, A.E.: Interventricular septal configuration as a predictor of right ventricular systolic hypertension in children. A cross-sectional echocardiographic study. Circulation, *68*:68, 1983.

158. Ryan, T., Petrovic, O., Dillon, J.C., Feigenbaum, H., Conley, M.J., and Armstrong, W.F.: An echocardiographic index for separation of right ventricular volume and pressure overload. J. Am. Coll. Cardiol., *5*:918, 1985.

159. Canale, J.M., Sahn, D.J., Allen, H.D., Goldberg, S.J., Valdez-Cruz, L.M., and Ovitt, T.W.: Factors affecting real-time, cross-sectional echocardiographic imaging of perimembranous ventricular septal defects. Circulation, *63*:689, 1981.

160. Gondi, B. and Nanda, N.C.: Two-dimensional echocardiographic features of atrial septal aneurysms. Circulation, *63*:452, 1981.

161. Wolf, W.J., Casta, A., and Sapire, D.W.: Atrial septal aneurysms in infants and children. Am. Heart J., *113*: 1149, 1987.

162. Hanley, P., Tajik, J., Hynes, J., Edwards, W., Reeder, G., Hagler, D., and Seward, J.: Diagnosis and classification of atrial septal aneurysm by two-dimensional echocardiography: Report of 80 consecutive cases. J. Am. Coll. Cardiol., *6*:1370, 1985.

163. Hauser, A.M., Timmis, G.C., Stewart, J.R., Ramos, R.G., Gangadharan, V., Westveer, D.C., and Gordon, S.: Aneurysm of the atrial septum as diagnosed by echocardiography: Analysis of 11 patients. Am. J. Cardiol., *53*:1402, 1984.

164. Wysham, D.G., McPherson, D.D., and Kerber, R.E.: Asymptomatic aneurysm of the interatrial septum. J. Am. Coll. Cardiol., 4:1311, 1984.

165. Alexander, M.D., Bloom, K.R., Hart, P., D'Silva, F., and Murgo, J.P.: Atrial septal aneurysm: A cause for midsystolic click. Report of a case and review of the literature. Circulation, 63:1186, 1981.

166. Mortera, C., Rissech, M., Payola, M., Miro, C., and Perich, R.: Cross sectional subcostal echocardiography: Atrioventricular septal defects and the short axis cut. Br. Heart J., 58:267, 1987.

167. Lipshultz, S.E., Sanders, S.P., Mayer, J.E., Colan, S.D., and Lock, J.E.: Are routine preoperative cardiac catheterization and angiography necessary before repair of ostium primum atrial septal defect? J. Am. Coll. Cardiol., 11:373, 1988.

168. Gutgesell, H.P. and Huhta, J.C.: Cardiac septation in atrioventricular canal defect. J. Am. Coll. Cardiol., 8:1421, 1986.

169. Hagler, D.J., Tajik, A.J., Seward, J.B., Mair, D., and Ritter, D.G.: Real-time wide-angle sector echocardiography: Atrioventricular canal defects. Circulation, 59:140, 1979.

170. Silverman, N.H., Zuberbuhler, J.R., and Anderson, R.H.: Atrioventricular septal defects: Cross-sectional echocardiographic and morphologic comparisons. Int. J. Cardiol., 13:309, 1986.

171. Kronik, G., Slany, J., and Moesslacher, H.: Contrast M-mode echocardiography in diagnosis of atrial septal defect in acyanotic patients. Circulation, 59:372, 1979.

172. Gullace, G., Savoia, M.T., Raviza, P., Knippel, M., and Ranzi, C.: Detection of atrial septal defect with left-to-right shunt by inferior vena cava contrast echocardiography. Br. Heart J., 47:445, 1982.

173. Valdes-Cruz, L.M., Pieroni, D.R., Roland, J.M.A., and Shematek, J.P.: Recognition of residual postoperative shunts by contrast echocardiographic techniques. Circulation, 55:148, 1977.

174. Valdes-Cruz, L.M., Pieroni, D.R., Roland, J.M.A., and Varghese, P.J.: Echocardiographic detection of intracardiac right-to-left shunts following peripheral vein injections. Circulation, 54:558, 1976.

175. VanHare, G.G. and Silverman, N.H.: Contrast two-dimensional echocardiography in congenital heart disease: Techniques, indications and clinical utility. J. Am. Coll. Cardiol., 13:673, 1989.

176. Santoso, T., Meltzer, R.S., Castellanos, S., Serruys, P.W., and Roelandt, J.: Contrast echocardiographic shunts may persist after atrial septal defect repair. Eur. Heart J., 4:129, 1983.

177. Franker, T.D., Harris, P.J., Behar, V.S., and Kisslo, J.A.: Detection and exclusion of interatrial shunts by two-dimensional echocardiography and peripheral venous injections. Circulation, 59:379, 1979.

178. Weyman, A.E., Wann, L.S., Caldwell, R.L., Hurwitz, R.A., Dillon, J.C., and Feigenbaum, H.: Negative contrast echocardiography: A new method for detecting left-to-right shunts. Circulation, 59:498, 1979.

179. Morimoto, K., Matsuzaki, M., Tohma, Y., Ono, S., Tanaka, N., Michishige, H., Murata, K., Anno, Y., and Kusukawa, R.: Diagnosis and quantitative evaluation of secundum-type atrial septal defect by transesophageal Doppler echocardiography. Am. J. Cardiol., 66:85, 1990.

180. Mehta, R.H., Helmcke, F., Nanda, N.C., Hsiung, M., Pacifico, A.D., and Hsu, T.L.: Transesophageal Doppler color flow mapping assessment of atrial septal defect. J. Am. Coll. Cardiol., 16:1010, 1990.

181. Hausmann, D., Daniel, W.G., Mügge, A., Ziemer, G., and Pearlman, A.S.: Value of transesophageal color Doppler echocardiography for detection of different types of atrial septal defects in adults. J. Am. Soc. Echocardiogr., 5:481, 1992.

182. Kronzon, I., Tunick, P.A., Freedberg, R.S., Trehan, N., Rosenzweig, B.P., and Schwinger, M.E.: Transesophageal echocardiography is superior to transthoracic echocardiography in the diagnosis of sinus venosus atrial septal defect. J. Am. Coll. Cardiol., 17:537, 1991.

183. Hiraishi, S., Agata, Y., Saito, K., Oguchi, K., Misawa, H., Fujino, N., and Horiguchi, Y.: Interatrial shunt flow profiles in newborn infants: A colour flow and pulsed Doppler echocardiographic study. Br. Heart J., 65:41, 1991.

184. Minagoe, S., Tei, C., Kisanuki, A., Arikawa, K., Nakazono, Y., Yoshimura, H., Kashima, T., and Tanaka, H.: Noninvasive pulsed Doppler echocardiographic detection of the direction of shunt flow in patients with atrial septal defect. Criculation, 71:745, 1985.

185. Pollick, C., Sullivan, H., Cujec, B., and Wilansky, S.: Doppler color-flow imaging assessment of shunt size in atrial septal defect. Circulation, 78:522, 1988.

186. Sherman, F.S., Sahn, D.J., Valdes-Druz, L.M., Chung, K.J., and Elias, W.: Two-dimensional Doppler color flow mapping for detecting atrial and ventricular septal defects. Herz, 12:212, 1987.

187. Dittman, H., Jacksch, R., Voelker, W., Karsch, K.R., and Seipel, L.: Accuracy of Doppler echocardiography in quantification of left to right shunts in adult patients with atrial septal defect. J. Am. Coll. Cardiol., 11:338, 1988.

188. Valdes-Cruz, L.M., Horowitz, S., Mesel, E., Sahn, D.J., Fisher, D.C., and Larson, D.: A pulsed Doppler echocardiographic method for calculating pulmonary and systemic blood flow in atrial level shunts: Validation studies in animals and initial human experience. Circulation, 69:80, 1984.

189. Kitabatake, A., Inoue, M., Asao, M., Ito, H., Masuyama, T., Tanouchi, J., Morita, T., Hori, M., Yoshima, H., Ohnishi, K., and Abe, H.: Noninvasive evaluation of the ratio of pulmonary to systemic flow in atrial septal defect by duplex Doppler echocardiography. Circulation, 69:73, 1984.

190. Jenni, R., Ritter, M., Vieli, A., Hirzel, H.O., Schmid, E.R., Grimm, J.G., and Turina, M.: Determination of the ratio of pulmonary blood flow to systemic blood flow by deviation of amplitude weighted mean velocity from continuous wave Doppler spectra. Br. Heart J., 61:167, 1989.

191. Cloez, J.L., Schmidt, K.G., Birk, E., and Silverman, N.H.: Determination of pulmonary to systemic blood flow ratio in children by a simplified Doppler echocardiographic method. J. Am. Coll. Cardiol., 11:825, 1988.

192. Freed, M.D., Nadas, A.S., Norwood, W.I., and Castaneda, A.R.: Is routine preoperative cardiac catheterization necessary before repair of secundum and sinus venosus atrial septal defects? J. Am. Coll. Cardiol., 4:333, 1984.

193. Shub, C., Tajik, J., Seward, J.B.V., Hagler, D.J., and Danielson, G.K.: Surgical repair of uncomplicated atrial septal defect without "routine" preoperative cardiac catheterization. J. Am. Coll. Cardiol., 6:49, 1985.

194. Huhta, J.C., Glasow, P., Murphy, D.J., Gutgesell, H.P., Ott, D.A., McNamara, D.G., and Smith, E.O.: Surgery

without catheterization for congential heart defects: Management of 100 patients. J. Am. Coll. Cardiol., *9*: 823, 1987.

195. Martin, G.R.: Increased prevalence of ventricular septal defects: Epidemic or improved diagnosis? Pediatrics, *83*: 200, 1992.

196. Soto, B., Becker, A.E., Moulaert, A.J., Lie, J.T., and Anderson, R.H.: Classification of ventricular septal defects. Br. Heart J., *43*:332, 1980.

197. Hornberger, L.K., Sahn, D.J., Krabill, K.A., Sherman, F.S., Swensson, R.E., Pesonen, E., Hagen-Ansert, S., and Chung, K.J.: Elucidation of the natural history of ventricular septal defects by serial Doppler color flow mapping studies. J. Am. Coll. Cardiol., *13*:1111, 1989.

198. Corone, P., Doyon, F., Gaudeau, S., Guerin, F., Vernant, P., Ducam, H., Rumeau-Rouquette, C., and Gaudeau, P.: Natural history of ventricular septal defect: A study involving 790 cases. Circulation, *55*:908, 1977.

199. Sharif, D.S., Huhta, J.C., Marantz, P., Hawkins, H.K., and Yoon, G.Y.: Two-dimensional echocardiographic determination of ventricular septal defect size: Correlation with autopsy. Am. Heart J., *117*:1333, 1989.

200. Helmcke, F., deSouza, A., Nanda, N.C., Villacosta, I., Gatewood, Jr., R., Colvin, E., and Soto, B.: Two-dimensional and color Doppler assessment of ventricular septal defect of congenital origin. Am. J. Cardiol., *63*:1112, 1989.

201. Capelli, H., Andrade, J.L., and Somerville, J.: Classification of the site of ventricular septal defect by two-dimensional echocardiography. Am. J. Cardiol., *51*:1474, 1983.

202. Andrade, J.L., Serino, W., DeLeval, M., and Somerville, J.: Two-dimensional echocardiographic assessment of surgically closed ventricular septal defect. Am. J. Cardiol., *52*:325, 1983.

203. Bierman, F.Z., Fellows, K., and Williams, R.G.: Prospective identification of ventricular septal defects in infancy using subxiphoid two-dimensional echocardiography. Circulation, *62*:807, 1980.

204. Cheatham, J.P., Latson, L.A., and Gutgesell, H.P.: Ventricular septal defect in infancy: Detection with two-dimensional echocardiography. Am. J. Cardiol., *47*:85, 1981.

205. Sutherland, G.R., Godman, M.J., Smallhorn, J.F., Guiterras, P., Anderson, R.H., and Hunter, S.: Ventricular septal defects. Two-dimensional echocardiographic and morphological correlations. Br. Heart J., *47*:316, 1982.

206. Schmidt, K.G., Cassidy, S.C., Silverman, N.H., and Stanger, P.: Doubly committed subarterial ventricular septal defects: Echocardiographic features and surgical implications. J. Am. Coll. Cardiol., *12*:1538, 1988.

207. Stevenson, J.G., Kawabori, I., Dooley, T., and Guntheroth, W.G.: Diagnosis of ventricular septal defect by pulsed Doppler echocardiography. Circulation, *58*:322, 1978.

208. Magherini, A., Azzolina, G., Wiechmann, V., and Fantini, F.: Pulsed Doppler echocardiography for diagnosis of ventricular septal defects. Br. Heart J., *43*:143, 1980.

209. Hatle, L. and Rokseth, R.: Noninvasive diagnosis and assessment of ventricular septal defect by Doppler ultrasound. Acta Med. Scand., *645*:47, 1981.

210. Linker, D.T., Rossvoll, O., Chapman, J.V., and Angelsen, B.A.J.: Sensitivity and speed of colour Doppler flow mapping compared with continuous wave Doppler for the detection of ventricular septal defects. Br. Heart J., *65*:201, 1991.

211. Ortiz, E., Robinson, P.J., Deanfield, J.E., Franklin, R., Macartney, F.J., and Wyse, R.K.H.: Localisation of ventricular septal defects by simultaneous display of superimposed colour Doppler and cross-sectional echocardiographic images. Br. Heart J., *54*:53, 1985.

212. Sommer, R.J., Golinko, R.J., and Ritter, S.B.: Intracardiac shunting in children with ventricular septal defect: Evaluation with Doppler color flow mapping. J. Am. Coll. Cardiol., *16*:1437, 1990.

213. Ludomirsky, A., Tani, L., Murphy, D.J., and Huhta, J.C.: Usefulness of color-flow doppler in diagnosing and in differentiating supracristal ventricular septal defect from right ventricular outflow tract obstruction. Am. J. Cardiol., *67*:194, 1991.

214. Ludomirsky, A., Huhta, J.C., Vick, G.W., Murphy, D.J., Danford, D.A., and Morrow, W.R.: Color Doppler detection of multiple ventricular septal defects. Circulation, *74*:1317, 1986.

215. Smallhorn, J.F., Tommasini, G., and Macartney, F.J.: Detection and assessment of straddling and overriding atrioventricular valves by two dimensional echocardiography. Br. Heart J., *46*:254, 1981.

216. Barron, J.V., Sahn, D.J., Valdes-Cruz, L.M., Lima, C.O., Grenadier, E., Allen, H.D., and Goldberg, S.J.: Two-dimensional echocardiographic evaluation of overriding and straddling atrioventricular valves associated with complex congenital heart disease. Am. Heart J., *107*:1006, 1984.

217. Rice, J.J.: Straddling atrioventricular valve: Two-dimensional echocardiographic diagnosis, classification and surgical implications. Am. J. Cardiol., *55*:505, 1985.

218. Sutherland, G.S., Smyllie, J.H., Ogilvie, B.C., and Keeton, B.R.: Colour flow imaging in the diagnosis of multiple ventricular septal defects. Br. Heart J., *62*:43, 1989.

219. Moises, V.A., Maciel, B.C., Hornberger, L.K., Murillo-Olivas, A., Valdes-Cruz, L.M., Sahn, D.J., and Weintraub, R.G.: A new method for noninvasive estimation of ventricular septal defect shunt flow by Doppler color flow mapping: Imaging of the laminar flow convergence region on the left septal surface. J. Am. Coll. Cardiol., *18*:824, 1991.

220. Garg, A., Shrivastava, S., Radhakrishnan, S., Dev, V., and Saxena, A.: Doppler assessment of interventricular pressure gradient across isolated ventricular septal defect. Clin. Cardiol., *13*:717, 1990.

221. Houston, A.B., Lim, M.K., Doig, W.B., Reid, J.M., and Coleman, E.N.: Doppler assessment of the interventricular pressure drop in patients with ventricular septal defects. Br. Heart J., *60*:50, 1988.

222. Silbert, D.R., Brunson, S.C., Schiff, R., and Diamant, S.: Determination of right ventricular pressure in the presence of a ventricular septal defect using continuous wave Doppler ultrasound. J. Am. Coll. Cardiol., *8*:379, 1986.

223. Murphy, D.J., Ludomirsky, A., and Huhta, J.C.: Continuous wave Doppler in children with ventricular septal defect: Noninvasive estimation of interventricular pressure gradient. Am. Heart J., *57*:428, 1986.

223a. Pieroni, D.R., Nishimura, R.A., Bierman, F.Z., Colan, S.D., Kaufman, S., Sanders, S.P., Seward, J.B., Tajik, A.J., Wiggins, J.W., and Zahka, K.G.: Second natural history study of congenital heart defects. Ventricular septal defect: Echocardiography. Circulation, *87 [suppl I]*: I-80, 1993.

224. Baron, J.V., Sahn, D.J., Valdes-Cruz, L.M., Grenadier, E., Allen, H.D., and Goldberg, S.J.: Two-dimensional echocardiographic features of ventricular septal aneu-

rysm paradoxically bulging into the left ventricular outflow tract. Am. Heart J., *104*:156, 1982.

225. Canale, J.M., Sahn, D.J., Valdes-Cruz, L.M., Allen, H.D., Goldberg, S.J., and Ovitt, T.W.: Accuracy of two-dimensional echocardiography in the detection of aneurysms of the ventricular septum. Am. Heart J., *101*:255, 1981.

226. Ramaciotti, C., Keren, A., and Silverman, N.H.: Importance of (perimembranous) ventricular spetal aneurysm in the natural history of isolated perimembranous ventricular septal defect. Am. J. Cardiol., *57*:268, 1986.

227. Rychik, J., Norwood, W.I., and Chin, A.J.: Doppler color flow mapping assessment of residual shunt after closure of large ventricular septal defects. Circulation, *84* (Suppl 3):III-153, 1991.

228. Mostow, N., Riggs, T., and Borkat, G.: Echocardiographic features of ventricular septal defect patch dehiscence. Am. Heart J., *102*:941, 1981.

229. Allwork, S.P.: Anatomical-embryological correlates in atrioventricular septal defects. Br. Heart J., *47*:419, 1982.

230. Mehta, S., Hirschfeld, S., Riggs, T., and Liebman, J.: Echocardiographic estimation of ventricular hypoplsia in complete atrioventricular canal. Circulation, *59*:888, 1979.

231. Heydarian, M., Griffith, B.P., and Zuberbuhler, J.R.: Partial atrioventricular canal associated with discrete subaortic stenosis. Am. Heart J., *109*:915, 1985.

232. Wenink, A.C.G., Ottenkamp, J., Guit, G.L., Draulans-Noe, Y., and Doornbos, J.: Correlation of morphology of the left ventricular outflow tract with two-dimensional Doppler echocardiography and magnetic resonance imaging in atrioventricular septal defect. Am. J. Cardiol., *63*:1137, 1989.

233. Carvalho, J.S., Rigby, M.L., Shinebourne, E.A., and Anderson, R.H.: Cross sectional echocardiography for recognition of ventricular topology in atrioventricular septal defect. Br. Heart J., *61*:285, 1989.

234. Arisawa, J., Morimoto, S., Ikezoe, J., Hamada, S., Kozuka, T., Sano, T., Ogawa, M., Matsuda, H., and Kawashima, Y.: Cross sectional echocardiographic anatomy of common atrioventricular valve in atrial isomerism. Br. Heart J., *62*:291, 1989.

235. Roberson, D.A., Muhiudeen, I.A., Silverman, N.H., Turley, K., Haas, G.S., and Cahalan, M.K.: Intraoperative transesophageal echocardiography of atrioventricular septal defect. J. Am. Coll. Cardiol., *18*:537, 1991.

236. Hiraishi, S., Fujino, N., Saito, K., Oguchi, K., Kadoi, N., Agata, Y., Horiguchi, Y., Hozumi, H., and Yashior, K.: Responsiveness of the ductus arteriosus to prostaglandin E1 assessed by combined cross sectional and pulsed Doppler echocardiography. Br. Heart J., *62*:140, 1989.

237. Cloez, J.L., Isaaz, K., and Pernot, C.: Pulsed Doppler flow characteristics of ductus arteriosus in infants with associated congenital anomalies of the heart or great arteries. Am. J. Cardiol., *57*:845, 1986.

238. Sahn, D.J. and Allen, H.D.: Real-time cross-sectional echocardiographic imaging and measurement of the patent ductus arteriosus in infants and children. Circulation, *58*:343, 1978.

239. Snider, A.R. and Silverman, N.H.: Suprasternal notch echocardiography: A two-dimensional technique for evaluating congenital heart disease. Circulation, *63*:165, 1981.

240. Huhta, J.C., Gutgesell, H.P., Latson, L.A., and Huffines, F.D.: Two-dimensional echocardiographic assessment of the aorta in infants and children with congenital heart disease. Circulation, *70*:417, 1984.

241. Stevenson, J.G., Kaoabori, I., and Guntheroth, W.G.: Pulsed Doppler echocardiographic diagnosis of patent ductus arteriosus: Sensitivity, specificity, limitations and technical features. Cathet. Cardiovasc. Diagn., *6*:255, 1980.

242. Barron, J.V., Sanches-Ugarte, T., Keirns, C., Gonzalez-Medina, A., and Vazquez-Sanches, J.: Calcification of patent ductus arteriosus detected by two-dimensional echocardiography. Am. Heart J., *114*:446, 1987.

243. Perez, J.E., Nordlicht, S.M., and Geltman, E.M.: Patent ductus arteriosus in adults: Diagnosis by suprasternal and parasternal pulsed Doppler echocardiography. Am. J. Cardiol., *53*:1473, 1984.

244. Takenaka, K., Sakamoto, T., Shiota, T., Amano, W., Igarashi, T., and Sugimoto, T.: Diagnosis of patent ductus arteriosus in adults by biplane transesophageal color Doppler flow mapping. Am. J. Cardiol., *68*:691, 1991.

245. Silverman, N.H., Lewis, A.B., and Heyman, M.A.: Echocardiographic assessment of ductus arteriosus shunt in premature infants. Circulation, *50*:821, 1974.

246. Barron, J.V., Sahn, D.J., Valdes-Cruz, L.M., Lima, C.O., Goldberg, S.J., Grenadier, E., and Allen, H.D.: Clinical utility of two-dimensional Doppler echocardiographic techniques for estimating pulmonary to systemic blood flow ratios in children with left-to-right shunting atrial septal defect, ventricular septal defect of patent ductus ateriosus. J. Am. Coll. Cardiol., *3*:169, 1984.

247. Vick, G.W.I., Huhta, J.C., and Gutgesell, H.P.: Assessment of the ductus arteriosus in preterm infants utilizing suprasternal two-dimensional/Doppler echocardiography. J. Am. Coll. Cardiol., *5*:973, 1985.

248. Milne, M.J., Sung, R.Y.T., Fok, T.F., and Crozier, I.G.: Doppler echocardiographic assessment of shunting via the ductus arteriosus in newborn infants. Am. J. Cardiol., *64*:102, 1989.

249. Hiraishi, S., Horiguchi, Y., Misawa, H., Oguchi, K., Kadoi, N., Fujino, N., and Yashiro, K.: Noninvasive Doppler echocardiographic evaluation of shunt flow dynamics of the ductus arteriosus. Circulation, *75*:1146, 1987.

250. Houston, A.B., Gnanapragasam, J.P., Lim, M.K., Doig, W.B., and Coleman, E.N.: Doppler ultrasound and the silent ductus arteriosus. Br. Heart J., *65*:97, 1991.

251. Musewe, N.N., Smallhorn, J.F., Benson, L.N., Burrows, P.E., and Freedom, R.M.: Validation of Doppler-derived pulmonary arterial pressure in patients with ductus arteriosus under different hemodynamic states. Circulation, *76*:1081, 1987.

252. Musewe, N.N., Poppe, D., Smallhorn, J.F., Hellman, J., Whyte, H., Smith, B., and Freedom, R.M.: Doppler echocardiographic measurement of pulmonary artery pressure from ductal Doppler velocities in the newborn. J. Am. Coll. Cardiol., *15*:446, 1990.

253. Stevenson, J.G., Kaoabori, I., and Guntheroth, W.G.: Noninvasive detection of pulmonary hypertension in patent ductus arteriosus by pulsed Doppler echocardiography. Circulation, *4*:113, 1979.

254. Serwer, G.A., Armstrong, B.E., and Anderson, P.A.W.: Noninvasive detection of retrograde descending aortic flow in infants using continuous wave Doppler ultrasonography. J. Pediatr., *97*:394, 1980.

255. Swensson, R.E., Valdes-Cruz, L.M., Sahn, D.J., Sherman, F.S., Chung, K.J., Scagnelli, S., and Hagen-Ansert, S.: Real-time Doppler color flow mapping for detec-

tion of patent ductus arteriosus. J. Am. Coll. Cardiol., 8:1105, 1986.

256. Liao, P-K., Su, W-J., and Hung, J-S.: Doppler echocardiographic flow characteristics of isolated patent ductus arteriosus: Better delineation by Doppler color flow mapping. J. Am. Coll. Cardiol., 12:1285, 1988.

257. Winter, F.S.: Persistent left superior vena cava. Survey of world literature and report of thirty additional cases. Angiology, 5:90, 1954.

258. Huhta, J.C., Smallhorn, J.F., Macartney, F.J., Anderson, R.H., and DeLeval, M.: Cross-sectional echocardiographic diagnosis of systemic venous return. Br. Heart J., 48:388, 1982.

259. Foale, R., Bourdillon, P.D., Somerville, J., and Rickards, A.: Anomalous systemic venous return: Recognition by two-dimensional echocardiography. Eur. Heart J., 4:186, 1983.

260. Snider, A.R., Ports, T.A., and Silverman, N.H.: Venous anomalies of the coronary sinus: Detection by M-mode, two-dimensional, and contrast echocardiography. Circulation, 60:721, 1979.

261. Cohen, B.E., Winer, H.E., and Kronzon, I.: Echocardiographic findings in patients with left superior vena cava and dilated coronary sinus. Am. J. Cardiol., 44:158, 1979.

262. Chaudhry, F. and Zabalgoitia, M.: Persistent left superior vena cava diagnosed by contrast transesophageal echocardiography. Am. Heart J., 122:1175, 1991.

263. Stümper, O., Barron, J.V., and Rijlaarsdam, M.: Assessment of anomalous systemic and pulmonary venous connections by transesophageal echocardiography in infants and children. Br. Heart J., 66:411, 1991.

264. Mascarenhas, E., Javier, R.P., and Samet, P.: Partial anomalous pulmonary venous connection and drainage. Am. J. Cardiol., 31:512, 1973.

265. Stewart, J.R., Schaff, H.V., Fortuin, N.J., and Brawley, R.K.: Partial anomalous pulmonary venous return with intact atrial septum. Thorax, 38:859, 1983.

266. Huhta, J.C., Gutgesell, H.P., and Nihill, M.R.: Crosssectional echocardiographic diagnosis of total anomalous pulmonary venous connection. Br. Heart J., 53:525, 1985.

267. Van der Velde, M.E., Parness, I.A., Colan, S.D., Spevak, P.J., Lock, J.E., Mayer, Jr., J.E., and Sanders, S.P.: Two-dimensional echocardiography in the pre- and postoperative management of totally anomalous pulmonary venous connection. J. Am. Coll. Cardiol., 18:1746, 1991.

268. Chin, A.J., Sanders, S.P., Sherman, F., Lang, P., Norwood, W.I., and Castaneda, A.R.: Accuracy of subcostal two-dimensional echocardiography in prospective diagnosis of total anomalous pulmonary venous connection. Am. Heart J., 113:1153, 1987.

269. Sahn, D.J., Allen, H.D., Lange, L.W., and Goldberg, S.J.: Cross-sectional echocardiographic diagnosis of the sites of total anomalous pulmonary venous drainage. Circulation, 60:1317, 1979.

270. Cooper, M.J., Teitel, D.F., Silverman, N.H., and Enderlein, M.A.: Study of the infradiaphragmatic total anomalous pulmonary venous connection with cross-sectional and pulsed Doppler echocardiography. Circulation, 70:412, 1984.

271. Paquet, M. and Gutgesell, H.: Echocardiographic features of total anomalous pulmonary venous connection. Circulation, 52:599, 1975.

272. Orsmond, G.S., Ruttenberg, H.S., Bessinger, F.B., and Miller, J.H.: Echocardiographic features of total anoma-

lous pulmonary venous connection to the coronary sinus. Am. J. Cardiol., 41:597, 1978.

273. Snider, A.R., Silverman, N.H., Turley, K., and Ebert, P.A.: Evaluation of infradiaphragmatic total anomalous pulmonary venous connection with two-dimensional echocardiography. Circulation, 66:1129, 1982.

274. Aziz, K.U., Paul, M.H., Bharati, S., Lev, M., and Shannon, K.: Echocardiographic features of total anomalous pulmonary venous drainage into the coronary sinus. Am. J. Cardiol., 42:108, 1978.

275. Smallhorn, J.F., Sutherland, G.R., Tommasini, G., Hunter, S., Anderson, R.H., and Macartney, F.J.: Assessment of total anomalous pulmonary venous connection by two-dimensional echocardiography. Br. Heart J., 46:613, 1981.

276. Smallhorn, J.F., Burrows, P., Wilson, G., Coles, J., Gilday, D.L., and Freedom, R.M.: Two-dimensional and pulsed Doppler echocardiography in the postoperative evaluation of total anomalous pulmonary venous connection. Circulation, 76:298, 1987.

277. Smallhorn, J.F. and Freedom, R.M.: Pulsed Doppler echocardiography in the preoperative evaluation of total anomalous pulmonary venous connection. J. Am. Coll. Cardiol., 8:1413, 1986.

278. Mehta, R.H., Jain, S.P., Nanda, N.C., Helmcke, F., and Sanyal, R.: Isolated partial anomalous pulmonary venous connection: Echocardiographic diagnosis and a new color Doppler method to assess shunt volume. Am. Heart J., 122:870, 1991.

279. Sreeram, N. and Walsh, K.: Diagnosis of total anomalous pulmonary venous drainage by Doppler color flow imaging. J. Am. Coll. Cardiol., 19:1577, 1992.

280. Romero-Cárdenas, A., Vargas-Barrón, J., Rylaarsdam, M., Stümper, O., Villegas, M., Bandín, M.A., Keirns, C., and Molina, J.: Total anomalous pulmonary venous return: Diagnosis by transesophageal echocardiography. Am. Heart J., 121:1831, 1991.

281. Maron, B.J., Leon, M.B., Swain, J.A., Cannon, R.O., and Pelliccia, A.: Prospective identification by two-dimensional echocardiography of anomalous origin of the left main coronary artery from the right sinus of Valsalva. Am. J. Cardiol., 68:140, 1991.

282. Piovesana, P., Corrado, D., Contessotto, F., Zampiero, A., Camponeschi, M., Lafisca, N., Verlato, R., and Pantaleoni, A.: Echocardiographic identification of anomalous origin of the left circumflex coronary artery from the right sinus of Valsalva. Am. Heart J., 119:205, 1990.

283. Gaither, N.S., Rogan, K.M., Stajduhar, K., Banks, A.K., Hull, R.W., Whitsitt, T., and Vernalis, M.D.: Anomalous origin and course of coronary arteries in adults: Identification and improved imaging utilizing transesophageal echocardiography. Am. Heart J., 122:69, 1991.

284. Samdarshi, T.E., Hill, D.L., and Nanda, N.C.: Transesophageal color Doppler diagnosis of anomalous origin of left circumflex coronary artery. Am. Heart J., 122:571, 1991.

285. Koh, K.K.: Confirmation of anomalous origin of the right coronary artery from the left sinus of Valsalva by means of transesophageal echocardiography. Am. Heart J., 122:851, 1991.

286. Jureidini, S.B., Appleton, R.S., Nouri, S., and Crawford, C.J.: Detection of coronary artery abnormalities in tetralogy of Fallot by two-dimensional echocardiography. J. Am. Coll. Cardiol., 14:960, 1989.

287. Berry, J.M., Einzig, S., Krabill, K.A., and Bass, J.L.: Evaluation of coronary artery anatomy in patients with

tetralogy of Fallot by two-dimensional echocardiography. Circulation, *78*:149, 1988.

288. Pasquini, L., Sanders, S.P., Parness, I.A., and Colan, S.D.: Diagnosis of coronary artery artery anatomy by two-dimensional echocardiography in patients with transposition of the great arteries. Circulation, *75*:557, 1987.

289. Oberhoffer, R.M., Ho, S.Y., and Anderson, R.H.: Coronary artery diameters in the heart with complete transposition of the great arteries. J. Am. Coll. Cardiol., *1516*: 1433, 1991.

290. Menahem, S. and Venables, A.W.: Anomalous left coronary artery from the pulmonary artery: A 15-year sample. Br. Heart J., *58*:378, 1987.

291. Koike, K., Musewe, N.N., Smallhorn, J.F., and Freedom, R.M.: Distinguishing between anomalous origin of the left coronary artery from the pulmonary trunk and dilated cardiomyopathy: Role of echocardiographic measurement of the right coronary artery diameter. Br. Heart J., *61*:192, 1989.

292. Rein, A.J.J.T., Colan, S.D., and Parness, I.A.: Regional and global left ventricular function in infants with anomalous origin of the left coronary artery from the pulmonary trunk: Preoperative and postoperative assessment. Circulation, *75*:115, 1987.

293. Caldwell, R.L., Hurwitz, R.A., and Girod, D.A.: Two-dimensional echocardiographic differentiation of anomalous left coronary artery from congestive cardiomyopathy. Am. Heart J., *106*:710, 1983.

294. Jureidini, S.B., Nouri, S., Crawford, C.J., Chen, S.C., Pennington, G., and Fiore, A.: Reliability of echocardiography in the diagnosis of anomalous origin of the left coronary artery from the pulmonary trunk. Am. Heart J., *122*:61, 1991.

295. Fisher, E.A.: Two-dimensional echocardiographic visualization of the left coronary artery in anomalous origin of the left coronary artery from the pulmonary artery. Circulation, *63*:698, 1981.

296. Sanders, S.P., Parness, I.A., and Colan, S.D.: Recognition of abnormal connections of coronary arteries with the use of Doppler color flow mapping. J. Am. Coll. Cardiol., *13*:922, 1989.

297. Schmidt, K.G., Cooper, M.J., Silverman, N.H., and Stanger, P.: Pulmonary artery origin of the left coronary artery: Diagnosis by two-dimensional echocardiography, pulsed Doppler ultrasound and color flow mapping. J. Am. Coll. Cardiol., *11*:396, 1988.

298. Ludomirsky, A., O'Laughlin, M.P., Reul, G.J., and Mullins, C.E.: Congenital aneurysm of the right coronary artery with fistulous connection to the right atrium. Am. Heart J., *119*:672, 1990.

299. Nishiguchi, T., Matsuoka, Y., Sennari, E., Okishima, T., Suzumiya, H., Akimoto, K., Takamura, K., Kawaguchi, K., Tashiro, S., Yamasaki, S., and Hayadawa, K.: Congenital coronary artery fistula: Diagnosis by two-dimensional Doppler echocardiography. Am. Heart J., *120*: 1244, 1990.

300. Lau, K. and Ng, Y.: Evaluation of coronary arterial fistula by color-coded Doppler echocardiography. Am. J. Cardiol., *64*:689, 1989.

301. Kimball, T.R., Daniels, S.R., Meyer, R.A., Knilans, T.K., Plowden, J.S., and Schwartz, D.C.: Color flow mapping in the diagnosis of coronary artery fistula in the neonate: Benefits and limitations. Am. Heart J., *117*:968, 1989.

302. Sahasakul, Y., Chaithiraphan, S., and Spiyoschati, S.: Diagnosis of a right coronary artery-left ventricular fis-

tula by cross sectional and Doppler echocardiography. Br. Heart J., *59*:593, 1988.

303. Miyatake, K., Okamoto, M., Kinoshita, N., Fusejima, K., Sakakibara, H., and Nimura, Y.: Doppler echocardiographic features of coronary arteriovenous fistula: Complementary roles of cross sectional echocardiography and the Doppler technique. Br. Heart J., *51*:508, 1984.

304. Slater, J., Lighty, G.W., Winer, H.E., Kahn, M.L., Kronzon, I., and Isom, O.W.: Doppler echocardiography and computed tomography in diagnosis of left coronary atriovenous fistula. J. Am. Coll. Cardiol., *4*:1290, 1984.

305. Pickoff, A.S.: Pulsed Doppler echocardiographic detection of coronary artery to right ventricular fistula. Pediatr. Cardiol., *2*:145, 1982.

306. Chia, B.I.: Two-dimensional and pulsed Doppler echocardiographic abnormalities in coronary artery-pulmonary artery fistula. Chest, *86*:901, 1984.

307. Cooper, M.J., Bernstein, D., and Silverman, N.H.: Recognition of left coronary artery fistula to the left and right ventricles by contrast echocardiography. J. Am. Coll. Cardiol., *6*:923, 1985.

308. Ching, K.J., Fulton, D.R., and Lapp, R.: One-year follow-up of cardiac and coronary artery disease in infants and children with Kawasaki disease. Am. Heart J., *115*: 1263, 1988.

309. Hiraishi, S.: Clinical course of cardiovascular involvement in the mucocutaneous lymph node syndrome. Relation between clinical signs of carditis and development of coronary arterial aneurysm. Am. J. Cardiol., *47*:323, 1981.

310. Arjunan, K., Daniels, S.R., and Meyer, R.A.: Coronary artery caliber in normal children and patients with Kawasaki disease but without aneurysms: An echocardiographic and angiographic study. J. Am. Coll. Cardiol., *8*:1119, 1986.

311. Hiraishi, S., Yashiro, K., and Kusano, S.: Noninvasive visualization of coronary arterial aneurysm in infants and young children with mucocutaneous lymph node syndrome with two-dimensional echocardiography. Am. J. Cardiol., *43*:1225, 1979.

312. Tatara, K. and Kusakawa, S.: Long-term prognosis of giant coronary aneurysm in Kawasaki disease: An angiographic study. J. Pediatr., *111*:705, 1987.

313. Ettedgui, J.A., Neches, W.H., and Pahl, E.: The role of cross-sectional echocardiography in Kawasaki disease. Cardiol. Young, *1*:221, 1991.

314. Bensky, A.S., Daniels, S.R., and Meyer, R.A.: Effects of stress on regional wall motion in children with Kawasaki disease. J. Am. Soc. Echocardiogr., *5*:315, 1992.

315. Issaz, K., Cloez, J.L., Marcon, F., Worms, A.M., and Pernot, C.: Is the aorta truly dextroposed in tetralogy of Fallot? A two-dimensional echocardiographic answer. Circulation, *73*:892, 1986.

316. Henry, W.L., Maron, B.J., and Griffith, J.M.: Differential diagnosis of anomalies of the great arteries by real-time two-dimensional echocardiography. Circulation, *51*: 283, 1975.

317. Hagler, D.J., Tajik, A.J., Seward, J.B., Mair, D.D., and Ritter, D.G.: Wide-angle two-dimensional echocardiographic profiles of conotruncal abnormalities. Mayo Clin. Proc., *55*:73, 1980.

318. Caldwell, R.L., Weyman, A.E., Hurwitz, R.A., Girod, D.A., and Feigenbaum, H.: Right ventricular outflow tract assessment by cross-sectional echocardiography in tetralogy of Fallot. Circulation, *59*:395, 1979.

319. Morris, D.C., Felner, J.M., Schlant, R.C., and Franch,

R.H.: Echocardiographic diagnosis of tetralogy of Fallot. Am. J. Cardiol., *36*:908, 1975.

320. Sanders, S.P., Bierman, F.Z., and Williams, R.G.: Conotruncal malformations: Diagnosis in infancy using subxiphoid 2-dimensional echocardiography. Am. J. Cardiol., *50*:1361, 1982.

321. Flanagan, M.F., Foran, R.B., VanPraagh, R., Jonas, R., and Sanders, S.P.: Tetralogy of Fallot with obstruction of the ventricular septal defect: Spectrum of echocardiographic findings. J. Am. Coll. Cardiol., *11*:386, 1988.

322. Segni, E.D., Einzig, S., Bass, J.L., and Edwards, J.E.: Congenital absence of the pulmonary valve associated with tetralogy of Fallot: Diagnosis by 2-dimensional echocardiography. Am. J. Cardiol., *51*:1798, 1983.

323. Musewe, N.N., Smallhorn, J.F., Moes, C.A.F., Freedom, R.M., and Trusler, G.A.: Echocardiographic evaluation of obstructive mechanism of tetralogy of Fallot with restrictive ventricular septal defect. Am. J. Cardiol., *61*: 664, 1988.

324. Marino, B., Franceschini, E., Ballerini, L., Marcelletti, C., and Thiene, G.: Anatomical-echocardiographic correlations in pulmonary atresia with intact ventricular septum. Use of subcostal cross-sectional views. Int. J. Cardiol., *11*:103, 1986.

325. Rowe, S.A., Zahka, K.G., Manolio, T.A., Horneffer, P.J., and Kidd, L.: Lung function and pulmonary regurgitation limit exercise capacity in postoperative tetralogy of Fallot. J. Am. Coll. Cardiol., *17*:461, 1991.

326. Horneffer, P.J., Zahka, K.G., Rowe, S.A., Manolio, T.A., Gott, V.L., Reitz, B.A., and Gardner, T.J.: Long-term results of total repair of tetralogy of Fallot in childhood. Ann. Thorac. Surg., *50*:179, 1990.

327. Vick, G.W. and Serwer, G.A.: Echocardiographic evaluation of the postoperative tetralogy of Fallot patient. Circulation, *58*:842, 1978.

328. George, L., Waldman, J.D., Mathewson, J.W., Kirkpatrick, S.E., Dappelbaum, S.J., and Turner, S.W.: Two-dimensional echocardiographic discrimination of normal from abnormal great artery relationships. Clin. Cardiol., *6*:327, 1983.

329. Henry, W.L., Maron, B.J., Griffith, J.M., Redwood, D.R., and Epstein, S.E.: Differential diagnosis of anomalies of the great arteries by real-time two-dimensional echocardiography. Circulation, *51*:283, 1975.

330. Daskalopoulos, D.A., Edwards, W.D., Driscoll, D.J., Seward, J.B., Tajik, A.J., and Hagler, D.J.: Correlation of two-dimensional echocardiographic and autopsy findings in complete transposition of the great arteries. Am. J. Cardiol., *2*:1151, 1982.

331. Chin, A.J., Yeager, S.B., Sanders, S.P., Williams, R.G., Bierman, F.Z., Burger, B.M., Norwood, W.I., and Castaneda, A.R.: Accuracy of prospective two-dimensional echocardiographic evaluation of left ventricular outflow tract in complete transposition of the great arteries. Am. J. Cardiol., *55*:759, 1985.

332. Bierman, F.Z. and Williams, R.G.: Prospective diagnosis of D-transposition of the great arteries in neonates by subxiphoid, two-dimensional echocardiography. Circulation, *60*:1496, 1979.

333. Allan, L.D., Leanage, R., Wainwright, R., Joseph, M.C., and Tynan, M.: Balloon atrial septostomy under two dimensional echocardiographic control. Br. Heart J., *47*: 41, 1982.

334. Ashfaq, M., Houston, A.B., Gnanapragasam, J.P., Lilley, S., and Murtagh, E.P.: Balloon atrial septostomy under echocardiographic control: Six years' experience

and evaluation of the practicability of cannulation via the umbilical vein. Br. Heart J., *65*:148, 1991.

335. Perry, L.W., Ruckman, R.N., Galioto, F.M., Shapiro, S.R., Potter, B.M., and Scott, L.P.: Echocardiographically assisted balloon atrial septostomy. Pediatr. Cardiol., *70*:403, 1982.

336. Roberson, D.A. and Silverman, N.H.: Malaligned outlet septum with subpulmonary ventricular septal defect and abnormal ventriculoarterial connection: A morphologic spectrum defined echocardiographically. J. Am. Coll. Cardiol., *16*:459, 1990.

337. Marino, B., deSimone, G., Pasquini, L., Giannico, S., Marcelletti, C., Ammirati, A., Guccione, P., Boldrini, R., and Ballerini, L.: Complete transposition of the great arteries: Visualization of left and right outflow tract obstruction using oblique subcostal two-dimensional echocardiography. Am. J. Cardiol., *55*:1140, 1985.

338. Pigott, J.D., Chin, A.J., and Weinberg, P.M.: Transposition of the great arteries with aortic arch obstruction. Anatomical review and report of surgical management. J. Thorac. Cardiovas. Surg., *94*:82, 1987.

339. Riggs, T.W., Muster, A.J., Aziz, K.U., Paul, M.H., Ilbawi, M., and Idriss, F.S.: Two-dimensional echocardiographic and angiocardiographic diagnosis of subpulmonary stenosis due to tricuspid valve pouch in complete transposition of the great arteries. J. Am. Cardiol., *1*:484, 1983.

340. Park, S.C., Neches, W.H., and Zuberbuhler, J.R.: Echocardiographic and hemodynamic correlation in transposition of the great arteries. Circulation, *57*:291, 1978.

341. Silverman, N.H., Payot, M., Stanger, P., and Rudolph, A.M.: The echocardiographic profile of patients after Mustard's operation. Circulation, *58*:1083, 1978.

342. Areias, J.C., Goldberg, S.J., Spitaels, S.E.C., and de Villeneuve, V.H.: An evaluation of range gated pulsed Doppler echocardiography for detecting pulmonary outflow tract obstruction in D-transposition of the great vessels. Am. Heart J., *96*:467, 1978.

343. Huhta, J.C.: Left ventricular wall thickness in complete transposition of the great arteries. J. Thorac. Cardiovas. Surg., *84*:97, 1982.

344. Martin, R.P., Qureshi, S.A., Ettedgui, J.A., Baker, E.J., O'Brien, B.J., Deverall, P.B., Yates, A.K., Maisey, M.N., Radley-Smith, R., Tynan, M., and Yacoub, M.H.: An evaluation of right and left ventricular function after anatomical correction and intra-atrial repair operations for complete transposition of the great arteries. Circulation, *82*:808, 1990.

345. Schmidt, K.G., Cloez, J.L., and Silverman, N.H.: Assessment of right ventricular performance by pulsed Doppler echocardiography in patients after intraatrial repair of aortopulmonary transposition in infancy or childhood. J. Am. Coll. Cardiol., *13*:1578, 1989.

346. Nascimento, R., Cunha, D.L., Bastos, P., VanZeller, P., and Rodrigues-Gomes, M.: Echo-Doppler study of right ventricular filling in asymptomatic patients with Senning operation for transposition of the great arteries. Am. J. Cardiol., *68*:693, 1991.

347. Carceller, A.M., Fouron, J.C., and Smallhorn, J.F.: Wall thickness, cavity dimensions, and myocardial contractility of the left ventricle in patients with simple transposition of the great arteries. A multicenter study of patients from 10 to 20 years of age. Circulation, *73*:622, 1986.

348. Ninomiya, K., Duncan, W.J., Cook, D.H., Olley, P.M., and Rowe, R.D.: Right ventricular ejection fraction and volumes after Mustard repair: Correlation of two dimen-

sional echocardiograms and cineangiograms. Am. J. Cardiol., 48:317, 1981.

349. Aziz, K.U., Paul, M.H., Bharati, S., Cole, R.B., Muster, A.J., Lev, M., and Idriss, F.S.: Two dimensional echocardiographic evaluation of Mustard operation for D-transposition of the great arteries. Am. J. Cardiol., 47:654, 1981.

350. Thompson, K. and Serwer, G.A.: Echocardiographic features of patients with and without residual defects after Mustard's procedure for transposition of the great vessels. Circulation, 64:1032, 1981.

351. Silverman, N.H. and Snider, A.R.: Two-dimensional Echocardiography in Congenital Heart Disease. Norwalk, CT, Appleton-Century-Crofts, 1982.

352. Silverman, N.H., Snider, R., Colo, J., Ebert, P.A., and Turley, K.: Superior venal caval obstruction after Mustard's operation: Detection by two-dimensional contrast echocardiography. Circulation, 64:392, 1981.

353. Smallhorn, J., Grow, R., Freedom, R., Trusler, G., Olley, P., Pacquet, M., Gibbons, J., and Vlad, P.: Pulsed Doppler echocardiographic assessment of the pulmonary venous pathway after the Mustard or Senning procedure for transposition of the great arteries. Circulation, 73:765, 1986.

354. Kaulitz, R., Stümper, O.F.W., Geuskens, R., Sreeram, N., Elzenga, N.J., Chang, C.K., Burns, J.E., Godman, M.J., Hess, J., and Sutherland, G.R.: Comparative values of the precordial and transesophageal approaches in the echocardiographic evaluation of atrial baffle function after an atrial correction procedure. J. Am. Coll. Cardiol., 16:686, 1990.

355. Takahashi, Y., Nakano, S., Shimazaki, Y., Kadoba, K., Taniguchi, K., Sano, T., Nakada, T., Tsuchitani, Y., Miyamoto, K., Matsuda, H., and Kawashima, Y.: Echocardiographic comparison of postoperative left ventricular contractile state between one- and two-stage arterial switch operation for simple transposition of the great arteries. Circulation, 84 (Suppl 3):III-180, 1991.

356. Gleason, M.M., Chin, A.J., Andrews, B.A., Barber, G., Helton, J.G., Murphy, J.D., and Norwood, W.I.: Two-dimensional and Doppler echocardiographic assessment of neonatal arterial repair for transposition of the great arteries. J. Am. Coll. Cardiol., 13:1320, 1989.

357. Martin, M.M., Snider, R., Bove, E.L., Serwer, G.A., Rosenthal, A., Peters, J., and Pollock, P.: Two-dimensional and Doppler echocardiographic evaluation after arterial switch repair in infancy for complete transposition of the great arteries. Am. J. Cardiol., 63:332, 1989.

358. Gibbs, J.L., Qureshi, S.A., Grieve, L., Webb, C., Smith, R.R., and Yacoub, M.H.: Doppler echocardiography after anatomical correction of transposition of the great arteries. Br. Heart J., 56:67, 1986.

359. Borow, K.M., Arensman, F.W., Webb, C., Radley-Smith, R., and Yacoub, M.H.: Assessment of the left ventricular contractile state after anatomic correction of transposition of the great arteries. Circulation, 69:106, 1984.

360. Colan, S.D., Trowitzsch, E., and Wernovsky, G.: Myocardial performance after arterial switch operation for transposition of the great arteries with intact ventricular septum. Circulation, 78:132, 1988.

361. Wernovsky, G., Hougen, T.J., and Walsh, E.P.: Midterm results after the arterial switch operation for transposition of the great arteries with intact ventricular septum: Clinical, hemodynamic, echocardiographic and electrophysiologic data. Circulation, 77:1333, 1988.

362. Allwork, S.P., Bentall, H.H., and Becker, A.E.: Congenitally corrected transposition: A morphologic study of 32 cases. Am. J. Cardiol., 38:910, 1976.

363. Lundstrom, U.: The natural and "unnatural" history of congenitally corrected transposition. Am. J. Cardiol., 65:1222, 1990.

364. Sutherland, G.R., Smallhorn, J.F., Anderson, R.H., Rigby, M.L., and Hunter, S.: Atrioventricular discordance. Cross-sectional echocardiographic morphological correlative study. Br. Heart J., 50:8, 1983.

365. Hagler, D.J., Tajik, A.J., Seward, J.B., Edwards, W.D., Mair, D.D., and Ritter, D.G.: Atrioventricular and ventriculoarterial discordance (corrected transposition of the great arteries). Mayo Clin. Proc., 56:591, 1981.

366. Meissner, M.D., Panidis, I.P., Eshaghpour, E., Mintz, G.S., and Ross, J.: Corrected transposition of the great arteries: Evaluation by two-dimensional and Doppler echocardiography. Am. Heart J., 111:599, 1986.

367. Carminati, M., Valsecchi, O., and Borghi, A.: Cross-sectional echocardiographic study of criss-cross hearts and superoinferior ventricles. Am. J. Cardiol., 59:114, 1987.

368. Marino, B., Sanders, S.P., Pasquini, L., Giannico, S., Parness, I.A., and Colan, S.D.: Two-dimensional echocardiographic anatomy in crisscross heart. Am. J. Cardiol., 58:325, 1986.

369. Marino, B., Sanders, S.P., Parness, I.A., and Colan, S.D.: Obstruction of right ventricular inflow and outflow in corrected transposition of the great arteries S,L,L: Two-dimensional echocardiographic diagnosis. J. Am. Coll. Cardiol., 8:407, 1986.

370. Celermajer, D.S., Seamus, C., Deanfield, J.E., and Sullivan, I.D.: Congenitally corrected transposition and Ebstein's anomaly of the systemic atrioventricular valve: Association with aortic arch obstruction. J. Am. Coll. Cardiol., 18:1056, 1991.

371. Macartney, F.J., Rigby, M.L., Anderson, R.H., Stark, J., and Silverman, N.H.: Double outlet right ventricle. Cross-sectional echocardiographic findings, their anatomical explanation and surgical relevance. Br. Heart J., 52:164, 1984.

372. DiSessa, T.G., Hagan, A.D., Pope, C., Samtoy, L., and Friedman, W.F.: Two-dimensional echocardiographic characteristics of double outlet right ventricle. Am. J. Cardiol., 44:1146, 1979.

373. Hagler, D.J., Tajik, A.J., Seward, J.B., Mair, D.D., and Ritter, D.G.: Double-outlet right ventricle: Wide-angle two-dimensional echocardiographic observations. Circulation, 50:104, 1981.

374. Ceballos, R., Soto, B., and Kirklin, J.W.: Truncus arteriosus. An anatomical-angiographic study. Br. Heart J., 49:589, 1983.

375. Rice, M.J., Seward, J.B., Hagler, D.J., Mair, D.D., and Tajik, A.J.: Definitive diagnosis of truncus arteriosus by two-dimensional echocardiography. Mayo Clin. Proc., 57:476, 1982.

376. Smallhorn, J.F., Anderson, R.H., and Macartney, F.J.: Two-dimensional echocardiographic assessment of communications between the ascending aorta and pulmonary trunk or individual pulmonary arteries. Br. Heart J., 47:563, 1982.

377. Marin-Garcia, J. and Tonkin, I.L.D.: Two-dimensional echocardiographic evaluation of persistent truncus arteriosus. Am. J. Cardiol., 50:1376, 1982.

378. Riggs, T.W. and Paul, M.H.: Two-dimensional echocardiographic prospective diagnosis of common truncus arteriosus in infants. Am. J. Cardiol., 50:1380, 1982.

379. Rao, P.S., Levy, J.M., Nikicicz, E., and Gilbert-Barness, E.F.: Tricuspid atresia: Association with persistent truncus arteriosus. Am. Heart J., 122:829, 1991.

380. Balaji, S., Burch, M., and Sullivan, I.D.: Accuracy of cross-sectional echocardiography in diagnosis of aorto-pulmonary window. Am. J. Cardiol., *67*:650, 1991.

381. Alboliras, E.T., Chin, A.J., Barber, G., Helton, J.G., and Pigott, J.D.: Detection of aortopulmonary window by pulsed and color Doppler echocardiography. Am. Heart J., *115*:900, 1988.

382. Rice, M.J., Seward, J.B., Hagler, D.J., Mair, D.D., and Tajik, A.J.: Visualization of aortopulmonary window by two-dimensional echocardiography. Mayo Clin. Proc., *8*:185, 1982.

383. Lange, L.W., Sahn, D.J., Allen, H.D., Ovitt, T.W., and Goldberg, S.J.: Cross-sectional echocardiography in hypoplastic left ventricle: Echocardiographic-angiographic-anatomic correlations. Pediatr. Cardiol., *2*:287, 1980.

384. Weinberg, P.M., Chin, A.J., Murphy, J.D., Pigott, J.D., and Norwood, W.I.: Postmortem echocardiography and tomographic anatomy of hypoplastic left heart syndrome after palliative surgery. Am. J. Cardiol., *58*:1228, 1986.

385. Bash, S.E., Huhta, J.C., Vick, G.W.I., Gutgesell, H.P., and Ott, D.A.: Hypoplastic left heart syndrome: Is echocardiography accurate enough to guide surgical palliation? J. Am. Coll. Cardiol., *7*:610, 1986.

386. Parikh, S.R., Hurwitz, R.A., Caldwell, R.L., and Waller, B.: Absent aortic valve in hypoplastic left heart syndrome. Am. Heart J., *119*:977, 1990.

387. Chin, T.K., Perloff, J.K., Williams, R.G., Jue, K., and Morhmann, R.: Isolated noncompaction of left ventricular myocardium: A study of eight cases. Circulation, *82*:507, 1990.

388. Conces, D.J., Ryan, T., and Tarver, R.D.: Noncompaction of ventricular myocardium: CT appearance. AJR Am. J. Roentgenol., *156*:717, 1991.

389. VanPraagh, R., Ongley, P.A., and Swan, H.J.C.: Anatomic types of single or common ventricle in man: Morphologic and geometric aspects of 60 necropsied cases. Am. J. Cardiol., *13*:367, 1964.

390. Anderson, R.H., Tynan, M., and Freedom, R.M.: Ventricular morphology in univentricular heart. Herz, *4*:184, 1979.

391. Anderson, R.H., Becker, A.E., and Freedom, R.M.: Problems in the nomenclature of the univentricular heart. Herz, *4*:97, 1979.

392. Huhta, J.C., Seward, J.B., Tajik, A.J., Hagler, D.J., and Edwards, W.D.: Two-dimensional echocardiographic spectrum of univentricular atrioventricular connection. J. Am. Coll. Cardiol., *5*:149, 1985.

393. Bevilacqua, M., Sanders, S.P., VanPraagh, S., Colan, S.D., and Parness, I.: Double-inlet single left ventricle: Echocardiographic anatomy with emphasis on the morphology of the atrioventricular valves and ventricular septal defect. J. Am. Coll. Cardiol., *18*:559, 1991.

394. Shiraishi, H. and Silverman, N.H.: Echocardiographic spectrum of double inlet ventricle: Evaluation of the interventricular communication. J. Am. Coll. Cardiol., *15*:1401, 1991.

395. Rigby, M.L., Anderson, R.H., Gibson, D., Jones, O.D.H., Joseph, M.C., and Shinebourne, E.A.: Two-dimensional echocardiographic categorisation of the univentricular heart. Br. Heart J., *46*:603, 1981.

396. Mair, D.D., Hagler, D.J., Julsrud, P.R., Puga, F.J., Schaff, H.V., and Danielson, G.K.: Early and late results of the modified Fontan procedure for double-inlet left ventricle: The Mayo Clinic experience. J. Am. Coll. Cardiol., *18*:1727, 1991.

397. Nakazawa, M., Aotsuka, H., Imai, Y., Kurosawa, H., Fukuchi, S., Satomi, G., and Takao, A.: Ventricular vol-ume characteristics in double-inlet left ventricle before and after septation. Circulation, *81*:1537, 1990.

398. Rao, P.S.: Atrioventricular canal mimicking tricuspid atresia: Echocardiographic and angiographic features. Br. Heart J., *58*:409, 1987.

399. Van Praagh, S., Vangi, V., Hee Sul, J., Metras, D., Parness, I., Castaneda, A.R., and Van Praagh, R.: Tricuspid atresia or severe stenosis with partial common atrioventricular canal: Anatomic data, clinical profile and surgical considerations. J. Am. Coll. Cardiol., *17*:932, 1991.

400. Anderson, R.H., Wilkinson, J.C., and Gerlis, M.: Atresia of the right ventricular orifice. Br. Heart J., *39*:414, 1977.

401. Rigby, M.L., Gibson, D.G., Joseph, M.C., Lincoln, J.C.R., Shinebourne, E.A., Shore, D.F., and Anderson, R.H.: Recognition of imperforate atrioventricular valves by two dimensional echocardiography. Br. Heart J., *47*:329, 1982.

402. Fyfe, D.A., Taylor, A.B., and Gillette, P.C.: Doppler echocardiographic confirmation of recurrent atrial septal defect stenosis in infants with mitral valve atresia. Am. J. Cardiol., *60*:410, 1987.

403. Andrade, J.L., Serino, W., DeLeval, M., and Somerville, J.: Two-dimensional echocardiographic evaluation of tricuspid hypoplasia in pulmonary atresia. Am. J. Cardiol., *53*:387, 1984.

404. Muhiudeen, I.A., Roberson, D.A., Silverman, N.H., Haas, G., Turley, K., and Cahalan, M.K.: Intraoperative echocardiography in infants and children with congenital cardiac shunt lesions: Transesophageal versus epicardial echocardiography. J. Am. Coll. Cardiol., *16*:1687, 1990.

405. Gussenhoven, E.J., VanHerwerden, L.A., Roelandt, J., Ligtvoet, K.M., Bos, E., and Witsenburg, M.: Intraoperative two-dimensional echocardiography in congenital heart disease. J. Am. Coll. Cardiol., *9*:565, 1987.

406. Sreeram, N., Kaulitz, R., Stümper, O.F.W., Hess, J., Quaegebeur, J.M., and Sutherland, G.R.: Comparative roles of intraoperative epicardial and early postoperative transthoracic echocardiography in the assessment of surgical repair of congenital heart defects. J. Am. Coll. Cardiol., *16*:913, 1990.

407. Hsu, Y.H., Santulli, T., Wong, A.L., Drinkwater, D., Laks, H., and Williams, R.G.: Impact of intraoperative echocardiography on surgical management of congenital heart disease. Am. J. Cardiol., *67*:1279, 1991.

408. Sutherland, G.R., Balaji, S., and Monro, J.L.: Potential value of intraoperative Doppler colour flow mapping in operations for complex intracardiac shunting. Br. Heart J., *62*:467, 1989.

409. Reed, K.L.: Cyanotic disease in the fetus: Intraoperative transesophageal versus epicardial ultrasound in surgery for congenital heart disease. J. Am. Soc. Echocardiogr., *3*:9, 1990.

410. Chang, A.C., Vetter, J.M., Gill, S.E., Franklin, W.H., Murphy, J.D., and Chin, A.J.: Accuracy of prospective two-dimensional/Doppler echocardiography in the assessment of reparative surgery. J. Am. Coll. Cardiol., *16*:903, 1990.

411. Allen, H.D., Sahn, D.J., and Lange, L.: Noninvasive assessment of surgical systemic to pulmonary artery shunts by range-gated pulsed Doppler echocardiography. J. Pediatr., *94*:395, 1979.

412. Stevenson, J.G., Kawabori, I., and Bailey, W.W.: Noninvasive evaluation of Blalock-Taussig shunts: Determination of patency and differentiation from patent ductus arteriosus by Doppler echocardiography. Am. Heart J., *106*:1121, 1983.

413. Fyfe, D.A., Currie, P.J., Seward, J.B., Tajik, A.J., Reeder, G.S., Mair, D.D., and Hagler, D.J.: Continuous-

wave Doppler determination of the pressure gradient across pulmonary artery bands: Hemodynamic correlation in 20 patients. Mayo Clin. Proc., *59*:744, 1984.

414. Fontan, F., Kirklin, J.W., Fernandez, G., Costa, F., Naftel, D.C., Tritto, F., and Blackstone, E.H.: Outcome after a "perfect" Fontan operation. Circulation, *81*:1520, 1990.

415. Hagler, D.J., Seward, J.B., Tajik, A.J., and Ritter, D.G.: Functional assessment of the Fontan operation: Combined M-mode, two-dimensional and Doppler echocardiographic studies. J. Am. Coll. Cardiol., *4*:756, 1984.

416. Penny, D.J. and Redington, A.N.: Doppler echocardiographic evaluation of pulmonary blood flow after the Fontan operation: The role of the lungs. Br. Heart J., *66*:372, 1991.

417. Penny, D.J., Rigby, M.L., and Redington, A.N.: Abnormal patterns of intraventricular flow and diastolic filling after the Fontan operation: Evidence for incoordinate ventricular wall motion. Br. Heart J., *66*:375, 1991.

418. Frommelt, P.C., Snider, A.R., Meliones, J.N., and Vermilion, R.P.: Doppler assessment of pulmonary artery flow patterns and ventricular function after the Fontan operation. Am. J. Cardiol., *68*:1211, 1991.

419. Qureshi, S.A., Richheimer, R., McKay, R., and Arnold, R.: Doppler echocardiographic evaluation of pulmonary artery flow after modified Fontan operation: Importance of atrial contraction. Br. Heart J., *64*:272, 1990.

420. Stümper, O., Sutherland, G.R., Geuskens, R., Roelandt, J.R.T.C., Bos, E., and Hess, J.: Transesophageal echocardiography in evaluation and management after a Fontan procedure. J. Am. Coll. Cardiol., *17*:1152, 1991.

421. Fyfe, D.A., Kline, C.H., Sade, R.M., Greene, C.A., and Gillette, P.C.: The utility of transesophageal echocardiography during and after Fontan operations in small children. Am. Heart J., *122*:1403, 1991.

422. Fyfe, D.A., Kline, C.H., Sade, R.M., and Gillette, P.C.: Transesophageal echocardiography detects thrombus formation not identified by transthoracic echocardiography after the Fontan operation. J. Am. Coll. Cardiol., *18*:1733, 1991.

423. Reeder, G.S., Currie, P.J., Fyfe, D.A., Hagler, D.J., Seward, J.B., and Tajik, A.J.: Extracardiac conduit obstruction: Initial experience in the use of Doppler echocardiography for noninvasive estimation of pressure gradient. J. Am. Coll. Cardiol., *4*:1006, 1984.

424. Meliones, J.N., Snider, R., Bove, E.L., Serwer, G.A., Peters, J., Lacina, S.J., Florentine, M.S., and Rosenthal, A.: Doppler evaluation of homograft valved conduits in children. Am. J. Cardiol., *64*:354, 1989.

425. Sahn, D.J.: Resolution and display requirements for ultrasound/Doppler evaluation of the heart in children, infants and unborn human fetus. J. Am. Coll. Cardiol., *5* (Suppl 1):12S, 1985.

426. Cyr, D.R., Guntheroth, W.G., and Mack, L.A.: A systematic approach to fetal echocardiography using real-time/two dimensional sonography. J. Ultrasound Med., *343*:350, 1986.

427. Wilson, N., Reed, K., Allen, H.D., Marx, G.R., and Goldberg, S.J.: Doppler echocardiographic observations of pulmonary and transvalvular velocity changes after birth and during the early neonatal period. Am. Heart J., *113*:750, 1987.

428. Linday, L.A., Ehlers, K.H., O'Loughlin, J.E., LaGamma, E.F., and Engle, M.A.: Noninvasive diagnosis of persistent fetal circulation versus congenital cardiovascular defects. Am. Heart J., *52*:847, 1983.

429. Azancot, A.: Analysis of ventricular shape by echocardiography in normal fetuses, newborns and infants. Circulation, *68*:1201, 1083.

430. Silverman, N.H. and Golbus, M.S.: Echocardiographic techniques for assessing normal and abnormal fetal cardiac anatomy. J. Am. Coll. Cardiol., *5*:20, 1985.

431. Groenenberg, I.A.L., Wladimiroff, J.W., and Hop, W.C.J.: Fetal cardiac and peripheral arterial flow velocity waveforms in intrauterine growth retardation. Circulation, *80*:1711, 1989.

432. Maulik, D., Nanda, N.C., and Saini, V.D.: Fetal Doppler echocardiography: Methods and characterization of normal and abnormal hemodynamics. Am. J. Cardiol., *53*:572, 1984.

433. Reed, K.L., Meijboom, E.J., and Sahn, D.J.: Cardiac Doppler flow velocities in human fetuses. Circulation, *73*:41, 1986.

434. Allan, L.D.: Prenatal screening for congenital heart disease. Br. Med. J., *292*:1717, 1988.

435. Kleinman, C.S., Hobbins, J.C., and Jaffe, C.C.: Echocardiographic studies of the human fetus: Prenatal diagnosis of congenital heart disease and cardiac dysrhythmias. Pediatrics, *65*:1059, 1980.

436. Silverman, N.H., Enderlein, M.A., and Stanger, P.: Recognition of fetal arrhythmias by echocardiography. JCU, *13*:255, 1985.

437. Gembruch, U., Knöpfle, G., Chatterjee, M., Bald, R., Redel, D.A., Födisch, H.-J., and Hansmann, M.: Prenatal diagnosis of atrioventricular canal malformations with up-to-date echocardiographic technology: Report of 14 cases. Am. Heart J., *121*:1489, 1991.

438. Machado, M.V.L., Crawford, D.C., Anderson, R.H., and Allan, L.D.: Atrioventricualr septal defect in prenatal life. Br. Heart J., *59*:352, 1988.

439. Allan, L.D., Chita, S.K., Anderson, R.H., Fagg, N., Crawford, D.C., and Tynan, M.J.: Coarctation of the aorta in prenatal life: An echocardiographic, anatomical, and functional study. Br. Heart J., *59*:356, 1988.

440. Robertson, M.A., Byrne, P.J., and Penkoske, P.A.: Perinatal management of critical aortic valve stenosis diagnosed by fetal echocardiography. Br. Heart J., *61*:365, 1989.

441. Angelini, A., Allan, L.D., Anderson, R.H., Crawford, D.C., Chita, S.K., and Ho, S.Y.: Measurements of the dimensions of the aortic and pulmonary pathways in the human fetus: A correlative echocardiographic and morphometric study. Br. Heart J., *60*:221, 1988.

442. Kenny, J.F., Plappert, T., Doubilet, P., Saltzman, D.H., Cartier, M., Zollars, L., Leatherman, G.F., and St. John Sutton, M.G.: Changes in intracardiac blood flow velocities and right and left ventricular stroke volumes with gestational age in the normal human fetus: A prospective Doppler echocardiographic study. Circulation, *74*:1208, 1986.

443. Sahn, D.J.: Prenatal ultrasound hypoplastic left heart syndrome in utero associated with hydrops fetalis. Am. Heart J., *104*:1368, 1982.

444. St. John Sutton, M., Gill, T., Plappert, T., Saltzman, D.H., and Doubilet, P.: Assessment of right and left ventricular function in terms of force development with gestational age in the normal human fetus. Br. Heart J., *66*:285, 1991.

445. Shime, J., Gresser, C.D., and Rakowski, H.: Quantitative two-dimensional echocardiographic assessment of fetal growth. Am. J. Obstet. Gynecol., *154*:294, 1986.

# 8

# Coronary Artery Disease

Probably no application for echocardiography is less well understood than its use as a diagnostic tool in patients with known or suspected coronary artery disease. Although clinicians commonly recognize the utility of echocardiography in examining patients with other forms of heart disease, they frequently fail to know the potential of this examination in patients with coronary artery disease.[1] With improvement in echocardiographic instruments, interest has increased in studying patients with coronary artery disease using echocardiography. The introduction of digital techniques for creating continuous loops and split-screen and quad-screen presentations should enhance the utility of echocardiography in these patients even further. Because of the high incidence of coronary artery disease and the increasing use of reperfusion, a major use for echocardiography should be in the examination of these patients.

The technical difficulties in examining patients with coronary artery disease have been emphasized in the past. With the improvement in echocardiographs, however, these difficulties have been reduced significantly. Improvement in transducer design, more sensitive pulsers and receivers, and enhanced gray scale are the advances in instrumentation that have improved the situation significantly. In addition, the availability of the apical windows in patients with coronary artery disease has made the two-dimensional echocardiographic examination infinitely more successful than previous efforts with M-mode echocardiography. Thus, in any echocardiographic laboratory, one should be able to examine over 90% of all patients with coronary artery disease.

## DETECTION OF ISCHEMIC MUSCLE

### Segmental Wall Abnormalities

One of the principal ways of detecting ischemic muscle is by noting abnormal motion of the ischemic segment. Both animal and clinical studies have documented that when the muscle becomes ischemic, its motion is altered almost immediately.[2-8] With the high sampling rate inherent in M-mode echocardiography, wall motion is recorded extremely well with this technique.[9] Figure 8–1 demonstrates an M-mode echocardiogram of a patient with obstruction of the proximal portion of the left anterior descending coronary artery. The motion of the

interventricular septum (LS) is negligible. The posterior left ventricular wall (EN) moves normally. Figure 8–2 demonstrates an M-mode echocardiogram in which the posterior left ventricular endocardium (EN) is hypokinetic, while septal motion (LS) is actually increased.

There are limitations to using wall motion as the sole criterion for ischemic muscle. The movement of any given segment of the ventricle is influenced by the adjacent muscle to which it is attached. For example, in a chamber with a dyskinetic ischemic segment, some of the adjacent normal tissue may be hypokinetic because its motion is influenced by the attached dyskinetic muscle. The reverse situation may also be true. If vigorously contracting normal muscle is next to an ischemic area, the hyperdynamic segment may pull the ischemic muscle toward the cavity, which may mask the abnormal perfusion. In general, when looking at motion abnormalities alone, the amount of ischemic muscle is usually overestimated.[10]

Probably a more specific finding for ischemic muscle is alteration in systolic thickening.[11-13] Normal myocardial muscle increases in thickness with systolic contraction. In Figure 8–1, the ischemic septum fails to thicken, whereas thickening is reduced in the ischemic posterior wall in Figure 8–2. With acute ischemia or infarction, one may actually note systolic thinning,[14-16] whereby the thickness of the left ventricular wall is greater in diastole than in systole (Fig. 8–3). Thus, the affected wall segment exhibits not only dyskinetic motion, but also systolic thinning, which is probably more specific for ischemia.

Although M-mode echocardiography was instrumental in demonstrating how echocardiography could be valuable in detecting ischemic muscle, the one-dimensional nature of the recording technique and the lack of spatial orientation made this technique limited for this application. Two-dimensional echocardiography is now the principle ultrasonic technique for detecting regional wall motion abnormalities in patients with coronary artery disease. Figure 8–4 demonstrates long-axis and four-chamber images of a patient with coronary artery disease who exhibits abnormal wall motion of the anterior septum in the long-axis view (*arrows*, LX-S) and similar dysfunction of the distal septum, apex, and apical lateral wall in the four-chamber view (*arrows*, 4C-S). Figure 8–5 shows the systolic frames from the long-axis, short-

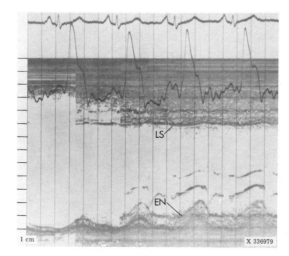

**Fig. 8–1.** Left ventricular echocardiogram of a patient with coronary artery disease and obstruction of the proximal portion of the left anterior descending coronary artery. The echo from the left side of the septum (LS) is actually paradoxical if not entirely flat toward the end of systole. Posterior left ventricular wall motion (EN) is reasonably normal.

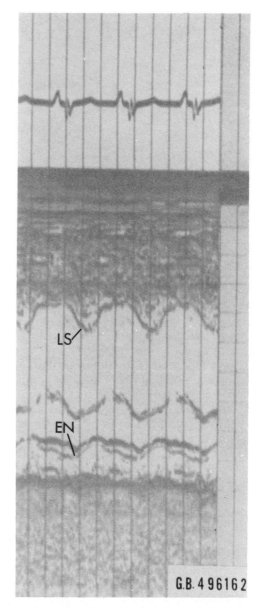

**Fig. 8–2.** M-mode echocardiogram through the left ventricle of a patient with an inferior wall myocardial infarction, demonstrating exaggerated motion of the interventricular septum (LS) with hypokinetic motion of the left ventricular endocardial echo (EN). (From Corya, B.C., et al.: Echocardiographic features of congestive cardiomyopathy compared with normal subjects in patients with coronary artery disease. Circulation, *49*:1153, 1974, by permission of the American Heart Association, Inc.)

axis, four-chamber, and two-chamber views of the same patient, which demonstrate the corresponding walls that are abnormal in this patient with anterior ischemia.

Wall motion abnormalities can also be demonstrated with a colorized regional wall motion scheme. Figure 8–6 shows a colorized display from the same patient as in Figures 8–4 and 8–5. Diastole (blue) is superimposed on systole (red). Normal wall motion is displayed as rims of red through the bluish gray background. Where no wall motion occurs (*arrows*), no rims of red are visualized. This colorized technique provides an opportunity to superimpose diastole and systole in a single still frame and helps to differentiate those wall segments that are or are not moving.

Figure 8–7 is another example of anterior wall ischemia, although in this situation, the proximal septum continues to move normally (*inward arrow*, LX-S) and the distal septum is moving abnormally (*outward arrow*). The normally moving proximal muscle and distal akinesis is also displayed in the four-chamber view (4C-S). Posterior-inferior ischemia is demonstrated in Figure 8–8. With this type of abnormality, the short-axis and two-chamber views best delineate the wall motion changes. In the short-axis view, the abnormal segments usually are from 6 o'clock to 9 o'clock if one were to describe the short axis as the face of a clock (SX-S, *arrows*). In the two-chamber examination, the abnormal segments involve the basal half of the inferior wall (2C-S, *arrows*).

One of the major advantages of two-dimensional echocardiography is that in many ways one can achieve a three-dimensional perspective of left ventricular regional function by simultaneously analyzing four different views. Figure 8–9 demonstrates the interrelationship between four common two-dimensional examinations. The long-axis, two-chamber, and four-chamber views are essentially longitudinal examinations from base to apex. The short-axis view is perpendicular to the longitudinal axis. The three longitudinal views divide the short axis into six segments. Using both short-axis and longitudinal views, one has the opportunity to visualize segments from more than one perspective.

Figure 8–10 shows the three longitudinal and three optional short-axis views. Using the relationship of these tomographic planes, a regional wall segment ap-

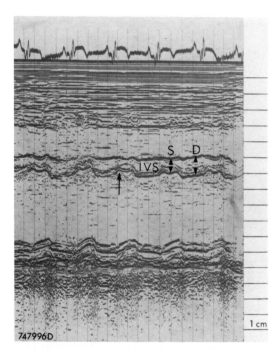

**Fig. 8–3.** M-mode echocardiogram of a patient with an acute anteroseptal myocardial infarction. The interventricular septum (IVS) is less thick in systole (S) than in diastole (D). In addition, septal motion is abnormal or dyskinetic (*arrow*).

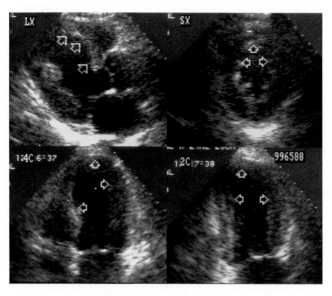

**Fig. 8–5.** Systolic two-dimensional echocardiogram in the long-axis (LX), short-axis (SX), four-chamber (4C) and two-chamber (2C) views of the same patient as noted in Figure 8–4. The short-axis examination shows akinesis in the anterior septum and free wall (*arrows*). 2C shows akinesis of the apical inferior wall, the apex, and the anterior wall (*arrows*).

proach can be used that divides the left ventricle into 16 segments. The left ventricle is divided into basal, mid, and apical thirds. Six segments are in the basal and mid sections and four segments are at the apex. One could record the 16 segments from either the three short-axis or three longitudinal views. The examinations are complementary and offer an opportunity to evaluate a given

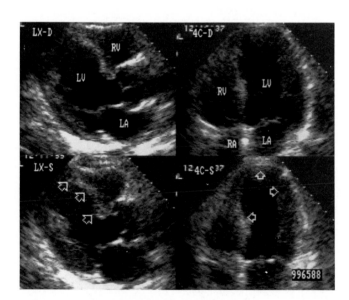

**Fig. 8–4.** Long-axis (LX) and four-chamber (4C) two-dimensional echocardiograms of a patient with an anterior myocardial infarction secondary to occlusion of the left anterior descending artery. In systole, the long-axis examination (LX-S) shows akinesis of the anterior septum (*arrows*). The four-chamber systolic view (4C-S) shows akinesis of the distal septum, apex, and apical lateral walls (*arrows*). LV = left ventricle; RV = right ventricle; LA = left atrium; RA = right atrium.

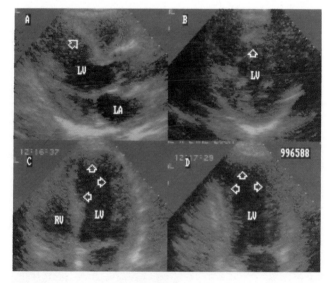

**Fig. 8–6.** Colorized regional wall study in the same patient whose standard echocardiograms were noted in Figures 8–4 and 8–5. Diastole (blue) is superimposed on systolic frames (red). A bright rim of red identifies those wall segments that are moving normally. In the area of abnormal wall motion (*arrows*), the rim of red is small or nonexistent. LV = left ventricle; LA = left atrium; RV = right ventricle.

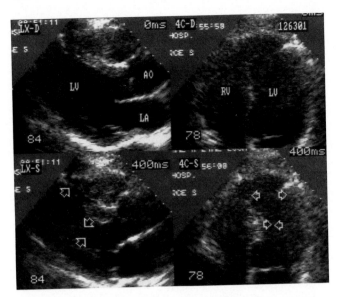

**Fig. 8–7.** Long-axis (LX) and four-chamber (4C) examination of another patient with an anterior infarction that resulted from obstruction of the left anterior descending coronary artery. In this patient, the obstruction is past the first septal perforator artery. Thus, the proximal septum, as seen in the long-axis systolic (LX-S) and four-chamber systolic (4C-S) views, continues to contract normally (*inward arrows*). The distal septum is akinetic (*outward arrows*). LV = left ventricle; AO = aorta; LA = left atrium; RV = right ventricle.

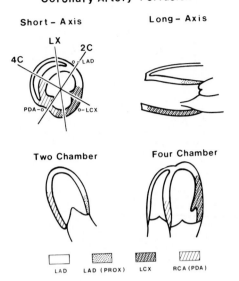

Relationship of Two-Dimensional Views And Coronary Artery Perfusion

**Fig. 8–9.** Diagram illustrating the relationship of two-dimensional echocardiographic views and coronary artery perfusion. 4C = four chamber; LX = long axis; 2C = two chamber; LAD = left anterior descending; LCX = left circumflex artery; RCA = right coronary artery; PDA = posterior descending artery.

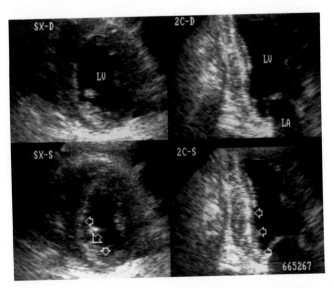

**Fig. 8–8.** Short-axis (SX) and two-chamber (2C) two-dimensional echocardiograms of a patient with an inferior myocardial infarction. In the short-axis systolic image (SX-S), the inferior wall (*arrows*) is akinetic. The two-chamber systolic image (2C-S) exhibits akinesis in the basal inferior segment (*arrows*). LV = left ventricle; LA = left atrium.

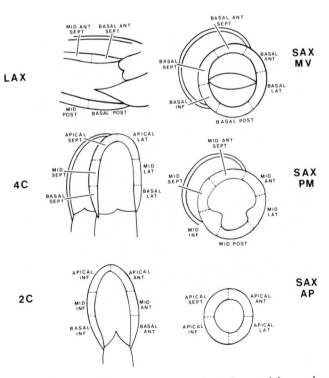

REGIONAL WALL SEGMENTS

**Fig. 8–10.** Diagram indicating how the left ventricle can be divided into 16 segments. One can identify these segments in a series of longitudinal views (LAX, 4C, 2C) or a series of short-axis views (SAX MV, SAX PM, SAX AP). The longitudinal and short-axis views overlap and complement each other.

segment in more than one view. The four apical segments are derived from the apical four- and two-chamber views. Because the parasternal long-axis examination does not visualize the apex, it does not contribute to evaluating the apex.

This regional wall segment approach has been adopted by the American Society of Echocardiography. A 20-segment scheme proved to be cumbersome and did not have the virtue of using the longitudinal or short-axis views interchangeably as one can with the 16-segment scheme.

Many investigators have recognized that wall motion is heterogeneous with regard to location and timing.[17–20] Certain areas of the normal left ventricle move more than others. In addition, the timing of motion may differ. Abnormal wall motion also may be characterized by alterations in both excursion and timing. Tardokinesis represents delay in wall motion and usually indicates abnormal function. This finding may not always be obvious in a real-time two-dimensional display. Digital techniques permit one to analyze only the first half of systole, at which time subtle wall motion abnormalities such as tardokinesis may be evident.

### Relationship of Wall Motion and Wall Thickening Abnormalities to Coronary Artery Perfusion

With the advent of coronary artery bypass surgery and coronary angioplasty, it has become increasingly important to know which coronary arteries are obstructed and where the obstructions are located. Many attempts have been made to look at the abnormally functioning myocardium in order to predict the location of the arterial obstructions. Two-dimensional echocardiography is probably as good a technique as there is for trying to make this assessment. Not all obstructed arteries produce wall motion changes, however. First of all, the obstruction may be partial and the ischemia may not be present in the resting state. In addition, collateral circulation can frequently preserve the function of the myocardium despite a severe or even total obstruction of the artery that normally perfuses the area. Thus, the lack of any wall motion abnormality does not exclude the possibility of an obstructed artery. On the other hand, when wall motion abnormalities do occur, one has a reasonable chance of predicting which vessel may be involved in the ischemic process.

Using correlative studies with coronary angiography and exercise echocardiography[21] and patients with acute myocardial infarction,[22] it has been possible to develop a scheme whereby certain areas of the two-dimensional echocardiogram can provide a reasonable prediction as to the arteries perfusing certain areas of the heart. Figure 8–9 demonstrates the approximate relationship between the standard two-dimensional echocardiographic views and coronary artery perfusion.

The parasternal long-axis view primarily visualizes the interventricular septum and the posterior left ventricular free wall. The septum seen in this view is the anterior interventricular septum and is almost invariably perfused by the left anterior descending coronary artery.

The basal centimeter or two of the interventricular septum are perfused by the first septal perforator, and thus one can frequently decide whether or not an obstruction in the left anterior descending coronary artery is before or after the first septal perforator. In Figure 8–4, the entire septum is akinetic because the obstruction of the left arterior descending artery is before the first septal perforator. The proximal septum moves normally in Figure 8–7, indicating that the first septal perforator is receiving blood either because the obstruction is past this artery or because the artery is receiving collateral flow.

The posterior left ventricular wall seen in the parasternal long-axis view is usually perfused by the left circumflex coronary artery. It is not routinely involved with the typical inferior myocardial infarction that results from an obstruction of flow to the posterior descending coronary artery.

In the short-axis view, areas of the myocardium perfused by all three main arteries can be detected. The left anterior descending coronary artery is located in the anterior groove between the attachment of the right ventricular and left ventricular free walls. This artery supplies the anterior portion of the left ventricular free wall as well as the anterior half of the interventricular septum. The posterior descending coronary artery is also predictably in the posterior groove between the attachment of the right ventricular and left ventricular free walls. This artery supplies blood to the posterior medial portion of the left ventricular free wall as well as to the posterior half of the interventricular septum. The amount of muscle perfused by the left circumflex artery can be variable. Usually, however, it supplies the posterior lateral portions of the short-axis view. The posterior descending coronary artery in usually a branch of the right coronary artery; with a left dominant system, the posterior descending coronary artery arises from the left circumflex artery.

The two-chamber apical view is somewhat comparable to the right anterior oblique view seen on contrast angiography. This particular examination visualizes myocardium supplied most exclusively by the left anterior descending and posterior descending coronary arteries. The posterior descending coronary artery represents the basal half or two thirds of the posterior wall in this view. The rest of the left ventricle is perfused by the left anterior descending coronary artery. The basal centimeter or two of the anterior wall are usually supplied from the proximal portion of the left anterior descending artery.

In the four-chamber view, muscle perfused by all three coronary arteries can again be visualized. The apex and the distal half or two thirds of the interventricular septum are supplied by the left anterior descending coronary artery. The proximal third of the septum is usually part of the posterior descending coronary artery distribution. The lateral free wall visualized in the four-chamber view is usually supplied by branches of the circumflex coronary artery.

Coronary anatomy is somewhat variable. The posterior descending artery is usually a branch of the right coronary artery, but it may be a part of the circumflex in a left dominant system. In addition, the relative sizes of the various arteries can differ from patient to patient. At least two areas of the echocardiogram can vary between different artery perfusions. The apical inferior segment can be perfused by either the left anterior descending artery or the posterior descending artery depending on the size of the individual arteries. The apical lateral wall may be perfused by the diagonal branch of the left anterior descending artery or by a branch of the circumflex artery. Usually, the left anterior descending artery is dominant and perfuses these two overlap areas.

### Quantitation of Ischemic Muscle

Many schemes are being used for quantitating regional myocardial dysfunction using echocardiography.[23–26] The current approach recommended by the American Society of Echocardiography is to use a wall scoring index based on the 16-segment approach.[25] Each segment is judged as to whether or not it is normal or abnormal based on a scheme giving a value of 1 for a normal segment, 2 for hypokinetic, 3 for akinetic, 4 for dyskinetic, and 5 for aneurysmal. The left ventricular score index is then derived by summing the scores and dividing by the number of segments evaluated. If a segment is not visualized, then it cannot be scored and is not included in the denominator. Obviously, if most of the segments are not visualized, then the score index is not reliable. Figure 8–11 shows a computer-generated report using a left ventricular score index. This particular program has one other feature, "percent normal muscle." This calculation is the percentage of the segments that were indicated as being normal. Another slight modification in this program is an indication for segments that are akinetic or dyskinetic with scar. Because the presence of scar has clinical value, it is useful to make that determination. Therefore, a score of 6 indicates that a segment is akinetic with scar and 7 is dyskinetic with scar. For the calculation of the motion score index, however, a segment designated as 6 is still given a value of 3 and dyskinetic with scar is still given a value of 4. The numbers 6 and 7 only note that these segments are not only akinetic or dyskinetic but they also are scarred.

Figure 8–12 shows another development using this basic approach. In this case, the left ventricle is presented as a bull's eye or "polar" display, with the 16 segments shown as a series of short-axis views as if viewed from the apex. This approach is convenient in that the entire ventricle can be displayed with one dia-

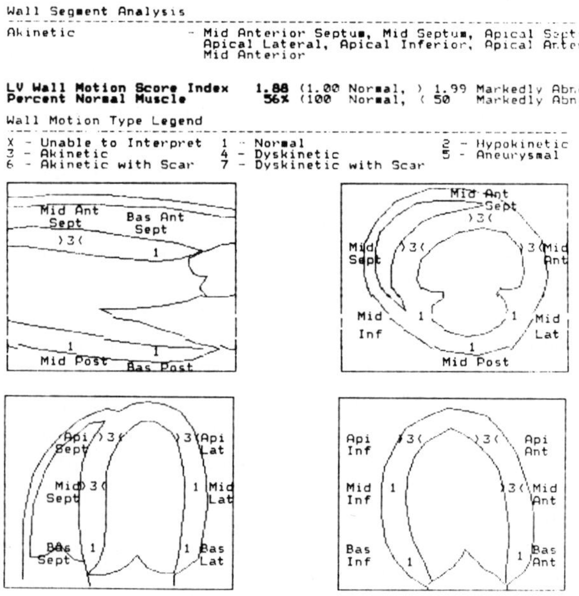

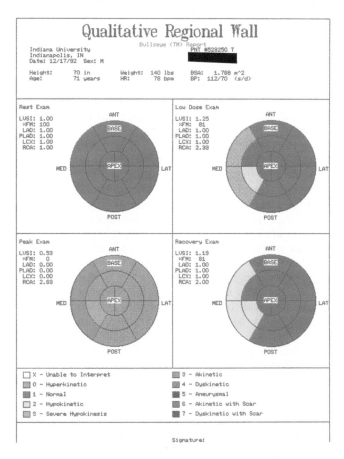

**Fig. 8–11.** A computer-generated regional wall motion report. The motion of the 16 segments are evaluated (1 = normal, 2 = hypokinetic, 3 = akinetic, 4 = dyskinetic, 5 = aneurysmal). Numbers 6 and 7 merely denote scarred segments. When generating the motion score index, a segment labeled 6 is given a value of 3 because it is akinetic. A segment designated 7 is given a value of 4 because it is dyskinetic. The motion score index is the average of all the scored segments. The percent normal muscle is that percentage of segments designated as normal.

**Fig. 8–12.** A computer-generated regional wall motion report whereby the left ventricle is represented by a bull's eye. The 16 segments are displayed as if visualizing the left ventricle from the apex. This type of report is particularly useful with a stress echocardiographic examination whereby the results of multiple studies are displayed on one sheet of paper. The colored segments facilitate interpretation of left ventricular wall motion. The motion score index is subdivided into coronary artery distributions as well as providing a global index. A value for hyperkinesis and severe hypokinesis is available.

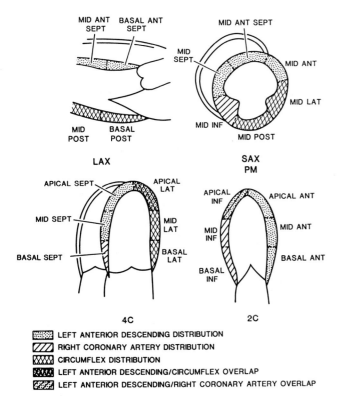

Fig. 8–13.  Diagram showing how the 16 segments are assigned to specific coronary arteries. The apical lateral and inferior apical segments (*cross-hatch*) are overlap segments. The apical lateral segment may be supplied by either the left anterior descending or circumflex arteries. If the segment is scored as abnormal, then the computer looks at how the apical septal segment is scored. If it too is abnormal, then the apical lateral segment is included in the anterior descending score. If the apical septum is normal and the mid lateral wall is abnormal, then the apical lateral segment is classified as circumflex. An abnormal apical inferior segment will be designated as left anterior descending if the apical septum on the four-chamber view is also abnormal. If the apical septum is normal and the basal inferior wall is abnormal, the apical inferior abnormality is classified as right coronary artery. (From Segar, D.S., et al.: Dobutamine stress echocardiography: Correlation with coronary lesion severity as determined by quantitative angiography. J. Am. Coll. Cardiol., *19*:1197, 1992.)

gram rather than with four. This feature is particularly useful when reporting stress echocardiograms. The use of color also makes the visualization and interpretation somewhat easier.

This report shows another feature. The segments are assigned to different coronary artery distributions so that one obtains both global and regional score indices. The segments are designated to an artery according to the scheme shown in Figure 8–13.[27] The two overlap areas, namely the apical septum and the apical lateral wall, are assigned to their appropriate arteries, depending on whether or not there are also wall motion changes in corresponding segments. For example, an abnormal apical inferior segment is assigned to the left anterior descending artery if the apical septum, which is invariably perfused by the left anterior descending artery, is also abnormal. If, however, the apical septum is normal

and the basal inferior wall is abnormal, then the apical inferior wall is assigned to the right coronary artery. A similar approach is taken for the apical lateral wall. If the apical lateral wall is abnormal and the apical septum is also abnormal, then the lateral wall segment is assigned to the left anterior descending artery. If, however, the apical septum is normal and the mid-lateral wall is abnormal, then an abnormal apical lateral wall is designated as part of the circumflex system.

With regional score indices, one can reintroduce hyperkinesis to the scheme. Many investigators still use hyperkinesis to generate a wall score index. Such a designation is particularly valuable in stress echocardiography, especially with pharmacologic stress. The problem with hyperkinesis and a global score index is that the hyperkinesis may mask wall motion abnormalities.[28,29] For example, if one had inferior wall akinesis and anterior wall hyperkinesis, then the score index may still be normal. If the akinetic inferior wall improves with reperfusion, the anterior wall will no longer be hyperkinetic, and the global score index will not change. Thus, the calculation will not reflect what actually takes place. With regional score indices, however, there is a reciprocal change in the left anterior descending and right coronary artery score indices, even though the global score index remains the same.

Many other schemes are being used for evaluating regional dysfunction with two-dimensional echocardiography. A 20-segment mapping technique has been used by one group of investigators.[30] This approach is sophisticated and requires making measurements of at least three short-axis and two longitudinal views. A computer then generates a surface map of the left ventricle. This technique has provided interesting information on the natural history of myocardial infarction,[31] but it is too tedious for routine clinical use. Other investigators have used as few as 9 segments.[32] The scoring system may also differ. Worsening function may be indicated as a decreasing number rather than as an increasing number. Despite these differences, the basic approach is similar. Except for the techniques that actually trace the recordings, the schemes are based on a qualitative evaluation of individual segments.

There are efforts to provide a more quantitative assessment of regional function. One can trace endocardial borders during diastole and systole and superimpose the two tracings to analyze regional ventricular dysfunction.[33–38] One of the issues raised with this approach is the necessity of having a reference system, because the heart may move or translate whereby diastole and systole are not properly superimposed. One option is to use a "floating reference." After one traces the endocardial borders, the computer calculates the center of the area or "mass" and superimposes the centers. Although this approach works well for normal ventricles, it tends to mask wall motion abnormalities.[38–40] Another alternative is to use a fixed external reference system. In this situation, one identifies an area of the heart that should not move and then superimposes the diastolic and systolic frames according to this reference.[39] The consensus is that with regional segmental disease, the fixed reference system appears to be more accurate.

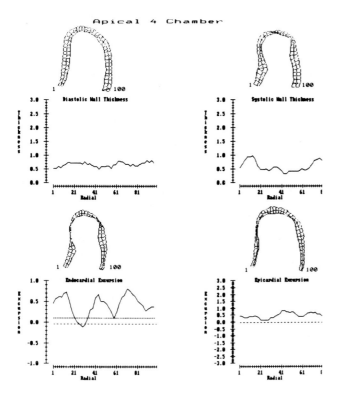

**Fig. 8–14.** Regional wall motion analysis using the centerline approach. This program requires tracing of the endocardial and epicardial walls in diastole and systole. The computer-generated report provides an analysis of diastolic and systolic wall thickness in 100 segments. In addition, both endocardial and epicardial excursion can be traced graphically.

The centerline method is a popular technique used in the angiographic laboratory.[41] With contrast left ventriculography, one traces the endocardial border in diastole and systole. The computer superimposes the two outlines and calculates the centerline between the two contours. The program then generates the deviation from that centerline of each of 100 segments. Figure 8–14

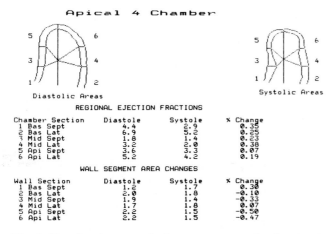

**Fig. 8–15.** Another quantitative assessment of regional wall function providing regional ejection fractions and wall segment area changes. This approach is based on tracing diastolic and systolic endocardial borders.

shows a similar approach using echocardiographic images. Because echocardiography can also trace the epicardium, a modification of the technique can be used to display wall thickness, as well as endocardial excursion. The chamber also can be divided into 6 regions instead of 100 segments. The computer program can then calculate regional ejection fractions or segment area changes (Fig. 8–15).

The centerline technique is probably the preferred method for the quantitative evaluation of regional wall function.[42] Needless to say, there are many limitations to this technique. First of all, the measurements are tedious, even with a computer. More importantly, it requires high-quality echocardiographic images for accurate measurements. Myocardial dropout, which is a common problem may make these measurements impossible. As a result, these calculations are primarily for investigational purposes and are rarely used for routine clinical evaluations.

## ASSESSMENT OF OVERALL PERFORMANCE OF THE ISCHEMIC LEFT VENTRICLE

The segmental nature of left ventricular dysfunction in patients with coronary artery disease has been the principal negative criticism of the standard M-mode dimensions used to evaluate left ventricular function. It was recognized early that the left ventricular dimensions using M-mode echocardiography would have significant problems in patients with segmental left ventricular dysfunction. In addition, clinicians have become impressed with the clinical utility of the ejection fraction as a means of evaluating left ventricular function in patients with coronary artery disease. As a result, physicians either have ignored echocardiography as a means for assessing left ventricular function in patients with coronary artery disease or have insisted on a measurement of ejection fraction.

Although the E point septal separation on the M-mode echocardiogram can provide an estimate of ejection fraction (see Chapter 3), its reliability in coronary artery disease is limited.[43,44] Investigators have therefore gone to two-dimensional echocardiography for attempts at measuring ejection fraction and left ventricular volumes in people with coronary artery disease. Most investigators have attempted to simulate the angiographic ejection fraction by using the apical two-chamber and four-chamber views for calculating left ventricular volumes and ejection fractions (Fig. 8–16).[45–48] They use standard angiographic area-length formulas or Simpson's rule for calculating volumes (see Chapter 3). Many authors have demonstrated that the ejection fraction can be predicted fairly well using two-dimensional echocardiography. It is also possible to use minor axis measurements to assess left ventricular function in patients with coronary artery disease (Fig. 8–16). The minor axis dimension of the base of the heart using the parasternal long-axis view and the minor axis area using the short-axis examination at the papillary muscle level (see Chapter 3) can assess both regional and global left ventricular function in patients with coronary artery disease. In

## Long-Axis        Short-Axis

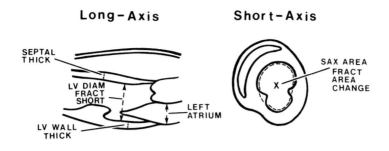

## Two Chamber        Four Chamber

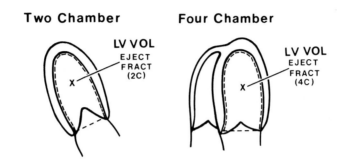

**Fig. 8–16.** Diagrams illustrating some of the quantitative measurements that can be obtained with two-dimensional echocardiography.

some aspects, the minor axis measurements have clinical advantages over the global ejection fraction. The minor axis dimensions and areas have regional information and can be better prognostic indicators, especially in patients with apical aneurysms.[49]

Figure 8–17 shows a long-axis study of a patient with a large old anterior myocardial infarction and a reduced global ejection fraction. Despite this poor global systolic function, the fractional shortening at the base of the heart is still within normal limits. The fact that the base

of the heart is still contracting normally means that this individual still has a functioning left ventricular "cuff," which carries a better prognosis than if the base of the heart is no longer functioning.[49] It is this type of regionalized systolic function that gives two-dimensional echocardiography its great value in evaluating patients with ischemic heart disease. Combining these regionalized systolic indices, such as fractional shortening and fractional area change, with a left ventricular score index for asymmetrically contracting ventricles, provides a

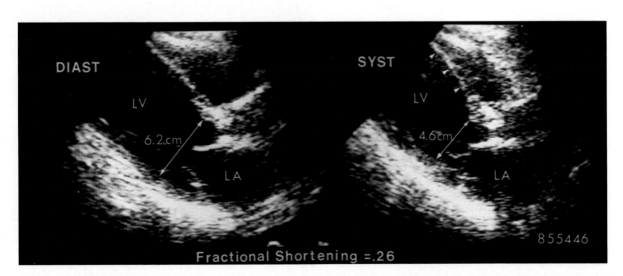

**Fig. 8–17.** Parasternal long-axis two-dimensional echocardiograms in diastole (DIAST) and systole (SYST) demonstrating how one obtains fractional shortening at the base of the left ventricle. In this patient, who has severe septal akinesis (*arrowheads*), the basal septum and posterior ventricular wall continue to move so that the fractional shortening is 0.26, which is still within normal limits. LV = left ventricle; LA = left atrium. (From Ryan, T., et al.: Quantitative two-dimensional echocardiographic assessment of patients undergoing left ventricular aneurysmectomy. Am. Heart J., *111*:715, 1986.)

powerful analysis of left ventricular function, which in many situations is better than a single, global ejection fraction.

Interest has been renewed in using the base of the heart, as viewed from the apical views, for an assessment of left ventricular function.[23] It has been recognized for many years that the heart contracts through its minor dimension and with the descent of the base toward the apex. Contrary to what is seen frequently with contrast and nuclear ventriculography, the normal apex moves very little. It is the base that acts as a piston to help propel blood. Figure 8–18 shows how the normal base moves toward the apex during the cardiac cycle. With anterior or posterior wall infarction, the corresponding annulus will move less than normal. This scheme permits both a global and regional analysis of left ventricular dysfunction.

Although M-mode echocardiography cannot accurately assess left ventricular volumes or ejection fractions, it can provide some hemodynamic information that can be helpful in patients with coronary artery disease. As noted in Chapter 4, mitral valve closure is related to altered left ventricular filling patterns.[50] Abnormal closure with atrial systole is a common finding in patients with coronary artery disease and elevated left ventricular diastolic pressure. Figure 8–19 demonstrates such a mitral valve in a patient with coronary artery disease. There is a distinct interruption in closure between the A and C points, with a plateau sometimes called a "B" bump. This finding has some prognostic value.[51–56]

Doppler echocardiography can also be useful in assessing global left ventricular function. As noted in Chapter 3, aortic velocities are useful in evaluating global systolic function. One can calculate mean or peak

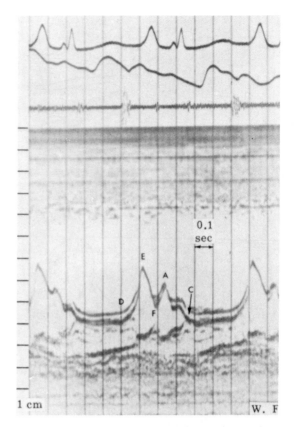

**Fig. 8–19.** Mitral valve echocardiogram of a patient with coronary artery disease and abnormal left ventricular function. The mitral valve closure between the A and C points is interrupted, and the A to C interval is prolonged.

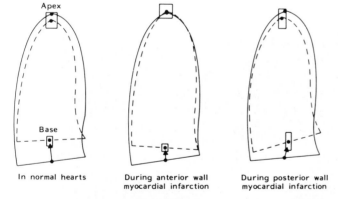

**Fig. 8–18.** Diagram showing how the base of the heart moves toward the apex. In normal hearts, the base moves uniformly toward the apex. With anterior infarction, the corresponding side of the annulus moves less than the other side, which is attached to normally contracting muscle. The reverse situation occurs with a posterior myocardial infarction. (From Assman, P.E., et al.: Two-dimensional echocardiographic analysis of the dynamic geometry of the left ventricle: The basis for an improved model of wall motion. J. Am. Soc. Echocardiogr., 6:396, 1988.)

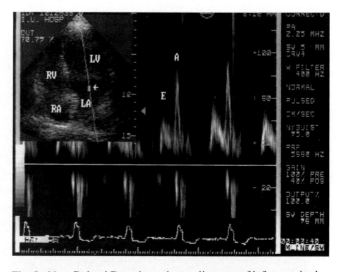

**Fig. 8–20.** Pulsed Doppler echocardiogram of left ventricular inflow in a patient with coronary artery disease. The initial inflow (E) is reduced and the velocity following atrial contraction (A) is increased. RV = right ventricle; LV = left ventricle; RA = right atrium; LA = left atrium.

acceleration or the time-velocity integral to provide an assessment of systolic function. Left ventricular inflow is commonly used to evaluate diastolic left ventricular performance. The pattern of diastolic flow is altered with myocardial ischemia. The principle change is a decrease in the E point and an increase in the A velocity (Fig. 8–20).[57–61] With left ventricular failure or significant mitral regurgitation, the E velocity increases and may exceed the A velocity.[62,62a] Abnormal flow patterns within the left ventricle have also been noted.[63–66] Blood tends to flow toward an area of dyskinesis.

## DETECTION OF REVERSIBLE ISCHEMIA

### Stress Echocardiography

It is well known that under resting conditions, patients with coronary artery disease may have normal left ventricular function. If no permanent myocardial damage has occurred and if the ventricle is not ischemic at the time of the examination, the routine echocardiographic study will not reflect any underlying coronary artery disease. Thus, there has been considerable interest for many years in combining echocardiography with stressful interventions that will produce ischemia.[67–82] Although in early studies investigators used M-mode echocardiography to evaluate stress-induced ischemia, all of the current examinations use two-dimensional echocardiography. Table 8–1 lists the types of stress echocardiography that are available. Most of the early exercise echocardiographic studies involved supine bicycle exercise.[21,68,69,74,83,84] Initially, the yield was only 70 to 80% with supine bicycle exercise. With advanced techniques and sophisticated tables, however, the yield is considerably higher.[85] There are, however, limitations to supine exercise. Leg fatigue is frequently a limiting factor, especially in older patients. Furthermore, the best echo-

**Table 8–1**
Stress Echocardiography

---

Exercise
  Post treadmill
  Supine bicycle
  Upright bicycle
Pharmacologic stress
  Adrenergic stimulation
    Dobutamine
    Isuprel
    Arbutamine
    Epinephrine
  Vasodilation
    Dypyridamole
    Adenosine
Pacing
  Esophageal
  Atrial
  Ventricular
Handgrip
Cold pressor

---

cardiographic images are usually obtained with the patient in the left lateral position rather than totally supine. Thus, the examination should be done so that the patient can role over either immediately after exercise or for the patient to be in that position during exercise.

Upright bicycle exercise has the advantage of less leg fatigue because the legs need not be supported against gravity.[72,86,87] More patients can tolerate this form of exercise and the level of exercise is greater. This technique however, is limited by the availability of acoustic windows. The parasternal approach is frequently unsatisfactory and one is restricted to either apical[87] or subcostal examinations.[86]

Treadmill exercise is the most popular form of stress testing in the United States. The principle problem with doing echocardiographic studies with the treadmill examination is the inability to obtain studies during the procedure; one must rely on the immediate post-treadmill examination.[75–78,88,89] Fortunately, treadmill exercise is the most vigorous form of stress. With stress-induced ischemia, a form of stunned myocardium occurs, and the recovery of ventricular function is delayed depending on the severity and duration of the ischemia.[90–92] As a result, with vigorous exercise, such as treadmill testing, one usually has several minutes during which wall motion abnormalities persist and can be recorded on the echocardiogram. With such an approach, one should try to complete the post-treadmill examination within 2 minutes. It should be emphasized, however, that the delay in recovery of ventricular function depends on the duration and severity of the ischemia. If one does not exercise the patient vigorously, one should not expect a long recovery time.[93]

With the treadmill echocardiographic approach, the patient is supine during the examination, and two parasternal and two apical views are obtained. The patient then exercises on the treadmill and then immediately returns to the examining table for the post-exercise examination.

One form of upright bicycle exercise is a modification of the treadmill approach. In this modified upright bicycle examination, the patient initially has a resting four-view examination while in the supine position.[87] The patient then sits on the bicycle and has another resting apical four-chamber and two-chamber examination. The subject then exercises. The apical views are recorded periodically throughout the examination. Just before termination of exercise, the apical two-chamber and four-chamber views are recorded. The patient then gets off of the bicycle and lies down on a table for an immediate post-exercise, supine four-view examination.

The technical advance that has made stress echocardiography practical is the introduction of digital recordings of echocardiograms.[88,89,94] By capturing a single cardiac cycle, one is able to overcome many of the technical limitations of examining an exercising individual. Respiratory interference from hyperventilation is a common problem during or immediately after exercise. The digital approach permits one to display the one cardiac cycle that does not contain respiratory interference. Furthermore, the digital technique allows one to display the resting and exercise cardiac images side by side for a better comparison.

Some of the details involved in digital echocardiographic recording are discussed in Chapters 1 and 2. A number of factors must be considered when performing stress echocardiography using digital recordings.[94] There are several ways of capturing the stress images. One can digitally record many if not all of the cardiac cycles during the stress examination. With this "full disclosure" approach, one then selects those cardiac cycles that are most representative and are artifact-free for comparison with the resting studies. Another approach is to record a series of four views intermittently during the examination. These four views are immediately reviewed. As soon as at least one satisfactory cardiac cycle is recorded, one then goes on to the next view. The intermittent four-view approach and the continuous "full disclosure" approach have their advantages and disadvantages, although both techniques seem to work satisfactorily and have been used in many different laboratories.

Figure 8–21 illustrates a parasternal long-axis two-dimensional echocardiogram of a normal individual before and immediately after treadmill exercise testing. Predictably, the systolic cavity becomes smaller as the vigor of ventricular contraction increases. Figure 8–22 demonstrates the short-axis view in the same patient. Virtual systolic cavity obliteration can again be seen fol-

lowing exercise. Figure 8–23 is from a patient with coronary artery disease. At rest, the parasternal long-axis view shows normal wall motion. The septum moves toward the left ventricular cavity during systole. After treadmill exercise, the interventricular septum is dyskinetic (*reverse arrows*). The proximal centimeter or two of the septum move normally. This patient had an obstructing lesion of the left anterior descending artery past the first septal perforator branch.

Figure 8–24 shows another exercise echocardiogram in a patient with an obstruction in the left anterior descending artery. This examination was performed with upright bicycle exercise. With the exercise echocardiogram, one can see akinesis of the entire interventricular septum (*arrows*) in both the long-axis and short-axis views. This illustration also provides some of the advances in digital stress echocardiography. The heart rates are indicated on the echocardiograms to assist in the interpretation. Furthermore, timers indicate when the examination was obtained. For example, both resting studies have a set of zeros on both lines, which means that the examination was before exercise started. With the exercise images, one can see that the patient exercised for 4 minutes and 4 seconds. The long-axis examination was obtained 34 seconds after exercise, and the short-axis study occurred 44 seconds after exercise. If these images had been obtained during exercise, the second line would have been a series of zeros. These

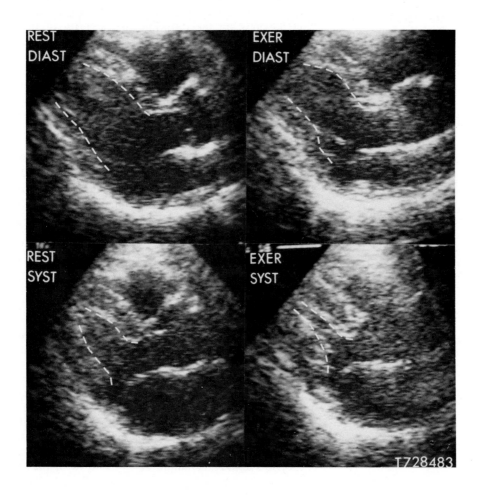

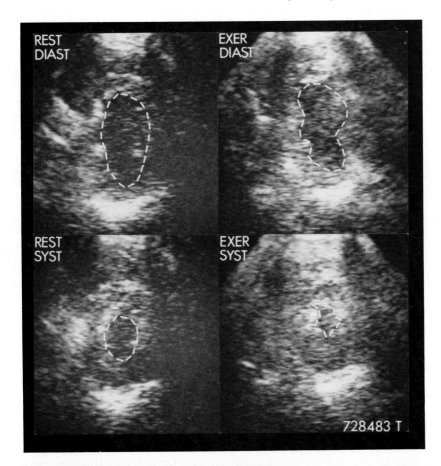

**Fig. 8–22.** Short-axis two-dimensional echocardiograms of a patient with no apparent heart disease before and after exercising on a treadmill. Following exercise the systolic cavity is extremely small (*dashed lines*).

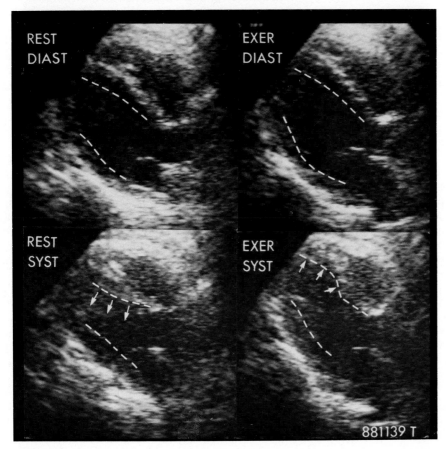

**Fig. 8–23.** Resting and immediate after exercise echocardiograms of a patient with an obstruction in the left anterior descending coronary artery. At rest, the septal motion is normal (*arrows*, REST, SYST). Immediately following exercise, the septum becomes dyskinetic (*reverse arrows*, EXER SYST).

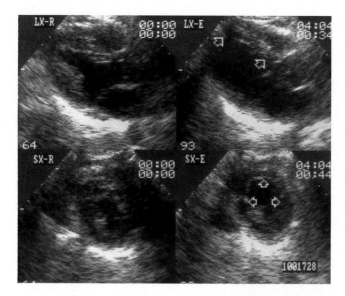

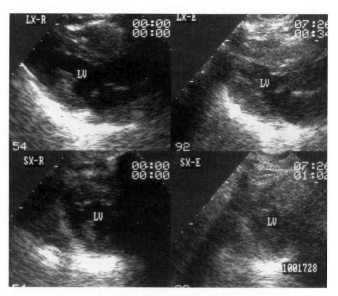

**Fig. 8–24.** Exercise echocardiogram of a patient with an obstruction in the proximal left anterior descending coronary artery. The long-axis (LX-R) and short-axis (SX-R) resting images are normal. With exercise, however, the long-axis (LX-E) and short-axis (SX-E) examinations reveal that the septum and anterior wall (*arrows*) become akinetic. The heart rate is indicated in the lower left corner of each image; the numbers in the upper right corner indicate the exercise duration (top) and the post-exercise duration (bottom). In this example, the long-axis examination was obtained at 34 seconds after exercise, the short-axis study was recorded 45 seconds after exercise.

**Fig. 8–25.** An exercise echocardiogram demonstrating a normal response. The individual exercised for 7 minutes, 26 seconds. At 34 seconds after exercise, the long-axis (LX-E) showed a hypercontractile left ventricle (LV). A similar result is shown in the short-axis exercise examination (SX-E). This exercise study is the post-angioplasty examination of the same patient whose positive stress test is noted in Figure 8–24.

timers assist greatly in the interpretation of the echocardiogram. If, for example, the second line had been 3 or 4 minutes, then the examination was done late after exercise stopped, and wall motion abnormalities may have already recovered.

The patient in Figure 8–24 had an obvious obstruction in the left anterior descending artery involving the entire septum. This proximal obstruction was noted at catheterization and successful angioplasty was performed. Figure 8–25 shows the follow-up exercise echocardiogram of the same patient. The resting studies look identical to the pre-angioplasty examination; however, the patient was able to exercise for 7 minutes and 26 seconds and the post-exercise images are now normal, showing hyperkinesis and cavity obliteration.

Exercise echocardiography is really the combination of two forms of stress testing.[95] The exercise component has useful clinical information, such as the duration of exercise, the patient's symptoms, and the electrocardiographic changes.[96] Many patients are not suitable for exercise testing, however. These individuals may be frail, may have severe peripheral vascular disease, or may have a sore groin because of a recent catheterization procedure. Thus, a stress testing program needs some form of nonexercise stress. Table 8–1 lists some of the forms of nonexercise stress testing that can be used with echocardiography. Handgrip and cold pressor tests are not practical. Handgrip alone does not produce

much stress;[97–100] it has been used in conjunction with pharmacologic testing.[101–104] Some investigators have used a more vigorous form of isometric exercise.[105] Cold pressor tests are painful and have poor patient acceptance.[75]

Both intracardiac and esophageal pacing have been used by numerous investigators.[73,106–108] Atrial pacing induces ischemia. The pacing technique has the advantage of offering a controlled form of stress that can be terminated immediately. Furthermore, one can theoretically examine the control and ischemic ventricle with identical heart rates, because when the pacemaker is turned off, the heart rate returns to baseline, even though the heart is still ischemic for a short period of time.[106] One can even evaluate the immediate post-pacing echocardiogram following ventricular pacing. As with every method, pacing has its advantages and disadvantages. Intracardiac pacing is invasive. Esophageal pacing is semi-invasive and is not without some discomfort to the patient.[108] Atropine may need to be added with atrial pacing, because one may develop heart block as the heart rate increases.

Pharmacologic stress testing is probably the most popular nonexercise form of stress echocardiography.[109–111] There are basically two approaches to performing pharmacologic stress with echocardiography.[112] Potent vasodilators, such as dipyridamole or adenosine, have been used with nuclear cardiology perfusion techniques. The potent vasodilators dilate the normal arteries at the expense of the obstructed arteries. As a result, blood is shunted toward the normal myocardium. The utility of this approach is understandable with a perfusion technique. For echocardiography to detect a wall motion abnormality, however, ischemica must be produced by a "steal phenomenon," whereby blood is shunted away from the obstructed arteries. Numerous investigators, primarily those working in Italy, have demonstrated that dipyridamole echocardiography is indeed an effective means of detecting ischemia.[113-121] Adenosine is also effective in inducing regional wall motion changes on the echocardiogram.[104,122,123] Patient symptoms are frequent with dipyridamole and adenosine, but the problems do not appear to be serious or life-threatening.[124,125]

The alternative pharmacologic approach is to use an adrenergic stimulating drug to simulate exercise.[126] Under these circumstances, ischemia is produced by increasing the heart rate and blood pressure as with exercise. The most popular pharmacologic agent is dobutamine.[27,128-136] This drug has a strong ionotropic and modest chronotropic effect on the heart. The safety and patient acceptance of dobutamine is good.[137-140] Transient arrhythmias or hypotension[139] are the most serious side effects, none of which have been life-threatening. The strong inotropic effect of dobutamine can produce intraventricular obstruction and hypotension,[141] which is quickly reversed by stopping the drug or giving a rapid acting beta-blocker. Dobutamine is usually given as an infusion with increasing doses. A common approach is to begin with 2.5 or 5 µg/kg/min for 3 minutes and then to increase the dose to 10, 20, 30, and as high as 50 µg/kg/min. If the chronotropic response is inadequate, up to 1.0 mg of atropine may be given.[142,143] Arbutamine is a new synthetic sympathomimetic drug being investigated for use in stress echocardiography.[144,145] The drug has a greater chronotropic effect than dobutamine.[146]

Figure 8–26 shows long-axis systolic echocardiograms at rest, low dose, peak dose, and post-dobuta-

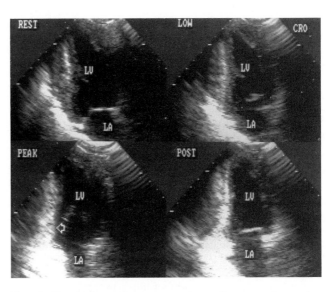

**Fig. 8–27.** Dobutamine stress echocardiogram of a patient with an obstruction in the right coronary artery. These serial two-chamber echocardiograms show akinesis (*arrow*) in the basal inferior wall during peak dose. LV = left ventricle; LA = left atrium.

mine. The heart rates are indicated on the recordings. As noted in this normal study, hyperkinesis and cavity obliteration occur with dobutamine. Figure 8–27 illustrates a dobutamine study in a patient who has an obstruction in the posterior descending artery. With the peak dose, akinesis of the basal posterior-inferior wall is noted (*arrow*). Figure 8–28 shows a colorized wall motion study of a dobutamine stress echocardiogram. The resting study is normal, with rims of red indicating

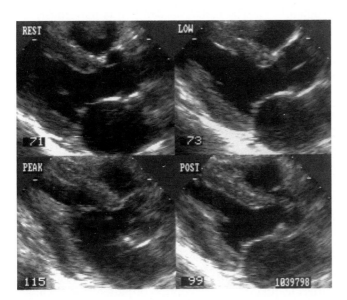

**Fig. 8–26.** A normal dobutamine stress echocardiogram. These long-axis systolic images show increasing hypercontractility and cavity obliteration as the test progresses from rest, low dose, and peak dose. The post-dobutamine examination demonstrates partial recovery of the hyperkinetic wall motion.

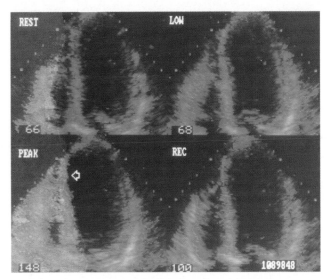

**Fig. 8–28.** Colorized regional wall analysis of a dobutamine stress echocardiogram in a patient with obstruction in the left anterior descending coronary artery. Normal wall motion is indicated by a rim of red outlined by the blue diastolic image. This rim of red virtually disappears (*arrow*) in the distal septum with peak dose. REC = recovery.

good wall motion throughout this four-chamber view. With the peak dobutamine dose, the distal septum becomes akinetic (*arrow*), appreciated with this colorized technique as absence of a red rim.

Occasionally, the heart translates, which means that the total heart moves from side to side. Such motion is particularly common with stress echocardiograms. Translation is highlighted with the colorized regional wall technique.[146a] In Figure 8–29, the patient underwent upright bicycle exercise, and the four-chamber resting and peak exercise views are displayed. The resting four-chamber view is normal, with uniform rims of red. In addition, the junction between the tricuspid and mitral annulus and the interventricular and interatrial septum does not move from right to left. This junction moves only base to apex or up and down. With exercise, the heart translates, and the junction between the septa and annula moves to the patient's right (EX-TR, *arrow*). Not only can the colorized technique make such translation apparent, but also the technique permits correction of the abnormality. One can move the digital images so that they are superimposed correctly (EX-COR, *up arrow*). Now the junction between the mitral and tricuspid annula is reoriented correctly. With correction, the septum is no longer displayed as dyskinetic but only akinetic.

Because nonexercise stress echocardiography does not have as much respiratory artifact, the digital recording technique is not as necessary for obtaining interpretable echocardiograms. The digital approach is still pre-ferred, however, because it greatly assists in the analysis of the echocardiogram.[147] The ability to see the resting and stress echocardiograms side by side is a great advantage. Furthermore, the wall motion changes can be subtle, and there is definitely a learning curve.[148] Sometimes, it is not sufficient to know if a segment contracts, but also when it contracts.[19] The digital approach assists in this analysis by looking at frame-by-frame changes. Occasionally, there is tardokinesis, i.e., wall motion is delayed. This abnormality is best detected by analyzing the first half of systole in a cine-loop. One may also be able to view the images in a "scan" loop, which goes from front to back, then back to front (i.e., cine-loop displaying frames 1 to 8 and then 8 to 1, etc., instead only 1 to 8). This display gives a more continuous appreciation of wall motion. Digital recordings also permit the use of such techniques as colorized regional wall analysis.

Nonexercise stress testing has been used with transesophageal echocardiography when transthoracic images are too poor to interpret.[149,150] Both pacing[151–153] and pharmacologic stress[154] have been used.

The sensitivity and specificity of stress echocardiography have been compared with that of coronary angiography[89,155,156] and nuclear cardiology.[157–168] Although definite differences exist between these examinations, in general, the specificity and sensitivity of stress echocardiography appears to be comparable to that of stress nuclear testing. Much of the popularity of stress echocardiography is based on the fact that the patients do not have to return for reperfusion testing, no ionizing radiation is involved, the results are immediately available, the tests are less costly, and exercise echocardiography does not require an intravenous injection.

One subgroup of patients in whom stress echocardiography has proved to be particularly valuable is women.[169,170] The electrocardiogram is notoriously inaccurate when used as a marker of ischemia in women. Thus, some form of stress imaging is frequently necessary in these patients. Stress nuclear testing is sometimes difficult in women in that the breast may interfere with accurate nuclear images. When tested against stress electrocardiography, the echocardiographic technique clearly appears to be more sensitive in all groups of patients.

An increasing number of articles in the literature demonstrate the prognostic value of stress echocardiography.[171–180c] Prognostic studies have been carried out in patients with stable coronary artery disease[175,179,180] or after a myocardial infarction.[181–185] The test is also proving valuable in assessing the risk of noncardiac surgery in patients with either known coronary artery disease or a high risk of having coronary artery disease.[172–174,186–189a]

Doppler echocardiography has also been used with stress testing for the evaluation of patients with known or suspected coronary artery disease. Most investigators have looked at aortic flow during or immediately after stress-induced ischemia.[97,190–200] Although the test indicates alterations in ventricular function with stress-induced ischemia, the examination is not sensitive;[197] it

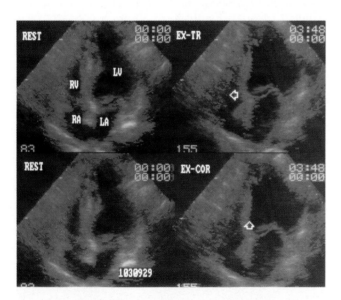

**Fig. 8–29.** Colorized regional wall study showing how cardiac translation can be corrected. In this exercise echocardiogram, the heart translates, whereby it moves to the patient's right (*arrow*) with peak exercise. Translation can be recognized by the junction of the tricuspid and mitral annulae moving either right to left or left to right. The digitized images can be reoriented so that the junction between the tricuspid and mitral annulae do not move sideways but only apically (*up arrow*) as is normal. After correction for translation (EX-COR), the interventricular septum is akinetic rather than dyskinetic, as seen in the translated exercise image (EX-TR).

identifies only those patients with severe coronary artery disease. In addition, the results do not provide any regional information. Investigators have also analyzed Doppler left ventricular inflow to assess the presence of ischemia following stress.[201–206b] One cannot use recordings with rapid heart rates because diastolic flow cannot be evaluated if diastole is too short. The diastolic changes persist, however, so that one can wait until the heart rate subsides before assessing the Doppler signal. As one would expect, ischemia produces a reduction in early diastolic flow. If, however, the patient developes significant ischemic mitral regurgitation, the early diastolic flow or E wave may be enhanced.[201] Again, the Doppler inflow recording is somewhat nonspecific and does not provide any regional information.

### Coronary Artery Spasm

Echocardiography has been used to monitor wall motion abnormalities in patients with coronary artery spasm or Prinzmetal's angina.[207–212] Figure 8–30 shows a series of coronary angiograms and M-mode echocardiograms in a patient with spasm of the left anterior descending artery.[208] With occlusion of the vessel, the septum becomes ischemic and barely moves. Septal motion

returns when blood again transverses the left anterior descending coronary artery (post ischemia). Investigators have used two-dimensional echocardiography to monitor wall motion changes in spontaneous vasospastic angina.[209,210] This type of angina has also been provoked by hyperventilation or ergonovine[210,213] and monitored with either M-mode or two-dimensional echocardiography. As expected, the ischemia produces prompt changes in wall motion and thickening with frequent dilatation of the left ventricle (Fig. 8–30). Following recovery from the anginal episode, wall motion and thickening of the affected area frequently become hyperdynamic.[207]

### Coronary Reperfusion

Digital echocardiography, with its ability to produce continuous loop images and side-by-side analysis, makes the evaluation of serial echocardiograms much easier and more accurate.[214–218] As a result, two-dimensional echocardiography is an excellent technique by which to note the effectiveness of reperfusion using bypass surgery, angioplasty, or thrombolysis.[219–228] Figure 8–31 shows long-axis and short-axis echograms of a patient who has anterior wall ischemia resulting from an

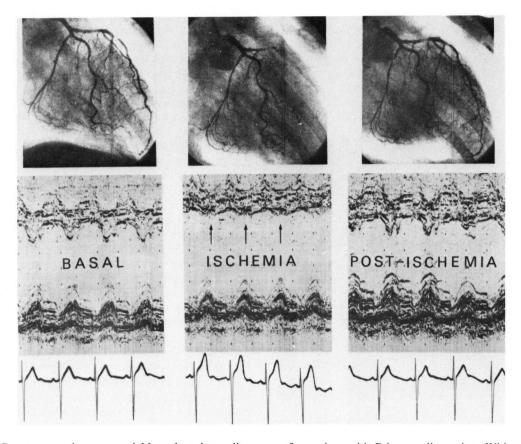

**Fig. 8–30.** Coronary angiograms and M-mode echocardiograms of a patient with Prinzmetal's angina. With spasm (middle records) the flow of blood through the left anterior descending coronary artery ceases, and septal motion is markedly reduced (*arrows*). Following ischemia flow returns to the left anterior descending coronary artery, and septal motion is normal. (From Distante, A., et al.: Transient changes in left ventricular mechanics during attacks of Prinzmetal's angina: An M-mode echocardiographic study. Am. Heart J., *107*:465, 1984.)

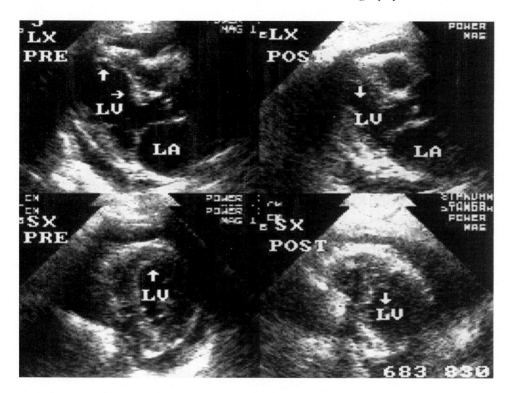

**Fig. 8–31.** Long-axis and short-axis two-dimensional echocardiograms of a patient with an occluded left anterior descending artery before (PRE) and after (POST) opening the artery with angioplasty. Before angioplasty, the septum and anterior walls (*reverse arrows*) are akinetic. These segments return to normal (*down arrows*) with reperfusion. LV = left ventricle; LA = left atrium. (From Feigenbaum, H.: Echocardiography. *In* Heart Disease, 4th Ed., Edited by E. Braunwald. Philadelphia, W.B. Saunders Co., 1992.)

obstructed left anterior descending artery. After opening the artery with angioplasty, significant improvement in anterior septal wall motion (POST) is noted. Figure 8–32 is a series of echocardiograms from the same patient demonstrating that the recovery of ventricular function may not be immediate. Figure 8–32A shows a long-axis

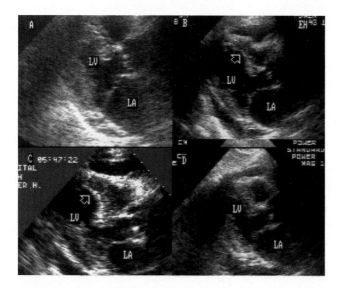

**Fig. 8–32.** Serial systolic long-axis echocardiograms of a patient with stable coronary artery disease (*A*) following an acute myocardial infarction (*B*), 5 days after re-opening the artery with angioplasty (*C*), and 6 weeks after reperfusion (*D*). The septum is clearly abnormal with the acute infarction (*arrow, B*) and 5 days after reperfusion (*arrow, C*). Some time between 5 days and 6 weeks, the septal motion returns to normal (*D*).

echocardiogram of this patient when she had stable coronary artery disease and a normal left ventricle. With an acute ischemic event, akinesis of the anterior septum occurs secondary to an obstruction in the left anterior descending artery. With reperfusion, an echocardiogram taken 5 days later (Fig. 8–32C) still shows the wall motion abnormality. The patient did well clinically and returned for a 6-week follow-up visit, at which time echocardiography revealed improvement in left ventricular function (Fig. 8–32D). This series of echocardiograms not only demonstrates the ability of echocardiography to document improvement in ventricular function with reperfusion, but also represents an excellent example of stunned myocardium whereby the return in function occurred sometime between 5 days and 6 weeks after reperfusion.[228a]

Figure 8–33 shows another example of improvement in ventricular function following reperfusion. The colorized regional wall study shows the lack of any wall motion before angioplasty (LX-PRE and 4C-PRE). After opening of the left anterior descending artery, one now sees a rim of red, indicating wall motion, in the postangioplasty examinations. In this example, the improvement in function is less dramatic, and a more sensitive technique for demonstrating the improvement is needed.

Experimental data show that reperfused myocardium becomes thicker whereas nonperfused muscle thins or is unchanged.[229] This observation has not yet been made clinically. The series of exercise echocardiograms noted in Figures 8–24 and 8–25 illustrates how one can use stress echocardiography to evaluate reperfusion[209–237a] or restenosis.[238,238a]

Stunned and hibernating myocardium are two recently recognized conditions that are proving to be im-

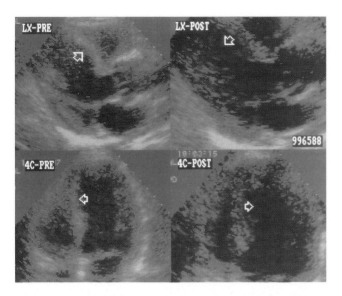

**Fig. 8–33.** Colorized wall motion of long-axis (LX) and four-chamber (4C) views of a patient before (PRE) and after (POST) reperfusion of a left anterior descending artery. There is either a small or nonexistent rim of red in the prereperfusion images (*reverse arrows*). With reperfusion, a small positive rim of red (*positive arrows*) can be visualized.

portant in patient management.[238b] Stunned myocardium is when ischemic muscle is reperfused and is still viable but not functioning.[239] Eventually, function spontaneously returns.[16,240] Hibernating myocardium is viable muscle that is nonfunctioning because of chronic ischemia.[241] Reperfusion may restore function. Serial echocardiograms can detect stunned and hibernating myocardium in a retrospective manner by observing improvement in ventricular function. There are efforts to use echocardiography to predict the return of ventricular function in stunned or hibernating myocardium. Nonfunctioning but viable muscle has been noted to contract with low-dose dobutamine stimulation.[242–246] Under these circumstances, one may predict return of function. Low-dose dipyridamole may have a similar application.[247] High-dose dipyridamole or dobutamine echocardiography may identify myocardium jeopardized by residual coronary obstructions following thrombolytic therapy.[248]

## MYOCARDIAL INFARCTION

### Detecting and Assessing Myocardial Infarction

Numerous experimental and clinical studies document that echocardiography is an excellent technique for detecting the early changes in function that occur with acute myocardial infarction.[249–251] All animal studies demonstrate prompt changes in wall motion and/or wall thickening immediately after coronary artery occlusion.[4,36,252–258] As with other forms of myocardial ischemia, changes in wall thickening provide a more accurate means than does wall motion to assess the presence

and extent of infarction.[36,253,255,258] There are obvious limitations to using wall motion in trying to predict infarct size. Noninfarcted, nonischemic muscle can be influenced by adjacent muscle, i.e., "tethering effect." Also, as already indicated, some myocardium may be "stunned." As a general rule, echocardiography tends to overestimate recent myocardial infarctions[259] and to underestimate old infarctions.[260] The explanation may in part be a result of stunning in the acute setting. The tethering effect of the normal muscle probably explains the underestimation with the old infarction.

Some question remains as to how large an infarction must be before it can be detected echocardiographically.[261,262] Experimental data would suggest that some subendocardial infarctions may not produce wall motion abnormalities because the amount of functioning muscle is still sufficient. Wall motion and wall thickening abnormalities noted on echocardiography correlate well with transmural infarctions (Q wave on the electrocardiogram).[263,264] Although there is some question as to how well myocardial function abnormalities correlate with non-Q wave or nontransmural infarctions,[13] one study showed that 10 of 12 patients with subendocardial nontransmural infarctions exhibited severe hypokinesis in the infarcted area.[265] In another study, only 2 of 6 patients with such infarctions exhibited wall motion abnormalities,[266] although all 6 patients showed abnormal wall thickening.

Despite the limitations of using echocardiography to quantitate the degree of myocardial dysfunction in the setting of acute infarction, the observation is that the echocardiographic evaluation of left ventricular function has important implications in patient management. Investigations show a good correlation of echocardiographic functional infarct size with studies using thallium,[267] ventriculography,[268–270] coronary angiography,[271] hemodynamics,[272] peak creatinine phosphokinase,[273] and nuclear ventriculography.[269]

Some differences are evident, in the literature as to whether or not wall motion abnormalities noted on the echocardiogram change with the natural history of infarction.[274–279] One group of authors say that 22% of hypokinetic segments and 12% of akinetic segments improve with time.[22] Only 5% of dyskinetic myocardium exhibit better motion. Other studies have indicated that the wall motion abnormalities are relatively constant and are present almost immediately after infarction occurred.[31,252,280] With the increased use of serial echocardiograms,[281] especially using digital, side-by-side techniques, all of these observations need to be re-evaluated.

One of the important uses of two-dimensional echocardiography in patients with myocardial infarction is not only to detect the presence and size of the myocardial infarction, but also to assess the status of the muscle not involved with the acute event.[273] The noninfarcted myocardium has important prognostic value. The number of obstructed coronary vessels can be predicted by looking at the areas remote to the infarction. Normally, the noninfarcted muscle becomes hyperkinetic in a compensatory fashion. This hyperkinesis occurs if the muscle is supplied by nonobstructed vessels. If the hyperkinesis fails to occur in remote areas, however, multivessel disease should be suspected.[22,282]

Attempts have been made to use echocardiography to identify acoustic changes in ischemic myocardial tissue.[283,283a] Scar tissue has been recognized for some time as producing thin, echogenic walls (Fig. 8–34).[284] Investigators have been using color-encoded two-dimensional echocardiography to help identify the echogenic scar after myocardial infarction.[285] An illustration of such a study is shown in Chapter 1 (see Tissue Identification). Digital image processing and measuring of pixel intensity is being studied as a means of identifying ischemic myocardium.[286] Integrated acoustic backscatter techniques are also being used to identify myocardial infarction.[287–289] One technique is based on the observation that the backscatter from normal muscle has a cyclic variation, decreasing with systole (Fig. 8–35). This cyclic variation disappears with ischemia (Fig. 8–36).

None of these investigational efforts have current clinical utility. The acoustic quantitation technique is probably the one that is under the most active investigation at present.

### Prognosis Following Myocardial Infarction

Echocardiography is proving to be an important tool for evaluating prognosis after myocardial infarction.[290–296] As expected, functional infarct size noted on the echocardiogram has good prognostic predictability.[297–301] Although a qualitative or semiquantitative assessment can easily be made by visually estimating the extent of abnormality, the dysfunction is probably assessed more objectively by tabulating a wall motion score index.[297–300] The prognosis also is determined to a large extent by the status of the noninfarcted muscle.[22,273] Doppler left ventricular inflow studies may also provide prognostic information.[302–304] A restrictive type of filling pattern with a tall E wave may indicate a high left ventricular diastolic pressure and a poor prognosis.

Patients who have chest pain and a normal two-dimensional echocardiogram either have no infarction or are going to have a relatively small infarction. This determination can be made in the emergency room.[305–310] Thus, echocardiography can play an important role in the triage of patients with chest pain. Ruling out a myocardial infarction in the emergency room can have great impact on medical costs of a given patient. If an echocardiogram can be obtained early after chest pain begins, it could help determine whether to begin thrombolytic therapy.

As mentioned previously, stress echocardiography is a useful examination for assessing prognosis after myocardial infarction.[181–183,311–315] Post-myocardial infarction patients who have positive stress echocardiograms have a higher incidence of ischemic events than those with a negative test.

## COMPLICATIONS OF MYOCARDIAL INFARCTION

### Infarct Extension and Expansion

Echocardiography can detect infarct extension whereby additional ischemic muscle becomes involved with the infarction process.[316] If one were to calculate percent normal muscle, this value would decrease while the wall motion score index would increase (get worse) with infarct extension. Infarct expansion is when the infarcted area dilates and becomes functionally more abnormal.[317–319] The regional score index would worsen but no change in percent functioning muscle would be noted.

Figure 8–37 shows serial systolic echocardiograms from a patient with an anterior myocardial infarction. Figure 8–37A shows a normally functioning ventricle when this patient has chronic angina before an infarction. With infarction a few days later (Fig. 8–37B), the anterior septum becomes akinetic (−). A couple of weeks later, the anterior septum is thin, dyskinetic, and dilated (Fig. 8–37C). This anterior septum exhibits scar

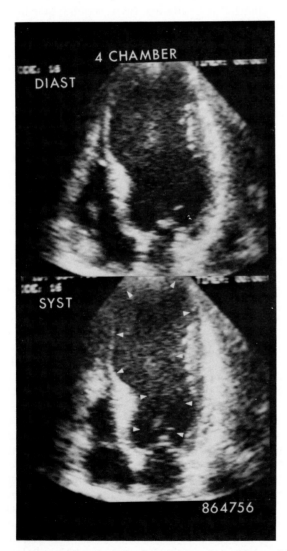

**Fig. 8–34.** Apical four-chamber views of a patient with a large myocardial infarction. Dilatation and decrease in thickness of the interventricular septum and apex (*reverse arrowheads*) are noted. The apical half of the left ventricular cavity is filled with echoes arising from stagnant blood.

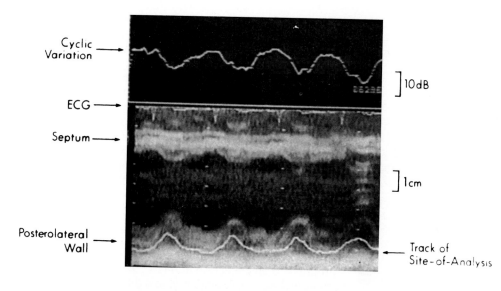

**Fig. 8–35.** Echocardiographic examination using integrated acoustic backscatter to distinguish normal from ischemic myocardium. In this recording of a normal posterolateral wall, one sees cyclic variation in the acoustic backscatter with the cardiac cycle. (From Milunski, M.R., et al.: Ultrasonic tissue characterization with integrated backscatter. Circulation, *80*:495, 1989, by permission of the American Heart Association, Inc.)

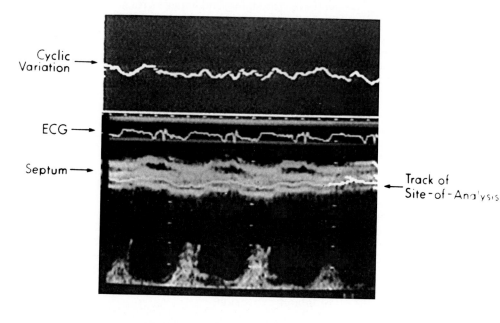

**Fig. 8–36.** Integrated acoustic backscatter image from a patient with an ischemic interventricular septum. The cyclic variation is gone in this ischemic muscle. (From Milunski, M.R., et al.: Ultrasonic tissue characterization with integrated backscatter. Circulation, *80*:495, 1989, by permission of the American Heart Association, Inc.)

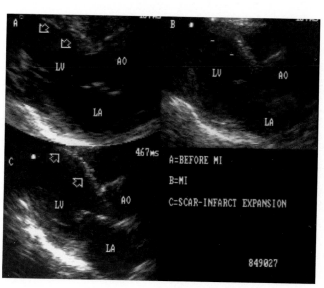

**Fig. 8–37.** Serial echocardiogram demonstrating a patient before myocardial infarction (*A*), during myocardial infarction (MI) (*B*), and with infarct expansion (*C*). Before the myocardial infarction, the septum motion moves normally (*inward arrows*). With the infarction, the interventricular septum shows no motion (−). Later, the interventricular septum became scarred, thin, and dilated (*outward arrows*). LV = left ventricle; AO = aorta; LA = left atrium.

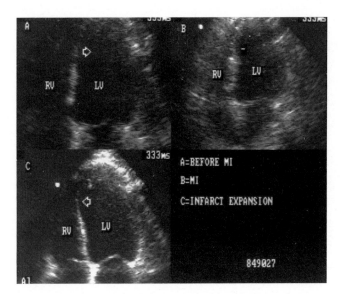

**Fig. 8–38.** Serial four-chamber echocardiograms of the same patient illustrated in Figure 8–37. Before the myocardial infarction (*A*), interventricular septal motion is normal (*inward arrow*). With the infarction (*B*), the distal septum becomes akinetic (− ). Later, the septum is thin and bulges (*outward arrow, C*) toward the right ventricle (RV). LV = left ventricle; MI = myocardial infarction.

formation and infarct expansion. Figure 8–38 shows four-chamber views of the same patient. Again, note the change in ventricular function with the development of the infarction (Fig. 8–38*B*). With infarct expansion (Fig. 8–38*C*), the distal septum becomes thin and bulges toward the right ventricle (*arrow*).

Numerous investigators have been studying the problem of infarct expansion. New therapeutic approaches try to limit the progression of this complication.[320–322] Infarct expansion can be assessed in many ways echocardiographically. Some investigators merely measure left ventricular volumes to note the presence of infarct expansion.[323,324] A relatively simple approach is to measure anterior and posterior segment lengths (Fig. 8–39).[319,325] With infarct expansion, the infarcted segment length increases. More sophisticated techniques for judging infarct expansion use a radius of curvature of the infarcted area.[326] When the damaged area dilates, the radius of curvature decreases as the segment bulges or becomes an aneurysm. Thus, the radius of curvature is one way of following infarct expansion. Another technique involves a surface map of the left ventricular endocardium.[317] Figure 8–40 shows an even more complicated approach to quantitating infarct expansion.[327] This technique attempts to provide a three-dimensional assessment of infarct size and shape. Needless to say, this relatively complicated technique is primarily for investigational purposes. One can also use various measurements of wall stress,[328] both global and regional, to try to assess infarct expansion. Infarct expansion may progress to an aneurysm and is a part of left ventricular "remodeling." Regional or global dilatation is the major factor in remodeling and impairs prognosis and function, in part by increasing myocardial wall stress, myocardial tension, and oxygen demand.

### Ventricular Aneurysm

Echocardiography has become one of the procedures of choice in detecting ventricular aneurysms after myocardial infarction.[329–337] The correlation between echocardiographic and angiographic detection of aneurysms is good. In fact, many workers feel that angiography is no longer necessary for the diagnosis of ventricular aneurysms.[333–335] In some situations, the echocardiographic definition of the aneurysm is superior than that noted with either angiography or radionuclide angiography.[331] Anterior infarctions more commonly produce aneurysms. Figure 8–34 reveals many of the characteristics of an anterior apical aneurysm: scar formation with loss of tissue in the infarcted area and dilatation of the damaged muscle. An aneurysm is in fact the end result of infarct expansion.

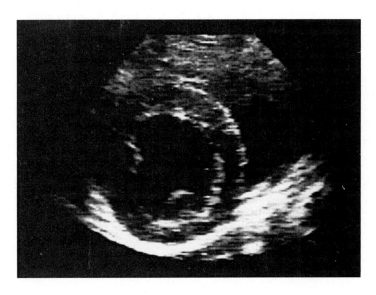

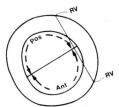

**Fig. 8–39.** A scheme whereby the short-axis left ventricular examination is divided into posterior and anterior halves for determining and quantitating infarct expansion. RV = right ventricle. (From Mehta, P.M., et al.: Functional infarct expansion, left ventricular dilatation, and isovolumnic relaxation time after coronary occlusion: Two-dimensional echocardiographic study. J. Am. Coll. Cardiol., *11*:632, 1988.)

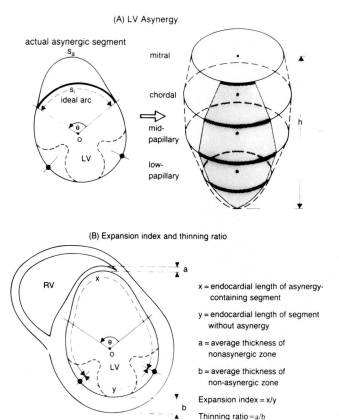

**Fig. 8–40.** A fairly elaborate scheme for measuring left ventricular asynergy and infarct expansion. (From Jugdutt, B.I. and Michorowski, E.L.: Role of infarct expansion in rupture of the ventricular septum after acute myocardial infarction: A two-dimensional echocardiographic study. Clin. Cardiol., *10*: 643, 1987.)

Another characteristic of an aneurysm is the abnormal flow of blood. Frequently, Doppler studies show a swirling pattern of blood flow in a large akinetic or dyskinetic aneurysm. Spontaneous contrast is commonly present next to large akinetic segments. Such spontaneous contrast is visible in the large apical akinetic area in Figure 8–34. The abnormal flow and/or spontaneous contrast may be the precursor of thrombus.

Figure 8–41 shows another patient with a large apical aneurysm. The aneurysm is visible in the four-chamber and two-chamber views. The aneurysm primarily involves the apex with preservation of proximal myocardial tissue. A larger aneurysm involving the entire anterior septum is noted in Figures 8–42 and 8–43. One again can identify the thin, dilated, aneurysmal wall in both the long-axis and four-chamber views.

Although most aneurysms occur at the apex and are the result of an anterior myocardial infarction, aneurysms associated with obstruction of the posterior descending coronary artery and inferior infarction also occur.[338] Figure 8–44 demonstrates an inferior aneurysm. The aneurysm (*arrowheads*) can be seen in the short-axis and two-chamber echocardiographic views. A much larger posterior aneurysm is illustrated in Figure 8–45. Figure 8–46 shows an even larger and more extensive posterior-inferior aneurysm. The massive extent of this abnormality can be seen in both the short-axis and two-chamber views. When an aneurysm involves much of the left ventricle and the remaining muscle dilates, the result is an ischemic cardiomyopathy.

These examples demonstrate that two-dimensional echocardiography can detect a variety of ventricular aneurysms. One of the major advantages of echocardiography is that wall thickness is routinely assessed. Thus, wall thinning, as well as dilatation, can be appreciated. The definition of an aneurysm can be disputed. Angiographically, one sees a bulge in the systolic or diastolic silhouette. Some of this bulge may merely be a result of loss of myocardial tissue and not true dilatation or bulging of the epicardial wall. Echocardiography provides the opportunity to differentiate between simple loss of tissue and actual bulging of ventricular walls.

In addition to establishing the existence and size of a ventricular aneurysm, echocardiography is particularly helpful in assessing the ventricular muscle not involved in the aneurysm. Early M-mode data demonstrated that the dimensions at the base of the heart could predict those patients who could survive aneurysmectomy. More recent data using two-dimensional measurements of the base of the heart support these observations.[49] It should come as no surprise that in patients with apical aneurysms, the echocardiographic measurements of the base of the heart have more prognostic value than the angiographic ejection fraction. Thus, two-dimensional minor axis measurements, which essentially assess the nonaneurysmal left ventricle, can be particularly useful in managing patients with ventricular aneurysms.

**Ventricular Pseudoaneurysm**

Echocardiography is an important tool for the detection of a pseudoaneurysm. Such a condition occurs in the event of rupture of the free wall of the left ventri-

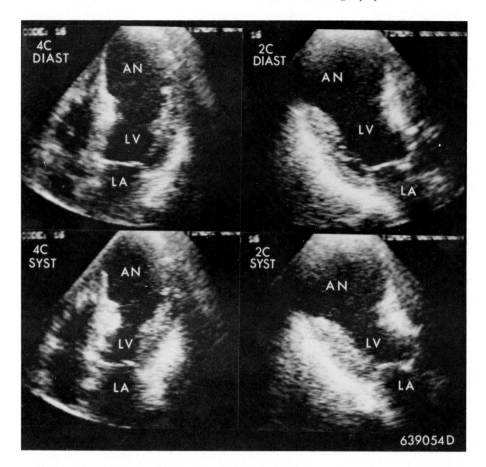

**Fig. 8–41.** Four-chamber (4C) and two-chamber (2C) two-dimensional echocardiograms of a patient with a large anterior apical aneurysm (AN). LV = left ventricle; LA = left atrium.

cle.[339–342] This complication is usually immediately fatal; however, in some reports of free wall rupture, two-dimensional echocardiography showed the trapped blood within the pericardium (Fig. 8–47).[341] If the patient survives the acute event, blood trapped within the pericardium produces a pseudoaneurysm, with the out-side wall being pericardium and clot rather than muscle. Two-dimensional echocardiography with Doppler enhancement is the procedure of choice for making this diagnosis.[343–356] Figure 8–48 illustrates an example of a pseudoaneurysm. This apical four-chamber view demonstrates an echo-free space originating from the lateral

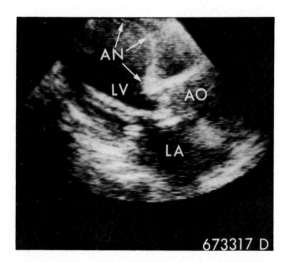

**Fig. 8–42.** Long-axis parasternal two-dimensional echocardiogram of a patient with coronary artery disease and an anteroseptal aneurysm (AN) of the interventricular septum. AO = aorta; LA = left atrium; LV = left ventricle.

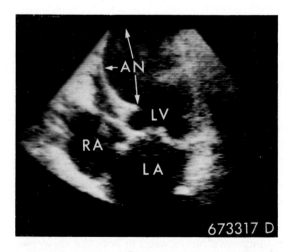

**Fig. 8–43.** Apical four-chamber two-dimensional echocardiogram of a patient with an aneurysm (AN) of the apical two thirds of the interventricular septum. LV = left ventricle; LA = left atrium; RA = right atrium.

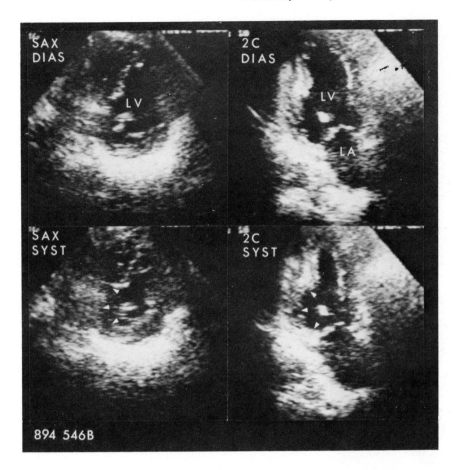

**Fig. 8–44.** Short-axis (SAX) and two-chamber (2C) two-dimensional echocardiograms of a patient with a posterior-inferior aneurysm (*arrowheads*). The wall of the aneurysm is irregular (2C DIAST and SYST). The irregularity is probably a result of echoes originating from small thrombi in the aneurysm. LV = left ventricle; LA = left atrium.

free wall of the left ventricle (PA). Figure 8–49 shows another patient with an even larger pseudoaneurysm, which was more posterior-lateral and could be detected in both the long-axis and four-chamber views.

Color flow imaging can be helpful with the diagnosis of pseudoaneurysm by detecting blood flowing in and out of the aneurysmal space (Fig. 8–50).[357–361] Figure 8–51 shows the spectral Doppler recording from a patient with a pseudoaneurysm. Contrast echocardiography, with injection of contrast medium into the left ventricle at cardiac catheterization, is an invasive technique used for diagnosis.[362] Some pseudoaneurysms are seen best with transesophageal echocardiography.[363,363a]

The echocardiographic criterion that differentiates a pseudoaneurysm from a true ventricular aneurysm is the width of the neck of the aneurysm. That portion of the pseudoaneurysm communicating with the left ventricular cavity is invariably smaller than the diameter of the pseudoaneurysm itself.[348,351] Another criterion for the echocardiographic diagnosis of pseudoaneurysm is the fact that, in systole, the cavity of the left ventricle gets smaller while the pseudoaneurysm frequently expands.[343–345,364,365] The color flow image can assist in this assessment as well.

The echocardiographic diagnosis of a pseudoaneurysm is clinically important because these aneurysms, contrary to true aneurysms, go on to rupture, with immediate death. Thus, the detection of a pseudoaneurysm can be an indication for prompt surgical intervention.

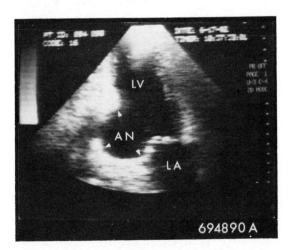

**Fig. 8–45.** Apical two-chamber two-dimensional echocardiogram of a patient with a very large posterior aneurysm (AN). LV = left ventricle; LA = left atrium.

## VENTRICULAR SEPTAL DEFECT

When the ruptured myocardium involves the interventricular septum, an acquired ventricular septal defect

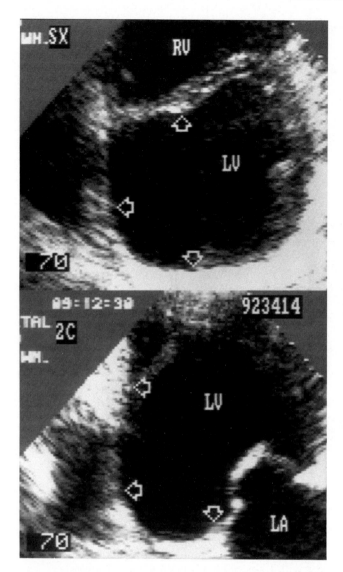

**Fig. 8–46.** Short-axis (SX) and two-chamber (2C) echocardiograms of a patient with a large posterior, inferior aneurysm (*arrows*). RV = right ventricle; LV = left ventricle; LA = left atrium.

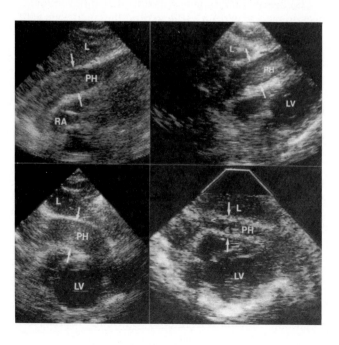

**Fig. 8–47.** Patient with a myocardial infarction and left ventricular free wall rupture who developed a pericardial hematoma (PH), which trapped the blood and prevented exsanguination. L = lung; RA = right atrium; LV = left ventricle. (From Brack, M., et al.: Two-dimensional echocardiographic characteristics of pericardial hematoma secondary to left ventricular free wall rupture complicating acute myocardial infarction. Am. J. Cardiol., 68:962, 1991.)

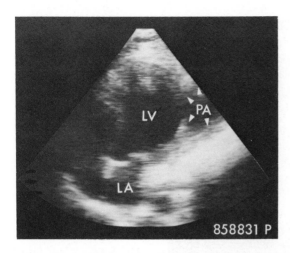

**Fig. 8–48.** Four-chamber two-dimensional echocardiogram of a patient with a pseudoaneurysm (PA) adjacent to the posterior lateral free wall of the left ventricle (LV). LA = left atrium.

develops. This complication of myocardial infarction can have devastating hemodynamic effects on the patient and, in many cases, can be fatal unless surgically corrected. Echocardiography is an ideal technique for the detection of this serious complication of myocardial infarction. Two-dimensional echocardiography offers the opportunity of directly visualizing the ruptured interventricular septum (Fig. 8–52).[366–368] Other authors have emphasized the finding of ventricular septal infarct expansion or aneurysm that invariably is present in patients with a ruptured ventricular septum.[369–374]

As expected, Doppler echocardiography is an excellent means of detecting a ruptured interventricular septum.[375] Figure 8–53 demonstrates a Doppler study in a patient with a ruptured ventricular septum.[376] Turbulent, high-velocity flow can be detected in systole on the right side of the interventricular septum in both the four-chamber and the short-axis views. Such a study can be reliable and specific for a ventricular septal defect.

The color flow Doppler examination offers an even more dramatic and probably more definitive examination of ventricular septal defects that occur after myocardial infarction.[377–379] Figure 8–54 demonstrates a

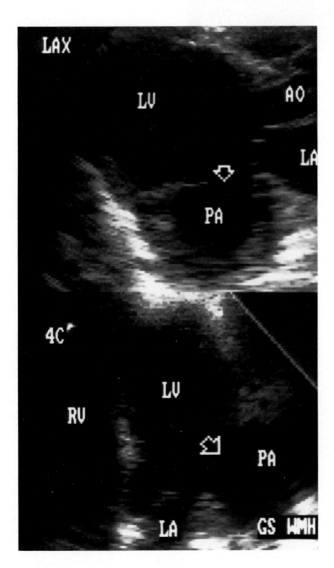

**Fig. 8–49.** Long-axis and four-chamber echocardiograms of a patient with a large posterior pseudoaneurysm (PA). The communication (*arrow*) between the left ventricle (LV) and the pseudoaneurysm can be identified in these views. AO = aorta; LA = left atrium; RV = right ventricle.

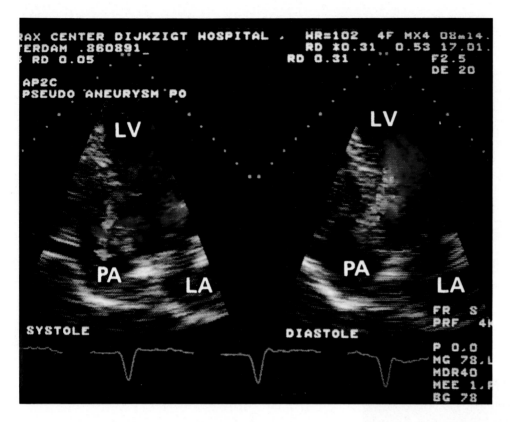

**Fig. 8–50.** Color flow imaging in a patient with a pseudoaneurysm (PA) allows identification of the flow passing from the left ventricle (LV) into the pseudoaneurysm. LA = left atrium. (From Sutherland, G.R., et al.: Advantages of colour flow imaging in the diagnosis of left ventricular pseudoaneurysm. Br. Heart J., *61*:62, 1989.)

color flow, two-dimensional Doppler echocardiogram of such a patient. Blood flowing from the left ventricle (LV) through the defect to the right side of the heart is demonstrated (*arrow*). A more complicated ventricular septal defect identified with color flow Doppler is illustrated in Figure 8–55. The rupture occurred in the basal portion of the interventricular septum after an inferior myocardial infarction. The blood then dissected through the septum and entered the right ventricle at a different location. It would be difficult to identify this situation without color flow imaging.

Color flow Doppler echocardiography is now the procedure of choice for detecting ventricular septal ruptures after myocardial infarction. These ruptures can occur in various locations. They accompany both anterior and inferior infarctions, frequently involve the apex, and may produce multiple defects. Rupture of a post-infarction aneurysm into the right atrium has been reported.[380]

Although transthoracic echocardiography is usually sufficient to diagnose a ruptured interventricular septum, the transesophageal examination may sometimes be helpful.[380a]

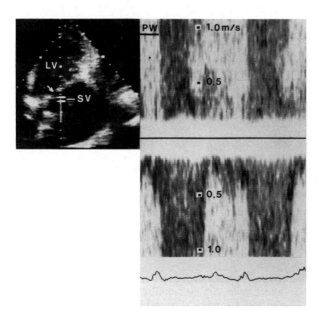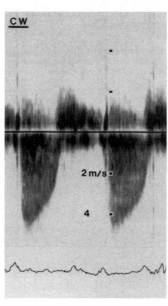

**Fig. 8–51.** Spectral Doppler recording with the sample volume (SV) in a pseudoaneurysm just beyond the communication (*arrow*) of the pseudoaneurysm and the left ventricle (LV). The pulsed Doppler (PW) recording shows the high-velocity aliasing systolic flow. The continuous wave (CW) recording shows the systolic velocity, which exceeds 4 m/sec. (From Bach, M., et al.: Diagnosis of left ventricular pseudoaneurysm using contrast and Doppler echocardiography. Am. Heart J., *118*:855, 1989.)

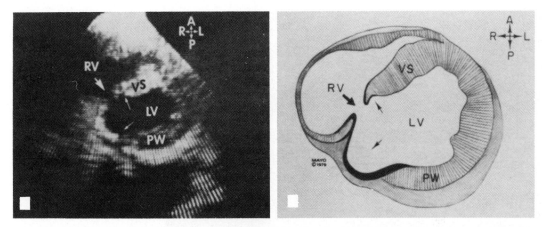

**Fig. 8–52.** Short-axis two-dimensional echocardiogram and diagram of a patient with a ruptured interventricular septum second-ary to a myocardial infarction. Note the aneurysmal bulging (*arrows*) of the ventricular septum (VS). In addition, echoes are discontinuous with communication between the right ventricle (RV) and the left ventricle (LV) at the site of the defect (*large arrow*). PW = posterior wall. (From Scanlan, J.G., Seward, J.B., and Tajik, A.J.: Visualization of ventricular septal rupture utilizing wide-angle, two-dimensional echocardiography. Mayo Clin. Proc., *54*:383, 1979.)

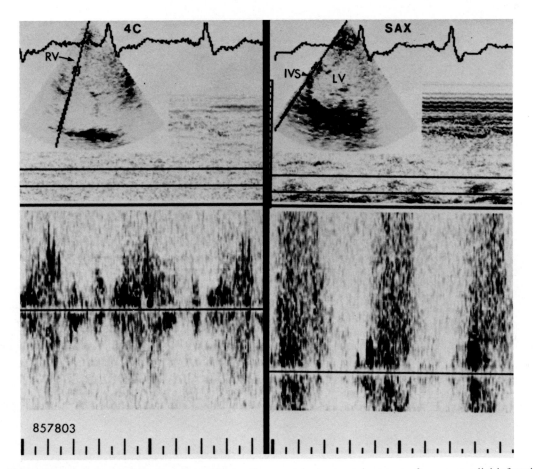

**Fig. 8–53.** Pulsed Doppler echocardiogram of a patient with a ventricular septal rupture after myocardial infarction. With the sample volume in the right ventricle (RV) near the interventricular septum (IVS), high-velocity systolic turbulent flow is recorded in both the four-chamber (4C) and short-axis (SAX) views. LV = left ventricle.

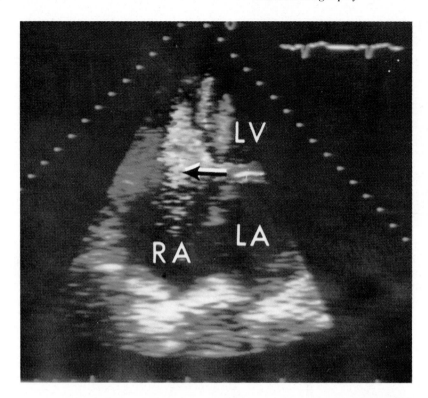

**Fig. 8–54.** Color flow mapping two-dimensional Doppler examination of a patient with a ventricular septal defect secondary to myocardial infarction. The abnormal flow (*arrow*) can be seen as an orange jet flowing from the left ventricle (LV) to the right side of the heart. RA = right atrium; LA = left atrium.

### Mural Thrombi

One of the most common complications of a myocardial infarction is the development of a mural thrombus. These thrombi usually occur adjacent to a dyskinetic area, which is commonly aneurysmally dilated. Two-dimensional echocardiography has become the procedure of choice in detecting mural thrombi.[381–384] In fact,

it has been used as a "gold standard" for numerous prospective studies to assess the incidence of mural thrombi and the development of systemic emboli.[385–394]

Most clots are involved with anterior infarctions and are usually located at the apex. Figure 8–56 demonstrates a fairly typical apical clot as seen in the apical four-chamber view.

Figure 8–57 shows some of the variety of clots that can be seen in the left ventricle after a myocardial infarction. In Figure 8–57*A*, one can identify a large apical thrombus in the left ventricle, as well as a small clot in the apical portion of the right ventricle. In Figure 8–57*B* and *C*, a more mobile clot with an echo-free center is

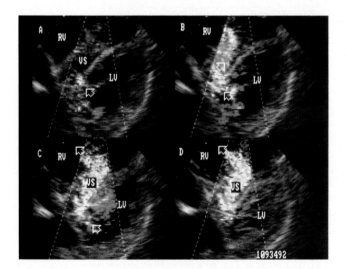

**Fig. 8–55.** Color flow Doppler study of a patient with a ruptured interventricular septum secondary to myocardial infarction. The rupture produces a dissection of the ventricular septum (VS). *A* shows how the rupture on the left side of the septum permits flow to enter the septum. Blood then dissects within the interventricular septum (*arrow, B*) and enters the right ventricle (RV) (*C* and *D*). LV = left ventricle.

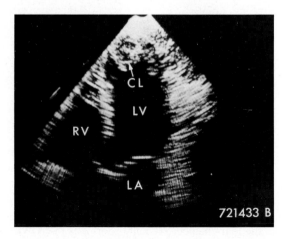

**Fig. 8–56.** Apical four-chamber two-dimensional echocardiogram of a patient with an apical clot (CL). LV = left ventricle; RV = right ventricle; LA = left atrium.

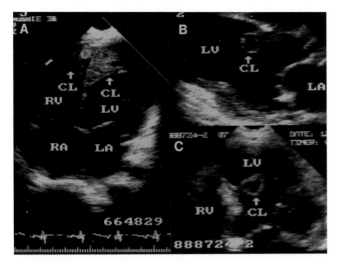

**Fig. 8–57.** Two-dimensional echocardiograms of two patients with mural thrombi secondary to myocardial infarction. *A* shows a clot (CL) in the apex of both the left ventricle (LV) and the right ventricle (RV). A smaller, mobile, echo-lucent clot attached to the interventricular septum is noted in *B* and *C*. LA = left atrium. (From Feigenbaum, H.: Echocardiography. *In* Heart Disease, 4th ed. Edited by E. Braunwald. Philadelphia, W.B. Saunders, Co., 1992.)

adjacent to an akinetic interventricular septum. The echo lucency probably represents a relatively fresh thrombus that has not totally solidified.

Although two-dimensional echocardiography is an excellent technique for detecting mural thrombi, there are some limitations. The clots can be subtle and must be differentiated from nonthrombotic echoes. Figure 8–58 demonstrates an apical clot that is not as striking as the one seen in Figure 8–56. The thrombus is less echogenic and could be missed by the casual observer. The apical clot in Figure 8–59 is even more subtle. The echoes are relatively faint, and the diagnosis is difficult because the clot does not protrude into the cavity of the left ventricle. It might be difficult to distinguish this echocardiogram from an off-axis four-chamber view that cuts through the wall of the left ventricle (Fig. 8–60).

Figure 8–61 is yet another example of an apical thrombus. This echocardiogram is more striking and fairly straightforward; however, the echocardiogram in Figure 8–62A is fairly similar to the one in Figure 8–61. The echoes near the apex of Figure 8–62A represent reverberations. Fortunately, the correct diagnosis can be made by noting the lack of any abnormal wall motion at the apex, which would make a thrombus unlikely. In addition, an extension of the reverberation during some of the echocardiographic views could be seen (Fig. 8–62B).

Clots are not limited to the cardiac apex. Figure 8–63 demonstrates a mural thrombus involving the interventricular septum. The thrombus can be seen lying along the wall of the interventricular septum, both in the long-axis and short-axis views. This echocardiogram is interesting in that it demonstrates another type of thrombus that can be seen echocardiographically, but also because one might have difficulty in distinguishing this thrombus from a hypertrophied interventricular septum. Possible confusion is most likely in the long-axis examination. The short-axis view should eliminate the possibility of

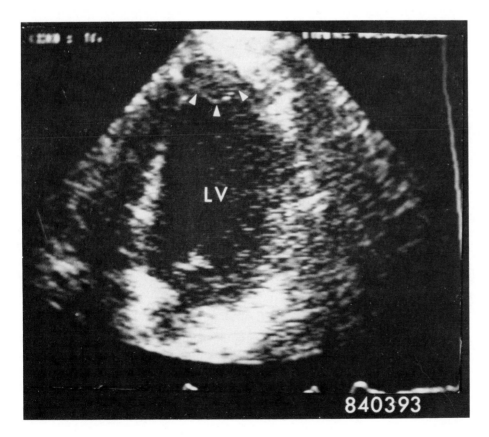

**Fig. 8–58.** Apical four-chamber two-dimensional echocardiogram of a patient with a small apical thrombus (*arrowheads*) associated with an akinetic apex. LV = left ventricle.

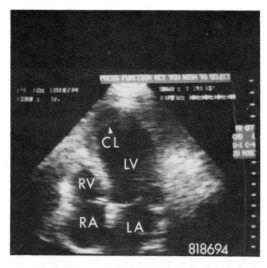

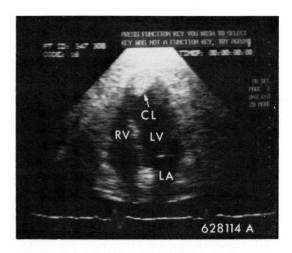

**Fig. 8–59.** Apical four chamber echocardiogram of a patient with a dilated apex and a mural clot (CL) layered along the apex. The clot is not very echogenic and only slightly distorts the outline of the left ventricular cavity (LV). RV = right ventricle; RA = right atrium; LA = left atrium.

**Fig. 8–61.** Four-chamber two-dimensional echocardiogram of a patient with a dense echogenic clot (CL) in the left ventricular apex. RV = right ventricle; LV = left ventricle; LA = left atrium.

a hypertrophied septum, since the clot does not involve all of the interventricular septum but instead lies against the anterior half of the interventricular septum and the anterior lateral wall.

Although clots usually occur with anterior myocardial infarctions, a thrombus can occasionally be seen in an inferior infarction, especially if an aneurysm develops. Figure 8–44 is an echocardiogram of a patient with a posterior aneurysm. On careful inspection, brighter echoes can be seen originating from thrombotic material within the aneurysm in the two-chamber view. Mural thrombi in the right ventricle have also been detected echocardiographically (Fig. 8–57).

The clinical questions being raised by the detection of mural thrombi with echocardiography are still unanswered. Several investigators have seen mural thrombi result in emboli;[386-388,390,394-399] however, there is no unanimity of opinion as to whether or not the presence of a mural thrombus is an indication for anticoagulation therapy and whether or not such therapy would in fact prevent systemic emboli.

As noted previously, echocardiography can also detect stagnant blood.[400] Several of the echocardiograms already illustrated demonstrate clouds of fuzzy, intracavitary echoes or spontaneous contrast adjacent to akinetic or dyskinetic walls. Figure 8–34, which is an apical four-chamber view of a patient with an anterior myocardial infarction, is a particularly good example of the intracavitary cloud of echoes that can be seen with stagnant blood. A similar example is noted in an animal study in Figure 8–64. An experimental myocardial infarction was induced that produced severe akinesis of the interventricular septum and dilatation of the left ventricular cavity. Within the cavity, a cloud of intracavitary echoes that frequently resembles "smoke" (*arrowheads*) can be detected. When the ligature around the obstructed coronary artery is removed, the wall motion returns to normal and the intracavitary "smoke" disappears. The exact mechanism for these intracavitary echoes is not clear. Somehow or other, the blood elements become echogenic. Rouleaux formation of the red cells is one possibility. This phenomenon could represent a precursor for intracavitary clots.

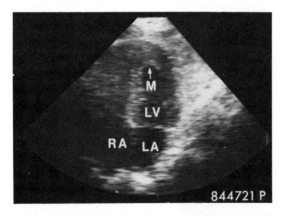

**Fig. 8–60.** Apical four-chamber two-dimensional echocardiogram of a patient who does not have an apical thrombus. The echocardiographic plane was tangential to the true left ventricular apex, making the apex look artifactually thick. Superficially the apical myocardium (M) resembles the apical clot noted in Fig. 8–59. LV = left ventricle; RA = right atrium; LA = left atrium.

### Mitral Regurgitation

At least three mechanisms are involved in the development of mitral regurgitation in a patient following an acute myocardial infarction.[401-403] One cause of mitral regurgitation is rupture of a papillary muscle.[403a] Such a complication can be detected with transthoracic[402,404] or transesophageal[406] echocardiography. Figure 8–65

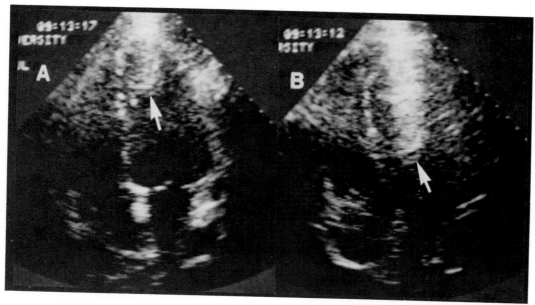

**Fig. 8–62.** Apical four-chamber echocardiograms of a patient who could be erroneously diagnosed as having an apical clot. The echocardiogram in *A* superficially resembles that in Figure 8–61, with the apical clot. The apparent clot (*arrow*), however, is secondary to a reverberation artifact. The reverberation is more obvious in *B* (*arrow*).

demonstrates a two-dimensional echocardiogram of a patient with a partial rupture of a papillary muscle. The separation of the papillary muscle can be detected (*arrow*). In one study of three patients with partial rupture of the papillary muscle, the actual defect could be seen on two-dimensional echocardiography in two of the three studies. In all three patients, M-mode criteria for a flail mitral valve could be detected.[405]

Another more common cause of mitral regurgitation in patients with myocardial infarction is fibrosis of the papillary muscle, with resultant foreshortening of the supporting structures of the mitral valve apparatus. Clo-

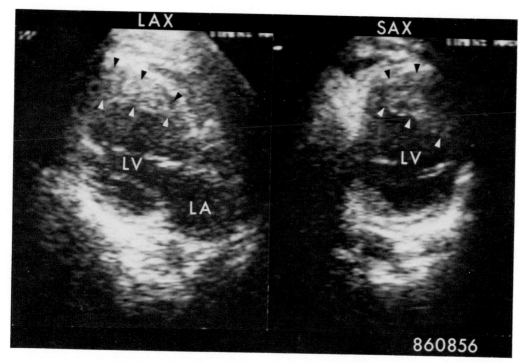

**Fig. 8–63.** Long-axis (LAX) and short-axis (SAX) two-dimensional echocardiograms of a patient with a mural thrombus along the anterior septum and anterior lateral wall (*arrowheads*). In the long-axis view, the thrombus could be mistaken for a thick interventricular septum. LV = left ventricle; LA = left atrium.

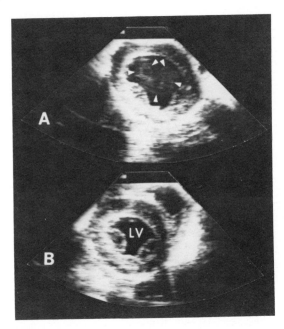

**Fig. 8–64.** Short-axis echocardiogram of a dog whose coronary artery was ligated and then released. When the artery was ligated (*A*), much of the left ventricular wall was akinetic and the cavity was filled with smoky echoes (*arrowheads*) produced by stagnant blood. When the artery was released (*B*), the wall motion returned to normal and the echogenic blood disappeared. LV = left ventricle.

sure of the mitral valve is now incomplete. The mitral leaflets do not approximate the mitral annulus in systole. Figure 8–66 demonstrates a patient with a scarred papillary muscle related to myocardial infarction and incomplete closure of the mitral valve.[407,408] This finding is probably one of the more common forms of papillary muscle dysfunction. This incomplete closure can be also noted in patients with a dilated cardiomyopathy. In this latter abnormality, migration of the papillary muscles occurs, which again foreshortens the supporting valve apparatus and prevents complete closure of the leaflets.

Mitral regurgitation can of course occur with myocardial ischemia and not necessarily infarction. Investigators have actually looked for mitral regurgitation with stress echocardiography using valvular regurgitation as a sign of ischemia.[201]

Although two-dimensional echocardiography is clearly the ultrasonic procedure of choice for detecting the cause of mitral regurgitation in a patient with coronary artery disease, Doppler echocardiography is better for detecting the presence and amount of regurgitation.

### Right Ventricular Infarction

Although the left ventricle is the principal chamber that is affected by coronary artery obstructive disease, there is increasing interest in the damage of the right ventricular chamber with the infarction process. The right ventricle is affected primarily when inferior infarction occurs. The situation usually arises when the proximal portion of the right coronary artery is obstructed,

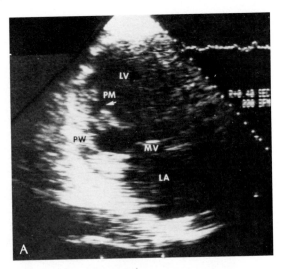

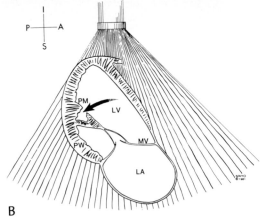

**Fig. 8–65.** Apical two-chamber echocardiogram (*A*) and diagram (*B*) of a patient with a partial rupture (*arrow*) of the papillary muscle (PM). LV = left ventricle; PW = posterior left ventricular wall; MV = mitral valve; LA = left atrium. (From Mishimura, R.A., Shub, C., and Tajik, A.J.: Two-dimensional echocardiographic diagnosis of partial papillary muscle rupture. Br. Heart J., *48*:598, 1982.)

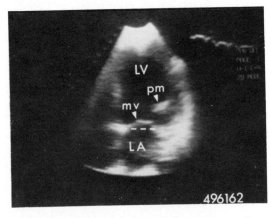

**Fig. 8–66.** Apical four-chamber echocardiogram of a patient with scarred papillary muscle and papillary muscle dysfunction. The papillary muscle (pm) is very echogenic, and during systole the mitral valve (mv) fails to reach the level of the mitral annulus (*dashed line*). LV = left ventricle; LA = left atrium.

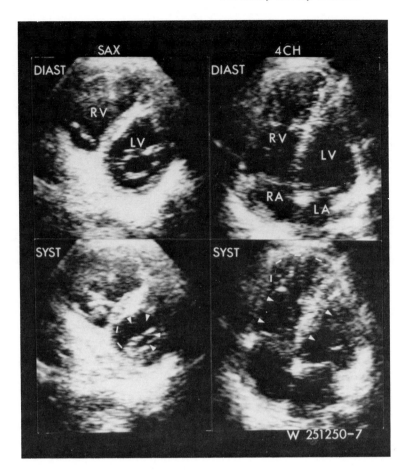

**Fig. 8–67.** Short-axis (SAX) and four-chamber (4CH) two-dimensional echocardiograms of a patient with an inferior myocardial infarction that is complicated by right ventricular infarction. The posterior-inferior wall is akinetic (*dashed line* SAX SYST). In addition, the apical half of the right ventricular free wall is akinetic (*dashed line* 4CH SYST). The right ventricle (RV) is also dilated. RA = right atrium; LV = left ventricle; LA = left atrium.

interrupting blood flow to the right ventricular branches as well as to the posterior descending coronary artery, which supplies the posterior-inferior wall of the left ventricle. The principal echocardiographic abnormalities noted with right ventricular infarction are abnormal motion of the right ventricular free wall[409–415] and right ventricular dilatation.[409,413,415–421] Figure 8–67 demonstrates short-axis and four-chamber views of a patient with an inferior myocardial infarction with involvement of the right ventricle. The typical posterior-inferior akinesis of the infarction can be seen in the short-axis view with akinesis in systole (*dashed line*). In the apical four-chamber view, the right ventricle is dilated, and, in systole, there is akinesis of the apical half of the right ventricle (*dashed line*).

Figure 8–68 shows a colorized regional wall echocardiogram of another patient with a right ventricular infarction. In the long-axis view (LX), one sees a normally functioning left ventricle. Rims of red represent left ventricular wall motion. The anterior right ventricular free wall, however, fails to move (*arrow*). The lack of a red rim identifies the right ventricular akinesis. The right ventricle is also dilated. The short-axis view shows the akinetic inferior segment of the left ventricle. In this case, the abnormal wall motion is subtle and barely visible (*arrow*). The four-chamber view again shows an akinetic right ventricular segment (*arrow*). Right ventricular dilatation is also noted. The two-chamber view

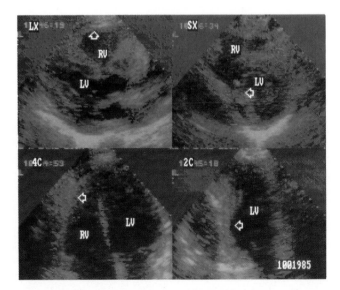

**Fig. 8–68.** Colorized regional wall display of a patient with a right ventricular myocardial infarction complicating an inferior infarction. The inferior wall abnormality can be seen in the two-chamber (2C) view in the basal inferior wall (*arrow*). The right ventricle (RV) is dilated in the four-chamber (4C) view. The long-axis (LX) and four-chamber (4C) examinations revealed that portions of the right ventricle fail to contract (no rim of red, *arrows*).

highlights the inferior infarction with akinesis (*arrow*) and hypokinesis of the basal inferior wall.

Aneurysm of the right ventricle has been noted echocardiographically.[409] As mentioned previously, thrombus in the right ventricle has also been detected.[418,422] Tricuspid regurgitation can be a complication of right ventricular infarction, and as a result abnormal interventricular septal motion may occur.[409] Right-to-left shunting through a probe patent foramen ovale has also been detected in patients with right ventricular infarction using contrast echocardiography.[423,424]

Besides the detection of right ventricular infarction, two-dimensional echocardiography can also demonstrate right ventricular free wall akinesis with exercise-induced ischemia.[425] Right atrial infarction has been detected with transesophageal echocardiography.[426] No Doppler evidence of right atrial contraction was recorded in this situation.

## EXAMINATION OF THE CORONARY ARTERIES

### Coronary Atherosclerosis

Although the primary value of echocardiography in patients with coronary artery disease is identifying myocardial abnormalities resulting from abnormal coronary artery blood flow, the ultrasonic technique can also be used to examine the coronary arteries directly.[427–435] Figure 8–69 demonstrates a transthoracic, short-axis two-dimensional study through the base of the heart demonstrating the left main (lm), the left circumflex (lcx), left anterior descending (lad), and diagonal (dg) arteries originating from the aorta (AO). Figure 8–70 depicts unusually large coronary arteries of a young adult with sickle cell disease. A normal right coronary artery can be seen in Figure 8–71. The curved nature of this artery usually does not permit it to be seen for any length in an individual frame. In Figure 8–71*A*, the origin of the right coronary artery (RCA) and the aorta (AO)

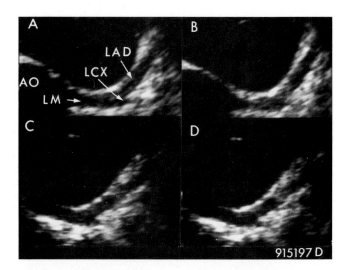

**Fig. 8–70.** Transthoracic examination of the left coronary artery in a patient with sickle cell disease. The patient has large, dilated coronary arteries. AO = aorta; LM = left main; LCX = left circumflex; LAD = left anterior descending. (From Feigenbaum, H.: Detection of coronary atherosclerosis by transthoracic echocardiography. *In* Echocardiography in Coronary Artery Disease. Edited by R.E. Kerber. Mt. Kisco, NY, Futura, 1988.)

are noted. The next frame (Fig. 8–71*B*) records the right coronary artery more distal to the aorta. Echograms in Fig. 8–71*C* and *D* demonstrate longer segments of the right coronary artery without identifying its connection with the aorta. Figure 8–72 shows normal left coronary arteries from the transesophageal approach. With this examination, the left circumflex artery is closer to the transducer than is the left anterior descending artery.

Figure 8–73 shows an example of a severely diseased left coronary artery. One can see "lumps and bumps" all along the walls of the arteries. This examination highlights the diffuse nature of this pathologic process. A

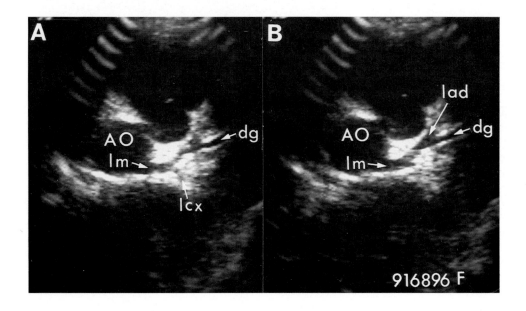

**Fig. 8–69.** Short-axis two-dimensional echocardiograms of a patient with a normal left coronary artery. AO = aorta; lm = left main coronary artery; lcx = left circumflex; dg = diagonal; lad = left anterior descending artery. (From Feigenbaum, H.: Echocardiography. *In* Heart Disease, 4th ed. Edited by E. Braunwald. Philadelphia, W.B. Saunders, Co., 1992.)

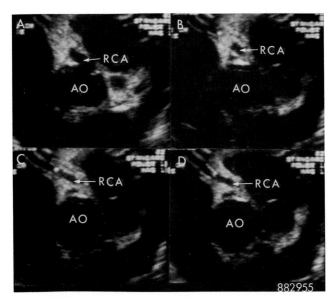

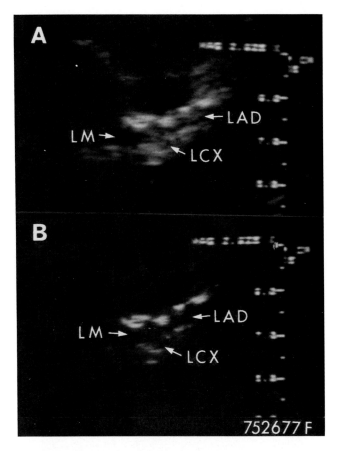

**Fig. 8–71.** Serial short-axis echocardiograms showing the right coronary artery (RCA) as it originates from the aorta (AO) and more distally (*B, C,* and *D*). (From Feigenbaum, H.: Detection of coronary atherosclerosis by transthoracic echocardiography. *In* Echocardiography in Coronary Artery Disease. Edited by R.E. Kerber. Mt. Kisco, NY, Futura, 1988.)

more isolated lesion in the left main coronary artery is demonstrated in Figure 8–74. The walls of the left main coronary artery are thickened and produce an obstruction (O) proximal to the origin of the left anterior descending (lad) and the left circumflex (lcx) arteries. Figure 8–75 shows a transesophageal echocardiographic recording of a patient with coronary artery disease.[436–438] In this case, the main pathologic lesion is at the junction between the left main (LM) and circumflex (CX) vessels. A smaller lesion is also visible within the circumflex artery. Color flow Doppler can be helpful by

**Fig. 8–73.** Transthoracic echocardiogram of the left coronary artery in a patient with diffuse, severe coronary artery disease. Multiple irregular echoes are noted on the walls of the left main (LM), the left anterior descending (LAD), and left circumflex (LCX) arteries. (From Feigenbaum, H.: Detection of coronary atherosclerosis by transthoracic echocardiography. *In* Echocardiography in Coronary Artery Disease. Edited by R.E. Kerber. Mt. Kisco, NY, Futura, 1988.)

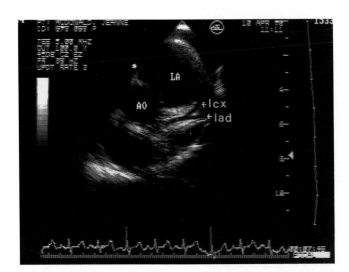

**Fig. 8–72.** Transesophageal echocardiogram of the proximal left coronary artery. LA = left atrium; AO = aorta; lcx = left circumflex; lad = left anterior descending.

demonstrating aliasing caused by acceleration of blood flow proximal to an obstructive lesion.[439–441a] This type of color flow Doppler examination of the coronary arteries is difficult with transthoracic echocardiography.

Although transthoracic and transesophageal echocardiography can demonstrate atherosclerotic lesions in the coronary arteries, the techniques are not widely used for this application. The transthoracic approach is technically demanding and depends on the instrument used. The transthoracic images demonstrated thus far were all obtained with a 5-MHz annular array transducer, which has a narrow beam. It takes this type of lateral resolution to visualize these small structures. Furthermore, the vessels are moving rapidly in and out of the examining plane. A digital recording, whereby one can isolate those frames that contain the artery, is also helpful.[435,442] One possible clinical application that may be useful is the differentiation between ischemic cardiomyopathy and idiopathic dilated cardiomyopathy.[442] These patients have a large heart, and the differential diagnosis is usually made with coronary angiography. If one is able to

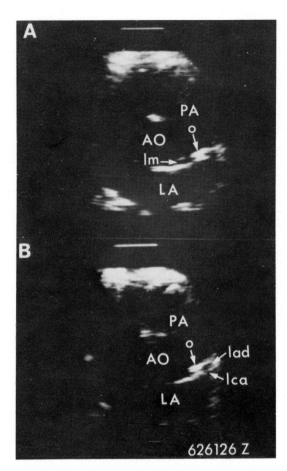

**Fig. 8–74.** Short-axis two-dimensional echocardiograms of a patient with atherosclerotic obstruction (o) just proximal to the bifurcation of the left main (lm) artery into its left anterior descending (lad) and left circumflex (lca) branches. AO = aorta; LA = left atrium; PA = pulmonary artery.

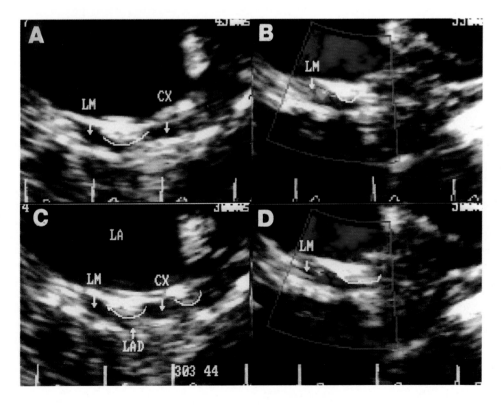

**Fig. 8–75.** Transesophageal echocardiogram of a patient with an obstructive lesion (*outline, A*) at the junction between the left main (LM) and the circumflex (CX) arteries. A second lesion (*outline, C*) is visible in the circumflex artery. Doppler flow (*B* and *D*) shows acceleration and aliasing in the left main artery proximal to the first stenotic lesion. LAD = left anterior descending.

visualize at least 2 cm of any coronary artery, the patient with ischemic cardiomyopathy should exhibit evidence of atherosclerosis. Because the probability is high that the arteries are diffusely diseased, a normal segment of coronary artery should exclude this possibility. The patients with idiopathic dilated cardiomyopathy will more likely have a completely normal arterial tree. Patients with cardiomyopathy are easier to examine transthoracically because the enlarged heart displaces the lung tissue that normally interferes with the coronary examination.

Despite the fact that the coronary arteries frequently are more easily visualized with the transesophageal approach,[443-445] this technique also has not achieved wide clinical popularity. Optimal visualization of the arteries is still somewhat limited, even with the biplane approach.[446] With the advent of omniplane transesophageal echocardiography, this situation may change.

Some investigators are using higher frequency transducers that are not commonly used in echocardiography. Linear array and curved array transducers, used primarily with peripheral vascular or abdominal ultrasonic examinations, have the advantage of using high frequencies, and thus have excellent resolution. Investigators have used a 7.5-MHz annual array transducer to visualize the middle and distal left anterior descending artery.[447,448] A high frequency linear array transducer can demonstrate internal mammary artery grafts.[449] Both imaging and Doppler techniques have been used in these examinations. Transesophageal echocardiography has also been used to visualize vein grafts.[450]

There is great interest in intracoronary ultrasonic visualization.[451-461a] Figure 8–76 shows an example of an intracoronary study in a patient with atherosclerosis in the left anterior descending coronary artery. The atherosclerotic disease is detected as a thickened, echogenic mass against the arterial wall (*arrows*). This technique provides exceptional visualization of coronary atherosclerosis. Data indicate that the ultrasonic approach is far more sensitive than routine coronary angiography.[452,462,462a] This examination has emphasized the diffuse nature of coronary atherosclerosis. Figure 8–77 shows varying degrees of coronary atherosclerosis as demonstrated by intravascular ultrasound.[463] Minimal atherosclerosis is noted in Figure 8–77A. One sees only a small thickening of the intima (*arrow*). More extensive intimal thickening is noted in Figure 8–77B. The cres-

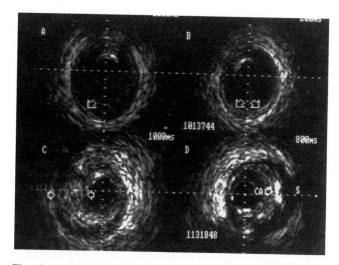

**Fig. 8–77.** Serial intracoronary ultrasonic images demonstrating different severities of coronary atherosclerosis: *A*, a small rim of thickened endothelium (*arrow*); *B*, larger amount of eccentric, endothelial thickening (*arrows*); *C*, a massive atherosclerotic plaque that is wider (*arrows*) than the residual lumen; *D*, calcification in the plaque (CA) produces shadowing (S).

cent-shaped intimal thickening can be seen on the posterior aspect of the artery (*arrows*). Extensive atherosclerosis is depicted in Figure 8–77C. The thick plaque (*arrows*) is actually larger than the residual lumen. Figure 8–77D shows calcification (CA) of an atherosclerotic plaque. As would be expected, shadowing (S) with loss of ultrasonic signal is seen behind the calcification.[464,465]

Various clinical applications have been suggested for this investigational technique.[463a-c] This examination is proving to be useful in the early detection of atherosclerosis in heart transplant patients.[466] Investigators are using intravascular ultrasound to monitor the effectiveness of coronary angioplasty,[464,467-474] especially atherectomy.[475-477a] Figure 8–78 shows an intravascular ultrasonic study of a patient before and after coronary atherectomy. The pre-atherectomy study (PRE) shows a thick atherosclerotic plaque (A). After the atherectomy, the bulk of the plaque is reduced (*arrows*). Intravascular ultrasound may prove useful in selecting which angioplasty catheter is proper for specific coronary lesions.

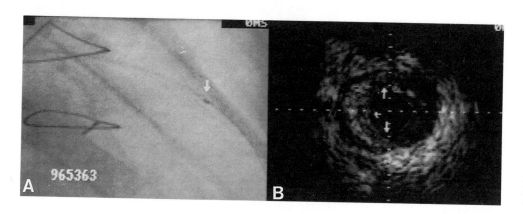

**Fig. 8–76.** Intracoronary ultrasonic examination with the ultrasonic device within the left anterior descending coronary artery. The location of the transducer (*arrow*) can be seen in the angiogram (*A*). The ultrasonic image (*B*) shows extensive atherosclerotic plaque (*arrows*) on the left hand side of the arterial wall.

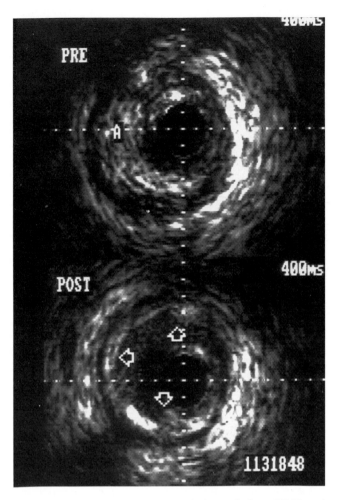

**Fig. 8–78.** Intracoronary ultrasonic image before (PRE) and after (POST) atherectomy and removal (*arrows*) of much of the pre-atherectomy atherosclerosis (A).

Because of the invasive and costly nature of this examination, widespread clinical applicability has yet to be determined. Ultrasonic devices with therapeutic features are being developed.[478,479] A catheter that has both a balloon and an ultrasonic transducer has been constructed for use in coronary angioplasty.[478]

Three-dimensional reconstruction of the intravascular ultrasonic examination enhances the display. Figure 8–79 shows how one can convert the two-dimensional intravascular ultrasonic examination into a three-dimensional display by pulling the catheter along the artery and continuously recording the images. In this patient, who has a coronary artery dissection and a stent, the three-dimensional display gives a dramatic demonstration of both the stent and the dissection flap within the coronary lumen. Unfortunately, there is some artifactual distortion with the three-dimensional reconstruction; the image suggests that the artery is straight when it in fact is curved.

Intraoperative epicardial echocardiography has been used to visualize the coronary arteries.[480–483,483a] This technique has been applied to judge the proper location and efficacy of bypass grafting.

Considerable interest has been generated in using Doppler techniques to investigate coronary blood flow. A small intracoronary Doppler transducer has been attached to a 3 French coronary artery guidewire for measuring coronary flow velocity (see Chapter 1).[484–495b] One way of using coronary flow velocity to investigate the coronary circulation is to assess coronary flow reserve. This measurement can be obtained by occluding a coronary artery and noting the hyperemic response. With normal circulation, after a 20-second coronary artery occlusion, the peak velocity will increase four to eight times.[484,486,487] One can also produce a hyperemic response by injecting a potent vasodilator, such as intracoronary papaverine or intravenous dipyridamole. Again, in a normal coronary artery, the peak velocity will increase four to eight times the resting value. A smaller increase would be indicative of abnormal coronary flow reserve and occurs with left ventricular hypertrophy or coronary atherosclerosis.

Investigators have also been looking at the timing of coronary flow for diagnostic clues of abnormal coronary circulation. Normal coronary flow primarily occurs during diastole. This diastolic predominance appears to be greater for the left coronary artery than for the right coronary artery.[487] Figure 8–80 shows Doppler velocity measurements proximal (*A*) and distal (*B*) to a 90% stenosis in the left anterior descending coronary artery.

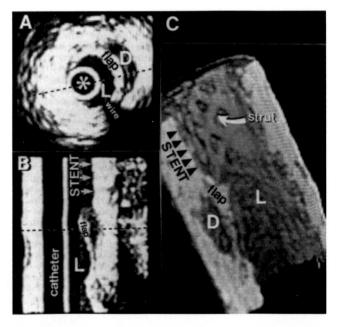

**Fig. 8–79.** Three-dimensional reconstruction of an intracoronary ultrasonic examination. The patient has a dissection (D) and an intracoronary stent inserted in the vessel. With three-dimensional reconstruction (*C*), a dramatic display of the struts of the stent can be appreciated. L = lumen. (Rosenfield, K., et al.: Three-dimensional reconstruction of human coronary artery and peripheral arteries from images recorded during two-dimensional intravascular ultrasound examination. *Circulation, 84*:1953, 1991, by permission of the American Heart Association.)

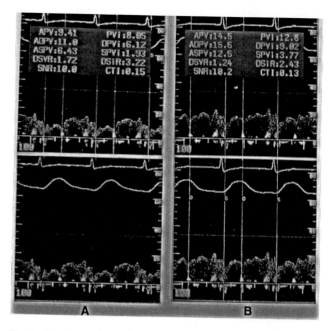
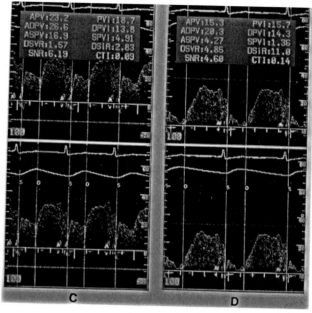

**Fig. 8–80.** Doppler velocity measurements using a Doppler tip catheter in the left anterior descending coronary artery proximal to a 90% stenosis (*A*) and distal to the stenosis (*B*). Normally, the diastolic velocity greatly exceeds the systolic velocity. Proximal to the obstruction, the diastolic velocity is only slightly higher than the systolic velocity, whereas distal to the obstruction, the two velocities are essentially equal. Two minutes after successful angioplasty (*C*), note a significant increase in the diastolic velocity and the diastolic/systolic velocity ratio. This difference is even greater 12 minutes after the angioplasty (*D*). The recording now resembles the normal coronary artery flow pattern. APV = time-averaged peak velocity; ADPV = average diastolic peak velocity; ASPV = average systolic peak velocity; DSVR = diastolic/systolic velocity ratio; SNR = signal to noise ratio; PVi = peak velocity integral; DPVi = diastolic peak velocity integral; SPVi = systolic peak velocity integral; DSiR = diastolic/systolic velocity integral ratio; CTI = peak tracing index. (From Segal, J., et al.: Alterations of phasic coronary artery flow velocity in humans during percutaneous coronary angioplasty. J. Am. Coll. Cardiol., *20*:276, 1992.)

These recordings demonstrate that proximal to the stenosis (Fig. 8–80*A*), the diastolic velocity is only slightly greater than the systolic velocity. Distal to the obstruction (Fig. 8–80*B*), the systolic and diastolic velocities are almost equal. After successful angioplasty, one can detect a substantial increase in diastolic velocity within 2 minutes (Fig. 8–80*C*). Twelve minutes after the angioplasty (Fig. 8–80*D*), the ratio between the diastolic and systolic velocities is large and the recording exhibits the usual normal coronary flow pattern.[489] Some investigators have noted that the ratio of systolic and diastolic coronary flow velocities can assist in the detection of coronary collateral flow using the Doppler guidewire technique.[492] Transthoracic[496,497] and transesophageal[498] Doppler recordings are also being used to measure coronary flow and flow reserve.

With the current interest in investigating the use of sonography to examine the coronary circulation, it is likely that echocardiography will play an increasingly important role in this aspect of coronary artery disease.

## KAWASAKI DISEASE

Although the echocardiographic examination of the coronary arteries was originally described for detecting atherosclerotic obstructive disease, a more generally accepted use of this examination is in patients with Kawasaki disease. This disease, which is also called mucocutaneous lymph node syndrome, has multiple coronary artery aneurysms as part of the syndrome. Although the disease is most common in Japan, it has been seen world-wide with increasing frequency. The reports of using two-dimensional echocardiography for detecting Kawasaki disease are numerous.[499–505]

Figures 8–82, 8–83, and 8–84 demonstrate a variety of coronary artery aneurysms that can be seen in this disease. This series of two-dimensional recordings not only shows the large number of aneurysms that can be detected with two-dimensional echocardiography, but also is an excellent means of locating the coronary arteries on two-dimensional echocardiographic examinations. Investigators studying this disease have developed many specialized echocardiographic views for visualizing almost the entire length of the major coronary arteries. Two-dimensional echocardiography is apparently an excellent technique for following these patients.[499] Although this problem has been seen primarily in children, cases of Kawasaki disease in adults have been reported.[506]

## CONGENITAL ANOMALIES OF THE CORONARY ARTERIES

Congenital malformations of the coronary arteries have been detected echocardiographically. The two major anomalies are fistulas and abnormal origin of the

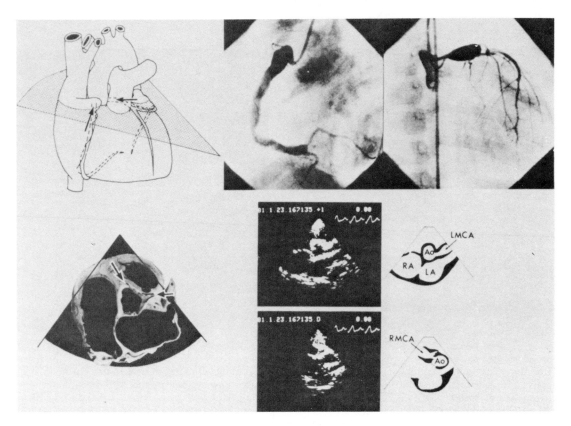

**Fig. 8–81.** Diagram, coronary angiograms, pathologic specimen, and two-dimensional echocardiograms of a patient with Kawasaki disease and aneurysms involving both the left main coronary artery (LMCA) and the right main coronary artery (RMCA). Ao = aorta; RA = right atrium; LA = left atrium. (From Satomi, G., et al.: Systematic visualization of coronary arteries by two-dimensional echocardiography in children and infants: Evaluation in Kawasaki's disease and coronary arteriovenous fistulas. Am. Heart J., *107*:497, 1984.)

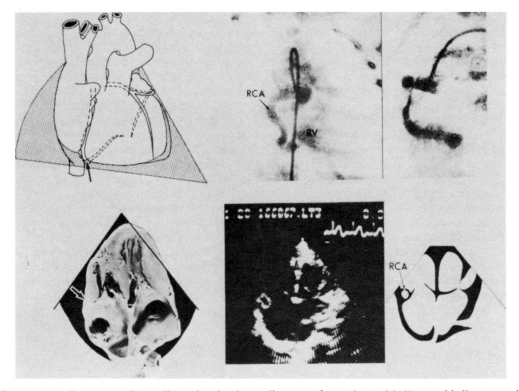

**Fig. 8–82.** Coronary angiograms and two-dimensional echocardiogram of a patient with Kawasaki disease and an aneurysm of the right coronary artery (RCA). The aneurysm is noted in the apical four-chamber view. (From Satomi, G., et al.: Systematic visualization of coronary arteries by two-dimensional echocardiography in children and infants: Evaluation in Kawasaki's disease and coronary arteriovenous fistulas. Am. Heart J., *107*:497, 1984.)

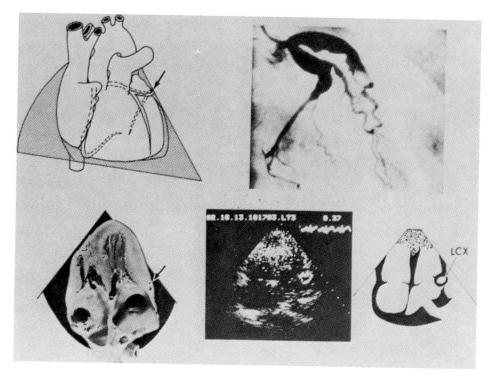

**Fig. 8–83.** Coronary arteriogram and two-dimensional echocardiogram of a patient with Kawasaki disease and aneurysmal dilatation of the left circumflex (LCX) artery. The aneurysm is noted in the apical four-chamber view along the lateral free wall between the left ventricle and the left atrium (*arrow*). (From Satomi, G., et al.: Systematic visualization of coronary arteries by two-dimensional echocardiography in children and infants: Evaluation in Kawasaki's disease and coronary arteriovenous fistulas. Am. Heart J., *107*:497, 1984.)

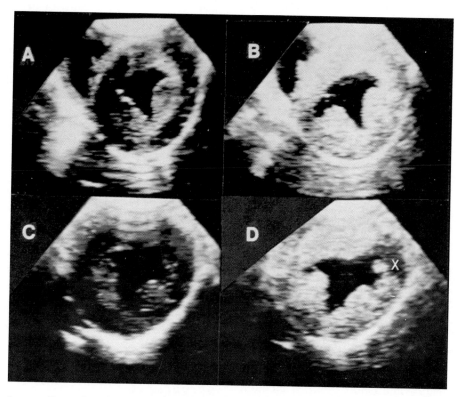

**Fig. 8–84.** Short-axis two-dimensional echocardiograms of a dog demonstrating the ability of contrast echocardiography to detect abnormalities of myocardial perfusion. Prior to ligation of a coronary artery (*A* and *B*), injection of contrast material in the root of the aorta produces a fairly uniform distribution of echoes within the myocardium. Following ligation of the coronary artery (*C* and *D*), the same injection produces a significant echo-free area (X) that corresponds to the site of the myocardial infarction.

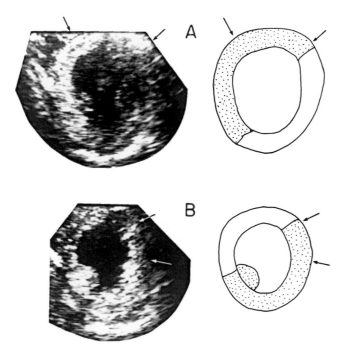

**Fig. 8–85.** Myocardial contrast study of a patient with an occluded left anterior descending (LAD) coronary artery and collateral fill from the right coronary artery. Injection of contrast material into the right coronary artery (RCA) (*A*) enhances the LAD distribution (*arrows*) through collaterals from the RCA. Injection of contrast material into the left main coronary artery (*B*) reveals the LAD bed (*arrows*) supplied by collaterals from the left circumflex. (From Sabia, P.J., et al.: Functional significance of collateral blood flow in patients with recent acute myocardial infarction: A study using myocardial contrast echocardiography. Circulation, *85*:2083, 1992, by permission of the American Heart Association, Inc.)

coronary arteries. These topics have already been covered in Chapter 7, Congenital Heart Disease.

## MYOCARDIAL PERFUSION USING CONTRAST ECHOCARDIOGRAPHY

The use of contrast echocardiography for assessing myocardial perfusion has been investigated for many years.[507–521] In this type of examination, contrast material is injected either into the root of the aorta or selectively into a coronary artery.[522] A variety of different contrast agents have been used with fairly similar results. Renewed interest in this application is stimulated by new commercially developed contrast agents, many of which pass through capillaries.[523] Figure 8–84 shows an animal experiment using the contrast myocardial perfusion technique before and after tying off a coronary artery. The short-axis two-dimensional echocardiogram prior to coronary ligation and before contrast medium is injected is shown in Figure 8–85A. With the introduction of contrast material, the myocardium becomes echogenic (*B*). The echogenicity is fairly uniform except for a small area at about 7 o'clock. The decrease in echoes may in part be a shadowing effect, because there

is also some loss of echoes posterior to that area. The post-coronary ligation echocardiograms are seen in Figure 8–83C and D. With the contrast injection, a new echo-free area (X) is visible in that portion of the myocardium served by the obstructed coronary artery. The ability to use this technique for detecting a totally obstructed coronary artery and the size of the resultant infarction is well documented.[507,513] Several techniques have been suggested for assessing perfusion in partially occluded arteries. Arrival time, washout curves, and peak intensity of the contrast material have provided reasonable results.[524–530] Vasodilators have been used with myocardial contrast echocardiography.[531,532] Reperfusion hyperemia has also been studied with this technique.[533] Investigators also use this approach to evaluate coronary flow reserve.[534]

Clinical applications for this use of contrast echocardiography have been studied in many laboratories. Because of the need to inject contrast medium directly in the coronary arteries or in the aortic root, this technique has been relegated to the cardiac catheterization laboratory[535] or the operating room. Under these situations, contrast echocardiography has proved to be valuable in assessing myocardial perfusion before and after reperfusion with either angioplasty[536–540] or bypass surgery.[541–543] The technique is proving to be useful in assessing the role and function of collateral vessels.[544–547] For example, Figure 8–85 shows an echocardiogram with injection of contrast material into the right coronary artery (*A*) of a patient with an occluded left anterior descending artery. The left anterior descending segments (*arrows*) are enhanced with contrast material from collaterals. Injecting contrast agents into the left main coronary artery (*B*) lights up more of the anterior descending myocardium from left circumflex collaterals. Some experimental data show that after thrombolysis, viable muscle will be enhanced with contrast material whereas nonviable myocardium will not.[548] Investigators are also examining the transmural distribution of contrast medium.[549]

Research in this area is active and new developments are appearing. A variety of digital techniques are being used to enhance the detection and quantitation of myocardial perfusion.[537] Investigators are looking at the gray levels and using digital subtraction approaches. Probably the greatest hope is the ability to use an intravenous injection of contrast material to visualize myocardial perfusion. With the use of new contrast agents that transverse capillaries comes some reason for optimism. To date, however, visualization of the myocardium after an intravenous injection is extremely faint, and even with computer enhancement, perfusion is difficult to detect.

## REFERENCES

1. Katz, A.S., Harrigan, P., and Parisi, A.F.: The value and promise of echocardiography in acute myocardial infarction and coronary artery disease. Clin. Cardiol., *15*:401, 1992.

2. Stefan, G. and Bing, R.J.: Echocardiographic findings in experimental myocardial infarction of the posterior left ventricular wall. Am. J. Cardiol., *30*:629, 1972.

3. Kerber, R.E., Marcus, M.L., Ehrhardt, J., Wilson, R., and Abboud, F.M.: Correlation between echocardiographically demonstrated segmental dyskinesis and regional myocardial perfusion. Circulation, *52*:1097, 1975.

4. Kerber, R.E. and Abboud, F.M.: Echocardiographic detection of regional myocardial infarction. Circulation, *47*:997, 1973.

5. Kerber, R.E., Marcus, M.L., Wilson, R., Ehrhardt, J., and Abboud, F.M.: Effects of acute coronary occlusion on the motion and perfusion of the normal and ischemic interventricular septum. Circulation, *54*:928, 1976.

6. Pezzano, A., Faletra, F., and Scarpini, S.: Echocardiographic evaluation during percutaneous transluminal coronary angioplasty. Cardiovasc. Imag., *1*:13, 1989.

7. Wohlgelernter, D., Jaffe, C.C., Cabin, H.S., Yeatman, L.A., and Cleman, M.: Silent ischemia during coronary occlusion produced by balloon inflation: Relation to regional myocardial dysfunction. J. Am. Coll. Cardiol., *10*:491, 1987.

8. Akasaka, T., Yoshikawa, J., Yoshida, K., Kato, H., Okumachi, F., Koizumi, K., Shiratori, K., Takao, S., Asaka, T., Shakudo, M., and Shono, H.: Mechanical and electrocardiographic sequence of coronary artery occlusion: An echocardiographic study during coronary angioplasty. J. Cardiogr., *16*:819, 1986.

9. Jacobs, J.J., Feigenbaum, H., Corya, B.C., and Phillips, J.F.: Detection of left ventricular asynergy by echocardiography. Circulation, *48*:263, 1973.

10. Weiss, J.L., Bulkley, B.H., Hutchins, G.M., and Mason, S.J.: Two dimensional echocardiographic recognition of myocardial injury in man: Comparison with postmortem studies. Circulation, *63*:401, 1981.

11. Gallagher, K.P., Kumada, T., Koziol, J.A., McKown, M.D., Kemper, W.S., and Ross, J.: Significance of regional wall thickening abnormalities relative to transmural myocardial perfusion in anesthetized dogs. Circulation, *62*:1266, 1980.

12. Traill, T.A.: Wall thickness changes considered as regional myocardial function in ischemic heart disease. Herz, *5*:275, 1980.

13. Torry, R.J., Myers, J.H., Adler, A.L., Liut, C.L., and Gallagher, K.P.: Effects of nontransmural ischemia on inner and outer wall thickening in the canine left ventricle. Am. Heart J., *122*:1292, 1991.

14. Pandian, N.G., Kieso, R.A., and Kerber, R.E.: Two dimensional echocardiography in experimental coronary stenosis. II. Relationship between systolic wall thinning and regional myocardial perfusion in severe coronary stenosis. Circulation, *66*:603, 1982.

15. Guth, B.D., White, F.C., Gallagher, K.P., and Bloor, C.M.: Decreased systolic wall thickening in myocardium adjacent to ischemic zones in conscious swine during brief coronary artery occlusion. Am. Heart J., *107*:458, 1984.

16. Charlat, M.L., O'Neill, P.G., Hartley, C.J., Roberts, R., and Bolli, R.: Prolonged abnormalities of left ventricular diastolic wall thinning in the "stunned" myocardium in conscious dogs: Time course and relation to systolic function. J. Am. Coll. Cardiol., *13*:185, 1989.

17. Weyman, A.E., Franklin, T.D., Hogan, R.D., Gillam, L.D., Wiske, P.S., Newell, J., Gibbons, E.F., and Foale, R.A.: Importance of temporal heterogeneity in assessing the contraction abnormalities associated with acute myocardial ischemia. Circulation, *70*:102, 1984.

18. Haendchen, R.V., Wyatt, H.L., Maurer, G., Zwehl, W., Bear, M., Meerbaum, S., and Corday, E.: Quantitation of regional cardiac function by two dimensional echocardiography. I. Patterns of contraction in the normal left ventricle. Circulation, *67*:1234, 1983.

19. Zeiher, A.M., Wollschlaeger, H., Bonzel, T., Kasper, W., and Just, H.: Hierarchy of levels of ischemia-induced impairment in regional left ventricular systolic function in man. Circulation, *76*:768, 1987.

20. Ross, J.: Assessment of ischemic regional myocardial dysfunction and its reversibility. Circulation, *74*:1186, 1986.

21. Takahashi, H., Bekki, H., Koga, Y., Utsu, F., Nagata, H., Itaya, M., Ohkita, Y., Itaya, K., Yoshioka, H., and Toshima, H.: Exercise two dimensional echocardiography: Correlation between exercise induced asynergy and coronary artery lesions. J. Cardiogr., *12*:347, 1982.

22. Stamm, R.B., Gibson, R.S., Bishop, H.L., Carabello, B.A., Beller, G.A., and Martin, R.P.: Echocardiographic detection of infarction: Correlation with the extent of angiographic coronary disease. Circulation, *67*:233, 1983.

23. Assmann, P.E., Slager, C.J., van der Borden, S.G., Dreysse, S.T., Tijssen, J.G.P., Sutherland, G.R., and Roelandt, J.R.: Quantitative echocardiographic analysis of global and regional left ventricular function: A problem revisited. J. Am. Soc. Echocardiogr., *3*:478, 1990.

24. Assmann, P.E., Slager, C.J., van der Borden, S.G., Sutherland, D.R., and Roelandt, J.R.: Reference systems in echocardiographic quantitative wall motion analysis with registration of respiration. J. Am. Soc. Echocardiogr., *4*:224, 1991.

25. Bourdillon, P.D.V., Broderick, T.M., Sawada, S.G., Armstrong, W.F., Ryan, T., Dillon, J.C., Fineberg, N.S., and Feigenbaum, H.: Regional wall motion index for infarct and noninfarct regions after reperfusion in acute myocardial infarction: Comparison with global wall motion index. J. Am. Soc. Echocardiogr., *2*:398, 1989.

26. Rifkin, R.D. and Koito, H.: Comparison with radionuclide angiography of two new geometric and four nongeometric models for echocardiographic estimation of left ventricular ejection fraction using segmental wall motion scoring. Am. J. Cardiol., *65*:1485, 1990.

27. Segar, D.S., Brown, S.E., Sawada, S.G., Ryan, T., and Feigenbaum, H.: Dobutamine stress echocardiography: Correlation with coronary lesion severity as determined by quantitative angiography. J. Am. Coll. Cardiol., *19*:1197, 1992.

28. Buda, A.J., Lefkowitz, C.A., and Gallagher, K.P.: Augmentation of regional function in nonischemic myocardium during coronary occlusion measured with two-dimensional echocardiography. J. Am. Coll. Cardiol, *16*:175, 1990.

29. Verani, M.S., Bolli, R., Tadros, S., Myers, M.L., Neto, S.B., Jain, A., Phillips, L., and Roberts, R.: Dissociation between global and regional systolic and disastolic ventricular function during coronary occlusion and reperfusion. Am. Heart J., *114*:687, 1987.

30. Guyer, D.E., Goale, R.A., Gillam, L.D., Wilkins, G.T., Guerrero, J.L., and Weyman, A.E.: An echocardiographic technique for quantifying and displaying the extent of regional left ventricular dyssynergy. J. Am. Coll. Cardiol., *8*:830, 1986.

31. Gillam, L.D., Franklin, T.D., Foale, R.A., Wiske, P.S., Guyer, D.E., Hogan, R.D., and Weyman, A.E.: The natural history of regional wall motion in the acutely infarcted canine ventricle. J. Am. Coll. Cardiol., *7*:1325, 1986.

32. Heger, J.J., Weyman, A.E., Wann, L.S., Rogers, E.W., Dillon, J.C., and Feigenbaum, H.: Cross-sectional echocardiographic analysis of the extent of left ventricular asynergy in acute myocardial infarction. Circulation, *61*: 1113, 1980.

33. Parisi, A.F., Moynihan, P.F., Folland, E.D., and Feldman, C.L.: Quantitative detection of regional left ventricular contraction abnormalities by two dimensional echocardiography. II. Accuracy in coronary artery disease. Circulation, *63*:761, 1981.

34. Sawada, H., Fujii, J., Kuboki, M., Watanabe, H., Aizawa, T., Ota, A., Kato, K., Onoe, M., and Kuno, Y.: Computer analysis of two dimensional echocardiogram for the quantitative evaluation of left ventricular asynergy in myocardial infarction. J. Cardiogr., *12*:65, 1982.

35. O'Boyle, J.E., Parisi, A.F., Nieminen, M., Kloner, R.A., and Khuri, S.: Quantitative detection of regional left ventricular contraction abnormalities by two dimensional echocardiography. Am. J. Cardiol., *51*:1732, 1983.

36. Fujii, J., Sawada, H., Aizawa, T., Kato, K., Onoe, M., and Kuno, Y.: Computer analysis of cross sectional echocardiogram for quantitative evaluation of left ventricular asynergy in myocardial infarction. Br. Heart J., *51*:139, 1984.

37. Schnittger, I., Fitzgerald, P.J., Gordon, E.P., Alderman, E.L., and Popp, R.L.: Computerized quantitative analysis of left ventricular wall motion by two dimensional echocardiography. Circulation, *70*:242, 1984.

38. Moynihan, P.F., Parisi, A.F., and Feldman, C.L.: Quantitative detection of regional left ventricular contraction abnormalities by two dimensional echocardiography. I. Analysis of methods. Circulation, *63*:752, 1981.

39. Clayton, P.D., Jeppson, G.M., and Klausner, S.C.: Should a fixed external reference system be used to analyze left ventricular wall motion? Circulation, *65*:1518, 1982.

40. Zoghbi, W.A., Charlat, M.L., Bolli, R., Zhu, W-X., Hartley, C.J., and Quinones, M.A.: Quantitative assessment of left ventricular wall motion by two-dimensional echocardiography: Validation during reversible ischemia in the conscious dog. J. Am. Coll. Cardiol., *11*:851, 1988.

41. McGillem, M.J., Mancini, J., DeBoe, S.F., and Buda, A.J.: Modification of the centerline method for assessment of echocardiographic wall thickening and motion: A comparison with areas of risk. J. Am. Coll. Cardiol., *11*:861, 1988.

42. Sheehan, F.H., Bolson, E.L., Dodge, H.T., Mathey, D.G., Schofer, J., and Woo, H-W.: Advantages and applications of the centerline method for characterizing regional ventricular function. Circulation, *74*:293, 1986.

43. D'Cruz, I.A., Lalmalani, G.G., Sambasivan, V., Cohen, H.C., and Glick, G.: The superiority of mitral E point-ventricular septum separation to other echocardiographic indicators of left ventricular performance. Clin. Cardiol., *2*:140, 1979.

44. Shea, P.M., Glover, M.U., Handler, J.B., Nelson, D.P., and Vieweg, W.V.R.: Novolumetric assessment of ventricular function by two dimensional echocardiography in patients with coronary artery disease. JCU, *11*:415, 1983.

45. Erbel, R., Schweizer, P., Meyer, J., Grenner, H., Krebs, W., and Effert, S.: Left ventricular volume and ejection fraction determination by cross-sectional echocardiography in patients with coronary artery disease: A prospective study. Clin. Cardiol., *3*:377, 1980.

46. Van Reet, R.E., Quinones, M.A., Poliner, L.R., Nelson, J.G., Waggoner, A.D., Kanon, D., Lubetkin, S.J., Pratt, C.M., and Winters, W.L.: Comparison of two dimensional echocardiography with gated radionuclide ventriculography in the evaluation of global and regional left ventricular function in acute myocardial infarction. J. Am. Coll. Cardiol., *3*:243, 1984.

47. Kan, G., Visser, C.A., Lie, K.I., and Durrer, D.: Measurement of left ventricular ejection fraction after acute myocardial infarction. A serial cross-sectional echocardiographic study. Br. Heart J., *51*:631, 1984.

48. Charuzi, Y., Davidson, R.M., Barrett, M.J., Beeder, C., Marshall, L.A., Loh, I.K., Prause, J.A., Meerbaum, S., and Corday, E.: Simultaneous assessment of segmental and global left ventricular function by two dimensional echocardiography in acute myocardial infarction. Clin. Cardiol., *6*:255, 1983.

49. Ryan, T., Petrovic, O., Armstrong, W.F., and Feigenbaum, H.: Quantitative two-dimensional echocardiographic assessment of patients undergoing left ventricular aneurysmectomy. Am. Heart J., *111*:714, 1986.

50. Konecke, L.L., Feigenbaum, H., Chang, S., Corya, B.C., and Fischer, J.C.: Abnormal mitral valve motion in patients with elevated left ventricular diastolic pressures. Circulation, *47*:989, 1973.

51. Corya, B.C., Rasmussen, S., Knoebel, S.B., and Feigenbaum, H.: Echocardiography in acute myocardial infarction. Am. J. Cardiol., *36*:1, 1975.

52. Corya, B.C., Rasmussen, S., Knoebel, S.B., and Feigenbaum, H.: M-mode echocardiography in evaluating left ventricular function and surgical risk in patients with coronary artery disease. Chest, *72*:181, 1977.

53. Dillon, J.C., Feigenbaum, H., Weyman, A.E., Corya, B.C., Peskoe, S., and Chang, S.: M-mode echocardiography in the evaluation of patients for aneurysmectomy. Circulation, *53*:657, 1976.

54. Shiotani, K., Sagara, T., Sugihara, M., Yamashita, K., Nawata, Y., Torii, S., Nishimoto, S., and Kawahira, K.: Echocardiographic evaluation of the prognosis during acute phase of myocardial infarction: Comparison with Te pyrophosphate and Tl chloride myocardial imagings. J. Cardiogr., *9*:285, 1979.

55. Saito, T.: Non-invasive assessment of left ventricular function and prognosis in acute myocardial infarction—clinical significance of B-B' step of the mitral valve in M-mode echocardiography. Jpn. Circ. J., *46*:1045, 1982.

56. Kondo, K., Shiina, A., Tsuchiya, M., Suzuki, H., Yaginuma, T., and Hosoda, S.: Hemodynamic significance of the A/E ratio and B-B' formation on the mitral valve echogram in patients with myocardial infarction. J. Cardiogr., *12*:861, 1982.

57. Koolen, J.J., Visser, C.A., David, G.K., Hoedemaker, G., Bot, H., van Wezel, H.B., and Dunning, A.J.: Transesophageal echocardiographic assessment of systolic and diastolic dysfunction during percutaneous transluminal coronary angioplasty. J. Am. Soc. Echocardiogr., *3*:374, 1990.

58. deBruyne, B., Lerch, R., Meier, B., Schlaepfer, H., Gabathuler, J., and Rutishauser, W.: Doppler assessment of left ventricular diastolic filling during brief coronary occlusion. Am. Heart J., *117*:629, 1989.

59. Humphrey, L.S., Topol, E.J., Rosenfeld, G.I., Borkon, A.M., Baumgartner, W.A., Gardner, T.J., Maruschak, G., and Weiss, J.L.: Immediate enhancement of left ventricular relaxation by coronary artery bypass grafting: Intraoperative assessment. Circulation, *77*:886, 1988.

60. Williamson, B.D., Lim, M.J., and Buda, A.J.: Transient left ventricular filling abnormalities (diastolic stunning

after acute myocardial infarction). Am. J. Cardiol., 66: 897, 1990.

61. Mathias, D.W., Wann, L.S., Sagar, K.B., and Klopfenstein, H.S.: The effect of regional myocardial ischemia on Doppler echocardiographic indexes of left ventricular performance: Influence of heart rate, aortic blood pressure, and the size of the ischemic zone. Am. Heart J., 116:953, 1988.

62. Oh, J.K., Ding, Z.P., Gersh, B.J., Bailey, K.R., and Tajik, A.J.: Restrictive left ventricular diastolic filling identifies patients with heart failure after acute myocardial infarction. J. Am. Soc. Echocardiogr., 5:497, 1992.

62a. Pipilis, A., Meyer, T.E., Ormerod, O., Flather, M., and Sleight, P.: Early and late changes in left ventricular filling after acute myocardial infarction and the effect of infarct size. Am. J. Cardiol., 70:1397, 1992.

63. Garrahy, P.J., Kwan, O.L., Booth, D.C., and DeMaria, A.N.: Assessment of abnormal systolic intraventricular flow patterns by Doppler imaging in a patient with left ventricular dyssynergy. Circulation, 82:95, 1990.

64. Chenzbraun, A., Keren, A., and Stern, S.: Doppler echocardiographic pattern of left ventricular filling in patients early after acute myocardial infarction. Am. J. Cardiol., 70:711, 1992.

65. Beppu, S., Izumi, S., Miyatake, K., Nagata, S., Park, Y-D., Sakakibara H., and Nimura, Y.: Abnormal blood pathways in left ventricular cavity in acute myocardial infarction. Circulation, 78:157, 1988.

66. Pennestri, F., Biasucci, L.M., Rinelli, G., Mongiardo, R., Lombardo, A., Rossi, E., Amico, C.M., Aquilina, O., and Loperfido, F.: Abnormal intraventricular flow patterns in left ventricular dysfunction determined by color Doppler study. Am. Heart J., 124:966, 1992.

67. Mason, S.J., Weiss, J.L., Weisfeldt, M.L., Garrison, J.B., and Fortuin, N.J.: Exercise echocardiography: Detection of wall motion abnormalities during ischemia. Circulation, 59:50, 1979.

68. Wann, L.S., Faris, J.V., Childress R.H., Dillon, J.C. Weyman, A.E., and Feigenbaum, H.: Exercise cross-sectional echocardiography in ischemic heart disease. Circulation, 60:1300, 1979.

69. Morganroth, J., Chen, C.C., David, D., Sawin, H.S., Naito, M., Parrotto, C., and Meixell, L.: Exercise cross-sectional echocardiographic diagnosis of coronary artery disease. Am. J. Cardiol., 47:20, 1981.

70. Maurer, G. and Nanda, N.C.: Two dimensional echocardiographic evaluation of exercise-induced left and right ventricular asynergy: Correlation with thallium scanning. Am. J. Cardiol., 48:720, 1981.

71. Mitamura, H., Ogawa, S., Hori, S., Yamazaki, H., Handa, S., and Nakamura, Y.: Two dimensional echocardiographic analysis of wall motion abnormalities during handgrip exercise in patients with coronary artery disease. Am. J. Cardiol., 48:711, 1981.

72. Crawford, M.H., Petru, M.A., Amon, W., Sorensen, S.G., and Vance, W.S.: Comparative value of two dimensional echocardiography and radionuclide angiography for quantitating changes in left ventricular performance during exercise limited by angina pectoris. Am. J. Cardiol., 53:42, 1984.

73. Takenaka, K., Sakamoto, T., Inoue, H., Amano, K., Hada, Y., Yamaguchi, T., Ishimitsu, T., Uchiyama, I., Kawahara, T., Murayama, M., Mashima, S., and Murao, S.: Pacing echocardiography: Regional wall motion, left ventricular dimension and R wave amplitude in patients with angina pectoris. Jpn. Heart J., 23:1, 1982.

74. Takahashi, H., Koga, Y., Itaya, M., Nagata, H., Itaya, K., Ohkita, Y., Bekki, H., Jinnouchi, J., Utsu, F., and Toshima, H.: Detection of exercise-induced left ventricular asynergy by two dimensional echocardiography. J. Cardiogr., 11:1193, 1981.

75. Gondi, B. and Nanda, N.C.: Cold pressor test during two dimensional echocardiography: Usefulness in detection of patients with coronary disease. Am. Heart J., 107:278, 1984.

76. Limacher, M.C., Quinones, M.A., Polner, L.R., Nelson, J.G., Winters, Jr., W.L., and Waggoner, A.D.: Detection of coronary artery disease with exercise two dimensional echocardiography. Circulation, 67:1211, 1983.

77. Robertson, W.S., Feigenbaum, H., Armstrong, W.F., Dillon, J.C., O'Donnell, J., and McHenery, P.W.: Exercise echocardiography: A clinically practical addition in the evaluation of coronary artery disease. J. Am. Coll. Cardiol., 2:1085, 1983.

78. Marwick, T.H., Nemec, J.J., Pashkow, F.J., Stewart, W.J., and Salcedo, E.E.: Accuracy and limitations of exercise echocardiography in a routine clinical setting. J. Am. Coll. Cardiol., 19:74, 1992.

79. Armstrong, W.F.: Exercise echocardiography: Phase II, convincing the skeptics. J. Am. Coll. Cardiol., 1:82, 1992.

79a. Mertes, H., Erbel, R., Nixdorff, U., Mohr-Kahaly, S., Wolfinger, D., and Meyer, J.: Stress echocardiography: A sensitive method for the detection of coronary artery disease. Herz, 16:355, 1991.

80. Agati, L., Arata, L., Luongo, R., Iacoboni, C., Renzi, M., Vizza, C.D., Penco, M., Fedele, F., and Dagianti, A.: Assessment of severity of coronary narrowings by quantitative exercise echocardiography and comparison with quantitative arteriography. Am. J. Cardiol., 67: 1201, 1991.

81. Oberman, A., Fan, P-H., Nanda, N.C., Lee, J.Y., Huster, W.J., Sulentic, J.A., and Storey, O.F.: Reproducibility of two-dimensional exercise echocardiography. J. Am. Coll. Cardiol., 14:923, 1989.

82. Marwick, T.H., Nemec, J.J., Torelli, J., Salcedo, E.E., and Stewart, W.J.: Extent and severity of abnormal left ventricular wall motion detected by exercise echocardiography during painful and silent ischemia. Am. J. Cardiol., 69:1483, 1992.

83. Ajisaka, R.: Role of exercise echocardiography as a predictor of coronary artery disease. Detection of exercise-induced asynergy by M-mode echocardiography. Jpn. Heart J., 24:161, 1983.

84. Fedele, F., Arata, L., Giannico, S., Oastore, L.R., DiRenzi, L., Penco, M., Agati, L., and Dagianti, A.: Echocardiography during ergometric tests in subjects with stable effort angina (author's transl.) G. Ital. Cardiol., 11:310, 1981.

85. Hecht, H.S., et al.: Digital supine bicycle stress echocardiography: A new technique for evaluating coronary artery disease. J. Am. Coll. Cardiol., 21:950, 1993.

86. Ginzton, L.E., Conant, R., Brizendine, M., Lee, F., Mena, I., and Laks, M.M.: Exercise subcostal two dimensional echocardiography: A new method of segmental wall motion analysis. Am. J. Cardiol., 53:805, 1984.

87. Presti, C.F., Armstrong, W.F., and Feigenbaum, H.: Comparison of echocardiography at peak exercise and after bicycle exercise in evaluation of patients with known or suspected coronary artery disease. J. Am. Soc. Echocardiogr., 1:119, 1988.

88. Crouse, L.J., Harbrecht, J.J., Vacek, J.L., Rosamond, T. L., and Kramer, P.H.: Exercise echocardiography as a screening test for coronary artery disease and correla-

tion with coronary arteriography. Am. J. Cardiol., *67*: 1213, 1991.

89. Sheikh, K.H., Bengtson, J.R., Helmy, S., Juarez, C., Burgess, R., Bashore, T.M., and Kisslo, J.: Relation of quantitative coronary lesion measurements to the development of exercise-induced ischemia assessed by exercise echocardiography. J. Am. Coll. Cardiol., *15*:1043, 1990.

90. Homans, D.C., Laxson, D.D., Sublett, E., Pavek, T., and Crampton, M.: Effect of exercise intensity and duration on regional function during and after exercise-induced ischemia. Circulation, *83*:2029, 1991.

91. Kloner, R.A., Allen, J., Cox, T.A., Zheng, Y., and Ruiz, C.E.: Stunned left ventricular myocardium after exercise treadmill testing in coronary artery disease. Am. J. Cardiol., *68*:329, 1991.

92. Athanasopoulos, G., Marsonis, A., Joshi, J., Oakley, C.M., and Nihoyannopoulos, P.: Significance of delayed recovery after digital exercise echocardiography. Br. Heart J., *66*:104, 1991.

93. About-Enein, H., Bengtson, J.R., Adams, D.B., Mostafa, M.A., Ibrahim, M.M., Hifny, A.A., and Sheikh, K.H.: Effect of the degree of effort on exercise echocardiography for the detection of restenosis after coronary artery angioplasty. Am. Heart J., *122*:430, 1991.

94. Feigenbaum, H.: Exercise echocardiography. J. Am. Soc. Echocardiogr., *1*:161, 1988.

95. Armstrong, W.F., O'Donnell, J., Dillon, J.C., McHenry, P.L., Morris, S.N., and Feigenbaum, H.: Complementary value of two-dimensional exercise echocardiography to routine treadmill exercise testing. Ann. Intern. Med., *105*:829, 1986.

96. Ryan, T., Segar, D.S., Sawada, S.G., Foltz, J., O'Donnell, J.A., and Feigenbaum, H.: Additive value of echocardiography to exercise electrocardiography for the detection of myocardial ischemia. Circulation, *86*:I-384, 1992 (Abstract).

97. Hayashi, K., Dote, K., Sunaga, Y., Sugiura, T., Iwasaka, T., and Inada, M.: Evaluation of preload reserve during isometric exercise testing in patients with old myocardial infarction: Doppler echocardiographic study. J. Am. Coll. Cardiol., *17*:106, 1991.

98. Ferrara, N., Vigorito, C., Leosco, D., Giordano, A., Abete, P., Longobardi, G., and Rengo, F.: Regional left ventricular mechanical function during isometric exercise in patients with coronary artery disease: Correlation with regional coronary blood flow changes. J. Am. Coll. Cardiol., *12*:1215, 1988.

99. Dawson, J.R. and Gibson, D.G.: Regional left ventricular wall motion in pacing induced angina. Br. Heart J., *59*: 309, 1988.

100. Iliceto, S., Amico, A., Marangelli, V., D'Ambrosio, G., and Rizzon, P.: Doppler echocardiographic evaluation of the effect of atrial pacing-induced ischemia on left ventricular filling in patients with coronary artery disease. J. Am. Coll. Cardiol., *11*:953, 1988.

101. Whitfield, S., Aurigemma, G., Pape, L., Leppo, J., Sweeney, A., Colgan, M., and Steuterman, S.: Two-dimensional Doppler echocardiographic correlation of dipyridamole-thallium stress testing with isometric handgrip. Am. Heart J., *121*:1367, 1991.

102. Mandysova, E., Niederle, P., Malkova, A., Feuereisl, R., Cervenka, V., Ascherman, M., and Mandys, F.: Usefulness of dipyridamole-handgrip echocardiography test for detecting coronary artery disease. Am. J. Cardiol., *67*:883, 1991.

103. Picano, E., Lattanzi, F., Masini, M., Distante, A., and

L'Abbate, A.: Does the combination with handgrip increase the sensitivity of dipyridamole-echocardiography test? Clin. Cardiol., *10*:37, 1987.

104. Tawa, C.B., Baker, W.B., Trakhtenbrolt, A., Desir, R., and Zoghbi, W.A.: Comparison of adenosine echocardiography (with and without handgrip) to exercise echocardiography in the detection of coronary artery disease. Circulation, *86*:I-863, 1992 (Abstract).

105. Fisman, E.Z., Ben-Ari, E., Pines, A., Drory, Y., Motro, M., and Kellermann, J.J.: Usefulness of heavy isometric exercise echocardiography for assessing left ventricular wall motion patterns late (≥6 months) after acute myocardial infarction. Am. J. Cardiol., *70*:1123, 1992.

106. Kondo, S., Meerbaum, S., Sakamaki, T., Shimoura, K., Tei, C., Shah, P.M., and Corday, E.: Diagnosis of coronary stenosis by two dimensional echocardiographic study of dysfunction of ventricular segments during and immediately after pacing. J. Am. Coll. Cardiol., *2*:689, 1983.

107. Chapman, P.D. and Wann, L.S.: Two-dimensional echocardiography during transesophageal pacing. Pract. Cardiol., *13*:105, 1987.

108. Matthews, R.V., Haskell, R.J., Ginzton, L.E., and Laks, M.M.: Usefulness of esophageal pill electrode atrial pacing with quantitative two-dimensional echocardiography for diagnosing coronary artery disease. Am. J. Cardiol., *64*:730, 1989.

109. Martin, T.W., Seaworth, J.F., Johns, J.P., Pupa, L.E., and Condos, W.R.: Comparison of adenosine, dipyridamole, and dobutamine in stress echocardiography. Ann. Intern. Med., *116*:190, 1992.

110. Distante, A., Moscarelli, E., Morales, M.A., Lattanzi, F., Reisenhofer, B., Lombardi, M., Picano, E., Rovai, D., and L'Abbate, A.: Pharmacological methods instead of exercise for the assessment of coronary artery disease. Echocardiography, *8*:99, 1991.

111. Previtali, M., Lanzarini, L., Ferrario, M., Tortorici, M., Mussini, A., and Montemartini, C.: Dobutamine versus dipyridamole echocardiography in coronary artery disease. Circulation, *83*:III-27, 1991.

112. Fung, A.Y., Gallagher, K.P., and Buda, A.J.: The physiologic basis of dobutamine as compared with dipyridamole stress interventions in the assessment of critical coronary stenosis. Circulation, *76*:943, 1987.

113. Picano, E. and Lattanzi, F.: Dipyridamole echocardiography. Circulation, *83*:III-19, 1991.

114. Pirelli, S., Danzi, G.B., Alberti, A., Massa, D., Piccalo, G., Faletra, F., Picano, E., Camplo, L., and DeVita, C.: Comparison of usefulness of high-dose dipyridamole echocardiography and exercise electrocardiography for detection of asymptomatic restenosis after coronary angioplasty. Am. J. Cardiol., *67*:1335, 1991.

115. Mazeika, P., Nihoyannopoulos, P., Joshi, J., and Oakley, C.M.: Evaluation of dipyridamole-Doppler echocardiography for detection of myocardial ischemia and coronary artery disease. Am. J. Cardiol., *68*:478, 1991.

116. Hattori, T., Uchiyama, T., Fujibayashi, Y., Sakamaki, T., Sato, Y., Kojima, M., and Kajiwara, N.: Ischemic heart disease evaluated using dipyridamole-stress two-dimensional echocardiography. J. Cardiol., *20*:589, 1990.

117. Fiorini, G., Prina, L., and dePonti, C.: Dipyridamole-echocardiography test in recent non-Q wave myocardial infarction. J. Appl. Cardiol., *5*:255, 1990.

118. Cohen, J.L., Greene, T.O., Alston, J.R., Wilchfort, S.D., and Kim, C.S.: Usefulness of oral dipyridamole digital echocardiography for detecting coronary artery disease. Am. J. Cardiol., *64*:385, 1989.

119. Picano, E., Masini, M., Lattanzi, F., Distante, A., and L'Abbate, A.: Role of dipyridamole-echocardiography test in electrocardiographically silent effort myocardial ischemia. Am. J. Cardiol., *58*:235, 1986.

120. Margonato, A., Chierchia, S., Cianflone, D., Smith, G., Crea, F., Davies, G.J., Maseri, A., and Foale, R.A.: Limitations of dipyridamole-echocardiography in effort angina pectoris. Am. J. Cardiol., *59*:225, 1987.

121. Picano, E.: High-dose dipyridamole echocardiography test: A new tool for the diagnosis of coronary artery disease. Pract. Cardiol., *14*:108, 1988.

122. Zoghbi, W.A., Cheirif, J., Kleiman, N.S., Verani, M.S., and Trakhtenbroit, A.: Diagnosis of ischemic heart disease with adenosine echocardiography. J. Am. Coll. Cardiol., *18*:1271, 1991.

123. Zoghbi, W.A.: Use of adenosine echocardiography for diagnosis of coronary artery disease. Am. Heart J., *122*:285, 1991.

124. Mazeika, P., Nihoyannopoulos, P., Joshi, J., and Oakley, C.M.: Uses and limitations of high dose dipyridamole stress echocardiography for evaluation of coronary artery disease. Br. Heart J., *67*:144, 1992.

125. Picano, E., Marini, C., and Pirelli, S.: Safety of intravenous high-dose dipyridamole echocardiography. Am. J. Cardiol., *70*:252, 1992.

126. Ferrara, N., Leosco, D., Longobardi, G., Abete, P., Papa, M., Vigorito, C., and Rengo, F.: Use of the epinephrine test in diagnosis of coronary artery disease. Am. J. Cardiol., *58*:256, 1986.

127. McNeill, A.J., Fioretti, P.M., El-Said, E.M., Salustri, A., deFeyter, P.J., and Roelandt, J.R.T.C.: Dobutamine stress echocardiography before and after coronary angioplasty. Am. J. Cardiol., *69*:740, 1992.

128. Mazeika, P.K., Nadazdin, A., and Oakley, C.M.: Dobutamine stress echocardiography for detection and assessment of coronary artery disease. J. Am. Coll. Cardiol., *19*:1203, 1992.

129. Sawada, S.G., Segar, D.S., Ryan, T., Dohan, A.M., Williams, R., and Feigenbaum, H.: Catecholamine stress echocardiography. Echocardiography, *9*:177, 1992.

130. Marcovitz, P.A. and Armstrong, W.F.: Accuracy of dobutamine stress echocardiography in detecting coronary artery disease. Am. J. Cardiol., *69*:1269, 1992.

131. Sawada, S.G., Segar, D.S., Ryan, T., Brown, S.E., Dohan, A.M., Williams, R., Fineberg, N.S., Armstrong, W.F., and Feigenbaum, H.: Echocardiographic detection of coronary artery disease during dobutamine infusion. Circulation, *83*:1605, 1991.

132. Mazeika, P., Nadazdin, A., and Oakley, C.M.: Detection of coronary disease by cross-sectional echocardiography during dobutamine stress. Br. Heart J., *66*:103, 1991.

133. Berthe, C., Pierard, L.A., Hiernaux, M., Trotteur, G., Lempereur, P., Karliner, J., and Kulbertus, H.E.: Predicting the extent and location of coronary artery disease in acute myocardial infarction by echocardiography during dobutamine infusion. Am. J. Cardiol., *58*:1167, 1986.

134. Martin, T.W., Seaworth, J.F., and Johns, J.P.: Comparison of exercise electrocardiography and dobutamine echocardiography. Clin. Cardiol., *15*:541, 1992.

135. Epstein, M., Gin, K., Sterns, L., and Pollick, C.: Dobutamine stress echocardiography: Initial experience of a Canadian centre. Can. J. Cardiol., *8*:273, 1992.

136. Salustri, A., Fioretti, P.M., Pozzoli, M.M., McNeill, A.J., and Roelandt, J.R.: Dobutamine stress echocardiography: Its role in the diagnosis of coronary artery disease. Eur. Heart J., *13*:70, 1992.

137. Martin, T.W., Seaworth, J.F., Johns, J.P., Pupa, L.E.,

and Condos, W.R.: Comparison of adenosine, dipyridamole, and dobutamine in stress echocardiography. Ann. Intern. Med., *116*:190, 1992.

138. Rosamond, T.L., Vacek, J.L., Hurwitz, A., Rowland, A.J., Beauchamp, G.D., and Crouse, L.J.: Hypotension during dobutamine stress echocardiography: Initial description and clinical relevance. Am. Heart J., *123*:403, 1992.

139. Mazeika, P.K., Nadazdin, A., and Oakley, C.M.: Clinical significance of abrupt vasodepression during dobutamine stress echocardiography. Am. J. Cardiol., *69*:1484, 1992.

140. Mertes, H., Sawada, S.G., Ryan, T., Segar, D.S., Kovacs, R., and Feigenbaum, H.: Symptoms, side effects and complications during dobutamine stress echocardiography: Experience in 1043 examinations. Circulation, *86*:I-126, 1992 (Abstract).

141. Pellikka, P.A., Oh, J.K., Bailey, K.R., Nichols, B.A., Monahan, K.H., and Tajik, A.J.: Dynamic intraventricular obstruction during dobutamine stress echocardiography. Circulation, *86*:1429, 1992.

142. McNeill, A.J., Fioretti, P.M., El-Said, E.M., Salustri, A., Forster, T., and Roelandt, J.R.T.C.: Enhanced sensitivity for detection of coronary artery disease by addition of atropine to dobutamine stress echocardiography. Am. J. Cardiol., *70*:141, 1992.

143. Pingitore, A., Reisenhofer, B., Chiaranda, S., Mattioli, R., Bellotti, P., Previtali, M., Quartacolosso, M., Gigli, G., Bibi, R., Heymann, J., Garyfallidis, X., and Picano, E.: Safety of dobutamine-atropine echocardiography: Preliminary results of a multicenter trial. Circulation, *86*:I-128, 1992 (Abstract).

144. Jaarsma, W. and Sutherland, G.: Computerized closed loop delivery of arbutamine, a new agent for the diagnosis of coronary artery disease. Circulation, *86*:I-126, 1992 (Abstract).

145. Ismail, G., Conant, S.R., Shapiro, S., Cao, T., French, W., and Ginzton, L.: Quantitative stress echocardiography: Comparison of exercise and pharmacologic stress with arbutamine. Circulation, *86*:I-127, 1992 (Abstract).

146. Hammond, H.K. and McKirnan, M.D.: Arbutamine is more effective than dobutamine as a diagnostic stress agent in a porcine model for myocardial ischemia. Circulation, *86*:I-126, 1992 (Abstract).

146a.Bates, J.R., Segar, D.S., Ryan, T., Sawada, S.G., Fitch, G.N., and Feigenbaum, H.: Colorized wall motion analysis to detect and correct for translation during upright bicycle stress echocardiography. J. Am. Coll. Cardiol., (Abstract). *21*:275A, 1993.

147. Cohen, J.L., Greene, T.O., Ottenweller, J., Binenbaum, S.Z., Wilchfort, S.D., Kim, C.S., and Alston, J.R.: Dobutamine digital echocardiography for detecting coronary artery disease. Am. J. Cardiol., *67*:1311, 1991.

148. Picano, E., Lattanzi, F., Orlandini, A., Marini, C., and L'Abbate, A.: Stress echocardiography and the human factor: The importance of being expert. J. Am. Coll. Cardiol., *17*:666, 1991.

149. Zabalgoitia, M., Gandhi, D.K., Abi-Mansour, P., Yarnold, P.R., Moushmoush, B., and Rosenblum, J.: Transesophageal stress echocardiography: Detection of coronary artery disease in patients with normal resting left ventricular contractility. Am. Heart J., *122*:1456, 1991.

150. Ehlert, F.A., Rosenblum, J., Gandhi, D.K., Buinevicius, R.P., and Zabalgoitia, M.: Evidence of hibernating myocardium by a new transesophageal echocardiographic technique. J. Am. Soc. Echocardiogr., *3*:420, 1990.

151. Hoffmann, R., Lambertz, H., Flachskampf, F.A., and

Hanrath, P.: Transesophageal echocardiography combined with atrial stimulation for detection of ischemia-induced wall motion impairment. Herz, *16*:367, 1991.

152. Lambertz, H., Kreis, A., Trumper, H., and Hanrath, P.: Simultaneous transesophageal echocardiography: A new method of stress echocardiography. J. Am. Coll. Cardiol., *16*:1143, 1990.

153. Kamp, O., DeCock, C.C., Kupper, A.J.F., Roos, J.P., and Visser, C.A.: Simultaneous transesophageal two-dimensional echocardiography and atrial pacing for detecting coronary artery disease. Am. J. Cardiol., *69*:1412, 1992.

154. Agati, L., Renzi, M., Sciomer, S., Vizza, D.C., Voci, P., Penco, M., Fedele, F., and Dagianti, A.: Transesophageal dipyridamole echocardiography for diagnosis of coronary artery disease. J. Am. Coll. Cardiol., *19*:765, 1992.

155. Armstrong, W.F., O'Donnell, J., Ryan, T., and Feigenbaum, H.: Effect of prior myocardial infarction and extent and location of coronary disease on accuracy of exercise echocardiography. J. Am. Coll. Cardiol., *10*:531, 1987.

156. Ryan, T., Vasey, C.G., Presti, C.F., O'Donnell, J.A., Feigenbaum, H., and Armstrong, W.F.: Exercise echocardiography: Detection of coronary artery disease in patients with normal left ventricular wall motion at rest. J. Am. Coll. Cardiol., *11*:993, 1988.

157. Galanti, G., Sciagra, R., Comeglio, M., Taddei, T., Bonechi, F., Giusti, F., Malfanti, P., and Bisi, G.: Diagnostic accuracy of peak exercise echocardiography in coronary artery disease: Comparison with thallium-201 myocardial scintigraphy. Am. Heart J., *122*:1609, 1991.

158. Ferrara, N., Bonaduce, D., Leosco, D., Longobardi, G., Abete, P., Morgano, G., Salvatore, M., and Rengo, F.: Two-dimensional echocardiographic evaluation of ventricular asynergy induced by dipyridamole: Correlation with thallium scanning. Clin. Cardiol., *9*:437, 1986.

159. Pozzoli, M.M.A., Fioretti, P.M., Salustri, A., Reijis, A.E.M., and Roelandt, J.R.T.C.: Exercise echocardiography and technetium-99m MIBI single-photon emission computed tomography in the detection of coronary artery disease. Am. J. Cardiol., *67*:350, 1991.

160. Jain, A., Suarez, J., Mahmarian, J.J., Zoghbi, W.A., Quinones, M., and Verani, M.S.: Functional significance of myocardial perfusion defects induced by dipyridamole using thallium-201 single-photon emission computed tomography and two-dimensional echocardiography. Am. J. Cardiol., *66*:802, 1990.

161. Nguyen, T., Heo, J., Ogilby, J.D., and Iskandrian, A.S.: Single photon emission computed tomography with thallium-201 during adenosine-induced coronary hyperemia: Correlation with coronary arteriography, exercise thallium imaging and two-dimensional echocardiography. J. Am. Coll. Cardiol., *16*:1375, 1990.

162. Pines, A.: Usefulness of immediate postexercise two-dimensional echocardiography in postmyocardial infarction patients without ischemic ECG changes in stress testing: Comparison with radionuclide angiography. Angiology, *40*:605, 1989.

163. Grayburn, P.A., Popma, J.J., Pryor, S.L., Walker, B.S., Simon, T.R., and Smitherman, T.C.: Comparison of dipyridamole-Doppler echocardiography to thallium-201 imaging and quantitative coronary arteriography in the assessment of coronary artery disease. Am. J. Cardiol., *63*:1315, 1989.

164. Marwick, T.H., Nemec, J.J., Stewart, W.J., and Salcedo, E.E.: Diagnosis of coronary artery disease using exercise echocardiography and positron emission tomography: Comparison and analysis of discrepant results. J. Am. Soc. Echocardiogr., *5*:231, 1992.

165. Amanullah, A.M., Lindvall, K., and Bevegard, S.: Exercise echocardiography after stabilization of unstable angina: Correlation with exercise Thallium-201 single photon emission computed tomography. Clin. Cardiol., *15*:585, 1992.

166. Quinones, M.A., Verani, M.S., Haichin, R.M., Mahmarian, J.J., Suarez, J., and Zoghbi, W.A.: Exercise echocardiography versus 201 T1 single photon emission computed tomography in evaluation of coronary artery disease. Circulation, *85*:1026, 1992.

167. Salustri, A., Pozzoli, M.M.A., Hermans, W., Ilmer, B., Cornel, J.H., Feijs, A.E.M., Roelandt, J.R.T.C., and Fioretti, P.M.: Relationship between exercise echocardiography and perfusion single-photon emission computed tomography in patients with single-vessel coronary artery disease. Am. Heart J., *124*:75, 1992.

168. Wynsen, J.C., Duchak, J.M., Smart, S.C., Pochis, W.T., Bamrah, V.S., and Sagar, K.B.: Dobutamine stress echocardiography versus dipyridamole SPECT isonitrile perfusion imaging for detection of coronary artery disease. Circulation, *86*:I-128, 1992 (Abstract).

169. Sawada, S.G., Ryan, T., Fineberg, N.S., Armstrong, W.F., Judson, W.E., McHenry, P.L., and Feigenbaum, H.: Exercise echocardiographic detection of coronary artery disease in women. J. Am. Coll. Cardiol., *14*:1440, 1989.

170. Masini, M., Picano, E., Lattanzi, F., Distante, A., and L'Abbate, A.: High dose dipyridamole-echocardiography test in women: Correlation with exercise-electrocardiography test and coronary arteriography. J. Am. Coll. Cardiol., *12*:682, 1988.

171. Severi, S. and Michelassi, C.: Prognostic impact of stress testing in coronary artery disease. Circulation, *83*:III-82, 1991.

172. Tischler, M.D., Lee, T.H., Hirsch, A.T., Lord, C.P., Goldman, L., Creager, M.A., and Lee, R.T.: Prediction of major cardiac events after peripheral vascular surgery using dipyridamole echocardiography. Am. J. Cardiol., *68*:593, 1991.

173. Lane, R.T., Sawada, S.G., Segar, D.S., Ryan, T., Lalka, S.G., Williams, R., Brown, S.E., Armstrong, W.F., and Feigenbaum, H.: Dobutamine stress echocardiography for assessment of cardiac risk before noncardiac surgery. Am. J. Cardiol., *68*:976, 1991.

174. Lalka, S.G., Sawada, S.G., Dalsing, M.C., Cikrit, D.F., Sawchuk, A.P., Kovacs, R.L., Segar, D.S., Ryan, T., and Feigenbaum, H.: Dobutamine stress echocardiography as a predictor of cardiac events associated with aortic surgery. J. Vasc. Surg., *15*:831, 1992.

175. Sawada, S.G., Ryan, T., Conley, M.J., Corya, B.C., Feigenbaum, H., and Armstrong, W.F.: Prognostic value of a normal exercise echocardiogram. Am. Heart J., *120*:49, 1990.

176. Picano, E., Severi, S., Michelassi, C., Lattanzi, F., Masini, M., Orsini, E., Distante, A., and L'Abbate, A.: Prognostic importance of dipyridamole-echocardiography test in coronary artery disease. Circulation, *80*:450, 1989.

177. Burger, A.J.: Progress in exercise two-dimensional echocardiography. Cardiovasc. Rev. Rep., *9*:45, 1988.

178. Amanullah, A.M. and Lindvall, K.: Predischarge exercise echocardiography in patients with unstable angina who respond to medical treatment. Clin. Cardiol., *15*:417, 1992.

179. Marcovitz, P.A., Bach, D.S., Shayna, V., and Armstrong, W.F.: An abnormal dobutamine echocardiogram

predicts death and myocardial infarction in the year following study. Circulation, *86:*I-789, 1992 (Abstract).

180. Usedom, J.E., Allen, S., Calvert, D., Arendell, G., and Vasey, C.G.: Prognostic significance of a normal exercise echocardiogram in patients with coronary artery disease. Circulation, *86:*I-789, 1992 (Abstract).

180a.Mazeika, P.K., Nadazdin, A., and Oakley, C.M.: Prognostic value of dobutamine echocardiography in patients with high pretest likelihood of coronary artery disease. Am. J. Cardiol., *71:*33–39, 1993.

180b.Mazeika, P.K., Nadazdin, A., and Oakley, C.M.: Prognostic value of dobutamine echocardiography in patients with high pretest likelihood of coronary artery disease. Am. J. Cardiol., *71:*33, 1993.

180c.Krivokapich, J., et al.: Prognostic usefulness of positive or negative exercise stress echocardiography for predicting coronary events in ensuing twelve months. Am. J. Cardiol., *71:*646, 1993.

181. Jaarsma, W., Visser, C.A., Kupper, A.J.F., Res, J.C.J., Van Eenige, M.J., and Ross, J.P.: Usefulness of two-dimensional exercise echocardiography shortly after myocardial infarction. Am. J. Cardiol., *57:*86, 1986.

182. Ryan, T., Armstrong, W.F., O'Donnell, J., and Feigenbaum, H.: Risk stratification following myocardial infarction using exercise echocardiography. Am. Heart J., *114:*1305, 1987.

183. Applegate, R.J., Dell'Italia, L.J., and Crawford, M.H.: Usefulness of two-dimensional echocardiography during low-level exercise testing early after uncomplicated myocardial infarction. Am. J. Cardiol., *60:*10, 1987.

184. Orlandini, A., Sclavo, M.G., Magaia, O., Seveso, G., Bolognese, L., Previtali, M., Margaria, F., Gandolfo, N., Chiaranda, S., Rosselli, P., Landi, P., Severi, S., Marini, C., and Picano, E.: The relative prognostic value of dipyridamole-echocardiography and coronary angiography early after uncomplicated acute myocardial infarction: Updated results of the EPIC study. Circulation, *86:*I-384, 1992 (Abstract).

185. Kuroda, T., Shiina, A., Yamasawa, M., Mitsuhashi, T., Seino, Y., Natsume, T., and Shimada, K.: Prognostic value of peak exercise 2-D echocardiographic analysis after acute myocardial infarction: A prospective 5-year follow-up study. Circulation, *86:*I-790, 1992 (Abstract).

186. Vincent, M., Marwick, T., D'Hondt, A-M., Granier, P., Verhelst, R., Melin, J., and Detry, J-M.: Prediction of perioperative events at vascular surgery: Selection of thallium scintigraphy or echocardiography with dipyridamole stress? Circulation, *86:*I-790, 1992 (Abstract).

187. Eichelberg, J.P., Schwarz, K.Q., Black, E.R., Green, R.M., and Ouriel, K.: Predictive value of dobutamine stress echocardiography before vascular surgery. Circulation, *86:*I-789, 1992 (Abstract).

188. Poldermans, D., Forster, T., Thomson, I.R., duBois, N.A.J.J., El-Said, E-S.M., van Urk, H., Roelandt, J.R.T.C., and Fioretti, P.M.: Dobutamine stress echocardiography for assessment of perioperative cardiac risk in patients undergoing major noncardiac vascular surgery. Circulation, *86:*I-11, 1992 (Abstract).

189. Pellikka, P.A., Oh, J.K., Roger, V.L., and Tajik, A.J.: Dobutamine stress echocardiography in aneurysmal disease. Circulation, *86:*I-128, 1992 (Abstract).

189a.Davila-Roman, V.G., et al.: Dobutamine stress echocardiography predicts surgical outcome in patients with an aortic aneurysm and peripheral vascular disease. J. Am. Coll. Cardiol., *21:*957, 1993.

190. Fisman, E.Z., Ben-Ari, E., Pines, A., Drory, Y., Shiner, R.J., Motro, M., and Kellerman, J.J.: Pronounced reduc-

tion of aortic flow velocity and acceleration during heavy isometric exercise in coronary artery disease. Am. J. Cardiol., *68:*485, 1991.

191. Kelly, T.A., Rothbart, R.M., Patrone, V.J., Watson, D.D., Weltman, A., and Gibson, R.S.: Continuous wave Doppler assessment of ascending aortic blood flow during exercise in normal volunteers and patients with suspected or known coronary artery disease. J. Appl. Cardiol., *5:*141, 1990.

192. Mehta, N., Bennett, D., Mannering, D., Dawkins, K., and Ward, D.E.: Usefulness of noninvasive Doppler measurements of ascending aortic blood velocity and acceleration in detecting impairment of the left ventricular functional response to exercise three weeks after acute myocardial infarction. Am. J. Cardiol., *58:*879, 1986.

193. Daley, P.J., Sagar, K.B., Collier, B., Kalbfleisch, J., and Wann, L.S.: Detection of exercise-induced changes in left ventricular performance by Doppler echocardiography. Br. Heart J., *58:*447, 1987.

194. Ihlen, H., Endresen, K., Golf, S., and Nitter-Hauge, S.: Cardiac stroke volume during exercise measured by Doppler echocardiography: Comparison with the thermodilution technique and evaluation of reproducibility. Br. Heart J., *58:*455, 1987.

195. Lazarus, M., Dang, T-Y., Gardin, J.M., Allfie, A., and Henry, W.L.: Evaluation of age, gender, heart rate and blood pressure changes and exercise conditioning on Doppler measured aortic blood flow acceleration and velocity during upright treadmill testing. Am. J. Cardiol., *62:*439, 1988.

196. Labovitz, A.J., Pearson, A.C., Chaitman, B.R., Byers, S.L., and Mrosek, D.G.: Doppler and two-dimensional echocardiographic assessment of left ventricular function before and after intravenous dipyridamole stress testing for detection of coronary artery disease. Am. J. Cardiol., *62:*1180, 1988.

197. Harrison, M.R., Smith, M.D., Friedman, B.J., and DeMaria, A.N.: Uses and limitations of exercise Doppler echocardiography in the diagnosis of ischemic heart disease. J. Am. Coll. Cardiol., *10:*809, 1987.

198. Miyashita, Y., Seki, K., Takahashi, I., Takayama, K., Hara, M., Nakatsuka, T., Yoshimura, S., and Furuhata, H.: Non-invasive evaluation of cardiac function by peak aortic flow acceleration (peak dF/dt) during exercise. Jpn. J. Med. Ultrasonics, *14:*1, 1987.

199. Daley, P.J., Sagar, K.B., Collier, B.D., Kalbfleisch, J., and Wann, L.S.: Detection of exercise-induced changes in left ventricular performance by Doppler echocardiography. Br. Heart J., *58:*447, 1987.

200. Bryg, R.J., Labovitz, A.J., Mehdirad, A., Williams, G.A., and Chaitman, B.R.: Effect of coronary artery disease on Doppler-derived parameters of aortic flow during upright exercise. Am. J. Cardiol., *58:*14, 1986.

201. Gonzalez, A., Naqvi, E., Tak, T., Choudhary, R.S., Rahimtoola, S.H., and Chandraratna, P.A.N.: Normalization of Doppler indices of diastolic dysfunction during pacing is a sign of ischemic mitral regurgitation. Am. Heart J., *121:*118, 1991.

202. Shahi, M., Nadazdin, A., and Foale, R.A.: Characteristics of left ventricular filling in coronary artery disease and myocardial ischemia after dipyridamole provocation. Br. Heart J., *65:*265, 1991.

203. Lombardo, A., Pennestri, F., Biasucci, L.M., Laurenzi, F., Vigna, C., Gimigliano, F., Rossi, E., Amico, C.M., Alecce, G., Rinelli, G., Nanna, M., and Loperfido, F.: Pulsed Doppler analysis of left ventricular systolic func-

tion during transesophageal atrial pacing in recent myocardial infarction. Cardiovasc. Imag., 2:233, 1990.

204. Iwase, M., Yokota, M., Maeda, M., Kamihara, S., Miyahara, T., Iwase, M., Hayashi, H., and Saito, H.: Noninvasive detection of exercise-induced markedly elevated left ventricular filling pressure by pulsed Doppler echocardiography in patients with coronary artery disease. Am. Heart J., 118:947, 1989.

205. Mitchell, G.D., Brunken, R.C., Schwaiger, M., Donohue, B.C., Krivokapich, J., and Child, J.S.: Assessment of mitral flow velocity with exercise by an index of stress-induced left ventricular ischemia in coronary artery disease. Am. J. Cardiol., 61:536, 1988.

206. Stoddard, M.F., Johnstone, J., Dillon, S., and Kupersmith, J.: The effect of exercise-induced myocardial ischemia on postischemic left ventricular diastolic filling. Clin. Cardiol., 15:265, 1992.

206a.Finkelhor, R.S., Ramer, C.L., Castellanos, M., Miron, S.D., and Teague, S.M.: Relation of exercise Doppler left ventricular filling to thallium lung uptake. Am. Heart J., 125:164–170, 1993.

206b.Finkelhor, R.S., et al. Relation of exercise Doppler left ventricular filling to thallium lung uptake. Am. Heart J., 125:164, 1993.

207. Egeblad, H., Vilhelmsen, R., and Mortensen, S.A.: Ischemic and postischemic ventricular wall motion abnormalities in Prinzmetal's angina provoked by hyperventilation. Am. Heart J., 104:1105, 1982.

208. Widlansky, S., McHenry, P.L., Corya, B.C., and Phillips, J.F.: Coronary angiography, echocardiographic, and electrocardiographic studies on a patient with variant angina due to coronary artery spasm. Am. Heart J., 90: 631, 1975.

209. Guazzi, M.D., Polese, A., Margrini, F., Olivari, M.T., Moruzzi, P., and Fiorentini, C.: Echocardiographic and hemodynamic correlates in Prinzmetal's angina pectoris: A case report. Angiology, 30:708, 1979.

210. Distante, A., Rovai, D., Picano, E., Moscarelli, E., Palombo, C., Morales, M.A., Michelassi, C., and L'Abbate, A.: Transient changes in left ventricular mechanics during attacks of Prinzmetal's angina: An M-mode echocardiographic study. Am. Heart J., 107:465, 1984.

211. Distante, A., et al.: Echocardiographic versus hemodynamic monitoring during attacks of variant angina pectoris. Am. J. Cardiol., 55:1319, 1985.

212. Rovai, D., et al.: Transient myocardial ischemia with minimal electrocardiographic changes: An echocardiographic study in patients with Prinzmetal's angina. Am. Heart J., 109:78, 1985.

213. Song, J-K., Park, S-W., Park, S-J., Kim, J-J., Doo, Y-C., and Lee, S.J-K.: Diagnostic values of intravenous ergonovine test with 2-dimensional echocardiography for induction of coronary vasospasm. Circulation, 86:I-127, 1992 (Abstract).

214. Broderick, T.M., Bourdillon, P.D.V., Ryan, T., Feigenbaum, H., Dillon, J.C., and Armstrong, W.F.: Comparison of regional and global left ventricular function by serial echocardiograms after reperfusion in acute myocardial infarction. J. Am. Soc. Echocardiogr., 2:315, 1989.

215. Bourdillon, P.D.V., Broderick, T.M., Sawada, S.G., Armstrong, W.F., Ryan, T., Dillon, J.C., Fineberg, N.S., and Feigenbaum, H.: Regional wall motion index for infarct and noninfarct regions after reperfusion in acute myocardial infarction: Comparison with global wall motion index. J. Am. Soc. Echocardiogr., 2:398, 1989.

216. Gentile, R., Armstrong, W., Bourdillon, P., Dillon, J., Ryan, T., and Feigenbaum, H.: Correlation between myocardial salvage and time of reperfusion with percutaneous transluminal coronary angioplasty in the setting of acute myocardial infarction: An echocardiographic study. Cardiovasc. Imaging, 1:24, 1989.

217. Bourdillon, P.D.V., Broderick, T.M., Williams, E.S., Davis, C., Dillon, J.C., Armstrong, W.F., Fineberg, N., Ryan, T., and Feigenbaum, H.: Early recovery of regional left ventricular function after reperfusion in acute myocardial infarction assessed by serial two-dimensional echocardiography. Am. J. Cardiol., 63:641, 1989.

218. Presti, C.F., Gentile, R., Armstrong, W.F., Ryan, T., Dillon, J.C., and Feigenbaum, H.: Improvement in regional wall motion after percutaneous transluminal coronary angioplasty during acute myocardial infarction: Utility of two-dimensional echocardiography. Am. Heart J., 115:1149, 1988.

219. Ellis, S.G., Henschke, C.I., Sandor, T., Wynne, J., Braunwald, E., and Kloner, R.A.: Time course of functional and biochemical recovery of myocardium salvaged by reperfusion. J. Am. Coll. Cardiol., 1:1047, 1983.

220. van den Berg, Jr., E.K., Popma, J.J., Dehmer, G.J., Snow, F.R., Lewis, S.A., Vetrovec, G.W., and Nixon, J.V.: Reversible segmental left ventricular dysfunction after coronary angioplasty. Circulation, 81:1210, 1990.

221. Lefkowitz, C.A., Pace, D.P., Gallagher, K.P., and Buda, A.J.: The effects of a critical stenosis myocardial blood flow, ventricular function, and infarct size after coronary reperfusion. Circulation, 77:915, 1988.

222. Otto, C.M., Stratton, J.R., Maynard, C., Althouse, R., Johannessen, K-A., and Kennedy, J.W.: Echocardiographic evaluation of segmental wall motion early and late after thrombolytic therapy in acute myocardial infarction: The Western Washington tissue plasminogen activator emergency room trial. Am. J. Cardiol., 65:132, 1990.

223. Ishii, K. and Degawa, T.: Left ventricular wall motion improvement after successful coronary reperfusion therapy in acute myocardial infarction: Prediction by two-dimensional echocardiography. J. Cardiol., 21:283, 1991.

224. White, H., Cross, D., Scott, M., and Norris, R.: Comparison of effects of thrombolytic therapy on left ventricular function in patients over with those under 60 years of age. Am. J. Cardiol., 67:913, 1991.

225. Touchstone, D.A., Beller, G.A., Mygaard, T.W., Tedesco, C., and Kaul, S.: Effects of successful intravenous reperfusion therapy on regional myocardial function and geometry in humans: A tomographic assessment using two-dimensional echocardiography. J. Am. Coll. Cardiol., 13:1506, 1989.

226. Uematsu, M., Masuyama, T., Nanto, S., Taniura, K., Naka, M., Taniura, T., Kimura, Y., Kodama, K., Tamai, J., Kitabatake, A., Inoue, M., and Kamada, T.: Coronary thrombolytic therapy in acute myocardial infarction: Time dependence of beneficial effects assessed by two-dimensional echocardiography. J. Cardiogr., 16:535, 1986.

227. Sone, T., Ishida, A., Sassa, H., Ikumura, Y., Yasuda, E., and Endo, T.: Reversible ischemic myocardial damage: Clinical observation using two-dimensional echocardiography. J. Cardiogr., 16:571, 1986.

228. Kumar, A., Minagoe, S., and Chandraratna, P.A.N.: Two-dimensional echocardiographic demonstration of restoration of normal wall motion after acute myocardial infarction. Am. J. Cardiol., 57:1232, 1986.

228a.Ito, H., et al.: Time course of functional improvement

in stunned myocardium in risk area in patients with reperfused anterior infarction. Circulation, *87*:355, 1993.

229. Friedman, G.H., Lee, M.S., Roth, S.L., Grunwald, A.M., and Bodenheimer, M.M.: Early and rapid prediction of patency of the infarct-related coronary artery by using left ventricular wall thickness as measured by two-dimensional echocardiography. J. Am. Coll. Cardiol., *20*:1599, 1992.

230. Yamasawa, M., Shiina, A., Fujita, T., Kuroda, T., Suzuki, O., Lino, T., Noda, T., Natsume, T., Haginuwa, T., and Hosoda, S.: Clinical use of exercise two-dimensional echocardiography for evaluating effects of percutaneous transluminal coronary angioplasty and coronary artery bypass graft. Jpn. J. Med. Ultrasonics, *18*:238, 1991.

231. Pirelli, S., Massa, D., Faletra, F., Piccalo, G., De Vita, C., Danzi, G.B., and Compolo, L.: Exercise electrocardiography versus dipyridamole echocardiography testing in coronary angioplasty. Circulation, *83*:III-38, 1991.

232. Bongo, A.S., Bolognese, L., Sarasso, G., Cernigliaro, C., Aralda, D., Carfora, A., Piccinino, C., Campi, A., Rossi, L., and Rossi, P.: Early assessment of coronary artery bypass graft patency by high-dose dipyridamole echocardiography. Am. J. Cardiol., *67*:133, 1991.

233. Biangini, A., Maffei, S., Baroni, M., Levantino, M., Comite, C., Russo, V., Salerno, L., Borzoni, G., Piacenti, M., and Salvatore, L.: Early assessment of coronary reserve after bypass surgery by dipyridamole transesophageal echocardiographic stress test. Am. Heart J., *120*:1097, 1990.

234. Picano, E., Pirelli, S., Marzilli, M., Faletra, F., Lattanzi, F., Campolo, L., Massa, D., Blberti, A., Gara, E., Distante, A., and L'Abbate, A.: Usefulness of high-dose dipyridamole echocardiographic test in coronary angioplasty. Circulation, *80*:807, 1989.

235. Labovitz, A.J., Lewen, M., Kern, M.J., Vandormael, M., Mrosek, D.G., Byers, S.L., Pearson, A.C., and Chaitman, B.R.: The effects of successful PTCA on left ventricular function: Assessment by exercise echocardiography. Am. Heart J., *117*:1003, 1989.

236. Broderick, T., Sawada, S., Armstrong, W.F., Ryan, T., Dillon, J.C., Bourdillon, P.D., and Feigenbaum, H.: Improvement in rest and exercise-induced wall motion abnormalities after coronary angioplasty: An exercise echocardiographic study. J. Am. Coll. Cardiol., *15*:591, 1990.

237. Crouse, L.J., Vacek, J.L., Beauchamp, G.D., Porter, C.B., Rosamond, T.L., and Kramer, P.H.: Exercise echocardiography after coronary artery bypass grafting. Am. J. Cardiol., *70*:572, 1992.

237a. Akosah, K.O., et al.: Ischemia-induced regional wall motion abnormality is improved after coronary angioplasty: Demonstration by dobutamine stress echocardiography. J. Am. Coll. Cardiol., *21*:584, 1993.

238. Hsiung, M.C., Roubin, G.S., and Nanda, N.C.: Usefulness of exercise echocardiography in the assessment of restenosis after intracoronary stenting. Circulation, *86*: I-789, 1992 (Abstract).

238a. Hecht, H.S., et al.: Usefulness of supine bicycle stress echocardiography for detection of restenosis after percutaneous transluminal coronary angioplasty. Am. J. Cardiol., *71*:293, 1993.

238b. Dilsizian, V., Bonow, R.O.: Current diagnostic techniques of assessing myocardial viability in patients with hibernating and stunned myocardium. Circulation, *87*: 1–20, 1993.

239. Bolli R.: Myocardial stunning in man. Circulation, *86*: 1671, 1992.

240. Preuss, K.C., Gross, G.J., Brooks, H.L., and Warltier, D.C.: Time course of recovery of "stunned" myocardium following variable periods of ischemia in conscious and anesthetized dogs. Am. Heart J., *114*:696, 1987.

241. Lewis, S.J., Sawada, S.G., Ryan T., Segar, D.S., Armstrong, W.F., and Feigenbaum, H.: Segmental wall motion abnormalities in the absence of clinically documented myocardial infarction: Clinical significance and evidence of hibernating myocardium. Am. Heart J., *121*: 1088, 1991.

242. Barilla, F., Gheorghiade, M., Alam, M., Khaja, F., and Goldstein, S.: Low-dose dobutamine in patients with acute myocardial infarction identifies viable but not contractile myocardium and predicts the magnitude of improvement in wall motion abnormalities in response to coronary revascularization. Am. Heart J., *122*:1522, 1991.

243. Movahed, A., Reeves, W.C., Rose, G.C., Wheeler, W.S., Jolly, S.R., Kearney, S., and Barnhill, P.E.: Dobutamine and improvement of regional and global left ventricular function in coronary artery disease. Am. J. Cardiol., *66*:375, 1990.

244. Pierard, L.A., DeLandsheere, C.M., Berthe, C., Rigo, P., and Kulbertus, H.E.: Identification of viable myocardium by echocardiography during dobutamine infusion in patients with myocardial infarction after thrombolytic therapy: Comparison with positron emission tomography. J. Am. Coll. Cardiol., *15*:1021, 1990.

245. Mengozzi, G., Lucignani, G., Mariani, M.A., Palagi, C., Landoni, C., Paolini, G., Biadi, O., Vanoli, G., Zuccari, M., Grossi, A., Mariani, M., and Fazio, F.: Identification of hibernating myocardium: A comparison between dobutamine-echocardiography and combined study of perfusion and metabolism. Circulation, *86*:I-383, 1992 (Abstract).

246. McGukin, J., Walsh, J., Tyson, I., Price, B., Davila-Roman, V., and Fontanet, H.: Detection of viable myocardium by dobutamine stress echocardiography validated by simultaneous dobutamine thallium imaging and by coronary angiography. Circulation, *86*:I-788, 1992 (Abstract).

247. Picano, E., Marzullo, P., Gigli, G., Reisenhofer, B., Parodi, O., Distante, A., and L'Abbate, A.: Identification of viable myocardium by dipyridamole-induced improvement in regional left ventricular function assessed by echocardiography in myocardial infarction and comparison with thallium scintigraphy at rest. Am. J. Cardiol., *70*:703, 1992.

248. Bolognese, L., Sarasso, G., Gongo, A.S., Rossi, L., Aralda, D., Piccinino, C., and Rossi, P.: Dipyridamole echocardiography test. A new tool for detecting jeopardized myocardium after thrombolytic therapy. Circulation, *84*:1100, 1991.

249. Lundgren, C., Bourdillon, P.D.V., Dillon, J.C., and Feigenbaum, H.: Comparison of contrast angiography and two-dimensional echocardiography for the evaluation of left ventricular regional wall motion abnormalities after acute myocardial infarction. Am. J. Cardiol., *65*:1071, 1990.

250. Kittleson, M.D., Knowlen, G.G., and Johnson, L.E.: Early and late global and regional left ventricular function after experimental transmural myocardial infarction: Relationships of regional wall motion, wall thickening, and global performance. Am. Heart J., *114*:70, 1987.

251. White, R.D., Cassidy, M.M., Cheitlin, M.D., Emilson,

B., Ports, T.A., Lim, A.D., Botvinick, E.H., Schiller, N.B., and Higgins, C.B.: Segmental evaluation of left ventricular wall motion after myocardial infarction: Magnetic resonance imaging versus echocardiography. Am. Heart J., *115*:166, 1988.

252. Reeder, G.S., Seward, J.B., and Tajik, A.J.: The role of two dimensional echocardiography in coronary artery disease. Mayo Clin. Proc., *57*:247, 1982.

253. Lieberman, A.N., Weiss, J.L., Jugdutt, B.I., Becker, L.C., Bulkley, B.H., Garrison, J.G., Hutchins, G.M., Kallman, C.A., and Weisfeldt, M.L.: Two dimensional wall motion and thickening to the extent of myocardial infarction in the dog. Circulation, *63*:739, 1981.

254. Wyatt, H.L., Meerbaum, S., Heng, M.K., Rit, J., Gueret, P., and Corday, E.: Experimental evaluation of the extent of myocardial dyssynergy and infarct size by two dimensional echocardiography. Circulation, *63*:607, 1981.

255. Nieminen, M., Parisi, A.F., O'Boyle, J.E., Folland, E.D., Khuri, S., and Kloner, R.A.: Serial evaluation of myocardial thickening and thinning in acute experimental infarction: Identification and quantification using two dimensional echocardiography. Circulation, *66*:174, 1982.

256. Blumenthal, D.S., Becker, L.C., Bulkley, B.H., Hutchins, G.M., Weisfeldt, M.L., and Weiss, J.L.: Impaired function of salvaged myocardium: Two dimensional echocardiographic quantification of regional wall thickening in the open-chest dog. Circulation, *67*:225, 1983.

257. Komasa, N., Tanimoto, M., Kimura, S., Yasutomi, N., Saito, Y., Yamamoto, T., Ikeoka, K., Makihata, S., Kawai, Y., and Iwasaki, T.: Echocardiography in superacute phase of myocardial infarction: An experimental study. J. Cardiogr., *12*:929, 1982.

258. Lieberman, A.N., Weiss, J.L., Jugdutt, B.I., Becker, L.C., Bulkley, B.H., Garrison, J.G., Hutchins, G.M., Kallman, C.A., and Weisfeldt, M.L.: Two dimensional echocardiography and infarct size: Relationship of regional wall motion and thickening to the extent of myocardial infarction in the dog. Circulation, *63*:739, 1981.

259. Force, T., Kemper, A., Perkins, L., Gilfoil, M., Cohen, C., and Parisi, A.F.: Overestimation of infarct size by quantitative two-dimensional echocardiography: The role of tethering and of analytic procedures. Circulation, *73*:1360, 1986.

260. Wilkins, G.T., Southern, J.F., Choong, C.Y., Thomas, J.D., Gallon, J.T., Guyer, D.E., and Weyman, A.E.: Correlation between echocardiographic endocardial surface mapping of abnormal wall motion and pathologic infarct size in autopsied hearts. Circulation, *77*:978, 1988.

261. Pandian, N.G., Skorton, D.J., Collins, S.M., Koyanagi, S., Kieso, R., Marcus, M.L., Kerber, R.E.: Myocardial infarct size threshold for two-dimensional echocardiographic detection: Sensitivity of systolic wall thickening and endocardial motion abnormalities in small versus large infarcts. Am. J. Cardiol., *55*:551, 1985.

262. Mann, D.L., Gillam, L.D., Mich, R., Foale, R., Newell, J.B., and Weyman, A.E.: Functional relation between infarct thickness and regional systolic function in the acutely and subacutely infarcted canine left ventricle. J. Am. Coll. Cardiol., *14*:481, 1989.

263. Koyanagi, S., Nabeyama, S., Ohzono, K., Takeshita, A., and Nakamura, M.: Wall motion abnormalities in Q wave and non-Q wave myocardial infarction in isolated left anterior descending coronary artery disease. J. Cardiogr., *16*:271, 1986.

264. Touchstone, D.A., Mygaard, T.W., and Kaul, S.: Correlation between left ventricular risk area and clinical,

265. Loh, I.K., Charuzi, Y., Beeder, C., Marshall, L.A., and Ginsburg, B.H.: Early diagnosis of nontransmural myocardial infarction by two dimensional echocardiography. Am. Heart J., *104*:963, 1982.

266. Henschek, C.I., Risser, T.A., Sandor, T., Hanlon, W.B., Neumann, A., and Wynne, J.: Quantitative computer-assisted analysis of left ventricular wall thickening and motion by two dimensional echocardiography in acute myocardial infarction. Am. J. Cardiol., *52*:960, 1983.

267. Nixon, J.V., Narahara, K.A., and Smitherman, T.C.: Estimation of myocardial involvement in patients with acute myocardial infarction by two dimensional echocardiography. Circulation, *62*:1248, 1980.

268. Kisslo, J.A., Robertson, D., Gilbert, B.W., von Ramm, O., and Behar, V.S.: A comparison of real-time, two-dimensional echocardiography and cineangiography in detecting left ventricular asynergy. Circulation, *55*:134, 1977.

269. Hecht, H.S., Taylor, R., Wong, M., and Shah, P.M.: Comparative evaluation of segmental asynergy in remote myocardial infarction by radionuclide angiography, two dimensional echocardiography, and contrast ventriculography. Am. Heart J., *101*:740, 1981.

270. Gentile, F., Greco, R., Siciliano, S., Violini, R., Marsico, L., Mininni, N., and Marsico, F.: Comparative accuracy of cross-sectional echocardiography and cineventriculography for left ventricular evaluation after myocardial infarction. G. Ital. Cardiol., *11*:1996, 1981.

271. Shibata, J., Takahashi, H., Itaya, M., Nagata, H., Itaya, K., Bekki, H., Koga, Y., Utsu, F., and Toshima, H.: Cross-sectional echocardiographic visualization of the infarcted site in myocardial infarction: Correlation with electrocardiographic and coronary angiographic findings. J. Cardiogr., *12*:885, 1982.

272. Heger, J.J., Weyman, A.E., Wann, L.S., Dillon, J.C., and Feigenbaum, H.: Cross-sectional echocardiography in acute myocardial infarction: Detection and localization of regional left ventricular asynergy. Circulation, *60*:531, 1979.

273. Gibson, R.S., Bishop, H.L., Stamm, R.B., Crampton, R.S., Beller, G.A., and Martin, R.P.: Value of early two dimensional echocardiography in patients with acute myocardial infarction. Am. J. Cardiol., *49*:1110, 1982.

274. Picard, M.H., Wilkins, G.T., Ray, P.A., and Weyman, A.E.: Progressive changes in ventricular structure and function during the year after acute myocardial infarction. Am. Heart J., *124*:24, 1992.

275. Picard, M.H., Wilkins, G.T., Ray, P.A., and Weyman, A.E.: Natural history of left ventricular size and function after acute myocardial infarction. Circulation, *82*:484, 1990.

276. Choong, C.Y., Gibbons, E.F., Hogan, R.D., Franklin, T.D., Nolting, M., Mann, D.L., and Weyman, A.E.: Relationship of functional recovery to scar contraction after myocardial infarction in the canine left ventricle. Am. Heart J., *117*:819, 1989.

277. Sabbah, H.N., Gheorghiade, M., Smith, S.T., Frank, D.M., and Stein, P.D.: Rate and extent of recovery of left ventricular function in patients following acute myocardial infarction. Am. Heart J., *114*:516, 1987.

278. Asinger, R.W., Mikell, F.L., Elsperger, J., Sharkey, S.W., Tilbury, T., Erlien, D., and Hodges, M.: Serial changes in left ventricular wall motion by two-dimen-

sional echocardiography following anterior myocardial infarction. Am. Heart J., *116*:50, 1988.

279. Mahias-Narvarte, H., Adams, K.F., and Willis, P.W.: Evolution of regional left ventricular wall motion abnormalities in acute Q and non-Q wave myocardial infarction. Am. Heart J., *113*:1369, 1987.

280. Visser, C.A., et al.: Detection and quantification of acute, isolated myocardial infarction by two dimensional echocardiography. Am. J. Cardiol., *47*:1020, 1981.

281. deSwaan, C., Cheriex, E.C., Braat, S.H.J.G., Stappers, J.L.M., and Wellens, H.J.J.: Improvement of systolic and diastolic left ventricular wall motion by serial echocardiograms in selected patients treated for unstable angina. Am. Heart J., *121*:789, 1991.

282. Parisi, A.F., Moynihan, P.F., Folland, E.D., Strauss, W.E., Sharma, G.V., and Sasahara, A.A.: Echocardiography in acute and remote myocardial infarction. Am. J. Cardiol., *46*:1205, 1980.

283. Fraker, T.D., Bingle, J.F., Wilkerson, R.D., Klingler, J.W., Weaver, M.T., and Andrews, L.T.: Acute myocardial ischemia detected in dogs by temporal variation in two-dimensional ultrasound gray level. Am. Heart J., *116*:398, 1988.

283a. Picano, E., Faletra, F., Marini, C., Paterni, M., Danzi, G.B., Lombardi, M., Campolo, L., Gigli, G., Landini, L., Pezzano, A., and Distante, A.: Increased echodensity of transiently asynergic myocardium in humans: A novel echocardiographic sign of myocardial ischemia. J. Am. Coll. Cardiol., *21*:199–207, 1993.

284. Gaasch, W.H. and Bernard, S.A.: The effect of acute changes in coronary blood flow on left ventricular end-diastolic wall thickness: An echocardiographic study. Circulation, *56*:593, 1977.

285. Parisi, A.F., Nieminen, M., O'Boyle, J.E., Moynihan, P.F., Khuri, S.F., Kloner, R.A., Folland, E.D., and Schoen, F.J.: Enhanced detection of the evolution of tissue changes after acute myocardial infarction using color-encoded two dimensional echocardiography. Circulation, *66*:764, 1982.

286. Tak, T., Visser, C., Rahimtoola, S.H., and Chandraratna, P.A.N.: Detection of acute myocardial infarction with digital image processing of two-dimensional echocardiogram. Am. Heart J., *124*:289, 1992.

287. Waggoner, A.D., Perez, J.E., Miller, J.G., and Sobel, B.E.: Differentiation of normal and ischemic right ventricular myocardium with quantitative two-dimensional integrated backscatter imaging. Ultrasound Med. Biol., *18*:249, 1992.

288. Vendenberg, B.F., Stuhlmuller, J.E., Rath, L., Kerber, R.E., Collins, S.M., Melton, H.E., and Skorton, D.J.: Diagnosis of recent myocardial infarction with quantitative backscatter imaging: Preliminary studies. J. Am. Soc. Echocardiogr., *4*:10, 1991.

289. Milunski, M.R., Mohr, G.A., Perez, J.E., Vered, Z., Wear, K.A., Gessler, C.J., Sobel, B.E., Miller, J.G., and Wickline, S.A.: Ultrasonic tissue characterization with integrated backscatter. Circulation, *80*:491, 1989.

290. Nishimura, R.A., Tajik, A.J., Shib, C., Miller, F.A., Ilstrup, D.M., and Harrison, C.E.: Role of two dimensional echocardiography in the prediction of in-hospital complications after acute myocardial infarction. J. Am. Coll. Cardiol., *4*:1080, 1984.

291. Bhatnagar, S.K., Al-Yusuf, A.R.: The role of prehospital discharge two-dimensional echocardiography in determining the prognosis of survivors of first myocardial infarction. Am. Heart J., *109*:472, 1985.

292. Jaarsma, W., Visser, C.A., van M.J.E., Verheugt, F.W.A., Kupper, A.J.F., and Roos, J.P.: Predictive value of two-dimensional echocardiographic and hemodynamic measurements on admission with acute myocardial infarction. J. Am. Soc. Echocardiogr., *1*:187, 1988.

293. Lavie, C.J. and Gersh, B.J.: Acute myocardial infarction: Initial manifestations, management, and prognosis. Mayo Clin. Proc., *65*:531, 1990.

294. Berning, J. and Steensgaard-Hansen, F.: Early estimation of risk by echocardiographic determination of wall motion index in an unselected population with acute myocardial infarction. Am. J. Cardiol., *65*:567, 1990.

295. Kloner, R.A. and Parisi, A.F.: Acute myocardial infarction: Diagnostic and prognostic applications of two-dimensional echocardiography. Circulation, *1*, July 1986–June 1988.

296. Launbjerg, J., Berning, J., Fruergaard, P., and Appleyard, M.: Sensitivity and specificity of echocardiographic identification of patients eligible for safe early discharge after acute myocardial infarction. Am. Heart J., *124*:846, 1992.

297. Horowitz, R.S. and Morganroth, J.: Immediate detection of early high-risk patients with acute myocardial infarction using two dimensional echocardiographic evaluation of left ventricular regional wall motion abnormalities. Am. Heart J., *103*:814, 1982.

298. Abrams, D.S., Starling, M.R., Crawford, M.H., and O'Rourke, R.A.: Value of noninvasive techniques for predicting early complications in patients with clinical class II acute myocardial infarction. J. Am. Coll. Cardiol., *2*:818, 1983.

299. Charuzi, Y., Davidson, R.M., Barrett, M.J., Beeder C., Marshall, L.A., Loh, I.K., Prause, J.A., Meerbaum, S., and Corday, E.: Simultaneous assessment of segmental and global left ventricular function by two-dimensional echocardiography in acute myocardial infarction. Clin. Cardiol. *6*:255, 1983.

300. Nishimura, R.A., Reeder, G.S., Miller, F.A., Ilstrup, D.M., Shub, C., Seward, J.B., and Tajik, A.J.: Prognostic value of predischarge two dimensional echocardiogram after acute myocardial infarction. Am. J. Cardiol., *53*:429, 1984.

301. Kan, G., Visser, C.A., Koolen, J.J., and Dunning, A.J.: Short and long-term predictive value of admission wall motion score in acute myocardial infarction. Br. Heart J., *56*:422, 1986.

302. Finkelhor, R.S., Sun, J-P., Castellanos, M., and Bahler, R.C.: Predicting left heart failure after a myocardial infarction: A preliminary study of the value of echocardiographic measures of left ventricular filling and wall motion. J. Am. Soc. Echocardiogr., *4*:215, 1991.

303. Delemarre, B.J., Visser, C.A., Bot, H., de Koning, H.J., and Dunning, A.J.: Predictive value of pulsed Doppler echocardiography in acute myocardial infarction. J. Am. Soc. Echocardiogr., *2*:102, 1989.

304. Finkelhor, R.S., Sun, J-P, and Bahlar, R.C.: Left ventricular filling shortly after an uncomplicated myocardial infarction as a predictor of subsequent exercise capacity. Am. Heart J., *119*:85, 1990.

305. Horowitz, R.S., Morganroth, J., Parrotto, C., Chen, C.C., Soffer, J., and Pauletto, F.J.: Immediate diagnosis of acute myocardial infarction by two dimensional echocardiography. Circulation, *65*:323, 1982.

306. Daly, K., Monaghan, M., Jackson, G., and Jewitt, D.E.: Cross-sectional echocardiography in the early detection of acute myocardial ischemia and infarction. Br. Heart J., *45*:610, 1981.

307. Berning, J., Launbjerg, J., and Appleyard, M.: Echocardiographic algorithms for admission and predischarge prediction of mortality in acute myocardial infarction. Am. J. Cardiol., 69:1538, 1992.

308. Sabia, P., Abbott, R.D., Afrookteh, A., Keller, M.W., Touchstone, D.A., and Kaul, S.: Importance of two-dimensional echocardiographic assessment of left ventricular systolic function inpatients presenting to the emergency room with cardiac-related symptoms. Circulation, 84:1615, 1991.

309. Peels, C.H., Visser, C.A., Kupper, A.J.F., Vizzer, F.C., and Roos, J.P.: Usefulness of two-dimensional echocardiography for immediate detection of myocardial ischemia in the emergency room. Am. J. Cardiol., 65:687, 1990.

310. Sasaki, H., Charuzi, Y., Beeder, C., Sugiki, Y., and Lew, A.S.: Utility of echocardiography for the early assessment of patients with nondiagnostic chest pain. Am. Heart J., 112:494, 1986.

311. Josephson, R.A., Weiss, J.L., Becker, L.C., and Shapiro, E.P.: Dipyridamole echocardiography in the detection of vulnerable myocardium in the early postinfarction period. J. Am. Soc. Echocardiogr., 2:324, 1989.

312. Bolognese, L., Sarasso, G., Gongo, A.S., Aralda, D., Piccinino, C., Rossi, L., and Rossi, P.: Stress testing in the period after infarction. Circulation, 83:III-32, 1991.

313. Bolognese, L., Sarasso, G., Aralda, D., Bondo, A.S., Rossi, L., and Rossi, P.: High dose dipyridamole echocardiography early after uncomplicated acute myocardial infarction: Correlation with exercise testing and coronary angiography. J. Am. Coll. Cardiol., 14:357, 1989.

314. Mannering, D., Cripps, T., Leech, G., Mehta, N., Valantine, H., Gilmour, S., and Bennett, E.D.: The dobutamine stress test as an alternative to exercise testing after acute myocardial infarction. Br. Heart J., 59:521, 1988.

315. Bolognese, L., Rossi, L., Sarasso, G., Prando, M.D., Bongo, A.S., Dellavesa, P., and Rossi, P.: Silent versus symptomatic dipyridamole-induced ischemia after myocardial infarction: Clinical and prognostic significance. J. Am. Coll. Cardiol., 19:953, 1992.

316. Isaacsohn, J.L., Earle, M.G., and Kemper, A.J., and Parisi, A.F.: Postmyocardial infarction pain and infarct extension in the coronary care unit: Role of two-dimensional echocardiography. J. Am. Coll. Cardiol., 11:246, 1988.

317. Picard, M.H., Wilkins, G.T., Gillam, L.D., Thomas, J.D., and Weyman, A.E.: Immediate regional endocardial surface expansion following coronary occlusion in the canine left ventricle: Disproportionate effects of anterior versus inferior ischemia. Am. Heart J., 121:753, 1991.

318. Weiss, J.L., Marino, P.N., and Shapiro, E.P.: Myocardial infarct expansion: Recognition, significance and pathology. Am. J. Cardiol., 68:35D, 1991.

319. Mehta, P.M., Alker, K.J., and Kloner, R.A.: Functional infarct expansion, left ventricular dilatation and isovolumic relaxation time after coronary occlusion: A two-dimensional echocardiographic study. J. Am. Coll. Cardiol., 11:630, 1988.

320. Oldroyd, K.G., Pye, M.P., Ray, S.G., Cobbe, S.M., and Dargie, H.J.: Early use of captopril to restrict myocardial infarct expansion. Cardiol. Board Rev., 9:67, 1992.

321. Jugdutt, B.I., Schwarz-Michorowski, B.L., and Khan, M.I.: Effect of long-term captopril therapy on left ventricular remodeling and function during healing of canine myocardial infarction. J. Am. Coll. Cardiol., 19:713, 1992.

322. Bonaduce, D., Petretta, M., Arrichiello, P., Conforti, G., Montemurro, V., Attisano, T., Bianchi, V., and Morgano, G.: Effects of captopril treatment on left ventricular remodeling and function after anterior myocardial infarction. J. Am. Coll. Cardiol., 19:858, 1992.

323. Marino, P., Destro, G., Barbieri, E., and Bicego, D.: Reperfusion of the infarct-related coronary artery limits left ventricular expansion beyond myocardial salvage. Am. Heart J., 123:1157, 1992.

324. Abernethy, M., Sharpe, N., Smith, H., and Gamble, G.: Echocardiographic prediction of left ventricular volume after myocardial infarction. J. Am. Coll. Cardiol., 17:1527, 1991.

325. Gottlieb, S.O., Becker, L.C., Weiss, J.L., Shapiro, E.P., Chandra, N.C., Flaherty, J.T., Gottlieb, S.H., Quyang, P., Mellits, E.D., Townsend, S.N., Weisfeldt, M.L., Healy, B., and Gerstenblith, G.: Nifedipine in acute myocardial infarction: An assessment of left ventricular function, infarct size, and infarct expansion. Br. Heart J., 59:411, 1988.

326. Force, T., Kemper, A., Leavitt, M., and Parisi, A.F.: Acute reduction in functional infarct expansion with late coronary reperfusion: Assessment with quantitative two-dimensional echocardiography. J. Am. Coll. Cardiol., 11:192, 1988.

327. Jugdutt, B.I.: Identification of patients prone to infarct expansion by the degree of regional shape distortion on an early two-dimensional echocardiogram after myocardial infarction. Clin. Cardiol., 13:28, 1990.

328. Nakano, K., Sugawara, M., Kato, T., Sasayama, S., Carabello, B.A., Asanoi, H., Umemura, J., and Koyanagi, H.: Regional work of the human left ventricle calculated by wall stress and the natural logarithm of reciprocal of wall thickness. J. Am. Coll. Cardiol., 12:1442, 1988.

329. Weyman, A.E., Peskoe, S.M., Williams, E.S., Dillon, J.C., and Feigenbaum, H.: Detection of left ventricular aneurysms by cross-sectional echocardiography. Circulation, 54:936, 1976.

330. Kambe, T., Nishimura, K., Hibi, N., Fukui, Y., Miwa, A., and Murase, M.: Real time observation of left ventricular aneurysm by B mode echocardiography. JCU, 6:405, 1978.

331. Sorensen, S.G., Crawford, M.H., Richards, K.L., Chaudhuri, T.K., and O'Rourke, R.A.: Non-invasive detection of ventricular aneurysm by combined two dimensional echocardiography and equilibrium radionuclide angiography. Am. Heart J., 104:145, 1982.

332. Amon, K.W. and Crawford, M.H.: Improved two dimensional echocardiographic technique for left ventricular aneurysm detection. JCU, 10:261, 1982.

333. Baur, H.R., Daniel, J.A., and Nelson, R.R.: Detection of left ventricular aneurysm on two dimensional echocardiography. Am. J. Cardiol., 50:191, 1982.

334. Gentile, F., Greco, R., Siciliano, S., Violini, R., Marsico, L., Mininni, N., and Marsico, F.: Comparative accuracy of cross-sectional echocardiography and cineventriculography for left ventricular evaluation after myocardial infarction. G. Ital. Cardiol., 11:1996, 1981.

335. Visser, C.A., Kan, G., David, G.K., Lie, K.I., and Durrer, D.: Echocardiographic-cineangiographic correlation in detecting left ventricular aneurysm: A prospective study of 422 patients. Am. J. Cardiol., 50:337, 1982.

336. Gueret, P., Farcot, J.C., Bardet, J., Boisante, L., Dubourg, O., Terdjman, M., Ferrier, A., Rigaud, M., and Bourdariaas, J.P.: Update on the study of true and false left ventricular aneurysms by two dimensional echocardiography. Arch. Mal Coeur, 75:1029, 1982.

337. Wong, M. and Shah, P.M.: Accuracy of two dimensional echocardiography in detecting left ventricular aneurysm. Clin. Cardiol., 6:250, 1983.

338. DePace, N.L., Dowinsky, S., Untereker, W., LeMole, G.M., Spagna, P.M., and Meister, S.G.: Giant inferior wall left ventricular aneurysm. Am. Heart J., 119:400, 1990.

339. Daikoku, S., Haze, K., Ogawa, H., Kawaguchi, M., Nonogi, H., Fukami, K., Sumiyoshi, T., and Hiramori, K.: Clinical and anatomical features of acute myocardial infarction associated with double rupture of the interventricular septum and ventricular free wall. J. Cardiol., 21:229, 1991.

340. Lopez-Sendon, J., Gonzalez, A., Lopez, De Sa E., Coma-Canella, I., Roldan, I., Dominguez, F., Maqueda, I., and Jadraque, L.M.: Diagnosis of subacute ventricular wall rupture after acute myocardial infarction: Sensitivity and specificity of clinical, hemodynamic and echocardiographic criteria. J. Am. Coll. Cardiol., 19:1145, 1992.

341. Brack, M., Asinger, R.W., Sharkey, S.W., Herzog, C.A., and Hodges, M.: Two-dimensional echocardiographic characteristics of pericardial hematoma secondary to left ventricular free wall rupture complicating acute myocardial infarction. Am. J. Cardiol., 68:961, 1991.

342. Pijls, N.H., Fast, J.H., van der Meer, J.J., and van der Werf, T.: Biventricular free wall rupture with extracardiac left-to-right shunt after myocardial infarction. Am. Heart J., 115:186, 1988.

343. Sears, T.D., Ong, Y.S., Starke, H., and Forker, A.D.: Left ventricular pseudoaneurysm identified by cross-sectional echocardiography. Ann. Intern. Med., 90:935, 1979.

344. Katz, R.J., Simpson, A., DiBianco, R., Fletcher, R.D., Bates, H.R., and Sauerbrunn, B.J.L.: Noninvasive diagnosis of left ventricular pseudoaneurysm: Role of two-dimensional echocardiography and radionuclide gated pool imaging. Am. J. Cardiol., 44:372, 1979.

345. Morcerf, F.P., Duarte, E.P., Salcedo, E.E., et al.: Echocardiographic findings in false aneurysm of the left ventricle. Cleve. Clin. Q., 43:71, 1976.

346. Alter, B.R., Lewis, M.E., Vargas, A., Rosenthal, S.P., and Chandarlapaty, S.K.C.: Noninvasive diagnosis of left ventricular pseudoaneurysm by radioangiography and echography. Am. Heart J., 101:236, 1981.

347. Dander, B., Zanolla, L., Nidasio, G.P., Buonanno, C., and Poppi, A.: M-mode and two dimensional echocardiographic diagnosis of pseudoaneurysm of the left ventricle (author's transl.). G. Ital. Cardiol., 11:686, 1981.

348. Gatewood, R.P., Jr. and Nanda, N.C.: Differentiation of left ventricular pseudoaneurysm with two dimensional echocardiography. Am. J. Cardiol., 46:869, 1980.

349. Glover, M.U., Hagan, A.D., Vieweg, W.V., and Ceretto, W.J.: Pseudoaneurysm of the left ventricle diagnosed by two dimensional echocardiography: Case report. Milit. Med., 146:696, 1981.

350. Levy, R., Rozanski, A., Charuzi, Y., Childs, W., Waxman, A., Corday, E., and Berman, D.S.: Complementary roles of two dimensional echocardiography and radionuclide ventriculography in ventricular pseudoaneurysm diagnosis. Am. Heart J., 102:1066, 1981.

351. Catherwood, E., Mintz, G.S., Kotler, M.N., Parry, W.R., and Segal, B.L.: Two dimensional echocardiographic recognition of left ventricular pseudoaneurysm. Circulation, 62:294, 1980.

352. Bansal, R.C., Pai, R.G., Hauck, A.J., and Isaeff, D.M.: Biventricular apical rupture and formation of pseudoaneurysm: Unique flow patterns by Doppler and color flow imaging. Am. Heart J., 124:497, 1992.

353. March, K.L., Sawada, S.G., Tarver, R.D., Kesler, K.A., and Armstrong, W.F.: Current concepts of left ventricular pseudoaneurysm: Pathophysiology, therapy, and diagnostic imaging methods. Clin. Cardiol., 12:531, 1989.

354. Otto, C.M. and Stratton, J.R.: Postinfarction left ventricular pseudoaneurysm: Echocardiographic diagnosis and prolonged survival in three patients. Clin. Cardiol., 11:189, 1988.

355. Saner, H.E., Asinger, R.W., Daniel, J.A., and Olson, J.: Two-dimensional echocardiographic identification of left ventricular pseudoaneurysm. Am. Heart J., 112:977, 1986.

356. Smeal, W.E., Dianzumba, S.B., and Joyner, C.R.: Evaluation of pseudoaneurysm of the left ventricle by echocardiography and pulsed Doppler. Am. Heart J., 113:1508, 1987.

357. Rueda, B., Panidis, I.P., Gonzales, R., and McDonough, M.: Left ventricular pseudoaneurysm: Detection and postoperative follow-up by color Doppler echocardiography. Am. Heart J., 120:990, 1990.

358. Tunick, P.A., Slater, W., and Kronzon, I.: The hemodynamics of left ventricular pseudoaneurysm: Color Doppler echocardiographic study. Am. Heart J., 117:1161, 1989.

359. Sutherland, G.R., Smyllie, J.H., and Roelandt, J.R.T.: Advantages of colour flow imaging in the diagnosis of left ventricular pseudoaneurysm. Br. Heart J., 61:59, 1989.

360. Roelandt, J.R.T.C., Sutherland, G.R., Yoshida, K., and Yoshikawa, J.: Improved diagnosis and characterization of left ventricular pseudoaneurysm by Doppler color flow imaging. J. Am. Coll. Cardiol., 12:807, 1988.

361. Schwarz, J., Hamad, N., Hernandez, G., DeCastro, C., Beard, E., Colley, D., and Hall, R.: Doppler color-flow echocardiographic recognition of left ventricular pseudoaneurysm. Am. Heart J., 116:1353, 1988.

362. Bach, M., Berger, M., Hecht, S.R., and Strain, J.E.: Diagnosis of left ventricular pseudoaneurysm using contrast and Doppler echocardiography. Am. Heart J., 118:854, 1989.

363. Burns, C.A., Paulsen, W., Arrowood, J.A., Tolman, D.E., Rose, B., Fabian, J.A., and Spratt, J.A.: Improved identification of posterior left ventricular pseudoaneurysms by transesophageal echocardiography. Am. Heart J., 124:796, 1992.

363a. Stoddard, M.F., et al.: Transesophageal echocardiography in the detection of left ventricular pseudoaneurysm. Am. Heart J., 125:534, 1993.

364. Geslin, P., P'ezard, P., Lhoste, P., and Tadei, A.: Noninvasive methods in the diagnosis of post-infarction false aneurysm. Apropos of a case. Arch. Mal Coeur, 73:1455, 1980.

365. Dander, B., Zanolla, L., Nidasio, G.P., Buonanno, C., and Poppi, A.: M-mode and two dimensional echocardiographic diagnosis of pseudoaneurysm of left ventricle. G. Ital. Cardiol., 11:686, 1981.

366. Chandraratna, P.A.N., Balachandran, P.K., Shah, P.M., and Hodges, M.: Echocardiographic observations on ventricular septal rupture complicating myocardial infarction. Circulation, 51:506, 1975.

367. Scanlan, J.G., Seward, J.B., and Tajik, A.J.: Visualization of ventricular septal rupture utilizing wide-angle two-dimensional echocardiography. Mayo Clin. Proc., 54:381, 1979.

368. Bishop, H.L., Gibson, R.S., Stamm, R.B., Beller, G.A., and Martin, R.P.: Role of two dimensional echocardiog-

raphy in the evaluation of patients with ventricular septal rupture postmyocardial infarction. Am. Heart J., *102*: 965, 1981.

369. Mintz, G.S., Victor, M.F., Kotler, M.N., Parry, W.R., and Segal, B.L.: Two dimensional echocardiographic identification of surgically correctable complications of acute myocardial infarction. Circulation, *64*:91, 1981.

370. Rogers, E.W., Glassman, R.D., Feigenbaum, H., Weyman, A.E., and Godley, R.W.: Aneurysms of the posterior interventricular septum with postinfarction ventricular septal defect. Echocardiographic identification. Chest, *78*:741, 1980.

371. Stephens, J.D., Giles, M.R., and Banim, S.O.: Ruptured postinfarction ventricular septal aneurysm causing congestive cardiac failure. Detection by two dimensional echocardiography. Br. Heart J., *46*:216, 1981.

372. Hodsden, J. and Nanda, N.C.: Dissecting aneurysm of the ventricular septum following acute myocardial infarction: diagnosis by real-time two dimensional echocardiography. Am. Heart J., *101*:671, 1981.

373. Jugdutt, B.I. and Michorowski, B.L.: Role of infarct expansion in rupture of the ventricular septum after acute myocardial infarction: A two-dimensional echocardiographic study. Clin. Cardiol., *10*:641, 1987.

374. Mascarenhas, D.A.N., Benotti, J.R., Daggett, W.M., Rifkin, R.D., Dave, R.D., and Spodick, D.H.: Postinfarction septal aneurysm with delayed formation of left-to-right shunt. Am. Heart J., *122*:226, 1991.

375. Miyatake, K., Okamoto, M., Kinoshita, N., Park, Y-D., Nagata, S., Izumi, S., Fusejima, K., Sakakibara, H., and Nimura, Y.: Doppler echocardiographic features of ventricular septal rupture in myocardial infarction. J. Am. Coll. Cardiol., *5*:182, 1985.

376. Eisenberg, P.R., Barzilai, B., and Perez, J.E.: Noninvasive detection by Doppler echocardiography of combined ventricular septal rupture and mitral regurgitation in acute myocardial infarction. J. Am. Coll. Cardiol., *4*:617, 1984.

377. Smyllie, J.H., Sutherland, G.R., Geuskens, R., Dawkins, K., Conway, N., and Roelandt, J.R.T.C.: Doppler color flow mapping in the diagnosis of ventricular septal rupture and acute mitral regurgitation after myocardial infarction. J. Am. Coll. Cardiol., *15*:1449, 1990.

378. Smyllie, J., Dawkins, K., Conway, N., and Sutherland, G.: Diagnosis of ventricular septal rupture after myocardial infarction: Value of colour flow mapping. Br. Heart J., *62*:260, 1989.

379. Amico, A., Iliceto, S., Rizzo, A., Cascella, V., and Risson, P.: Color Doppler findings in ventricular septal dissection following myocardial infarction. Am. Heart J., *117*:195, 1989.

380. Doig, J.C., Au, J., Dark, J.H., and Furniss, S.S.: Postinfarction communication between a left ventricular aneurysm and the right atrium. Eur. Heart J., *13*:1006, 1992.

380a. Ballal, R.S., Sanyal, R.S., Nanda, N.C., and Mahan, E.F.: Usefulness of transesophageal echocardiography in the diagnosis of ventricular septal rupture secondary to acute myocardial infarction. Am. J. Cardiol., *71*:367, 1993.

381. van den Bos, A.A., Bletter, W.B., and Hagemeijer, F.: Progressive development of left ventricular thrombus: Detection and evolution studied with echocardiographic techniques. Chest, *74*:307, 1978.

382. DeMaria, A.N., Bommer, W., Neumann, A., Grehl, T., Weinart, L., DeNardo, S., Amsterdam, E.A., and Mason, D.T.: Left ventricular thrombi identified by cross-sectional echocardiography. Ann. Intern. Med., *90*:14, 1979.

383. Meltzer, R.S., Guthaner, D., Rakowski, H., Popp, R.L., and Martin, R.P.: Diagnosis of left ventricular thrombi by two-dimensional echocardiography. Br. Heart J., *42*: 261, 1979.

384. Reeder, G.S., Tajik, A.J., and Seward, J.B.: Left ventricular mural thrombus. Two dimensional echocardiographic diagnosis. Mayo Clin. Proc., *56*:82, 1981.

385. Asinger, R.W., Mikell, F.L., Elsperger, J., and Hodges, M.: Incidence of left-ventricular thrombosis after acute transmural myocardial infarction. Serial evaluation by two dimensional echocardiography. New Engl. J. Med., *305*:297, 1981.

386. Friedman, M.J., Carlson, K., Marcus, F.I., and Woolfenden, J.M.: Clinical correlations in patients with acute myocardial infarction and left ventricular thrombus detected by two dimensional echocardiography. Am. J. Med., *72*:894, 1982.

387. Arvan, S.: Left ventricular mural thrombi secondary to acute myocardial infarction: predisposing factors and embolic phenomenon. JCU, *11*:467, 1983.

388. Bhatnagar, S.K. and Al Yusuf, A.R.: Left ventricular thrombi after acute myocardial infarction. Postgrad. Med. J., *59*:495, 1983.

389. Benichou, M., Aubry, J., Larbi, M.B., Romani, A., Chiche, G., Egre, A., Djiane, P., Bory, M., and Serradimigni, A.: Detection of left intraventricular thrombi in the acute phase of myocardial infarction by two dimensional echocardiography. Apropose of 103 cases. Arch. Mal Coeur, *76*:1012, 1983.

390. Keating, E.C., Gross, S.A., Schlamowitz, R.A., Glassman, J., Mazur, J.H., Pitt, W.A., and Miller, D.: Mural thrombi in myocardial infarctions. Prospective evaluation by two dimensional echocardiography. Am. J. Med., *74*:989, 1983.

391. Visser, C.A., Kan, G., Lie, K.I., and Durrer, D.: Left ventricular thrombus following acute myocardial infarction: A prospective serial echocardiographic study of 96 patients. Eur. Heart J., *4*:333, 1983.

392. Tramarin, R., Pozzoli, M., and Vecchio, C.: Left ventricular thrombosis in recent myocardial infarction. An echocardiographic study. G. Ital. Cardiol., *12*:397, 1982.

393. Weinreich, D.J., Burke, J.F., and Pauletto, F.J.: Left ventricular mural thrombi complicating acute myocardial infarction. Ann. Intern. Med., *100*:789, 1984.

394. Johannessen, K.A., Nordrehaug, J.E., and Von Der Lippe, G.: Left ventricular thrombosis and cerebrovascular accident in acute myocardial infarction. Br. Heart J., *51*:553, 1984.

395. Arvan, S. and Plehn, J.: Embolization of a left ventricular mural thrombus: verification by two dimensional echocardiography. Arch. Intern. Med., *142*:1952, 1982.

396. Kessler, K.M., Cotler, R.P., Bilsker, M.S., and Meyerberg, R.J.: Narrow-based left ventricular thrombus. Am. J. Cardiol., *53*:645, 1984.

397. Arvan, S.: Persistent intracardiac thrombi and systemic embolization despite anticoagulant therapy. Am. Heart J., *109*:178, 1985.

398. Visser, C.A., Kan, G., Meltzer, R.S., Dunning, A.J., Roelandt, J., VanCorler, M., DeKoning, H.: Embolic potential of left ventricular thrombus after myocardial infarction: A two-dimensional echocardiographic study of 119 patients. J. Am. Coll. Cardiol., *5*:1276, 1985.

399. Jugdutt, B.I., Sivaram, C.A., Wortman, C., Trudell, C., and Penner, P.: Prospective two-dimensional echocar-

diographic evaluation of left ventricular thrombus and embolism after acute myocardial infarction. J. Am. Coll. Cardiol., *13*:554, 1989.

400. Mikell, F.L., Asinger, R.W., Eisperger, J., Anderson, W.R., and Hodges, M.: Regional stasis of blood in the dysfunctional left ventricle: echocardiographic detection and differentiation from early thrombosis. Circulation, *66*:755, 1982.

401. Kono, T., Sabbah, H.N., Rosman, H., Slam, M., Jafri, S., Stein, P.D., and Goldstein, S.: Mechanism of functional mitral regurgitation during acute myocardial ischemia. J. Am. Coll. Cardiol., *19*:1101, 1992.

402. Barzilai, B., Gessler, C., Perez, J.E., Schaab, C., and Jaffe, A.S.: Significance of Doppler-detected mitral regurgitation in acute myocardial infarction. Am. J. Cardiol., 220:1988.

403. Bhatnagar, S.K. and Yusuf, A.R.: Significance of a mitral regurgitation systolic murmur complicating a first acute myocardial infarction in the coronary care unit—assessment by colour Doppler flow imaging. Eur. Heart J., *12*:1211, 1991.

403a.Hanlon, J.T., et al.: Echocardiography recognition of partial papillary muscle rupture. J. Am. Soc. Echocardiogr., *6*:101, 1993.

404. Nishimura, R.A., Shub, C., and Tajik, A.J.: Two dimensional echocardiographic diagnosis of partial papillary muscle rupture. Br. Heart J., *48*:598, 1982.

405. Nishimura, R.A., Schaff, H.V., Shub, C., Gersh, B.J., Edwards, W.D., and Tajik, A.J.: Papillary muscle rupture complicating acute myocardial infarction: Analysis of 17 patients. Am. J. Cardiol., *51*:373, 1983.

406. Stoddard, M.F., Keedy, D.L., and Kupersmith, J.: Transesophageal echocardiographic diagnosis of papillary muscle rupture complicating acute myocardial infarction. Am. Heart J., *120*:690, 1990.

407. Godley, R.W., Wann, L.S., Rogers, E.W., Feigenbaum, H., and Weyman, A.E.: Incomplete mitral leaflet closure in patients with papillary muscle dysfunction. Circulation, *63*:565, 1981.

408. Hayakawa, M., Inoy, T., Kawanishi, H., Kaku, K., Kumaki, T., Toh, S., and Fukuzaki, H.: Two dimensional echocardiographic findings of patients with papillary muscle dysfunction. J. Cardiogr., *12*:137, 1982.

409. D'Arcy, B. and Nanda, N.C.: Two dimensional echocardiographic features of right ventricular infarction. Circulation, *65*:167, 1982.

410. Fogelfeld, L., Hertzeanu, H., Gil, I., and Almog, C.: Right myocardial infarction with predominant right ventricular dysfunction. Isr. J. Med. Sci., *16*:859, 1980.

411. Elkayam, U., Halprin, S.L., Frishman, W., Strom, J., and Cohen, M.N.: Echocardiographic findings in cardiogenic shock due to right ventricular myocardial infarction: Cathet. Cardiovasc. Diagn., *5*:289, 1979.

412. Lopez-Sendon, J., Garcia-Fernandez, M.A., Coma-Canella I., Yanguela, M.M., and Banuelos, F.: Segmental right ventricular function after acute myocardial infarction: Two dimensional echocardiographic study in 63 patients. Am. J. Cardiol., *51*:390, 1983.

413. Baigrie, R.S., Haw, A., Morgan, C.D., Bakowski, H., Drobac, M., and McLaughlin, P.: The spectrum of right ventricular involvement in inferior wall myocardial infarction: A clinical, hemodynamic and noninvasive study. J. Am. Coll. Cardiol., *1*:1396, 1983.

414. Panidis, I.P., Kotler, M.N., Mintz, G.S., Ross, J., Ren, J.-F., Herling, I., and Kutalek, S.: Right ventricular function in coronary artery disease as assessed by two dimensional echocardiography. Am. Heart J., *107*:1187, 1984.

415. Cecchi, F., Zupprioli, A., Favilli, S., DiBari, M., Vannucci, A., Oini, R., and Marchionni, N.: Echocardiographic features of right ventricular infarction. Clin. Cardiol., 7:405, 1984.

416. Ferranti, E., Caputo, V., Gulla, S., and Latini, S.: Right ventricle myocardial infarction: Scintigraphic and echocardiographic findings. A case report. G. Ital. Cardiol., *11*:2249, 1981.

417. Kaul, S., Hopkins, J.M., and Shah, P.M.: Chronic effects of myocardial infarction on right ventricular function: A noninvasive assessment. J. Am. Coll. Cardiol., *2*:607, 1983.

418. Jugdutt, B.I., Sussex, B.A., Sivaram, C.A., and Rossall, R.E.: Right ventricular infarction: Two dimensional echocardiographic evaluation. Am. Heart J., *107*:505, 1984.

419. Goldberger, J.J., Himelman, R.B., Wolfe, C.L., and Schiller, N.B.: Right ventricular infarction: Recognition and assessment of its hemodynamic significance by two-dimensional echocardiography. J. Am. Soc. Echocardiogr., 4:140, 1991.

420. Chuttani, K., Sussman, H., and Pandian, N.G.: Echocardiographic evidence that regional right ventricular dysfunction occurs frequently in anterior myocardial infarction. Am. Heart J., *122*:850, 1991.

421. Bellamy, G.R., Rasmussen, H.H., Nasser, F.N., Wiseman, J.C., and Cooper, R.A.: Value of two-dimensional echocardiography, electrocardiography, and clinical signs in detecting right ventricular infarction. Am. Heart J., *112*:304, 1986.

422. Stowers, S.A., Lieboff, R.H., Wasserman, A.G., Katz, R.J., Bren, G.B., and Hsu, I.: Right ventricular thrombus formation in association with acute myocardial infarction: Diagnosis by two dimensional echocardiography. Am. J. Cardiol., *52*:912, 1983.

423. Manno, B.V., Bemis, C.E., Carver, J., and Mintz, G.S.: Right ventricular infarction complicated by right to left shunt. J. Am. Coll. Cardiol., *1*:554, 1983.

424. Rietveld, A.P., Merrman, L., Essed, C.E., Trimbos, J.B.M.J., and Hagemeijer, F.: Right to left shunt, with severe hypoxemia, at the atrial level in a patient with hemodynamically important right ventricular infarction. J. Am. Coll. Cardiol., *2*:766, 1983.

425. Maurer, G. and Nanda, N.C.: Two dimensional echocardiographic evaluation of exercise-induced left and right ventricular asynergy: Correlation with thallium scanning. Am. J. Cardiol., *48*:720, 1981.

426. Hilton, T.C., Pearson, A.C., Serota, H., Dressler, F.A., and Kern, M.J.: Right atrial infarction and cardiogenic shock complicating acute myocardial infarction: Diagnosis by transesophageal echocardiography. Am. Heart J., *120*:427, 1990.

427. Weyman, A.E., Feigenbaum, H., Dillon, J.C., Johnston, K.W., and Eggleton, R.C.: Noninvasive visualization of the left main coronary artery by cross-sectional echocardiography. Circulation, *54*:169, 1976.

428. Ribeiro, P., Shapiro, L.M., Gonzalex, A., Thompson, G.R., and Oakley, C.M.: Cross sectional echocardiographic assessment of the aortic root and coronary ostial stenosis in familial hypercholesterolemia. Br. Heart J., *50*:432, 1983.

429. Block, P.J. and Popp, R.L.: Detecting and excluding significant left main coronary artery narrowing by echocardiography. Am. J. Cardiol., *55*:937, 1985.

430. Rink, L.D., Feigenbaum, H., Godley, R.W., Weyman, A.E., Dillon, J.C., Phillips, J.F., and Marshall, J.E.: Echocardiographic detection of left main coronary artery obstruction. Circulation, 65:719, 1982.

431. Kenny, A. and Shapiro, L.M.: Transthoracic high-frequency two-dimensional echocardiography, Doppler and color flow mapping to determine anatomy and blood flow patterns in the distal left anterior descending coronary artery. Am. J. Cardiol., 69:1265, 1992.

432. Presti, C.F., Feigenbaum, H., Armstrong, W.F., Ryan, T., and Dillon, J.C.: Digital two-dimensional echocardiographic imaging of the proximal left anterior descending coronary artery. Am. J. Cardiol., 60:1254, 1987.

433. Douglas, P.S., Fiolkoski, J., Berko, B., and Reichek, N.: Echocardiographic visualization of coronary artery anatomy in the adult. J. Am. Coll. Cardiol., 11:565, 1988.

434. Vered, Z., Katz, M., Rath, S., Har-Zahav, Y., Battler, A., Benjamin, P., and Neufeld, H.N.: Two-dimensional echocardiographic analysis of proximal left main coronary artery in humans. Am. Heart J., 112:972, 1986.

435. Ryan, T., Armstrong, W.F., and Feigenbaum, H.: Two-dimensional echocardiographic assessment of left main coronary artery obstruction. Cardiol. Board Rev., 3:90, 1986.

436. Katz, E.S., Tunick, P.A., and Kronzon, I.: Observations of coronary flow augmentation and balloon function during intraaortic balloon counterpulsation using transesophageal echocardiography. Am. J. Cardiol., 69:1635, 1992.

437. Varma, V., Nanda, N.C., Soto, B., Roubin, G.S., Bajaj, R., Jain, S., and Sanyal, R.S.: Transesophageal echocardiographic demonstration of proximal right coronary artery dissection extending into the aortic root. Am. Heart J., 123:1055, 1992.

438. Yoshida, K., Yoshikawa, J., Hozumi, T., Yamaura, Y., Akasaka, T., Fukaya, T., and Kato, H.: Detection of left main coronary artery stenosis by transesophageal color Doppler and two-dimensional echocardiography. Circulation, 81:1271, 1990.

439. Yamagishi, M., Yasu, T., Ohara, K., Kuro, M., and Miyatake, K.: Detection of coronary blood flow associated with left main coronary artery stenosis by transesophageal Doppler color flow echocardiography. J. Am. Coll. Cardiol., 17:87, 1991.

440. Kyo, S., Takamoto, S., Matsumura, M., Yokote, Y., and Omoto, R.: Visualization of coronary blood flow by transesophageal Doppler color flow mapping. J. Cardiogr., 16:831, 1986.

441. Zwicky, P., Daniel, W.G., Mugge, A., and Lichtlen, P.R.: Imaging of coronary arteries by color-coded transesophageal Doppler echocardiography. Am. J. Cardiol., 62:639, 1988.

441a. Yamada, S., et al.: Transesophageal Doppler echocardiographic imaging and blood flow measurements for the diagnosis of stenotic left coronary arteries. J. Cardiol., 21:539, 1991.

442. Sawada, S.G., Ryan, T., Segar, D., Atherton, L., Fineberg, N., Davis, C., and Feigenbaum, H.: Distinguishing ischemic cardiomyopathy from nonischemic dilated cardiomyopathy with coronary echocardiography. Am. Heart J., 19:1223, 1992.

443. Reichert, S.L.A., Visser, C.A., Koolen, J.J., Chapman, J.V., Angelsen, B.A.J., Meyne, N.G., and Dunning, A.J.: Transesophageal examination of the left coronary artery with a 7.5-MHz annular array two-dimensional color flow Doppler tranduces. J. Am. Soc. Echocardiogr., 3:118, 1990.

444. Pearce, F.B., Sheikh, K.H., deBruijn, N.P., and Kisslo, J.: Imaging of the coronary arteries by transesophageal echocardiography. J. Am. Soc. Echocardiogr., 2:276, 1989.

445. Iliceto, S., Marangelli, V., Memmola, C., and Rizzon, P.: Transesophageal Doppler echocardiography evaluation of coronary blood flow velocity in baseline conditions and during dipyridamole-induced coronary vasodilation. Circulation, 83:61, 1991.

446. Samdarshi, T.E., Nanda, N.C., Gatewood, Jr., R.P., Ballal, R.S., Chang, L.K., Singh, H.P., Nath, H., Kriklin, J.K., and Pacifico, A.D.: Usefulness and limitations of transesophageal echocardiography in the assessment of proximal coronary artery stenosis. J. Am. Coll. Cardiol., 19:572, 1992.

447. Ross, Jr., J.J., Mintz, G.S., and Chandrasekaran, K.: Transthoracic two-dimensional of the distal left anterior descending coronary artery. J. Am. Coll. Cardiol., 15:373, 1990.

448. Faletro, F., Cipriani, M., Corno, R., Cali, G., Mantero, A., Cantoni, S., Formentini, A., Danzi, G.B., and Pezzano, A.: Transthoracic high frequency echocardiographic detection of atherosclerotic lesions in the descending portion of the left coronary artery. J. Am. Soc. Echocardiogr., In press.

449. Kyo, S., Matsumura, M., Takamoto, S., Yokote, Y., and Omoto, R.: Visualization of internal mammary artery bypass graft flow using a linear color flow mapping system with a convex type transducer. J. Cardiol., 19:1, 1989.

450. Dzavik, V., Lemay, M., and Chan, K-L.: Echocardiographic diagnosis of an aortocoronary venous bypass graft aneurysm. Am. Heart J., 118:619, 1989.

451. Jain, S.P., Roubin, G.S., Nanda, N.C., Dean, L.S., Agrawal, S.K., and Pinheiro, L.: Intravascular ultrasound imaging of saphenous vein graft stenosis. Am. J. Cardiol., 69:133, 1992.

452. St. Goar, F.G., Pinto, F.J., Alderman, E.L., Fitzgerald, P.J., Stinson, E.B., Billingham, M.E., and Popp, R.L.: Detection of coronary atherosclerosis in young adult hearts using intravascular ultrasound. Circulation, 86:756, 1992.

453. Liebson, P.R. and Klein, L.W.: Intravascular ultrasound in coronary atherosclerosis: A new approach to clinical assessment. Am. Heart J., 123:1643, 1992.

454. Mintz, G.S., Potkin, B.N. Cooke, P.H., Stark, K.S., Kent, K.M., Satler, L.F., Pichard, A.D., and Leon, M.B.: Intravascular ultrasound imaging in a patient with unstable angina. Am. Heart J., 123:1692, 1992.

455. Keren, G., Douek, P., Oblon, C., Bonner, R.F., Pichard, A.D. and Leon, M.B.: Atherosclerotic saphenous vein grafts treated with different interventional procedures assessed by intravascular ultrasound. Am. Heart J., 124:198, 1992.

456. Yock, P.G., Linker, D.T., and Angelsen, B.A.J.: Two-dimensional intravascular ultrasound: Technical development and initial clinical experience. J. Am. Soc. Echocardiogr., 2:296, 1989.

457. Pandian, N.G., Kreis, A., and O'Donnell, T.: Intravascular ultrasound estimation of arterial stenosis. J. Am. Soc. Echocardiogr., 2:390, 1989.

458. Tobis, J.M., Mallery, J., Mahon, D., Lehmann, K., Zalesky, P., Griffith, J., Gessert, J., Moriuchi, M., McRae, M., Dwyer, M-L., Greep, N., and Henry, W.L.: Intravascular ultrasound imaging of human coronary arteries in vivo. Circulation, 83:913, 1991.

459. Nissen, S.E., Gurley, J.C., Grines, C.L., Booth, D.C., McClure, R., Berk, M. Fischer, C., and DeMaria, A.N.:

Intravascular ultrasound assessment of lumen size and wall morphology in normal subjects and patients with coronary artery disease. Circulation, *84*:1087, 1991.

460. Anderson, M.H., Simpson, I.A., Katritsis, D., Davies, M.J., and Ward, D.E.: Intravascular ultrasound imaging of the coronary arteries: An in vitro evaluation of measurement of area of the lumen and atheroma characterisation. Br. Heart J., *68*:276, 1992.

461. Davies, S.W., Winterton, S.J., and Rothman, M.T.: Intravascular ultrasound to assess left main stem coronary artery lesion. Br. Heart J., *68*:524, 1992.

461a. Hodgson, J.M., et al.: Intracoronary ultrasound imaging: Correlation of plaque morphology with angiography, clinical syndrome and procedural results in patients undergoing coronary angioplasty. J. Am. Coll. Cardiol., *21*:35, 1993.

462. Sheikh, K.H., Harrison, J.K., Harding, M.B., Himmelstein, S.I., Kisslo, K.B., Davidson, C.J., and Bashore, T.M.: Detection of angiographically silent coronary atherosclerosis by intracoronary ultrasonography. Am. Heart J., *121*:1803, 1991.

462a. Hodgson, J.M., Reddy, K.G., Suneja, R., Nair, R.N., Lesnefsky, E.J., and Sheehan, H.M.: Intracoronary ultrasound imaging: Correlation of plaque morphology with angiography, clinical syndrome and procedural results in patients undergoing coronary angioplasty. J. Am. Coll. Cardiol., *21*:35–44, 1993.

463. Nakatani, S., Yamagishi, M., Takaki, H., Haze, K., and Miyatake, K.: Quantitative assessment of coronary artery stenosis by intravascular Doppler catheter technique. Circulation, *85*:1786, 1992.

463a. Garrand, T.J., et al.: Intravascular ultrasound diagnosis of a coronary artery pseudoaneurysm following percutaneous transluminal coronary angioplasty. Am. Heart J., *125*:880, 1993.

463b. Essop, A.R., et al.: The surgical implications of endoluminal coronary ultrasound. Am. Heart J., *125*:882, 1993.

463c. Nishimura, R.A., Higano, S.T., and Holmes, D.R., Jr: Use of intracoronary ultrasound imaging for assessing left main coronary artery disease. Mayo Clin. Proc., *68*:134, 1993.

464. Fitzgerald, P.J., Ports, T.A., and Yock, P.G.: Contribution of localized calcium deposits to dissection after angioplasty. Circulation, *86*:64, 1992.

465. Mintz, G.S., Douek, P., Pichard, A.D., Kent, K.M., Satler, L.F., Popma, J.J., and Leon, M.B.: Target lesion calcification in coronary artery disease: An intravascular ultrasound study. J. Am. Coll. Cardiol., *20*:1149, 1992.

466. St. Goar, F.G., Pinto, F.J., Alderman, E.L., Valantine, H.A., Schroeder, J.S., Gao, S-Z., Stinson, E.B., and Popp, R.L.: Intracoronary ultrasound in cardiac transplant recipients. Circulation, *85*:979, 1992.

467. Honye, J., Mahon, D.J., Jain, A., White, C.J., Ramee, S.R., Wallis, J.B., Al-Zarka, A., and Tobis, J.M.: Morphological effects of coronary balloon angioplasty in vivo assessed by intravascular ultrasound imaging. Circulation, *85*:1012, 1992.

468. Keren, G., Pichard, A.D., Kent, K.M., Satler, L.F., and Leon, M.B.: Failure or success of complex catheter-based interventional procedures assessed by intravascular ultrasound. Am. Heart J., *123*:200, 1992.

469. Yock, P.G., Fitzgerald, P.J., Linker, D.T., and Angelsen, B.A.J.: Intravascular ultrasound guidance for catheter-based coronary interventions. J. Am. Coll. Cardiol., *17*:39B, 1991.

470. Werner, G.S., Sold, G., Buchwald, A., Kreuzer, H., and Wiegand, V.: Intravascular ultrasound imaging of human coronary arteries after percutaneous transluminal angioplasty: Morphologic and quantitative assessment. Am. Heart J., *122*:212, 1991.

471. Potkin, B.N., Keren, G., Mintz, G.S., Douek, P.C., Picard, A.D., Satler, L.F., Kent, K.M., and Leon, M.B.: Arterial responses to balloon coronary angioplasty: An intravascular ultrasound study. J. Am. Coll. Cardiol., *20*:942, 1992.

472. Tenaglia, A.N., Buller, C.E., Kisslo, K.B., Phillips, H.R., Stack, R.S., and Davidson, C.J.: Intracoronary ultrasound predictors of adverse outcomes after coronary artery interventions. J. Am. Coll. Cardiol., *20*:1385, 1992.

473. Mintz, G.S., Potkin, B.N., Keren, G., Satler, L.F., Pichard, A.D., Kent, K.M., Popma, J.J., and Leon, M.B.: Intravascular ultrasound evaluation of the effect of rotational atherectomy in obstructive atherosclerotic coronary artery disease. Circulation, *86*:1383, 1992.

474. Gerber, T.C., Erbel, R., Gorge, G., Ge, J., Rupprecht, H-J., and Meyer, J.: Classification of morphologic effects of percutaneous transluminal coronary angioplasty assessed by intravascular ultrasound. Am. J. Cardiol., *70*:1546, 1992.

475. Jackman, Jr., J.D., Hermiller, J.B., Sketch, Jr., M.H., Davidson, C.J., Tcheng, J.E., Phillips, H.R., and Stack, R.S.: Combined rotational and directional atherectomy guided by intravascular ultrasound in an occluded vein graft. Am. Heart J., *124*:214, 1992.

476. Tenaglia, A.N., Buller, C.E., Kisslo, K.B., Stack, R.S., and Davidson, C.J.: Mechanisms of balloon angioplasty and directional coronary atherectomy as assessed by intracoronary ultrasound. J. Am. Coll. Cardiol., *20*:685, 1992.

477. Kimura, B.J., Fitzgerald, P.J., Sudhir, K., Amidon, T.M., Strunk, B.L., and Yock, P.G.: Guidance of directed coronary atherectomy by intracoronary ultrasound imaging. Am. Heart J., *124*:1365, 1992.

477a. De Lezo, J.S., et al.: Intracoronary ultrasound assessment of directional coronary atherectomy: Immediate and follow-up findings. J. Am. Coll. Cardiol., *21*:298, 1993.

478. Isner, J.M., Rosenfield, K., Losordo, D.W., Rose, L., Langevin, Jr., R.E., Razvi, S., and Kosowsky, B.D.: Combination balloon-ultrasound imaging catheter for percutaneous transluminal angioplasty. Circulation, *84*:739, 1991.

479. Yock, P.G., Fitzgerald, P.J., Jang, Y.-T., McKenzie, J., Belef, M., Starksen, N., White, N.W., Linker, D.T., and Simpson, J.B.: Initial trials of a combined ultrasound imaging/mechanical atherectomy catheter. J. Am. Coll. Cardiol., *15*:105A, 1990 (Abstract).

480. Isringhaus, H.: Epicardial coronary artery imaging. Echocardiography, *7*:253, 1990.

481. McPherson, D.D., Sirna, S.J., Hiratzka, L.F., Thorpe, L., Armstrong, M.L., Marcus, M.L., and Kerber, R.E.: Coronary arterial remodeling studied by high-frequency epicardial echocardiography: An early compensatory mechanism in patients with obstructive coronary atherosclerosis. J. Am. Coll. Cardiol., *17*:79, 1991.

482. McPherson, D.D. and Kerber, R.E.: New insights into the pathophysiology of coronary arteries by epicardial high frequency echocardiography. J. Am. Soc. Echocardiogr., *2*:284, 1989.

483. Hiratzka, L.F., McPherson, D.D., Brandt, B., Lamberth, W.C., Sirna, S., Marcus, M.L., and Kerber, R.E.: The role of intraoperative high-frequency epicardial

echocardiography during coronary artery revascularization. Circulation, 76:V-33, 1987.

483a. McPherson, D.D., Johnson, M.R., Collins, S.M., Kieso, R.A., Marcus, M.L., and Kerber, R.E.: Validation by high-frequency epicardial echocardiography of a new method of analyzing coronary angiography quantitatively in coronary artery disease. Am. J. Cardiol., 71:28–32, 1993.

484. Wilson, R.F., Laughlin, D.E., Ackell, P.H., Chilian, W.M., Holida, M.D., Hartley, C.J., Armstrong, M.L., Marcus, M.L., and White, C.W.: Transluminal, subselective measurement of coronary artery blood flow velocity and vasodilator reserve in man. Circulation, 72:82, 1985.

485. Sibley, D.H., Millar, H.D., Hartley, C.J., and Whitlow, P.L.: Subselective measurement of coronary-blood flow velocity using a steerable Doppler catheter. J. Am. Coll. Cardiol., 8:1332, 1986.

486. Wilson, R.F. and White, C.W.: Measurement of maximal coronary flow reserve: A technique of assessing the physiologic significance of coronary arterial lesions in humans. Herz., 12:163, 1987.

487. Marcus, M.L., Rossen, J.D., Simonetti, I., and Winniford, M.D.: Applications of Doppler techniques to the measurement of coronary flood flow reserve in patients. In Echocardiography in Coronary Artery Disease. Edited by R.E. Kerber. Mt. Kisco, NY, Futura, 1988.

488. Grayburn, P.A., Willard, J.E., Haagen, D.R., Brickner, M.E., Alvarez, L.G., and Eichhorn, E.J.: Measurement of coronary flow using high-frequency intravascular ultrasound imaging and pulsed Doppler velocimetry: In vitro feasibility studies. J. Am. Soc. Echocardiogr., 5:5, 1992.

489. Segal, J., Kern, M.J., Scott, N.A., King, III, S.B., Doucette, J.W., Heuser, R.R., Ofili, E., and Siegel, R.: Alterations of phasic coronary artery flow velocity in humans during percutaneous coronary angioplasty. J. Am. Coll. Cardiol., 20:276, 1992.

490. Rossen, J.D., Oskarsson, H., Stenberg, R.G., Braun, P., Talman, C.L., and Winniford, M.D.: Simultaneous measurement of coronary flow reserve by left anterior descending coronary artery Doppler and great cardiac vein thermodilution methods. J. Am. Coll. Cardiol., 20:402, 1992.

491. Doucette, J.W., Corl, D., Payne, H.M., Flynn, A.E., Goto, M., Nassi, M., and Segal, J.: Validation of a Doppler guide wire for intravascular measurement of coronary artery flow velocity. Circulation, 85:1899, 1992.

492. Ofili, E., Kern, M.J., Tatineni, S., Deligonul, U., Aguirre, F., Serota, H., and Labovitz, A.J.: Detection of coronary collateral flow by a Doppler-tipped guide wire during coronary angioplasty. Am. Heart J., 122:221, 1991.

493. Yamagishi, M., Hotta, D., Tamai, J., Nakatani, S., and Miyatake, K.: Validity of catheter-tip Doppler technique in assessment of coronary flow velocity and application of spectrum analysis method. Am. J. Cardiol., 67:758, 1991.

494. Sudhir, K., Hargrave, V.K., Johnson, E.L., Aldea, G., Mori, H., Ports, T.A., and Yock, P.G.: Measurement of volumetric coronary blood flow with a Doppler catheter: Validation in an animal model. Am. Heart J., 124:870, 1992.

495. Kern, M.J., Deligonul, U., Vandormael, M., Labovitz, A., Gudipati, C.V., Gabliani, G., Bodet, J., Shah, Y., and Kennedy, H.L.: Impaired coronary vasodilator reserve in the immediate postcoronary angioplasty period: Analysis of coronary artery flow velocity indexes and regional cardiac venous efflux. J. Am. Coll. Cardiol., 13:860, 1989.

495a. Ofili, E.O., et al.: Analysis of coronary blood flow velocity dynamics in angiographically normal and stenosed arteries before and after endolumen enlargement by angioplasty. J. Am. Coll. Cardiol., 21:308, 1993.

495b. Thompson, M.A., Deychak, Y.A., and Segal, J.: Doppler-tipped guide wire assessment of retrograde coronary artery flow distal to a total occlusion and its reversal after laser recanalization. Am. Heart J., 125:526, 1993.

496. Ross, Jr., J.J., Ren, J-F., Land, W., Chandrasekaran, K., and Mintz, G.S.: Transthoracic high frequency (7.5 MHz) echocardiographic assessment of coronary vascular reserve and its relation to left ventricular mass. J. Am. Coll. Cardiol., 16:1393, 1990.

497. Fusejima, K., Takahara, Y., Sudo, Y., Murayama, H., Masuda, Y., and Inagaki, Y.: Comparison of coronary hemodynamics in patients with internal mammary artery and saphenous vein coronary artery bypass grafts: A noninvasive approach using combined two-dimensional and Doppler echocardiography. J. Am. Coll. Cardiol., 15:131, 1990.

498. Yamagishi, M., Miyatake, K., Beppu, S., Kumon, K., Suzuky, S., Tanaka, N., and Nimura, Y.: Assessment of coronary blood flow by transesophageal two-dimensional pulsed Doppler echocardiography. Am. J. Cardiol., 62:641, 1988.

499. Harada, K., Uesato, T., Toyoda, H., Usami, H., and Okada, T.: Acute febrile mucocutaneous lymph node syndrome with multiple aneurysms: Report of a case. Pediatr. Cardiol., 4:215, 1983.

500. Saito, A., Nojima, K., Ueda, K., and Nakano, H.: New approach to visualize the left coronary artery using two dimensional echocardiography. J. Cardiogr., 12:963, 1982.

501. Satomi, G., Nakamura, K., Narai, S., and Takao, A.: Systematic visualization of coronary arteries by two dimensional echocardiography in children and infants: Evaluation in Kawasaki's disease and coronary arteriovenous fistulas. Am. Heart J., 107:497, 1984.

502. Ichinose, E., Eto, Y., Takechi, T., Yoshioka, F., and Kato, H.: Two dimensional echocardiographic study of coronary artery lesion in Kawasaki disease: A new approach to visualize the right coronary artery: J. Cardiogr., 12:111, 1982.

503. Meyer, R.A.: Echocardiography in Kawasaki disease. J. Am. Soc. Echocardiogr., 2:269, 1989.

504. Ghung, K.J., Fulton, D.R., Lapp, R., Spector, S., and Sahn, D.J.: One-year follow-up of cardiac and coronary artery disease in infants and children with Kawasaki disease. Am. Heart J., 115:1263, 1988.

505. Vogel, M., Smallhorn, J.F., and Freedom, R.M.: Serial analysis of regional left ventricular wall motion by two-dimensional echocardiography in patients with coronary artery enlargement after Kawasaki disease. J. Am. Coll. Cardiol., 20:915, 1992.

506. Takagi, S., Oshimi, K., Sumiya, M., Gonda, N., Kano, S., Takaku, F., Miyata, K., and Yaginuma, T.: Adult onset mucocutaneous lymph node syndrome with coronary aneurysm. Am. Heart J., 101:852. 1981.

507. Armstrong, W.F., West, S.R., Mueller, T.M., Dillon, J.C., and Feigenbaum, H.: Assessment of location and size of myocardial infarction with contrast-enhanced echocardiography. J. Am. Coll. Cardiol., 2:63, 1983.

508. Kemper, A.J., O'Boyle, J.E., Sharma, S., Cohen, C.A., Kloner, R.A., Khuri, S.F., and Parisi, A.F.: Hydrogen

peroxide contrast-enhanced two dimensional echocardiography: Real-time in vivo delineation of regional myocardial perfusion. Circulation, *68*:603, 1983.

509. Ten Cate, F.J., Drury, J.K., Meerbaum, S., Noordsy, J., Feinstein, S., Shah, P.M., and Corday, E.: Myocardial contrast two dimensional echocardiography: Experimental examination at different coronary flow levels. J. Am. Coll. Cardiol., *3*:1219, 1984.

510. Yasui, K., Matsumoto, M., Shimazu, T., Maeda, T., Nakajima, S., Fukushima, M., Hori, M., Inoue, M., Abe, H., Satoh, H., and Minamino, T.: Visualization of intramyocardial blood flow distribution with contrast echomyocardiography. J. Cardiogr., *12*:895, 1982.

511. Tei, C., Sakamaki, T., Shah, P.M., Meerbaum, S., Shimoura, K., Kondo, S., and Corday, E.: Myocardial contrast echocardiography: A reproducible technique of myocardial opacification for identifying regional perfusion deficits. Circulation, *67*:585, 1983.

512. Armstrong, W.F., Mueller, T.M., Kinney, E.L., Tickner, E.G., Dillon, J.C., and Feigenbaum, H.: Assessment of myocardial perfusion abnormalities with contrast-enhanced two dimensional echocardiography. Circulation, *66*:166, 1982.

513. Kaul, S., et al.: Contrast echocardiography in acute myocardial ischemia: I. In vivo determination of total left ventricular "area at risk." J. Am. Coll. Cardiol., *4*:1272, 1984.

514. Cheirif, J., Desir, R.M., Bolli, R., Mahmarian, J.J., Zoghbi, W.A., Verani, M.S., and Quinones, M.A.: Relation of perfusion defects observed with myocardial contrast echocardiography to the severity of coronary stenosis: Correlation with thallium-201 single-photon emission tomography. J. Am. Coll. Cardiol., *19*:1343, 1992.

515. Rovai, D., Lombardi, M., Ghelardini, G., Marzilli, M., Taddei, L., Michelassi, C., Distante, A., DeMaria, A.N., and L'Abbate, A.: Discordance between responses of contrast echo intensity to increased flow rate in human coronary circulation and in vitro. Am. Heart J., *124*:398, 1992.

516. Vandenberg, B.F.: Myocardial perfusion and contrast echocardiography: Review and new perspectives. Echocardiography, *8*:65, 1991.

517. Kemper, A., Force, T., Filfoil, M., Perkins, L.A., and Parisi, A.F.: Topographic correspondence of contrast echocardiographic perfusion mapping and myocardial infarct extent after varying durations of coronary occlusion. J. Am. Soc. Echocardiogr., *1*:104, 1988.

518. Kaul, S., Kelly, P., Oliner, J.D., Glasheen, W.P., Keller, M.W., and Watson, D.D.: Assessment of regional myocardial blood flow with myocardial contrast two-dimensional echocardiography. J. Am. Coll. Cardiol., *13*:468, 1989.

519. Lim, Y-J., Nanto, S., Masuyama, T., Kodama, K., Ikeda, T., Kitabatake, A., and Kamada, T.: Visualization of subendocardial myocardial ischemia with myocardial contrast echocardiography in humans. Circulation, *79*:233, 1989.

520. Keller, M.W., Glasheen, W., Teja, K., Gear, A., and Kaul, S.: Myocardial contrast echocardiography without significant hemodynamic effects or reactive hyperemia: A major advantage in the imaging of regional myocardial perfusion. J. Am. Coll. Cardiol., *12*:1039, 1988.

521. Kaul, S., Glasheen, W., Ruddy, T.D., Pandian, N.G., Weyman, A.E., and Okada, R.D.: The importance of defining left ventricular area at risk in vivo during acute myocardial infarction: An experimental evaluation with myocardial contrast two-dimensional echocardiography. Circulation, *75*:1249, 1987.

522. Reisner, S.A., Ong, L.S., Lichtenberg, G.S., Amico, A.F., Shapiro, J.R., Allen, M.N., and Meltzer, R.S.: Myocardial perfusion imaging by contrast echocardiography with use of intracoronary sonicated albumin in humans. J. Am. Coll. Cardiol., *14*:660, 1989.

523. Keller, M.W., Segal, S.S., Kaul, S., and Duling, B.: The behavior of sonicated albumin microbubbles within the microcirculation: A basis for their use during myocardial contrast echocardiography. Circulation Res., *65*:458, 1989.

524. Maurer, G., Ong, K., Haendchen, R., Torres, M., Tei, C., Wood, F., Meerbaum, S., Shah, P., and Corday, E.: Myocardial contrast two dimensional echocardiography: Comparison of contrast disappearance rates in normal and underperfused myocardium. Circulation, *69*:418, 1984.

525. Tei, C., Kondo, S., Meerbaum, S., Ong, K., Maurer, G., Wood, F., Sakamaki, T., Shimoura, K., Corday, E., and Shah, P.M.: Correlation of myocardial echo contrast disappearance rate ("washout") and severity of experimental coronary stenosis. J. Am. Coll. Cardiol., *3*:39, 1984.

526. Kemper, A.J., Nickerson, D., Boyle, III, C.C., Saleh, R., and Parisi, A.F.: Quantifying changes in regional myocardial perfusion with aortic contrast echocardiography. J. Am. Soc. Echocardiogr., *2*:36, 1989.

527. Vandenberg, B.F., Kieso, R., Fox-Eastham, K., Chilian, W., and Kerber, R.E.: Quantitation of myocardial perfusion by contrast echocardiography: Analysis of contrast gray level appearance variables and intracyclic variability. J. Am. Coll. Cardiol., *13*:200, 1989.

528. Shapiro, J.R., Reisner, S.A., Amico, A.F., Kelly, P.F., and Meltzer, R.S.: Reproducibility of quantitative myocardial contrast echocardiography. J. Am. Coll. Cardiol., *15*:602, 1990.

529. Cheirif, J., Zoghbi, W.A., Raizner, A.E., Minor, S.T., Winters, W.L., Klein, M.S., DeBauche, T.L., Lewis, J.M., Roberts, R., and Quinones, M.A.: Assessment of myocardial perfusion in humans by contrast echocardiography. I. Evaluation of regional coronary reserve by peak contrast intensity. J. Am. Coll. Cardiol., *11*:735, 1988.

530. Rovai, D., Ghelardini, G., Lombardi, M., Trivella, M.G., Nevola, E., Taddei, L., Michelassi, C., Distante, A., DeMaria, A.N., and L'Abbate, A.: Myocardial washout of sonicated iopamidol reflects coronary blood flow in the absence of autoregulation. J. Am. Coll. Cardiol., *20*:1417, 1992.

531. Cheirif, J., Zoghbi, W.A., Bolli, R., O'Neill, P.G., Hoyt, B.D., and Quinones, M.A.: Assessment of regional myocardial perfusion by contrast echocardiography. II. Detection of changes in transmural and subendocardial perfusion during dipyridamole-induced hyperemia in a model of critical coronary stenosis. J. Am. Coll. Cardiol., *14*:1555, 1989.

532. Keller, M.W., Glasheen, W., Smucker, M.L., Burwell, L.R., Watson, D.D., and Kaul, S.: Myocardial contrast echocardiography in humans. II. Assessment of coronary blood flow reserve. J. Am. Coll. Cardiol., *12*:925, 1988.

533. Armstrong, W.F. and Gage, S.W.: Evaluation of reperfusion hyperemia with myocardial contrast echocardiography. J. Am. Soc. Echocardiogr., *1*:322, 1988.

534. Reisner, S.A., Ong, L.S., Fitzpatrick, P.G., Lichtenberg, G.S., Sullebarger, J.T., Allen, M.N., and Meltzer, R.S.: Evaluation of coronary flow reserve using myocardial contrast echocardiography in humans. Eur. Heart J., *13*:389, 1992.

534a.Porter, T.R., et al.: Myocardial contrast echocardiography for the assessment of coronary blood flow reserve: validation in humans. J. Am. Coll. Cardiol., *21*:349, 1993.

535. Feinstein, S.B., Lang, R.M., Dick, C., Neumann, A., Al-Sadir, J., Chua, K.G., Carroll, J., Feldman, T., and Borow, K.M.: Contrast echocardiography during coronary arteriography in humans: Perfusion and anatomic studies. J. Am. Coll. Cardiol., *11*:59, 1988.

536. Grill, H.P., Brinker, J.A., Taube, J.C., Walford, G.D., Midei, M.G., Flaherty, J.T., and Weiss, J.L.: Contrast echocardiography mapping of collateralized myocardium in humans before and after coronary angioplasty. J. Am. Coll. Cardiol., *16*:1594, 1990.

537. Reisner, S.A., Ong, L.S., Lichtenberg, G.S., Shapiro, J.R., Amico, A.F., Allen, M.N., and Meltzer, R.S.: Quantitative assessment of the immediate results of coronary angioplasty by myocardial contrast echocardiography. J. Am. Coll. Cardiol., *13*:852, 1989.

538. Griffin, B., Timmis, A.D., Henderson, R.A., and Sowton, E.: Contrast perfusion echocardiography: Identification of area at risk of dyskinesis during percutaneous transluminal coronary angioplasty. Am. Heart J., *114*:497, 1987.

539. Lang, R.M., Feinstein, S.B., Feldman, T., Neumann, A., Chua, K.G., and Borow, K.M.: Contrast echocardiography for evaluation of myocardial perfusion: Effects of coronary angioplasty. J. Am. Coll. Cardiol., *8*:232, 1986.

540. Spotnitz, W.D. and Kaul, S.: Intraoperative assessment of myocardial perfusion using contrast echocardiography. Echocardiography, *7*:209, 1990.

541. Keller, M.W., Spotnitz, W.D., Matthew, T.L., Glasheen, W.P., Watson, D.D., and Kaul, S.: Intraoperative assessment of regional myocardial perfusion using quantitative myocardial contrast echocardiography: An experimental evaluation. J. Am. Coll. Cardiol., *16*:1267, 1990.

542. Mudra, H., Zwehl, W., Klauss, V., Kreuzer, E., Haufe, M.C., Angermann, C., and Theisen, K.: Intraoperative myocardial contrast echocardiography for assessment of regional bypass perfusion. Am. J. Cardiol., *66*:1077, 1990.

543. Spotnitz, W.D., Keller, M.W., Watson, D.D., Nolan, S.P., and Kaul, S.: Success of internal mammary bypass grafting can be assessed intraoperatively using myocardial contrast echocardiography. J. Am. Coll. Cardiol., *12*:196, 1988.

544. Sabia, P.J., Powers, E.R., Jayaweera, A.R., Ragosta, M., and Kaul, S.: Functional significance of collateral blood flow in patients with recent acute myocardial infarction. Circulation, *85*:2080, 1992.

545. Spotnitz, W.D., Matthew, T.L., Keller, M.W., Powers, E.R., and Kaul, S.: Intraoperative demonstration of coronary collateral flow using myocardial contrast two-dimensional echocardiography. Am. J. Cardiol., *65*:1259, 1990.

546. Lim, Y.-J., Nanto, S., Masuyama, T., Kodama, K., Kohama, A., Kitzbatake, A., and Kamada, T.: Coronary collaterals assessed with myocardial contrast echocardiography in healed myocardial infarction. Am. J. Cardiol., *66*:556, 1990.

547. Widimsky, P., Cornel, J.H., and Ten Cate, F.J.: Evaluation of collateral blood flow by myocardial contrast-enhanced echocardiography. Br. Heart J., *59*:20, 1988.

548. Ito, H., Tomooka, T., Sakai, N., Yu, H., Higashino, Y., Fujii, K., Masuyama, T., Kitabatake, A., and Minamino, T.: Lack of myocardial perfusion perfusion immediately after successful thrombolysis. Circulation, *85*:1699, 1992.

549. Kaul, S., Jayaweera, A.R., Glasheen, W.P., Villanueva, F.S., Gutgesell, H.P., and Spotnitz, W.D.: Myocardial contrast echocardiography and the transmural distribution of flow: A critical appraisal during myocardial ischemia not associated with infarction. J. Am. Coll. Cardiol., *20*:1992.

550. Monaghan, M.J., Quigley, P.J., Metcafe, J.M., Thomas, S.D., and Jewitt, D.E.: Digital subtraction contrast echocardiography: A new method for the evaluation of regional myocardial perfusion. Br. Heart J. *59*:12, 1988.

# 9

# Diseases of the Myocardium

An assortment of diseases primarily affect the myocardium. The list of known factors or agents that can alter myocardial function is growing. Our understanding of these abnormalities has broadened, largely as a result of proven diagnostic procedures such as echocardiography. This chapter includes a description of some of the echocardiographic findings in patients with primary myocardial abnormalities.

## HYPERTROPHIC CARDIOMYOPATHY

Echocardiography has not only become an important means of detecting hypertrophic cardiomyopathy, but also has greatly enhanced our understanding of the pathogenesis and pathophysiology of this cardiomyopathy. Because of echocardiography's unique ability to evaluate cardiac morphology and function, this technique has become the procedure of choice for the diagnosis of hypertrophic cardiomyopathy. Although certain findings in this disease state are characteristic, variability is great and the versatility of the echocardiographic examination is extremely valuable in assessing the many manifestations of hypertrophic cardiomyopathy.

### Asymmetric Hypertrophy

A characteristic feature of hypertrophic cardiomyopathy is hypertrophy of the interventricular septum disproportionate to the free wall of the left ventricle.[1-8] Figure 9–1 shows a two-dimensional echocardiogram of a patient with hypertrophic cardiomyopathy who has a septum (S) that is larger than the posterior ventricular wall (PW). Figure 9–2 is another example of a hypertrophied interventricular septum (IVS). In this case, the septal hypertrophy extends to the apex (Fig. 9–2B). The four-chamber view is another excellent examination for identifying a hypertrophied interventricular septum (Fig. 9–3).

Septal hypertrophy has become so characteristic of hypertrophic cardiomyopathy that the term asymmetric septal hypertrophy, or ASH, has at times been used synonymously with this abnormality. With greater experience, it has become apparent that a variety of hypertrophic patterns associated with this cardiomyopathy is the rule rather than the exception. Although the septum is usually hypertrophied, the degree and the location of the hypertrophy can vary greatly.[9-13] Figure 9–4 shows septal hypertrophy involving the proximal and middle portion of the septum. The apex is relatively thin and uninvolved with the hypertrophic process. Figure 9–5 shows echocardiographic frames and diagrams of a patient in whom the hypertrophied septum is limited only to the proximal portion of that structure. A type of hypertrophic cardiomyopathy involving the posterior wall and not the septum has been described.[14] Figure 9–6 shows another form of hypertrophic cardiomyopathy whereby the apex is primarily involved in the hypertrophic process.[15-21a] The basal portion of the septum and posterior wall are relatively uninvolved. Figure 9–7 shows another form of hypertrophic myopathy in which the entire left ventricle is involved fairly uniformly. One sees massive hypertrophy of both the septum and free wall with complete cavity obliteration in systole. Thus, although asymmetric septal hypertrophy is the usual manifestation of hypertrophic cardiomyopathy, multiple forms of hypertrophy and each type can present in different ways.

The age of the patient is a factor in the clinical course of hypertrophic cardiomyopathy. Cardiomyopathy of the young patient[22,23] can be totally different from what is noted in the elderly individual.[24-27] In the older patient, one must be careful not to interpret proximal septal hypertrophy as hypertrophic myopathy.[26] The so-called "sigmoid septum" may produce an outflow obstruction and simulate either hypertrophic myopathy or fixed aortic stenosis (see Chapter 6).

Because of the various forms of asymmetric hypertrophy, two-dimensional echocardiography is clearly the ultrasonic examination of choice for making this diagnosis; however, M-mode echocardiography is still used for assessing septal and posterior wall thickness. Figure 9–8 shows a fairly typical patient with a septum that is considerably thicker than the posterior left ventricular free wall. The M-mode technique for measuring septal thickness is less accurate than two-dimensional echocardiography, not only because of the varied forms of septal hypertrophy, but also because of some of the limitations in measuring septal thickness with an M-mode recording. Figure 9–9 shows an attempt at an M-mode measurement of septal thickness. In this particular case, the M-mode cursor is clearly tangential to the septum and the thickness measurement is artifactually too large. The cursor could have been directed more toward the apex

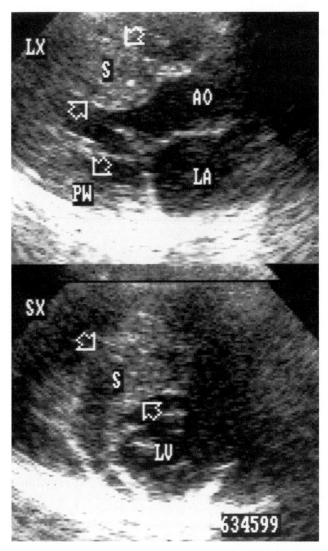

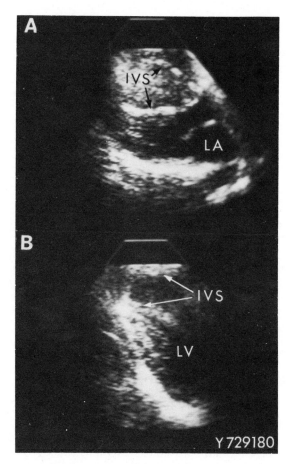

**Fig. 9–2.** Parasternal long-axis two-dimensional echocardiograms of a patient with asymmetric septal hypertrophy. Marked hypertrophy can be seen in the basal, *A*, and apical, *B*, parts of the interventricular septum (IVS). LA = left atrium; LV = left ventricle.

**Fig. 9–1.** Long-axis (LX) and short-axis (SX) two-dimensional echocardiograms of a patient with hypertrophic cardiomyopathy. The thickened interventricular septum (S) is significantly thicker than the posterior left ventricular free wall (PW). AO = aorta; LA = left atrium; LV = left ventricle.

to get a more accurate measurement, but even then it is unlikely that the M-mode cursor could have been directed perpendicularly through the septum. Thus, any measurement would have been erroneously large.

Left ventricular hypertrophy, even asymmetric hypertrophy, is not specific for hypertrophic cardiomyopathy. Patients with hypertension may produce hypertrophy that simulates hypertrophic cardiomyopathy.[28–32] Patients undergoing hemodialysis may also exhibit asymmetric septal hypertrophy.[33,34] The appearance of the heart in some athletes may be confused with hypertrophic cardiomyopathy.[35] Even aortic stenosis may produce asymmetric septal hypertrophy and simulate hypertrophic cardiomyopathy.[36] Newborn infants of diabetic mothers may show a form of hypertrophy that mimics hypertrophic cardiomyopathy.[37–39] Tumors invading the interventricular septum can simulate hyper-

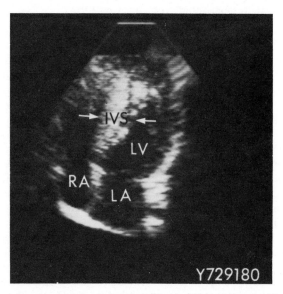

**Fig. 9–3.** Apical four-chamber view of the patient in Figure 9–2. Note that the hypertrophied interventricular septum (IVS) is thickest in the apical half of the septum. LV = left ventricle; RA = right atrium; LA = left atrium.

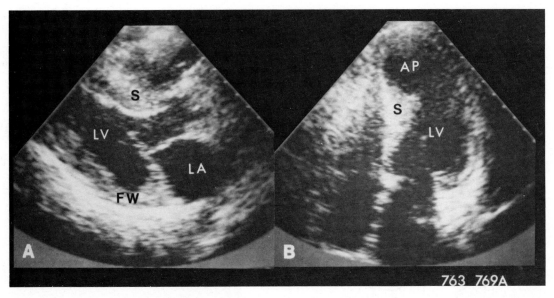

**Fig. 9–4.** Long-axis (*A*) and apical four-chamber (*B*) echocardiograms of a patient with hypertrophic cardiomyopathy whose hypertrophy primarily involves the proximal two thirds of the interventricular septum (S). The apex (AP) is spared from the hypertrophic process. LV = left ventricle; FW = left ventricular free wall; LA = left atrium.

trophic myopathy.[40,41] Even a mural thrombus positioned against the interventricular septum could masquerade as a thickened interventricular septum (Fig. 9–10).[42] A patient with a myocardial infarction involving the posterior left ventricular wall may have a relatively thin posterior wall compared to the septum.[43]

In addition to the ability of two-dimensional echocardiography to measure the thickness of the cardiac walls, several echocardiographers have noticed a change in the acoustic properties of the septal echoes in patients with hypertrophic cardiomyopathy.[44–46] This finding is most distinct in the intramyocardial echoes from the septum in Figures 9–11 and 9–12. Figure 9–11 shows two bright oval echoes in the interventricular septum. A similar example is seen in Figure 9–12 whereby the intraseptal echoes are more linear. These intramyocardial echoes

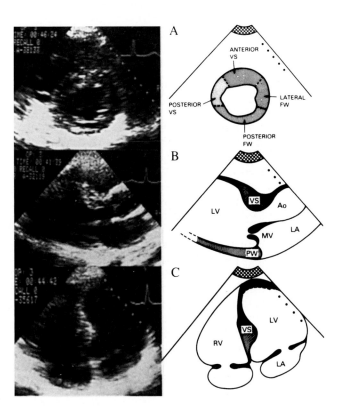

**Fig. 9–5.** Diagrams and echocardiograms of a patient with relatively mild hypertrophic cardiomyopathy. The hypertrophied septum (VS) is limited to the proximal portion of the interventricular septum. FW = free wall; PW = posterior wall; LV = left ventricle; AO = aorta; LA = left atrium; MV = mitral valve; RV = right ventricle. (From Spirito, P., et al.: Severe functional limitation in patients with hypertrophic cardiomyopathy and only mild localized left ventricular hypertrophy. J. Am. Coll. Cardiol., *8*:539, 1986.)

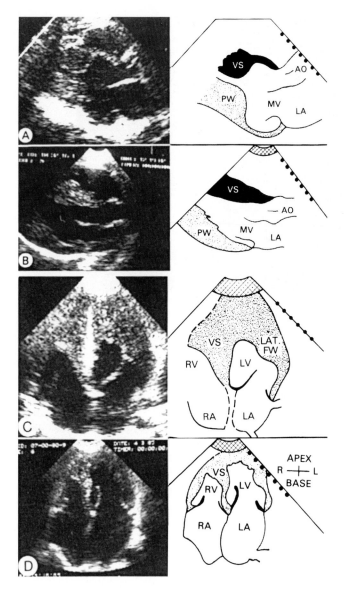

**Fig. 9–6.** Echocardiograms of patients with apical hypertrophic cardiomyopathy. *A* shows a striking demarcation between the thin, proximal, normal septum and the apical half (VS), which is hypertrophied. The posterior ventricular wall (PW) is also hypertrophied. In *B,* the left ventricle is more gradually hypertrophied toward the apex. Apical hypertrophy is seen in *C.* The hypertrophied ventricular septum and lateral free wall (LAT FW) obliterate the apex. In *D,* the apical hypertrophy is modestly thicker than the basal portion of the left ventricle. AO = aorta; MV = mitral valve; LA = left atrium; RV = right ventricle; RA = right atrium. (From Louie, E.K. and Maron, B.J.: Apical hypertrophic cardiomyopathy: Clinical and two-dimensional echocardiographic assessment. Ann. Intern. Med., *106*:667, 1987.)

are sometimes called "speckling."[45,47] The pathologic or histologic significance of this finding is uncertain. It is tempting to correlate the peculiar echo pattern with the histologic finding of myocardial fiber disarray; however, there is no proof that the two observations are related.

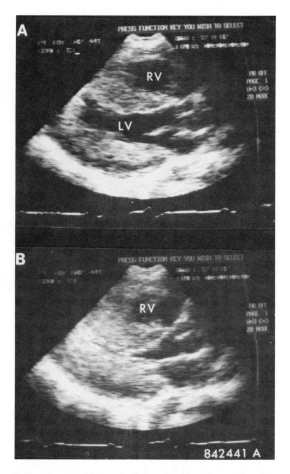

**Fig. 9–7.** Long-axis two-dimensional echocardiogram of a patient with hypertrophic cardiomyopathy who exhibits uniform hypertrophy of the entire left ventricle (LV). RV = right ventricle; A = diastole; B = systole.

## Left Ventricular Outflow Obstruction

A common accompaniment to hypertrophic cardiomyopathy is dynamic obstruction of the left ventricular outflow tract. When such a hemodynamic alteration occurs, the term used to describe this entity is hypertrophic obstructive cardiomyopathy (HOCM) or idiopathic hypertrophic subaortic stenosis (IHSS). Echocardiography has played an important role in the identification and understanding of this obstruction. Figure 9–13 illustrates how the hypertrophic left ventricle contracts. In Figure 9–13*A,* one sees the hypertrophied mid-septum at end diastole. As systole progresses (Fig. 9–13*B*), the mitral valve apparatus moves toward the interventricular septum and produces what has been called systolic anterior motion of the mitral valve, or SAM. Toward the end of systole (Fig. 9–13*C*), the hypertrophied septum frequently isolates the apical portion of the ventricle (A) from the body of the left ventricular cavity (LV). At end systole (Fig. 9–13*D*), the apical two thirds of the ventricle is obliterated. With these dynamic forces in action, it is not surprising that hypertrophic cardiomyopathy produces some striking and unusual hemodynamic alterations.

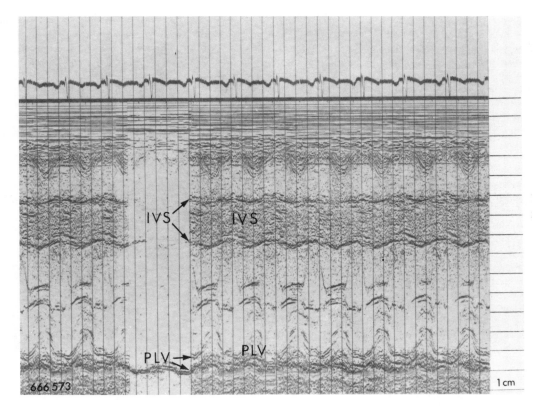

**Fig. 9–8.** M-mode echocardiogram of a patient with asymmetric septal hypertrophy. The interventricular septum (IVS) is much thicker than the posterior left ventricular wall (PLV). The echoes from the interventricular septum also have a different appearance than those from the myocardium of the posterior left ventricular wall. (From Feigenbaum, H.: Echocardiography. *In* Heart Disease. Edited by E. Braunwald. Philadelphia, W.B. Saunders Co., 1980.)

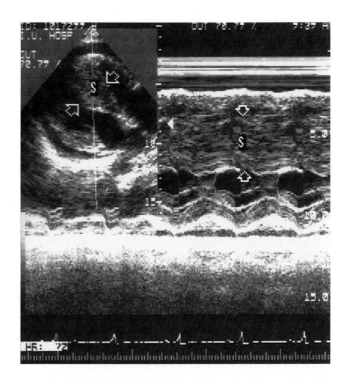

**Fig. 9–9.** M-mode echocardiogram of a patient with hypertrophic cardiomyopathy. The M-mode cursor traverses the interventricular septum (S) tangentially so that the M-mode thickness (*small arrows*) is greater than the actual thickness (*large arrows*, two-dimensional image).

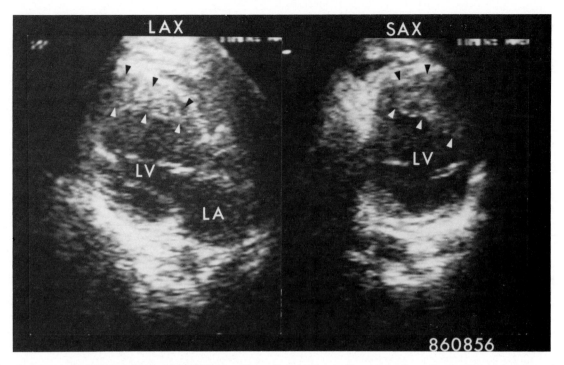

**Fig. 9–10.** Long-axis (LAX) and short-axis (SAX) two-dimensional echocardiograms of a patient with a mural thrombus (*arrowheads*) along the anterior septum and anterior lateral wall. In the long-axis view the thrombus can simulate a thickened interventricular septum. LV = left ventricle; LA = left atrium.

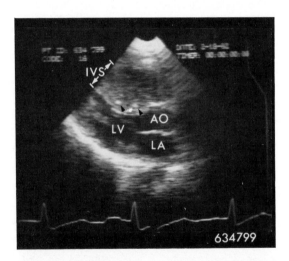

**Fig. 9–11.** Long-axis two-dimensional echocardiogram of a patient with hypertrophic cardiomyopathy. Two bright oval echoes (*arrowheads*) can be seen. LV = left ventricle; LA = left atrium; AO = aorta.

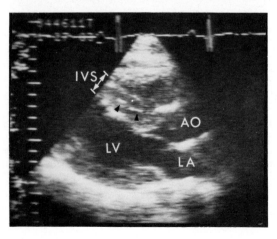

**Fig. 9–12.** Long-axis two-dimensional echocardiogram of a patient with hypertrophic cardiomyopathy. Two linear bright echoes (*arrowheads*) can be seen within the septum. LV = left ventricle; AO = aorta; LA = left atrium.

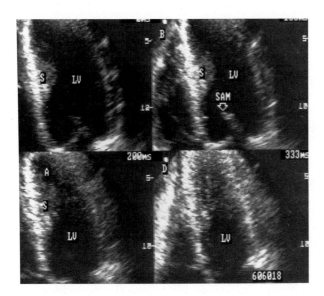

**Fig. 9–13.** Serial frames during a cardiac cycle of a patient with hypertrophic cardiomyopathy. The hypertrophied mid-interventricular septum (S) is noted at end diastole (*A*). In mid-ventricular systole (*B*), the tip of the mitral valve points toward the interventricular septum (SAM). Toward the end of systole (*C*), the hypertrophied septum isolates the apex (A) from the body of the left ventricle (LV). At end systole (*D*), the apical half of the left ventricle is obliterated.

The most frequent and most easily recognized functional abnormality with hypertrophic cardiomyopathy is the development of left ventricular outflow tract obstruction. The echocardiographic hallmark of this abnormality is the development of systolic anterior motion of the mitral valve, or SAM.[48,49] Figure 9–14 shows a two-dimensional echocardiogram illustrating SAM in both the long-axis and four-chamber views. Basically, one sees curling of the mitral valve apparatus toward the septum in systole. Transesophageal echocardiography can be used to identify SAM (Fig. 9–15). The transesophageal approach also can be used to identify the hypertrophied septum (VS), turbulent flow within the left ventricular outflow tract (Fig. 9–15C), and the commonly accompanying mitral regurgitation (MR).[50–52]

Probably the best way to identify SAM is with M-mode echocardiography (Fig. 9–16). Because of excellent temporal resolution, the M-mode examination demonstrates the motion of the mitral apparatus toward the interventricular septum. This tracing shows that the leaflet moves anteriorly toward the interventricular septum shortly after the onset of systole and then returns to its normal position just before the onset of ventricular diastole. This echocardiographic observation not only provides another diagnostic tool for this important clinical abnormality but also helps establish at least one possible mechanism for the obstruction of the left ventricular outflow tract. This echocardiographic finding provides evidence that the mitral valve apparatus plays a role in obliterating the left ventricular outflow tract and probably contributes to the pressure gradient found below the aortic valve.[53,54]

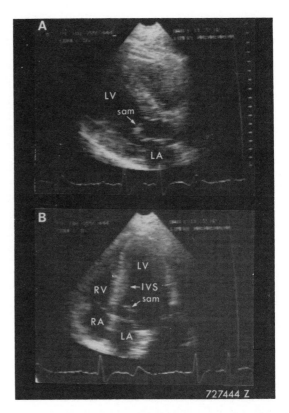

**Fig. 9–14.** Long-axis (*A*) and apical four chamber (*B*) echocardiograms of a patient with hypertrophic cardiomyopathy and a prominent systolic anterior motion (sam) of the anterior mitral leaflet. LV = left ventricle; LA = left atrium; RV = right ventricle; RA = right atrium; IVS = interventricular septum.

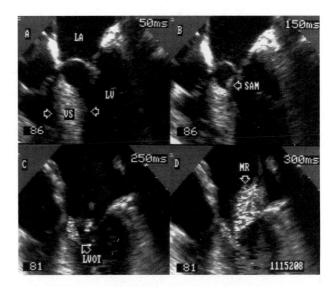

**Fig. 9.15.** Transesophageal echocardiographic examination of a patient with hypertrophic cardiomyopathy. The end-diastolic frame (*A*) identifies the hypertrophied interventricular septum (*arrows*, VS). In mid-systole (*B*), one can see systolic anterior motion of the mitral valve (SAM). Black and white Doppler flow imaging shows high-velocity flow in the left ventricular outflow tract (LVOT, *C*) and a high velocity mitral regurgitation jet (MR, *D*).

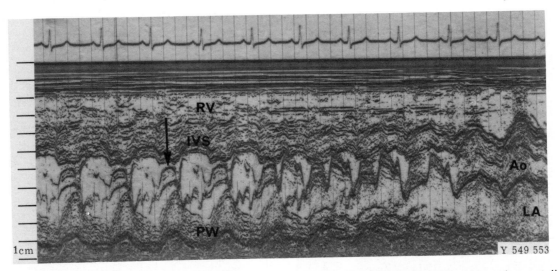

**Fig. 9–16.** M-mode echocardiographic scan of a patient with hypertrophic subaortic stenosis demonstrating systolic anterior motion (*arrow*) of the mitral valve. RV = right ventricle; IVS = interventricular septum; PW = posterior left ventricular wall; AO = aorta; LA = left atrium. (From Chang, S.: Echocardiography: Techniques and Interpretation, ed. 2. Philadelphia, Lea & Febiger, 1981.)

Several investigators have indicated that the pattern of SAM can predict the degree of obstruction.[55] These authors have found that the closer the leaflet comes to the septum and the longer the leaflet is in apposition to the septum, the greater is the severity of the obstruction. Although some question remains as to the quantitative aspect of this observation,[56–58] it is generally accepted that when the SAM touches the interventricular septum and becomes flat, a high degree of obstruction likely exists.[53] If the leaflet merely moves upward, may or may not come close to the septum, and drops backward quickly, then a lesser degree of obstruction probably exists.[59] With the current availability of Doppler techniques for more accurate assessment of pressure gradients, the quantitative aspect of the M-mode findings is probably moot; however, it is still useful to observe the M-mode appearance of the mitral valve apparatus to correlate the finding with hemodynamics observations noted with Doppler techniques.

The outflow obstruction in patients with hypertrophic

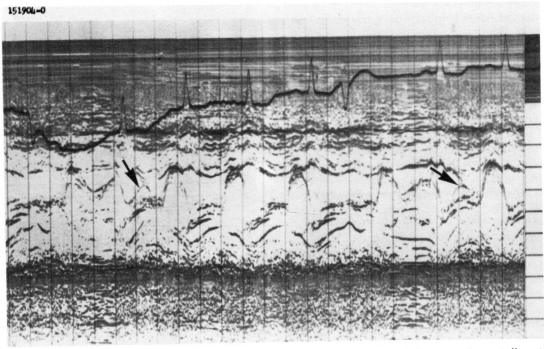

**Fig. 9–17.** Mitral valve echocardiogram of a patient with hypertrophic subaortic stenosis in whom the systolic anterior motion (*arrows*) only occurs following a premature ventricular systole.

cardiomyopathy is classically dynamic and may not always be present at rest.[60,61] This feature is one of the hallmarks of this abnormality. Figure 9–17 demonstrates that the SAM (*arrow*) may only occur after the compensatory pause following a premature ventricular systole.[62] During a sinus beat, mitral motion during systole is grossly normal. The production of a subaortic pressure gradient after a compensatory or long pause[63] has been one of the recognized features of hypertrophic obstructive cardiomyopathy. Thus, efforts to bring out the abnormal mitral valve motion are occasionally necessary to identify patients with the disease. Provocation, such as a Valsalva maneuver, the use of amyl nitrite, intravenous isoproterenol, or even a noninvasively induced premature ventricular systole[62] brings out systolic anterior motion of the mitral valve that may be absent at rest.

It must be remembered that the mitral valve is attached to the mitral annulus, which is an integral part of the left ventricle. Motion exhibited by the mitral valve is in part related to any motion of the mitral annulus and/or left ventricular wall. For example, in any condition in which posterior ventricular wall motion is exaggerated, motion of the systolic component of the mitral valve echoes is exaggerated. This phenomenon may occur in any situation in which paradoxic septal motion is present. When the septum is moving abnormally, one frequently finds a "compensatory" exaggerated motion of the opposing left ventricular wall. Such motion is commonly noted in patients with right ventricular volume overload[52] and possibly in those individuals with ventricular aneurysm and anterior wall dyskinesis.[65] One must also be careful not to misinterpret aortic wall motion superimposed on mitral valve motion as SAM. A

true SAM should return to the baseline prior to the onset of ventricular diastole.

Dynamic outflow obstruction does not only occur with asymmetric septal hypertrophy. The M-mode echocardiogram in Figure 9–18 shows systolic anterior mitral motion (*arrow*); however, the interventricular septum (IVS) and posterior left ventricular wall (PW) are both hypertrophied. Thus, dynamic left ventricular outflow obstruction may occur with concentric hypertrophy.[66] Figure 9–19 shows another example of subaortic obstruction and SAM in a patient with concentric left ventricular hypertrophy. In addition, the patient has pericardial effusion, illustrating that other accompanying problems frequently bring out the subaortic obstruction.[67] Pericardial effusion seems to be one condition that is associated with hypertrophic subaortic stenosis.[68–70] Anemia and hypovolemia are also noted to occur with this condition.[56] Correcting the secondary problem may relieve the obstruction. Another entity associated with hypertrophic subaortic stenosis is mitral annulus calcification, especially in the elderly.[24] The relationship between these two abnormalities is not understood.[71]

Some patients show SAM with no evidence of hypertrophic cardiomyopathy.[72–81] Figure 9–20A shows a patient with aortic stenosis and insufficiency with predominant insufficiency. There is no evidence of asymmetric hypertrophy; however, the posterior left ventricular wall and the septum are thicker than normal, and generalized ventricular hypertrophy is present because of aortic valve disease. Some anterior motion of the mitral valve can be noted in early systole (*arrow*). Even with provocation, no evidence of subaortic obstruction was identified at cardiac catheterization. In addition, the sur-

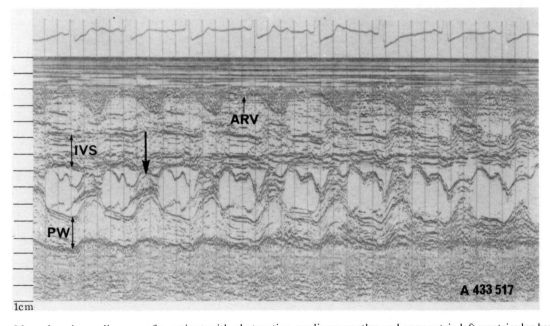

**Fig. 9–18.** M-mode echocardiogram of a patient with obstructive cardiomyopathy and concentric left ventricular hypertrophy. Systolic anterior motion of the mitral valve (*arrow*) can be seen obstructing the left ventricular outflow tract. The thickness of the interventricular septum (IVS) and posterior left ventricular wall (PW) are approximately equal. ARV = anterior right ventricular wall.

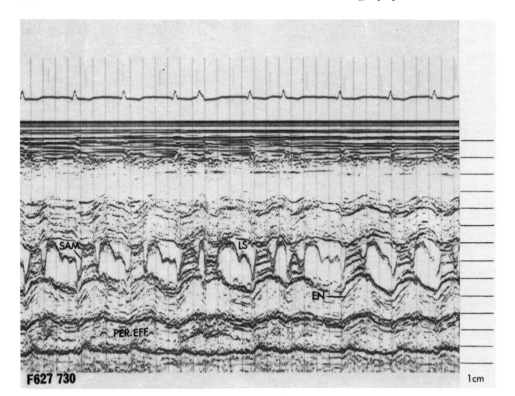

**Fig. 9–19.** M-mode echocardiogram of a patient with concentric left ventricular hypertrophy and systolic anterior motion (SAM) of the mitral valve producing outflow obstruction. The patient also has significant pericardial effusion (PER, EFF.). LS = left side of septum; EN = posterior left ventricular endocardium.

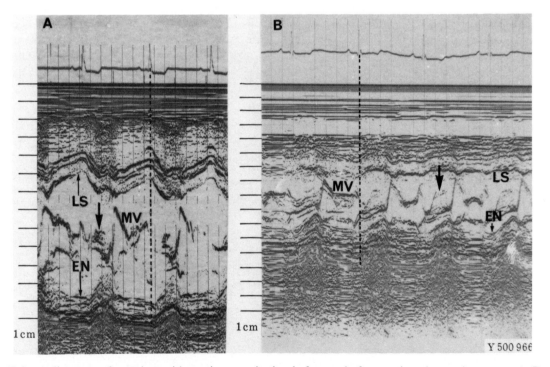

**Fig. 9–20.** Echocardiograms of a patient with aortic regurgitation before and after aortic valve replacement. *A,* Preoperative view of systolic anterior motion (*arrow*). *B,* Postoperative view of even more striking systolic anterior motion (*arrow*). Hypertrophic subaortic stenosis was not evident prior to or at the time of surgery. LS = left septum; MV = mitral valve; EN = posterior left ventricular endocardium.

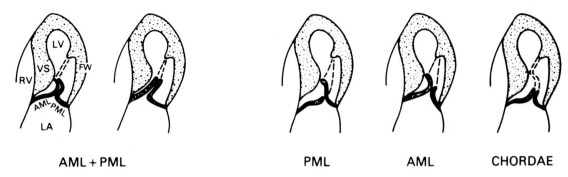

AML + PML        PML      AML      CHORDAE

**Fig. 9–21.** Diagram demonstrating the various parts of the mitral valve apparatus that can encroach on the left ventricular outflow tract and produce possible obstruction. AML = anterior mitral leaflet; PML = posterior mitral leaflet; LV = left ventricle; VS = ventricular septum; RV = right ventricle; FW = left ventricular free wall; LA = left atrium. (From Spirito, R. and Baron, B.J.: Patterns of systolic anterior motion of the mitral valve in hypertrophic cardiomyopathy: Assessment by two-dimensional echocardiography. Am. J. Cardiol., *54*:1039, 1984.)

geon could not find any evidence of hypertrophic sub-aortic stenosis at the time the aortic valve was replaced. Figure 9–20*B* shows the postoperative echocardiogram. The left ventricle is considerably smaller, and there is abnormal septal motion, which is commonly seen after any surgical procedure; however, the abnormal systolic motion of the mitral valve (*arrow*) is still present and may even be exaggerated postoperatively.[82]

The finding of SAM in patients without the clinical syndrome of asymmetric septal hypertrophy raises a question of whether the mitral motion might be a non-specific reaction to ventricular hypertrophy or to any distortion of the ventricular cavity.[69,83,84] The coexistence of dynamic subaortic obstruction is well recognized with fixed outflow obstructions[85–89] and in such conditions as transposition of the great arteries.[90,91] Even patients with mitral valve prolapse have an element of SAM (see Chapter 6).[92–95] Dynamic left ventricular out-

flow obstruction has also been noted with an anomalous papillary muscle that inserted directly into the mitral leaflet.[96,97]

There are many theories as to how SAM is produced.[98] Some authors think that the SAM may be produced by various parts of the mitral valve apparatus.[99,100] In some cases, the echocardiographic finding is produced by a combination of both the anterior and posterior leaflets (Fig. 9–21).[101,102] At other times, it may involve only one leaflet or the other and, in some patients, only the chordae. Some investigators hypothesize that obstruction is produced only when the leaflets produce the SAM. If only the chordae are involved, no dynamic obstruction occurs. Yet other authorities feel that the hypertrophied papillary muscles are involved in the obstructive process in some situations (Fig. 9–22).[103,104] Other theories involving the production of SAM include a Venturi effect of the blood flowing across

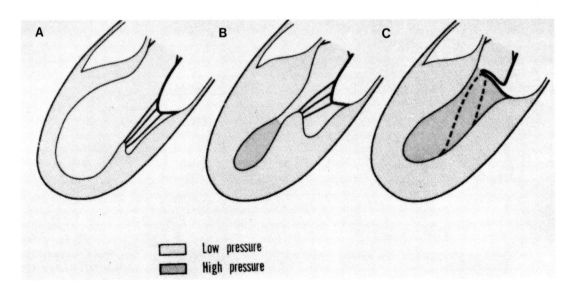

Low pressure
High pressure

**Fig. 9–22.** Diagram illustrating two sites for obstruction in patients with hypertrophic obstructive cardiomyopathy. In *B*, the site of obstruction is at the level of a hypertrophied papillary muscle and interventricular septum. In *C*, the obstruction occurs with the mitral valve leaflets opposing the hypertrophied septum. (From Nagata, et al.: Mechanism of systolic anterior motion of the mitral valve and site of intraventricular pressure gradient in hypertrophic obstructive cardiomyopathy. Br. Heart J., *49*: 234, 1983.)

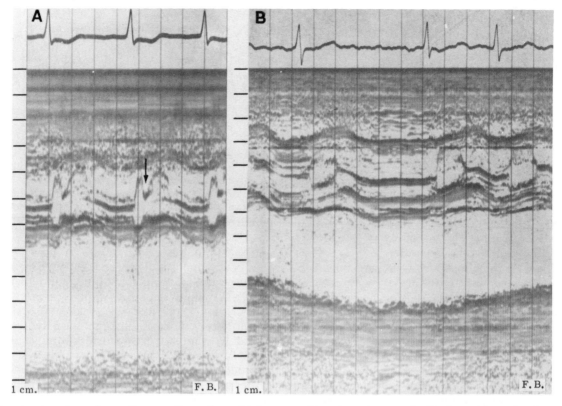

**Fig. 9–23.** Aortic valve echocardiogram of a patient with hypertrophic subaortic stenosis. During midsystole, the aortic valve closes (*arrow*) secondary to the subvalvular obstruction and reopens before diastole begins. Following the use of propranolol, the systolic closure of the aortic valve is not apparent (*B*). (From Feigenbaum, H.P: Clinical applications of echocardiography. Prog. Cardiovasc. Dis., *14*:531, 1972.)

the hypertrophied septum; both positive and reverse Venturi effects have been mentioned. Other investigators have suggested that malposition of the papillary muscles is a major factor in permitting the mitral valve apparatus to oppose the septum.[49] The displacement of the valve apparatus is also thought to be a principle

cause for the frequently seen mitral regurgitation that occurs with hypertrophic cardiomyopathy.

Aortic valve motion can indicate an alteration in aortic blood flow in patients with dynamic subaortic obstruction.[105-108] Figure 9–23 shows an M-mode aortic valve echocardiogram of a patient with hypertrophic obstruc-

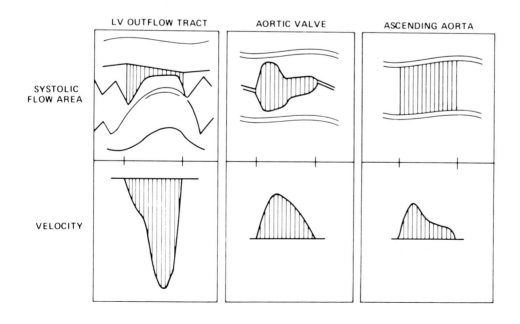

**Fig. 9–24.** Diagrams demonstrating the typical M-mode tracings (upper recordings) and Doppler velocities (lower tracings) of the left ventricular outflow tract, the aortic valve, and the ascending aorta with hypertrophic obstructive cardiomyopathy. (From Yock, P.G., Hatle, L., and Popp, R.L.: Patterns and timing of Doppler-detected intracavitary and aortic flow in hypertrophic cardiomyopathy. J. Am. Coll. Cardiol., *8*:1055, 1986.)

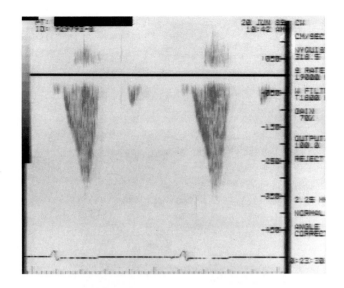

**Fig. 9–25.** Continuous wave Doppler aortic flow of a patient with hypertrophic obstructive cardiomyopathy. The late peaking velocity is typical of dynamic obstruction of the left ventricular outflow tract.

tive cardiomyopathy. Mid-systolic closure (*arrow*) of the anterior leaflet can be identified. Following relief of the obstruction with propranolol (Fig. 9–23B), the systolic closure is no longer present.

Spectral Doppler echocardiography is the procedure of choice for determining the presence and severity of left ventricular outflow tract obstruction.[109-112] Figure 9–24 diagrammatically shows the Doppler recordings corresponding to the M-mode echocardiographic findings. The classic continuous wave (CW) left ventricular outflow Doppler recording shows a relatively slow increase in velocity in early systole, which then picks up speed and peaks late in systole.[113] This velocity pattern corresponds nicely with the SAM on the M-mode echocardiogram.[114] Figure 9–25 is a characteristic continuous wave Doppler recording of the left ventricular outflow tract showing the late peaking velocity in a patient with dynamic subaortic obstruction. The aortic valve flow and ascending aortic flow correlate with the corresponding M-mode tracings (Fig. 9–24).

Figures 9–26 and 9–27 provide evidence that the continuous wave Doppler velocities accurately reflect the hemodynamic obstruction. In Figure 9–26, the classic late peaking velocity tracing with a maximum velocity of 4 M/sec corresponds nicely with a 67-mm gradient at the time of cardiac catheterization. Figure 9–27 demonstrates how a more severe form of obstruction following a premature ventricular systole produces a high velocity, which again compares well with the hemodynamic gradient. It should be noted that the shape of the velocity curve will change as the obstruction becomes more holosystolic. In Figure 9–27, late systolic peaking is not evident as this severe form of obstruction produces a holosystolic gradient. Figure 9–28 illustrates the variety of continuous wave Doppler left ventricular outflow tract

recordings that can occur with hypertrophic cardiomyopathy. In Figures 9–28A and 9–28B, an initial rapid rise in velocity is followed by a slowing and then a rapid rise to a late peak. With increasing obstruction, the late systolic peaking becomes less pronounced. In Figure 9–28F, one sees a holosystolic gradient with more severe obstruction.

Figure 9–29 shows a technical problem with continuous wave Doppler recordings in a patient with hypertrophic cardiomyopathy. Because these patients commonly have mitral regurgitation[115] as well as the left ventricular outflow tract obstruction, one must be careful to differ-

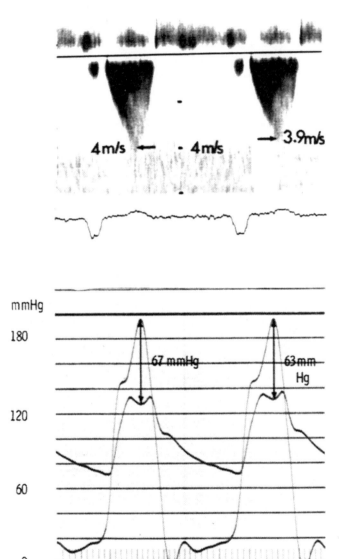

**Fig. 9–26.** Simultaneous continuous wave Doppler and catheter pressure recordings in a patient with hypertrophic obstructive cardiomyopathy. The peak velocities of 4 M/sec and 3.9 M/sec correspond to a Doppler-derived gradient of 64 and 61 mm Hg. These values correlate well with the measured peak catheter gradients of 67 and 63 mm Hg. (From Sasson, Z., et al.: Doppler echocardiographic determination of the pressure gradient in hypertrophic cardiomyopathy. J. Am. Coll. Cardiol., *11*:754, 1988.)

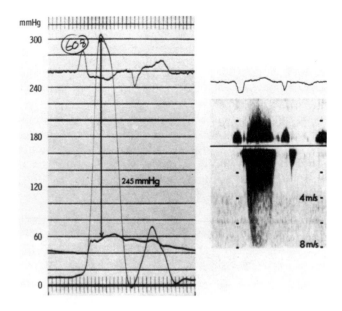

**Fig. 9–27.** Simultaneous pressure and Doppler recordings of a patient with severe obstruction of the left ventricular outflow tract secondary to hypertrophic obstructive cardiomyopathy. The cardiac cycle represents a post-extrasystolic beat. The peak velocity of 8 M/sec produces a Doppler gradient of 256 mm Hg, which corresponds well with the measured gradient of 245 mm Hg. (From Sasson, Z., et al.: Doppler echocardiographic determination of the pressure gradient in hypertrophic cardiomyopathy. J. Am. Coll. Cardiol., *11*:754, 1988.)

entiate the Doppler recording of the two abnormalities. It is possible to register the mitral regurgitation and the outflow obstruction simultaneously (Fig. 9–29). As long as one records the classical late systolic peaking velocity, one can be reasonably certain that the outflow tract is being recorded; however, as already noted, with marked obstruction, the gradient is more holosystolic and may be difficult to distinguish from mitral regurgitation. Therefore, technical care is necessary to avoid confusing the outflow tract recording with mitral regurgitation. Continuous wave Doppler recordings with two-dimensional imaging may help eliminate this confusion.

Color flow Doppler helps to identify the location of the obstructing lesion.[116–118] Figure 9–30 shows acceleration and aliasing of blood flow in the middle of the left ventricular cavity (*arrow*). The blood accelerates as it approaches the subaortic obstruction. Past the obstruction and proximal to the aortic valve, one can detect turbulent blood flow.

The right ventricle may also be involved with hypertrophic cardiomyopathy. Dynamic obstruction in the right ventricular outflow can be a component of this abnormality.[119–122] Figure 9–31 shows a Doppler recording of a patient who had hypertrophic myopathy with obstruction of the right ventricular outflow tract. The peak velocity is nearly 5 M/sec. A secondary velocity of about 2.5 M/sec (*arrow*) is noted proximal to the major obstruction. In both cases, there is late peaking of the velocity envelopes.

Finding abnormal diastolic blood flow with the cardio-

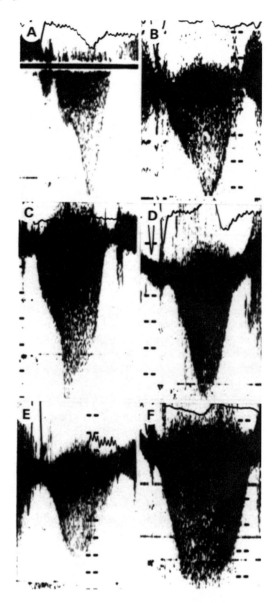

**Fig. 9–28.** Continuous wave Doppler recordings from six patients with hypertrophic obstructive cardiomyopathy demonstrating the variability in waveforms that can occur with this abnormality. In *A*, *B*, and *C*, the brief initial rise in velocity is relatively rapid and is followed by a more gradual increase in velocity to achieve a peak in mid-systole. This pattern produces an asymmetric leftward concave shape to the recording. In *D*, *E*, and *F*, the rise in velocity is more gradual and the wave form is more symmetric. (From Panza, J.A., et al.: Utility of continuous wave Doppler echocardiography in the non-invasive assessment of left ventricular outflow tract pressure gradient in patients with hypertrophic cardiomyopathy. J. Am. Coll. Cardiol., *19*:97, 1992.)

myopathic process is not surprising.[123–129] Figure 9–32 illustrates the common patterns of left ventricular inflow that are seen clinically. Because abnormal left ventricular relaxation and elevated left ventricular diastolic pressures commonly occur with hypertrophic cardiomyopathy, the pattern in Figure 9–32*B* is observed in these patients. The diastolic filling patterns, however, can be

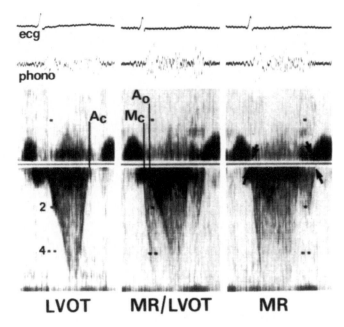

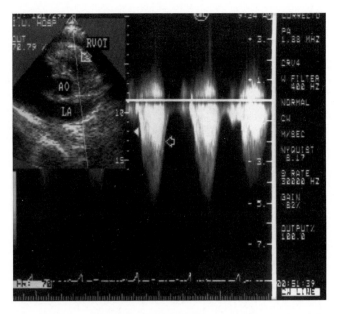

**Fig. 9–29.** Continuous wave Doppler recordings from a patient with hypertrophic cardiomyopathy showing how the left ventricular outflow tract (LVOT) recordings can be confused with the mitral regurgitation (MR) jet commonly present in these patients. Overlapping recordings (MR/LVOT) can be obtained with the ultrasonic beam in an intermediate position. $A_c$ = aortic closure; $A_o$ = aortic opening; $M_c$ = mitral closure. (From Yock, E.G., Hatle, L., and Popp, R.L.: Patterns and timing of Doppler-detected intracavitary and aortic flow in hypertrophic cardiomyopathy. J. Am. Coll. Cardiol., 8:1052, 1986.)

**Fig. 9–31.** Continuous wave Doppler recording in the right ventricular outflow tract of a patient with hypertrophic cardiomyopathy and obstruction of the right ventricular outflow tract. The peak Doppler velocity is approximately 5 M/sec. One can also visualize a smaller velocity (*arrow*), which peaks at about 2.5 M/sec. RVOT = right ventricular outflow tract; AO = aorta; LA = left atrium.

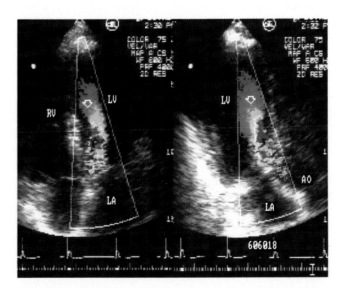

**Fig. 9–30.** Color flow Doppler study of a patient with hypertrophic obstructive cardiomyopathy. Blood flowing within the left ventricular outflow tract accelerates (*arrows*) and then aliases as it approaches the subvalvular obstruction. High-velocity turbulent flow occurs within the left ventricular outflow tract at and distal to the obstruction. RV = right ventricle; LV = left ventricle; LA = left atrium; AO = aorta.

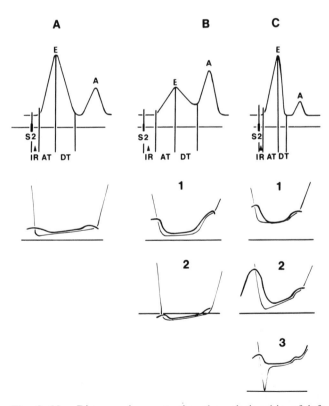

**Fig. 9–32.** Diagram demonstrating the relationship of left ventricular inflow velocities and left ventricular and left atrial pressures in normal subjects (*A*), in patients with abnormal left ventricular relaxation or low filling pressures (*B*), and in patients with elevated left ventricular filling pressures, mitral regurgitation, or restrictive physiology (*C*).

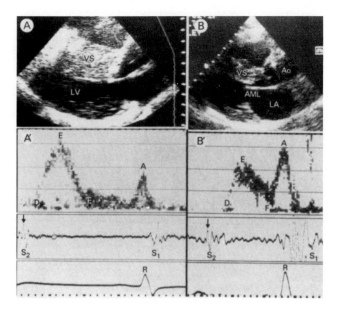

**Fig. 9-33.** Two-dimensional echocardiograms and pulsed Doppler left ventricular inflow velocities of two patients with hypertrophic cardiomyopathy. The patient in *A* has a massively thickened interventricular septum (VS), yet the Doppler velocities exhibit a relatively normal pattern. The patient in *B* has a lesser degree of hypertrophy, and the Doppler velocity shows a typical abnormal relaxation pattern. LV = left ventricle; AO = aorta; LA = left atrium; AML = anterior mitral leaflet. (From Spirito, P. and Maron, B.J.: Relation between extent of left ventricular hypertrophy and diastolic filling abnormalities in hypertrophic cardiomyopathy. J. Am. Coll. Cardiol., *15*:811, 1990.)

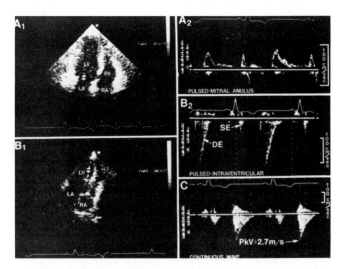

**Fig. 9-34.** Pulsed Doppler recordings at the mitral annulus ($A_1$ and $A_2$), at the middle of the left ventricular cavity ($B_1$ and $B_2$), and continuous wave Doppler (*C*). The recordings were all obtained from an apical transducer position. The velocity at the mitral annulus is normal. At the middle ventricular level, brief systolic emptying (SE) of the apical cavity is followed by a diastolic high-velocity jet from apex to base, indicative of further diastolic emptying (DE) of the apical cavity through a narrow intraventricular channel. Continuous wave Doppler shows mitral inflow velocity and a high diastolic velocity jet in the opposite direction. LA = left atrium; LV = left ventricle; PKV = peak jet velocity; RA = right atrium; RV = right ventricle. (From Zoghbi, W.A., et al.: Mid cavity obstruction in apical hypertrophy: Doppler evidence of diastolic intraventricular gradient with higher apical pressure. Am. Heart J., *116*:1471, 1988.)

quite variable.[130] Figure 9-33 shows two examples of patients with hypertrophic cardiomyopathy who had unexpected mitral flow velocities. In the patient with massive septal hypertrophy, one would expect an abnormal relaxation pattern, yet the tracing was relatively normal. In Figure 9-33*B*, a patient with lesser degree of hypertrophy has the more typical abnormal relaxation pattern.

Many reasons account for the different patterns of mitral inflow. Mitral regurgitation would increase the early filling phase and is commonly present with hypertrophic myopathy. In addition, the various ways in which the left ventricle hypertrophies may also influence whether or not a relaxation or restrictive type of pattern dominates.

A somewhat uniquely abnormal diastolic Doppler pattern in hypertrophic cardiomyopathy occurs because the apex is frequently isolated from the body of the left ventricle during the contraction process (Fig. 9-13). As a result, with early diastole, blood may actually flow from the apex into the body of the ventricle. Figure 9-34 shows an example of intracavity, high-velocity diastolic flow as blood leaves the apex and moves toward the outflow tract. A variety of these peculiar intracavitary flow phenomena has been reported.[131-136]

#### Evaluation of Therapy

Echocardiography can be helpful in assessing the benefits of medical or surgical therapy of hypertrophic car-

diomyopathy.[137-146] Figure 9-23 shows how aortic valve motion changes as obstruction is relieved with medical therapy. Figure 9-35 shows the echocardiographic findings in a patient before and after surgical septal myectomy. In the M-mode echocardiogram, one can appreciate the absence of SAM postoperatively (E). In the short-axis view, one sees the site of the myectomy (*arrows*) as the septal contour is altered. The long-axis view (F) may show a similar finding or just widening of the outflow tract. The color Doppler study (G) demonstrates disappearance of the turbulent jet in the left ventricular outflow tract. Echocardiography is now used frequently during surgery for hypertrophic cardiomyopathy.[147] The examination can be helpful in guiding the surgeon and judging the effectiveness of repair before closing the chest.[148,149]

### IDIOPATHIC DILATED CARDIOMYOPATHY

Patients with idiopathic dilated cardiomyopathy are characterized by dilated, poorly contracting left ventricles and echocardiographic signs of low cardiac output and high intracardiac pressures.[150-152] Figure 9-36 shows the hallmarks of dilated cardiomyopathy. The left ventricle is dilated and little difference is noted between diastole and systole. All of the systolic indices, whether

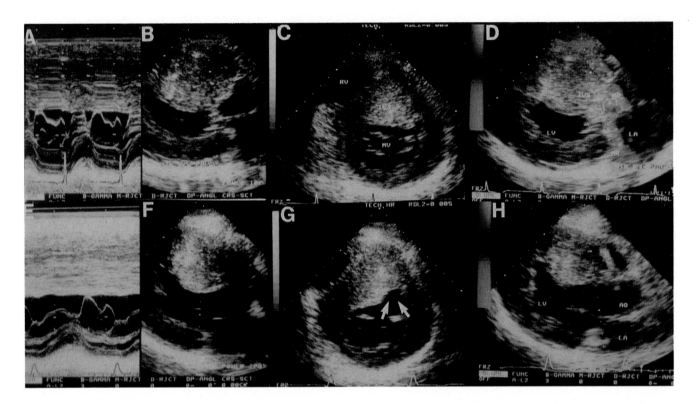

**Fig. 9–35.** Study from a patient with hypertrophic obstructive cardiomyopathy (*A–D*) who underwent successful septal myectomy (*E–H*). Preoperatively, severe systolic anterior motion (SAM) with prolonged septal contact was present, as evident in the M-mode (*A*) and long-axis (*B*) images. Circumferential extent of septal hypertrophy can be seen in the parasternal short-axis view at the level of the mitral leaflet (*C*). Color flow imaging (*D*) revealed high-velocity outflow tract jet and eccentric posteriorly directed jet of mitral regurgitation. Postoperatively, the myectomy site can be seen (*G, arrows*), resulting in widening of the outflow tract (*F* and *G*) with regression of SAM (*E*) and disappearance of turbulent outflow and mitral regurgitant jets (*H*). (From Rakowski, H., et al.: Echocardiographic and Doppler assessment of hypertrophic cardiomyopathy. J. Am. Soc. Echocardiogr., *1*:45, 1988.)

one measures fractional shortening, fractional area change, or ejection fraction, are reduced. Wall thickness remains normal and global dysfunction is fairly generalized. With increased left ventricular filling pressures and usually mitral regurgitation, left atrial dilatation is common in association with this abnormality (Fig. 9–36).

Figure 9–37 is a typical left ventricular M-mode echocardiogram from a patient with dilated cardiomyopathy.[153,154] The left ventricle is dilated and both the septal and posterior ventricular walls move poorly; however, wall thickness is within normal limits. Following a premature atrial systole and a prolonged diastolic pause, abnormal closure of the mitral valve can be noted (*arrow*). Some authors emphasize the characteristic shape of the left ventricle in patients with dilated cardiomyopathy. The dilatation is primarily in the short axis rather than in the length, and thus the left ventricle becomes spherical.[155–157] In a form of mildly dilated cardiomyopathy, patients have a significant decrease in systolic function but dilatation of the left ventricle is not a prominent feature.[158] This entity is another form of idiopathic cardiomyopathy.

Mitral inflow is invariably abnormal in these patients with severe myocardial dysfunction.[159–163] The usual

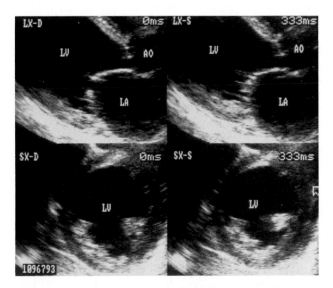

**Fig. 9–36.** Long-axis and short-axis two-dimensional echocardiograms of a patient with a dilated cardiomyopathy. The left ventricle (LV) and left atrium (LA) are both dilated. Little difference in size of the left ventricular cavity is noted from diastole (LX-D and SX-D) and systole (LX-S and SX-S).

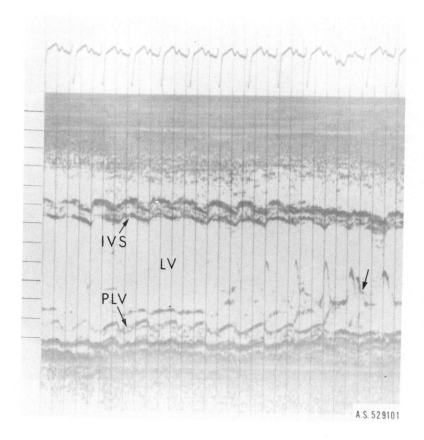

A.S. 529101

**Fig. 9–37.** M-mode echocardiogram of the left ventricle in a patient with congestive cardiomyopathy. The left ventricle (LV) is dilated, and the motion of the interventricular septum (IVS) and posterior left ventricular wall (PLV) is markedly reduced. Following a premature atrial systole and a prolonged diastolic pause, abnormal closure of the mitral valve (*arrow*) can be noted.

pattern, especially early in the disease state, is abnormal relaxation similar to that shown in Figure 9–32B. As mitral regurgitation or elevated left ventricular diastolic pressures occur, however, the abnormal relaxation pattern may progress toward the abnormal compliance (Fig. 9–32C) variety, with a tall E wave and small A wave,[160,164] which usually carries a poor prognosis.[165] During this progression, one may recognize a pattern of "pseudonormalization."

With a dilated, poorly contracting left ventricle, it is not surprising that abnormal flow patterns are recognized within the left ventricle.[164–169] This abnormal flow may be exhibited as spontaneous contrast (Fig. 9–38) or as a swirling pattern of blood flow, especially in the apical half of the left ventricle (Fig. 9–39). As might be expected, these patients have a high incidence of mural thrombi.[170–173] Left atrial spontaneous contrast and thrombi are also found in patients with idiopathic dilated cardiomyopathy.[173a]

It is not always easy to distinguish idiopathic dilated cardiomyopathy from a severely dilated dysfunctional left ventricle associated with coronary artery disease. Although idiopathic dilated myopathy usually has diffuse symmetric hypokinesis, regional abnormalities may also occur. With significant mitral regurgitation, septal motion may be enhanced and the posterolateral walls may be disproportionately hypokinetic. Efforts at distinguishing idiopathic from ischemic cardiomyopathy using regional wall motion as a criterion have been disappointing. If patients have scarred walls, one can be certain that ischemic disease is the principal etiologic factor.

Another recent attempt has been to examine the coronary arteries ultrasonically.[174] If atheroscleortic disease is found within the walls of the proximal coronary arteries, then the probability is extremely high that the cardiomyopathic state is related to coronary artery disease (see Chapter 8).

A common finding with dilated cardiomyopathy is incomplete closure of the mitral valve or "papillary muscle dysfunction" (Fig. 9–40).[175] This finding likely contributes to the common presence of mitral regurgitation.[176]

One form of cardiomyopathy primarily involves the right ventricle.[177,178] The echocardiogram shows typical findings of a right ventricular volume overload. Uhl's disease is also a type of right ventricular dysplasia or myopathy. Massive right ventricular dilatation is again noted.[179,180] These patients may have diastolic opening of the pulmonary valve or delayed closure of the tricuspid valve.[181]

## RESTRICTIVE CARDIOMYOPATHY

Restrictive cardiomyopathy is a form of cardiac pathophysiology that includes a number of different disease states. Patients with an infiltrative cardiomyopathy, such as amyloidosis, glycogen storage disease, or thalassemia can produce this type of physiologic picture. Cardiac transplant rejection is another entity that is indistinguishable from the clinical findings noted in this group of patients. There is also an idiopathic form of restrictive

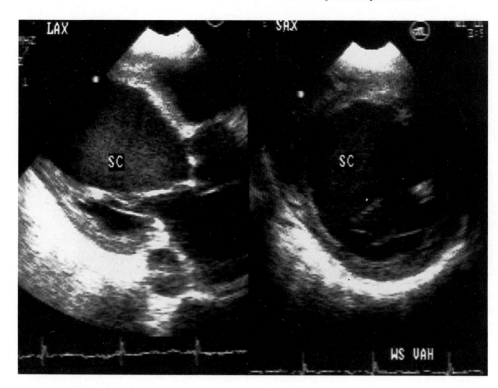

**Fig. 9–38.** A patient with dilated cardiomyopathy exhibiting spontaneous contrast (SC) within this dilated, poorly moving left ventricle. LAX = long axis; SAX = short axis.

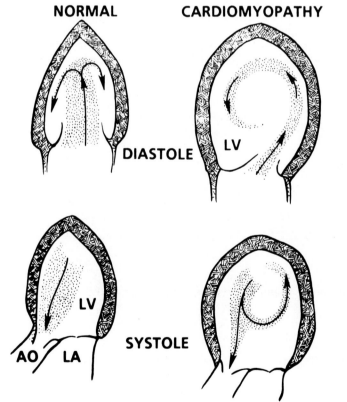

**Fig. 9–39.** Diagram showing the patterns of left ventricular inflow (upper drawings) and left ventricular outflow (lower drawings) of a normal subject and a patient with a dilated cardiomyopathy. The unidirectional normal inflow and outflow in the normal subject contrasts with a swirling flow pattern as blood enters the left ventricle (LV) in the patient with cardiomyopathy. With ejection, some of the blood may be directed back toward the apex rather than having all of the blood enter the aorta (AO) as is normal. LA = left atrium. (From D'Cruz, I.A. and Sharaf, I.S.: Patterns of flow within the dilated cardiomyopathic left ventricle: Color flow Doppler observations. Echocardiography, 8:228, 1991.)

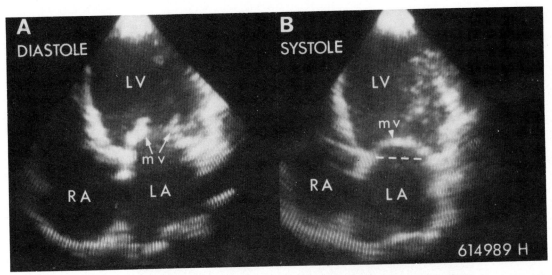

**Fig. 9–40.** Apical four-chamber two-dimensional echocardiogram of a patient with congestive cardiomyopathy. The size of the left ventricle (LV) changes little from diastole (*A*) to systole (*B*). In addition, there is incomplete closure of the mitral valve (mv) in systole. The closed leaflets fail to reach the plane of the mitral annulus (*dotted line*). RA = right atrium; LA = left atrium.

cardiomyopathy. The hallmark of restrictive physiology is abnormal compliance of the left ventricle with rapid inflow and abrupt cessation of flow early in diastole.[182-188] The typical mitral flow velocity curve is characterized by Figure 9–32C. The left atrial and left ventricular pressures are identified in Figure 9–32C-3. An early diastolic drop is followed by a rise in the left ventricular pressure giving the classical "dip and plateau"

or "square root sign." These hemodynamics produce a short isovolumic relaxation time (IR), a tall E wave, and a short deceleration time (DT).[185,186] Atrial velocity is also suppressed because of restricted ability of the ventricle to fill with atrial systole. As a result, the E to A ratio is high.

Figure 9–41 shows mitral and tricuspid flow velocities in a patient with restrictive cardiomyopathy. The tall

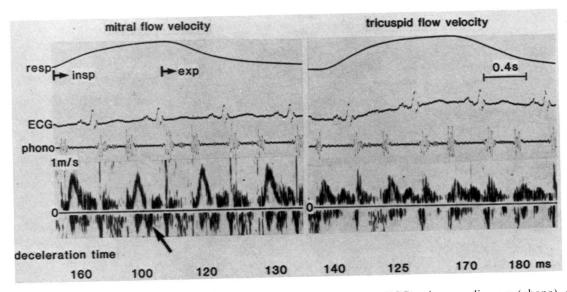

**Fig. 9–41.** Simultaneous recordings of respiration (resp), the electrocardiogram (ECG), phonocardiogram (phono), and mitral and tricuspid pulsed Doppler tracings in a patient with restrictive cardiomyopathy. There is minimal respiratory variation in peak early mitral flow velocity with respiration and a relatively low flow velocity with atrial contraction. The mitral deceleration time is short, and shortens further (bottom values) during inspiration, with mid-diastolic reversal of flow (diastolic regurgitation, *arrow*) seen at the same time. The early tricuspid flow velocity also shows inspiratory shortening of the deceleration time with only a moderate increase in peak velocity, and no decrease in early velocity is noted on the first beat of expiration. (From Hatle, L.K., et al.: Differentiation of constrictive pericarditis and restrictive cardiomyopathy by Doppler echocardiography. Circulation, 79:357, 1989.)

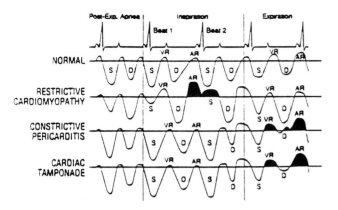

**Fig. 9–42.** Drawings showing the pulsed Doppler hepatic venous flow profile during different phases of respiration from a normal subject and in patients with restrictive cardiomyopathy, constrictive pericarditis, and cardiac tamponade. In restrictive cardiomyopathy, inspiratory decrease and/or flow reversal occurs during systole (*shaded area*) and at the time of atrial contraction (AR). In constrictive pericarditis and cardiac tamponade, decrease of forward diastolic flow and reversal are at the time of atrial contraction (AR). D = diastolic forward flow; S = systolic forward flow; VR = end systolic or V wave-related reverse flow. (From Bansal, R.C. and Chandrarsekaran, K.: Role of echocardiography and Doppler techniques in the evaluation of pericardial diseases. Echocardiography, 6:313, 1989.)

early diastolic velocity and short late diastolic velocities are readily recognized in the mitral flow. Also, a short time interval between the second heart sound and the onset of mitral flow indicates a short isovolumic relaxation time. This tracing also points out a reversal of flow in mid-diastole (*arrow*). This hemodynamic finding will produce diastolic mitral regurgitation, which is a characteristic finding of restrictive physiology. Respiratory variation in the flow velocities of both the tricuspid and mitral valves is minimal, a distinguishing feature from constrictive pericarditis, which has a similar physiologic picture but greater respiratory variation.

Venous velocities in restrictive cardiomyopathy also have fairly characteristic patterns.[186–188] Figure 9–42 diagrammatically shows hepatic venous flow velocities with normal physiology, restrictive cardiomyopathy, constrictive pericarditis, and cardiac tamponade. The distinguishing feature between normal and restrictive cardiomyopathy is the increase in diastolic velocities. The normal systolic velocity is slightly higher than the diastolic velocity. Systolic velocity is labeled as X and diastolic velocity as Y by some authors. The increased diastolic velocity would go along with the tall E wave seen in the mitral and tricuspid velocities. This diagram also notes an increase in atrial flow reversal, especially with inspiration.

Figure 9–43 shows the pulmonary venous flow velocities as recorded with transesophageal echocardiography of normal flow (PV-N), with restrictive cardiomyopathy (PV-R), and with constrictive pericarditis (PV-CP). Again, one sees an increase in the diastolic velocities (Y) with restrictive cardiomyopathy. The discrepancy

between normal and restrictive myopathy ratios of systolic and diastolic (X and Y) velocities is fairly striking. The X to Y ratio of restrictive cardiomyopathy also differs from constrictive pericarditis (Fig. 9–43, PV-CP).

The Doppler findings with restrictive cardiomyopathy can be subtle. In certain disease states, the physiology may vary. For example, with amyloidosis, which is a classic example of restrictive cardiomyopathy, early stages of this disease may produce abnormal left ventricular relaxation with a mitral flow pattern characterized by a short E wave and tall A wave. Accompanying hemodynamic factors, such as mitral regurgitation,

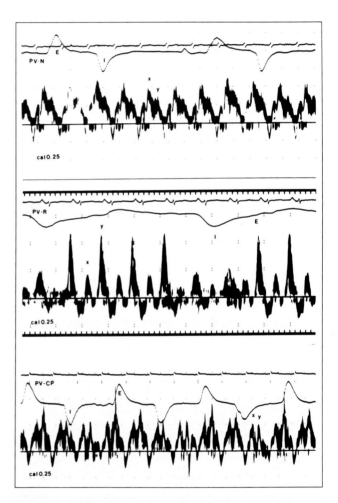

**Fig. 9–43.** Transesophageal pulsed Doppler recordings of pulmonary venous flow in a normal patient (PV-N, *A*), a patient with restrictive cardiomyopathy (PV-R, *B*), and a patient with constrictive pericarditis (PV-CP, *C*). Pulmonary venous systolic flow velocity (x) and diastolic flow velocity (y), both toward the left atrium, are inscribed above the baseline. Inspiration (I) is indicated by a negative deflection and expiration (E) is indicated by a positive deflection using nasal capnometry. The electrocardiogram is positioned at the top of each strip trace recording. (From Schiavone, W.A., Calafiore, P.A., and Salcedo, E.E.: Transesophageal Doppler echocardiographic demonstration of pulmonary venous flow velocity in restrictive cardiomyopathy and constrictive pericarditis. Am. J. Cardiol., 63:1286, 1989.)

elevated filling pressures, and elevated preload or afterload, will influence these inflow patterns. Furthermore, arrhythmias, especially atrial fibrillation whereby no atrial contraction occurs, clearly alter these Doppler patterns.

Digitized M-mode recordings are also being used to evaluate restrictive cardiomyopathy.[189] One sees abrupt filling of the left ventricle with cessation of flow in diastole. One again distinguishes this pattern from constrictive pericarditis by noting a lack of respiratory variation.

## INFILTRATIVE CARDIOMYOPATHY

Infiltrative cardiomyopathy is a term used for a group of diseases, many of which are metabolic in nature, whereby the cardiac muscle is infiltrated by abnormal substances. The abnormalities reported to produce myocardial changes that can be detected with echocardiography include amyloidosis,[190-200] iron overload from multiple transfusions,[201-205] hemachromatosis,[206] thalassemia, sarcoidosis,[207-209] glycogen storage disease or Pompei's disease,[210-213] and mucolipidosis.[214-216] Some of these diseases, such as glycogen storage disease, are also classified as "storage" rather than "infiltrative" cardiomyopathy.

The most common type of infiltrative cardiomyopathy in the echocardiographic literature is amyloid heart disease,[217] which has several characteristic echocardiographic features.[218,219] Figure 9–44 shows many of the classic manifestations of amyloid heart disease as noted on the two-dimensional echocardiogram.[220] The amyloid apparently infiltrates all parts of the heart; there-

fore, thickening of all myocardial walls and valves is noted. Figure 9–44 shows a hypertrophied interventricular septum and posterior left ventricular wall. Note also thickening of the aortic, mitral, and tricuspid valves. A somewhat unique, but not always universal, feature is thickening of the interatrial septum. The thickened interatrial septum is frequently seen best in the subcostal view. Figure 9–45 shows another patient with amyloid heart disease who has thick right and left ventricular walls and interatrial septum.

The M-mode echocardiogram also exhibits a fairly characteristic examination. Figure 9–46 demonstrates a thickened right ventricular wall, interventricular septum, and posterior left ventricular wall. There is also a small pericardial effusion, which is fairly common with this infiltrative myopathy. The left ventricle is not di-

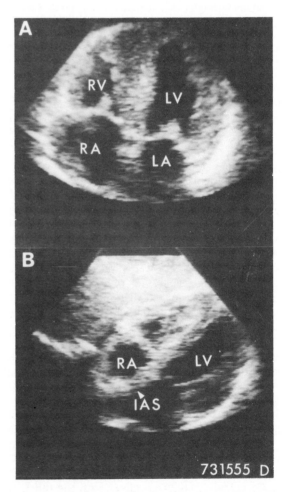

**Fig. 9–45.** Four-chamber, *A,* and subcostal, *B,* two-dimensional echocardiograms of a patient with hereditary amyloidosis. The four-chamber view demonstrates markedly hypertrophied cardiac walls, especially the interventricular septum and the free wall of the right ventricle. The tricuspid and mitral valve leaflets are also thickened. The left ventricular (LV) and right ventricular (RV) cavities are small. The subcostal examination demonstrates the thickened interatrial septum (IAS), which may occur in amyloid heart disease. RA = right atrium; LA = left atrium.

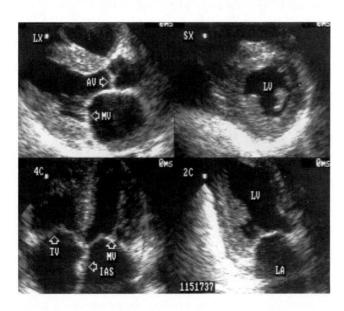

**Fig. 9–44.** Two-dimensional echocardiogram of a patient with amyloid heart disease. All of the cardiac walls and valves are thickened and echogenic. LX = long axis; SX = short axis; 4C = four chamber; 2C = two chamber; AV = aortic valve; MV = mitral valve; LV = left ventricle; TV = tricuspid valve; IAS = interatrial septum; LA = left atrium.

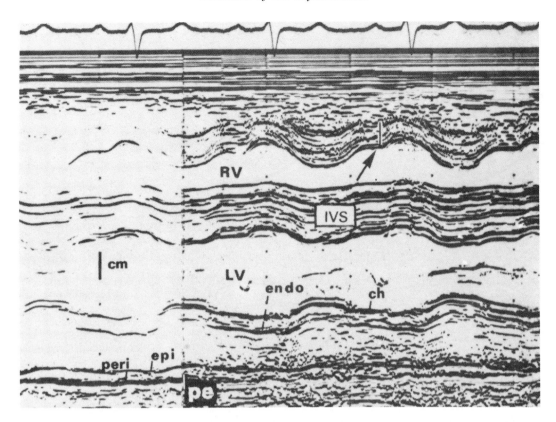

**Fig. 9–46.** M-mode echocardiogram of a patient with amyloid cardiomyopathy. The thickened anterior right ventricular wall (RV) measures 10 mm in diastole (*arrow*). The interventricular septum (IVS) and the posterior left ventricular wall between the endocardium (endo) and epicardium (epi) are hypertrophied. The motion of both ventricular walls is reduced, and the overall cavity size is normal. There is a small pericardial effusion (pe). LV = left ventricle: Ch = chordae. (From Child, J.S., Krivokapich, J., and Abbasi, A.S: Increased right ventricular wall thickness on echocardiography in amyloid infiltrative cardiomyopathy. Am. J. Cardiol., *44*:1391, 1979.)

lated, and systolic function usually remains intact until late in the course of the disease.

As with most infiltrative cardiomyopathies, filling of the left ventricle is abnormal. As a result, left atrial dilatation is commonly associated with this problem (Fig. 9–44). In addition, left ventricular inflow or mitral Doppler recordings are altered in some way.[221–225] The classic mitral flow in a patient with amyloid heart disease is the restrictive type (Fig. 9–32C). In fact, amyloid heart disease is frequently used as the typical example of restrictive cardiomyopathy. It has been noted, however, that in the early stages of the disease, the flow pattern is actually of the abnormal left ventricular relaxation type (Fig. 9–32B). As the disease progresses, pseudonormalization of mitral flow can be detected.[222] Amyloidosis also involves the right ventricle and produces similarly abnormal right ventricular inflow patterns.[226]

Besides making the diagnosis of amyloid heart disease, echocardiography is proving to be important as a prognostic indicator. Left ventricular systolic and diastolic function can be assessed fairly accurately with echocardiography. When M-mode and two-dimensional echocardiography show reduced systolic function, the prognosis is poor. Furthermore, when diastolic flow changes from abnormal relaxation to the restrictive form, one is entering a later stage of the disease.

Two-dimensional echocardiography is also being used to make a specific tissue diagnosis.[227,228] In Figure 9–45, one can identify "patchy amorphous, high-intensity echoes" in the left ventricular myocardium.[193–197,200] This type of myocardial echo is fairly characteristic if not diagnostic for amyloid heart infiltration, especially of the hereditary type. Figure 9–47 diagrammatically illustrates some of the types of intramyocardial echoes that have been recognized in various conditions.[229] Type IIA is the typical two-dimensional echocardiographic appearance of patients with infiltrative cardiomyopathy, such as amyloidosis. Type I consists of a uniform, fine echo pattern throughout the myocardium or else a generalized myocardial echolucency, as noted by the area near the posterior wall (PW). The type I pattern is seen with concentric hypertrophy, as in hypertension or aortic stenosis. Type IIB intramyocardial echoes are commonly seen with hypertrophic cardiomyopathy. The last type (IIC) consists of localized, echo-dense thin walls that result from myocardial infarction (see Chapter 8).

Many of the other infiltrative cardiomyopathies,[230–232] such as Pompei's disease and many of the hematologic abnormalities,[233–235] produce nonspecific echocardiographic findings. The walls are usually thickened and may be somewhat more echo-reflective. Cavity size is usually normal, and ventricular function is

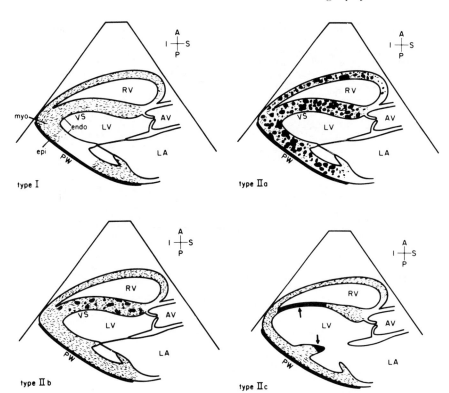

**Fig. 9–47.** Diagram demonstrating some of the types of myocardial echoes noted in diseases affecting the myocardium (see text for details). (From Bhondari, A.K. and Nanda, N.C.: Myocardial texture characterization by two-dimensional echocardiography. Am. J. Cardiol., *51*:817, 1983.)

reduced late in the disease. The hypertrophied walls may look like concentric hypertrophy or even asymmetric septal hypertrophy. Some patients with mucopolysaccharid storage abnormalities may produce an echocardiographic appearance that is similar to hypertrophic cardiomyopathy. Investigators have been using quantitative ultrasonic analysis to detect myocardial changes with thalassemia major and iron overload.[235a]

One form of infiltrative cardiomyopathy that has somewhat more characteristic echocardiographic findings is cardiac sarcoidosis.[236–237] Figure 9–48 shows an

example of a patient with cardiac sarcoidosis. A characteristic feature is localized thinning and dilatation of the left ventricle. The involved area of the left ventricle is usually toward the base. In Figure 9–48, one sees thinning of the basal portion of the inferolateral wall (*open arrow*) and papillary muscle (*closed arrow*). This recording would resemble an inferior lateral myocardial infarction with scar and a shallow aneurysm. Figure 9–49 shows another example of cardiac sarcoidosis. Again,

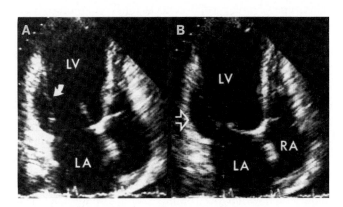

**Fig. 9–48.** Apical four-chamber view during diastole (*A*) and systole (*B*) in a patient with cardiac sarcoidosis demonstrating a dilated left ventricular cavity and a thinned, akinetic basal inferior wall (*open arrow*) and papillary muscle (*closed arrow*), which resulted in severe mitral regurgitation. LV = left ventricle; LA = left atrium; RA = right atrium. (From Burstow, D.J., et al.: Two-dimensional echocardiographic findings in systemic sarcoidosis. Am. J. Cardiol., *63*:480, 1989.)

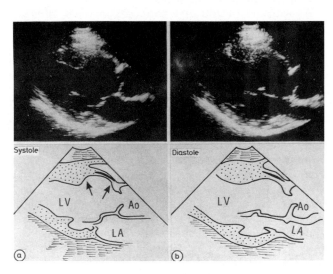

**Fig. 9–49.** Long-axis systolic (*a*) and diastolic (*b*) views of a patient with sarcoidosis. The proximal septum (*arrows*) is thin and dilated. LV = left ventricle; AO = aorta; LA = left atrium. (From Valantine, E.H., et al.: Sarcoidosis: A pattern of clinical and morphological presentation. Br. Heart J., *57*: 256, 1987.)

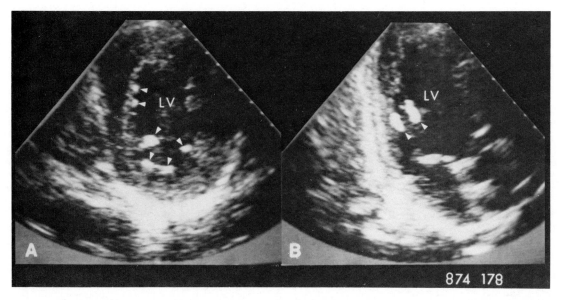

**Fig. 9–50.** Short-axis (*A*) and apical two-chamber (*B*) two-dimensional echocardiograms of a patient with endomyocardial disease and eosinophilia. Numerous echogenic areas (*arrowheads*) can be seen throughout the left ventricular endocardium. LV = left ventricle.

one sees thinning of the proximal portion of the left ventricle. In this case, it involves the proximal septum. As with all cardiomyopathies, sarcoidosis produces abnormal left ventricular filling.[238]

## FIBROPLASTIC CARDIOMYOPATHY

Numerous authors have described the echocardiographic findings of endomyocardial fibrosis.[239–249] These patients may have the clinical signs of primary congestive cardiomyopathy or a restrictive form of cardiomyopathy with abnormal filling. Pathologically, a layer of fibrosis surrounds the endocardium. Endomyocardial fibrosis may occur with or without eosinophilia. Figure 9–50 shows a two-dimensional echocardiogram of a patient who has endomyocardial disease and eosinophilia.[250,251] Numerous echogenic areas are evident along the endocardium and the mitral valve apparatus. Figure 9–51 shows another example of eosinophilic endocardial fibrosis.[252] In this patient, the right ventricle is the chamber primarily involved. One can see massive fibrosis in the right ventricular cavity. The hemodynamic effect is to make the right ventricle virtually nonfunctioning and a passive conduit. An interesting Doppler finding is that with right atrial contraction, the pressure is transmitted directly into the pulmonary artery. Thus, one sees increased flow in the pulmonary artery with atrial contraction (Fig. 9–52).

Figure 9–53 diagrammatically shows the many manifestations of endocardial myocardial fibrosis that can involve either or both ventricles. Obliteration of the apex is a fairly characteristic finding with this problem. Figure 9–54 shows an M-mode echocardiogram before and after surgical removal of the endocardial fibrous tissue. The right ventricular cavity dimension is improved

and is the most striking finding in this recording. The left ventricular cavity also increases but to a lesser degree. Because of abnormal ventricular filling, the atria are almost always dilated in this disorder.[245] These patients are also susceptible to cardiac thrombi and peripheral embolization.[248,253]

## MYOCARDIAL DISEASE ASSOCIATED WITH NEUROMUSCULAR DISORDERS

An assortment of neuromuscular abnormalities have associated myocardial malfunction. Many of these car-

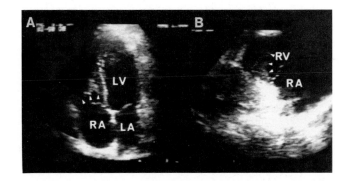

**Fig. 9–51.** Two-dimensional echocardiogram from the apical four-chamber view (*A*) and parasternal long-axis view of the right ventricular inflow tract (*B*) demonstrating a large mass filling the right ventricular cavity (*arrowheads*) in a patient with hypereosinophilic syndrome. LV = left ventricle; LA = left atrium; RA, right atrium; RV, right ventricle. (From Presti, C., Ryan, T., and Armstrong, W.F.: Two-dimensional and Doppler echocardiographic findings in hypereosinophilic syndrome. Am. Heart J., *114*:173, 1987.)

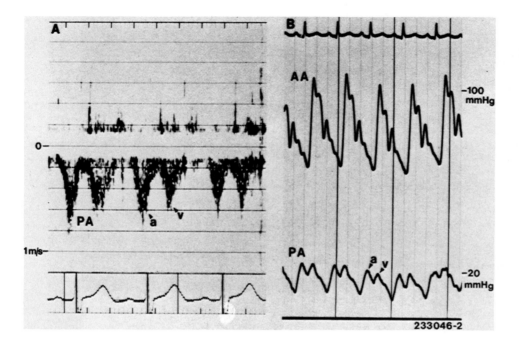

**Fig. 9–52.** Pulsed Doppler pulmonary artery velocities (*A*) and aortic and pulmonary artery pressures (*B*) in the same patient with hypereosinophilic syndrome whose two-dimensional recording is shown in Figure 9–51. Pulmonary artery flow is biphasic with a substantial portion of the flow occurring during atrial systole (a) and relatively less flow during ventricular systole (v). A corresponding large A wave in the pulmonary artery pressure is noted (a). AA = ascending aorta; PA = pulmonary artery. (From Presti, C., Ryan, T., and Armstrong, W.F.: Two-dimensional and Doppler echocardiographic findings in hypereosinophilic syndrome. Am. Heart J., *114*: 173, 1987.)

diac abnormalities have been detected echocardiographically.[254–269] The neuromuscular entities include Friedreich's ataxia and muscular dystrophy.[270,271] Echocardiographic findings are relatively nonspecific and primarily consist of left ventricular hypertrophy and dysfunction. The conditions may present as concentric hypertrophy, dilated cardiomyopathy, or asymmetric hypertrophy resembling hypertrophic cardiomyopathy.[272,273] Figure 9–55 shows a two-dimensional echocardiogram of a patient with Friedreich's ataxia. One can appreciate generalized hypertrophy with the septum somewhat thicker than the posterior ventricular wall. Similar findings have been noted with familial neurofibromatosis and Duchenne's cardiomyopathy.[274,275]

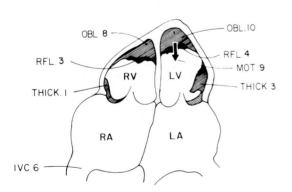

**Fig. 9–53.** Drawing illustrating the two-dimensional echocardiographic findings in patients with endomyocardial disease. THICK = thickening; MOT = altered motion; OBL = obliteration; RFL = reflecting clot; LA = left atrium; IVC = inferior vena cava. (From Acquatella, H., et al.: Value of two-dimensional echocardiography in endomyocardial disease with and without eosinophilia. Circulation, *67*:1219, 1983.)

## CARDIAC ABNORMALITIES AND INFECTIOUS AGENTS

A variety of infectious agents or presumed infectious agents have been known to affect the heart. Vitral myocarditis is possibly the most prevalent of these entities.[276] The viral etiology is frequently not confirmed and is only presumed. This problem is thought to be one of the causes of idiopathic dilated cardiomyopathy. The echocardiographic findings are usually nonspecific and polymorphic.[277–281] One may see a dilated or hypertrophied ventricle. Both left ventricular dysfunction and right ventricular dysfunction may be noted. Regional wall motion abnormalities can also be detected.[280,281] One may see both abnormal relaxation or restrictive type of filling abnormalities in these patients.

On rare occasion, tuberculosis can invade the myocardium and present as a restrictive cardiomyopathy.[282] Tuberculosis has also been reported to produce a submitral left ventricular aneurysm.[283] The infectious agent for Kawasaki disease may also involve the myocardium. Characteristically, Kawasaki cardiac manifestation involves the coronary arteries (see Chapter 8); however, left ventricular dysfunction in addition to coronary abnormalities may also be present.[284–288]

Patients with human immunodeficiency virus (HIV) infection or AIDS frequently have cardiac abnormalities.[289] This involvement is probably a direct viral infection of the myocardium.[290–293] These individuals may have left ventricular dilatation and impaired systolic function.[293a] Pericardial effusion is another common finding in patients with AIDS.

Some infectious diseases of the heart are not commonly seen in the United States and produce characteristic echocardiographic findings. Chagas is an infectious myocarditis seen primarily in South America.[294–298] The findings may be nonspecific, although localized aneu-

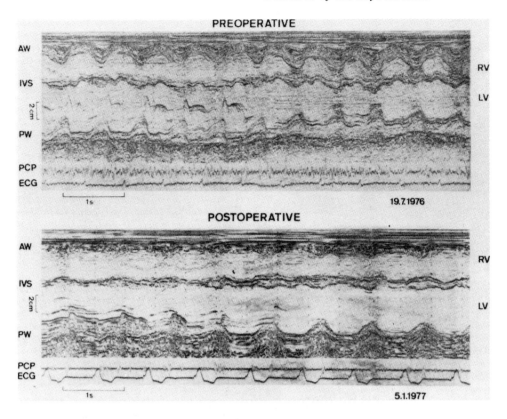

PREOPERATIVE

AW

IVS

2 cm

PW

PCP

ECG

1s

RV

LV

19.7.1976

POSTOPERATIVE

AW

IVS

2 cm

PW

PCP
ECG

1s

RV

LV

5.1.1977

**Fig. 9–54.** Pre- and postoperative M-mode echocardiograms in a patient with biventricular endomyocardial fibrosis. Endocardial thickening of the right ventricular anterior wall with systolic obliteration of the right ventricular cavity toward the apex can be seen in the preoperative echocardiogram. Endocardial 'fibrosis of the left ventricular posterior wall is found toward the left ventricular apex. The postoperative recording shows diminution of the right anterior wall and left posterior endocardial thickening. The systolic obliteration of the right ventricular cavity is no longer present following surgery. AW = anterior wall; IVS = interventricular septum; PW = posterior wall; PCP = phonocardiogram; ECG = electrocardiogram; RV = right ventricle; LV = left ventricle. (From Hess, O.M., et al.: Pre- and postoperative findings in patients with endomyocardial fibrosis. Br. Heart J., *40*:406, 1978.)

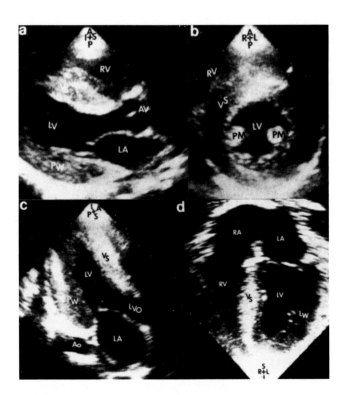

**Fig. 9–55.** Two-dimensional echocardiograms from a patient with Friedreich's ataxia showing symmetric thickening of the ventricular septum (VS) and left ventricular posterior wall (PW/LW) with prominent papillary muscles (PM). The left ventricular outflow tract (LVO) is widely patent in systole. *a* = parasternal long-axis view; *b* = short-axis view at the papillary muscles; *c* = apical long-axis view; *d* = apical four-chamber view; RV = right ventricle: LV = left ventricle; AV = aortic valve; LA = left atrium; Ao = aorta; RA = right atrium. (From Alboliaris, E.T., et al.: Spectrum of cardiac involvement in Friedreich's ataxia: Clinical, electrocardiographic and echocardiographic observations. Am. J. Cardiol., *58*:521, 1986.)

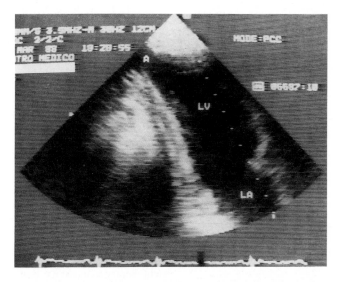

**Fig. 9–56.** Apical two-chamber echocardiogram showing a typical Chagas' left ventricular (LV) "narrow neck" apical aneurysm (A). The abnormality could not be seen using the four-chamber view. LV = left ventricle; LA = left atrium. (From Acquatella, H.: Echocardiographic overview of Chagas' disease and endomyocardial fibrosis: Diagnostic implications for nontropic countries. Echocardiography, 6:137, 1989.)

rysms, especially involving the apex and having a "narrow neck," are fairly typical in patients with this abnormality. Figure 9–56 shows such a patient who exhibits a "narrow neck" apical aneurysm.

Cardiac echinococcosis is another infectious process involving the heart.[299–301] With this entity, hydatid cysts may be found within the heart. Figure 9–57 shows a patient with a large hydatid cyst involving the right ventricle. The postoperative tracing shows the cyst is reduced.

## MYOCARDIAL DYSFUNCTION AND TOXIC AGENTS

A variety of toxic agents are known to produce abnormal cardiac function. These agents include venom,[302] alcohol,[303–307] cocaine,[308–310] and several drugs including doxorubicin.[311–317] The earliest manifestation of this type of toxic myocardiopathy is impaired filling of the early abnormal relaxation type (Fig. 9–32B). With more advanced toxicity, abnormal systolic function and left ventricular dilatation may be manifest.

## CARDIAC ABNORMALITIES RESULTING FROM TRAUMA

A variety of cardiac problems can occur because of trauma.[318–323b] Trauma has been noted to change the acoustic properties of the myocardium.[319] Frequently, this injury results in disruption of the valve or wall. Septal defects,[323–327] pseudoaneurysms,[328–330] ruptured papillary muscles and other forms of valvular regurgitation on both the right and left side,[331–333] and fistulas

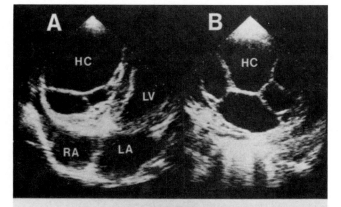

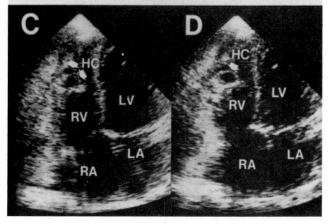

**Fig. 9–57.** Preoperative apical views of a patient with a large hydatid cyst within the right ventricle (*A* and *B*). The postoperative echocardiograms (*C* and *D*) show only two small remaining cysts in the right ventricular walls. HC = hydatid cyst; LV = left ventricle; LA = left atrium; RA = right atrium; RV = right ventricle. (From Oliver, J.M., et al.: Two-dimensional echocardiographic features of echinococcosis of the heart and great vessels. Clinical and surgical implications. Circulation, 78:331, 1988.)

from the aorta to the right atrium[334,335] have all been reported to occur after trauma. A fairly dramatic consequence of trauma is noted in Figure 9–58. This patient had an atrial septal hematoma form after blunt chest trauma.[336] One sees a huge echocardiographic mass attached to the interatrial septum. A left ventricular thrombus has also been detected following blunt chest trauma.[336a]

Electrical trauma or electrocution has also been noted to produce cardiac abnormalities.[337–339] These findings are frequently regional wall motion abnormalities.

## EFFECT OF SYSTEMIC ILLNESSES ON THE HEART

In a large number of studies, echocardiography was used to follow systemic medical problems that may have an effect on the heart. Echocardiography is used frequently to follow the effects of systemic hypertension on left ventricular function.[340–346] Left ventricular hypertrophy and alterations of systolic and diastolic func-

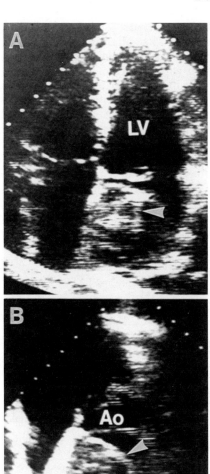

**Fig. 9–58.** Four-chamber (*A*) and short-axis (*B*) two-dimensional echocardiogram of a patient who developed a large hematoma (*arrows*) of the interatrial septum as a result of blunt chest trauma. LV = left ventricle; Ao = aorta. (From Rowe, S.K. and Porter, C.B.: Atrial septal hematoma: Two-dimensional echocardiographic findings after blunt chest trauma. Am. Heart J., *114*:651, 1987.)

tion are major complications of hypertension. Thus, echocardiography appears to be the procedure of choice in monitoring these individuals. The echocardiogram not only has diagnostic value but also is proving to be a powerful prognostic indicator of future morbid events.[342,347]

Many people have been evaluating diabetic patients to see the effect of this disease on the heart.[348–350] Diabetes appears to alter left ventricular diastolic function.[350a] Abnormal left ventricular relaxation recorded by Doppler echocardiography has been recognized by numerous investigators.[351–354] A form of left ventricular hypertrophy, septal hypertrophy, and SAM in children of diabetic mothers is an entity that simulates hypertrophic cardiomyopathy.[36–38]

Patients with other endocrine disorders, such as hypothyroidism and acromegaly, have also been reported to show echocardiographic changes. Acromegaly produces cardiomegaly, with concentric left ventricular hypertrophy and occasional dilatation.[268,355–359] Some patients exhibit septal hypertrophy and simulate hypertrophic myopathy.[358] Although left ventricular mass is invariably increased, systolic function appears to be normal.[359]

Some authors have demonstrated a reversible form of cardiomyopathy in patients with hypothyroidism.[360,361] Left ventricular dilatation and decreased systolic function have been noted to improve with treatment of the hypothyroidism.

Other systemic problems that affect the heart include lupus erythematosus.[362–365] This problem frequently produces pericardial effusion, but it may also present with left ventricular hypertrophy and impaired left ventricular function. Both systolic and diastolic dysfunction have been reported with this systemic illness.[366] Acute rheumatic fever will also produce a form of myocarditis that involves not only the valves but also the myocardium.

Carcinoid heart disease classically involves the right side of the heart and is characterized by restricted motion of the tricuspid and pulmonary valves; however,

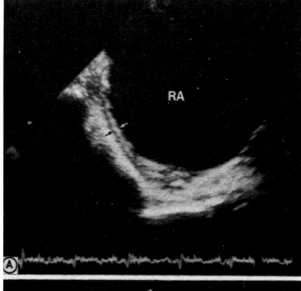

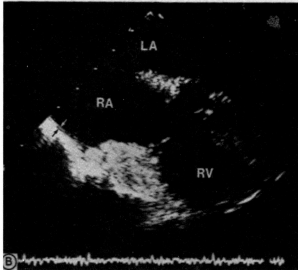

**Fig. 9–59.** Transesophageal echocardiographic recording of the right atrium (RA) in a patient with carcinoid heart disease (*A*) and a patient with a normal right atrium (*B*). The right atrial free wall is significantly thicker in the patient with carcinoid heart disease. LA = left atrium; RV = right ventricle. (From Lundin, L., et al.: Transesophageal echocardiography improves the diagnostic value of cardiac ultrasound in patients with carcinoid heart disease. Br. Heart J., *64*:193, 1990.)

it has also been noted, especially with transesophageal echocardiography, that the walls of the right side of the heart are also involved.[367,368] Figure 9–59 shows a transesophageal echocardiogram whereby the right atrial wall is thickened in a patient with carcinoid heart disease.

## CARDIAC TRANSPLANTATION

Echocardiography is being used to follow patients with orthotopic heart transplants. Several authors have reported abnormal findings with cardiac rejection.[369–378] Although increased diastolic left ventricular wall thick-

ness has been reported,[379–381] the principle manifestation appears to be alterations in ventricular filling.[382–384a] The typical finding is evidence of a restricted filling pattern with rejection. Figure 9–60 shows serial Doppler recordings of a patient with no rejection and with moderate rejection. With mitral flow, one can see the characteristic restrictive pattern with a tall E wave, short deceleration time, and a relatively small atrial component.

Figure 9–61 illustrates another set of serial mitral valve Doppler studies in a patient after cardiac transplantation. The upper recording shows mild evidence of rejection, with a tall E wave and short A wave. Several weeks later, with more severe rejection, one can see abolition of the A wave, and the E wave is even taller. Serial tricuspid Doppler recordings from the same patient are seen in Figure 9–62. In the earlier study, tricus-

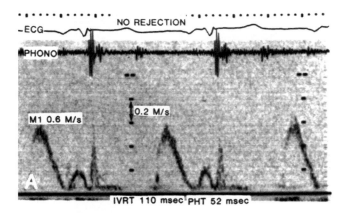

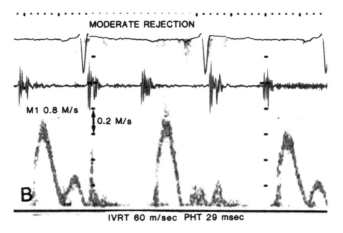

**Fig. 9–60.** Mitral flow velocity curves using pulsed wave Doppler in transplant recipients with no rejection (*A*) and with moderate acute rejection (*B*). With rejection, the isovolumic relaxation time (IVRT) is 60 msec; without rejection, it is 110 msec. The pressure half-time (PHT) decreases from 52 to 29 msec with rejection. M1 = peak early mitral flow velocity; M2 = peak mitral velocity after mitral systole. (From Gibbons, R.S.: Doppler echocardiography for rejection surveillance in the cardiac allograft recipient. J. Am. Soc. Echocardiogr., *4*:97, 1991.)

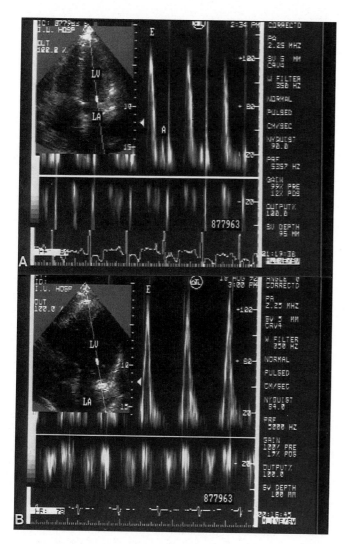

**Fig. 9–61.** Serial pulsed Doppler mitral valve velocity recordings of a patient after cardiac transplantation before (*A*) and during (*B*) rejection. With rejection, the small atrial velocity (A) disappears and the early diastolic velocity (E) increases. LV = left ventricle; LA = left atrium.

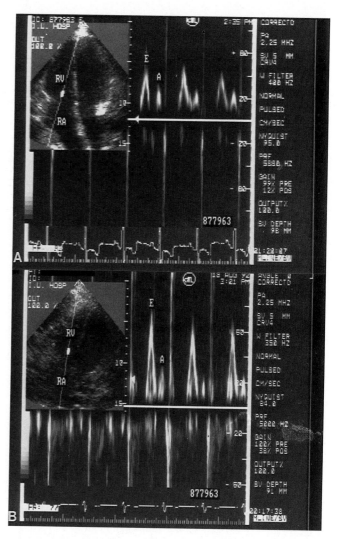

**Fig. 9–62.** Serial pulsed Doppler tricuspid valve velocities in the same patient whose mitral valve recording is shown in Figure 9–61. Before rejection, the tricuspid velocities profile is relatively normal, with a moderately taller E velocity than A velocity (*A*). With rejection (*B*), the early velocity is significantly elevated, increasing the E to A ratio. RV = right ventricle; RA = right atrium.

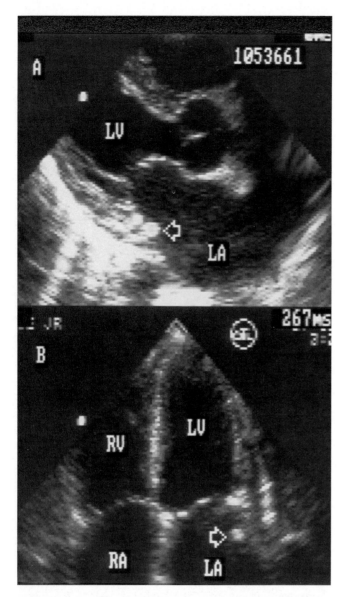

**Fig. 9–63.** Long-axis (*A*) and four-chamber (*B*) echocardiograms of a patient after cardiac transplantation. The junction (*arrows*) between the recipient and donor left atria can be noted. LV = left ventricle; LA = left atrium; RV = right ventricle; RA = right atrium.

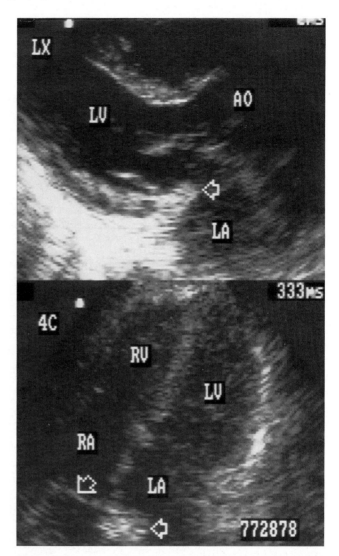

**Fig. 9–64.** Two-dimensional echocardiograms taken in the long-axis (LX) and four-chamber (4C) views of a cardiac transplantation patient whose suture line between the donor and recipient left atria is unusually large, simulating a pathologic mass (*small arrows*). The suture line between the donor and recipient right atria can also be seen (*large arrow*). LV = left ventricle; AO = aorta; LA = left atrium; RV = right ventricle; RA = right atrium.

pid flow has a fairly normal E to A ratio. With more severe rejection, however, a striking change in the E to A ratio can be noted.

Abnormal Doppler recordings in transplant rejection have been noted by several investigators. Forward systolic superior vena caval flow is said to be diminished with rejection.[385] The reliability of all of these findings, however, is still somewhat questionable.[385a] Most authorities agree that the best way to use Doppler measurements is by following a given patient and looking for changes in the recordings.

M-mode recordings of altered left ventricular filling have also been used to identify rejection.[384] Investigators are attempting to identify transplant rejection by

noting acoustic changes in the myocardium.[386] Pericardial effusion is another problem that occurs in transplant patients.[387] As discussed in the chapter on coronary artery disease (Chapter 8), transplanted hearts have a form of accelerated coronary atherosclerosis. Intracoronary ultrasound is being used to study and hopefully to help to manage this problem.

A characteristic finding following cardiac transplantation stems from the fact that these patients have atria from both donor and recipient hearts. This situation produces interesting atrial patterns that can be seen on the electrocardiogram and on Doppler recordings. In addition, one can frequently see fairly prominent echoes from the suture lines attaching the two atria.[388] Figure 9–63 shows a fairly typical example of the echoes that originate from the suture line. Occasionally, these echoes can be fairly large and simulate a pathologic mass. Figure 9–64 shows an example of a fairly large, echo-producing mass from the suture line.

## REFERENCES

1. Abbasi, A.S., MacAlpin, R.N., Eber, L.M., and Pearce, M.L.: Echocardiographic diagnosis of idiopathic hypertrophic cardiomyopathy without outflow obstruction. Circulation, *46*:897, 1972
2. Henry, W.L., Clark, C.E., Roberts, W.C., Morrow, A.G., and Epstein, S.E.: Difference in distribution of myocardial abnormalities in patients with obstructive and non-obstructive asymmetric septal hypertrophy (ASH): Echocardiographic and gross anatomic findings. Circulation, *50*:447, 1974.
3. Henry, W.L., Clark, C.E., and Epstein, S.E.: Asymmetric septal hypertrophy: The unifying link in the IHSS disease spectrum: Observation regarding its pathogenesis, pathophysiology, and course. Circulation, *47*:827, 1973.
4. vanDorp, W.G., Ten Cate, F.J., Vletter, W.B., Dohmen, H., and Roelandt, J.: Familial prevalence of asymmetric septal hypertrophy. Eur. J. Cardiol., *4/3*:349,1976.
5. Henry, W.L., Clark, C.E., and Epstein, S.E.: Asymmetric septal hypertrophy (ASH): Echocardiographic identification of the pathognomonic anatomic abnormality of IHSS. Circulation, *47*:225, 1973.
6. Sayaya, J., Longo, M.R., and Schlant, R.C.: Echocardiographic interventricular septal wall motion and thickness: Study in health and disease. Am. Heart J., *87*:681, 1974.
7. Maron, B.J., Henry, W.L., Clark, C.E., Redwood, D.R., Roberts, W.C., and Epstein, S.E.: Asymmetric septal hypertrophy in childhood. Circulation, *53*:9, 1976.
8. Schweizer, P., Hanrath, P., Bleifield, W., and Effert, S.: Echocardiographic criteria of asymmetrical hypertrophy of the ventricular septum without outflow tract obstruction. Dtsch. Med. Wochensch., *100*:2189, 1975.
9. Shapiro, L.M. and McKenna, W.J.: Distribution of left ventricular hypertrophy in hypertrophic cardiomyopathy: A two dimensional echocardiographic study. J. Am. Coll. Cardiol., *2*:437, 1983.
10. Maron, B.J., Gottdiener, J.S., Bonow, R.O., and Epstein, S.E.: Hypertrophic cardiomyopathy with unusual locations of left ventricular hypertrophy undetectable by M-mode echocardiography. Identification by wide-angle two dimensional echocardiography. Circulation, *63*:409, 1981.
11. Belenkie, I., MacDonald, R.P.R., and Smith, E.R.: Localized septal hypertrophy: Part of the spectrum of hypertrophic cardiomyopathy or an incidental echocardiographic finding? Am. Heart J., *115*:385, 1988.
12. Spirito, P., Maron, B.J., Bonow, R.O., and Epstein, S.E.: Severe functional limitation in patients with hypertrophic cardiomyopathy and only mild localized left ventricular hypertrophy. J. Am. Coll. Cardiol., *8*:537, 1986.
13. Spirito, P. and Maron, B.J.: Hypertrophic cardiomyopathy with mild left ventricular hypertrophy. Cardiol. Board Review, *4*:119, 1987.
14. Lewis, J.F. and Maron, B.J.: Hypertrophic cardiomyopathy characterized by marked hypertrophy of the poste-

15. rior left ventricular free wall: Significance and clinical implications. J. Am. Coll. Cardiol., *18*:421, 1991.
15. Maron, B.J., Bonow, R.O., Seshagiri, T.N.R., Roberts, W.C., and Epstein, S.E.: Hypertrophic cardiomyopathy with ventricular septal hypertrophy localized to the apical region of the left ventricle (apical hypertrophic cardiomyopathy). Am. J. Cardiol., *49*:1838, 1982.
16. Steingo, L., Dansky, R., Pocock, W.A., and Barlow, J.B.: Apical hypertrophic nonobstructive cardiomyopathy. Am. Heart J., *104*:635, 1982.
17. Kereiakes, D.J., Anderson, D.J., Crouse, L., and Chatterjee, K.: Apical hypertrophic cardiomyopathy, Am. Heart J., *106*:855, 1983.
18. Keren, G., et al.: Apical hypertrophic cardiomyopathy: Evaluation by noninvasive and invasive techniques in 23 patients. Circulation, *71*:45, 1985.
19. Webb, J.G., Sasson, Z., Rakowski, H., Liu, P., and Wigle, E.D.: Apical hypertrophic cardiomyopathy: Clinical follow-up and diagnostic correlates. J. Am. Coll. Cardiol., *15*:83, 1990.
20. Louie, E.K. and Maron, B.J.: Apical hypertrophic cardiomyopathy: Clinical and two-dimensional echocardiographic assessment. Ann. Intern. Med., *106*:663, 1987.
21. Nakamura, T., Matsubara, K., Furukawa, K., Kitamura, H., Azuma, A., Sugihara, H., Katsume, H., Nakagawa, M., Miyao, K., and Kunishige, H.: Apical sequestration in hypertrophic cardiomyopathy: Its clinical features and pathophysiology. J. Cardiol., *21*:361, 1991.
21a. Ko, Y-L., Lei, M-H., Chiang, F-T., Chen, J-J., Kuan, P., and Lien, W-P.: Apical hypertrophic cardiomyopathy of the Japanese type: Occurrence with familial hypertrophic cardiomyopathy in a family. Am. Heart J., *124*:1626, 1992.
22. Meyer, R.A.: Cardiomyopathy in the young. J. Am. Soc. Echocardiogr., *1*:88, 1988.
23. Panza, J.A., Maris, T.J., and Maron, B.J.: Development and determinants of dynamic obstruction to left ventricular outflow in young patients with hypertrophic cardiomyopathy. Circulation, *85*:1398, 1992.
24. Fay, W.P., Taliercio, C.P., Ilstrup, D.M., Tajik, A.J., and Gersh, B.J.: Natural history of hypertrophic cardiomyopathy in the elderly. J. Am. Coll. Cardiol., *16*:821, 1990.
25. Lewis, J.F. and Maron, B.J.: Elderly patients with hypertrophic cardiomyopathy: A subset with distinctive left ventricular morphology and progressive clinical course late in life. A. Am. Coll. Cardiol., *13*:36, 1989.
26. Agatston, A.S., Polakoff, R., Hippogoankar, R., Schnur, S., and Samet, P.: The significance of increased left ventricular outflow tract velocities in the elderly measured by continuous wave Doppler. Am. Heart J., *117*:1320, 1989.
27. Lever, H.M., Karam, R.F., Currie, P.J., and Healy, B.P.: Hypertrophic cardiomyopathy in the elderly. Circulation, *79*:580, 1989.
28. Doi, Y.L., Deanfield, J.E., McKenna, W.J., Dargie, H.J., Oakley, C.M., and Goodwin, J.F.: Echocardiographic differentiation of hypertensive heart disease and hypertrophic cardiomyopathy. Br. Heart J., *44*:395, 1980.
29. Smolenskii, A.V.: Asymmetric hypertrophy of the myocardium in patients with hypertension (echocardiographic data). Kardiologiia, *23*:69, 1983.
30. Pearson, A.C., Gudipati, C.V., and Labovitz, A.J.: Systolic and diastolic flow abnormalities in elderly patients with hypertensive hypertrophic cardiomyopathy. J. Am. Coll. Cardiol., *12*:989, 1988.

31. Harrison, M.R., Grigsby, C.G., Souther, S.K., Smith, M.D., and DeMaria, A.N.: Midventricular obstruction associated with chronic systemic hypertension and severe left ventricular hypertrophy. Am. J. Cardiol., *68*: 761, 1991.

32. Schmieder, R.E., Messerli, F.H., Nunez, B.D., Garavaglia, G.E., and Frohlich, E.D.: Hemodynamic, humoral and volume findings in systemic hypertension with isolated ventricular septal hypertrophy. Am. J. Cardiol., *62*:1053, 1988.

33. Bernardi, D., Bernini, L., Cini, G., Ghione, S., and Bonechi, I.: Asymmetric septal hypertrophy and sympathetic overactivity in normotensive hemodialyzed patients. Am. Heart J., *109*:539, 1985.

34. Abbasi, A.S., Slaughter, J.C., and Allen M.W.: Asymmetric septal hypertrophy in patients on long-term hemodialysis. Chest, *74*:548, 1978.

35. Lewis, J.F., Spirito, P., Pelliccia, A., and Maron, B.J.: Usefulness of Doppler echocardiographic assessment of diastolic filling in distinguishing ''athlete's heart'' from hypertrophic cardiomyopathy. Br. Heart J., *68*:296, 1992.

36. Hess, O.M., Schneider, J., Turina, M., Carroll, J.D., Rothlin, M., and Krayenbuehl, H.P.: Asymmetric septal hypertrophy in patients with aortic stenosis: An adaptive mechanism or a coexistence of hypertrophic cardiomyopathy? J. Am. Coll. Cardiol., *1*:783, 1983.

37. Gutgesell, H.P., Mullins, C.E., Gillette, P.C., et al.: Transient hypertrophic subaortic stenosis in infants of diabetic mothers. J. Pediatr., *89*:120, 1976.

38. Holliday, H.L.: Hypertrophic cardiomyopathy in infants of poorly-controlled diabetic mothers. Arch. Dis. Child., *56*:258, 1981.

39. Lusson, J.R., Gaulme, J., Raynaud, E.J., and Cheynel, J.: Asymmetrical hypertrophic cardiomyopathy in neonates of diabetic mothers. Arch. Fr. Pediatr., *39*:433, 1982.

40. Cabin, H.S., Costello, R.M., Vasudevan, C., Maron, B.J., and Roberts, W.C.: Cardiac lymphoma mimicking hypertrophic cardiomyopathy. Am. Heart J., *104*:466, 1981.

41. Isner, J.M., Falcone, M.W., Virmani, R., and Roberts, W.C.: Cardiac sarcoma causing ''ASH'' and simulating coronary heart disease. Am. J. Med., *66*:1025, 1979.

42. Pollick, C., Koipillai, C., Howard, R., and Rakowski, H.: Left ventricular thrombus demonstrating canalization and mimicking asymmetric septal hypertrophy on echocardiographic study. Am Heart J., *104*:641, 1982.

43. Stern, A., Kessler, K.M., Hammer, W.J., Kreulen, T.H., and Spann, J.F.: Septal-free wall disproportion in inferior infarction: The echocardiographic differentiation from hypertrophic cardiomyopathy. Circulation, *58*:700, 1978.

44. Bulkley, B.H., Weisfeldt, M.L., and Hutchins, G.M.: Asymmetric septal hypertrophy and myocardial fiber disarray: Features of normal, developing, and malformed hearts. Circulation, *56*:292, 1977.

45. Martin, R.P., Rakowski, H., French, J., and Popp, R.L.: Idiopathic hypertrophic subaortic stenosis viewed by wide-angle, phased-array echocardiography. Circulation, *59*:1206, 1979.

46. Lattanzi, F., Spirito, P., Picano, E., Mazzarisi, A., Landini, L., Distante, A., Vecchio, C., and L'Abbate, A.: Quantitative assessment of ultrasonic myocardial reflectivity in hypertrophic cardiomyopathy. J. Am. Coll. Cardiol., *17*:1085, 1991.

47. Massay, R.J., Logan-Sinclair, R.B., Bamber, J.C., and Gibson, D.G.: Quantitative effects of speckle reduction on cross sectional echocardiographic images. Br. Heart J., *62*:298, 1989.

48. Ballester, M., Rickards, A., Rees, S., and McDonald, L.: Systolic anterior motion of the mitral valve in hypertrophic cardiomyopathy. A cross-sectional echocardiographic study. Eur. Heart J., *4*:846, 1983.

49. Jiang, L., Levine, R.A., King, M.E., and Weyman, A.E.: An integrated mechanism for systolic anterior motion of the mitral valve in hypertrophic cardiomyopathy based on echocardiographic observations. Am. Heart J., *113*: 633, 1987.

50. Pridie, R.B. and Oakley, C.M.: Mechanism of mitral regurgitation in hypertrophic obstructive cardiomyopathy. Br. Heart J., *32*:203, 1970.

51. Hasegawa, I., Sakamoto, T., Hada, Y., Takenaka, K., Amano, K., Takahashi, H., Takahashi, T., Suzuki, J., Shiota, T., and Sugimoto, T.: Relationship between mitral regurgitation and left ventricular outflow obstruction in hypertrophic cardiomyopathy. J. Am. Soc. Echocardiogr., *2*:177, 1989.

52. Widimsky, P., Ten Cate, F.J., Vletter, W., and van Herwerden, L.: Potential applications for transesophageal echocardiography in hypertrophic cardiomyopathies. J. Am. Soc. Echocardiogr., *5*:163, 1992.

53. Henry, W.L., Clark, C.E., Griffith, J.M., and Epstein, S.E.: Mechanism of left ventricular outflow obstruction in patients with obstructive asymmetric septal hypertrophy (idiopathic hypertrophic subaortic stenosis). Am. J. Cardiol., *35*:337, 1975.

54. Gustavson, A., Liedholm, H., and Tylen, U.: Hypertrophic cardiomyopathy: A correlation between echocardiography, angiographic, and hemodynamic findings. Ann Radiol. (Paris), *20*:419, 1977.

55. Pollick, C., Radowski, H., and Wigle, E.D.: Muscular subaortic stenosis: The quantitative relationship between systolic anterior motion and the pressure gradient. Circulation, *69*:43, 1984.

56. Rossen, R.M., Goodman, D.J., Ingham, R.E., and Popp, R.L.: Echocardiographic criteria in the diagnosis of idiopathic hypertrophic subaortic stenosis. Circulation, *50*: 747, 1974.

57. Feizi, O. and Emanuel, R.: Echocardiographic spectrum of hypertrophic cardiomyopathy. Br. Heart J., *37*:1286, 1975.

58. King, J.F., DeMaria, A.N., Miller, R.R., Hilliard, G.K., Zelis, R., and Mason, D.T.: Markedly abnormal mitral valve motion without simultaneous intraventricular pressure gradient due to uneven mitral-septal contact in idiopathic hypertrophic subaortic stenosis. Am. J. Cardiol., *34*:360, 1974.

59. Henry, W.L., Clark, E.E., Glancy, D.L., and Epstein, S.E.: Echocardiographic measurement of the left ventricular outflow gradient in idiopathic hypertrophic subaortic stenosis. N. Engl. J. Med., *288*:989, 1973.

60. Shah, P.M., Gramiak, R., and Kramer, D.H.: Ultrasound localization of left ventricular outflow obstruction in hypertrophic obstructive cardiomyopathy. Circulation, *40*: 3, 1969.

61. Shah, P.M., Gramiak, R., Adelman, A.G., and Wigle, E.D.: Role of echocardiography in diagnostic and hemodynamic assessment of hypertrophic subaortic stenosis. Circulation, *44*:891, 1971.

62. Angoff, G.H., Wistran, D., Sloss, L.J., Markis, J.E., Come, P.C., Zoll, P.M., and Cohn, P.F.: Value of a noninvasively induced ventricular extrasystole during echocardiographic and phonocardiographic assessment of pa-

tients with idiopathic hypertrophic subaortic stenosis. Am. J. Cardiol., *42*:919, 1978.

63. Come, P.C., Riley, M.F., and Miklozek, C.L.: Echocardiographic evidence of increased obstruction following long cycle lengths in atrial fibrillation in patients with hypertrophic cardiomyopathy. JCU, *12*:241, 1984.

64. Tajik, A.J., Gau, G.T., and Schattenberg, T.T.: Echocardiographic pseudo IHSS pattern in atrial septal defect. Chest, *62*:324, 1972.

65. Greenwald, J., Yap, J.F., Franklin, M., and Lichtman, A.M.: Echocardiographic mitral systolic motion in left ventricular aneurysm. Br. Heart J., *37*:684, 1975.

66. Maron, B.J., Gottidiener, J.S., Roberts, W.C., Henry, W.L., Savage, D.D., and Epstein, S.E.: Left ventricular outflow tract obstruction due to systolic anterior motion of the anterior mitral leaflet in patients with concentric left ventricular hypertrophy. Circulation, *57*:527, 1978.

67. Deligonul, U., Uppstrom, E., Penick, W., Seacord, L., Kern, M.J.: Dynamic left ventricular outflow tract obstruction induced by pericardial tamponade during acute anterior myocardial infarction. Am. Heart J., *121*:190, 1991.

68. Levisman, J.A.: Systolic anterior motion of the mitral valve due to hypovolemia and anemia. Chest, *70*:687, 1976.

69. Buckley, B.H. and Fortuin, J.J.: Systolic anterior motion of the mitral valve without asymmetric septal hypertrophy. Chest, *69*:694, 1976.

70. Schulman, P., Come, P.C., Isaacs, R., and Radvany, P.: Left ventricular outflow obstruction induced by tamponade in hypertrophic cardiomyopathy. Chest, *80*:110, 1981.

71. Kronzon, I. and Glassman, E.: Mitral ring calcification in idiopathic hypertrophic subaortic stenosis. Am. J. Cardiol., *42*:60, 1978.

72. Wei, J.Y., Weiss, J.L., and Bulkley, B.H.: The heterogeneity of hypertrophic cardiomyopathy: An autopsy and one-dimensional echocardiographic study. Am. J. Cardiol., *45*:24, 1980.

73. Crawford, M.H., Groves, B.M., and Horwitz, L.D.: Dynamic left ventricular outflow tract obstruction and systolic anterior motion of the mitral valve in the absence of asymmetric septal hypertrophy. Am. J. Med., *65*:703, 1978.

74. Mintz, G.S., Kotler, M.N., Segal, B.L., and Parry, W.R.: Systolic anterior motion of the mitral valve in the absence of asymmetric septal hypertrophy. Circulation, *57*:256, 1978.

75. Boughner, D.R., Rakowski, H., and Wigle, E.D.: Mitral valve systolic anterior motion in the absence of hypertrophic cardiomyopathy. Circulation, *58*:916, 1978.

76. Drobinsky, G., Botreau-Roussel, P., and Grosgogeat, Y.: An echocardiographic trap: Protosystolic advance of the mitral valve in normal subjects. Nouv. Presse Med., *5*:1914, 1976.

77. Gardin, J.M., Stephanides, L.M., Kordecki, S., and Talano, J.V.: Systolic anterior motion in the absence of asymmetric septal hypertrophy: A buckling phenomenon of the chordae tendinae. Circulation (Suppl. II), *58*:121, 1978. (Abstract)

78. Gardin, J.M., Talano, J.V., Stephanides, L., Fizzano, J., and Lesch, M.: Systolic anterior motion in the absence of asymmetric septal hypertrophy. A buckling phenomenon of the chordae tendineae. Circulation, *63*:181, 1981.

79. Lindvall, K. and Herrlin, B.: Mitral annulus calcification, systolic anterior motion of the anterior mitral leaflet and outflow obstruction in two patients without hypertrophic cardiomyopathy. An echocardiographic report. Acta Med. Scand., *209*:513, 1981.

80. Maron, B.J., Gottdiener, J.S., and Perry, L.W.: Specificity of systolic anterior motion of anterior mitral leaflet for hypertrophic cardiomyopathy. Br. Heart J., *45*:206, 1981.

81. McKenna, W.J., Stewart, J.T., Nihoyannopoulos, P., McGinty, F., and Davies, M.J.: Hypertrophic cardiomyopathy without hypertrophy: Two families with myocardial disarray in the absence of increased myocardial mass. Br. Heart J., *63*:287, 1990.

82. Thompson, R., Ahmed, M., Pridie, R., and Yacoub, M.: Hypertrophic cardiomyopathy after aortic valve replacement. Am. J. Cardiol., *45*:33, 1980.

83. Maron, B.J., Epstein, S.E., Bonow, R.O., Wyngaarden, M.K., and Wesley, Y.E.: Obstructive hypertrophic cardiomyopathy associated with minimal left ventricular hypertrophy. Am. J. Cardiol., *53*:377, 1984.

84. Wei, J.Y., Weiss, J.L., and Bulkley, B.H.: Nonspecificity of the echocardiographic diagnosis of idiopathic hypertrophic subaortic stenosis: A clinicopathologic study. Circulation (Suppl. II), *58*:237, 1978. (Abstract)

85. Maron, B.J., Gottdiener, J.S., Roberts, W.C., Hammer, W.J., and Epstein, S.E.: Nongenetically transmitted disproportionate ventricular outflow obstruction. Br. Heart J., *41*:345, 1979.

86. Harrison, E.E., Sbar, S.S., Martin, H., and Pupello, D.F.: Coexisting right and left hypertrophic subvalvular stenosis and fixed left ventricular outflow obstruction due to aortic valve stenosis. Am. J. Cardiol., *40*:133, 1977.

87. Bloom, K.R., Meyer, R.A., Bove, K.E., and Kaplan, S.: The association of fixed and dynamic left ventricular outflow obstruction. Am. Heart J., *89*:586, 1975.

88. Krueger, S.K., Hofschire, P.J., and Forker, A.D.: Echocardiographic features of combined hypertrophic and membranous subvalvular aortic stenosis: A case report. JCU, *4*:31, 1976.

89. Hanrath, P., von Essen, R., Bleifeld, W., and Effert, S.: Idiopathic hypertrophic subaortic stenosis in aortic valve disease—diagnosis using echocardiography. Z. Kardiol., *65*:964, 1976.

90. Aziz, K.U., Paul, M.H., Idriss, F.S., Wilson, A.D., and Master, A.J.: Clinical manifestations of dynamic left ventricular outflow tract stenosis in infants with d-transposition of the great arteries with intact ventricular septum. Am. J. Cardiol., *44*:290, 1979.

91. DiSessa, T.G., Childs, W., Ti, C., and Friedman, W.F.: Systolic anterior motion of the mitral valve in a one day old infant with d-transposition of the great vessels. JCU, *6*:186, 1978.

92. Yokota, Y., Kawanishi, H., Ohmori, K., Oda, A., Inoh, T., and Fukuzaki, H.: Studies on systolic anterior motion (SAM) pattern in idiopathic mitral valve prolapse by echocardiography. J. Cardiogr., *9*:259, 1979.

93. Kessler, K.M., Anzola, E., Sequeira, R., Serafini, A.N., and Myerburg, R.J.: Mitral valve prolapse and systolic anterior motion: A dynamic spectrum. Am. Heart J., *105*:685, 1983.

94. Panza, J.A. and Maron, B.J.: Simultaneous occurrence of mitral valve prolapse and systolic anterior motion in hypertrophic cardiomyopathy. Am. J. Cardiol., *67*:404, 1991.

95. Petrone, R.K., Klues, H.G., Panza, J.A., Peterson, E.E., and Maron B.J.: Coexistence of mitral valve prolapse in a consecutive group of 528 patients with hyper-

trophic cardiomyopathy assessed with echocardiography. J. Am. Coll. Cardiol., 20:55, 1992.

96. Roldan, C.A., Gurule, F.T., and Shively, B.K.: Anomalous papillary muscle producing dynamic left ventricular outflow tract obstruction. J. Am. Soc. Echocardiogr. 4: 267, 1991.

97. Klues, H.G., Roberts, W.C., and Maron, B.J.: Anomalous insertion of papillary muscle directly into anterior mitral leaflet in hypertrophic cardiomyopathy. Significance in producing left ventricular outflow obstruction. Circulation, 84:1188, 1991.

98. Jinnouchi, J., Yoshioka, H., Koga, Y., and Toshima, H.: Mechanism of outflow obstruction in hypertrophic cardiomyopathy with asymmetric septal hypertrophy: Two-dimensional echocardiographic study. J. Cardiogr. 7:23, 1977.

99. Rodger, J.C.: Motion of mitral apparatus in hypertrophic cardiomyopathy with obstruction. Br. Heart J., 38:732, 1976.

100. Shah, P.M., Taylor, R.D., and Wong, M.: Abnormal mitral valve coaptation in hypertrophic obstructive cardiomyopathy: Proposed role in systolic anterior motion of mitral valve. Am. J. Cardiol., 48:258, 1981.

101. Maron, B.J., Harding, A.M., Spirito, P., Roberts, W.C., and Waller, B.F.: Systolic anterior motion of the posterior mitral leaflet: A previously unrecognized cause of dynamic subaortic obstruction in patients with hypertrophic cardiomyopathy. Circulation, 68:282, 1983.

102. Spirito, P. and Maron, B.J.: Patterns of systolic motion of the mitral valve in hypertrophic cardiomyopathy: Assessment by two dimensional echocardiography. Am. J. Cardiol., 54:1039, 1984.

103. Isshiki, T., Umeda, T., and Machii, K.: Cross-sectional echocardiographic study on the papillary muscles in hypertrophic cardiomyopathy. J. Cardiogr., 8:631, 1978.

104. Nagata, S., Nimura, Y., Beppu, S., Park, Y.D., and Sakakibara, H.: Mechanism of systolic anterior motion of mitral valve and site of interventricular pressure gradient in hypertrophic obstructive cardiomyopathy. Br. Heart J., 49:234, 1983.

105. Doi, Y.L., McKenna, W.J., Gehrke, J., Oakley, C.M., and Goodwin, J.F.: M-mode echocardiography in hypertrophic cardiomyopathy: Diagnostic criteria and prediction of obstruction. Am. J. Cardiol., 45:6, 1980.

106. Feigenbaum, H.: Clinical applications of echocardiography. Prog. Cardiovasc. Dis., 14:531, 1972.

107. Gramiak, R. and Shah, P.M.: Cardiac ultrasonography: A review of current applications. Radiol. Clin. North Am., 9:469, 1971.

108. Sakurai, S. and Tanaka, H.: Temporal relationship between early systolic closure of the aortic valve and aortic flow: Experimental study with and without systolic anterior motion of the mitral valve. Am. Heart J., 112:113, 1986.

109. Panza, J.A., Petrone, R.K., Fananapazir, L., and Maron, B.J.: Utility of continuous wave Doppler echocardiography in the noninvasive assessment of left ventricular outflow tract pressure gradient in patients with hypertrophic cardiomyopathy. J. Am. Coll. Cardiol., 19:91, 1992.

110. Rakowski, H., Sasson, Z., and Wigle, E.D.: Echocardiography and Doppler assessment of hypertrophic cardiomyopathy. J. Am. Soc. Echocardiogr., 1:31, 1988.

111. Come, P.C., Riley, M.F., Carl, L.V., and Lorell, B.: Doppler evidence that true left ventricular-to-aortic pressure gradients exist in hypertrophic cardiomyopathy. Am. Heart J., 116:1253, 1988.

112. Sasson, Z., Yock, P.G., Hatle, L.K., Alderman, E.L., and Popp, R.L.: Doppler echocardiographic determination of the pressure gradient in hypertrophic cardiomyopathy. J. Am. Coll. Cardiol., 11:752, 1988.

113. Cogswell, T.L., Sagar, K.B., and Wann, L.S.: Left ventricular ejection dynamics in hypertrophic cardiomyopathy and aortic stenosis: Comparison with the use of Doppler echocardiography. Am. Heart J., 113:110, 1987.

114. Lin, C-S., Chen, K-S., Lin, M-C., Fu, M-C., and Tang, S-M.: The relationship between systolic anterior motion of the mitral valve and the left ventricular outflow tract Doppler in hypertrophic cardiomyopathy. Am. Heart J., 122:1671, 1991.

115. Kinoshita, N., Nimura, Y., Ikamoto, M., Miyatake, K., Nagata, S., and Sakakibara, H.: Mitral regurgitation in hypertrophic cardiomyopathy. Noninvasive study by two dimensional Doppler echocardiography. Br. Heart J., 49:574, 1983.

116. Hoit, B.D., Penonen, E., Dalton, N., and Sahn, D.J.: Doppler color flow mapping studies of jet formation and spatial orientation in obstructive hypertrophic cardiomyopathy. Am. Heart J., 117:1119, 1989.

117. Nishimura, R.A., Tajik, A.J., Reeder, G.S., and Seward, J.B.: Evaluation of hypertrophic cardiomyopathy by Doppler color flow imaging: Initial observations. Mayo Clin. Proc., 61:631, 1986.

118. Schwammental, E., Block, M., Schwartzkopff, B., Losse, B., Borggrefe, M., Schulte, H.D., Bircks, W., and Breithardt, G.: Prediction of the site and severity of obstruction in hypertrophic cardiomyopathy by color flow mapping and continuous wave Doppler echocardiography. J. Am. Coll. Cardiol., 20:964, 1992.

119. Matsumoto, H., Fukuda, H., Kado, H., Yasui, H., Honda, S., and Ishida, T.: A case of idiopathic hypertrophic obstructive cardiomyopathy causing severe right ventricular outflow tract obstruction in infancy. Jpn. Heart J., 24:757, 1983.

120. VonDoenhoff, L.J. and Nanda, N.C.: Obstruction within the right ventricular body: Two dimensional echocardiographic features. Am. J. Cardiol., 51:1498, 1983.

121. Cardiel, E.A., Alonso, M., Delcan, J.L., and Menarguez, L.: Echocardiographic sign of right-sided hypertrophic obstructive cardiomyopathy. Br. Heart J., 40:1321, 1978.

122. Brik, H, Meller, J., Bahler, A.S., Herman, M.V., and Teichholz, L.E.: Systolic anterior motion of the tricuspid valve in idiopathic hypertrophic subaortic stenosis. JCU, 6:121, 1978.

123. Nihoyannopoulos, P., Karatasakis, G., Frenneaux, M., McKenna, W.J., and Oakley, C.M.: Diastolic function in hypertrophic cardiomyopathy: Relation to exercise capacity. J. Am. Coll. Cardiol., 19:536, 1992.

124. Silverman, P.R., Ten Cate, F.J., Serruys, P.W., and Roelandt, J.R.T.C.: Abnormal diastolic flow patterns in hypertrophic cardiomyopathy: Evaluation by simultaneous Doppler echocardiography, cineangiography, and hemodynamics. J. Am. Soc. Echocardiogr., 2:346, 1989.

125. Okushi, H., Oki, T., Tominaga, T., Ishimoto, T., Uchida, T., Fukuda, N., Mikawa, T., Irahara, K., Asai, M., and Mori, H.: Mode of left ventricular diastolic filling in hypertrophic cardiomyopathy as studied by pulsed Doppler echocardiography and multigated blood pool scan. J. Cardiogr., 16:585, 1986.

126. Maron, B.J., Spirito, P., Green, K.J., Wesley, Y.E., Bonow, R.O., and Arce, J.: Noninvasive assessment of left ventricular diastolic function by pulsed Doppler echocardiography in patients with hypertrophic cardiomyopathy. J. Am. Coll. Cardiol., 10:733, 1987.

127. Shapiro, L.M. and Gibson, D.G.: Patterns of diastolic

dysfunction in left ventricular hypertrophy. Br. Heart J., *59*:438, 1988.

128. Gidding. S.S., Snider, A.R., Rocchini, A.P., Peters, J., and Farnsworth, R.: Left ventricular diastolic filling in children with hypertrophic cardiomyopathy: Assessment with pulsed Doppler echocardiography. J. Am. Coll. Cardiol., *8*:310, 1986.

129. Takenaka, K., Dabestani, A., Gardin, J.M., Russell, D., Clark, S., Allfie, A., and Henry, W.L.: Left ventricular filling in hypertrophic cardiomyopathy: A pulsed Doppler echocardiography study. J. Am. Coll. Cardiol., *7*: 1263, 1986.

130. Spirito, P. and Maron, B.J.: Relation between extent of left ventricular hypertrophy and diastolic filling abnormalities in hypertrophic cardiomyopathy. J. Am. Coll. Cardiol., *15*:808, 1990.

131. Nakamura, T., Matsubara, K., Furukawa, K., Azuma, A., Sugihara, H., Katsume, H., and Nakagawa, M.: Diastolic paradoxic jet flow in patients with hypertrophic cardiomyopathy: Evidence of concealed apical asynergy with cavity obliteration. J. Am. Coll. Cardiol., *19*:516, 1992.

132. Seiler, C., Jenni, R., and Krayenbuehl, H.P.: Intraventricular blood flow during isovolumetric relaxation and diastole in hypertrophic cardiomyopathy. J. Am. Soc. Echocardiogr., *4*:247, 1991.

133. Ando, H., Imaizumi, T., Urabe, Y., Takeshita, A., and Nakamura, M.: Apical segmental dysfunction in hypertrophic cardiomyopathy: Subgroup with unique clinical features. J. Am. Coll. Cardiol., *16*:1579, 1990.

134. Zoghbi, W.A., Haichin, R.N., and Quinones, M.A.: Midcavity obstruction in apical hypertrophy: Doppler evidence of diastolic intraventricular gradient with higher apical pressure. Am. Heart J., *116*:1469, 1988.

135. Blazer, D., Kotler, M.N., Parry, W.R., Wertheimer, J., and Nakhjavan, F.K.: Noninvasive evaluation of mid-left ventricular obstruction by two-dimensional and Doppler echocardiography flow Doppler echocardiography. Am. Heart J., *114*:1162, 1987.

136. Yock, P.G., Hatle, L., and Popp, R.L.: Patterns and timing of Doppler-detected intracavitary and aortic flow in hypertrophic cardiomyopathy. J. Am. Coll. Cardiol., *8*: 1047, 1986.

137. Schapira, J.N., Stemple, D.R., Martin, R.P., Rakowski, H., Stinson, E.B., and Popp, R.L.: Single and two-dimensional echocardiographic visualization of the effects of septal myectomy in idiopathic hypertrophic subaortic stenosis. Circulation, *58*:850, 1978.

138. Spirito, P., Maron, B.J., and Rosing, D.R.: Morphologic determinants of hemodynamic state after ventricular septal myotomy-myectomy in patients with obstructive hypertrophic cardiomyopathy: M-mode and two dimensional echocardiographic assessment. Circulation, *70*: 984, 1984.

139. Popp, R.L. and Harrison, D.C.: Ultrasound in the diagnosis and evaluation of therapy of idiopathic hypertrophic subaortic stenosis. Circulation, *40*:905, 1969.

140. Bolton, R.M., Jr., King, J.F., Polumbo, R.A., Mason, D., Pugh, D.M., Reis, R.L., and Dunn, M.I.: The effects of operation on the echocardiographic features of idiopathic hypertrophic subaortic stenosis. Circulation, *50*: 897, 1974.

141. Hardarson, T. and Curiel, R.: Study of clinical pharmacology of hypertrophic obstructive cardiomyopathy by noninvasive diagnostic investigation. Br. Heart J., *35*: 865, 1973.

142. Shah, P.M., Gramiak, R., Adelman, A.G., and Wigle,

E.D.: Echocardiographic assessment of the effects of surgery and propranolol on the dynamics of outflow obstruction and hyperpranolol on the dynamics of outflow obstruction and hypertrophic subaortic stenosis. Circulation, *45*:516, 1972.

143. Roberts, C.S., Gertz, S.D., Klues, H.G., Cannon, III, R.O., Maron, B.J., McIntosh, C.L., and Roberts, W.C.: Appearance of or persistence of severe mitral regurgitation without left ventricular outflow obstruction after partial ventricular septal myotomy-myectomy in hypertrophic cardiomyopathy. Am. J. Cardiol., *68*:1726, 1991.

144. Masuyama, T., Nellessen, U., Stinson, E., and Popp, R.L.: Improvement in left ventricular diastolic filling by septal myectomy in hypertrophic cardiomyopathy. J. Am. Soc. Echocardiogr., *3*:196, 1990.

145. Sherrid, M., Delia, E., and Dwyer, E.: Oral disopryamide therapy for obstructive hypertrophic cardiomyopathy. Am. J. Cardiol., *62*:1085, 1988.

146. Iwase, M., Sotobata, I., Takagi, S., Miyaguchi, K., Xiao, H., Jing, H., and Yokota, M.: Effects of Diltiazem on left ventricular diastolic behavior in patients with hypertrophic cardiomyopathy: Evaluation with exercise pulsed Doppler echocardiography. J. Am. Coll. Cardiol., *9*: 1099, 1987.

147. Stewart, W.J., Schiavone, W.A., Salcedo, E.E., Lever, H.M., Cosgrove, E.M., and Gill, C.C.: Intraoperative Doppler echocardiography in hypertrophic cardiomyopathy: Correlations with the obstructive gradient. J. Am. Coll. Cardiol., *10*:327, 1987.

148. Marwick, T.H., Stewart, W.J., Lever, H.M., Lytle, B.W., Rosenkranz, E.R., Duffy, C.I., and Salcedo, E.E.: Benefits of intraoperative echocardiography in the surgical management of hypertrophic cardiomyopathy. J. Am. Coll. Cardiol., *20*:1066, 1992.

149. Grigg, L.E., Wigle, E.D., Williams, W.G., Daniel, L.B., and Rakowski, H.: Transesophageal Doppler echocardiography in obstructive hypertrophic cardiomyopathy: Clarification of pathophysiology and importance in intraoperative decision making. J. Am. Coll. Cardiol., *20*:42, 1992.

150. Goldberg, S.J., Valdes-Cruz, L.M., Sahn, D.J., and Allen, H.D.: Two dimensional echocardiographic evaluation of dilated cardiomyopathy in children. Am. J. Cardiol., *52*:1244, 1983.

151. Gardin, J.M., Iseri, L.T., Elkayam, U., Tobis, J., Childs, W., Burn, C.S., and Henry, W.L.: Evaluation of dilated cardiomyopathy by pulsed Doppler echocardiography. Am. Heart J., *106*:1057, 1983.

152. Shah, P.M.: Echocardiography in congestive or dilated cardiomyopathy. J. Am. Soc. Echocardiogr., *1*:20, 1988.

153. Corya, B.C., Feigenbaum, H., Rasmussen, S., and Black, M.J.: Echocardiographic features of congestive cardiomyopathy compared with normal subjects and patients with coronary artery disease. Circulation, *49*:1153, 1974.

154. Ghafour, A.S. and Gutgesell, H.P.: Echocardiographic evaluation of left ventricular function in children with congestive cardiomyopathy. Am. J. Cardiol., *44*:1332, 1979.

155. D'Cruz, I.A., Daly, D.P., and Shroff, S.G.: Left ventricular shape and size in dilated cardiomyopathy: Quantitative echocardiographic assessment. Echocardiography, *8*:187, 1991.

156. D'Cruz, I.A., Shroff, S.G., Janicki, J.S., Jain, A., Reddy, H.K., and Lakier, J.B.: Differences in the shape of the normal, cardiomyopathic, and volume overloaded

human left ventricle. J. Am. Soc. Echocardiogr., *2*:408, 1989.

157. Douglas, P.S., Morrow, R., Ioli, A., and Reichek, N.: Left ventricular shape, afterload and survival in idiopathic dilated cardiomyopathy. J. Am. Coll. Cardiol., *13*: 311, 1989.

158. Keren, A., Billingham, M.E., and Popp, R.L.: Features of mildly dilated congestive cardiomyopathy compared with idiopathic restrictive cardiomyopathy and typical dilated cardiomyopathy. J. Am. Soc. Echocardiogr., *1*:78, 1988.

159. Lavine, S.J.: Left ventricular diastolic function in idiopathic cardiomyopathy: Doppler hemodynamic corrections. Echocardiography, *8*:151, 1991.

160. St. Goar, F.G., Masuyama, T., Alderman, E.L., and Popp, R.L.: Left ventricular diastolic dysfunction in end-stage dilated cardiomyopathy: Simultaneous Doppler echocardiography and hemodynamic evaluation. J. Am. Soc. Echocardiogr., *4*:349, 1991.

161. Xiao, H.B., Lee, C.H., and Gibson, D.G.: Effect of left bundle branch block on diastolic function in dilated cardiomyopathy. Br. Heart J., *66*:443, 1991.

162. Vanoverschelde, J-L., Raphael, D.A., Roberrt, A.R., and Cosyns, J.R.: Left ventricular filling in dilated cardiomyopathy: Relation to functional class and hemodynamics. J. Am. Coll. Cardiol., *15*:1288, 1990.

163. Lavine, S.J. and Arends, D.: Importance of the left ventricular filling pressure on diastolic filling in idiopathic dilated cardiomyopathy. Am. J. Cardiol., *64*:61, 1989.

164. Hayakawa, M., Yokota, Y., Kumaki, T., Fujitani, K., Kurogane, K., Takeuchi, M., Kawanishi, H., Inoh, T., and Tukuzaki, H.: Intracardiac flow pattern in dilated cardiomyopathy studied with pulsed Doppler echocardiography. J. Cardiogr., *13*:317, 1983.

165. Shen, W.F., Tribouilloy, C., Rey, J-L., Baudhuin, J-J., Boey, S., Duffosse, H., and Lesbre, J-P.: Prognostic significance of Doppler-derived left ventricular diastolic filling variables in dilated cardiomyopathy. Am. Heart J., *124*:1524, 1992.

166. D'Cruz, I.A. and Sharaf, I.S.: Patterns of flow within the dilated cardiomyopathic left ventricle: Color flow Doppler observations. Echocardiography, *8*:227, 1991.

167. Jacobs, L.E., Kotler, M.N., and Parry, W.R.: Flow patterns in dilated cardiomyopathy: A pulsed-wave and color flow Doppler study. J. Am. Soc. Echocardiogr., *3*: 294, 1990.

168. Delemarre, B.J., Bot, H., Visser, C.A., and Dunning, A.J.: Pulsed Doppler echocardiographic description of a circular flow pattern in spontaneous left ventricular contrast. J. Am. Soc. Echocardiogr., *1*:114, 1988.

169. Fennestri, F., Biasucci, L.M., Rinelli, G., Mongiardo, R., Lombardo, A., Rossi, E., Amico, C.M., Aquilina, O., and Loperfido, F.: Abnormal intraventricular flow patterns in left ventricular dysfunction determined by color Doppler study. Am. Heart J., *124*:966, 1992.

170. Suzuki, S., Yanagisawa, M., Yano, S., Itoh, K., and Kotohda, K.: Cross-sectional echocardiographic findings of left ventricular thrombi in a ten-year-old patient with cardiomyopathy. Jpn. Heart J., *20*:675, 1979.

171. Arita, M., Ueno, Y., and Masuyama, Y.: Detection of intracardiac thrombi in a case of cardiomyopathy by two dimensional echocardiography. Br. Heart J., *47*:397, 1982.

172. Gottdiener, J.S., Gay, J.A., VanVoorhees, L., DiBianco, R., and Fletcher, R.D.: Frequency and embolic potential of left ventricular thrombus in dilated cardiomy-opathy: assessment by two dimensional echocardiography. Am. J. Cardiol., *52*:1281, 1983.

173. Falk, R.H., Foster, E., and Coats, M.H.: Ventricular thrombi and thromboembolism in dilated cardiomyopathy: A prospective follow-up study. Am. Heart J., *123*: 136, 1992.

173a. Siostrzonek, P., Kuppensteiner, R., Gossinger, H., Zangeneh, M., Heinz, G., Kreiner, G., Stumpflen, A., Buxbaum, P., Ehringer, H., and Mosslacher, H.: Hemodynamic and hemorheologic determinants of left atrial spontaneous echo contrast and thrombus formation in patients with idiopathic dilated cardiomyopathy. Am. Heart J., *125*:430, 1993.

174. Sawada, S.G., Ryan, T., Segar, D., Atherton, L., Fineberg, N., Davis, C., and Feigenbaum, H.: Distinguishing ischemic cardiomyopathy from nonischemic dilated cardiomyopathy with coronary echocardiography. J. Am. Coll. Cardiol., *19*:1223, 1992.

175. Godley, R.W., Wann, L.S., Rogers, E.W., Feigenbaum, H., and Weyman, A.E.: Incomplete mitral leaflet closure in patients with papillary muscle dysfunction. Circulation, *63*:565, 1981.

176. Bruss, J., Jacobs, L.E., and Kotler, M.N.: Mechanism of mitral regurgitation in dilated cardiomyopathy. Echocardiography, *8*:219, 1991.

177. Fitchett, D.H., Sugrue, D.D., MacArthur, C.G., and Oakley, C.M.: Right ventricular dilated cardiomyopathy. Br. Heart J., *51*:25, 1984.

178. Foale, R.A., Nihoyannopoulos, P., Ribeiro, P., McKenna, W.J., Oakley, C.M., Krikler, D.M., and Rowland, E.: Right ventricular abnormalities in ventricular tachycardia of right ventricular origin: Relation to electrophysiological abnormalities. Br. Heart J., *56*:45, 1986.

179. Laurent, J.M., Lablanche, J.M., Tilmant, P.Y., Marache, P., Folliot, J.F., and Ducloux, G.: Right ventricular dysplasia: Uhl's disease. Echocardiography and tomodensitometry study. A propos of a case in an adult. Ann. Cardiol. Angiol., *32*:191, 1983.

180. Hayakawa, M., Yokota, Y., Kumaki, T., Fujitani, K., Kurogane, K., Ito, Y., Kawanishi, H., Inoh, T., and Fukuzaki, H.: Two dimensional echocardiographic findings in a case of arrhythmogenic right ventricular dysplasia. J. Cardiogr., *13*:453, 1983.

181. Higuchi, S., Caglar, N.M., Shimada, R., Yamada, A., Takeshita, A., and Nakamura, M.: Sixteen-year follow-up of arrhythmogenic right ventricular dysplasia. Am. Heart. J., *108*:1363, 1984.

182. Vaitkus, P.T. and Kussmaul, W.G.: Constrictive pericarditis versus restrictive cardiomyopathy: A reappraisal and update of diagnostic criteria. Am. Heart J., *122*:1431, 1991.

183. Izumi, S., Miyatake, K., Beppu, S., Yamagishi, M., Akiyama, T., Hiroaka, H., Yamamoto, K., Suzuki, S., Nagata, S., Sakakibara, H., and Nimura, Y.: Doppler echocardiographic features of the atrial and ventricular filling modes and their significance in restrictive myocardial diseases. J. Cardiol., *20*:311, 1990.

184. Hirota, Y., Shimizu, G., Kita, Y., Nakayama, Y., Suwa, M., Kawamura, K., Nagata, S., Sawayama, T., Izumi, T., Nakano, T., Toshima, H., and Sekiguchi, M.: Spectrum of restrictive cardiomyopathy: Report of the national survey in Japan. Am. Heart J., *120*:188, 1990.

185. Spirito, P., Lupi, G., Melevendi, C., and Vecchio, C.: Restrictive diastolic abnormalities identified by Doppler echocardiography in patients with thalassemia major. Circulation, *82*:88, 1990.

186. Hatle, L.K., Appleton, C.P., and Popp, R.L.: Differentiation of constrictive pericarditis and restrictive cardiomyopathy by Doppler echocardiography. Circulation, *79*: 357, 1989.

187. Schiavone, W.A., Calafiore, P.A., and Salcedo, E.E.: Transesophageal Doppler echocardiographic demonstration of pulmonary venous flow velocity in restrictive cardiomyopathy and constrictive pericarditis. Am. J. Cardiol., *63*:1286, 1989.

188. Appleton, C.P., Hatle, L.K., and Popp, R.L: Demonstration of restrictive ventricular physiology by Doppler echocardiography. J. Am. Coll. Cardiol., *11*:757, 1988.

189. Morgan, J.M., Raposo, L., Clague, J.C., Chow, W.H., and Oldershaw, P.J.: Restrictive cardiomyopathy and constrictive pericarditis: Non-invasive distinction by digitised M mode echocardiography. Br. Heart J., *61*:29, 1989.

190. Child, J.S., Krivokapich, J., and Abbasi, A.S.: Increased right ventricular wall thickness on echocardiography in amyloid infiltrative cardiomyopathy. Am. J. Cardiol., *44*: 1391, 1979.

191. Giles, T.D., Leon-Galindo, J., and Burch, B.E.: Echocardiographic findings in amyloid cardiomyopathy. South. Med. J., *71*:1393, 1978.

192. Child, J.S., Levisman, J.A., Abbasi, A.S., and MacAlpin, R.N.: Echocardiographic manifestations of infiltrative cardiomyopathy: A report of seven cases due to amyloid. Chest, *70*:726, 1976.

193. Chiaramida, S.A., Goldman, M.A., Zema, M.J., Pizzarello, R.A., and Goldberg, H.M.: Real-time cross-sectional echocardiographic diagnosis of infiltrative cardiomyopathy due to amyloid. JCU, *8*:58, 1980.

194. Nomeir, A.M. and Watts, L.E.: Amyloid heart disease. South. Med. J., *74*:1412, 1981.

195. Siqueira-Filho, A.G., Cunha, C.L., Tajik, A.J., Seward, J.B., Schattenberg, T.T., and Giuliani, E.R.: M-mode and two dimensional echocardiographic features in cardiac amyloidosis. Circulation, *63*:188, 1981.

196. Pi'erard, L., Verhaugt, F.W., Meltzer, R.S., and Roelandt, J.: Echocardiographic aspects of cardiac amyloidosis. Acta Cardiol., *36*:455, 1981.

197. Choo, M.H., Gwee, H.M., Tan, Y.O., LaBrooy, S., Choo, I.H., and Chia, B.L.: Cardiac amyloidosis—diagnosis by two dimensional echocardiography. Ann. Acad. Med. Singapore, *11*:98, 1982.

198. Noma, S., Akaishi, M., Murayama, A., Akiyama, H., Ogawa, S., Handa, S., Nakamura, Y., Sohma, Y., Hosoda, Y., and Gotoh, M.: Echocardiographic findings of a patient with cardiac amyloidosis and ventricular outflow obstruction. J. Cardiogr., *12*:267, 1982.

199. Roberts, W.C. and Waller, B.F.: Cardiac amyloidosis causing cardiac dysfunction: Analysis of 54 necropsy patients. Am. J. Cardiol., *52*:137, 1983.

200. Nicolosi, G.L., Pavan, D., Lestuzzi, C., Burelli, C., Zardo, F., and Zanuttini, D.: Prospective identification of patients with amyloid heart disease by two dimensional echocardiography. Circulation, *70*:432, 1984.

201. Henry, W.L., Nienhuis, A.W., Wiener, M., Miller, D.R., Canale, V.C., and Piomelli, S.: Echocardiographic abnormalities in patients with transfusion-dependent anemia and secondary myocardial iron deposition. Am. J. Med., *64*:547, 1978.

202. Mir, M.A.: Evidence for non-infiltrative cardiomyopathy in acute leukaemia and lymphoma: A clinical and echocardiographic study. Br. Heart J., *40*:725, 1978.

203. Valdes-Cruz, L.M., Reinecke, C., Rutkowski, M., Du-
dell, G.G., Goldberg, S.J., Allen, H.D., Sahn, D.J., and Piomelli, S.: Preclinical abnormal segmental cardiac manifestations of thalassemia major in children on transfusion-chelation therapy: Echographic alterations of left ventricular posterior wall contraction and relaxation patterns. Am. Heart J., *103*:505, 1982.

204. Leon, M.B., Borer, J.S., Bacharach, S.L., Green, M.V., Benz, Jr., E.J., Griffith, P., and Nienhuis, A.W.: Detection of early cardiac dysfunction in patients with severe beta-thalassemia and chronic iron overload. N. Engl. J. Med., *301*:1143, 1979.

205. Kremastinos, D.T., Toutouzas, P.K., Vyssoulis, G.P., Venetis, C.A., and Avgoustakis, D.G.: Iron overload and left ventricular performance in beta thalassemia. Acta Cardiol., *39*:29, 1984.

206. Candell-Riera, J., Lu, L., Seres, L., Gonzalez, J.B., Batile, J., Permanyer-Miralda, G., Garcia-del-Castillo, H., and Soler-Soler, J.: Cardiac hemochromatosis: Beneficial effects of iron removal therapy. Am. J. Cardiol., *52*: 824, 1983.

207. Lorell, B., Alderman, E.L., and Mason, J.W.: Cardiac sarcoidosis. Am. J. Cardiol., *42*:143, 1978.

208. Capin, D., McDonough, M., and James, F.: Cardiac sarcoidosis. A case with unusual manifestation. Arch. Intern. Med., *143*:142, 1983.

209. Kaplan, S.D., Chartash, E.K., Pizzarello, R.A., and Furie, R.A.: Cardiac manifestations of the antiphospholipid syndrome. Am. Heart J., *124*:1331, 1992.

210. Rees, A., Elbl, F., Minhas, K., and Solinger, R.: Echocardiographic evidence of outflow tract obstruction in Pompe's disease (glycogen storage disease of the heart). Am. J. Cardiol., *37*:1103, 1976.

211. Bass, J.L., Shrivastava, S., Grabowski, G.A., Desnick, R.J., and Moller, J.H.: The M-mode echocardiogram in Fabry's disease. Am. Heart J., *100*:807, 1980.

212. Gussenhoven, W.J., Busch, H.F., Kleijer, W.J., and DeVilleneuve, V.H.: Echocardiographic features in the cardiac type of glycogen storage disease. II. Eur. Heart J., *4*:41, 1983.

213. Olson, L.J., Reeder, G.S., Noller, K.L., Edwards, W.D., Howell, R.R., and Michels, V.V.: Cardiac involvement in glycogen storage disease. III. Morphologic and biochemical characterization with endomyocardial biopsy. Am. J. Cardiol., *53*:980, 1984.

214. Satoh, Y., Sakamoto, K., Fujibayashi, Y., Uchiyama, T., Kajiwara, N., and Hatano, M.: Cardiac involvement in mucolipidosis. Importance of noninvasive studies for detection of cardiac abnormalities. Jpn. Heart J., *24*:149, 1983.

215. Cohen, I.S., Fluri-Lundeen, J., and Wharton, T.P.: Two dimensional echocardiographic similarity of Fabry's disease to cardiac amyloidosis: A function of ultrastructural analogy? JCU, *11*:437, 1984.

216. Pressly, T.A., Franklin, J.O., Alpert, M.A., Reams, G.P., and Taylor, L.M.: Cardiac valvular involvement in Tangier disease. Am. Heart J., *113*:200, 1987.

217. Cueto-Garcia, L., et al.: Echocardiographic features of amyloid ischemic heart disease. Am. J. Cardiol., *55*:606, 1985.

218. Simons, M. and Isner, J.M.: Assessment of relative sensitivities of noninvasive tests for cardiac amyloidosis in documented cardiac amyloidosis. Am. J. Cardiol., *69*: 425, 1992.

219. Falk, R.H., Plehn, J.F., Deering, T., Schick, E.C., Boinay, P., Rubinow, A., Skinner, M., and Cohen, A.S.: Sensitivity and specificity of the echocardiographic fea-

tures of cardiac amyloidosis. Am. J. Cardiol., *59*:418, 1987.

220. Picano, E., Pinamonti, B., Ferdeghini, E.M., Landini, L., Slavich, G., Orlandini, A., Marini, C., Lattanzi, F., and Camerini, F.: Two-dimensional echocardiography in myocardial amyloidosis. Echocardiography, *8*:253, 1991.

221. Klein, A.L. and Tajik, A.J.: Doppler assessment of diastolic function in cardiac amyloidosis. Echocardiography, *8*:233, 1991.

222. Klein, A.L., Hatle, L.K., Taliercio, C.P., Oh, J.K., Kyle, R.A., Gerz, M.A., Bailey, K.R., Seward, J.B., and Tajik, A.J.: Prognostic significance of Doppler measures of diastolic function in cardiac amyloidosis. Circulation, *83*:808, 1991.

223. Klein, A.L., Hatle, L.K., Taliercio, C.P., Taylor, C.L., Kyle, R.A., Bailey, K.R., Seward, J.B., and Tajik, A.J.: Serial Doppler echocardiographic follow-up of left ventricular diastolic function in cardiac amyloidosis. J. Am. Coll. Cardiol., *16*:1135, 1990.

224. Klein, A.L., Hatle, L.K., Burstwo, D.J., Seward, J.B., Kyle, R.A., Bailey, K.R., Luscher, T.F., Gertz, M.A., and Tajik, A.J.: Doppler characterization of left ventricular diastolic function in cardiac amyloidosis. J. Am. Coll. Cardiol., *13*:1017, 1989.

225. Kinoshita, O., Hongo, M., Yamada, H., Misawa, T., Kono, J., Okubo, S., and Ikeda, S.: Impaired left ventricular diastolic filling in patients with familial amyloid polyneuropathy: A pulsed Doppler echocardiographic study. Br. Heart J., *61*:198, 1989.

226. Klein, A.L., Hatle, L.K., Burstow, D.J., Taliercio, C.P., Seward, J.B., Kyle, R.A., Bailey, K.R., Gertz, M.A., and Tajik, A.J.: Comprehensive Doppler assessment of right ventricular diastolic function in cardiac amyloidosis. J. Am. Coll. Cardiol., *15*:99, 1990.

227. Pinamonti, B., Picano, E., Ferdeghini, E.M., Lattanzi, F., Slavich, G., Landini, L., Camerini, F., Benassi, A., Distante, A., and L'Abbate, A.: Quantitative texture analysis in two-dimensional echocardiography: Application to the diagnosis of myocardial amyloidosis. J. Am. Coll. Cardiol., *14*:666, 1989.

228. Chandrasekaran, K., Aylward, P.E., Fleagle, S.R., Burns, T.L., Seward, J.B., Tajik, A.J., Collins, S.M., and Skorton, D.J.: Feasibility of identifying amyloid and hypertrophic cardiomyopathy with the use of computerized quantitative texture analysis of clinical echocardiographic data. J. Am. Coll. Cardiol., *13*:832, 1989.

229. Bhondari, A.K. and Nanda, N.C.: Myocardial texture characterization by two dimensional echocardiography. Am. J. Cardiol., *51*:817, 1983.

230. Seifert, B.L., Snyder, M.S., Klein, A.A., O'Loughlin, J.E., Magid, M.S., and Engle, M.A.: Development of obstruction to ventricular outflow and impairment of inflow in glycogen storage disease of the heart: Serial echocardiographic studies from birth to death at 6 months. Am. Heart J., *123*:239, 1992.

231. Gross, D.M., Williams, J.C., Caprioli, C., Dominquez, B., Howell, R.R.: Echocardiographic abnormalities in the mucopolysaccharide storage diseases. Am. J. Cardiol., *61*:170, 1988.

232. Klein, A.L., Oh, J.K., Miller, F.A., Seward, J.B., and Tajik, A.J.: Two-dimensional and Doppler echocardiographic assessment of infiltrative cardiomyopathy. J. Am. Soc. Echocardiogr., *1*:48, 1988.

233. Spirito, P., Lupi, G., Melevendi, C., and Vecchio, C.: Restrictive diastolic abnormalities identified by Doppler echocardiography in patients with thalassemia major. Circulation, *82*:88, 1990.

234. Canale, C., Terrachini, V., Vallebona, A., Bruzzone, F., Masperone, M.A., and Caponnetto, S.: Thalassemic cardiomyopathy: Echocardiographic difference between major and intermediate thalassemia at rest and during isometric effort: Yearly follow-up. Clin. Cardiol., *11*:563, 1988.

235. Rahko, P.S., Salerni, R., and Uretsky, B.F.: Successful reversal by chelation therapy of congestive cardiomyopathy due to iron overload. J. Am. Coll. Cardiol., *8*:436, 1986.

235a. Lattanzi, F., Bellotti, P., Picano, E., Chiarella, F., Mazzarisi, A., Melevendi, C., Forni, G., Landini, L., Distante, A., and Vecchio, C.: Quantitative ultrasonic analysis of myocardium in patients with thalassemia major and iron overload. Circulation, *87*:748, 1993.

236. Burstow, D.J., Tajik, A.J., Bailey, K.R., DeRemee, R.A., and Taliercio, C.P.: Two-dimensional echocardiographic findings in systemic sarcoidosis. Am. J. Cardiol., *63*:478, 1989.

237. Valantine, H., McKenna, W.J., Nihoyannopoulos, P., Mitchell, A., Foale, R.A., Davies, M.J., and Oakley, C.M.: Sarcoidosis: A pattern of clinical and morphological presentation. Br. Heart J., *57*:256, 1987.

238. Tan, L-B., Dickie, S., and McKenna, W.J.: Left ventricular diastolic characteristics of cardiac sarcoidosis. Am. J. Cardiol., *58*:1126, 1986.

239. Hess, O.M., Turina, M., Senning, A., Goebel, N.H., Scholer, Y., and Krayenbuehl, H.P.: Pre- and postoperative findings in patients with endomyocardial fibrosis. Br. Heart J., *40*:406, 1978.

240. Chew, C.Y.C., Ziady, G.M., Raphael, M.J., Nellen, M., and Oakley, C.M.: Primary restrictive cardiomyopathy: Non-trophical endomyocardial fibrosis and hypereosinophilic heart disease. Br. Heart J., *39*:399, 1977.

241. Di'enot, B., Ekra, A., and Bertrand, E.: Echocardiographic changes in 10 cases of left constrictive endomyocardial fibrosis isolated or bilateral with left-sided predominance. Arch. Mal Coeur, *74*:1063, 1981.

242. Candell-Riera, J., Permanyer-Meralda, G., and Soler-Soler, J.: Echocardiographic findings in endomyocardial fibrosis. Chest *82*:88, 1982.

243. George, B.O., Gaba, F.E., and Talabi, A.I.: M-mode echocardiographic features of endomyocardial fibrosis. Br. Heart J., *48*:222, 1982.

244. Acquatella, H.: Two dimensional echocardiography in endomyocardial disease. Postgrad. Med. J., *59*:157, 1983.

245. Acquatella, H., Schiller, N.B., Puigbo, J.J., Gomez-Mancebo, J.R., Suarez, C., and Acquatella, G.: Value of two dimensional echocardiography in endomyocardial disease with and without eosinophilia. A clinical and pathologic study. Circulation, *67*:1219, 1983.

246. Vijayaraghavan, G., Davies, J., Sadanandan, S., Spry, C.J.F., Gibson, D.G., and Goodwin, J.F.: Echocardiographic features of tropical endomyocardial disease in South India. Br. Heart J. *50*:450, 1983.

247. Carceller, A.M., Maroto, E., and Fouron, J-C.: Dilated and contracted forms of primary endocardial fibroelastosis: A single fetal disease with two stages of development. Br. Heart J., *63*:311, 1990.

248. Wiseman, M.N., Giles, M.S., and Camm, A.J.: Unusual echocardiographic appearance of intracardiac thrombi in a patient with endomyocardial fibrosis. Br. Heart J., *56*:179, 1986.

249. Ribeiro, P.A., Muthusamy, R., and Duran, C.M.G.: Right-sided endomyocardial fibrosis with recurrent pulmonary emboli leading to irreversible pulmonary hypertension. Br. Heart J., *68*:326, 1992.

250. Smith, M.D., Metcalf, M., DeMaria, A.N., Hendren, W.G., Walter, P.F., and Jones, E.L.: Hypereosinophilic syndrome resulting in aortic and mitral stenosis: A case requiring double valve replacement. Am. Heart J., *117*: 475, 1989.

251. Naito, H., Nakatsuka, M., Yuki, K., and Yamada, H.: Giant left ventricular thrombi in the hypereosinophilic syndrome: Report of two cases. J. Cardiogr., *16*:475, 1986.

252. Presti, C., Ryan, T., and Armstrong, W.F.: Two-dimensional and Doppler echocardiographic findings in hypereosinophilic syndrome. Am. Heart J., *114*:172, 1987.

253. Gottdiner, J.S., Maron, B.J., Schooley, R.T., Harley, J.B., Roberts, W.C., and Fauci, A.S.: Two dimensional echocardiographic assessment of the idiopathic hypereosinophilic syndrome. Circulation, 67:572, 1983.

254. Eterovic, I., Angelini, P., Leechman, R., and Cooley, D.A.: Obliterative restrictive endomyocardial fibrosis: A Surgical approach. Cardiovasc. Dis., *6*:66, 1979.

255. Björkem, G., Lundström, N.R., Wallentin, I., and Carlgren, L.E.: Endocardial fibroelastosis with predominant involvement of left atrium. Possibility of diagnosis by noninvasive methods. Br. Heart J., *46*:331, 1981.

256. Davies, J., Gibson, D.G., Foale, R., Heer, K., Spry, D.J.F., Oakley, C.M., and Goodwin, J.F.: Echocardiographic features of eosinophilic endomyocardial disease. Br. Heart J., *48*:434, 1982.

257. Davies, J., Spry, D.J., Sapsford, R., Olsen, E.G., DePerez, G., Oakley, C.M., and Goodwin, J.F.: Cardiovascular features of 11 patients with eosinophilic endomyocardial disease. Q.J. Med. *52*:23, 1983.

258. Bletry, O., Scheuble, C., Careze, P., Masquet, C., and Priollet, P.: Cardiac manifestations of the hypereosinophilic syndrome. The value of two dimensional echocardiography (12 cases). Arch. Mal Coeur, *77*:633, 1984.

259. Shimada, H., Inoue, M., Tamura, T., Ishihara, T., Kanemitsu, H., and Ishikawa, K.: Echocardiograms in progressive muscle dystrophy. J. Cardiogr., *8*:689, 1978.

260. Van der Hausaert, L.G. and Dumoulin, M.: Hypertrophic cardiomyopathy in Friedreich's ataxia. Br. Heart J., *38*:1291, 1976.

261. Goldberg, S.J., Feldman, L., Reinecke, C., Stern, L.Z., Sahn, D.J., and Allen, H.D.: Echocardiographic determination of contraction and relaxation measurements of the left ventricular wall in normal subjects and patients with muscular dystrophy. Circulation, *62*:1061, 1980.

262. Maione, S., Filla, A., Teti, G., Giumta, A., Serino, C., DeFalco, F.A., Mansi, D., and Campanella, G.: Cardiac abnormalities in Friedreich's ataxia patients and first-degree relatives. Evidence of hypertrophic cardiomyopathy in obligate heterozygotes. Acta Neurol., *35*:354, 1980.

263. St. John Sutton, M.G., Olukotun, A.Y., Tajik, A.J., Lovett, J.L., and Giuliani, E.R.: Left ventricular function in Friedreich's ataxia. Br. Heart J., *44*:309, 1980.

264. Weiss, E., Kronzon, I., Winer, H.E., and Berger, A.R.: Case report: Echocardiographic observations in patients with Friedreich's ataxia. Am. J. Med. Sci., *282*:136, 1981.

265. Gottdiener, J.S., Hawley, R.J., Maron, B.J., Bertorini, T.F., and Engle, W.K.: Characteristics of the cardiac hypertrophy in Friedreich's ataxia. Am. Heart J., *103*:525, 1982.

266. Farah, M.G., Evans, E.B., and Vignos, P.J.: Echocardiographic evaluation of left ventricular function in Duchenne's muscular dystrophy. Am. J. Med., *69*:248, 1980.

267. Goldberg, S.J., Stern, L.Z., Feldman, L., Allen, H.D., Sahn, D.J., and Valdes-Cruz, L.M.: Serial two dimensional echocardiography in Duchenne muscular dystrophy. Neurology, *32*:1101, 1982.

268. Goldberg, S.J., Stern, L.Z., Feldman, L., Sahn, D.J., Allen, H.D., and Valdes-Cruz, L.M.: Serial left ventricular wall measurements in Duchenne's muscular dystrophy. J. Am. Coll. Cardiol., *2*:136, 1983.

269. Hiromasa, S., Ikeda, T., Kubota, K., Hattori, N., Nishimura, M., Watanabe, Y., Maldonado, C., Palakurthy, P.R., and Kupersmith, J.: Myotonic dystrophy: Ambulatory electrocardiogram, electrophysiologic study, and echocardiographic evaluation. Am. Heart J., *113*:1482, 1987.

270. Child, J.S., Perloff, J.K., Bach, P.M., Wolfe, A.D., Perlman, S., and Kark, R.A.P.: Cardiac involvement in Friedreich's ataxia: A clinical study of 75 patients. J. Am. Coll. Cardiol., *7*:1370, 1986.

271. Alboliras, E.T., Shub, C., Gomez, M.R., Edwards, W.D., Hagler, D.J., Reeder, G.S., Seward, J.B., and Tajik, A.J.: Spectrum of cardiac involvement in Friedreich's ataxia: Clinical, electrocardiographic and echocardiographic observations. Am. J. Cardiol., *58*:518, 1986.

272. Fitzpatrick, A.P. and Emanuel, R.W.: Familial neurofibromatosis and hypertrophic cardiomyopathy. Br. Heart J., *60*:247, 1988.

273. Alboliras, E.T., Shub, C., Gomez, M.R., Edwards, W.D., Hagler, D.J., Reeder, G.S., Seward, J.B., and Tajik, A.J.: Spectrum of cardiac involvement in Friedreich's ataxia: Clinical, electrocardiographic and echocardiographic observations. Am. J. Cardiol., *58*:518, 1986.

274. Miyoshi, K.: Echocardiographic evaluation of fibrous replacement in the myocardium of patients with Duchenne muscular dystrophy. Br. Heart J., *66*:452, 1991.

275. Moise, N.S., Valentine, B.A., Brown, C.A., Erb, H.N., Beck, K.A., Cooper, B.J., and Gilmour, R.F.: Duchenne's cardiomyopathy in a canine model: Electrocardiographic and echocardiographic studies. J. Am. Coll. Cardiol., *17*:812, 1991.

276. Nieminen, M.S., Keikkila, J., and Karjalainen, J.: Echocardiography in acute infectious myocarditis: Relation to clinical and electrocardiographic findings. Am. J. Cardiol., *53*:1331, 1984.

277. Baba, Y., Konishi, H., Kawaratani, H., and Takemoto, K.: Echocardiographic features of severe acute infectious myocarditis. Jpn. J. Med. Ultrasonics, *17*:74, 1990.

278. Weinhouse, E., Wanderman, K.L., Sofer, S., Gussarsky, Y., and Gueron, M.: Viral myocarditis simulating dilated cardiomyopathy in early childhood: Evaluation by serial echocardiography. Br. Heart J., *56*:94, 1986.

279. Arvan, S. and Manalo, E.: Sudden increase in left ventricular mass secondary to acute myocarditis. Am. Heart J., *116*:200, 1988.

280. Laurenceau, J.L., Cereze, P., and Dumesnil, J.G.: Echocardiographic monitoring of myocarditis: Detection of regional dysfunction. Coeur Med. Interne, *18*:451, 1979.

281. Pinamonti, B., Alberti, E., Cigalotto, A., Dreas, L., Salvi, A., Silvestri, F., and Camerini, F.: Echocardiographic findings in myocarditis. Am. J. Cardiol., *62*:285, 1988.

282. Bali, H.K., Wahi, S., Sharma, B.K., Anand, I.S., Datta, B.N., and Wahi, P.L.: Myocardial tuberculosis presenting as restrictive cardiomyopathy. Am. Heart J., *120*:703, 1990.

283. Daxini, B.V., Mandke, J.V., and Sharma, S.: Echocardiographic recognition of tubercular submitral left ven-

tricular aneurysm extending into left atrium. Am. Heart J., *119*:970, 1990.

284. Chung, K.J., Fulton, D.R., Lapp, R., Spector, S., and Sahn, D.J.: One-year follow-up of cardiac and coronary artery disease in infants and children with Kawasaki disease. Am. Heart J., *115*:1263, 1988.

285. Newburger, J.W., Sanders, S.P., Burns, J.C., Parness, I.A., Beiser, A.S., and Colan, S.D.: Left ventricular contractility and function in Kawasaki syndrome. Circulation, *79*:1237, 1989.

286. Ichida, F., Fatica, N.S., O'Loughlin, J.E., Snyder, M.S., Ehlers, K.H., and Engle, M.A.: Correlation of electrocardiographic and echocardiographic changes in Kawasaki syndrome. Am. Heart J., *116*:812, 1988.

287. Newburger, J.W., Sanders, S.P., Burns, J.C., Parness, I.A., Beiser, A.S., and Colan, S.D.: Left ventricular contractility and function in Kawasaki syndrome. Circulation, *79*:1237, 1989.

288. Chung, K.J., Fulton, D.R., Lapp, R., Spector, S., and Sahn, D.J.: One-year follow-up of cardiac and coronary artery disease in infants and children with Kawasaki disease. Am. Heart J., *115*:1263, 1988.

289. Fink, L., Reichele, N., and Sutton, M.G.S.J.: Cardiac abnormalities in acquired immune deficiency syndrome. Am. J. Cardiol., *54*:1161, 1984.

290. Blanchard, D.G., Hagenhoff, C., Chow, L.C., McCann, H.A., and Dittrich, H.C.: Reversibility of cardiac abnormalities in human immunodeficiency virus (HIV)-infected individuals: A serial echocardiographic study. J. Am. Coll. Cardiol., *17*:1270, 1991.

291. Himelman, R.B., Chung, W.S., Chernoff, D.N., Schiller, N.B., and Hollander, H.: Cardiac manifestations of human immunodeficiency virus infection: A two-dimensional echocardiographic study. J. Am. Coll. Cardiol., *13*:1030, 1989.

292. Reilly, J.M., Dunnion, R.E., Anderson, D.W., O'Leary, T.J., Simmons, J.T., Lane, H.C., Fauci, A.S., Roberts, W.C., Virmani, R., and Parrillo, J.E.: Frequency of myocarditis, left ventricular dysfunction and ventricular tachycardia in the acquired immune deficiency syndrome. Am. J. Cardiol., *62*:789, 1988.

293. Webb, J.G., Chan-Yan, C., and Kiess, M.C.: Cardiac dysfunction associated with the acquired immunodeficiency syndrome (AIDS). Clin. Cardiol., *11*:423, 1988.

293a. Jacob, A.J., Sutherland, G.R., Bird, A.G., Brettle, R.P., Ludlam, C.A., McMillan, A., and Boon, N.A.: Myocardial dysfunction in patients infected with HIV: Prevalence and risk factors. Br. Heart J., *68*:549, 1992.

294. Ortiz, J., Matsumoto, A.Y., Monaco, C.A.F., Barretto, A.C.P.: Echocardiography in Chagas' Disease. Echocardiography, *3*:41, 1986.

295. Acquatella, H., Schiller, N.B., Puigbo, J.J., Giordano, H., Suarez, J.A., Casai, H., Arreaza, N., Valecillos, R., and Hirschhaut, E.: M-mode and two dimensional echocardiography in chronic Chagas' heart disease. Circulation, *62*:787, 1980.

296. Castagnino, H.E., Joïg, M.E., and Thompson, A.C.: Ventricular aneurysms in chronic Chagas' cardiopathy. J. Cardiovasc. Surg., *23*:28, 1982.

297. Acquatella, H.: Echocardiographic overview of Chagas' disease and endomyocardial fibrosis: Diagnostic implications for nontropical countries. Echocardiography, *6*:137, 1989.

298. Acquatella, H. and Schiller, N.B.: Echocardiographic recognition of Chagas disease and endomyocardial fibrosis. J. Am. Soc. Echocardiogr., *1*:60, 1988.

299. Oliver, J.M., Sotillo, J.F., Dominguez, F.J., Lopez, de Sa E., Calvo, L., Salvador, A., and Paniagua, J.M.: Two-dimensional echocardiographic features of echinococcosis of the heart and great blood vessels. Circulation, *78*:327, 1988.

300. Desnos, M., Brochet, E., Cristofini, P., Cosnard, G., Keddari, M., Mostefai, M., and Gay, J.: Polyvisceral echinococcosis with cardiac involvement imaged by two-dimensional echocardiography, computed tomography and nuclear magnetic resonance imaging. Am. J. Cardiol., *59*:383, 1987.

301. Lanzoni, A.M., Barrios, V., Moya, J.L., Epeldegui, A., Celemin, D., Lafuente, C., and Asin-Cardiel, E.: Dynamic left ventricular outflow obstruction caused by cardiac echinococcosis. Am. Heart J., *124*:1083, 1992.

301a. Rey, M., Alfonso, F., Torrecilla, E.G., McKenna, W.J., Balaguer, J., Alvarez, L., Rabago, P., Rabago, G., and Nihoyannopoulos, P.: Diagnostic value of two-dimensional echocardiography in cardiac hydatid disease. Eur. Heart J., *12*:1300, 1991.

302. Kumar, E.B., Soomro, R.S., Hamdani, A.A., and Shimy, N.E.: Scorpion venom cardiomyopathy. Am. Heart J., *123*:725, 1992.

303. Houda, N., Mori, T., Takeuchi, M., Yamamoto, N., Morita, N., Sugawa, M., Nakano, T., and Takezawa, H.: Echocardiographic evaluation of cardiac involvement in patients with chronic alcoholism. Cardiography, *13*:551, 1983.

304. Kupari, M., Koskinen, P., and Suokas, A.: Left ventricular size, mass and function in relation to the duration and quantity of heavy drinking in alcoholics. Am. J. Cardiol., *67*:274, 1991.

305. Kupari, M., Koskinen, P., Hynynen, M., Salmenpera, M., and Ventila, M.: Acute effects of ethanol on left ventricular diastolic function. Br. Heart J., *64*:29, 1990.

306. Kupari, M., Koshinen, P., Suokas, A., and Ventila, M.: Left ventricular filling impairment in asymptomatic chronic alcoholics. Am. J. Cardiol., *66*:1473, 1990.

307. Kupari, M. and Koshinen, P.: Comparison of the cardiotoxicity of ethanol in women versus men. Am. J. Cardiol., *70*:645, 1992.

308. Chokshi, S.K., Moore, R., Pandian, N.G., and Isner, J.M.: Reversible cardiomyopathy associated with cocaine intoxication. Ann. Intern. Med., *111*:1039, 1989.

309. Mendelson, M.A. and Chandler, J.: Postpartum cardiomyopathy associated with maternal cocaine abuse. Am. J. Cardiol., *70*:1092, 1992.

310. Chakko, S., Fernandez, A., Mellman, T.A., Milanes, F.J., Kessler, K.M., and Myerburg, R.J.: Cardiac manifestations of cocaine abuse: A cross-sectional study of asymptomatic men with a history of long-term abuse of "crack cocaine." J. Am. Coll. Cardiol., *20*:1168, 1992.

310a. Om, A, Ellahham, S., and Ornato, J.P.: Reversibility of cocaine-induced cardiomyopathy. Am. Heart J., *124*:1639, 1992.

311. Shuman, R.D., Ettinger, D.S., Abeloff, M.D., Livengood, S.V., and Fortuin, N.J.: Comparative analysis of noninvasive cardiac parameters in the detection and evaluation of Adriamycin cardiotoxicity. Johns Hopkins Med. J., *148*:57, 1981.

312. Hutter, J.J., Jr., Sahn, D.G., Woolfenden, J.M., and Carnahan, Y.: Evaluation of the cardiac effects of doxorubicin by serial echocardiography. Am. J. Dis. Child., *135*:653, 1981.

313. Borow, K.M., Henderson, I.C., Neuman, A., Colan, S., Grady, S., Papish, S., and Goorin, A.: Assessment of left ventricular contractility in patients receiving doxorubicin. Ann. Intern. Med., *99*:750, 1983.

314. Goldberg, S.J., Hutter, J.J., Jr., Feldman, L., and Goldberg, S.M.: Two sensitive echocardiographic techniques for detecting doxorubicin toxicity. Med. Pediatr. Oncol., *11*:172, 1983.

315. Marchandise, B., Schroeder, E., Bosly, A., Doyen, C., Weynants, P., and Kremer, R.: Early detection of doxorubicin cardiotoxicity: Interest of Doppler echocardiographic analysis of left ventricular filling dynamics. Am. Heart J., *118*:92, 1989.

316. Klewer, S.E., Goldberg, S.J., Donnerstein, R.L., Berg, R.A., Hutter, Jr., J.J.: Dobutamine stress echocardiography: A sensitive indicator of diminished myocardial function in asymptomatic Doxorubicin-treated long-term survivors of childhood cancer. J. Am. Coll. Cardiol., *19*: 394, 1992.

317. Stoddard, M.F., Seeger, J., Liddell, N.E., Hadley, T.J., Sullivan, D.M., and Kupersmith, J.: Prolongation of isovolumetric relaxation time as assessed by Doppler echocardiography predicts doxorubicin-induced systolic dysfunction in humans. J. Am. Coll. Cardiol., *20*:62, 1992.

318. Hermoni, Y., Engel, P.J., and Gallant, T.E.: Sequelae of injury to the heart caused by multiple needles. J. Am. Coll. Cardiol., *8*:1226, 1986.

319. Skorton, D.J., Collins, S.M., Nichols, J., Pandian, N.G., Bean, J.A., and Kerber, R.E.: Quantitative texture analysis in two dimensional echocardiography—application to the diagnosis of experimental myocardial contusion. Circulation, *68*:217, 1983.

320. Miller, F.A., Seward, J.B., Gersh, B.J., Tajik, A.J., and Mucha, P.: Two dimensional echocardiographic findings in cardiac trauma. Am. J. Cardiol., *50*:1022, 1982.

321. Lambertz, H., Rustige, J., Sechtem, U., and Von Essen, R.: Heart lesions caused by blunt trauma. Echocardiographic follow-up studies. Dtsch. Med. Wochenschr., *109*:218, 1984.

322. King, R.M., Mucha, P., Jr., Seward, J.B., Gersh, B.J., and Farnell, M.B.: Cardiac contusion: A new diagnostic approach utilizing two dimensional echocardiography. J. Trauma, *23*:6120, 1983.

323. Boland, M.J., Martin, H.F., and Ball, R.M.: Nonpenetrating traumatic ventricular septal defect: Two-dimensional echocardiographic and angiographic findings. Am. J. Cardiol., *55*:1242, 1985.

323a. Schiavone, W.A., Ghumrawi, B.K., Catalzno, D.R., Haver, D.W., Pipitone, A.J., L'Hommedieu, R.H., Keyser, P.H., and Tsai, A.R.: The use of echocardiography in the emergency management of nonpenetrating traumatic cardiac rupture. Ann. Emerg. Med., *20*:1248, 1991.

323b. Plummer, D., Brunette, D., Asinger, R., and Ruiz, E.: Emergency department echocardiography improves outcome in penetrating cardiac injury. Ann. Emerg. Med., *21*:709, 1992.

324. Wilson, V.E., Kirsch, M.M., Starkey, T.D., and Armstrong, W.F.: Left ventricular to right atrial septal defect secondary to blunt thoracic trauma diagnosed by transesophageal echocardiography. Echocardiography, *8*:363, 1991.

325. Clyne, C.A., Aurigemma, G., Sweeney, A., Pezzella, A.T., Paraskos, J., and Pape, L.: Traumatic intracardiac communication: Detection by color flow mapping. J. Am. Soc. Echocardiogr., *2*:342, 1989.

326. Wilson, V.E., Kirsch, M.M., Starkey, T.D., and Armstrong, W.F.: Left ventricular to right atrial septal defect secondary to blunt thoracic trauma diagnosed by transesophageal echocardiography. Echocardiography, *8*:363, 1991.

327. Ilia, R., Goldfarb, B., Wanderman, K.L., and Gueron, M.: Spontaneous closure of a traumatic ventricular septal defect after blunt trauma documented by serial echocardiography. J. Am. Soc. Echocardiogr., *5*:203, 1992.

328. Ettedgui, J.A., Altman, C.A., and Santoro, A.M.: Echocardiographic diagnosis of left ventricular pseudoaneurysm in a child after cardiopulmonary bypass. J. Am. Soc. Echocardiogr., *4*:491, 1991.

329. Matsumoto, A.Y., Ortiz, J., and Nanda, N.C.: Left ventricular pseudoaneurysm due to penetrating injury of the chest: An echocardiographic diagnosis. Am. Heart J., *115*:1134, 1988.

330. Ettedgui, J.A., Altman, C.A., and Santoro, A.M.: Echocardiographic diagnosis of left ventricular pseudoaneurysm in a child after cardiopulmonary bypass. J. Am. Soc. Echocardiogr., *4*:491, 1991.

331. Hilton, T., Mezei, L., and Pearson, A.C.: Delayed rupture of tricuspid papillary muscle following blunt chest trauma. Am. Heart J., *119*:1410, 1990.

332. Dodd, D.A., Johns, J.A., and Graham, T.P.: Transient severe mitral and tricuspid regurgitation following blunt chest trauma. Am. Heart J., *114*:652, 1987.

333. Linka, A., Ritter, M., Turina, M., and Jenni, R.: Acute tricuspid papillary muscle rupture following blunt chest trauma. Am. Heart J., *124*:799, 1992.

334. Kamiya, H., Hanaki, Y., Kojima, S., Ohsugi, S., Ohno, M., Ina, H., Hayase, S., Hiramatsu, H., and Horiba, M.: Fistula between noncoronary sinus of Valsalva and right atrium after blunt chest trauma. Am. Heart J., *114*:429, 1987.

335. Clyne, C.A., Aurigemma, G., Sweeney, A., Pezzella, A.T., Paraskos, J., and Pape, L.: Traumatic intracardiac communication: Detection by color mapping. J. Am. Soc. Echocardiogr., *2*:342, 1989.

336. Rowe, S.K. and Porter, C.B.: Atrial septal hematoma: Two-dimensional echocardiographic findings after blunt chest trauma. Am. Heart J., *114*:650, 1987.

336a. Rechavia, E., Imbar, S., Birnbaum, Y., Strasberg, B., and Sclarovsky, S.: Protruding left ventricular thrombus formation following blunt chest trauma. Am. Heart J., *125*:893, 1993.

337. Ku, C-S., Lin, S-L., Hsu, T-L., Wang, S-P., and Chang, M-S.: Myocardial damage associated with electrical injury. Am. Heart J., *118*:621, 1989.

338. Xenopoulos, N., Movahed, A., Hudson, P., and Reeves, W.C.: Myocardial injury in electrocution. Am. Heart J., *122*:1481, 1991.

339. Messina, A.G., Paranicas, M., Katz, B., Markowitz, J., and Yao, F.S.: Effect of electroconvulsive therapy on the electrocardiogram and echocardiogram. Anesth. Analg., *75*:511, 1992.

340. Ganau, A., Devereux, R.B., Roman, M.J., DeSimone, G., Pickering, T.G., Saba, P.S., Vargiu, P., Simongini, I., and Laragh, J.H.: Patterns of left ventricular hypertrophy and geometric remodeling in essential hypertension. J. Am. Coll. Cardiol., *19*:1550, 1992.

341. Pearson, A.C., Gudipati, C., Nagelhout, D., Sear, J., Cohen, J.D., Labovitz, A.J., Mrosek, D., and St. Vrain, J.: Echocardiographic evaluation of cardiac structure and function in elderly subjects with isolated systolic hypertension. J. Am. Coll. Cardiol., *17*:422, 1991.

342. Siegel, D., Cheitlin, M.D., Black, D.M., Seeley, D., Hearst, N., and Hulley, S.B.: Risk of ventricular arrhythmias in hypertensive men with left ventricular hypertrophy. Am. J. Cardiol., *65*:742, 1990.

343. Szlachcic, J., Tubau, J.F., O'Kelly, B., and Massie, B.M.: Correlates of diastolic filling abnormalities in hy-

pertension: A Doppler echocardiographic study. Am. Heart J., *120*:386, 1990.

344. Blake, J., Devereux, R.B., Herrold, E.M., Jason, M., Fisher, J., Borer, J.S., and Laragh, J.H.: Relation of concentric left ventricular hypertrophy and extracardiac target organ damage to supranormal left ventricular performance in established essential hypertension. Am. J. Cardiol., *62*:246, 1988.

345. DeSimone, G., DiLorenzo, L., Moccia, D., Costantino, G., Buonissimo, S., and DeDivitiis, O.: Hemodynamic hypertrophied left ventricular patterns in systemic hypertension. Am. J. Cardiol., *60*:1317, 1987.

346. Masuyama, T., Lee, J-M., Yamamoto, K., Tanouchi, J., Hori, M., and Kamada, T.: Analysis of pulmonary venous flow velocity patterns in hypertensive hearts: Its complementary value in the interpretation of mitral flow velocity patterns. Am. Heart J., *124*:983, 1992.

347. Casale, P.N., Devereux, R.B., Milner, M., Zullo, G., Harshfield, G.A., Pickering, T.G., and Laragh, J.H.: Value of echocardiographic measurement of left ventricular mass in predicting cardiovascular morbid events in hypertensive men. Ann. Intern. Med., *105*:173, 1985.

348. Friedman, N.E., Levitsky, L.L., Edidin, D.V., Vitullo, D.A., Lacina, S.J., and Chiemmongkoltip, P.: Echocardiographic evidence for impaired myocardial performance in children with type I diabetes mellitus. Am. J. Med., *73*:846, 1982.

349. Perez, J.E., McGill, J.B., Santiago, J.V., Schechtman, K.B., Waggoner, A.D., Miller, J.G., and Sobel, B.E.: Abnormal myocardial acoustic properties in diabetic patients and their correlation with the severity of disease. Am. Heart J., *19*:1154, 1992.

350. Zarich, S.W. and Nesto, R.W.: Diabetic cardiomyopathy. Am. Heart J., *118*:1000, 1989.

350a. Hiramatsu, K., Ohara, N., Shigematsu, S., Aizawa, T., Ishihara, F., Niwa, A., Yamada, T., Naka, M., Momose, A., and Yoshizawa, K.: Left ventricular filling abnormalities in non-insulin dependent diabetes mellitus and improvement by a short-term glycemic control. Am. J. Cardiol., *70*:1185, 1992.

351. Riggs, T.W. and Transue, D.: Doppler echocardiographic evaluation of left ventricular diastolic function in adolescents with diabetes mellitus. Am. J. Cardiol., *65*:899, 1990.

352. Sampson, M.J., Chambers, J.B., Sprigings, D.C., and Drury, P.L.: Abnormal diastolic function in patients with type 1 diabetes and early nephropathy. Br. Heart J., *64*:266, 1990.

353. Zarich, S.W., Arbuckle, B.E., Cohen, L.R., Roberts, M., and Nesto, R.W.: Diastolic abnormalities in young asymptomatic diabetic patients assessed by pulsed Doppler echocardiography. J. Am. Coll. Cardiol., *12*:114, 1988.

354. Sakura, E., Okamoto, M., Yokote, Y., Shimamoto, H., Yamagata, T., Amioka, H., Hashimoto, M., Takahashi, M., Tsuchioka, Y., Matsuura, H., and Kajiyama, G.: Analysis of inflow and ejection flow dynamics of the left ventricle in diabetics. Jpn. J. Med. Ultrasonics, *13*:10, 1986.

355. Mather, H.M., Boyd, M.H., and Jenkins, J.S.: Heart size and function in acromegaly. Br. Heart J., *41*:697, 1979.

356. Smallridge, R.C., Rajfer, S., Davia, J., and Schaaf, M.: Acromegaly and the heart: An echocardiographic study. Am. J. Med., *66*:22, 1979.

357. Gsanady, M., Gaspar, L., Hogye, M., and Gruber, N.: The heart in acromegaly: An echocardiographic study. Int. J. Cardiol., *2*:349, 1983.

358. Bertoni, P.D., DiMichele, R., Canziani, R., and Morandi, G.: Acromegalic cardiomyopathy: An echocardiographic study. G. Ital. Cardiol., *13*:152, 1983.

359. O'Keefe, J.C., Grant, S.J., Wiseman, J.C., Stiel, J.N., Wilmshurst, E.G., Cooper, R.A., and Edwards, A.C.: Acromegaly and the heart—echocardiographic and nuclear imaging studies. Aust. N.Z. Med., *12*:603, 1982.

360. Santos, A.D., Miller, R.P., Mathew, P.K., Wallace, W.A., Cave, W.T., Jr., and Hinojosa, L: Echocardiographic characterization of the reversible cardiomyopathy of hypothyroidism. Am. J. Med., *68*:675, 1980.

361. Fouron, J.C., Bourgin, J.H., Letarte, J., Dussault, J.H., Ducharme, G., and Davignon, A.: Cardiac dimensions and myocardial function of infants with congenital hypothyroidism. An echocardiographic study. Br. Heart J., *47*:584, 1982.

362. Doherty, III, N.E.: Echocardiographic findings in systemic lupus erythematosus. Am. J. Cardiol., *61*:1144, 1988.

363. Enomoto, K., Kaji, Y., Mayumi, T., Tsuda, Y., Kanaya, S., Nagasawa, K., Fujino, T., and Niho, Y.: Frequency of valvular regurgitation by color Doppler echocardiography in systemic lupus erythematosus. Am. J. Cardiol., *67*:209, 1991.

364. Leung, W-H., Wong, K-L., Lau, C-P., Wong, C-K., Cheng, C-H., and Tai, Y-T.: Doppler echocardiographic evaluation of left ventricular diastolic function in patients with systemic lupus erythematosus. Am. Heart J., *120*:82, 1990.

365. Roldan, C.A., Shively, B.K., Lau, C.C., Furule, F.T., Smith, E.A., and Crawford, M.H.: Systemic lupus erythematosus valve disease by transesophageal echocardiography and the role of antiphospholipid antibodies. J. Am. Coll. Cardiol., *20*:1127, 1992.

366. Sasson, Z., Rasooly, Y., Chow, C.W., Marshall, S., and Urowitz, M.B.: Impairment of left ventricular diastolic function in systemic lupus erythematosus. Am. J. Cardiol., *69*:1629, 1992.

367. Lundin, L., Landelius, J., Andren, B., and Oberg, K.: Transesophageal echocardiography improves the diagnostic value of cardiac ultrasound in patients with carcinoid heart disease. Br. Heart J., *64*:190, 1990.

368. Lundin, L., Norheim, I., Landelius, J., Oberg, K., and Theodorsson-Norheim, E.: Carcinoid heart disease: Relationship of circulating vasoactive substances to ultrasound-detectable cardiac abnormalities. Circulation, *77*:264, 1988.

369. Fan, P., Kirklin, J.K., Naftel, D.C., Bourge, R.C., Nanda, N.C., Hsiung, M.C., White-Williams, C., and Smith, S.: Application of echocardiographic color flow Doppler mitral regurgitation to the diagnosis of acute cardiac transplant rejection. Echocardiography, *9*:169, 1992.

370. Lambertz, H., Sigmund, M., Hoffman, R., Flachskampf, F.A., Messmer, B.J., and Hanrath, P.: Transesophageal Doppler analysis of pulmonary venous flow in cardiac transplant recipients. Am. Heart J., *121*:623, 1991.

371. Valantine, H.A., Hatle, L.K., Appleton, C.P., Gibbons, R., and Popp, R.L.: Variability of Doppler echocardiographic indexes of left ventricular filling in transplant recipients and in normal subjects. J. Am. Soc. Echocardiogr., *3*:276, 1990.

372. Gibbons, R.S.: Doppler echocardiography for rejection surveillance in the cardiac allograft recipient. J. Am. Soc. Echocardiogr., *4*:97, 1991.

373. Brockway, B.A.: Echocardiography and cardiac transplantation: A literature review and practical approach. J. Am. Soc. Echocardiogr., *2*:425, 1989.

374. Reynolds, T. and Halfman-Franey, M.: The role of the cardiac sonographer in the evaluation of the heart transplant recipient. J. Am. Soc. Echocardiogr., *2*:431, 1989.

375. Paulsen, W., Magid, N., Sagar, K., Hastillo. A., Wolfgang, T.C., Lower, R.R., and Hess, M.L.: Left ventricular function of heart allografts during acute rejection: An echocardiographic assessment. J. Heart Transplant., *4*: 525, 1985.

376. Cladellas, M., Abadal, M.L., Pons-llado, G., Ballester, M., Carreras, F., Obrador, D., Garcia-moll, M., Padro, J.M., Aris, A., and Caralps, J.M.: Early transient multivalvular regurgitation detected by pulsed Doppler in cardiac transplantation. Am. J. Cardiol., *58*:1122, 1986.

377. Frommelt, M.A., Snider, A.R., Crowley, D.C., Meliones, J.N., and Heidelberger, K.P.: Echocardiographic indexes of allograft rejection in pediatric cardiac transplant recipients. J. Am. Soc. Echocardiogr., *5*:41, 1992.

378. Sagar, K.B., Hastillo, A., Wolfgang, T.C., Lower, R.R., and Hess, M.L.: Left ventricular mass by M-mode echocardiography in cardiac transplant patients with acute rejection. Circulation, *64*:217, 1981.

379. Melvin, K.R., Pollick, C., Hunt, S.A., McDougall, R., Goris, M.L., Oyer, P., Popp, R.L., and Stinson, E.B.: Cardiovascular physiology in a case of heterotopic cardiac transplantation. Am. J. Cardiol., *49*:1301, 1982.

380. Mannaerts, H.F.J., Balk, A.H.M.M., Simoons, B.M.L., Tijssen, J., van der Borden, S.G., Zondervan, P., Sutherland, G.R., and Roelandt, J.R.T.C.: Changes in left ventricular function and wall thickness in heart transplant recipients and their relation to acute rejection: An assessment by digitised M Mode echocardiography. Br. Heart J., *68*:356, 1992.

381. Desruennes, M., Corcos, T., Cabrol, A., Gandjbakhch, I., Pavie, A., Leger, P., Eugene, M., Bors, V., and Cabrol, C.: Doppler echocardiography for the diagnosis of acute caradiac allograft rejection. J. Am. Coll. Cardiol., *12*:63, 1988.

382. Valantine, H.A., Appleton, C.P., Hatle, L.K., Hunt, S.A., Billingham, M.E., Shumway, N.E., Stinson, E.B., and Popp, R.L.: A hemodynamic and Doppler echocardiographic study of ventricular function in long-term cardiac allograft recipients. Circulation, *79*:66, 1989.

383. Valantine, H.A., Oldershaw, P.J., Fowler, M.B., Gibson, D.G., Hatle, L., Hunte, S.A., Billingham, M.E., Stinson, E.B., and Popp, R.L.: Changes in Doppler and M-mode echocardiographic indices of left ventricular function during acute cardiac allograft rejection. Br. Heart J., *57*:86, 1987.

384. Stork, T., Mockel, M., Eichstadt, H., Walkowiak, T., Siniawski, H., Muller, R., Hetzer, R., and Hochrein, H.: Noninvasive diagnosis of cardiac allograft rejection by means of pulsed Doppler and M-mode ultrasound. J. Ultrasound Med., *10*:569, 1991.

384a. Valantine, H.A., Yeoh, T.K., Gibbons, R., McCarthy, P., Stinson, E.B., Gillingham, M.E., and Popp, R.L.: Sensitivity and specificity of diastolic indexes for rejection surveillance: Temporal correlation with endomyocardial biopsy. J. Heart Lung Transplant., *10*:757, 1991.

385. Simmonds, M.B., Lythall, D.A., Slorach, C., Ilsley, C.D.J., Mitchell, A.G., and Yacoub, M.H.: Doppler examination of superior vena caval flow for the detection of acute cardiac rejection. Circulation, *85*:II-259, 1992.

385a. Spes, C.H., Schnaack, S.D., Schutz, A., Gokel, J.M., Kemkes, B.M., Theisen, K., and Angermann, C.E.: Serial Doppler echocardiographic assessment of left and right ventricular filling for non-invasive diagnosis of mild acute cardiac allograft rejection. Eur. Heart J., *13*:889, 1992.

386. Masuyama, T., Valantine, H.A., Gibbons, R., Schnittger, I., and Popp, R.L.: Serial measurement of integrated ultrasonic backscatter in human cardiac allografts for the recognition of acute rejection. Circulation, *81*:829, 1990.

387. Valantine, H.A., Hunt, S.A., Gibbons, R., Billingham, M.E., Stinson, E.B., and Popp, R.L.: Increasing pericardial effusion in cardiac transplant recipients. Circulation, *79*:603, 1989.

388. Starling, R.C., Baker, P.B., Hirsch, S.C., Myerowitz, P.D., Galbraith, T.A., and Binkley, P.F.: An echocardiographic and anatomic description of the donor-recipient atrial anastomosis after orthotopic cardiac transplantation. Am. J. Cardiol., *64*:109, 1989.

# 10

# Pericardial Disease

## PERICARDIAL EFFUSION

### Detection of Pericardial Fluid

The technique that probably provided much of the impetus for the development of echocardiography in the United States was the detection of pericardial effusion.[1-5] Because a harmless, bedside examination for pericardial effusion has obvious clinical advantages, this technique has become one of the most popular applications of diagnostic ultrasound. The theory behind the echocardiographic technique for the detection of pericardial effusion is simple. Normally, the pericardial sac is only a potential space, and the heart is in direct contact with the surrounding structures. In the presence of pericardial effusion, this potential space fills with relatively echo-free fluid, which separates the heart from the surrounding pericardium.

Figure 10–1 demonstrates four two-dimensional echocardiographic views of a patient with a large pericardial effusion. The relatively echo-free pericardial fluid (PE) can be seen surrounding the heart in the long-axis (A), short-axis at the papillary muscle level (B), short-axis at the base (C), and the apical four-chamber views (D). The accumulation of pericardial fluid is primarily anterior with this large effusion. The heart seems to settle or drop posteriorly into this huge, fluid-filled sac.

Figure 10–2 shows an example of a moderately large pericardial effusion. In these long-axis and short-axis views, one sees that the fluid primarily collects posteriorly. The anterior pericardial effusion (arrow) is a smaller space and is not as echo-free because of near field clutter. In this patient, the echocardiographic diagnosis of pericardial effusion depends primarily on the posterior collection of the fluid. Some of the earlier radiographic techniques for making this diagnosis primarily detected anterior fluid. Whether or not the heart "floats" or "sinks" with pericardial effusion seems to depend on the amount of the fluid. As noted in Figure 10–1, if one has a large pericardial effusion, the heart seems to settle posteriorly with a greater accumulation of fluid anteriorly. With lesser amounts of effusion, one sees more fluid posteriorly than anteriorly. Figure 10–3 shows one possible explanation for the early accumulation of fluid posteriorly. In this two-dimensional echocardiogram, one again sees a large posterior pericardial effusion. The short-axis view reveals that the fluid accumulates primarily in the posterior cul-de-sac and then along the lateral border of the heart.

Where the fluid collects is probably a function of how the pericardium can expand rather than whether the heart sinks or floats. The posterior cul-de-sac and the lateral walls are more expandable. These areas offer less resistance to stretching of the pericardium, providing an area where fluid initially collects. Later, when the effusion increases and totally surrounds the heart, the heart can move freely and may settle posteriorly within the fluid.

Although the first ultrasonic description of pericardial effusion showed only anterior fluid,[6] the usual echocardiographic technique has emphasized the detection of pericardial fluid posterior to the left ventricle, because anterior fluid may be neglible with small effusions and relatively echo-free spaces anteriorly have been a potential source of false-positive evidence of effusion.[7-10] Epicardial fat, for example, may produce an echo-free space anteriorly that can be mistaken for pericardial fluid. Any separation between the heart and the anterior chest wall can cause confusion. Thus, unless one is suspicious of a loculated anterior effusion, it is wise not to make a diagnosis of pericardial effusion on the basis of an anterior echo-free space without some evidence of posterior fluid.

M-mode echocardiography is still a useful technique for the detection of pericardial fluid.[2,11-14] Figure 10–4 demonstrates an M-mode study showing an echo-free pericardial space both anterior to the right ventricular wall and behind the posterior left ventricular wall. Some of the echo-free space extends behind the left atrium.

Transthoracic echocardiography is almost always sufficient to detect pericardial effusion. Transesophageal echocardiography, however, can also make this diagnosis.[15,16] Pericardial effusion is not one of the major indications for a transesophageal study, unless the transthoracic examination is technically unsatisfactory, as may occur after cardiac surgery. Intravascular ultrasound represents a possible alternative ultrasonic technique for the diagnosis of pericardial effusion in specific clinical situations. Cardiac perforation with resultant pericardial effusion is a complication that may occur in a cardiac catheterization laboratory. When this situation occurs, one usually brings a standard echocardiograph into the catheterization laboratory and obtains a transthoracic echocardiogram. This environment, however, is not

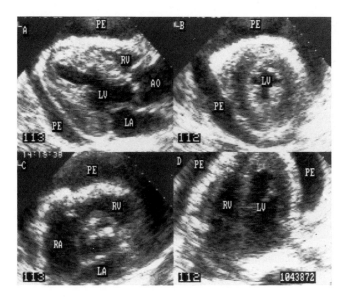

**Fig. 10–1.** Long-axis (*A*), short-axis at the papillary muscle (*B*), short-axis at the base of the heart (*C*), and apical four-chamber (*D*) two-dimensional echocardiograms of a patient with a large pericardial effusion (PE). The relatively echo-free fluid can be seen surrounding the heart in all views. RV = right ventricle; LV = left ventricle; AO = aorta; LA = left atrium; RA = right atrium.

ideal for high-quality transthoracic echocardiography. It is frequently difficult to place the patient on the left side for optimal ultrasonic visualization. Furthermore, some delay and inconvenience may be associated with bringing the equipment to the laboratory that may already be filled with equipment. Investigators using intravascular ultrasonic catheters have shown that such a device in the right atrium will easily detect pericardial fluid.[17] Figure 10–5 shows an intravascular ultrasonic study demonstrating an echo-free space between the right atrial wall and the parietal pericardium.

Pericardial fluid may not always collect uniformly around the heart. As already noted, the fluid may collect relatively more anteriorly or posteriorly. In some situations, especially after cardiac surgery, adhesions in certain areas of the pericardium may produce loculated pericardial effusion.[15,18] Under these circumstances, the usual diagnostic criteria for the circumferential accumulation of pericardial fluid do not hold. Two-dimensional echocardiography is essential for the detection of loculated effusion. Figure 10–6 shows an example of loculated effusion along the right atrial border. This diagnosis can be difficult. The use of contrast echocardiography can assist in identifying an extracardiac echo-free space.[19] As stated, this situation frequently occurs in the postoperative state.[20,21] This particular echocardiogram also shows compression of the right atrial wall, which is one of the signs of cardiac tamponade (see subsequent discussion). Another interesting finding in this echocardiogram is that the pericardial compression forced a probe patent foramen ovale to open and produce right-left shunting, as demonstrated by contrast echoes moving from the right atrium into

the left side of the heart.[22,22a,22b] Loculated pericardial fluid may also be suspected when there is distention of the oblique pericardial sinus behind the left atrium.[23]

Transesophageal echocardiography is helpful in identifying loculated fluid, especially if not all areas of the heart are seen with the transthoracic examination.[20,21] This situation is again common after cardiac surgery because bandages on the chest, residual intrathoracic air, ventilators, and the inability of a patient to roll over may all interfere with the ability to obtain a satisfactory transthoracic examination.

### Differentiation Between Pericardial and Pleural Effusions

Left pleural effusion is not a frequent problem in the echocardiographic diagnosis of pericardial effusion, be-

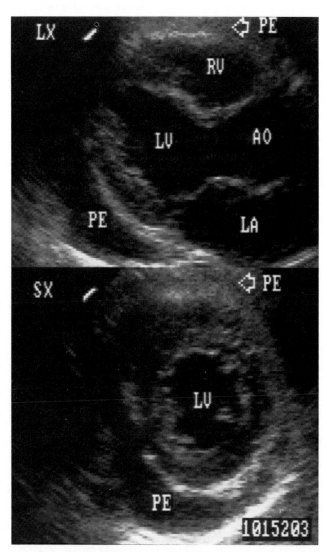

**Fig. 10–2.** Long-axis (LX) and short-axis (SX) two-dimensional echocardiograms of a patient with moderate pericardial effusion. The fluid (PE) is seen primarily posteriorly. The anterior pericardial effusion is smaller and more echogenic in part because of near field clutter. RV = right ventricle; LV = left ventricle; AO = aorta; LA = left atrium.

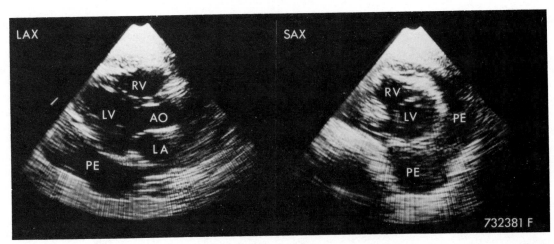

**Fig. 10–3.** Long-axis (LAX) and short-axis (SAX) two-dimensional echocardiograms of a patient with a large pericardial effusion. The pericardial effusion (PE) can be seen accumulating posteriorly and laterally. RV = right ventricle; LV = left ventricle; AO = aorta; LA = left atrium.

cause fluid usually accumulates along the pleural surface rather than in the retrocardiac space. Retrocardiac pleural effusions can occur, however. The patient in Figure 10–7 has both pericardial effusion and pleural effusion posteriorly. In the long-axis view (Fig. 10–7A), the pericardial effusion (PE) tapers as it approaches the left atrium (LA). A helpful echocardiographic sign for differentiating pleural from pericardial effusion is that the descending aorta is separated from the left atrium by pericardial effusion but not by pleural effusion.[24,25] Thus, in Figure 10–7, the echo-free space from the pericardial effusion is between the aorta and the left atrium,

whereas the pleural effusion is posterior to the aorta. Figure 10–8 demonstrates a patient with a large retrocardiac pleural effusion. No pericardial effusion is seen, and the descending aorta (DA) lies between the pleural effusion and the left atrium (LA). There is no echo-free space between the aorta and the left atrium.

## Quantitation of Pericardial Fluid

With routine echocardiography, one usually makes a qualitative assessment of the amount of pericardial fluid. Figure 10–1 is an example of a large pericardial effusion.

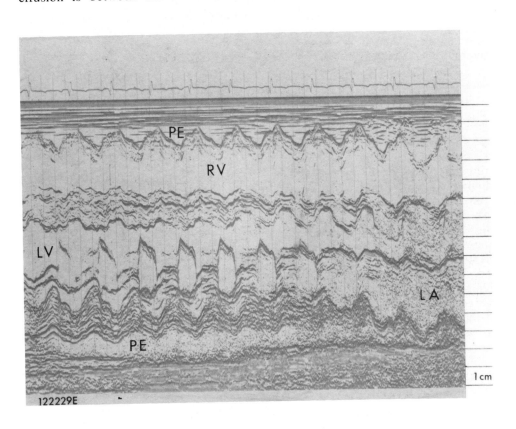

**Fig. 10–4.** M-mode scan of a patient with pericardial effusion. The pericardial effusion (PE) behind the left ventricle (LV) decreases as the ultrasonic beam is directed toward the left atrium (LA). RV = right ventricle.

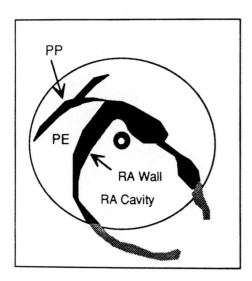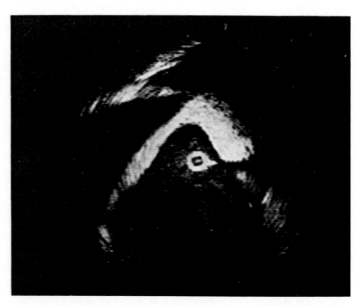

**Fig. 10–5.** Intracardiac echocardiographic image recorded with the ultrasound positioned within the right atrium (RA) in a patient with pericardial effusion. The catheter is represented as a small circular signal in the center of the recording. Pericardial effusion (PE) is seen as an echo-free space between the right atrial wall and the parietal pericardium (PP). (From Weintraub, A.R., et al.: Intracardiac two-dimensional echocardiography in patients with pericardial effusion in cardiac tamponade. J. Am. Soc. Echocardiogr., *4*:572, 1991.)

The amount of fluid is determined by the size of the echo-free space surrounding the heart. Figure 10–2 would be an example of a moderate effusion. Note the fairly large echo-free space posteriorly and only a small echo-free space anteriorly. Figure 10–9 provides an example of a small pericardial effusion. The fluid is seen as a small echo-free rim posteriorly and hardly any fluid anteriorly. Some authors have used a semiquantitative approach to judge the amount of pericardial effusion.[26] Effusions that totally surround the heart and are at least 1 cm in width have been designated as large effusions. A moderate effusion is classified as one that surrounds the heart but is 1 cm or less at its greatest width, and a small effusion is one that is only localized posteriorly

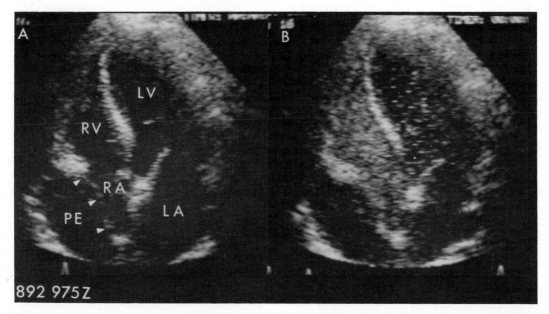

**Fig. 10–6.** (*A*) Apical four-chamber two-dimensional echocardiogram of a patient with a loculated pericardial effusion (PE) next to the right atrium (RA). The pericardial fluid compresses the right atrial free wall (*arrowheads*). An intravenous contrast injection (*B*) shows echogenic contrast filling of the right side of the heart. A small amount of contrast material passes into the left side of the heart through a probe patent foramen ovale. There is no contrast in the echo-free pericardial effusion. RV = right ventricle; LV = left ventricle; LA = left atrium.

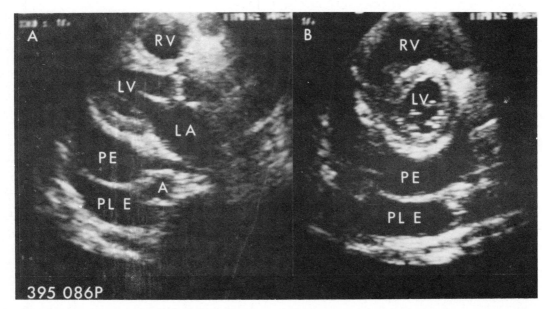

**Fig. 10–7.** Long-axis (*A*) and short-axis (*B*) two-dimensional echocardiograms of a patient with pericardial effusion (PE) and pleural effusion (PL E). In the long-axis view, the aorta (A) lies between the two bodies of fluid. RV = right ventricle; LV = left ventricle; LA = left atrium.

and usually is 1 cm or less in width. These authors noted that quantitating the effusion in this fashion in hospitalized patients provided prognostic value that was better than the echocardiographic signs of tamponade.[26]

Several efforts have been made to use both M-mode and two-dimensional echocardiography to quantitate pericardial effusion.[27–29] The techniques basically attempt to calculate the volume of the pericardial sac and subtract the volume of the heart. Figure 10–10 shows a diagram of how one might theoretically quantitate pericardial effusion from a two-dimensional echocardiographic examination.[30] By obtaining major and minor dimensions of the pericardium in the apical four-cham-

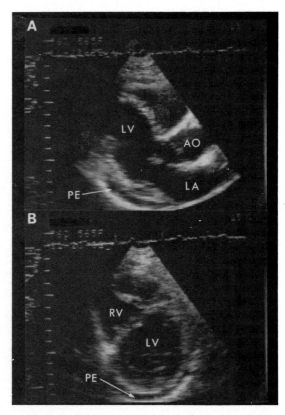

**Fig. 10–9.** Long-axis (*A*) and short-axis (*B*) two-dimensional echocardiograms of a patient with a small pericardial effusion (PE) posterior to the left ventricle (LV). AO = aorta; LA = left atrium; RV = right ventricle.

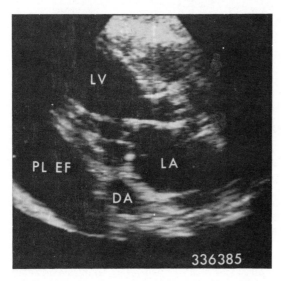

**Fig. 10–8.** Long-axis two-dimensional echocardiogram of a patient with a large retrocardiac pleural effusion (PL EF). LV = left ventricle; LA = left atrium; DA = descending aorta.

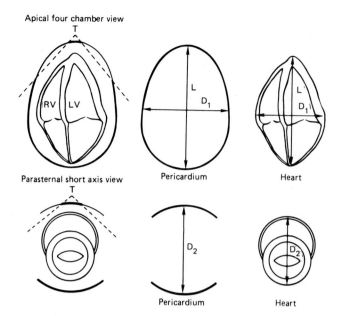

Fig. 10–10. Diagram demonstrating how one may quantitate pericardial effusion by calculating the volume of the pericardium and subtracting the volume of the heart. The pericardial volume can be obtained by obtaining the length (L) and one minor dimension ($D_1$) from the apical four-chamber view and the other minor dimension ($D_2$) from the short-axis view. A similar calculation of the cardiac volume can be obtained from the four-chamber and two-chamber views. (From D'Cruz, I.A. and Hoffman, P.K.: A new cross-sectional echocardiographic method for estimating the volume of large pericardial effusion. Br. Heart J., 66:449, 1991.)

ber and short-axis views and then deriving cardiac dimensions in the same views, one can calculate volume of the pericardium and subtract the volume of the heart to determine the volume of pericardial fluid. The M-mode technique is similar except that one uses single linear pericardial and cardiac dimensions to make the volume calculations.[27]

## Cardiac Tamponade

A long list of echocardiographic signs have been described in patients with cardiac tamponade. The echocardiographic sign that appears to be most popular and has withstood the test of time is collapse of the cardiac chambers in diastole.[31–36] The most common finding is diastolic invagination of the right ventricular[31,32,37–39] and/or right atrial wall during diastole (Fig. 10–11).[40–42] In this illustration, one sees that the right ventricular free wall is compressed (*arrow*) in the long-axis view. The wall literally collapses against the interventricular septum. A similar phenomenon occurs with the right atrial free wall (*arrow*, 4C view). The short-axis views in Figure 10–12 demonstrate invaginations of the right ventricular free wall (*arrowhead*) in early diastole.

M-mode echocardiography may detect the right ventricular diastolic collapse more easily than the two-dimensional examination.[31,32] The timing of the collapse is more apparent on the M-mode recording. Figure 10–13

illustrates an example of diastolic collapse of the right ventricle (*arrow*). Timing of the collapse can be made by correlating it with mitral valve opening or septal and posterior ventricular wall motion. Figure 10–14 shows that right ventricular collapse can even be seen from an apical view in some individuals. Figure 10–15 provides another example of right atrial collapse. One can appreciate the fact that the right atrial collapse occurs in diastole with a normally shaped right atrial cavity in systole. The duration of right atrial collapse may relate to the severity of the tamponade.

Ample data show the reliability of right ventricular and right atrial collapse for the detection of cardiac tamponade. It must be emphasized that tamponade is a clinical syndrome and is usually defined by certain findings at the bedside. It has been noted that the echocardiographic signs may precede the clinical manifestations in

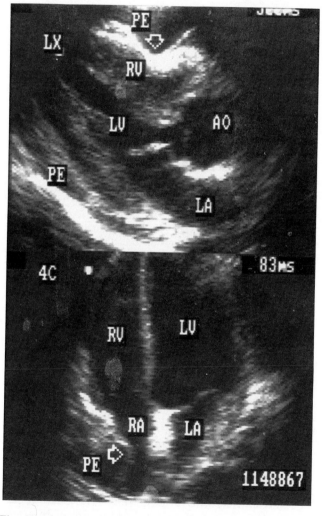

Fig. 10–11. Long-axis (LX) and four-chamber (4C) two-dimensional echocardiographic views of a patient with pericardial effusion (PE) and cardiac tamponade. The long-axis view shows diastolic collapse of the right ventricular wall (*arrow*); the four-chamber view shows collapse of the right atrial free wall (*arrow*). RV = right ventricle; LV = left ventricle; AO = aorta; LA = left atrium; RA = right atrium.

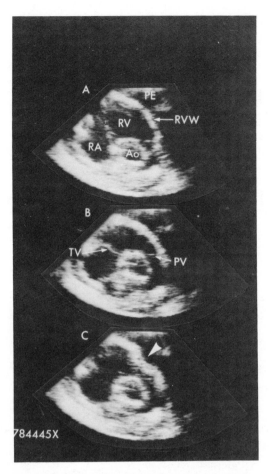

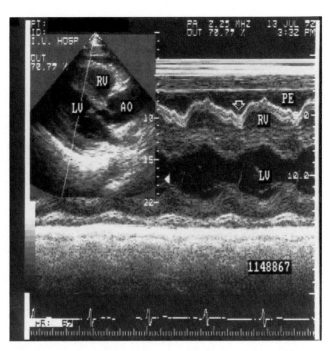

**Fig. 10–13.** M-mode echocardiogram demonstrating diastolic collapse (*arrow*) of the right ventricular free wall in a patient with pericardial effusion (PE) and cardiac tamponade. RV = right ventricle; LV = left ventricle; AO = aorta.

**Fig. 10–12.** Short-axis two-dimensional echocardiograms of a patient with pericardial effusion and cardiac tamponade. Early diastolic indentation of the right ventricular free wall (*arrowhead*) is noted (*C*). The right ventricular free wall (RVW) has a normal configuration at end diastole (*A*) and end systole (*B*). PE = pericardial effusion; RV = right ventricle; RA = right atrium; Ao = aorta; TV = tricuspid valve; PV = pulmonary valve. (From Armstrong, W.F., et al.: Diastolic collapse of the right ventricle with cardiac tamponade: An echocardiographic study. Circulation, *65*:1491, 1982, by permission of the American Heart Association, Inc.)

tamponade, so in some cases, right ventricular and right atrial collapse may be precursors of tamponade rather than actual manifestations of this problem.[34,36] In general, right atrial collapse is more sensitive but slightly less specific than right ventricular collapse.

There are a few important exceptions to the use of right-sided collapse for diagnosing tamponade. One situation whereby right ventricular collapse is absent in the presence of tamponade is when pressure is elevated in the right ventricle with resultant right ventricular hypertrophy. The usual explanation for collapse of the right ventricular and atrial free walls is that these low pressure chambers have thin walls and are easily compressible with elevated pericardial pressure. This hypothesis would explain why collapse may not occur if the right ventricular pressure is significantly elevated.[43] In one report, a patient had tamponade and right-sided col-

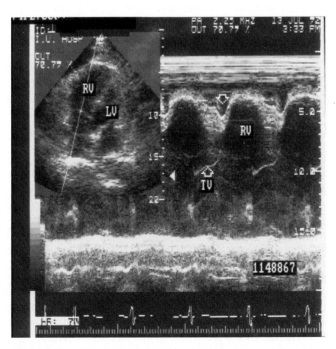

**Fig. 10–14.** M-mode echocardiogram showing diastolic collapse of the right ventricular free wall (*arrow*) in a recording made from the apical four-chamber transducer location. RV = right ventricle; LV = left ventricle; TV = tricuspid valve.

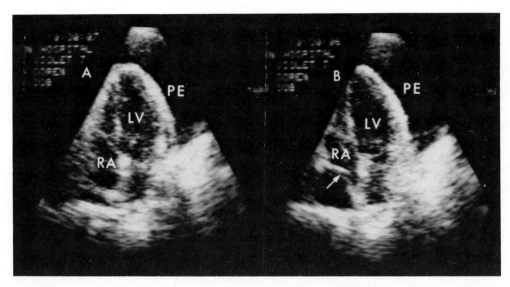

**Fig. 10–15.** Apical four-chamber two-dimensional echocardiograms of a patient with a large pericardial effusion (PE) and collapse (*arrow*) of the right atrial (RA) free wall during diastole (*B*). LV = left ventricle.

lapse; however, with transfusion and an increase in the right-sided filling pressures, the right-sided collapse disappeared.[44] Patients with right ventricular infarction and pericardial effusion may have marked dilatation of the right ventricle, and again, there may be failure to collapse appropriately with effusion and tamponade.[45]

Low pressure tamponade is when blood volume is low and clinical evidence of tamponade may be absent. Under these circumstances, right ventricular and atrial collapse will still be present and their detection may be critical in making the proper evaluation.[46] As already mentioned, however, transfusion may increase the right ventricular and atrial pressures to the point that the right-sided collapse may disappear.[44] There is a report of a patient with low pressure cardiac tamponade in whom the right heart collapse was not present.[47] The tamponade was associated with a localized pericardial effusion, which explained the lack of right atrial or ventricular collapse. The correct diagnosis of tamponade was made by the Doppler signs for hemodynamic compromise. False-positive right ventricular collapse has been reported in the presence of pleural effusions.[48]

Left atrial or left ventricular collapse may also be present in a patient with pericardial effusion.[43,49,50] As one would predict, this situation usually occurs when pressures in the left atrium and left ventricle are relatively low. Figure 10–16 shows an example of left atrial collapse in a patient with cardiac tamponade. Note the obvious pericardial effusion lateral to the left atrium. One can see progressive invagination of the left atrial free wall (*arrowheads*) in this four-chamber view. Figure 10–17 demonstrates an example of left ventricular diastolic collapse.[51–53] A huge posterior pericardial effusion is visible. As with the right ventricular wall, the diastolic collapse occurs in early diastole with normalization of the wall in late diastole. Left ventricular collapse has also been reported in association with pleural effusion.[54]

Left ventricular and/or left atrial collapse is a possibility when the fluid accumulates eccentrically or it is loculated. Figure 10–18 shows a post-operative patient who had a large loculated pericardial effusion next to the left ventricle. The fluid produced compression or diastolic collapse of the left ventricular free wall (*arrow*) with clinical tamponade.

Inferior vena cava plethora with blunted respiratory variation is another important sign of cardiac tamponade.[55,56] Figure 10–19 shows a patient with inferior vena cava dilatation that does not vary with respiration. This particular patient happened to have constrictive pericarditis, but the physiologic findings are identical to those of cardiac tamponade.

Spectral Doppler has been used by many investigators to identify cardiac tamponade.[57–64] The technique primarily involves Doppler recordings of mitral, tricuspid, and/or systemic venous tracings together with the phases of respiration. Pulmonary venous flow also has been analyzed in persons with tamponade.[65] Figure 10–20 shows that in the normal situation, respiratory variation of mitral flow is minimal. With cardiac tamponade, however, inspiration produces a decrease in left-sided filling and reduced early diastolic velocity through the mitral valve. To be certain that this change in velocity is not just positional and reflects differences in location of the sample volume with respiration, it is advisable to measure isovolumic relaxation time as well as total amplitude of the early diastolic velocity. Figure 10–21 demonstrates the mitral flow velocity in another patient with tamponade. With tamponade, inspiration produces a dramatic decrease in early diastolic mitral velocity and prolongation of the isovolumic relaxation time. During expiration, the isovolumic relaxation time shortens and the initial mitral velocity increases.

Systemic venous Doppler flow is also helpful in making the diagnosis of cardiac tamponade. Figure 10–22 diagrammatically shows pulsed Doppler, hepatic venous

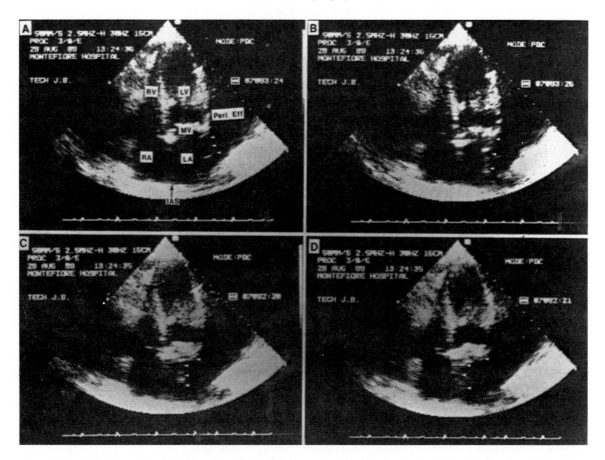

**Fig. 10–16.** Serial frames from a cardiac cycle of a patient with pericardial effusion and collapse of the left atrial free wall (*arrowheads*). The left atrium (LA) is fully distended late in diastole (*A*). Left atrial compression begins after atrial contraction (*B*) and becomes most marked in early systole (*C* and *D*). RV = right ventricle; LV = left ventricle; MV = mitral valve; RA = right atrium; LA = left atrium; IAS = interatrial septum. (From Fusman, B., et al.: Isolated collapse of left-sided heart chambers in cardiac tamponade: Demonstration by two-dimensional echocardiography. Am. Heart J., *121*:614, 1991.)

flow profiles in a variety of different states. With normal physiology, the systolic velocity is slightly higher than the diastolic velocity, and there are small ventricular and atrial reverse flows. With cardiac tamponade, the systolic and diastolic flows are reduced with expiration, and reverse flow with atrial contraction is increased (Fig. 10–22). In Figure 10–21, hepatic venous flow is virtually absent with expiration.

One use of the Doppler technique for detecting cardiac tamponade is that if respiratory variation in venous and transvalvular flow does not change with pericardiocentesis, one must be suspicious of effusive constrictive pericarditis. Figure 10–23 shows an example of a patient who had pericardial effusion and clinical tamponade. Following pericardiocentesis, the respiratory variation in mitral and hepatic venous flow persisted. This finding provided evidence of underlying constriction. Only after pericardiectomy did the mitral and hepatic venous flows normalize.

Respiratory variations can also be seen with M-mode echocardiography.[66–68] With inspiration comes an abrupt and dramatic increase in right ventricular dimensions at the expense of the left ventricle (Fig. 10–24). A

decrease in the mitral diastolic slope is also noted with inspiration. The separation of the mitral leaflets is decreased, suggesting decreased mitral valve flow and left ventricular stroke volume with inspiration. This reciprocal filling of the ventricles is similar to the findings in Doppler recordings and is indicative of cardiac filling whereby expansion of the left and right ventricular free walls is limited by the pericardial fluid and pressure. As will be discussed subsequently, constrictive pericarditis can produce the same phenomenon. Figure 10–25 is another M-mode echocardiogram of a patient with pericardial effusion and cardiac tamponade. The diastolic right ventricular dimension at end-expiration ($RV_e$) is small.[67,69] In early studies with M-mode echocardiography, investigators emphasized that a right ventricular end-diastolic dimension of 2 cm or less was indicative of cardiac tamponade.[70] Figure 10–25 also demonstrates right ventricular diastolic collapse, which is the more popular finding for tamponade. The postpericardiocentesis M-mode recording of the same patient in Figure 10–25 is noted in Figure 10–26. One detects a larger right ventricular dimension, and the diastolic right ventricular free wall collapse is gone.

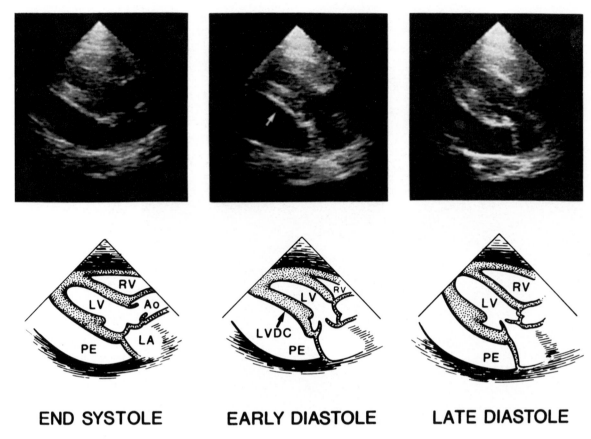

**END SYSTOLE**          **EARLY DIASTOLE**          **LATE DIASTOLE**

**Fig. 10–17.** Serial echocardiographic images in the parasternal long-axis view obtained postoperatively from a patient with a large posterior pericardial effusion (PE) and tamponade. The right ventricle (RV) is adherent to the anterior chest wall. The contour of the posterior left ventricular wall (LV) is normal at end systole. During early diastole, however, the left ventricular posterior wall invaginates inward (*arrow*) and exhibits LV diastolic collapse (LVDC). By late diastole, the left ventricle has resumed its normal contour. LA = left atrium; Ao = aorta; RV = right ventricle; LV = left ventricle. (From Chauttani, K., et al.: Left ventricular diastolic collapse: An echocardiographic sign of regional cardiac tamponade. Circulation, *83*:2002, 1991, by permission of the American Heart Association, Inc.)

Loculated pericardial effusions can also produce localized tamponade. These conditions frequently are iatrogenic and may occur following surgery[71] or after mediastinal irradiation.[72] Under these circumstances, generalized signs of tamponade may not be present.

Transient "pseudohypertrophy" of the left ventricle has been reported in patients with tamponade.[73,73a] This finding has not been confirmed.

With a combination of two-dimensional, M-mode, and Doppler echocardiography, the ultrasonic examination should be reliable in detecting hemodynamic compromise resulting from pericardial effusion and should identify patients who are in frank cardiac tamponade or who are susceptible to clinical tamponade. When there is underlying left ventricular dysfunction, relatively small effusions may produce many of the echocardiographic findings of tamponade.[74]

### Cardiac Motion in Patients with Pericardial Effusion

Early in the use of echocardiography to detect pericardial effusion, it became apparent that cardiac motion is frequently altered in patients with large effusions.[75,76]

Figure 10–27 shows long-axis and four-chamber echocardiograms of a patient with a large pericardial effusion and clinical tamponade. The long-axis diastolic frame (Fig. 10–27A) shows the large posterior pericardial effusion. With diastole, not only is there diastolic collapse of the right ventricular free wall (*arrow*), but also the entire heart moves anteriorly and the posterior pericardial space increases as the heart moves anteriorly within the pericardial sac. The four-chamber systolic (Fig. 10–27C) and diastolic (Fig. 10–27D) frames again show how the heart moves from right to left within the large fluid-filled pericardium. Figure 10–28 is a short-axis echocardiographic examination again demonstrating how the heart moves anteriorly with diastole in a patient with a large pericardial effusion.

This excessive cardiac motion associated with large pericardial effusions was first detected with M-mode echocardiography. Figure 10–29 demonstrates an M-mode echocardiogram of a patient with a large effusion showing striking cardiac displacement throughout the cardiac cycle: posterior motion of the heart with systole and upward or anterior motion with diastole. Occasionally, with the older M-mode technique, cardiac motion

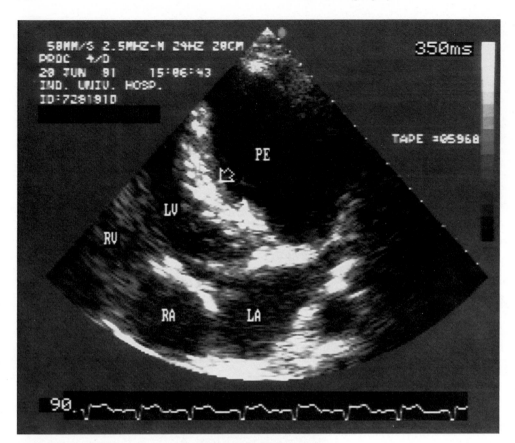

**Fig. 10–18.** Apical four-chamber echocardiogram of a patient with a large loculated pericardial effusion (PE) that causes collapse (*arrow*) of the free wall of the left ventricle (LV). RV = right ventricle; RA = right atrium; LA = left atrium.

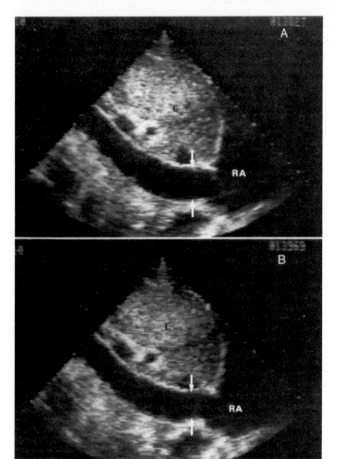

**Fig. 10–19.** A patient with inferior vena cava dilatation that does not vary with inspiration. Little difference is noted in the width of the inferior vena cava (*arrows*) with inspiration (*A*) and expiration (*B*). This finding is compatible with either cardiac tamponade or constrictive pericarditis. L = left atrium; RA = right atrium. (From Himelman, R.B., et al.: Septal bounce vena cava plethora, and pericardial adhesion: Informative two-dimensional echocardiographic signs of pericardial constriction. J. Am. Soc. Echocardiogr., *1*:333, 1988.)

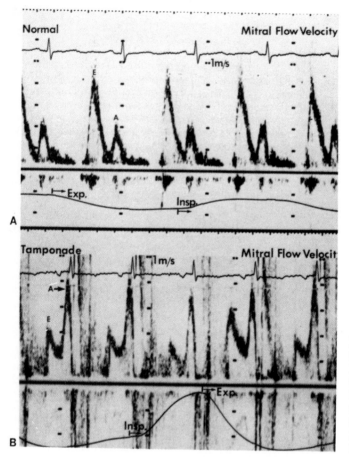

**Fig. 10–20.** Mitral flow velocity profiles from a normal control subject (*A*) and from a patient with cardiac tamponade (*B*). Minimal if any respiratory variation in mitral flow is evident in the normal subject. With tamponade, the first beat after the beginning of inspiration produces a decrease in the height of the early diastolic E velocity, and with the onset of expiration, there is an increase in this early diastolic velocity. (From Burstow, D.J., et al.: Cardiac tamponade: Characteristic Doppler observations. Mayo Clin. Proc., *64*:316, 1989.)

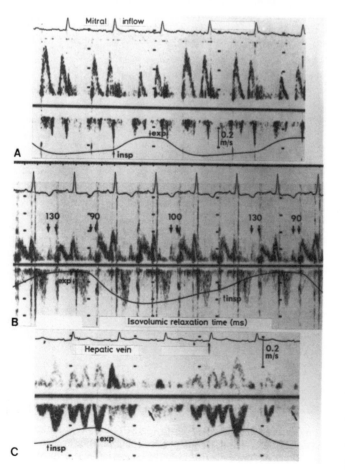

**Fig. 10–21.** Pulsed Doppler recordings of mitral inflow and hepatic venous flow in a patient with cardiac tamponade. *A* demonstrates how the early diastolic flow velocity decreases with inspiration and increases with expiration. *B* shows how the isovolumic relaxation time decreases with the onset of expiration and increases with inspiration. With expiration (*C*), there is a decrease in the hepatic venous flow. (From Hayes, S.N., Freeman, W.K., and Gersh, B.J.: Low pressure cardiac tamponade: Diagnosis facilitated by Doppler echocardiography. Br. Heart J., *63*:137, 1990.)

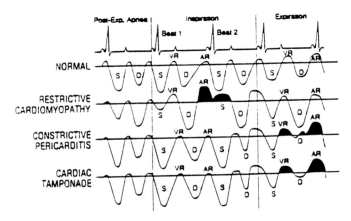

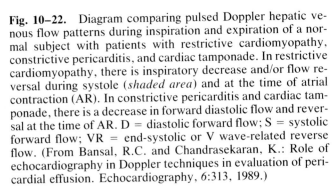

**Fig. 10–22.** Diagram comparing pulsed Doppler hepatic venous flow patterns during inspiration and expiration of a normal subject with patients with restrictive cardiomyopathy, constrictive pericarditis, and cardiac tamponade. In restrictive cardiomyopathy, there is inspiratory decrease and/or flow reversal during systole (*shaded area*) and at the time of atrial contraction (AR). In constrictive pericarditis and cardiac tamponade, there is a decrease in forward diastolic flow and reversal at the time of AR. D = diastolic forward flow; S = systolic forward flow; VR = end-systolic or V wave-related reverse flow. (From Bansal, R.C. and Chandrasekaran, K.: Role of echocardiography in Doppler techniques in evaluation of pericardial effusion. Echocardiography, 6:313, 1989.)

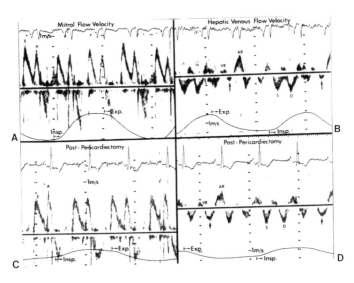

**Fig. 10–23.** Mitral and hepatic venous flow velocity profiles after pericardiocentesis (*A* and *B*) and after pericardiectomy (*C* and *D*) from a patient with cardiac tamponade in whom effusive-constrictive pericarditis was present at thoracotomy. Note persistent respiratory variation in mitral flow and substantial expiratory decrease in diastolic forward flow (*arrows*) in hepatic venous flow after pericardiocentesis (*A* and *B*). After pericardiectomy, respiratory variation in mitral flow velocity is minimal, and the velocity of hepatic venous diastolic forward flow (*arrows*) during expiration (Exp) is now normal. (From Berstow, D.J., et al.: Cardiac tamponade: Characteristic Doppler observations. Mayo Clin. Proc., *64*:322, 1989.)

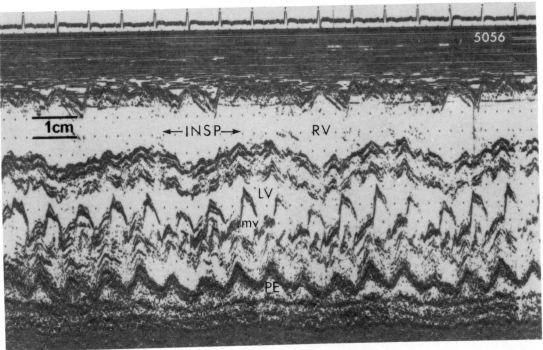

**Fig. 10–24.** M-mode echocardiogram of a patient with cardiac tamponade. During inspiration (INSP), the size of the right ventricle (RV) suddenly increases, and the size of the left ventricle (LV) decreases as the interventricular septum moves posteriorly. The total amplitude and opening of the mitral valve (mv) also decrease with inspiration. PE = pericardial effusion.

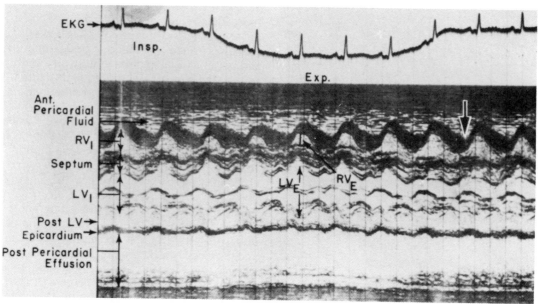

**Fig. 10–25.** M-mode echocardiogram of a patient with pericardial effusion and cardiac tamponade. During expiration, the right ventricle ($RV_E$) is diminished. Note also posterior motion of the right ventricular wall in diastole (*large arrow*). INSP = inspiration; Exp = expiration; $LV_E$ = left ventricle with expiration. (From Settle, H.P., et al.: Echocardiographic study of cardiac tamponade. Circulation, 56:951, 1977, by permission of the American Heart Association, Inc.)

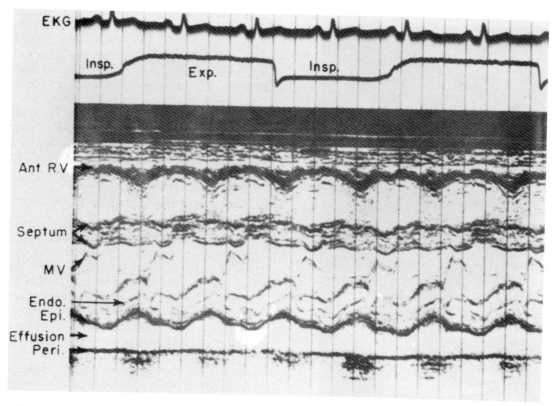

**Fig. 10–26.** Echocardiogram of the patient in Figure 10–25 after pericardiocentesis and relief of the cardiac tamponade. With removal of the pericardial fluid, the size of the right ventricle increases, the respiratory variation decreases, and the amount of posterior pericardial effusion decreases. The abnormal diastolic motion of the right ventricular wall seen in Figure 10–25 is no longer present. RV = right ventricle; MV = mitral valve; Endo = endocardium; Epi = epicardium; Peri = pericardium; Insp = inspiration; Exp = expiration. (From Settle, H.P., et al.: Echocardiographic study of cardiac tamponade. Circulation, 56: 951, 1977, by permission of the American Heart Association, Inc.)

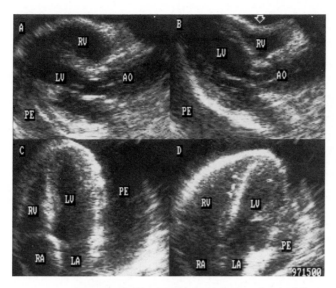

**Fig. 10–27.** Parasternal long-axis (*A* and *B*) and apical four-chamber (*C* and *D*) two-dimensional views of a patient with a large pericardial effusion and a "swinging heart." The long-axis view demonstrates how the heart moves in an anterior-posterior direction; the four-chamber view reveals right-left cardiac translation. This patient also has diastolic collapse of the right ventricle (*arrow*). RV = right ventricle; LV = left ventricle; AO = aorta; PE = pericardial effusion; RA = right atrium; LA = left atrium.

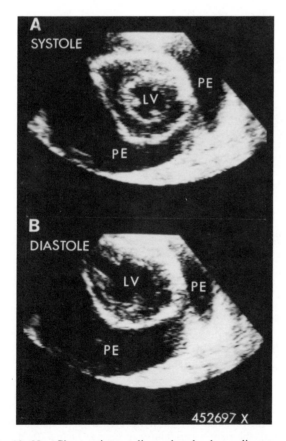

**Fig. 10–28.** Short-axis two-dimensional echocardiogram of a patient with a large pericardial effusion, demonstrating the shift in cardiac position from systole to diastole. PE = pericardial effusion; LV = left ventricle.

in patients with large pericardial effusions so distorted the echocardiogram that it was difficult to make the proper diagnosis. Figure 10–30 shows a patient with massive, principally anterior pericardial effusion. The amount of cardiac motion greatly distorts the pattern of cardiac echoes, making their identity difficult.

If one analyzes the pattern of motion in Figure 10–19, it is noted that the cycle of cardiac motion corresponds to two electrocardiographic cardiac cycles. In most areas, the QRS complex changes slightly as the position of the heart is altered by excessive motion.[75,76] Figure 10–31*A* shows another example of massive pericardial effusion whereby the entire heart is moving so that its position varies with every other electrical depolarization. The height of the electrocardiographic R wave alternates. With removal of a small amount of pericardial fluid (Fig. 10–31*B*), the alternating cardiac motion stops and the electrocardiographic alternation, or electrical alternans, also ceases. This echocardiographic finding in patients with pericardial effusion was instrumental in establishing the mechanism for electrical alternation in patients with pericardial effusion.[75–79]

Most of the patients, at least the adults, who exhibit excess cardiac motion on the echocardiogram have a pericardial effusion related to a malignancy.[80] Another cause is chronic tuberculous pericarditis, although this etiologic factor is not as common. A possible explanation for why these conditions produce excessive cardiac motion is because a "swinging heart" requires a large, chronically accumulated pericardial effusion and a minimum of adhesions. The bloody fluid, with its possibly increased lubricity, may permit the heart to move more freely. In children, swinging of the heart with pericardial effusion may be seen in association with benign viral pericarditis as well as malignancies.

As echocardiography has become more readily available and patients with pericardial effusion are detected sooner, the massive pericardial effusions that produce excessive cardiac motion and echocardiographic alternation are decreasing in frequency.

### Etiology of Pericardial Effusion

Clues can be obtained from the echocardiogram as to the possible etiology of pericardial effusion.[81,82] Some investigators have noted that grossly bloody pericardial effusions are relatively echogenic.[83,84] This finding might be expected because stagnant red cells should reflect more echoes than clear, serous pericardial fluid. The echogenicity of the fluid may be even greater if there is clot formation within the pericardial space.[85] Occasionally, spontaneous echoes have been noted within the pericardial fluid.[85a] In some cases, this finding is caused by gas-forming infection.[86,87] In other situations, the etiology of the spontaneous echoes has not been determined. Figure 10–32 shows an example of spontaneous echoes within pericardial fluid associated with pneumopericardium.[88] Frank clot within the pericardial sac is seen in Figure 10–33. The clot is obviously echogenic. In this case, the clot was detected with transesophageal echocardiography. One can also appreciate how the clot produces compression of the right atrium.

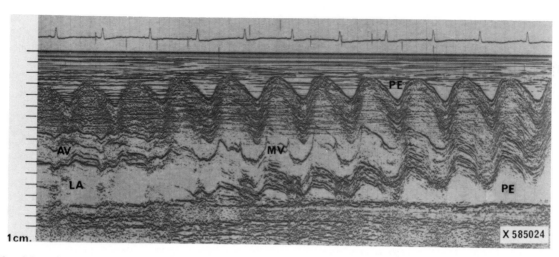

**Fig. 10-29.** M-mode scan of a patient with a large pericardial effusion. Note how the posterior echo-free space increases as the ultrasonic beam approaches the cardiac apex. The entire heart is moving vigorously, distorting the motion of all cardiac echoes. PE = pericardial effusion; MV = mitral valve; AV = aortic valve; LA = left atrium. (From Bonner, A.J., et al.: An unusual precordial pulse and sound associated with large pericardial effusion. Chest, *68:*829, 1975.)

A common cause of pericardial effusion is neoplastic involvement of the pericardium.[89,90] As already mentioned, excessive cardiac motion may be one of the clues that pericardial effusion is related to a neoplasm. Figure 10-34 shows a patient with a malignancy who had metastases to the visceral pericardium (*arrowhead, arrows*). These structures can be detected as echogenic masses attached to the visceral pericardium.[89] Figure 10-35 shows another example of a localized mass along the visceral pericardium. In this patient, the mass (M) is

seen in both the long-axis and short-axis views. Frequently, one detects only a thickened and sometimes irregular pericardium. Figure 10-36, identifies a patient with a thickened visceral pericardium. "Lumps and bumps" are visible all along the pericardium of this patient with malignant effusion.

Neoplasm adjacent to the pericardium can frequently be detected echocardiographically. Figure 10-37 shows a patient with a cystic mass (*arrowheads*) adjacent to the parietal pericardium. Pericardial effusion (PE) is also

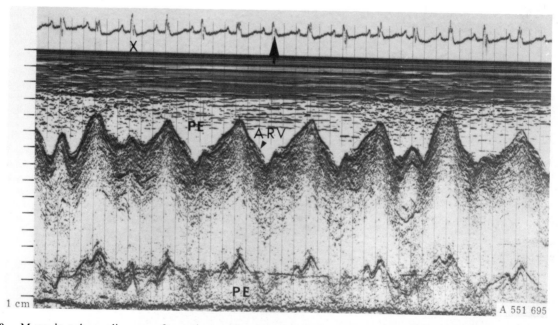

**Fig. 10-30.** M-mode echocardiogram of a patient with a massive pericardial effusion (PE). The anterior pericardial space is unusually large, and the echoes from the anterior right ventricular wall (ARV) are very echo-producing. The entire tracing is distorted because of excessive motion, and identification of the cardiac echoes can be confusing. The motion of the cardiac echoes is out of sequence with the electrocardiogram, which is distorted because of positional changes of the heart. The QRS marked X is different from that marked by an arrow. (From Chang, S.: M-mode Echocardiographic Techniques and Pattern Recognition. Philadelphia, Lea & Febiger, 1976.)

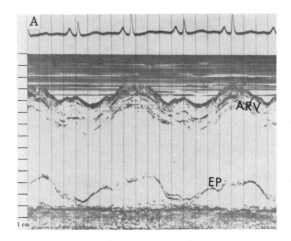

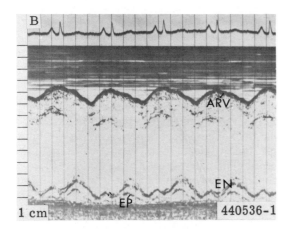

**Fig. 10–31.**  Echocardiogram of a patient with massive pericardial effusion. *A*, The anterior right ventricular echo (ARV) and the posterior left ventricular epicardial echo (EP) move essentially in similar directions. The position of the heart is slightly different with each cardiac cycle. The corresponding electrocardiogram shows classic electrical alternation. *B*, Following removal of some of the pericardial effusion, the cardiac excursions are synchronous with each electrical depolarization. Electrical alternation is no longer present. EN = posterior left ventricular endocardium.

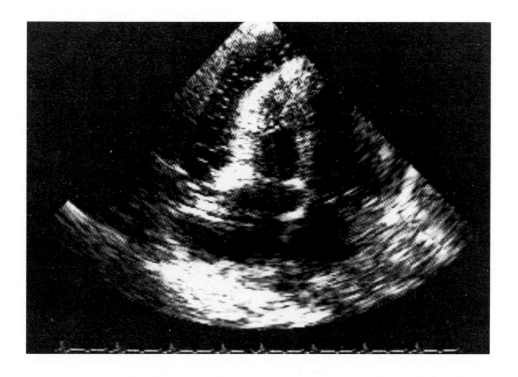

**Fig. 10–32.**  Two-dimensional echocardiogram illustrating echogenic bubbles within the pericardial space resulting from pneumopericardium. (From Bedotto, J.B., et al.: Echocardiographic diagnosis of pneumopericardium and hydropneumopericardium. J. Am. Soc. Echocardiogr., *1*:339, 1988.)

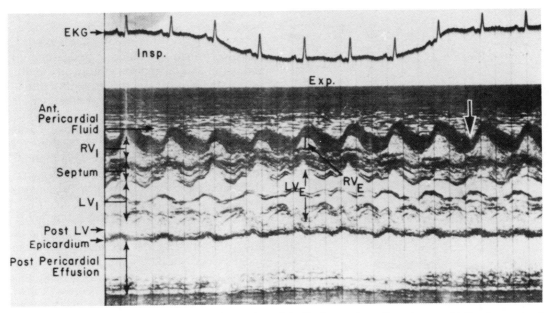

**Fig. 10–25.** M-mode echocardiogram of a patient with pericardial effusion and cardiac tamponade. During expiration, the right ventricle (RV$_E$) is diminished. Note also posterior motion of the right ventricular wall in diastole (*large arrow*). INSP = inspiration; Exp = expiration; LV$_E$ = left ventricle with expiration. (From Settle, H.P., et al.: Echocardiographic study of cardiac tamponade. Circulation, *56*:951, 1977, by permission of the American Heart Association, Inc.)

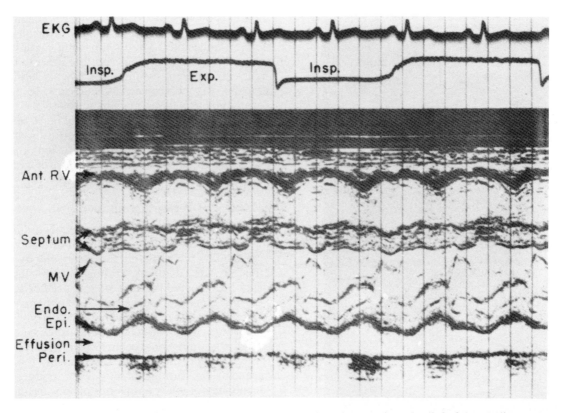

**Fig. 10–26.** Echocardiogram of the patient in Figure 10–25 after pericardiocentesis and relief of the cardiac tamponade. With removal of the pericardial fluid, the size of the right ventricle increases, the respiratory variation decreases, and the amount of posterior pericardial effusion decreases. The abnormal diastolic motion of the right ventricular wall seen in Figure 10–25 is no longer present. RV = right ventricle; MV = mitral valve; Endo = endocardium; Epi = epicardium; Peri = pericardium; Insp = inspiration; Exp = expiration. (From Settle, H.P., et al.: Echocardiographic study of cardiac tamponade. Circulation, *56*: 951, 1977, by permission of the American Heart Association, Inc.)

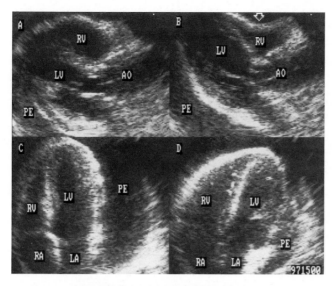

**Fig. 10–27.** Parasternal long-axis (*A* and *B*) and apical four-chamber (*C* and *D*) two-dimensional views of a patient with a large pericardial effusion and a "swinging heart." The long-axis view demonstrates how the heart moves in an anterior-posterior direction; the four-chamber view reveals right-left cardiac translation. This patient also has diastolic collapse of the right ventricle (*arrow*). RV = right ventricle; LV = left ventricle; AO = aorta; PE = pericardial effusion; RA = right atrium; LA = left atrium.

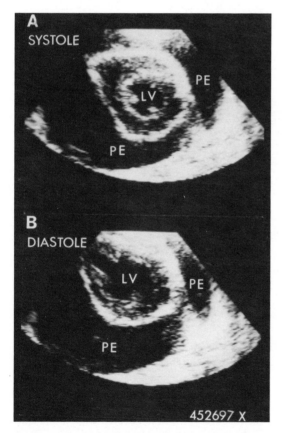

**Fig. 10–28.** Short-axis two-dimensional echocardiogram of a patient with a large pericardial effusion, demonstrating the shift in cardiac position from systole to diastole. PE = pericardial effusion; LV = left ventricle.

in patients with large pericardial effusions so distorted the echocardiogram that it was difficult to make the proper diagnosis. Figure 10–30 shows a patient with massive, principally anterior pericardial effusion. The amount of cardiac motion greatly distorts the pattern of cardiac echoes, making their identity difficult.

If one analyzes the pattern of motion in Figure 10–19, it is noted that the cycle of cardiac motion corresponds to two electrocardiographic cardiac cycles. In most areas, the QRS complex changes slightly as the position of the heart is altered by excessive motion.[75,76] Figure 10–31A shows another example of massive pericardial effusion whereby the entire heart is moving so that its position varies with every other electrical depolarization. The height of the electrocardiographic R wave alternates. With removal of a small amount of pericardial fluid (Fig. 10–31B), the alternating cardiac motion stops and the electrocardiographic alternation, or electrical alternans, also ceases. This echocardiographic finding in patients with pericardial effusion was instrumental in establishing the mechanism for electrical alternation in patients with pericardial effusion.[75–79]

Most of the patients, at least the adults, who exhibit excess cardiac motion on the echocardiogram have a pericardial effusion related to a malignancy.[80] Another cause is chronic tuberculous pericarditis, although this etiologic factor is not as common. A possible explanation for why these conditions produce excessive cardiac motion is because a "swinging heart" requires a large, chronically accumulated pericardial effusion and a minimum of adhesions. The bloody fluid, with its possibly increased lubricity, may permit the heart to move more freely. In children, swinging of the heart with pericardial effusion may be seen in association with benign viral pericarditis as well as malignancies.

As echocardiography has become more readily available and patients with pericardial effusion are detected sooner, the massive pericardial effusions that produce excessive cardiac motion and echocardiographic alternation are decreasing in frequency.

### Etiology of Pericardial Effusion

Clues can be obtained from the echocardiogram as to the possible etiology of pericardial effusion.[81,82] Some investigators have noted that grossly bloody pericardial effusions are relatively echogenic.[83,84] This finding might be expected because stagnant red cells should reflect more echoes than clear, serous pericardial fluid. The echogenicity of the fluid may be even greater if there is clot formation within the pericardial space.[85] Occasionally, spontaneous echoes have been noted within the pericardial fluid.[85a] In some cases, this finding is caused by gas-forming infection.[86,87] In other situations, the etiology of the spontaneous echoes has not been determined. Figure 10–32 shows an example of spontaneous echoes within pericardial fluid associated with pneumopericardium.[88] Frank clot within the pericardial sac is seen in Figure 10–33. The clot is obviously echogenic. In this case, the clot was detected with transesophageal echocardiography. One can also appreciate how the clot produces compression of the right atrium.

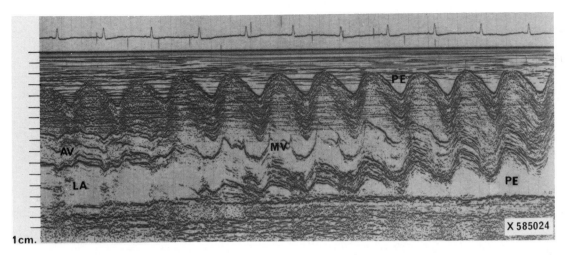

**Fig. 10–29.** M-mode scan of a patient with a large pericardial effusion. Note how the posterior echo-free space increases as the ultrasonic beam approaches the cardiac apex. The entire heart is moving vigorously, distorting the motion of all cardiac echoes. PE = pericardial effusion; MV = mitral valve; AV = aortic valve; LA = left atrium. (From Bonner, A.J., et al.: An unusual precordial pulse and sound associated with large pericardial effusion. Chest, *68*:829, 1975.)

A common cause of pericardial effusion is neoplastic involvement of the pericardium.[89,90] As already mentioned, excessive cardiac motion may be one of the clues that pericardial effusion is related to a neoplasm. Figure 10–34 shows a patient with a malignancy who had metastases to the visceral pericardium (*arrowhead, arrows*). These structures can be detected as echogenic masses attached to the visceral pericardium.[89] Figure 10–35 shows another example of a localized mass along the visceral pericardium. In this patient, the mass (M) is

seen in both the long-axis and short-axis views. Frequently, one detects only a thickened and sometimes irregular pericardium. Figure 10–36, identifies a patient with a thickened visceral pericardium. "Lumps and bumps" are visible all along the pericardium of this patient with malignant effusion.

Neoplasm adjacent to the pericardium can frequently be detected echocardiographically. Figure 10–37 shows a patient with a cystic mass (*arrowheads*) adjacent to the parietal pericardium. Pericardial effusion (PE) is also

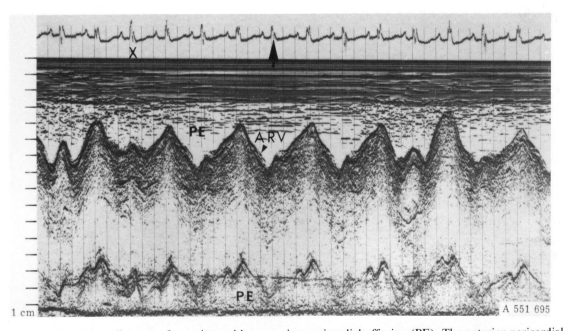

**Fig. 10–30.** M-mode echocardiogram of a patient with a massive pericardial effusion (PE). The anterior pericardial space is unusually large, and the echoes from the anterior right ventricular wall (ARV) are very echo-producing. The entire tracing is distorted because of excessive motion, and identification of the cardiac echoes can be confusing. The motion of the cardiac echoes is out of sequence with the electrocardiogram, which is distorted because of positional changes of the heart. The QRS marked X is different from that marked by an arrow. (From Chang, S.: M-mode Echocardiographic Techniques and Pattern Recognition. Philadelphia, Lea & Febiger, 1976.)

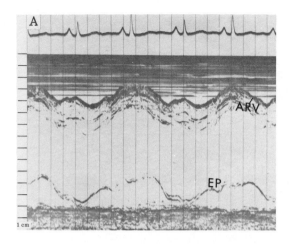

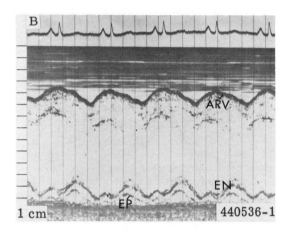

**Fig. 10–31.** Echocardiogram of a patient with massive pericardial effusion. *A*, The anterior right ventricular echo (ARV) and the posterior left ventricular epicardial echo (EP) move essentially in similar directions. The position of the heart is slightly different with each cardiac cycle. The corresponding electrocardiogram shows classic electrical alternation. *B*, Following removal of some of the pericardial effusion, the cardiac excursions are synchronous with each electrical depolarization. Electrical alternation is no longer present. EN = posterior left ventricular endocardium.

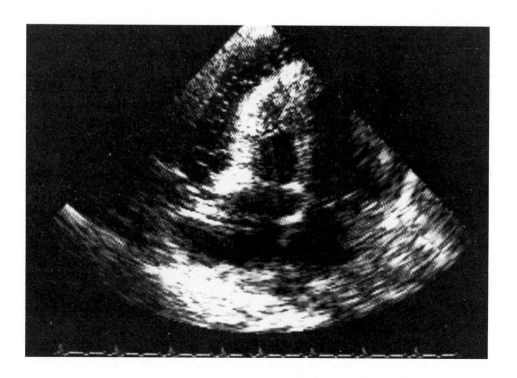

**Fig. 10–32.** Two-dimensional echocardiogram illustrating echogenic bubbles within the pericardial space resulting from pneumopericardium. (From Bedotto, J.B., et al.: Echocardiographic diagnosis of pneumopericardium and hydropneumopericardium. J. Am. Soc. Echocardiogr., *1*:339, 1988.)

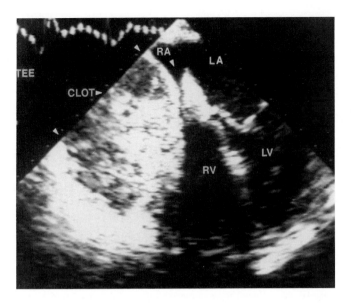

**Fig. 10–33.** Transesophageal echocardiogram showing a massive clot that severely compresses the right atrium (RA). LA = left atrium; RV = right ventricle; LV = left ventricle. (From Kochar, G.S., et al.: Right atrial compression in postoperative cardiac patients: Detection by transesophageal echocardiography. J. Am. Coll. Cardiol., *16*:513, 1990.)

present. A pericardial cyst,[92] a teratoma,[93,94] and a pheochromocytoma[95] have been detected within the pericardial sac with two-dimensional echocardiography.

Fibrinous stranding can provide a dramatic two-dimensional echocardiogram (Fig. 10–38).[96,96a] Visualization of these strands waving in the fluid produces a striking real-time echocardiographic study. Frequently, however, the fibrous strands are subtle (Fig. 10–39). In this patient, the strands are less echogenic, and one must look at multiple views to see them. The strands are not as mobile and seem to be firmly attached to both visceral and parietal pericardial layers.

## Pericardiocentesis

Several reports demonstrate the value of using echocardiography to assist in monitoring pericardiocentesis. M-mode echocardiography was used.[97] The technique was helpful in identifying the location of the needle by injecting saline or pericardial fluid through the needle, thereby creating a contrast echocardiogram (Fig. 10–40). If contrast echoes are noted within the pericardial space, the location of the needle is not intracardiac. Two-dimensional echocardiography is now used for monitoring pericardiocentesis.[98–102] This examination

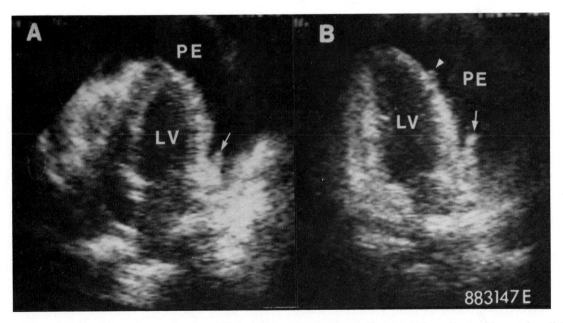

**Fig. 10–34.** Four-chamber (*A*) and two-chamber (*B*) two-dimensional echocardiograms of a patient with a pericardial effusion (PE) secondary to metastatic malignancy. Two implants (*arrows* and *arrowhead*) can be noted on the surface of the pericardium. LV = left ventricle.

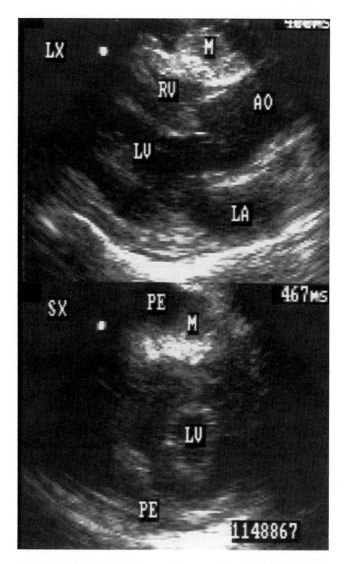

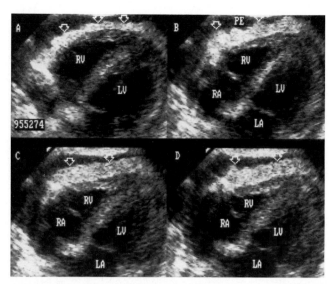

**Fig. 10–36.** Serial frames from a subcostal four-chamber examination of a patient with pericardial effusion (PE) and a thickened pericardium. "Lumps and bumps" (*arrows*) can be seen along the thickened visceral pericardium attached to the right ventricular free wall. RV = right ventricle; LV = left ventricle; RA = right atrium; LA = left atrium.

the needle. The blind, subcostal approach may not be the best approach for a given patient. An anterior pericardiocentesis is frequently preferable, but it may be hazardous without echocardiographic assistance. Physicians are also using echocardiography to monitor percutaneous pericardial biopsy.[106]

## ACUTE PERICARDITIS

Unless acute pericarditis is associated with pericardial effusion, the echocardiogram may be normal in patients with this abnormality. The sonographic examination may be helpful in a patient with known or suspected

**Fig. 10–35.** Echogenic mass (M) attached to the visceral pericardium of the right ventricular free wall. The mass can be seen in both the long-axis (LX) and short-axis (SX) views. RV = right ventricle; LV = left ventricle; AO = aorta; LA = left atrium; PE = pericardial effusion.

may be combined with contrast injections to assist in locating the point of the needle and noting the extent of the pericardial fluid. In one report, a negative contrast effect was produced by blood leaking into the pericardial space from a stab wound.[99] This finding helped to locate the site of the laceration. Pericardiocentesis-induced intrapericardial thrombi and intramyocardial hematomas[103] have also been noted echocardiographically.[104,105] It is not easy to identify the tip of the pericardiocentesis needle, even with two-dimensional echocardiography.[102] The shaft of the needle is not difficult to see, but one cannot be certain that the entire needle is being visualized.

Monitoring pericardiocentesis echocardiographically gives more latitude to the physician performing the procedure and added safety to the patient. Knowing the location of the fluid provides better options for inserting

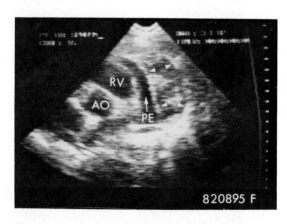

**Fig. 10–37.** Short-axis two-dimensional echocardiogram through the base of the heart in a patient with pericardial effusion (PE) and a cystic mass (*arrowheads*) adjacent to the parietal pericardium. RV = right ventricle; AO = aorta.

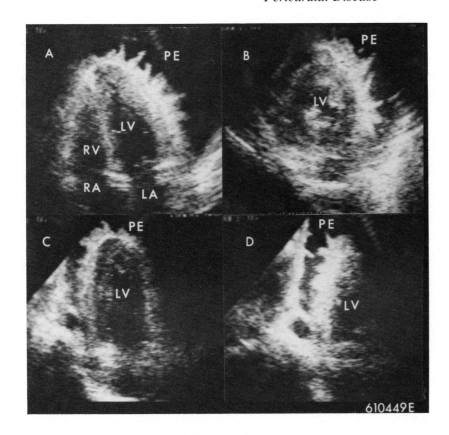

**Fig. 10–38.** Apical four-chamber (*A*), short-axis (*B*), apical two-chamber (*C*), and modified two-chamber (*D*) views of a patient with fibrinous pericarditis. The pericardial effusion (PE) is filled with fibrinous strands attached to the pericardium. RV = right ventricle; LV = left ventricle; RA = right atrium; LA = left atrium.

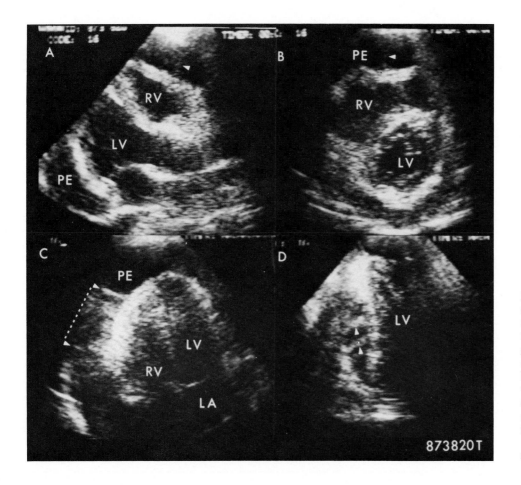

**Fig. 10–39.** Long-axis (*A*), short-axis (*B*), four-chamber (*C*), and two-chamber (*D*) two-dimensional echocardiograms of a patient with pericardial effusion (PE) and fibrous strands between the visceral and parietal pericardia. In some views, the fibrous strands (*arrowheads*) are subtle. RV = right ventricle; LV = left ventricle; LA = left atrium.

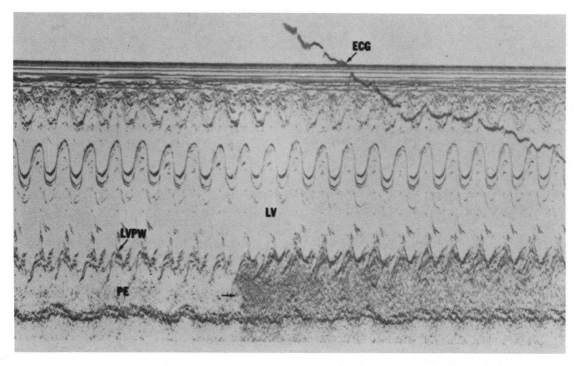

**Fig. 10–40.** Echocardiogram taken during pericardiocentesis, at which time contrast material was injected into the pericardial sac. The echo-producing contrast (*arrow*) can be seen in the space occupied by the pericardial effusion (PE). LV = left ventricle; LVPW = left ventricular posterior wall. (From Chandraratna, P.A.N., et al.: Echocardiographic contrast studies during pericardiocentesis. Ann. Intern. Med., *87*:199, 1977.)

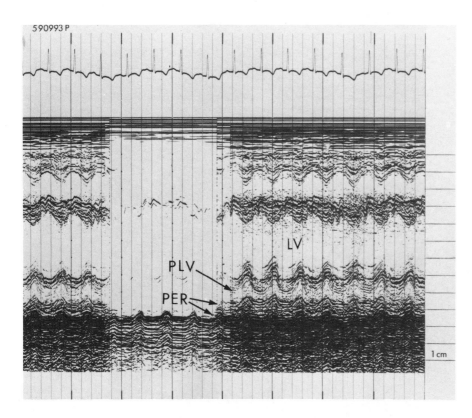

**Fig. 10–41.** M-mode echocardiogram of a patient with a thickened pericardium. A band of dense echoes originating from the pericardium (PER) can be seen posterior to the relatively echo-free space of the posterior left ventricular myocardium (PLV). All pericardial echoes move synchronously and exhibit the same amplitude of motion as the epicardium of the posterior left ventricular wall. LV = left ventricle.

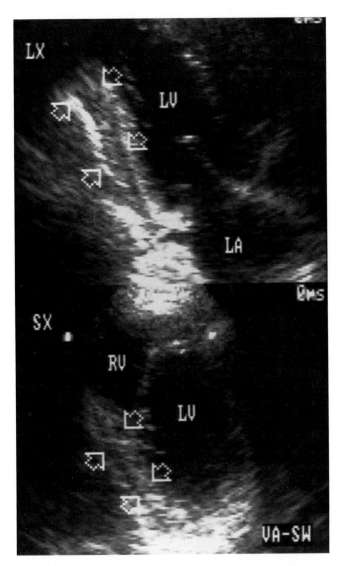

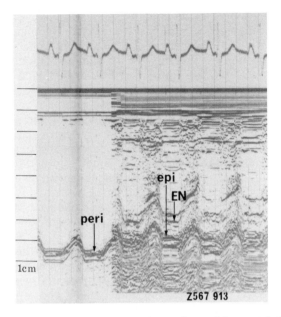

**Fig. 10–43.** Echocardiogram of a patient with constrictive pericarditis. Filling abruptly ceases in early diastole with virtually flat endocardial (EN), epicardial (epi), and pericardial (peri) echoes during the latter two thirds of diastole. The distance between the epicardial and pericardial echoes is thought to represent the thickness of the pericardium.

**Fig. 10–42.** Apical long-axis (LX) and short-axis (SX) two-dimensional echocardiograms of a patient with a thickened pericardium and constrictive pericarditis. The thickened pericardium (*arrows*) can be seen along the posterior wall of the left ventricle (LV) in the long-axis view and the left ventricle and right ventricle (RV) in the short-axis view. LA = left atrium.

acute pericarditis because finding pericardial fluid enhances the diagnosis. On the other hand, failure to find pericardial effusion or any other echocardiographic abnormality does not exclude the possibility of acute pericarditis.

## THICKENED PERICARDIUM

It is relatively easy to detect a thickened pericardium in the presence of pericardial effusion.[107,108] Several examples of obviously thickened pericardia have been illustrated (see Figs. 10–1, 10–34, 10–36, and 10–38). The major difficulty encountered with echocardiography is in the detection of a thickened pericardium without an

effusion. Such an abnormality has been described with both M-mode and two-dimensional echocardiography,[109,110] although the reliability of this echocardiographic diagnosis is questionable. Figure 10–41 demonstrates an M-mode echocardiogram with a strikingly thickened pericardium. The pericardium is echogenic and is closely adherent to the posterior left ventricular wall. No intervening fluid is present. One cannot be absolutely certain that the apparently thickened pericardium is not an echogenic pericardial effusion with adhesions; however, the recording does not represent an uncomplicated pericardial effusion. The intensity of the pericardial echoes certainly is suggestive of something other than homogeneous pericardial fluid. Figure 10–42 shows a two-dimensional echocardiogram of a patient with a thickened pericardium and constriction. In these long-axis and short-axis views, one can see a linear, bright echo that is 1 cm or so away from the posterior ventricular myocardium. This echo and the left ventricular epicardial echo represent the borders of the thickened pericardium (*arrows*).

Despite isolated reports of the utility of echocardiography in detecting a thickened pericardium, other imaging methods, such as computerized tomography, are probably superior and more reliable for this diagnosis. As a result, echocardiography is not used routinely for this purpose.

## CONSTRICTIVE PERICARDITIS

Although echocardiography is not reliable in detecting a thickened pericardium, many echocardiographic signs are indicative of constrictive pericarditis.[111] M-mode echocardiography is still a fairly useful technique for determining this diagnosis.[112-120] One M-mode sign of constriction is a flattening of the mid- and late diastolic motion of the left ventricular free wall. Figure 10–43 demonstrates an echocardiogram of a patient with constrictive pericarditis. The systolic and early diastolic motion of the posterior left ventricular wall and pericardium are normal; however, after early ventricular filling, the left ventricular wall abruptly stops and becomes flat. No gradual downward motion is noted in mid-diastole or with atrial systole. This finding in patients with constrictive pericarditis has been noted by many investigators,[115,118,120,121] some of whom used digitized M-mode recordings.[122] The sign, however, is not pathognomonic for constriction.

A rapid early diastolic, or E to F, slope of the mitral valve has also been noted in patients with constrictive pericarditis.[109,116,117] Figure 10–44 illustrates two mitral valve recordings from the same patient whose tracings appear in Figure 10–43. There is rapid and early closure of the mitral valve (Fig. 10–44B). At other times, a more normal mitral valve can be appreciated (Fig. 10–44A). The rapid, early ventricular filling can also be noted on an M-mode recording of the aorta.[112] Under these circumstances, there is a sharp downward motion of the posterior aortic root in early diastole. All of these M-mode signs reflect early, rapid filling of the left ventricle and abrupt cessation of filling caused by the constricting effect of the thickened pericardium.

Interventricular septal motion may also be abnormal in patients with constrictive pericarditis.[113,114,116,123]

Figure 10–40 shows an example of this abnormal septal motion. The principle finding is an exaggerated anterior motion of the septum with atrial filling. Because the posterior free wall of the left ventricle is unable to expand properly, an increase in left ventricular volume with atrial systole produces a displacement of the septum toward the lower pressure right ventricle. The anterior motion of the left septum (LS) occurs at the end of the electrocardiographic P wave (*arrow*). This timing should be distinguished from that which occurs with a right ventricular volume overload. In the latter situation, the brisk anterior septal motion occurs after the onset of depolarization.

Another M-mode sign of constrictive pericarditis involving the interventricular septum is a double component of septal motion during atrial systole.[113,114] Before the abrupt anterior motion that occurs at the end of the P wave (*arrow*) (Fig. 10–45), one sees posterior displacement of the septum at the middle of the P wave (Fig. 10–46). This atrial systolic notch is in addition to an early diastolic notch, which is an exaggeration of the normal diastolic dip with early ventricular filling. An early diastolic notch can also be seen in Figure 10–45. The changes in interventricular septal motion are a result of the interrelationship of right and left ventricular pressures and filling of a heart whose free walls cannot expand because of the constricting pericardium.[91]

Yet another M-mode echocardiographic finding in patients with constrictive pericarditis is premature opening of the pulmonary valve.[112,118,124,125] Figure 10–47 demonstrates a pre- and postpericardiectomy pulmonary valve echocardiogram in a patient with constriction.

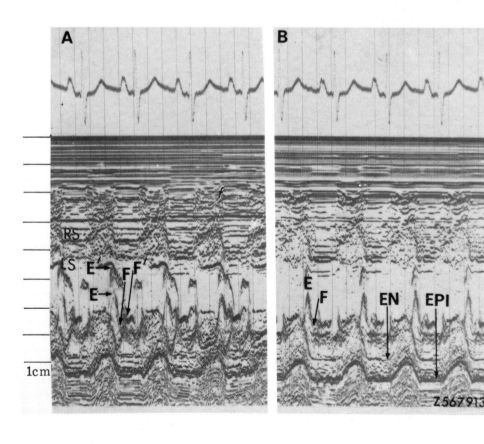

**Fig. 10–44.** Mitral valve and left ventricular echocardiograms of the patient in Figure 10–43. Several echoes are from the mitral valve, one of which closes rapidly with a steep diastolic closing slope (E–F). Another mitral valve echo shows a slightly slower slope (E'–F'). The echocardiograms again show flat motion of the left ventricular echoes during diastole. RS = right side of septum; LS = left side of septum; EN = posterior left ventricular endocardium; EPI = posterior left ventricular epicardium.

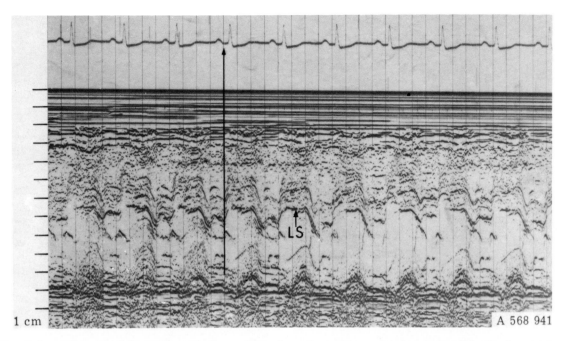

**Fig. 10–45.** Echocardiogram of the interventricular septum of a patient with constrictive pericarditis. During atrial systole and before ventricular depolarization (*arrow*), there is a brisk anterior motion of the septum (LS) that remains anterior throughout ventricular ejection. The septum then moves downward or posteriorly with ventricular relaxation.

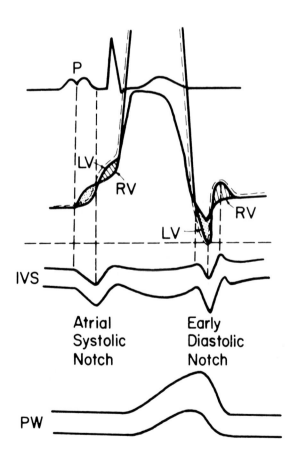

**Fig. 10–46.** Diagram illustrating the interventricular septal (IVS) motion in patients with constrictive pericarditis. The atrial systolic notch and early diastolic notch are thought to be a result of the interrelationship of the left ventricular (LV) and right ventricular (RV) pressures. P = electrocardiographic P wave; PW = posterior left ventricular wall. (From Tei, C., et al.: Atrial systolic notching on the interventricular septal echogram: An echocardiographic sign of constrictive pericarditis. J. Am. Coll. Cardiol., *1*:907, 1983.)

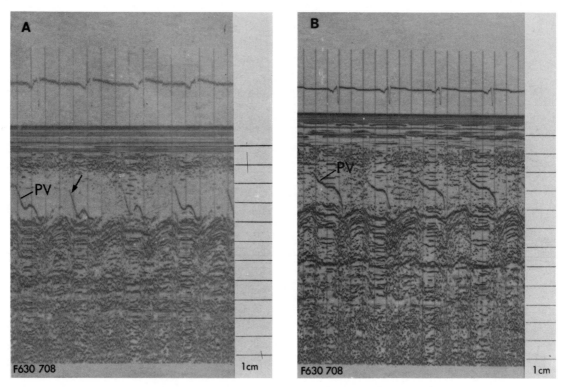

**Fig. 10–47.** Pulmonary valve echocardiograms from a patient with constrictive pericarditis before and after surgical removal of the pericardium. *A*, Preoperatively, there is a rapid downward motion (*arrow*) of the pulmonary valve (PV) prior to atrial systole. *B*, Postoperatively, there is only the normal gradual posterior motion of the pulmonary valve during diastole.

Prior to surgical removal of the thickened pericardium, there is a brisk, downward opening motion of the pulmonary valve (*arrow*) before the electrocardiographic P wave. This premature opening presumably results from an increase in right ventricular diastolic pressure in mid-diastole. The right ventricular pressure rises abruptly and transiently exceeds the pulmonary artery pressure, permitting opening of the pulmonary valve. After relief of the constriction (Fig. 10–47*B*), the premature opening of the valve is no longer seen.[118,124] This echocardiographic finding is not common and probably indicates an elevation of right ventricular diastolic pressure.

Of several two-dimensional echocardiographic signs of pericardial constriction,[126] a dilated inferior vena cava without respiratory variation (Fig. 10–19) is one of the more common findings. This sign is indicative of high pressure in the right atrium and is thus nonspecific. Figure 10–48 shows another two-dimensional echocardiographic sign of pericardial constriction. In this case, the abnormal motion of the interventricular septum noted on the M-mode tracing can be detected on the two-dimensional echocardiogram. The apical four-chamber view reveals a to-and-fro motion of the interventricular septum in a heart that is encased in a rigid pericardial covering. In real time, the septal motion appears as a "septal bounce."[126] Displacement of the interatrial septum toward the left atrium with inspiration is another reported sign of constrictive pericarditis.[127] Another sign relies on looking at the relationship of the visceral and parietal pericardia with two-dimensional echocardi-

ography. Normally, one can see the two structures sliding over each other. In patients with constrictive pericarditis, these two layers of tissue are adherent and do not move independently.[126] One group of authors has noted that the angle between the posterior left ventricular wall and posterior left atrium is decreased with pericardial constriction (Fig. 10–49).[128] The theory behind this sign is that the thickened, constricting pericardium affects the posterior left ventricle more than the posterior left atrium. Thus, the posterior left atrial wall can expand at a more acute angle to the left ventricular wall. The reliability of this sign has yet to be determined.

Considerable interest has been generated in using Doppler recordings to make the diagnosis of constrictive pericarditis.[129,130] The Doppler signs are similar to those noted in persons with cardiac tamponade. Figure 10–50 shows Doppler recordings before and after a pericardiectomy. With constriction, early mitral flow is reduced with the onset of inspiration. In addition, the isovolumic relaxation time (IVRT) is prolonged. With expiration, mitral flow returns to normal and the IVRT shortens. A reciprocal relationship exists with tricuspid flow. With the onset of expiration (*arrows*), early tricuspid flow is diminished. Both of these flow patterns are normalized after pericardiectomy (Fig. 10–50*B*).

Systemic venous flow is also altered in the presence of constrictive pericarditis.[129] In Figure 10–22, the hepatic venous flow appears to be similar in cardiac tamponade and in constrictive pericarditis. In this diagram, the systolic flow velocity is somewhat larger than the diastolic

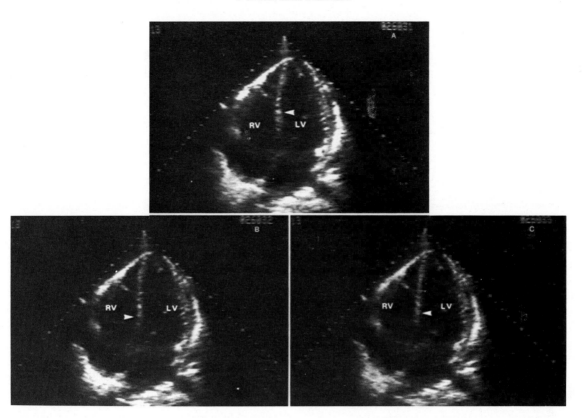

**Fig. 10–48.** Sequential frames from an apical four-chamber examination in a patient with constrictive pericarditis. Arrowheads show rapid to and fro changes in septal curvature, which appears as a "septal bounce" in real time. RV = right ventricle; LV = left ventricle. (From Himelman, R.B., et al.: Septal bounce vena cava plethora, and pericardial adhesion: Informative two-dimensional echocardiographic signs in the diagnosis of pericardial constriction. J. Am. Soc. Echocardiogr., *1*:333, 1988.)

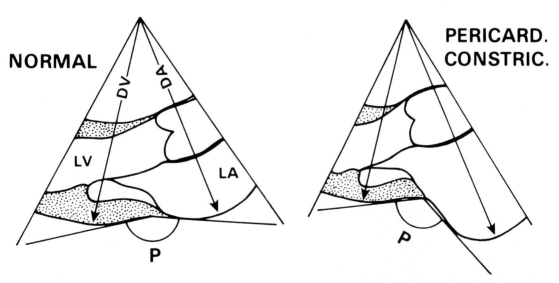

**Fig. 10–49.** Diagram showing how the angle (P) and the distances from the transducer to the posterior left atrial wall (DA) and the left ventricular wall (DV) can be used to differentiate the normal relationship of the posterior left ventricular and the left atrial walls from that with pericardial constriction. With pericardial constriction, the angle P is smaller and the difference between DA and DV is greater than in normal subjects. LV = left ventricle; LA = left atrium. (From D'Cruz, I.A., et al.: Abnormal left ventricular-left atrial posterior wall contour: A new two-dimensional echocardiographic sign in constrictive pericarditis. Am. Heart J., *118*:129, 1989.)

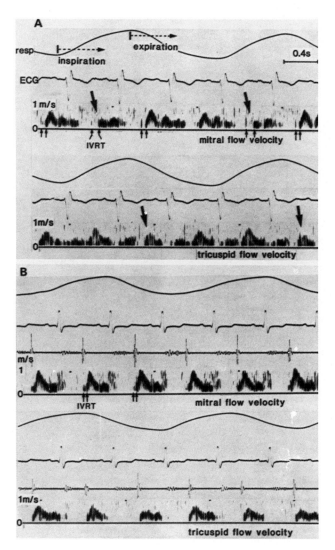

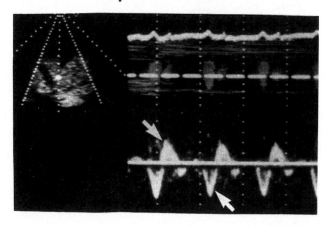

## PERICARDIAL CONSTRICTION

### hepatic vein

### RA pressure

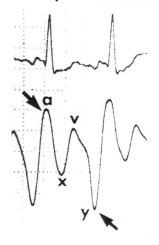

**Fig. 10–50.** Mitral and tricuspid flow velocity recordings in a patient before and after pericardiectomy for constrictive pericarditis. With constriction (*A*), early mitral flow is reduced (*arrow*) with the onset of inspiration. In addition, the isovolumic relaxation time (IVRT) is prolonged. With expiration, mitral flow returns to normal and the IVRT shortens. There is a reciprocal relationship with tricuspid flow. After pericardiectomy (*B*), the flow patterns return to normal and little variation is noted with respiration. (From Hatle, L.K., et al.: Differentiation of constrictive pericarditis and restrictive cardiomyopathy by Doppler echocardiography. Circulation, *79:* 357, 1989, by permission of the American Heart Association, Inc.)

**Fig. 10–51.** Pulsed Doppler recording of hepatic venous flow and right atrial (RA) pressure in a patient with pericardial constriction. The pulsed Doppler recording mirrors the right atrial pressure tracing. The arrows point to the prominent *a* wave (with flow reversal) and to a deep y descent (with increased forward flow) and the corresponding changes in the right atrial pressure. (From Gupta, M.K. and Sasson, Z.: The mechanisms and importance of tricuspid regurgitation and hepatic pulsations in dilated cardiomyopathy: A review. Echocardiography, *8:*199, 1991.)

velocity in both constrictive pericarditis and cardiac tamponade. Other investigators, however, have suggested that the diastolic flow exceeds the systolic flow in patients with constrictive pericarditis. Figure 10–51 shows an example of hepatic venous flow and right atrial pressure in a patient with pericardial constriction. Note a downward, early diastolic flow or Y descent. The early systolic, downward motion is barely seen. The other striking finding is reversal of flow with atrial systole (*arrow*).

Unfortunately, the literature is still somewhat confusing regarding the use of Doppler recordings to differentiate cardiac tamponade from constriction and restrictive cardiomyopathy. The systemic venous pattern with increased diastolic flow is similar to what other authors have recognized with restrictive cardiomyopathy. The major differentiating feature is the lack of respiratory variation with restrictive cardiomyopathy versus tamponade and constrictive pericarditis. It should be noted, however, that other conditions, such as chronic obstructive lung disease, also produce respiratory variation in Doppler recordings. A possible differentiating point is that with constrictive pericarditis, the respiratory changes occur with the first cardiac beat following the onset of inspiration or expiration. With lung disease, the changes are more gradual, occurring later in the respiratory cycle.[131]

Figure 10–52 is from a study distinguishing restrictive cardiomyopathy from constrictive pericarditis using pulmonary venous flow.[131,132] In this illustration, the systolic and diastolic flow velocities are about equal with constriction, whereas with restrictive cardiomyopathy, the diastolic flow velocity is considerably higher than the systolic velocity.

In summary, there are numerous echocardiographic signs for constrictive pericarditis.[133] No one finding is pathognomonic for the entity. It is best to initiate a complete echocardiographic study including M-mode, Doppler, and two-dimensional techniques. One should try to find as many of the signs of constriction as possible. Certainly the greater the number of such findings, the higher the likelihood of a correct diagnosis.

## PERICARDIAL CYSTS

In a few reports, echocardiography was used to identify pericardial cysts.[92] This abnormality usually occurs at the right atrial border and is in an area frequently difficult to detect with a transthoracic echocardiographic study. Theoretically, transesophageal echocardiography may be able to detect this abnormality more readily. On the other hand, the radiographic diagnosis is reasonably clear and echocardiography is not often the technique chosen to make the differential diagnosis. Figure 10–53 shows one example of a pericardial cyst that was more posterior and lateral than usual. One can detect the echo-free space readily on the long-axis and short-axis examinations. This entity can be distinguished from pericardial effusion because it is more localized and has a spherical configuration.

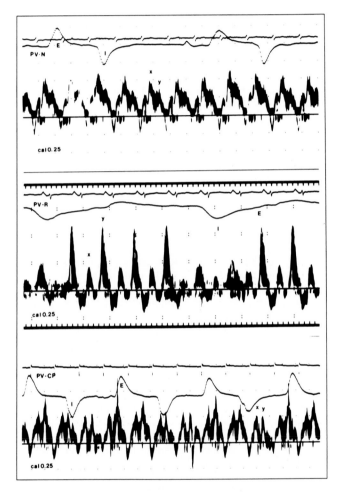

**Fig. 10–52.** Transesophageal pulsed Doppler recordings of pulmonary venous flow velocities in a patient with normal flow (PV-N, *A*), a patient with restrictive cardiomyopathy (PV-R, *B*), and a patient with constrictive pericarditis (PV-CP, *C*). Pulmonary venous systolic flow velocity (x) and diastolic flow velocity (y) are both toward the left atrium and are inscribed above the baseline. Inspiration (I) is indicated by a negative deflection and expiration (E) is indicated by a positive deflection using nasal capnometry. The electrocardiogram is positioned at the top of each recording (see text for details). (From Schiavone, W.A., et al.: Transesophageal Doppler echocardiographic demonstration of pulmonary venous flow velocity in restrictive cardiomyopathy and constrictive pericarditis. Am. J. Cardiol., *63*:1286, 1989.)

## ABSENT PERICARDIUM

The normal pericardium exerts considerable influence on cardiac motion. Besides providing stability to the location of the heart within the chest, the pericardium also limits dilatation of the chambers. After surgical removal of the pericardium, the heart frequently expands. Posterior left ventricular wall motion may become exaggerated. Patients who have congenital absence of the left pericardium also exhibit excessive motion of the poste-

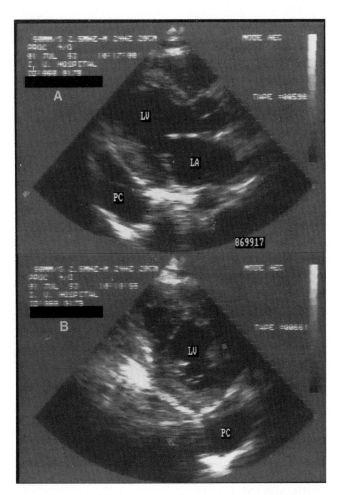

**Fig. 10–53.** Long-axis (*A*) and short-axis (*B*) echocardiograms of a patient with a pericardial cyst (PC) posterior to the left ventricular wall. LV = left ventricle; LA = left atrium.

rior left ventricular wall.[134,135] One of the consequences is that excessive cardiac motion can influence the pattern of motion of the entire heart. The heart also shifts to the left, often leaving more of the right ventricle visible than is usual on a routine left parasternal echocardiogram. The resultant excessive cardiac motion distorts the cardiac echoes, especially affecting the interventricular septum. With ventricular systole, the exaggerated posterior left ventricular wall motion produces anterior displacement of the interventricular septum. Thus, with congenital absence of the left pericardium, one notes dilatation of the right ventricle, excessive posterior left ventricular wall motion, and paradoxic motion of the interventricular septum. These findings may simulate right ventricular volume overload.[104] Fortunately, other clinical and echocardiographic signs help with the differential diagnosis.

With partial absence of the pericardium, the left side of the heart is usually uncovered by the pericardial defect. The left atrium can protrude through the missing pericardial tissue. As a result, an enlarged left atrial appendage[136] or even a left atrial aneurysm[137–139] may be

present. Both abnormalities have been detected with two-dimensional echocardiography.

## REFERENCES

1. Feigenbaum, H., Waldhausen, J.A., and Hyde, L.P.: Ultrasound diagnosis of pericardial effusion. JAMA, *191*: 107, 1965.
2. Feigenbaum, H., Zaky, A., and Waldhausen, J.A.: Use of ultrasound in the diagnosis of pericardial effusion. Ann. Intern. Med., *65*:443, 1966.
3. Goldberg, B.B., Ostrum, B.J., and Isard, J.J.: Ultrasonic determination of pericardial effusion. JAMA, *202*:103, 1967.
4. Klein, J.J. and Segal, B.L.: Pericardial effusion diagnosed by reflected ultrasound. Am. J. Cardiol., *22*:57, 1968.
5. Moss, A. and Bruhn, F.: The echocardiogram: An ultrasound technic for the detection of pericardial effusion. N. Engl. J. Med., *274*:380, 1966.
6. Edler, I.: Diagnostic use of ultrasound in heart disease. Acta Med. Scand., *308*:32, 1955.
7. Rifkin, R.D., Isner, J.M., Carter, B.L., and Bankoff, M.S.: Combined posteroanterior subepicardial fat simulating the echocardiographic diagnosis of pericardial effusion. J. Am. Coll. Cardiol., *3*:1333, 1984.
8. Wada, T., Honda, M., and Matsuyama, S.: Extra echo spaces: Ultrasonography and computerized tomography correlations. Br. Heart J., *47*:430, 1982.
9. Isner, J.M., Carter, B.L., Roberts, W.C., and Bankoff, M.S.: Subepicardial adipose tissue producing echocardiographic appearance of pericardial effusion. Am. J. Cardiol., *51*:565, 1983.
10. Savage, D.D., Garrison, R.J., Brand, F., Anderson, S.J., Castelli, W.P., Kannel, W.B., and Feinlieb, M.: Prevalence and correlates of posterior extra echocardiographic spaces in a free-living population based sample (the Framingham Study). Am. J. Cardiol., *51*:1207, 1983.
11. Feigenbaum, H.: Echocardiographic diagnosis of pericardial effusion. Am. J. Cardiol., *26*:475, 1970.
12. Abbasi, A.S., Ellis, N., and Flynn, J.U.: Echocardiographic M-scan technique in the diagnosis of pericardial effusion. JCU, *1*:300, 1973.
13. Lemire, F., Tajik, A.J., Giuliani, E.R., Gau, G.T., and Schattenberg, T.T.: Further echocardiographic observations in pericardial effusion. Mayo Clin. Proc., *51*:13, 1976.
14. Tajik, A.J.: Echocardiography in pericardial effusion. Am. J. Med., *63*:29, 1977.
15. Simpson, I.A., Munsch, C., Smith, E.E.J., and Parker, D.J.: Pericardial haemorrhage causing right atrial compression after cardiac surgery: Role of transesophageal echocardiography. Br. Heart J., *65*:355, 1991.
16. Torelli, J., Marwick, T.H., and Salcedo, E.E.: Left atrial tamponade: Diagnosis by transesophageal echocardiography. J. Am. Soc. Echocardiogr., *4*:413, 1991.
17. Weintraub, A.R., Schwartz, S.L., Smith, J., Hsu, T-L., and Pandian, N.G.: Intracardiac two-dimensional echocardiography in patients with pericardial effusion and cardiac tamponade. J. Am. Soc. Echocardiogr., *4*:571, 1991.
18. Alfonso, F., Zamorano, J., Castanon, J., Gil-Aguado, M., Rodrigo, J.L., Macaya, C., and Zarco, P.: Postoperative pericardial hematoma causing localized cardiac tam-

ponade and presenting echocardiographically as a right atrial mass. Am. Heart J., *122*:252, 1991.

19. Nootens, M., Ford, K., and Devries, S.: Utility of contrast echocardiography in the evaluation of a suspected right atrial mass. Am. J. Cardiol., *69*:833, 1992.

20. Beppu, S., Ikegami, K., Tanaka, N., Kumon, K., Izumi, S., Nakajima, S., Nakatani, S., Miyatake, K., and Nimura, Y.: Cardiac tamponade as a complication of open heart surgery: The clinical significance and diagnostic value of transesophageal echocardiography. J. Cardiol., *21*:124, 1991.

21. Kochar, G.S., Jacobs, L.E., and Kotler, M.N.: Right atrial compression in postoperative cardiac patients: Detection by transesophageal echocardiography. J. Am. Coll. Cardiol., *16*:511, 1990.

22. Thompson, R.C., Finck, S.J., Leventhal, J.P., and Safford, R.E.: Right-to-left shunt across a patent foramen ovale caused by cardiac tamponade: Diagnosis by transesophageal echocardiography. Mayo Clin. Proc., *66*:391, 1991.

22a. Musselman, D.R., Dehmer, G.J., Hoffman, Jr., B.J., and Hinderliter, A.L.: Localized right atrial tamponade and right-to-left shunting as a complication of pericarditis after myocardial infarction. Am. Heart J., *125*:241, 1983.

22b. Musselman, D.R., Dehmer, G.J., Hoffman, B.J., and Hinderliter, A.L.: Localized right atrial tamponade and right-to-left shunting as a complication of pericarditis after myocardial infarction. Am. Heart J., *125*:241, 1993.

23. D'Cruz, I.A., Macander, P.J., Gross, C.M., and Pai, G.M.: Distention of the oblique pericardial sinus in tamponade due to loculated posterior pericardial effusion. Am. J. Cardiol., *65*:1520, 1990.

24. Haaz, W.S., Mintz, G.S., Kotler, M.N., Parry, W., and Segal, B.L.: Two dimensional echocardiographic recognition of the descending thoracic aorta: Value in differentiating pericardial from pleural effusion. Am. J. Cardiol., *46*:739, 1980.

25. Lewandowski, B.J., Jaffer, N.M., and Winsberg, F.: Relationship between the pericardial and pleural spaces in cross-sectional imaging. JCU, *9*:271, 1981.

26. Eisenberg, M.J., Oken, K., Guerrero, S., Saniei, M.A., and Schiller, N.B.: Prognostic value of echocardiography in hospitalized patients with pericardial effusion. Am. J. Cardiol., *70*:934, 1992.

27. Horowitz, M.S., Schultz, C.S., Stinson, E.B., Harrison, D.C., and Popp, R.L.: Sensitivity and specificity of echocardiographic diagnosis of pericardial effusion. Circulation, *50*:239, 1974.

28. Parameswaran, R. and Goldberg, H.: Echocardiographic quantitation of pericardial effusion. Chest, *83*:767, 1983.

29. D'Cruz, I., Prabhu, R., Cohen, H.C., and Glick, G.: Potential pitfalls in quantification of pericardial effusions by echocardiography. Br. Heart J., *39*:529, 1977.

30. D'Cruz, I.A. and Hoffman, P.K.: A new cross sectional echocardiographic method for estimating the volume of large pericardial effusions. Br. Heart J., *66*:448, 1991.

31. Shina, S., Yaginuma, T., Kondo, K., Kawai, N., and Hosoda, S.: Echocardiographic evaluation of impending cardiac tamponade. J. Cardiogr., *9*:555, 1979.

32. Armstrong, W.F., Schilt, B.F., Helper, D.J., Dillon, J.C., and Feigenbaum, H.: Diastolic collapse of the right ventricle with tamponade: An echocardiographic study. Circulation, *65*:1491, 1982.

33. Reydel, B., and Spodick, D.H.: Frequency and significance of chamber collapses during cardiac tamponade. Am. Heart J., *119*:1160, 1990.

34. Aebischer, N., Shurman, A.J., and Sharma, S.: Late localized tamponade causing superior vena cava syndrome: An unusual complication of aortic valve replacement. Am. Heart J., *115*:1130, 1988.

35. Conrad, S.A. and Byrnes, T.J.: Diastolic collapse of the left and right ventricles in cardiac tamponade. Am. Heart J., *115*:475, 1988.

36. Levine, M.J., Lorell, B.H., Diver, D.J., and Come, P.C.: Implications of echocardiographically assisted diagnosis of pericardial tamponade in contemporary medical patients: Detection before hemodynamic embarrassment. J. Am. Coll. Cardiol., *17*:59, 1991.

37. Leimgruber, P.P., Klopfenstein, S., Wann, L.S., and Brooks, H.L.: The hemodynamic derangement associated with right ventricular diastolic collapse in cardiac tamponade: An experimental echocardiographic study. Circulation, *68*:612, 1983.

38. Williams, G.J. and Partridge, J.B.: Right ventricular diastolic collapse: An echocardiographic sign of tamponade. Br. Heart J., *49*:292, 1983.

39. Siengh, S., et al.: Right ventricular and right atrial collapse in patients with cardiac tamponade—a combined echocardiographic and hemodynamic study. Circulation, *70*:966, 1984.

40. Gillam, L.D., Guyer, D.E., Gibson, T.C., King, M.E., Marshall, J.E., and Weyman, A.E.: Hydrodynamic compression of the right atrium: A new echocardiographic sign of cardiac tamponade. Circulation, *68*:294, 1983.

41. Shono, H., Yoshikawa, J., Yoshida, K., Kato, H., Okumachi, F., Shiratori, K., Koizumi, K., Takao, S., Asaka, T., and Akasada, T.: Value of right ventricular and atrial collapse in identifying cardiac tamponade. J. Cardiogr., *16*:627, 1986.

42. Kronzon, I., Cohen, M.L., and Winer, H.E.: Diastolic atrial compression: A sensitive echocardiographic sign of cardiac tamponade. J. Am. Coll. Cardiol., *2*:770, 1983.

43. Brodyn, N.E., Rose, M.R., Prior, F.P., and Haft, J.I.: Left atrial diastolic compression in a patient with a large pericardial effusion and pulmonary hypertension. Am. J. Med., *88*:1, 1990.

44. Tunick, P.A., Nachamie, M., and Kronzon, I.: Reversal of echocardiographic signs of pericardial tamponade by transfusion. Am. Heart J., *119*:199, 1990.

45. Hoit, B.D. and Fowler, N.O.: Influence of acute right ventricular dysfunction on cardiac tamponade. J. Am. Col. Cardiol., *18*:1787, 1991.

46. Labib, S.B., Udelson, J.E., and Pandian, N.G.: Echocardiography in low pressure cardiac tamponade. Am. J. Cardiol., *63*:1156, 1989.

47. Hayes, S.N., Freeman, W.K., and Gersh, B.J.: Low pressure cardiac tamponade: Diagnosis facilitated by Doppler echocardiography. Br. Heart J., *63*:136, 1990.

48. Vaska, K., Wann, L.S., Sagar, K., and Klopfenstein, H.S.: Pleural effusion as a cause of right ventricular diastolic collapse. Circulation, *86*:609, 1992.

49. Fusman, B., Schwinger, M.E., Charney, R., Ausubel, K., and Cohen, M.V.: Isolated collapse of left-sided heart chambers in cardiac tamponade: Demonstration by two-dimensional echocardiography. Am. Heart J., *121*:613, 1991.

50. Torelli, J., Marwick, T.H., and Salcedo, E.E.: Left atrial tamponade: Diagnosis by transesophageal echocardiography. J. Am. Soc. Echocardiogr., *4*:413, 1991.

51. D'Cruz, I.A. and Kleinman, D.: Extracardiac causes of

paradoxical motion of the left ventricular wall. Am. Heart J., *115*:473, 1988.

52. Lee, R.T., Bhatia, S.J.S., Kirshenbaum, J.M., and Friedman, P.L.: Left ventricular tamponade: Echocardiographic and hemodynamic manifestations. Clin. Cardiol., *12*:102, 1989.

53. Chuttani, K., Pandian, N.G., Mohanty, P.K., Rosenfield, K., Schwartz, S.L., Udelson, J.E., Simonetti, J., Kusay, B.S., and Caldeira, M.E.: Left ventricular diastolic collapse. An echocardiographic sign of regional cardiac tamponade. Circulation, *83*:1999, 1991.

54. Kisanuki, A., Shono, H., Kiyonaga, K., Kawataki, M., Otsuji, Y., Minagoe, S., Nakao, S., Nomoto, K., and Tanaka, H.: Two-dimensional echocardiographic demonstration of left ventricular diastolic collapse due to compression by pleural effusion. Am. Heart J., *122*:1173, 1991.

55. Himelman, R.B., Kircher, B., Rockey, D.C., and Schiller, N.B.: Inferior vena cava plethora with blunted respiratory response: A sensitive echocardiographic sign of cardiac tamponade. J. Am. Coll. Cardiol., *12*:1470, 1988.

56. Eisenberg, M.J. and Schiller, N.B.: Bayes' Theorem and the echocardiographic diagnosis of cardiac tamponade. Am. J. Cardiol., *68*:1242, 1991.

57. Byrd, B.F. and Linden, R.W.: Superior vena cava Doppler flow velocity patterns in pericardial disease. Am. J. Cardiol., *65*:1464, 1990.

58. Hayes, S.N., Freeman, W.K., and Gersh, B.J.: Low pressure cardiac tamponade: Diagnosis facilitated by Doppler echocardiography. Br. Heart J., *63*:136, 1990.

59. Appleton, C.P., Hatle, L.K., and Popp, R.L.: Cardiac tamponade and pericardial effusion: Respiratory variation in transvalvular flow velocities studied by Doppler echocardiography. J. Am. Coll. Cardiol., *11*:1020, 1988.

60. Leeman, D.E., Levine, M.J., and Come, P.C.: Doppler echocardiography in cardiac tamponade: Exaggerated respiratory variation in transvalvular blood flow velocity integrals. J. Am. Coll. Cardiol., *11*:572, 1988.

61. Burstow, D.J., Oh, J.K., Bailey, K.R., Seward, J.B., and Tajik, A.J.: Cardiac tamponade: Characteristic Doppler observations. Mayo Clin. Proc., *64*:312, 1989.

62. Gonzalez, M.S., Basnight, M.A., Appleton, C.P., Carucci, M., Henry, C., and Olajos, M.: Experimental pericardial effusion: Relation of abnormal respiratory variation in mitral flow velocity to hemodynamics and diastolic right heart collapse. J. Am. Coll. Cardiol., *17*:239, 1991.

63. Reynertson, S.I., Konstadt, S.N., Louie, E.K., Segil, L., Rao, T.L.K., and Scanlon, P.J.: Alterations in transesophageal pulsed Doppler indexes of filling of the left ventricle after pericardiotomy. J. Am. Coll. Cardiol., *18*:1655, 1991.

64. Schutzman, J.J., Obarski, T.P., Pearce, G.L., and Klein, A.L.: Comparison of Doppler and two-dimensional echocardiography for assessment of pericardial effusion. Am. J. Cardiol., *70*:1353, 1992.

65. Hoit, B.D. and Ramrakhyani, K.: Pulmonary venous flow in cardiac tamponade: Influence of left ventricular dysfunction and the relation to pulsus paradoxus. J. Am. Soc. Echocardiogr., *4*:559, 1991.

66. Nanda, N.C., Gramiak, R., and Gross, C.M.: Echocardiography of cardiac valves in pericardial effusion. Circulation, *54*:500, 1976.

67. D'Cruz, I.A., Cohen, H.C., Prabbu, R., and Glick, G.: Diagnosis of cardiac tamponade by echocardiography:

Changes in mitral valve motion and ventricular dimensions, with special reference to paradoxical pulse. Circulation, *52*:460, 1975.

68. Settle, H.P., Adolph, R.J., Fowler, N.O., Engel, P., Agruss, N.S., and Levenson, N.I.: Echocardiographic study of cardiac tamponade. Circulation, *56*:951, 1977.

69. Armstrong, W.F., Feigenbaum, H., and Dillon, J.C.: Acute right ventricular dilation and echocardiographic volume overload following pericardiocentesis for relief of cardiac tamponade. Am. Heart J., *107*:1266, 1984.

70. Schiller, N.B. and Botvinick, E.H.: Right ventricular compression as a sign of cardiac tamponade: An analysis of echocardiographic ventricular dimensions and their clinical implications. Circulation, *56*:774, 1977.

71. Simpson, I.A., Munsch, C., Smith, E.E.J., and Parker, D.J.: Pericardial hemorrhage causing right atrial compression after cardiac surgery: Role of transesophageal echocardiography. Br. Heart J., *65*:355, 1991.

72. Gheorghiade, M., Cheek, B.H., and Chakko, S.C.: Isolated right heart tamponade following mediastinal irradiation. Am. Heart J., *112*:167, 1986.

73. Segni, E.D., Beker, B., Arbel, Y., Bakst, A., Dean, H., Levi, A., Kaplinsky, E., and Klein, H.O.: Left ventricular pseudohypertrophy in pericardial effusion as a sign of cardiac tamponade. Am. J. Cardiol., *66*:508, 1990.

73a. DiSegni, E., Feinberg, M.S., Sheinowitz, M., Motro, M., Battler, A., Kaplinsky, E., and Vered, Z.: Left ventricular pseudohypertrophy in cardiac tamponade: An echocardiographic study in a canine model. J. Am. Coll. Cardiol., *21*:1286, 1993.

74. Hoit, B.D., Gabel, M., and Fowler, N.O.: Cardiac tamponade in left ventricular dysfunction. Circulation, *82*:1370, 1990.

75. Feigenbaum, H., Zaky, A., and Grabhorn, L.: Cardiac motion in patients with pericardial effusion: A study using ultrasound cardiography. Circulation, *34*:611, 1966.

76. Krueger, S.K., Zucker, R.P., Dzindzio, B.S., and Forker, A.D.: Swinging heart syndrome with predominant anterior pericardial effusion. JCU, *4*:113, 1976.

77. Gabor, G.E., Winsberg, F., and Bloom, H.S.: Electrical and mechanical alternation in pericardial effusion. Chest, *59*:341, 1971.

78. Yuste, P., Torres, Carballada, M.A., and Miguel Alonso, J.L.: Mechanism of electric alternans in pericardial effusion: Study with ultrasonics. Arch. Inst. Cardiol. Mex., *45*:197, 1975.

79. Rinkenberger, R.L., Polumbo, R.A., Bolton, M.R., and Dunn, M.: Mechanism of electrical alternans in patients with pericardial effusion. Cathet. Cardiovasc. Diagn., *4*:63, 1978.

80. Ratib, O. and Perrenoud, J.J.: Demonstration of electrical and mechanical alternans in malignant pericardial effusion with 2-D echocardiography. JCU, *12*:501, 1984.

81. Hinds, S.W., Reisner, S.A., Amico, A.F., and Meltzer, R.S.: Diagnosis of pericardial abnormalities by 2D-echo: A pathology-echocardiography correlation in 85 patients. Am. Heart J., *123*:143, 1992.

82. Martin, R.P., Bowden, R., Filly, K., and Popp, R.L.: Intrapericardial abnormalities in patients with pericardial effusion: Findings by two-dimensional echocardiography. Circulation, *61*:568, 1980.

83. Lopez-Sendon, J., et al.: Identification of blood in pericardial cavity in dogs by two-dimensional echocardiography. Am. J. Cardiol., *53*:1194, 1984.

84. Lopez-Sendon, J., Garcia-Fernandez, M.A., Coma-Canella, I., Silvestre, J., deMiguel, E., Jadraque, L. Martin: Identification of blood in the pericardial cavity in dogs

by two dimensional echocardiography. Am. J. Cardiol., *53*:1194, 1984.

85. Schuster, A.H. and Nanda, N.C.: Pericardiocentesis induced intrapericardial thrombus: Detection by two dimensional echocardiography. Am. Heart J., *104*:308, 1982.

85a. D'Cruz, I.A., Holman, M.S., and Childers, L.S.: Spontaneous mobile contrast echoes in pericardial effusion. Am. Heart J., *120*:1472, 1990.

86. Ku, C-S., Hsiung, M-C., Hsu, T-L., Ding, Y-A., and Shieh, S-M.: Spontaneous contrast in the pericardial sac caused by gas-forming organisms. J. Am. Soc. Echocardiogr., *4*:67, 1991.

87. Mantana, A., Marvric, Z., Vukas, D., and Beg-Zec, Z.: Spontaneous contrast echoes in pericardial effusion: Sign of gas-producing infection. Am. Heart J., *124*:521, 1992.

88. Bedotto, J.B., McBride, W., Abraham, M., and Taylor, A.L.: Echocardiographic diagnosis of pneumopericardium and hydropneumopericardium. J. Am. Soc. Echocardiogr., *1*:359, 1988.

89. Chandraratna, P.A.N. and Aronow, W.S.: Detection of pericardial metastases by cross-sectional echocardiography. Circulation, *63*:54, 1981.

90. Frohwein, S.C., Karalis, D.G., McQuillan, J.M., Ross, J.J., Mintz, G.S., and Chandrasekaran, K.: Preoperative detection of pericardial angiosarcoma by transesophageal echocardiography. Am. Heart J., *122*:874, 1991.

91. Chandraratna, P.A.N. and Aronow, W.S.: Detection of pericardial metastases by cross-sectional echocardiography. Circulation, *63*:197, 1981.

92. Hynes, J.K., Tajik, A.J., Osborn, M.J., Orszulak, T.A., and Seward, J.B.: Two dimensional echocardiographic diagnosis of pericardial cyst. Mayo Clin. Proc., *58*:60, 1983.

93. Farooki, Z.W., Arciniegas, E., Hakimi, M., Clapp, S., Jackson, W., and Green, E.W.: Real-time echocardiographic features of intrapericardial teratoma. JCU, *10*:125, 1982.

94. Seguin, J.R., Coulon, P.L., Perez, M., Grolleau-Raoux, R., and Chaptal, P.A.: Echocardiographic diagnosis of an intrapericardial teratoma in infancy. Am. Heart J., *113*:1239, 1987.

95. Rosamond, T.L., Hamburg, M.S., Vacek, J.L., and Borkon, A.M.: Intrapericardial pheochromocytoma. Am. J. Cardiol., *70*:700, 1992.

96. Lam, D. and Rapaport, E.: Two-dimensional echocardiographic demonstration of intrapericardial fibrinous strands in rheumatoid pericarditis. Am. Heart J., *114*:442, 1987.

96a. Chiaramida, S.A., Goldman, M.A., Zema, M.J., Pizzarello, R.A., and Goldberg, H.M.: Echocardiographic identification of intrapericardial fibrous strands in acute pericarditis with pericardial effusion. Chest, *77*:85, 1980.

97. Chandraratna, P.A.N., First, J., Langevin, E., and O'Dell, R.: Echocardiographic contrast studies during pericardiocentesis. Ann. Intern. Med., *87*:199, 1977.

98. Callahan, J.A., Seward, J.B., Tajik, A.J., Holmes, D.R. Jr., Smith, B.C., Reeder, G.S., and Miller, F.A., Jr.: Pericardiocentesis assisted by two dimensional echocardiography. J. Thorac. Cardiovasc. Surg., *85*:877, 1983.

99. Chandraratna, P.A.N., Reid, C.L., Nimalasuriya, A., Kawanishi, D., and Rahimtoola, S.H.: Application of two dimensional contrast studies during pericardiocentesis. Am. J. Cardiol., *52*:1120, 1983.

100. Dubourg, O., Ferrier, A., Gueret, P., Farcot, J.C., Terdjman, M., Rocha, P., and Bourdarias, J.P.: Two dimensional contrast echocardiography during the drainage of hemopericardium with tamponade. Presse Med., *12*:2225, 1983.

101. Konishi, T., Anzai, T., and Kanazawa, N.: Pericardial puncture under the ultrasonic cardiotomographic guidance: Application of pericardial effusion. J. Cardiogr., *12*:181, 1982.

102. Preis, L.K., Taylor, G.J., and Martin, R.P.: Traumatic pericardiocentesis: Two dimensional echocardiographic visualization of an unfortunate event. Arch. Intern. Med., *142*:2327, 1982.

103. Meliones, J.N., Snider, R., Beekman, R.H., Bengur, A.R., and Bogaards, M.A.: Echocardiographic detection of pericardiocentesis-induced subepicardial and intramyocardial hematoma. Am. J. Cardiol., *64*:820, 1989.

104. Calabrese, P., Iliceto, S., and Rizzon, P.: Pericardiocentesis-induced intrapericardial thrombus: Visualization of thrombus formation and spontaneous internal lysis by two-dimensional echocardiography. JCU, *13*:49, 1985.

105. Lin, C.S., Jan, Y.I., Chen, H.Y., Hou, S.H., and Kuo, C.C.: Two-dimensional echocardiographic detection of pericardiocentesis-induced intrapericardial thrombus. Chest, *86*:787, 1984.

106. Selig, M.B.: Percutaneous pericardial biopsy under echocardiographic guidance. Am. Heart J., *122*:879, 1991.

107. Blickman, J.G., Dunlop, R.W., and Fulton, D.R.: Diagnostic implications of the echocardiographically demonstrated pericardial peel. Am. Heart J., *119*:965, 1990.

108. Alio-Bosch, J., Candell-Riera, J., Monge-Rangel, L., and Soler-Soler, J.: Intrapericardial echocardiographic images and cardiac constriction. Am. Heart J., *121*:207, 1991.

109. Schnittger, I., Bowden, R.E., Abrams, J., and Popp, R.L.: Echocardiography: Pericardial thickening and constrictive pericarditis. Am. J. Cardiol., *42*:388, 1978.

110. Chandraratna, P.A.N. and Imaizumi, T.: Echocardiographic diagnosis of thickened pericardium. Cardiovasc. Med., *3*:1279, 1978.

111. Hiroyama, N., Matsuzaki, M., Anno, Y., Toma, Y., Tamitani, M., Maeda, T., Konishi, M., Okada, K., Tanaka, N., Suetsugu, M., Ono, S., and Kusukawa, R.: Echocardiography in a case of acute tuberculous pericarditis which progressed to constrictive pericarditis. J. Cardiogr., *16*:501, 1986.

112. Chandraratna, P.A.N., Aronow, W.S., and Imaizumi, T.: Role of echocardiography in detecting the anatomic and physiologic abnormalities of constrictive pericarditis. Am. J. Med. Sci., *283*:141, 1982.

113. Pool, P.E., Seagren, S.C., Abbasi, A.S., Charuzi, Y., and Kraus, R.: Echocardiographic manifestations of constrictive pericarditis: Abnormal septal motion. Chest, *68*:684, 1975.

114. Candell-Riera, J., DelCastillo, G., Permanyer-Miralda, G., and Soler-Soler, J.: Echocardiographic features of the interventricular septum in chronic constrictive pericarditis. Circulation, *57*:1154, 1978.

115. D'Cruz, I.A., Levinsky, R., Anagnostopoulos, C., and Cohen, H.C.: Echocardiographic diagnosis of partial pericardial constriction of the left ventricle. Radiology, *127*:755, 1978.

116. Yamamoto, T., Makihata, S., Yasutomi, N., Tanimoto, M., Ando, H., Iwasaki, T., Yorifuji, S., Shimizu, Y., and Miyamoto, T.: Echocardiographic and impedance cardiographic manifestations of constrictive pericarditis. J. Cardiogr., *8*:719, 1978.

117. Matsuo, H., Kitabatake, A., Matsumoto, M., Hamanaka, Y., Beppu, S., Nagata, S., Tamai, M., Ohara,

T., Senda, S., and Nimura, Y.: Echocardiographic manifestation of constrictive pericarditis and pericarditis with effusion. Cardiovasc. Sound Bull., *5*:173, 1975.

118. Nishimoto, M., Tanaka, C., Oku, H., Ikuno, Y., Kawai, S., Furukawa, K., Takeuchi, K., and Shiota, K.: Presystolic pulmonary valve opening in constrictive pericarditis. J. Cardiogr., *7*:55, 1977.

119. Tei, C., Child, J.S., Tanaka, H., and Shah, P.M.: Atrial systolic notch on the interventricular septal echogram. An echocardiographic sign of constrictive pericarditis. J. Am. Coll. Cardiol., *1*:907, 1983.

120. Voelkel, A.G., Pietro, D.A., Folland, E.D., Fisher, M.L., and Parisi, A.F.: Echocardiographic features of constrictive pericarditis. Circulation, *58*:871, 1978.

121. Cohen, M.V. and Greenberg, M.A.: Constrictive pericarditis: Early and late complication of cardiac surgery. Am. J. Cardiol., *43*:657, 1979.

122. Morgan, J.M., Raposo, L., Claque, J.C., Chow, W.H., and Oldershaw, P.J.: Restrictive cardiomyopathy and constrictive pericarditis: Non-invasive distinction by digitised M mode echocardiography. Br. Heart J., *59*:629, 1988.

123. Gibson, T.C., Grossman, W., McLaurin, L.P., Moos, S., and Craige, E.: An echocardiographic study of the interventricular system in constrictive pericarditis. Br. Heart J., *38*:738, 1976.

124. Wann, L.S., Weyman, A.E., Dillon, J.C., and Feigenbaum, H.: Premature pulmonary valve opening. Circulation, *55*:128, 1977.

125. Hada, Y., Sakamoto, T., Hayashi, T., Ichiyasu, H., and Amano, K.: Echocardiogram of normal pulmonary valve: Physiological data and effect of atrial contraction on the valve motion. Jpn. Heart J., *18*:421, 1977.

126. Himelman, R.B., Lee, E., and Schiller, N.B.: Septal bounce, vena cava plethora, and pericardial adhesion: Informative two-dimensional echocardiographic signs in the diagnosis of pericardial constriction. J. Am. Soc. Echocardiogr., *1*:333, 1988.

127. Vilacosta, I., Calvar, A.S.R., Prieto, E.I., Recio, M.G., and Elbal, L.M.: Transesophageal echocardiographic features of the atrial septum in constrictive pericarditis. Am. J. Cardiol., *68*:271, 1991.

128. D'Cruz, I.A., Dick, A., Gross, C.M., Hand, C.R., and Lalmalani, G.G.: Abnormal left ventricular-left atrial posterior wall contour: A new two-dimensional echocardiographic sign in constrictive pericarditis. Am. Heart J., *118*:128, 1989.

129. von Bibra, H., Schober, K., Jenni, R., Busch, R., Sebening, H., and Blomer, H.: Diagnosis of constrictive pericarditis by pulsed Doppler echocardiography of the hepatic vein. Am. J. Cardiol., *63*:483, 1989.

130. Hatle, L.K., Appleton, C.P., and Popp, R.L.: Differentiation of constrictive pericarditis and restrictive cardiomyopathy by Doppler echocardiography. Circulation, *79*: 357, 1989.

131. Schiavone, W.A., Calafiore, P.A., Currie, P.J., and Lytle, B.W.: Doppler echocardiographic demonstration of pulmonary venous flow velocity in three patients with constrictive pericarditis before and after pericardiectomy. Am. J. Cardiol., *63*:145, 1989.

132. Schiavone, W.A., Calafiore, P.A., and Salcedo, E.E.: Transesophageal Doppler echocardiographic demonstration of pulmonary venous flow velocity in restrictive cardiomyopathy and constrictive pericarditis. Am. J. Cardiol., *63*:1286, 1989.

133. Vaitkus, P.T. and Kussmaul, W.G.: Constrictive pericarditis versus restrictive cardiomyopathy: A reappraisal and update of diagnostic criteria. Am. Heart J., *122*:1431, 1991.

134. Payvandi, M.N. and Kerber, R.E.: Echocardiography in congenital and acquired absence of pericardium. Circulation, *53*:86, 1976.

135. Hermann, H., Raizner, A.E., Chahine, R.A., et al.: Congenital absence of the left pericardium: An unusual palpation finding and echocardiographic demonstration of the defect. South. Med. J., *69*:1222, 1976.

136. Ruys, F., Paulus, W., Stevens, C., and Brutsaert, D.: Expansion of the left atrial appendage is a distinctive cross-sectional echocardiographic feature of congenital defect of the pericardium. Eur. Heart J., *4*:738, 1983.

137. Goebel, N. and Jenni, R.: Aneurysms of the left atrium in pericardial defect. Z. Kardiol., *72*:696, 1983.

138. Candan, I., Erol, C., and Sonel, A.: Cross sectional echocardiographic appearance in presumed congenital absence of the left pericardium. Br. Heart J., *55*:405, 1986.

139. Vargas-Barron, J., Sanchez-Ugarte, T., Keirns, C., Vazquez-Sanchez, J., Fernandez-Vazquez, F., and Barragan, R.: The differential diagnosis of partial absence of left pericardium and congenital left atrial aneurysm. Am. Heart J., *118*:1348, 1989.

# 11

# Cardiac Masses

With the advent of two-dimensional and especially transesophageal echocardiography, the detection of masses in and around the heart has become one of the major uses of echocardiography.[1-8] Some masses, such as vegetations and left ventricular thrombi, have already been discussed in previous chapters.

## NORMAL VARIANTS

Before discussing the detection of pathologic masses within the heart, the normal variants that can mimic abnormal intracardiac masses should be reviewed.[9,9a] Many of these structures were discussed in Chapter 2. The normal moderator band within the right ventricle can occasionally be misinterpreted as a pathologic structure (Fig. 11–1).[10] The moderator band is best seen in the apical four-chamber view. The echoes from this structure are at the apical third of the right ventricular cavity. Because the right ventricle is normally trabeculated, right ventricular hypertrophy accentuates these trabeculations and may produce confusing echocardiograms. Occasionally, prominent left ventricular trabeculations may cause confusion.[11]

Figure 11–1 also illustrates how the lateral wall of the left atrium can impinge on the cavity and produce what might be interpreted as an abnormal left atrial mass. Such echoes are usually ignored, except when one is examining a patient for a suspected source of systemic emboli. Under these circumstances, one begins to notice subtle echoes that normally are not even appreciated. The eustachian valve in the right atrium may be prominent in some individuals (Fig. 11–2).[12,13] Occasionally, a eustachian valve is large enough to produce obstruction to flow. Figure 11–3 shows multiple views of a patient with an unusually large eustachian valve. The inferior vena cava (Fig. 11–3D) is dilated, suggesting that the eustachian valve may be impeding blood flow from the inferior vena cava to the right atrium. The patient was otherwise asymptomatic, and nothing further was done.[12]

The eustachian valve can be seen readily with transesophageal echocardiography. Figure 11–4 illustrates horizontal and longitudinal views of the eustachian valve between the right atrium and the inferior vena cava. The structure is usually membranous, undulates, and needs to be distinguished from a pathologic mass.

Another nonpathologic entity that may be seen in the right atrium is the Chiari network.[14,15] These fine filamentous structures are remnants of developmental structures within the right atrium. Figure 11–5 shows multiple views of patients with such a Chiari network (arrows). The filamentous structures move about within the right atrium and are in different locations in each of the frames. This type of structure is appreciated better in a real-time examination, especially with a transesophageal echocardiogram (Fig. 11–6).[16,17]

The right atrial wall is frequently irregular with prominent trabeculations or pectinate muscles. These structures are occasionally seen with transthoracic echocardiography; however, with the high resolution available with transesophageal echocardiography, these structures may be fairly striking (Fig. 11–7). Figure 11–7B demonstrates a large muscle band within the right atrium that can again cause confusion. One can distinguish normal muscle from a pathologic mass by withdrawing the probe and scanning the heart toward the base so that the normal wall begins to surround the superior vena cava and separates the great vein from the right atrial appendage. The chambers on the right side of the heart are usually more trabeculated than those on the left. Occasionally, however, a highly trabeculated atrial appendage may be difficult to distinguish from a thrombus (Fig. 11–7A).

## MASSES OF QUESTIONABLE CLINICAL SIGNIFICANCE

Several structures recognized echocardiographically probably have no clinical significance in most cases. One such entity is false tendons within the left ventricle.[18] These echocardiographic structures traverse the left ventricular cavity and can be multiple (Fig. 11–8); they can be seen in any view of the left ventricle (Fig. 11–9). Occasionally, false tendons are extremely prominent and produce a confusing echocardiogram (Fig. 11–10). The clinical significance of these structures is uncertain, although they rarely produce any symptoms.[19-21]

Fat can accumulate in a variety of places within the heart. This accumulation can produce what appears to be an echogenic mass. The interatrial septum is a site that tends to accumulate fat. Lipomatous hypertrophy of

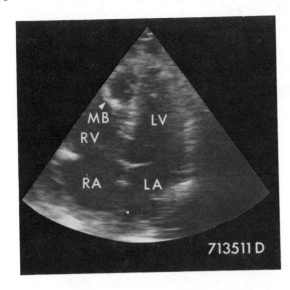

**Fig. 11–1.** Apical four-chamber two-dimensional echocardiogram of a patient with a prominent moderator band (MB) in the right ventricle (RV). LV = left ventricle; RA = right atrium; LA = left atrium.

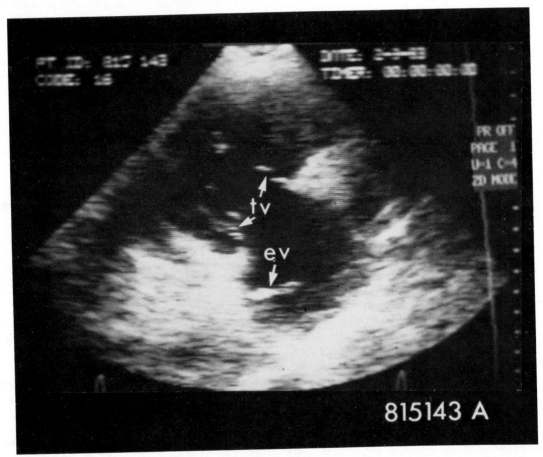

**Fig. 11–2.** Parasternal long-axis echocardiogram of the right ventricular inflow tract demonstrating a prominent eustachian valve (ev). tv = tricuspid valve.

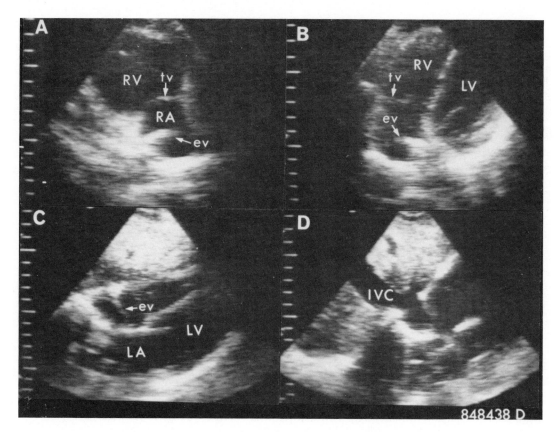

**Fig. 11–3.** Two-dimensional echocardiograms of a patient with an unusually large eustachian valve (ev). The valve can be seen in the long-axis view of the right ventricular inflow tract *(A)*, the apical four-chamber view *(B)*, and the subcostal four-chamber view *(C)*. The inferior vena cava (IVC) is dilated *(D)*. RV = right ventricle; tv = tricuspid valve; RA = right atrium; LV = left ventricle; LA = left atrium.

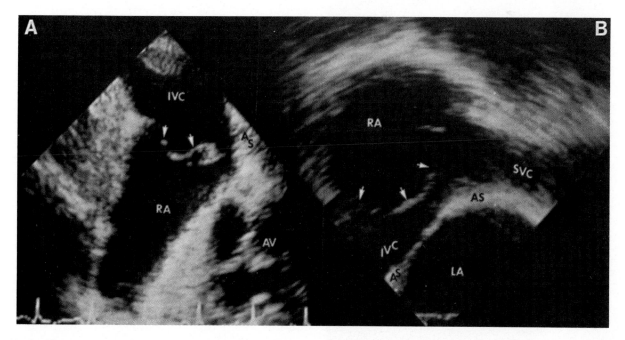

**Fig. 11–4.** Transesophageal echocardiographic examination of a prominent eustachian valve. In the horizontal plane *(A)*, the valve *(arrows)* can be seen at the junction between the orifice of the inferior vena cava (IVC) and the right atrium (RA). The structure is usually membranous and undulates with cardiac action. In the longitudinal plane *(B)*, the eustachian membrane *(arrows)* is again between the right atrium (RA) and inferior vena cava and separates the body of the right atrium from the interatrial septum (AS). Occasionally, the membrane can be mistaken for a mass or thrombus. LA = left atrium; SVC = superior vena cava. (From Seward, J.B., et al.: Critical appraisal of transesophageal echocardiography: Limitations, pitfalls, and complications. J. Am. Soc. Echocardiogr., 5:288, 1992.)

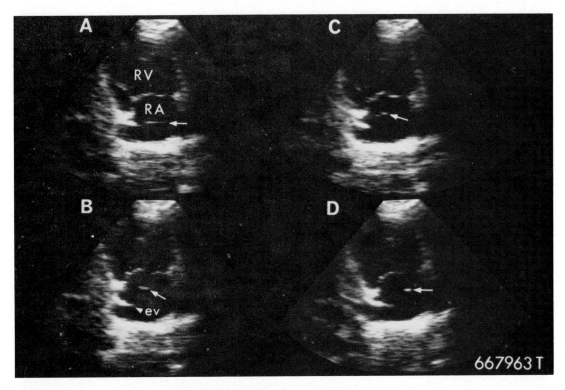

**Fig. 11–5.** Two-dimensional echocardiogram of a patient with a Chiari network. Echoes originating from the filamentous structures *(arrows)* move randomly within the right atrium (RA). RV = right ventricle; ev = eustachian valve.

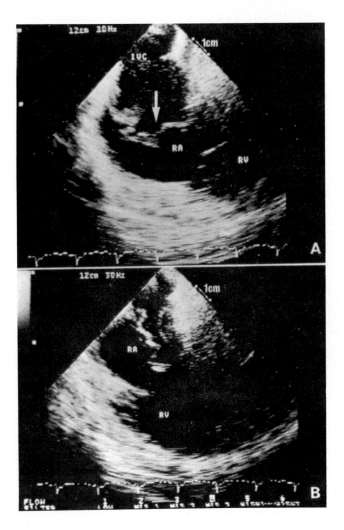

**Fig. 11–6.** Biplane transesophageal echocardiographic examination of a Chiari's network *(arrow)* within the right atrium (RA). IVC = inferior vena cava; RV = right ventricle. (From Cujec, B., et al.: Identification of Chiari's network with transesophageal echocardiography. J. Am. Soc. Echocardiogr., 5: 98, 1992.)

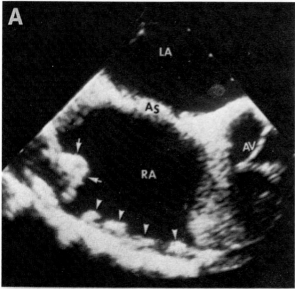

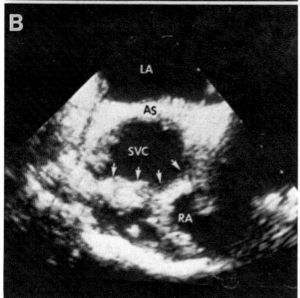

**Fig. 11–7.** Transesophageal echocardiographic examination showing right atrial (RA) trabeculations or pectinate muscles *(arrowheads)* and muscular bands *(arrows)*. The right atrium is more trabeculated (i.e., pectinate muscles) than the left atrium (LA). A highly trabeculated atrial appendage may be difficult to distinguish from thrombus. This example is from a patient with an atrial septal defect in whom the atrial musculature is hypertrophied. In *A*, there is a larger muscle band *(arrows)* commonly visualized at the orifice of the superior vena cava. *B* demonstrates that the identity of the normal atrial muscle bundle can be obtained by slow withdrawal of the transesophageal scope in the horizontal plane. Normal muscle encircles the superior vena caval orifice (SVC), separating it from the right atrial appendage. AS = atrial septum; AV = aortic valve. (From Seward, J.B., et al.: Critical appraisal of transesophageal echocardiography: Limitations, pitfalls, and complications. J. Am. Soc. Echocardiogr., 5:288, 1992.)

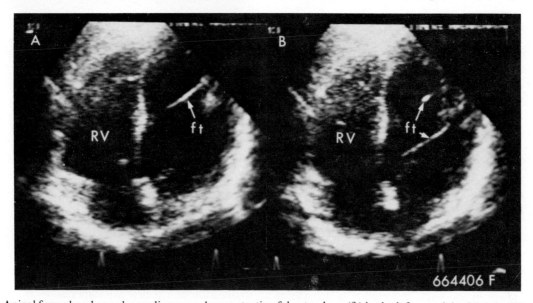

**Fig. 11–8.** Apical four-chamber echocardiograms demonstrating false tendons (ft) in the left ventricle. Slightly different examining planes *(A)* and *(B)* record several false tendons. RV = right ventricle.

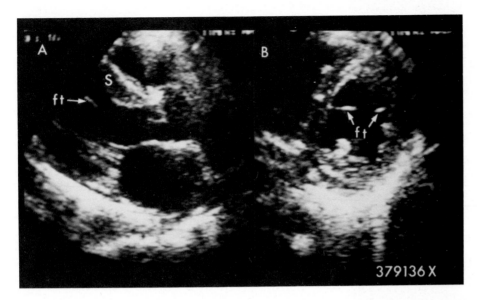

**Fig. 11–9.** Long-axis *(A)* and short-axis *(B)* two-dimensional echocardiograms of a patient with a false tendon (ft) in the left ventricle. In the long-axis view, *(A)*, the abnormal echo can cause some confusion as to its relationship to the interventricular septum (S). In the short-axis view *(B)*, the structure (ft) can be seen traversing the cavity of the ventricle.

the interatrial septum can produce a fairly characteristic echocardiogram,[21a–24] as shown in Figure 11–11. The septum is unusually thick. The fat within the structure is echogenic. The fossa ovalis is frequently spared by fat infiltration, resulting in an actual doughnut-shaped hypertrophy of the interatrial septum (Fig. 11–12). Figure 11–13 shows the transesophageal echocardiographic examination of a lipomatous atrial septum.[25] A dumbbell-shaped configuration of the interatrial septum with thick, fat-laden echoes surrounding a thin echo at the level of the fossa ovalis[21b] is fairly characteristic. The interatrial septal fat may involve the right atrial wall.[25a]

Fat may also be present in other areas of the heart. The partition between the left upper pulmonary vein and the left atrial appendage may accumulate fat, creating a mass-like appearance on a transesophageal echocardiogram (Fig. 11–14). The proximal part of the wall is usu-

ally thin and the distal portion is thicker and more bulbous. The tricuspid annulus may also accumulate fat and produce a mass-like effect echocardiographically. Figure 11–15 shows a transesophageal echocardiogram of a fat-laden tricuspid annulus that appears as an echogenic mass between the right atrium and the right ventricle. Yet another location for fat to accumulate is in the transverse sinus between the left atrium, the ascending aorta, and the pulmonary artery (Fig. 11–16). This structure can be mistaken for a mass within the left atrium.

Aneurysms of the interatrial septum have been noted by many investigators.[26–31] Figure 11–17 shows a patient with an atrial septal aneurysm. The aneurysm is usually at the level of the foramen ovale. In this particular patient, the aneurysm bulges toward the right atrium in diastole and toward the left atrium in systole. The

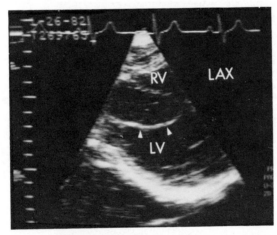

**Fig. 11–10.** Long-axis (LAX) two-dimensional echocardiogram of a patient with an unusually prominent left ventricular false tendon *(arrowheads)*. Such an echo can produce a confusing echocardiogram and might be incorrectly considered part of the interventricular septum. RV = right ventricle; LV = left ventricle.

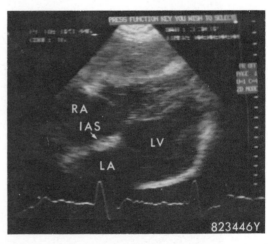

**Fig. 11–11.** Subcostal four-chamber two-dimensional echocardiogram of a patient with lipomatous hypertrophy of the interatrial septum (IAS). RA = right atrium; LA = left atrium; LV = left ventricle.

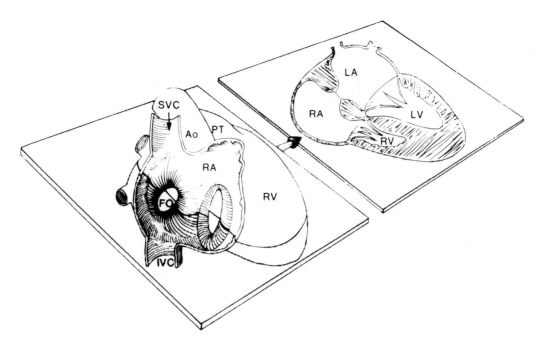

**Fig. 11–12.** Diagram demonstrating how lipomatous hypertrophy of the interatrial septum frequently spares the fossa ovalis (FO) so that the two-dimensional echocardiogram of the atrial septum gives a "dumbbell" appearance. SVC = superior vena cava; IVC = inferior vena cava; RA = right atrium; Ao = aorta; PT = pulmonary trunk; RV = right ventricle; RA = right atrium; LA = left atrium; LV = left ventricle. (From Fyke, F.E., III, et al.: Diagnosis of lipomatous hypertrophy of the atrial septum by two-dimensional echocardiography. J. Am. Coll. Cardiol., *1*:1352, 1983.)

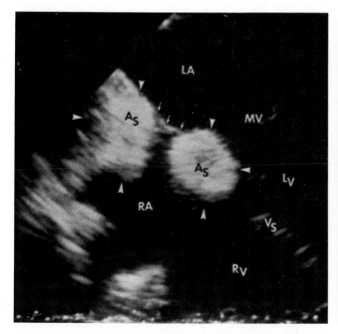

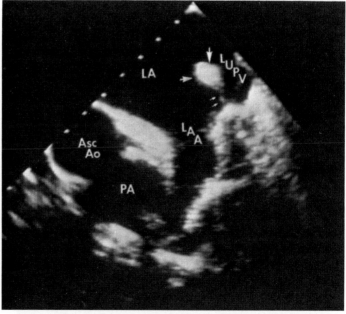

**Fig. 11–13.** Transesophageal echocardiographic study of a patient with a lipomatous atrial septum. The atrial septum (AS) is inundated with echogenic fatty tissue. The membrane of the fossa ovalis *(small arrows)* is spared. LA = left atrium; MV = mitral valve; LV = left ventricle; VS = ventricular septum; RA = right atrium; RV = right ventricle. (From Seward, J.B., et al.: Critical appraisal of transesophageal echocardiography: Limitations, pitfalls, and complications. J. Am. Soc. Echocardiogr., *5*:288, 1992.)

**Fig. 11–14.** Infiltration of the normal partition *(small arrows)* between the left upper pulmonary vein (LUPV) and left atrial appendage (LAA) with fat, producing a pseudomass *(large arrows)*. This normal variant can be striking with a transesophageal echocardiographic examination. LA = left atrium; ASC Ao = ascending aorta; PA = pulmonary artery. (From Seward, J.B., et al.: Critical appraisal of transesophageal echocardiography: Limitations, pitfalls, and complications. J. Am. Soc. Echocardiogr., *5*:288, 1992.)

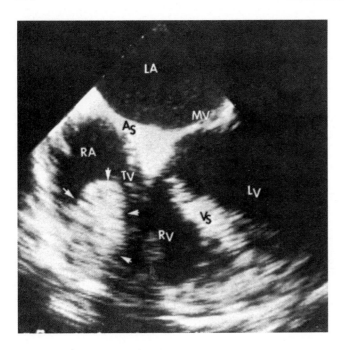

**Fig. 11–15.** Transesophageal examination showing infiltration of fat within the tricuspid annulus *(arrows)* between the right atrium (RA) and the right ventricle (RV). LA = left atrium; TV = tricuspid valve; MV = mitral valve; LV = left ventricle; RV = right ventricle; VS = ventricular septum. (From Seward, J.B., et al.: Critical appraisal of transesophageal echocardiography: Limitations, pitfalls, and complications. J. Am. Soc. Echocardiogr., 5:288, 1992.)

confusing echocardiogram can sometimes be clarified by the use of a right-sided contrast echocardiogram that outlines the aneurysm as it bulges into the right atrium. Transesophageal echocardiography can detect the atrial septal aneurysms with greater clarity and precision (Fig. 11–18).[32,32a]

Although an atrial septal aneurysm is commonly considered a benign condition, greater experience and investigation has shown that this condition is associated with a higher incidence of shunting through the interatrial septum.[33,34] Using contrast and Doppler flow esophageal echocardiography, various investigators have shown that up to 90% of these aneurysms have a potential right-to-left shunt. Figure 11–19 demonstrates a transesophageal examination of an atrial septal aneurysm whereby a contrast injection reveals a small right-to-left shunt. At least two cases of thrombi forming within an atrial septal aneurysm have increased the pos-

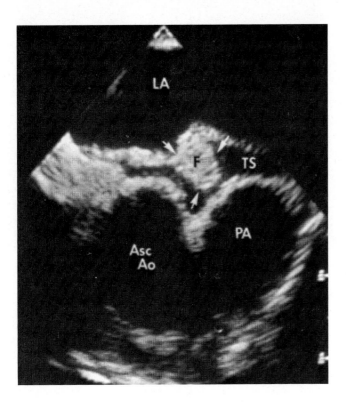

**Fig. 11–16.** A transesophageal echocardiogram showing pericardial fat (F) within the transverse sinus (TS). This pericardial reflection, which lies between the left atrium (LA) and the ascending aorta (Asc Ao) and pulmonary artery (PA), can accumulate fat and appear as a pseudomass. (From Seward, J.B., et al.: Critical appraisal of transesophageal echocardiography: Limitations, pitfalls, and complications. J. Am. Soc. Echocardiogr., 5:288, 1992.)

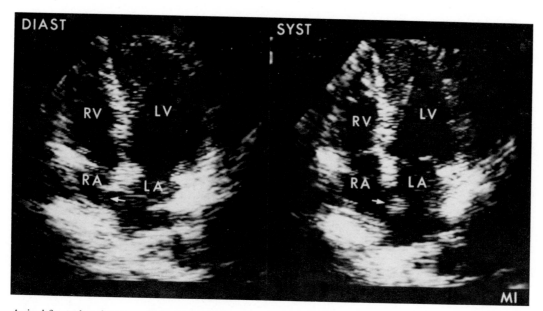

**Fig. 11–17.** Apical four-chamber two-dimensional echocardiograms of a patient with an aneurysm of the interatrial septum. In diastole, the redundant aneurysmal septum *(arrow)* moves toward the right atrium (RA). In systole, the floppy aneurysm reverses its direction *(arrow)* and moves toward the left atrium (LA). RV = right ventricle; LV = left ventricle.

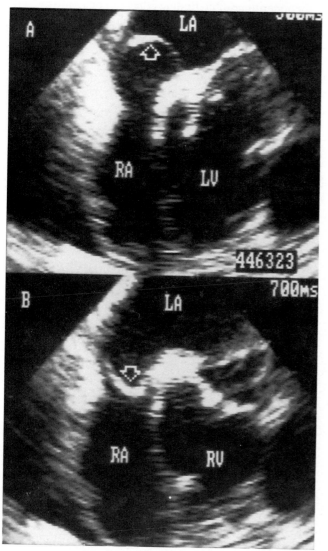

**Fig. 11–18.** Transesophageal echocardiogram illustrating an atrial septal aneurysm or "floppy septum." This examination demonstrates how the redundant septal tissue bulges back and forth *(arrows)* between the left atrium (LA) and right atrium (RA). LV = left ventricle; RV = right ventricle.

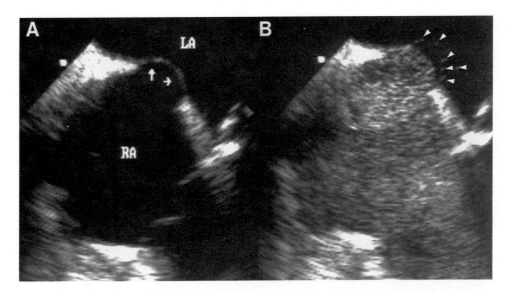

**Fig. 11–19.** Transesophageal echocardiographic examination of an atrial septal aneurysm *(arrows, A)* with a small number of contrast bubbles *(arrowheads, B)* appearing in the left atrium (LA) following a right-sided contrast injection. RA = right atrium.

sibility that these anomalies may be the source of systemic emboli.[35,36] Thus, although the entity is usually benign, there are potential clinical problems that must be appreciated with an atrial septal aneurysm.

As noted in Chapter 10, transplant patients have a prominent echo from the suture line between the donor and recipient left atria (Fig. 11–20).[37] These echoes can be prominent but rarely cause any clinical difficulty. A remnant of the common pulmonary vein has been

noted echocardiographically as another "pseudo-mass."[38]

Echocardiographic findings that can be confused with pathologic masses are not always limited to echogenic abnormalities. Echo-free spaces can also be confused as cystic or fluid-filled space-occupying lesions. Figure 11–21 shows two possible situations in which one might mistake echo-free areas as pathologic conditions. The right atrial appendage, which is rarely seen with trans-

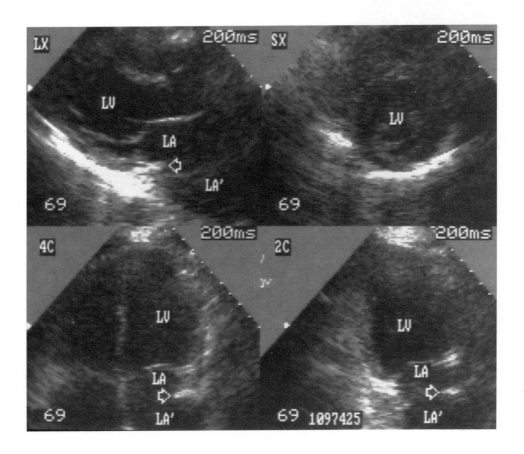

**Fig. 11–20.** Long-axis (LX), short-axis (SX), four-chamber (4C), and two-chamber (2C) examinations of a patient after cardiac transplantation. The junction between the donor (LA) and recipient (LA') left atria can be visualized *(arrows)*. LV = left ventricle.

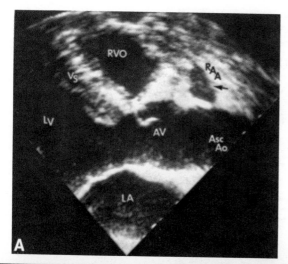

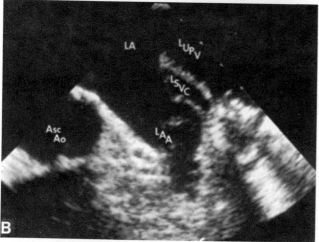

**Fig. 11–21.** Transesophageal echocardiographic examination showing the right atrial appendage (RAA) in the longitudinal plane *(A)*. The echo-free right atrial appendage is noted anterior to the ascending aorta (Asc Ao). A persistent superior vena cava (LSVC) will appear as an echo-free space between the left upper pulmonary vein (LUPV) and the left atrial appendage (LAA, *B*). The persistent left superior vena cava can be identified by color flow Doppler and usually with an associated dilated coronary sinus. LA = left atrium; LV = left ventricle; RVO = right ventricular outflow; AV = aortic valve. (From Seward, J.B., et al.: Critical appraisal of transesophageal echocardiography: Limitations, pitfalls, and complications. J. Am. Soc. Echocardiogr., 5:288, 1992.)

thoracic echocardiography, can be seen fairly routinely with a transesophageal examination. This echo-free space appears anterior to the ascending aorta and needs to be identified as a normal structure. An anomalous left superior vena cava may also cause confusion, especially with transesophageal echocardiography. This anomalous vessel will be seen between the left upper pulmonary vein and the left atrial appendage. The entity can usually be identified by color flow Doppler as well as the presence of a dilated coronary sinus, which is characteristic of an anomalous left superior vena cava. A contrast injection in a left upper extremity vein will opacify the coronary sinus and confirm the diagnosis.

Other pseudocardiac masses include a hiatus hernia, a diaphragmatic hernia,[38a] or a descending aortic aneurysm, which may impinge on the heart and be misinterpreted.

## PRIMARY CARDIAC NEOPLASMS

The most common primary cardiac neoplasm is the myxoma.[39–42] The diagnosis of a left atrial myxoma has been one of the principal uses of echocardiography since the introduction of the technique.[43–53] Figure 11–22

shows long-axis and apical four-chamber views of a fairly typical example of a left atrial myxoma. This patient also happens to have an atrial septal aneurysm. It is interesting that the aneurysm does not move back and forth between the right and left atria as in Figure 11–17 because the high left atrial pressure keeps the aneurysm bulging into the right atrium throughout the cardiac cycle.

The classic left atrial myxoma is a mobile echogenic mass that is in the body of the left atrium in systole and passes through the mitral orifice in diastole. These patients commonly have mitral valve obstruction and symptoms that simulate those of mitral stenosis. Occasionally, one will detect a left atrial myxoma that is not near the mitral orifice and is otherwise clinically silent (Fig. 11–23). This patient happened to have aortic valve disease, and the myxoma was detected as part of a routine follow-up echocardiogram for this condition.

M-mode echocardiography was the first technique used to detect left atrial myxomas. Figure 11–24 demonstrates an M-mode scan of a patient with a fairly typical mobile left atrial tumor. One sees a cloud of tumor echoes (T) behind the anterior leaflet of the mitral valve (MV). In this patient, the echo-producing mass almost

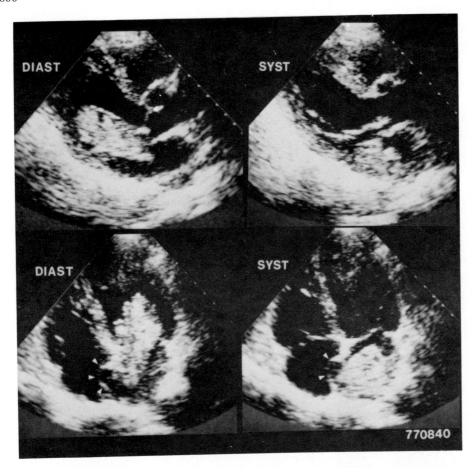

**Fig. 11–22.** Long-axis and apical four-chamber two-dimensional echocardiograms in diastole and systole in a patient with a left atrial myxoma and an atrial septal aneurysm. The septal aneurysm *(arrowheads)* can be seen bulging toward the right atrium in both diastole and systole.

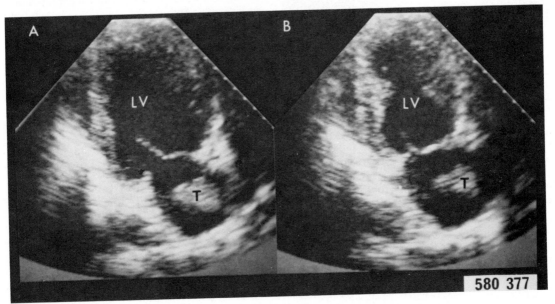

**Fig. 11–23.** Apical two-chamber echocardiograms in diastole *(A)* and systole *(B)* of a patient with a left atrial myxoma (T) that is not near the mitral orifice and is immobile. LV = left ventricle.

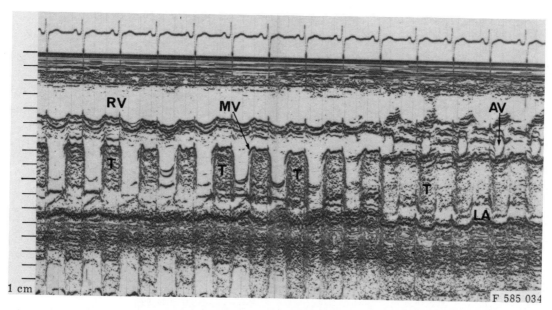

**Fig. 11–24.** M-mode scan of a patient with a left atrial myxoma. The tumor echoes (T) are visible behind the anterior leaflet of the mitral valve (MV) during diastole and almost completely fill the left atrium (LA) during ventricular systole. RV = right ventricle; AV = aortic valve. (From Chang, S.: Echocardiography: Techniques and Interpretation, ed. 2. Philadelphia, Lea & Febiger, 1981.)

completely fills the mitral valve throughout diastole. Directing the ultrasonic beam into the left atrium, one can follow the echo-producing mass into the left atrium and see how it practically fills the entire left atrial cavity. Only a small posterior echo-free space is not filled with tumor. The aortic valve, which shows signs of decreased blood flow, is anterior to the tumor-filled left atrium.

Although it is usually possible to detect left atrial myxomas with transthoracic echocardiography, the trans-

esophageal examination produces spectacular images of left atrial masses, especially a left atrial myxoma.[54–56] A huge left atrial myxoma virtually filling the left atrial cavity can be seen in the transesophageal echocardiogram in Figure 11–25. A smaller myxoma is seen in Figure 11–26. Although this pedunculated mobile tumor was seen on the transthoracic echocardiogram, the tumor was relatively faint. Such a tumor could be missed in a patient who was not easy to examine echocardio-

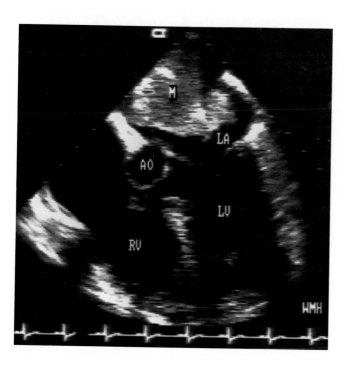

**Fig. 11–25.** Transesophageal echocardiogram showing a huge mass (M) within the left atrium (LA). AO = aorta; LV = left ventricle; RV = right ventricle.

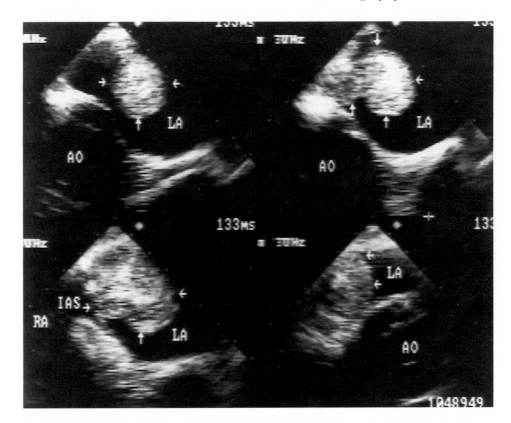

Fig. 11–26. Serial transesophageal echocardiograms of a relatively small left atrial myxoma *(arrows)*. The myxoma can be seen attached to the interatrial septum (IAS) at lower left. AO = aorta; LA = left atrium; RA = right atrium. (From Feigenbaum, H.: Echocardiography. *In* Heart Disease. 4th Ed. Edited by E. Braunwald. Philadelphia, W.B. Saunders, Co., 1992.)

graphically. The transesophageal examination not only offers a higher sensitivity for detecting left atrial tumors, but also permits a clearer picture of the attachment or stalk of the tumor and a more precise characterization of the size, shape, and location of the mass. Figure 11–27 shows a myxoma that originates near the

mitral annulus. The tumor almost appears as if it were connected to the valve itself. Actually, it is connected to the lower portion of the atrial septum near the mitral annulus. Virtually every cardiac surgeon would appreciate a transesophageal echocardiogram before surgery to make certain that the exact nature and location of the

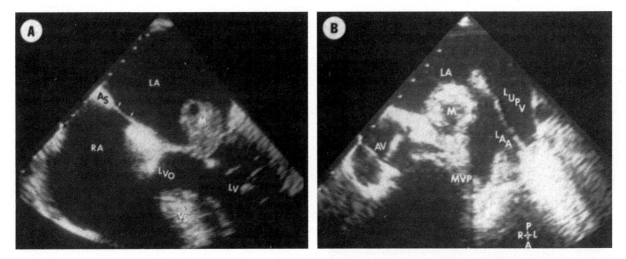

Fig. 11–27.    Transesophageal echocardiographic study of a left atrial myxoma that originates near the mitral annulus. The tumor appears almost as if it is attached to the valve itself. The myxoma (M) actually connects to the lower portion of the atrial septum near the mitral annulus. LA = left atrium; RA = right atrium; LVO = left ventricular outflow; LV = left ventricle; VS = ventricular septum; AV = aortic valve; MVP = mitral valve prolapse; LAA = left atrial appendage; LUPV = left upper pulmonary vein. (From Reeder, G.S., et al.: Transesophageal echocardiography in cardiac masses. Mayo Clin. Proc., 66:1103, 1991.)

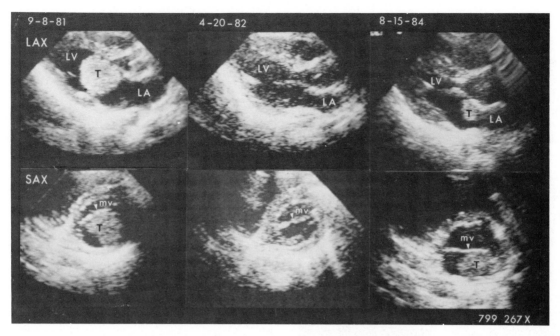

**Fig. 11–28.** Serial two-dimensional echocardiograms in long-axis (LAX) and short-axis (SAX) views of a patient with a recurrent left atrial myxoma. The tumor (T) is striking on 9/8/81. It is not present in the postoperative echocardiogram (4/20/82); however on 8/15/84, a small tumor (T) can again be seen in the left atrium (LA). LV = left ventricle; mv = mitral valve.

tumor is known prior to thoracotomy. Rare cases of multiple myxomas may also be detected more readily with the transesophageal approach.

One of the obvious advantages of echocardiography is its ability to provide serial studies. On rare occasions, the left atrial tumor, recurs.[57-60] Figure 11–28 is a set of serial echocardiograms of a patient who had a classic left atrial myxoma. The postoperative echocardiogram was essentially normal; however, several years later, the patient had evidence of systemic emboli. On the echocardiogram, one can see recurrence of the tumor near the location of the original myxoma. In this patient, the myxoma was not malignant. Echocardiography can also be used to follow any change in size of a tumor.[61-63]

Unusual left atrial myxomas have been reported. Hemorrhage within the left atrial myxoma has been noted echocardiographically.[64,65] Infection on the myxoma has been detected with transesophageal echocardiography.[66] The transesophageal technique has also been used to identify cystic left atrial myxomas.[1,67]

The right atrium is the second most common location for a myxoma. Numerous such neoplasms have been detected echocardiographically.[50,68-77] Figure 11–29 shows a fairly typical two-dimensional echocardiogram of a large right atrial tumor that lies within the right atrium in systole and passes through the tricuspid valve into the right ventricle in diastole. Multiple right atrial myxomas have been reported.[75] Biatrial myxomas are less common but have also been described.[78-82] Figure 11–30 demonstrates an M-mode scan of a patient with biatrial myxomas. The left atrial tumor shows the classic M-mode findings with a mass of echoes posterior to the anterior mitral leaflet (AM). Note the small echo-free

gap between the mitral leaflet and the tumor mass at the onset of diastole. This small, echo-free gap is useful in differentiating a mobile tumor that follows the movement of blood from a mass of echoes that attach to the valve itself. The echoes from the right-sided tumor (R) appear within the right ventricle in diastole. Again, transesophageal echocardiography may provide spectacular images of right atrial myxomas.[83]

Myxomas may also involve the ventricles.[84-90] Figure 11–31 demonstrates a large myxoma originating from the left ventricle.[84] Figure 11–32 shows a transesophageal echocardiogram of a patient with a left ventricular myxoma. These tumors can be clinically silent and may be detected as an incidental finding.[90] In this particular example, the tumor actually had two lobes. On rare occasion, a left ventricular myxoma will obstruct the left ventricular outflow tract.[89]

Myxomas on the right side of the heart can be so large that it is difficult to know the origin of the mass.[89-92] Figure 11–33 shows a huge tumor occupying almost the entire right side of the heart. The mass obstructed the tricuspid valve and produced massive hemodynamic changes. A smaller, more mobile right ventricular tumor is noted in Figure 11–34. This tumor stays within the right ventricular cavity and was noted to be mobile on the real-time echocardiographic study.

Naturally, a myxoma that obstructs a valve orifice will produce appropriate Doppler findings of valve orifice stenosis.[93,94]

An assortment of other neoplasms primarily affect the heart and can be detected echocardiographically.[95-102] Rhabdomyomas and rhabdomyosarcomas are relatively common neoplasms, especially in infants.[103-113] These

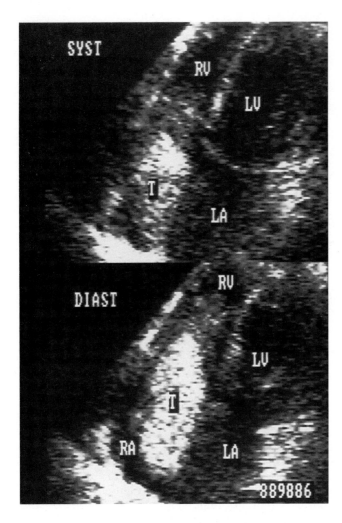

**Fig. 11–29.** Transthoracic apical four-chamber examination of a patient with a large right atrial myxoma. The tumor (T) resides in the right atrium in systole and passes through the tricuspid orifice into the right ventricle in diastole (DIAST). RV = right ventricle; RA = right atrium; LV = left ventricle; LA = left atrium.

tumors tend to involve the ventricles. In one report, the sarcoma produced mitral stenosis.[114] A left ventricular fibroma has also been described in the echocardiographic literature.[107] The fibroma may primarily involve the interventricular septum.[115] Lymphomas involving the papillary muscles and the mitral valves have been seen on both transthoracic and transesophageal two-dimensional echocardiograms.[116–121] Figure 11–35 shows

an example of a patient with a lymphoma that involves both the left and right ventricles. An interesting feature of this tumor is that the center of the echogenic mass appears relatively echo-free. The tumors were in fact solid lymphomas.

An interesting neoplasm noted by several investigators is a papillary fibroelastoma.[122–127] This small pedunculated, benign tumor can occur in almost any part of

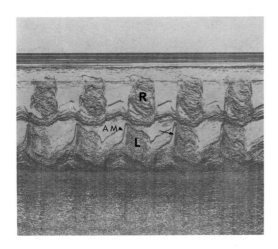

**Fig. 11–30.** M-mode echocardiogram of a patient with biatrial myxomas. The right tumor (R) appears in the right ventricle during diastole. The left tumor (L) is posterior to the anterior mitral leaflet (AM) in diastole. A small echo-free gap is evident *(arrow)* between the mitral leaflet and the left atrial tumor in early diastole.

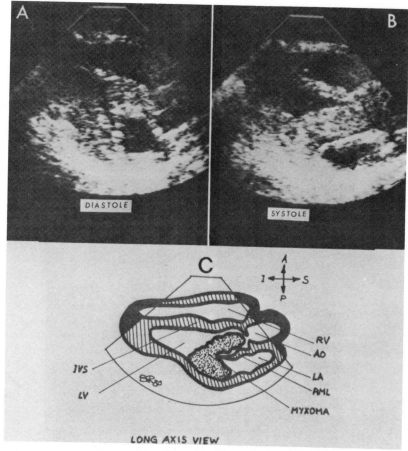

**Fig. 11–31.** Diastolic *(A)* and systolic *(B)* long-axis echocardiograms and a diagram *(C)* of a patient with a large left ventricular myxoma. IVS = interventricular septum; LV = left ventricle; RV = right ventricle; AO = aorta; LA = left atrium; PML = posterior mitral leaflet. (From Mazer, M.S., and Harrigan, P.: Left ventricular myxoma; M-mode and two-dimensional echocardiographic features. Am. Heart J., *104*:875, 1982.)

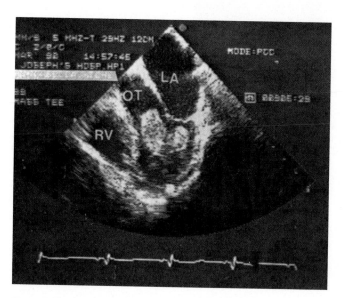

**Fig. 11–32.** Transesophageal echocardiogram of a bilobed left ventricular myxoma. LA = left atrium; OT = outflow tract; RV = right ventricle. (From Wrisley, D., et al.: Left ventricular myxoma discovered incidentally by echocardiography. Am. Heart J., *121*:1554, 1991.)

the heart. Figure 11–36 shows a two-dimensional echocardiogram and a diagram of one of these small tumors attached to the mural leaflet of the mitral valve. Similar tumors have been noted attached to the aortic valve, tricuspid valve, and walls of the ventricles. The clinical significance of these tumors is unclear. One group of investigators suggested elective surgical resection once the lesions are seen echocardiographically,[124] because they can produce systemic embolization.[128]

## NONCARDIAC NEOPLASMS INVADING THE HEART

A host of neoplasms may involve the heart, either through metastases or by direct extension of the primary lesion. Tumors may travel up the inferior vena cava into the right side of the heart. Leiomyomata from uterine neoplasms have been demonstrated to invade the right side of the heart.[129-133] These tumors may even obstruct the tricuspid valve.[133] Renal cell carcinoma may involve the right side of the heart via the inferior vena cava.[134] Colon cancer has also been noted to metastasize to the

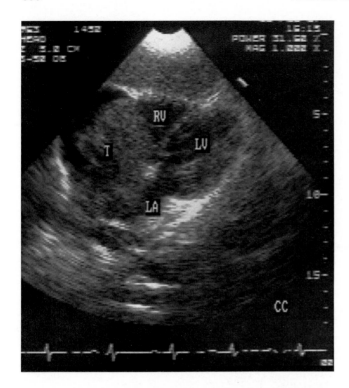

**Fig. 11–33.** A massive right heart tumor (T) practically fills the entire right atrium and right ventricle. RV = right ventricle; LV = left ventricle; LA = left atrium.

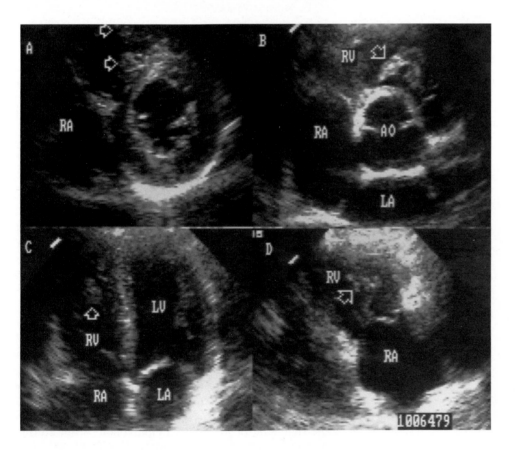

**Fig. 11–34.** Highly mobile right ventricular tumor *(arrows)*. The tumor is seen in multiple locations in the short-axis at the papillary muscle *(A)*, the short-axis at the base of the heart *(B)*, the apical four-chamber *(C)*, and the long-axis right ventricular inflow *(D)* examinations. RA = right atrium; RV = right ventricle; LV = left ventricle; LA = left atrium.

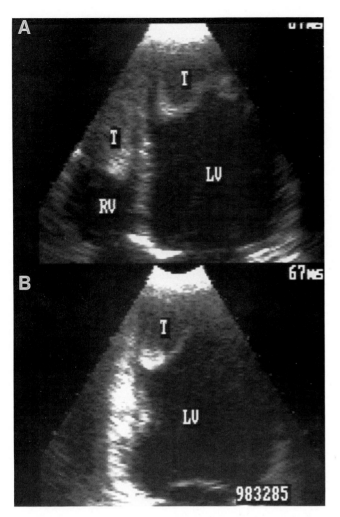

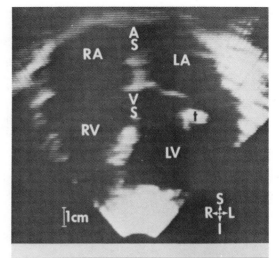

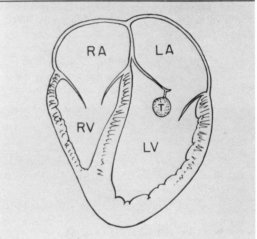

**Fig. 11–35.** Apical four-chamber *(A)* and two-chamber *(B)* views of a patient with a lymphoma involving both the right ventricle (RV) and the left ventricle (LV). The tumor (T) in the left ventricle has a relatively echolucent center.

**Fig. 11–36.** Apical four-chamber two-dimensional echocardiogram and diagram of a patient with a papillary fibroelastoma (t) attached to the mitral valve. The two-dimensional view is inverted in this illustration. RA = right atrium; AS = atrial septum; LA = left atrium; RV = right ventricle; VS = ventricular septum; LV = left ventricle. (From Shub, C., Tajik, A.J., Seward, J.B., Edwards, W.D., Pruitt, R.D., Orsyulak, T.A., and Pluth, J.R.: Cardiac papillary fibroelastomas: Two dimensional echocardiographic recognition. Mayo Clin. Proc., 56:629, 1981.)

heart.[135] Several other metastatic neoplasms have been noted.[135–145] Many of these tumors metastasize to the right side of the heart.[132,146–151] Occasionally, a nonneoplastic mass, such as an intramyocardial hematoma, may present as a pseudotumor of the right ventricle.[152]

## EXTRACARDIAC MASSES

A variety of extracardiac masses have been detected echocardiographically,[153–163] including mediastinal tumors,[153,164–169] pericardial tumors,[156,158,159,164–167, 170–173] intrathoracic neoplasms,[155,171,174] and pericardial cysts.[175] Pericardial cysts were described in Chapter 10. Figure 11–37 demonstrates a large posterior mediastinal mass that distorts the left atrium. Even the esophagus can compress the heart and present as an extracardiac mass.[176–178] Figure 11–38 shows an anterior mediastinal mass in the long-axis and four-chamber views. The echogenic mass clearly distorts the anterior left ventricular wall. The four-chamber view is misshapened as the left ventricle is compressed by this echogenic mass.

Transesophageal echocardiography can be extremely helpful in detecting mediastinal or extracardiac masses. Figure 11–39 shows a solid mass infiltrating the aortic wall and superior vena cava. Figure 11–40 shows a mediastinal mass that is encasing the right pulmonary artery and superior vena cava. The normal circular superior vena cava is now triangular because of the compression of the tumor. Figure 11–41 demonstrates an extracardiac mass in a patient who also has a pericardial effusion. The mass is cystic and is probably responsible for the pericardial fluid. Transesophageal echocardiography has also been of value in detecting a pericardial angiosarcoma.[179] Figure 11–42 shows transthoracic *(A)* and transesophageal *(B)* examinations of a cystic mass posterior to the left atrium.

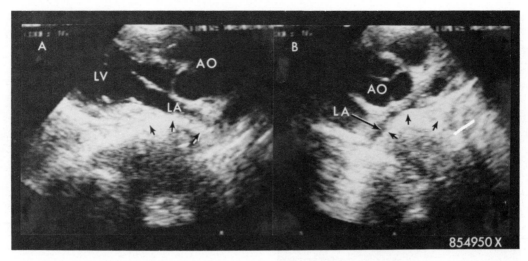

**Fig. 11–37.** Long-axis *(A)* and short-axis *(B)* two-dimensional echocardiograms of a patient with a posterior mediastinal mass *(arrows)* compressing the left atrium (LA). LV = left ventricle; AO = aorta.

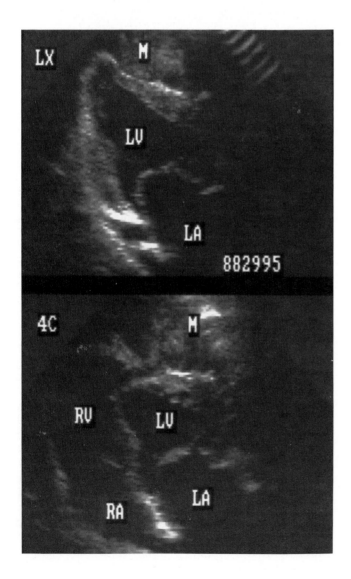

**Fig. 11–38.** Long-axis (LX) and four-chamber (4C) views of a patient with a large anterior mediastinal mass (M). LV = left ventricle; LA = left atrium; RV = right ventricle; RA = right atrium.

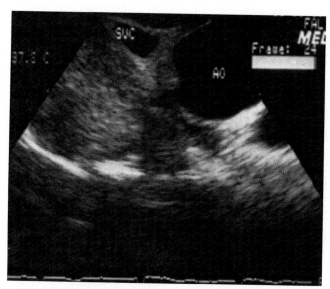

**Fig. 11–39.** Transesophageal echocardiographic examination demonstrating a solid mass infiltrating the aortic wall and the superior vena cava. SVC = superior vena cava; AO = aorta. (From Faletra, F., et al.: Transesophageal echocardiography in the evaluation of mediastinal masses. J. Am. Soc. Echocardiogr., *5*:183, 1992.)

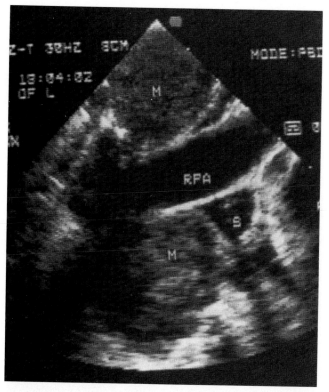

**Fig. 11–40.** Transesophageal echocardiographic examination demonstrating a mediastinal mass (M) that encases the right pulmonary artery (RPA) and superior vena cava (S). The normal circular superior vena cava is now distorted to assume the shape of a triangle, which is consistent with compression of the vessel. (From Dawkins, P.R., et al.: Use of transesophageal echocardiography in the assessment of mediastinal masses and superior vena cava obstruction. Am. Heart J., *122*:1470, 1991.)

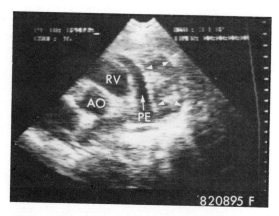

**Fig. 11–41.** Short-axis two-dimensional echocardiogram through the base of the heart of a patient with a cystic mass *(arrowheads)* adjacent to the pericardium. There is also a small pericardial effusion (PE). RV = right ventricle; AO = aorta.

## INTRACARDIAC THROMBI

Many of the intracardiac thrombi have been discussed in previous chapters. Thrombi associated with myocardial infarction (see Chapter 8), cardiomyopathy (see Chapter 9), and mitral valve disease (see Chapter 6) have been mentioned. Large, bright, irregular, mobile thrombi are fairly easy to detect echocardiographically. Immobile mural thrombi can cause difficulties in echocardiographic interpretation. Figure 11–43 illustrates some of the various left ventricular thrombi that can be seen echocardiographically. Figure 11–43 shows a small apical thrombus that is difficult to see and must be distinguished from near field clutter that commonly can be present. A flat mural thrombus along the interventricular septum, such as in Figure 11–43, may also be confusing and sometimes is misinterpreted as a thickened interventricular septum. Larger and more pedunculated and protruding clots, such as in Figure 11–43*B* and *D*, are more readily identified echocardiographically.

Color flow Doppler may be used to differentiate the blood pool from a mural thrombus.[180] It is also possible that the new contrast agents that traverse the pulmonary capillaries may also help to identify a mural thrombus in questionable cases.

The shape and mobility of the clot seem to have some relationship to the possibility of embolization.[181–184] The flat immobile clots, such as in Figure 11–43*A* and *C*, have less tendency to embolize. Those clots that protrude into the cavity, however, especially in views other than just the apical views, and those that are mobile, such as in Figure 11–43*D*, are prone to produce emboli. Figure 11–44 shows a patient with a highly mobile clot that is of the type that will most likely embolize. This somewhat pedunculated, highly mobile clot can be seen in all cardiac views. The center of the mass is relatively echo-free, suggesting liquifaction of the thrombus.

Extensive thrombus formation within the left ventricular cavity can produce a change in the size of the left ventricular cavity. Figure 11–45 shows a massive throm-

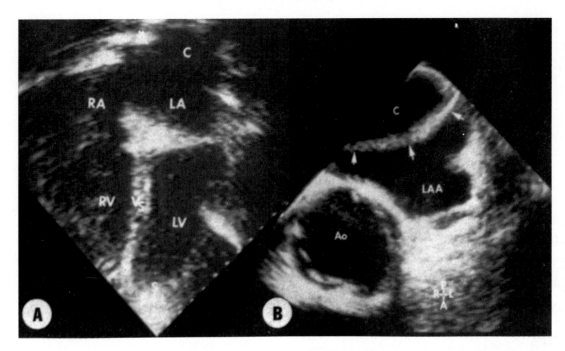

**Fig. 11–42.** Transthoracic *(A)* and transesophageal *(B)* echocardiogram of a cystic lesion *(C)* posterior to the left atrium. The transesophageal echocardiogram shows compression *(arrows)* of the left atrium by the cyst. RA = right atrium; RV = right ventricle; LV = left ventricle; LA = left atrium; Ao = aorta; LAA = left atrial appendage. (From Reeder, G.S., et al.: Transesophageal echocardiography in cardiac masses. Mayo Clin. Proc., *66*:1107, 1991.)

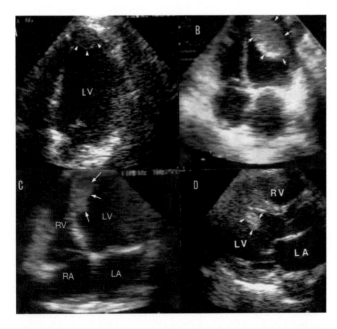

**Fig. 11–43.** Echocardiograms demonstrating a variety of different left ventricular thrombi *(arrows)* that can be identified echocardiographically. The thrombi in *A* and *C* are relatively flat and adherent to the walls. The thrombus in *B* is large and protrudes into the cavity of the left ventricle. *D* demonstrates a relatively small, more mobile thrombus attached to the interventricular septum. LV = left ventricle; RV = right ventricle; RA = right atrium; LA = left atrium.

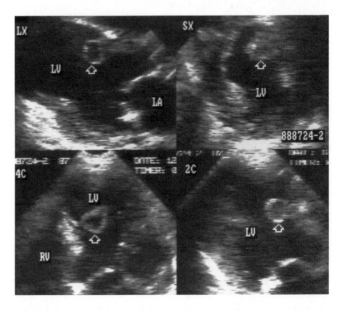

**Fig. 11–44.** Long-axis (LX), short-axis (SX), four-chamber (4C), and two-chamber (2C) views of a patient with a mobile thrombus *(arrows)* attached to the interventricular septum. The thrombus is echolucent, suggesting liquifaction of the center.

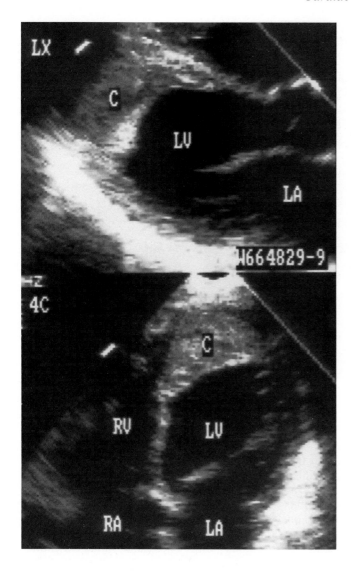

**Fig. 11–45.** Massive apical clot (C) that functionally amputates the apex in the long-axis (LX) and four-chamber (4C) views. LV = left ventricle; LA = left atrium; RV = right ventricle; RA = right atrium.

bus involving the apical third that effectively amputates that part of the left ventricle. The clot essentially decreases left ventricular volume by one third. Spontaneous contrast may occur in the same situation in which thrombus is likely to form,[185] such as in patients with dilated cardiomyopathies or akinetic walls resulting from large infarctions. Figure 11–46 shows a patient with a dilated cardiomyopathy in whom spontaneous contrast is seen in both the long-axis and short-axis views. It is possible to see both echogenic clot as well as spontaneous contrast in the same echocardiogram.[186] A rare case of left ventricular mural thrombus and normal ventricular function in a patient with ulcerative colitis has been reported.[187]

Using only transthoracic echocardiography, left atrial thrombi are somewhat difficult to assess.[188,189] Large clots within the body of the left atrial cavity have been noted by numerous individuals. Figure 11–47 shows three views of a fairly large left atrial thrombus. This clot involved a large portion of the left atrial free wall. This type of abnormality is fairly easy to diagnose with transthoracic two-dimensional echocardiography. Fig-

ure 11–48 shows a slightly more subtle left atrial thrombus. This clot is again quite large; however, the quality of the echoes is not much different than the echoes seen with stagnant blood within the left atrium. This thrombus is more subtle and can be difficult to detect, especially if the clot exhibits no mobility.

Transesophageal echocardiography has revolutionized the ability of the echocardiographer to detect left atrial thrombi.[190] Left atrial clots frequently form in the left atrial appendage. This area is difficult to see with transthoracic echocardiography.[191] With transesophageal studies, however, the appendage is readily apparent and clots within this structure can be detected with reliability. Figure 11–49 shows two patients with left atrial thrombi. One can see the echogenic mass in various locations within the left atrial appendage. Transesophageal echocardiography is now the procedure of choice for detecting or excluding left atrial thrombi. In several types of patients, left atrial clots are particularly hazardous. This situation includes individuals who have atrial fibrillation and are to undergo electrical cardioversion or patients who are to have mitral balloon valvuloplasty.

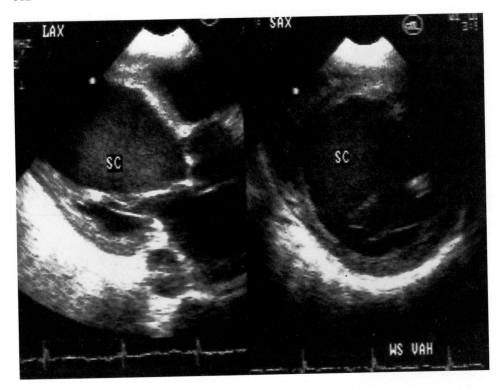

**Fig. 11–46.** Long-axis(LAX) and short-axis (SAX) examinations of a patient with a dilated cardiomyopathy and spontaneous contrast (SC) in the left ventricle.

In both cases, it is important to know whether or not left atrial clots are present. Transesophageal echocardiography is now being used routinely to rule out the presence of such clots.[192,193] The examination is also being used to determine the incidence or frequency of left atrial thrombi in patients with idiopathic or ischemic dilated cardiomyopathy.[194]

Occasionally, left atrial clots are virtually adherent to the mitral valve and do not reside in much of the atrial chamber. Figure 11–50 shows an example of a patient

with mitral stenosis and a left atrial thrombus. The clot is adherent to the mitral orifice and probably contributes to the obstruction of blood through the mitral valve. With the advent of transesophageal echocardiography, multiple types of left atrial clots have been described.[195] An example of a highly mobile, freely moving left atrial thrombus seen with transesophageal echocardiography is demonstrated in Figure 11–51. An unattached, freely moving clot within the left atrium is often called a left atrial ball thrombus.[196–201] The transesophageal exami-

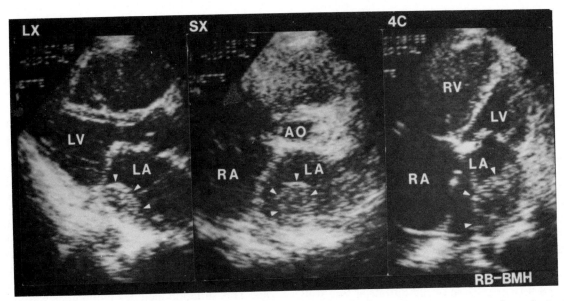

**Fig. 11–47.** Long-axis (LA), short-axis (SX) and four-chamber (4C) two-dimensional echocardiograms of a patient with a large clot *(arrowheads)* in the left atrium (LA). LV = left ventricle; AO = aorta; RA = right atrium.

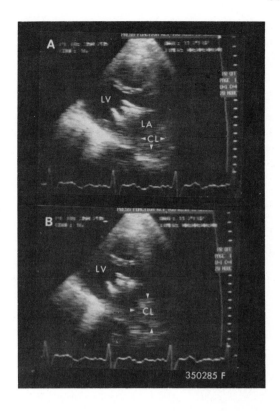

**Fig. 11–48.** Two long-axis views of a patient with a large clot (CL) in the left atrium (LA). This clot is not nearly as echogenic as the one noted in Figure 11–47. LV = left ventricle.

nation provides numerous opportunities to see this clot move throughout the left atrium. One can identify some cystic structures within the middle of the mass. Also, spontaneous contrast is evident in the vicinity of the left atrial appendage. Left atrial clots obstructing pulmonary veins have been detected with transesophageal echocardiography.[202]

Clots in all cardiac chambers can be detected fairly easily with echocardiography, especially now with the availability of the transesophageal technique.[202a] Figure 11–52 shows a patient with thrombus in both left and right ventricular apices. The right ventricular clot can be seen in the apical four-chamber view and the parasternal, right ventricular outflow view.

Because of the high-frequency transducers that are used with transesophageal echocardiography, spontaneous contrast is readily apparent with this examination.[203–207] Figure 11–53 shows two examples of patients who exhibit spontaneous contrast with dilated left atria. As commonly noted, the spontaneous contrast is accompanied by more solid echogenic thrombi. Figure 11–53

shows spontaneous contrast in a patient who also has a mobile linear clot attached to the atrial wall *(arrow)*. In Figure 11–53*B*, an echogenic clot *(small arrow)* is attached to the junction between the left atrial appendage and the body of the left atrium. In addition, the atrial appendage is filled with a mass of echoes *(large arrow)* that is more dense than the spontaneous contrast within the cavity of the left atrium but less dense than the solid echogenic thrombus. This intermediary state may be a more gelatinous form of early thrombus formation.[208,209] Spontaneous contrast has been noted in the left atrium after cardiac transplantation.[210]

Right atrial clots have been noted by numerous investigators.[211–217] These clots are particularly important because they frequently are precursors of pulmonary emboli.[218–223] The clots usually form within systemic veins and pass through the right atrium. They may be trapped temporarily in the right atrium and right ventricle as they traverse the right side of the heart.[224] Figure 11–54 shows an example of a large clot passing between the right atrium and the right ventricle. These clots are usu-

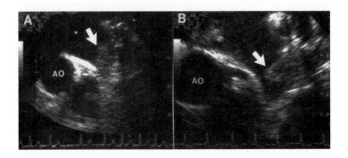

**Fig. 11–49.** Transesophageal echocardiograms of two patients with thrombi in the left atrial appendage. In *A*, the thrombus *(arrow)* completely fills the left atrial appendage. In *B*, the thrombus *(arrow)* is attached to the lateral wall of the appendage. LA = left atrium. (From Pollick, C. and Taylor, D.: Assessment of left atrial appendage function by transesophageal echocardiography: Implications for the development of thrombus. Circulation, *84*:226, 1991, by permission of the American Heart Association, Inc.)

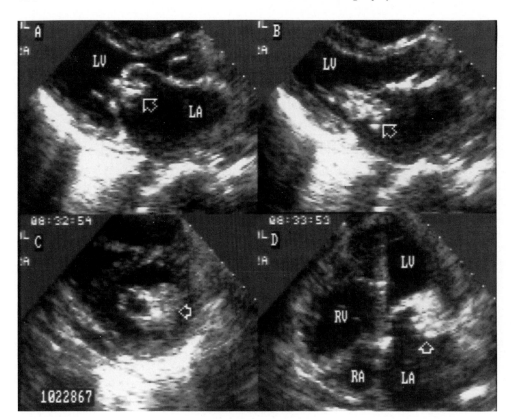

**Fig. 11–50.** Echocardiograms of a patient with mitral stenosis and a thrombus adherent to the mitral leaflets. The long-axis *(A and B)*, short-axis *(C)*, and four-chamber *(D)* views demonstrate the echogenic thrombus *(arrows)* adherent to the domed, stenotic mitral valve. LV = left ventricle; RV = right ventricle; RA = right atrium; LA = left atrium.

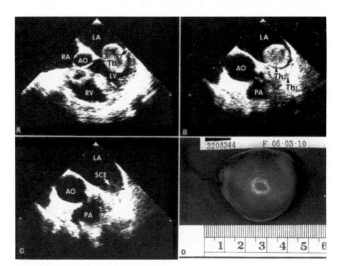

**Fig. 11–51.** Transesophageal echocardiographic views and pathologic specimen of a patient with a highly mobile, spherical thrombus (Th) within the left atrium. *A* shows an echofree center, likely a result of cystic structures within the thrombus. *B* shows a second thrombus (Th₁) within the left atrial appendage. *C* shows spontaneous contrast (SCE) within the left atrium. The surgical specimen is noted in *D*. (From Kuo, C.T., et al.: Left atrial ball thrombus in non-rheumatic atrial fibrillation diagnosed by transesophageal echocardiography. Am. Heart J., *123*:1396, 1992.)

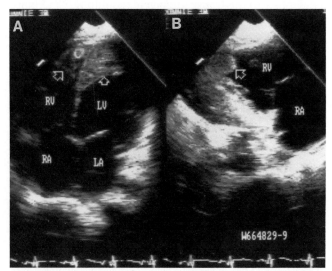

**Fig. 11–52.** Four-chamber *(A)* and long-axis right ventricular inflow *(B)* echocardiograms of a patient with thrombus *(arrows)* in the apex of the left ventricle (LV) and the right ventricle (RV). The right ventricular thrombus has a different appearance in the two views.

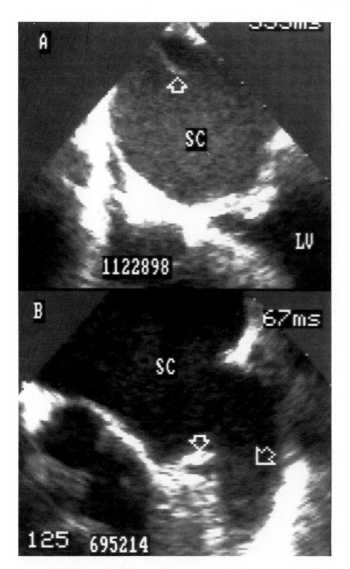

**Fig. 11–53.** Transesophageal echocardiograms of two patients with spontaneous contrast (SC) and formed thrombi *(arrows)* in the left atrium. In *A,* the thrombus is linear and mobile. In *B,* a clot *(small arrow)* is attached at the junction of the left atrial appendage and the body of the left atrium. A less dense echogenic mass *(large arrow)* is faintly seen within the left atrial appendage. LV = left ventricle.

ally highly mobile and potentially dangerous as they pass into the lungs. Transesophageal echocardiography can provide fairly dramatic images of these thrombi.[225] Figure 11–55 shows transverse and longitudinal plane examinations of a patient with a huge, mobile right atrial thrombus. The thrombus is multilobulated. Several authors have emphasized the ability to see these clots more readily with transesophageal rather than transthoracic echocardiography.

Clots in the pulmonary artery are potentially lethal.[226–230] Figure 11–56 shows a patient with repeated pulmonary emboli. One readily identifies the dilated right ventricle and right atrium that result from long-standing pulmonary hypertension. In addition, visualiz-

ation of the pulmonary artery in the short-axis view reveals an echogenic thrombus *(arrow)* within the main pulmonary artery. As one would predict, the transesophageal approach allows visualization of pulmonary artery emboli with even greater clarity.[231–235] Figure 11–57 shows an example of a thrombus within the right pulmonary artery. The mass occupies approximately 40% of the diameter of the right pulmonary artery and was consistent with a fresh thrombus.

The transesophageal examination also offers an opportunity to detect thrombus in the systemic veins.[236,237] Figure 11–58 shows a thrombus within the superior vena cava that extends into the right atrium. Several examples of superior vena cava thrombus have been detected with the transesophageal echocardiographic examination. The thrombus can be seen at various levels of the superior vena cava using this esophageal approach.

## OTHER MASSES

A variety of other entities present as masses on echocardiograms. Some of these conditions, such as vegeta-

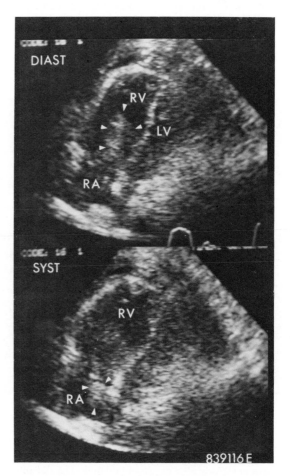

**Fig. 11–54.** Apical four-chamber two-dimensional echocardiograms of a patient with a large thrombus *(arrowheads)* in the right atrium (RA) and right ventricle (RV). The clot moves back and forth between the right atrium and right ventricle from diastole to systole. LV = left ventricle.

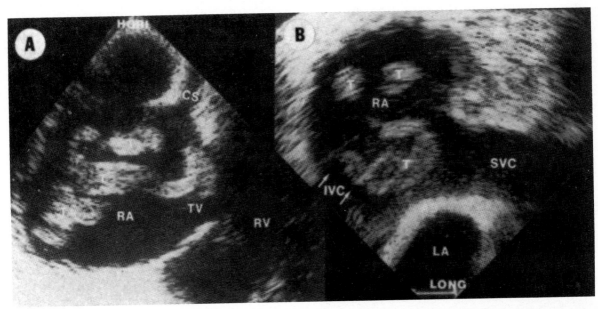

**Fig. 11–55.** Transverse *(A)* and longitudinal *(B)* transesophageal echocardiograms of a patient with a large, irregularly shaped thrombus (T) within the right atrium (RA). The multilobulated thrombus is consistent with a "string" thrombus from peripheral embolization. CS = coronary sinus; TV = tricuspid valve; RV = right ventricle; IVC = inferior vena cava; SVC = superior vena cava; LA = left atrium. (From Reeder, G.S., et al.: Transesophageal echocardiography in cardiac masses. Mayo Clin. Proc., *66*:1105, 1991.)

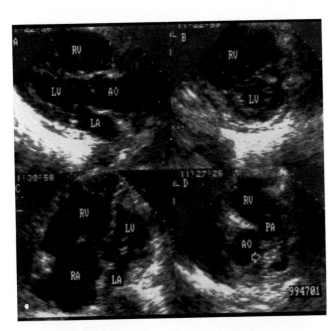

**Fig. 11–56.** Two-dimensional echocardiograms of a patient with repeated pulmonary emboli. A dilated right ventricle (RV) can be seen in the long-axis *(A)*, the short-axis at the papillary muscle level *(B)*, and the apical four-chamber *(C)* views. The right atrium (RA) is also massively dilated. The flat interventricular septum *(B)* indicates a pressure overload of the right ventricle. In the short-axis view at the base of the heart *(D)*, one can see an echogenic thrombus *(arrow)* within the pulmonary artery (PA). LV = left ventricle; AO = aorta; LA = left atrium.

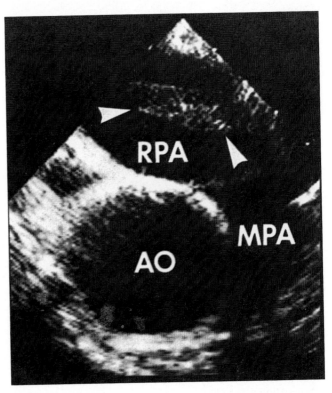

**Fig. 11–57.** Transesophageal echocardiogram demonstrating a large thrombus *(arrows)* within the right pulmonary artery (RPA). AO = aorta; MPA = main pulmonary artery. (From Klein, A.L., et al.: Visualization of acute pulmonary emboli by transesophageal echocardiography. J. Am. Soc. Echocardiogr., *3*:414, 1990.)

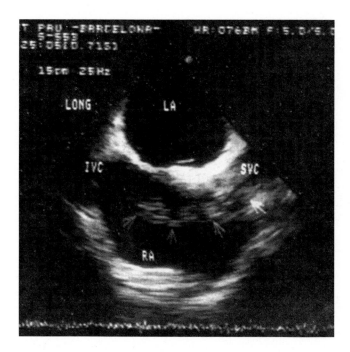

**Fig. 11–58.** A large thrombus *(arrows)* extending from the superior vena cava (SVC) into the right atrium (RA) as seen with a transesophageal echocardiographic study. LA = left atrium; IVC = inferior vena cava. (From Guindo, J., et al.: Fibrinolytic therapy for superior vena cava and right atrial thrombus: Diagnosis and follow-up with biplane transesophageal echocardiography. Am. Heart J. *124*:512, 1992.)

tions or other infectious problems, have been discussed in the appropriate chapters. Post-traumatic hematomas have also been described (see Chapter 9). Hemangiomas have been noted echocardiographically.[238,239] Some of these entities produce spectacular echocardiograms. An interesting abnormality is an echinococcal cyst,[240–242] which was described in Chapter 9. This entity is rare in the United States but may be seen in other parts of the world. Figure 11–59 shows a two-dimensional echocardiogram of an echinococcal cyst in the heart. This multiseptate cyst frequently involves the interventricular septum and can greatly distort the echocardiogram.[241,243]

## ULTRASONIC TISSUE TYPING OF CARDIAC MASSES

Attempts have been made to identify the type of cardiac mass according to ultrasonic tissue typing.[244–248] One technique involves digital analysis of gray levels from the mass.[244] Another approach is to use color-encoded two-dimensional echocardiography to highlight the differences in gray level of the various abnormalities.[245] These techniques apparently can help to distinguish a neoplasm from a thrombus.[246] This application, however, has yet to be substantiated and is not a part of routine echocardiographic assessment.

## MANMADE OBJECTS IN THE HEART

A number of manmade objects can be seen in and around the heart. Intracardiac catheters are the most common objects seen echocardiographically.[249–261] Figure 11–60 shows an apical four-chamber view of a patient with a catheter in the right ventricle. The fairly bright linear echo can be seen in this view. Figure 11–61 shows a similar patient, with a catheter detected in the subcostal four-chamber examination.[262] The ability to recognize these iatrogenic masses is important so that they are not confused with some pathologic condition. Occasionally, the catheters, especially pacemaker catheters, may perforate one of the cardiac

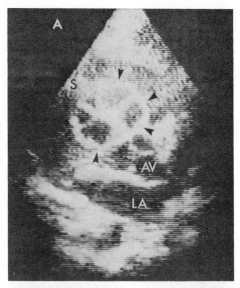

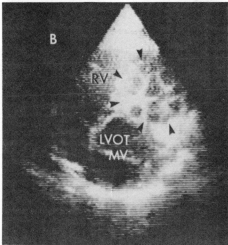

**Fig. 11–59.** Long-axis *(A)* and short-axis *(B)* two-dimensional echocardiograms of a patient with an echinococcal cyst *(arrowheads)*. The multiseptated cystic structure involves the anterior septum (S). AV = aortic valve; LA = left atrium; RV = right ventricle; LVOT = left ventricular outflow tract; MV = mitral valve. (From Limacher, M.C., et al.: Cardiac echinococcal cyst. Diagnosis by two-dimensional echocardiography. J. Am. Coll. Cardiol., *2*:574, 1983.)

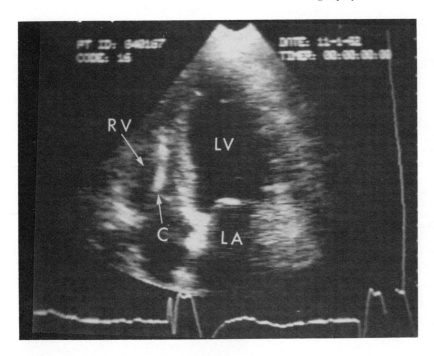

**Fig. 11–60.** Apical four-chamber two-dimensional echocardiogram of a patient with a catheter (C) in the right ventricle (RV). LV = left ventricle; LA = left atrium.

walls.[252,254,263–267] These catheters may also have clots attached to them, which can be seen on the echocardiogram.[268–270] An infected transvenous pacemaker has been identified with transesophageal echocardiography.[270a] A rare case of "cardiac strangulation" from the epicardial pacemaker has been reported.[271] Figure 11–62 shows a transesophageal echocardiographic demonstration of an intraaortic balloon in the descending aorta.[272] One can appreciate the closed *(A)* and open balloon *(B)*. Interestingly, a large atherosclerotic plaque was visible nearby *(C)*.

The ability to see these catheters ultrasonically permits one to use echocardiography instead of fluoroscopy to monitor catheter placement.[273] In addition, investigators have been using echocardiography to assist with myocardial biopsies.[274–277] Monitoring the biotome may be particularly helpful during right ventricular biopsies to avoid damaging the tricuspid valve apparatus.

More pathologic manmade objects, such as needles[278] and bullets,[261,278a,278b] have been reported. One of the features of a metallic object, such as a bullet, is the striking reverberations produced by this highly reflective object. Figure 11–63 shows echocardiograms of a patient with a bullet in the heart. The most striking finding is

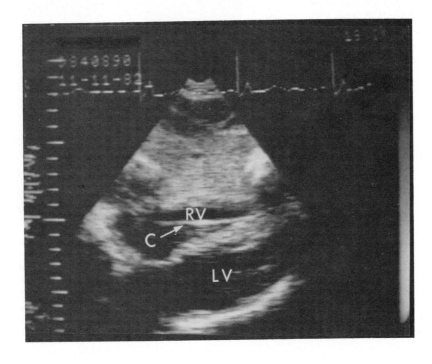

**Fig. 11–61.** Subcostal four-chamber echocardiogram of a patient with a catheter (C) in the right ventricle (RV). LV = left ventricle.

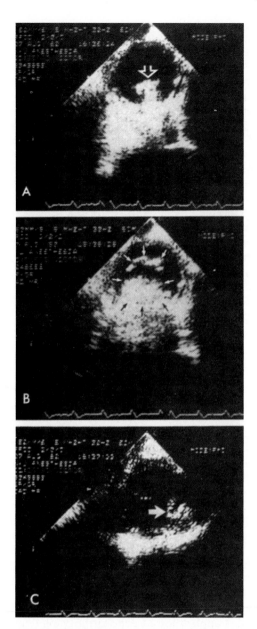

**Fig. 11–62.** Transesophageal echocardiograms of the descending aorta in a patient with an intraaortic balloon. The collapsed balloon *(arrow)* is noted in *A*. The inflated balloon in *B* is indicated by the small arrows. *C* shows a large atherosclerotic plaque *(large arrow)* near the site of the balloon. (From Katz, E.S., Tunick, P.A., and Kronzon, I.: Observations of coronary flow augmentation and balloon function during intraaortic balloon counterpulsation using transesophageal echocardiography. Am. J. Cardiol., *69*:1636, 1992.)

the long reverberation trailing away from the foreign body. This reverberation becomes a useful artifact to identify a highly reflective but small object.

Occasionally, the foreign body is not as reflective and is seen merely as an echogenic mass within the heart. Figure 11–64 shows the echocardiogram of a patient who had a small pellet lodged within the heart at the junction between the right ventricular annulus and the interventricular septum. The echogenic mass again pro-

duces a "comet-like" reverberation superimposed on the interatrial septum.

## PROBE PATENT FORAMEN OVALE

Although a probe patent foramen ovale does not produce an intracardiac mass, this entity may be the conduit

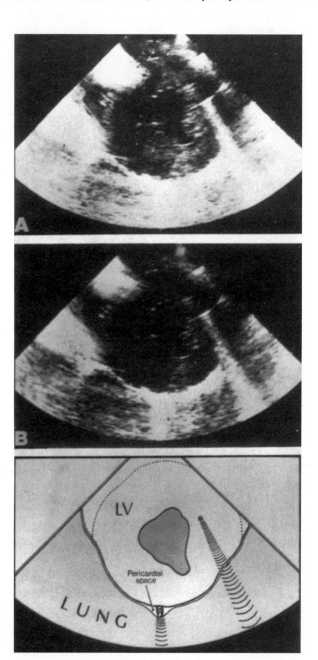

**Fig. 11–63.** High-gain *(A)* and low-gain *(B)* recordings and a diagram of a patient with gunshot wounds within the heart. The bullets are identified best with the low-gain setting and visualization of a comet-like reverberation behind the two foreign bodies. LV = left ventricle. (From Reeves, W.C., et al.: Utility of precordial, epicardial, and transesophageal two-dimensional echocardiography in the detection of intracardiac foreign bodies. Am. J. Cardiol., *64*:408, 1989.)

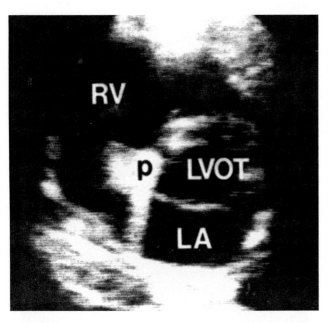

**Fig. 11–64.** Parasternal, short-axis view showing a pellet (p) and its comet-like reverberation between the left ventricular outflow tract (LVOT), the left atrium (LA), and the right ventricle (RV). (From Fyfe, D.A., et al.: Preoperative localization of an intracardiac foreign body by two-dimensional echocardiography. Am. Heart J., *113*:211, 1987.)

for the passage of a mass from the systemic veins into the systemic arteries. As a result, looking for a probe patent foramen ovale is a common reason for ordering an echocardiogram. With the advent of transesophageal echocardiography, especially using contrast enhancement and Doppler flow imaging, the ultrasonic examination is proving to be sensitive and reliable for identifying a probe patent foramen ovale.[279,279a] Figure 11–65

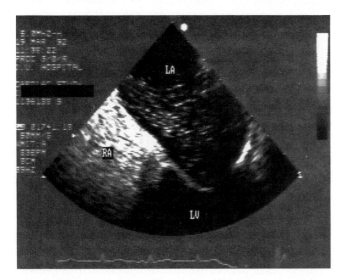

**Fig. 11–65.** Transesophageal echocardiogram of a patient with a probe patent foramen ovale. An intravenous contrast injection demonstrates shunting from the right atrium (RA) to the left atrium (LA). LV = left ventricle.

shows a positive right-to-left contrast-enhanced study with transesophageal echocardiography in a patient with a probe patent foramen ovale. In a variety of studies, it has been noted that people with systemic emboli have a higher incidence of a probe patent foramen ovale;[280] however, direct proof of cause and effect between the presence of the defect and a systemic embolus is not great.[280a] Patients with a mobile or dilated foramen ovale seem to have a higher incidence of potential shunt.[280b] Instances of finding clot lodged within or passing through a patent foramen ovale have been reported, but these have been few.[281,282] The best means for detecting a patent foramen ovale is to perform a transesophageal echocardiographic study and a systemic venous contrast injection. Injecting the contrast material during a Valsalva maneuver or cough[282a] helps to open the patent foramen. Once a probe patent defect is discovered, its management depends on the clinical situation. Debate continues as to how often this abnormality is responsible for a systemic embolus.

## SUMMARY

The identification of cardiac masses is one of the most important uses of two-dimensional transthoracic and transesophageal echocardiography. The individuals performing and interpreting echocardiograms must be extremely careful in making the diagnosis of a pathologic mass within the heart. Erroneous diagnoses can lead to serious mismanagement of the patient. One certainly does not want to overlook a potentially lethal situation, such as a myxoma or right atrial thrombus. On the other hand, one does not want to subject an individual to unnecessary cardiac surgery on the basis of an echocardiographic artifact or normal variant. Looking for echocardiographic masses is occasionally like taking a Rorschach test. When examining a patient with a systemic embolus, one seems to find all sorts of peculiar echoes that could conceivably be sources for emboli. Thus, although this application of echocardiography can be extremely rewarding when a potentially curable cardiac abnormality is found, it can also be frustrating when recording echoes that are difficult to explain.[283] The fact remains that in patients who have no evidence of a cardiac abnormality, finding the source of an embolus with an echocardiogram is still a low probability.[284–286a] Frequently, one will find a peculiar, unexplained echo or a common entity such as a probe patent foramen ovale that will only add speculation and confusion as to whether or not this finding is related to the embolic event.[287] Therefore, any discussion of the sonographic detection of cardiac masses must always end with a word of caution.[288]

## REFERENCES

1. Mugge, A., Daniel, W.G., Haverich, A., and Lichtlen, P.R.: Diagnosis of noninfective cardiac mass lesions by

two-dimensional echocardiography. Circulation, *83*:70, 1991.

2. Reeder, G.S., Khandheria, B.K., Seward, J.B., and Tajik, A.J.: Transesophageal echocardiography and cardiac masses. Mayo Clin. Proc., *66*:1101, 1991.

3. Black, J.W., Hopkins, A.P., Lee, L.C.L., Jacobson, B.M., and Walsh, W.F.: Role of transesophageal echocardiography in evaluation of cardiogenic embolism. Br. Heart J., *66*:302, 1991.

4. Pearson, A.C., Labovitz, A.J., Tatineni, S., and Gomez, C.R.: Superiority of transesophageal echocardiography in detecting cardiac sources of embolism in patients with cerebral ischemia of uncertain etiology. J. Am. Coll. Cardiol., *17*:66, 1991.

5. Fyfe, D.A., Kline, C.H., Sade, R.M., and Gillette, P.C.: Transesophageal echocardiography detects thrombus formation not identified by transthoracic echocardiography after the Fontan operation. J. Am. Coll. Cardiol., *18*:1733, 1991.

6. Alam, M. and Sun, I.: Transesophageal echocardiographic evaluation of left atrial mass lesions. J. Am. Soc. Echocardiogr., *4*:323, 1991.

7. Alam, M., Sun, I., and Smith, S.: Transesophageal echocardiographic evaluation of right atrial mass lesions. J. Am. Soc. Echocardiogr., *4*:331, 1991.

8. Herrera, C.J., Mehlman, D.J., Hartz, R.S., Talano, J.V., and McPherson, D.D.: Comparison of transesophageal and transthoracic echocardiograph for diagnosis of right-sided cardiac lesions. Am. J. Cardiol., *70*:964, 1992.

9. Safety Monitoring Committee, Echocardiography Committee, Writing Committee: Predictors of Thromboembolism in Atrial Fibrillation: II. Echocardiographic Features of Patients at Risk. Ann. Intern. Med., *116*:6, 1992.

9a. Stoddard, M.F., Liddell, N.E., Longacker, R.A., and Dawkins, P.R.: Transesophageal echocardiography: Normal variants and mimickers. Am. Heart J., *124*:1587, 1992.

10. Keren, A., Billingham, M.E., and Popp, R.L.: Echocardiographic recognition and implications of ventricular hypertrophic trabeculations and aberrant bands. Circulation, *70*:836, 1984.

11. Boyd, M.T., Seward, J.B., Tajik, A.J., and Edwards, W.D.: Frequency and location of prominent left ventricular trabeculations at autopsy in 474 normal human hearts: Implications for evaluation of mural thrombi by two-dimensional echocardiography. J. Am. Coll. Cardiol., *9*: 323, 1987.

12. Leon, M., Pechacek, L.W., Solana, L.G., Massumkhani, A., and Colley, D.A.: Identification of a prominent eustachian valve by means of contrast two dimensional echocardiography. Texas Heart Institute J., *10*:219, 1983.

13. Schrem, S.S., Freedberg, R.S., Gindea, A.J., and Kronzon, I.: The association between unusually large eustachian valves and atrioventricular valvular prolapse. Am. Heart J., *120*:204, 1990.

14. Werner, J.A., Cheitlin, M.D., Gross, B.W., Speck, S.M., and Ivey, T.D.: Echocardiographic appearance of the Chiari network: Differentiation from right-heart pathology. Circulation, *63*:1104, 1981.

15. Cloez, J.L., Neimann, J.L., Chivoret, G., Danchin, N., Bruntz, J.F., Godenir, J.P., and Faivre, G.: Echocardiographic rediscovery of an anatomical structure: The Chiari network. A propos of 16 cases. Arch. Mal Coeur. *76*:1284, 1983.

16. Cujec, B., Mycyk, T., and Khouri, M.: Identification of Chiari's network with transesophageal echocardiography. J. Am. Soc. Echocardiogr., *5*:96, 1992.

17. Katz, E.S., Freedberg, R.S., Rutkovsky, L., Martin, J.C., and Kronzon, I.: Identification of an unusual right atrial mass as a Chiari network by biplane transesophageal echocardiography. Echocardiography, *9*:273, 1992.

18. Luetmer, P.H., Edwards, W.D., Seward, J.B., and Tajik, A.J.: Incidence and distribution of left ventricular false tendons: An autopsy study of 483 normal human hearts. J. Am. Coll. Cardiol., *8*:179, 1986.

19. Sethuraman, K.R., Sriram, R., and Balachandar, J.: Left ventricular false tendons: Echocardiographic incidence in India and clinical importance. Int. J. Cardiol., *6*:385, 1984.

20. Malouf, J., Gharzuddine, W., and Kutayli, F.: A reappraisal of the prevalence and clinical importance of left ventricular false tendons in children and adults. Br. Heart J., *55*:587, 1986.

20a. Brenner, J.I., Baker, K., Ringel, R.E., and Berman, M.A.: Echocardiographic evidence of left ventricular bands in infants and children. J. Am. Coll. Cardiol., *3*: 1515, 1984.

20b. Perry, L.W., Ruckman, R.N., Shapiro, S.R., Kuehl, K.S., Galioto, F.M. and Scott, L.P.: Left ventricular false tendons in children: Prevalence as detected by two dimensional echocardiography and clinical significance. Am. J. Cardiol., *52*:1264, 1983.

20c. Vered, Z., Meltzer, R.S., Benjamin, P., Motro, M., and Neufeld, H.N.: Prevalence and significance of false tendons in the left ventricle as determined by echocardiography. Am. J. Cardiol., *53*:330, 1984.

21. Suwa, M., Hirota, Y., Kaku, K., Yoneda, Y., Nakayama, A., Kawamura, K., and Doi, K.: Prevalence of the coexistence of left ventricular false tendons and premature ventricular complexes in apparently healthy subjects: A prospective study in the general population. J. Am. Coll. Cardiol., *12*:910, 1988.

21a. Fyke, III, F.E., Tajik, A.J., Edwards, W.D., and Seward, J.B.: Diagnosis of lipomatous hypertrophy of the interatrial septum by two dimensional echocardiography. J. Am. Coll. Cardiol., *1*:1352, 1983.

21b. Seward, J.B., Khandheria, B.K., Oh, J.K., Freeman, W.K., and Tajik, A.J.: Critical appraisal of transesophageal echocardiography: Limitations, pitfalls, and complications. J. Am. Soc. Echocardiogr., *5*:288, 1992.

22. Kindman, L.A., Wright, A., Tye, T., Seale, W., and Appleton, C.: Lipomatous hypertrophy of the interatrial septum: Characterization by transesophageal and transthoracic echocardiography, magnetic resonance imaging, and computed tomography. J. Am. Soc. Echocardiogr., *1*:450, 1988.

23. Applegate, P.M., Tajik, A.J., Ehman, R.L., Julsrud, P.R., and Miller, F.A.: Two-dimensional echocardiographic and magnetic resonance imaging observations in massive lipomatous hypertrophy of the atrial septum. Am. J. Cardiol., *59*:489, 1987.

24. Jornet, A., Batalla, J., Uson, M., Mallol, A., Reig, J., Petit, M.: Lipomatous hypertrophy of the interatrial septum. Echocardiography, *9*:501, 1992.

25. Pochis, W.T., Saeian, K., and Sagar, K.B.: Usefulness of transesophageal echocardiography in diagnosing lipomatous hypertrophy of the atrial septum with comparison to transthoracic echocardiography. Am. J. Cardiol., *70*: 396, 1992.

25a. Cohen, I.S. and Raiker, K.: Atrial lipomatous hypertrophy: Lipomatous atrial hypertrophy with significant involvement of the right atrial wall. J. Am. Soc. Echocardiogr., 6:30, 1993.

26. Kong, C.W. and Chan, W.: The echocardiographic fea-

tures of an aneurysm of the inter-atrial septum. Angiology, *35*:188, 1984.

27. Canny, M., Drobinski, G., Thomas, D., Gautier, J.C., Awada, A., Leclerc, J.P., Gong, L., Chane-Woon-Ming, M., and Gandjbakhch, I.: Interatrial septal aneurysm. Echocardiographic diagnosis. Arch. Mal Coeur, *77*:337, 1984.

28. Wysham, D.G., McPherson, D.D., and Kerber, R.E.: Asymptomatic aneurysm of the interatrial septum. J. Am. Coll. Cardiol., *4*:1311, 1984.

29. Gallet, B., et al.: Atrial septal aneurysm—A potential cause of systemic embolism. Br. Heart J., *53*:292, 1985.

30. Smith, A.J., Panidis, I.P., Berger, S., and Gonzales, R.: Large atrial septal aneurysm mimicking a cystic right atrial mass. Am. Heart J., *120*:714, 1990.

31. Belkin, R.N. and Kisslo, J.: Atrial septal aneurysm: Recognition and clinical relevance. Am. Heart J., *120*:948, 1990.

32. Yeoh, J.K., Appelbe, A.F., and Martin, R.P.: Atrial septal aneurysm mimicking a right atrial mass on transesophageal echocardiography. Am. J. Cardiol., *68*:827, 1991.

32a. Schneider, B., Hofmann, T., Meinertz, T., and Hanrath, P.: Diagnostic value of transesophageal echocardiography in atrial septal aneurysm. Int. J. Card. Imaging, *8*:143, 1992.

33. Burstow, D.J., McEniery, P.T., and Stafford, E.G.: Fenestrated atrial septal aneurysm: Diagnosis by transesophageal echocardiography. J. Am. Soc. Echocardiogr., *3*:499, 1990.

34. Schneider, B., Hanrath, P., Vogel, P., and Meinertz, T.: Improved morphologic characterization of atrial septal aneurysm by transesophageal echocardiography: Relation to cerebrovascular events. J. Am. Coll. Cardiol., *16*:1000, 1990.

35. Pearson, A.C., Nagelhout, D., Castello, R., Gomez, C.R., and Labovitz, A.J.: Atrial septal aneurysm and stroke: A transesophageal echocardiographic study. J. Am. Coll. Cardiol., *18*:1223, 1991.

36. Zabalgoitia-Reyes, M., Herrera, C., Gandhi, D.K., Mehlman, D.J., McPherson, D.D., and Talano, J.V.: A possible mechanism for neurologic ischemic events in patients with atrial septal aneurysm. Am. J. Cardiol., *66*:761, 1990.

37. Starling, R.C., Baker, P.B., Hirsch, S.C., Myerowitz, P.D., Galbraith, T.A., and Binkley, P.F.: An echocardiographic and anatomic description of the donor-recipient atrial anastomosis after orthoptopic cardiac transplantation. Am. J. Cardiol., *64*:109, 1989.

38. Manning, W.J., Waksmonski, C.A., and Riley, M.F.: Remnant of the common pulmonary vein mistaken for a left atrial mass: Clarification by transesophageal echocardiography. Br. Heart J., *68*:4, 1992.

38a. Movsowitz, H.D., Jacobs, L.E., Movsowitz, C., Kotler, M.N., and Ioli, A.W.: Transesophageal echocardiographic evaluation of a transthoracic echocardiographic pitfall: A diaphragmatic hernia mimicking a left atrial mass. J. Am. Soc. Echocardiogr. *6*:104, 1993.

39. Fyke, F.E., III, et al.: Primary cardiac tumors: Experience with 30 consecutive patients since the introduction of two-dimensional echocardiography. J. Am. Coll. Cardiol., *5*:1465, 1985.

40. Vargas-Barron, J., Romero-Cardenas, A., Villegas, M., Keirns, C., Gomez-Jaume, A., Delong, R., and Malo-Camacho, R.: Transthoracic and transesophageal echocardiographic diagnosis of myxomas in the four cardiac cavities. Am. Heart J., *121*:931, 1991.

41. Nomeir, A-M., Watts, L.E., Seagle, R., Joyner, C.R., Corman, C., and Prichard, R.W.: Intracardiac myxomas: Twenty-year echocardiographic experience with review of the literature. J. Am. Soc. Echocardiogr., *2*:139, 1989.

42. Pechacek, L.W., Gonzalez-Camid, F., Hall, R.J., Garcia, E., deCastro, C.M., Leachman, R.D., and Montiel-Amoroso, G.: The echocardiographic spectrum of atrial myxoma: A ten-year experience. Texas Heart Institute J., *12*:179, 1986.

43. Bass, N.M. and Sharratt, G.P.: Left atrial myxoma diagnosed by echocardiography with observations on tumour movement. Br. Heart J., *35*:1332, 1973.

44. Effert, S. and Domanig, E.: The diagnosis of intraatrial tumor and thrombi by the ultrasonic echo method. German Med. Mth., *4*:1, 1959.

45. Finegan, R.E. and Harrison, D.C.: Diagnosis of left atrial myxoma by echocardiography. N. Engl. J. Med., *282*:1022, 1970.

46. Gustafson, A., Edler, I., Dahlback, O., Kaude, J., and Persson, S.: Left atrial myxoma diagnosed by ultrasound cardiography. Angiology, *24*:554, 1973.

47. Kostis, J.B. and Moghadam, A.N.: Echocardiographic diagnosis of left atrial myxoma. Chest, *58*:550, 1970.

48. Popp, R.L. and Harrison, D.C.: Ultrasound in the diagnosis of atrial tumor. Ann. Intern. Med., *71*:785, 1969.

49. Schattenberg, T.T.: Echocardiographic diagnosis of left atrial myxoma. Mayo Clin. Proc., *43*:620, 1968.

50. Wolfe, S.B., Popp, R.L., and Feigenbaum, H.: Diagnosis of atrial tumors by ultrasound. Circulation, *39*:615, 1969.

51. Abdulla, A.M., Stefadouros, M.A., Mucha, E., Moore, H.V., and O'Malley, G.A.: Left atrial myxoma: Echocardiographic diagnosis and determination of size. JAMA, *238*:510, 1977.

52. Perry, L.S., King, J.F., Zeft, H.O., Manley, J.C., Gross, C.M., and Wann, L.S.: Two dimensional echocardiography in the diagnosis of left atrial myxoma. Br. Heart J., *45*:667, 1981.

53. Moses, H.W. and Nanda, N.C.: Real time two dimensional echocardiography in the diagnosis of left atrial myxoma. Chest *78*:788, 1980.

54. Reeves, W.C. and Chitwood, W.R., Jr.: Assessment of left atrial myxoma using transesophageal two-dimensional echocardiography and color flow Doppler. Echocardiography, *6*:547, 1989.

55. Salmon, K., Decoodt, P., and Capon, A.: Detection of a left atrial myxoma by systematic transesophageal echocardiography in stroke. Am. Heart J., *122*:580, 1991.

56. Obeid, A.I., Marvasti, M., Parker, F., and Rosenberg, J.: Comparison of transthoracic and transesophageal echocardiography in diagnosis of left atrial myxoma. Am. J. Cardiol., *63*:1006, 1989.

57. Winer, H.E., Kronzon, I., Fox, A., Hines, G., Trehan, N., Antapol, S., and Reed, G.: Primary cardiac chondro-myxosarcoma—clinical and echocardiographic manifestations: A case report. J. Thorac. Surg., *74*:567, 1977.

58. Zackia, A.H., Weber, D.J., Ramsey, C., and Wong, B.: Recurrence of left atrial myxoma. J. Cardiovasc. Surg. (Torino), *25*:467, 1974.

59. Hada, Y., Takahashi, T., Takenaka, K., Sakamoto, T., and Murao, S.: Recurrent multiple myxomas. Am. Heart J., *107*:1280, 1984.

60. Pavlides, G.S., Levin, R.N., and Hauser, A.M.: Left ventricular recurrence of a resected left atrial myxoma. Am. Heart J., *117*:1390, 1989.

61. Pochis, W.T., Wingo, M.W., Cinquegrani, M.P., and Sagar, K.R.: Echocardiographic demonstration of rapid

growth of a left atrial myxoma. Am. Heart J., *122*:1781, 1991.

62. Ahern, T., Chandrasekaran, K., Minta, G.S., and Ross, J.: Detection of growth of an atrial myxoma after aortic valve replacement. Am. Heart J., *118*:1062, 1989.

63. Roudaut, R., Gosse, P., and Dallocchio, M.: Rapid growth of a left atrial myxoma shown by echocardiography. Br. Heart J., *58*:413, 1987.

64. Rahilly, G.T. and Nanda, N.C.: Two dimensional echographic identification of tumor hemorrhages in atrial myxomas. Am. Heart J., *101*:237, 1981.

65. Bryhn, M., Gustafson, A., and Stubbe, I.: Two dimensional echocardiography in the diagnosis of hemorrhages in a left atrial myxoma. Acta Med. Okayama, *212*:433, 1982.

66. Tunick, P.A., Fox, A.C., Culliford, A., Levy, R., and Kronzon, I.: The echocardiographic recognition of an atrial myxoma vegetation. Am. Heart J., *119*:679, 1990.

67. Thier, W., Schluter, M., Krebber, .-J., Polonius, M.-J., Kloppel, G., Becker, K., and Hanrath, P.: Cysts in left atrial myxomas identified by transesophageal cross-sectional echocardiography. Am. J. Cardiol., *51*:1793, 1983.

68. Harbold, N.B., Jr. and Gau, G.T.: Echocardiographic diagnosis of right atrial myxoma. Mayo Clin. Proc., *48*:284, 1973.

69. Farooki, Z.Q., Green, E.W., and Arciniegas, E.: Echocardiographic pattern of right atrial tumour motion. Br. Heart J., *38*:580, 1976.

70. Pernod, J., Piwnica, A., and Duret, J.C.: Right atrial myxoma: An echocardiographic study. Br. Heart J., *40*:201, 1978.

71. Meyers, S.N., Shapiro, S.E., Barresi, V., et al.: Right atrial myxoma with right to left shunting and mitral valve prolapse. Am. J. Med., *62*:308, 1977.

72. Frishman, W., Factor, S., Jordon, A., Hellman, C., El-kayam, U., LeJemtel, T., Strom, J., Unschuld, H., and Becker, R.: Right atrial myxoma: Unusual clinical presentation and atypical glandular histology. Circulation, *59*:1070, 1979. (Case report)

73. Atsuchi, Y., Nagai, Y., Nakamura, K., et al.: Echocardiographic diagnosis of prolapsing right atrial myxoma. Jpn. Heart J., *17*:798, 1976.

74. Pores, I.H., Abel, R.M., Gray, L., and Jacobs, G.P.: Giant right atrial myxoma with rheumatic mitral valve disease. Angiology, *35*:313, 1984.

75. Gladden, J.R., Dreiling, R.J., Gollub, S.B., Bixler, T.J., and Dunn, M.I.: Two dimensional echocardiographic features of multiple right atrial myxomas. Am. J. Cardiol., *52*:1364, 1983.

76. Chaptal, P.A., Grolleau, R., Ferrière, M., Renevier, D., and Nègre, G.: Myxomas of the right atrium. Arch. Mal Coeur, *73*:1479, 1980.

77. Panidis, I.P., Kotler, M.N., Mintz, G.S., and Ross, J.: Clinical and echocardiographic features of right atrial masses. Am. Heart J., *107*:745, 1984.

78. Fitterer, J.D., Spicer, M.J., and Nelson, W.P.: Echocardiographic demonstration of bilateral atrial myxomas. Chest, *70*:282, 1976.

79. Nicholson, K.G., Prior, A.L., Norman, A.G., Naik, D.R., and Kennedy, A.: Bilateral atrial myxomas diagnosed preoperatively and successfully removed. Br. Med. J., *2*(6084):440, 1977.

80. Gustafson, A.G., Edler, I.G., and Dahlback, O.K.: Bilateral atrial myxomas diagnosed by echocardiography. Acta Med. Scand., *201*:391, 1977.

81. Tway, K.P., Shah, A.A., and Rahimtoola, S.H.: Multiple bilateral myxomas demonstrated by two dimensional echocardiography. Am. J. Med., *71*:896, 1981.

82. Dittmann, H., Voelker, W., Karsch, K.R., and Seipel, L.: Bilateral atrial myxomas detected by transesophageal two-dimensional echocardiography. Am. Heart J., *118*:172, 1989.

83. Rey, M., Tunon, J., Compres, H., Rabago, R., Fraile, J., and Rabago, P.: Prolapsing right atrial myxoma evaluated by transesophageal echocardiography. Am. Heart J., *122*:875, 1991.

84. Mazer, M.S. and Harrigan, P.R.: Left ventricular myxoma: M-mode and two dimensional echocardiographic features. Am. Heart J., *104*:875, 1982.

85. Abramowitz, R., Majdan, J.F., Plzak, L.F., and Berger, B.C.: Two dimensional echocardiographic diagnosis of separate myxomas of both the left atrium and left ventricle. Am. J. Cardiol., *53*:379, 1984.

86. Fukui, H., et al.: Left ventricular myxoma with special reference to diagnostic approach: Report of a case. J. Cardiogr., *12*:545, 1982.

87. Viswanathan, B., Luber, J.M., Jr., and Bell-Thomson, J.: Right ventricular myxoma. Ann. Thorac. Surg., *39*:280, 1985.

88. Fagan, Jr., L.F., Castello, R., Barner, H., Moran, M., and Labovitz, A.J.: Transesophageal echocardiographic diagnosis of recurrent right ventricular myxoma 2 years after excision of right atrial myxoma. Am. Heart J., *120*:1456, 1990.

89. Rosenzweig, A., Harrigan, P., and Popvic, A.D.: Left ventricular myxoma simulating aortic stenosis. Am. Heart J., *117*:962, 1989.

90. Wrisley, D., Rosenberg, J., Giambartolomei, A., Levy, I., Turiello, C., and Antonini, T.: Left ventricular myxoma discovered incidentally by echocardiography. Am. Heart J., *121*:1554, 1991.

91. Turlapati, R.V., Jacobs, L.E., and Kotler, M.N.: Right atrial myxoma causing total destruction of the tricuspid valve leaflets. Am. Heart J., *120*:1227, 1990.

92. Gultekin, N., Doger, H., Turkoglu, C., Ozturk, S., Gokhan, N., and Demiroglu, C.: Giant right atrial thrombus causing right ventricular inflow and outflow obstruction. Am. Heart J., *116*:1367, 1988.

93. Goli, V.D., Thadani, U., Thomas, S.R., Voyles, W.F., and Teague, S.M.: Doppler echocardiographic profiles in obstructive right and left atrial myxomas. J. Am. Coll. Cardiol., *9*:701, 1987.

94. Gorcsan, III, J., Blanc, M.S., Reddy, P.S., and Marrone, G.C.: Hemodynamic diagnosis of mitral valve obstruction by left atrial myxoma with transesophageal continuous wave Doppler. Am. Heart J., *124*:1109, 1992.

95. Shechter, M., Glikson, M., Agranat, O., and Motro, M.: Echocardiographic demonstration of mitral block caused by left atrial spindle cell sarcoma. Am. Heart J., *123*:232, 1992.

96. Pinamonti, B., Sinagra, G., Slavich, G., Calucci, F., Manzini, V.D., Bussani, R., and Silvestri, F.: Echocardiographic and Doppler findings in primary sarcoma of the pulmonary artery. Echocardiography, *9*:155, 1992.

97. Chu, K-M., Hsiung, M-C., Wang, D-J., and Shieh, S-M.: Malignant fibrous histiocytoma of the heart with cerebral metastasis: A transesophageal echocardiographic demonstration. Echocardiography, *6*:517, 1989.

98. Pasquale, M., Katz, N.M., Caruso, A.C., Bearb, M.E., and Bitterman, P.: Myxoid variant of malignant fibrous histiocytoma of the heart. Am. Heart J., *122*:248, 1991.

99. Farooki, Z.Q., Chang, C.H., Jackson, W.L., Clapp,

S.K., Hakimi, M., Arciniegas, E., and Pinsky, W.W.: Intracardiac teratoma in a newborn. Clin. Cardiol., *11*: 642, 1988.

100. Morishita, T., Yamazaki, J., Ohsawa, H. Uchi, T., Kawamura, Y., Okuzumi, K., Nakano, H., Wakakura, M., Okamoto, K., Koyama, N., and Komatsu, H.: Malignant schwannoma of the heart. Clin. Cardiol., *11*:126, 1988.

101. Hui, G., McAllister, H.A., and Angelini, P.: Left atrial paraganglioma: Report of a case and review of the literature. Am. Heart J., *113*:1230, 1987.

102. McKenney, P.A., Moroz, K., Haudenschild, C.C., Shemin, R.J., and Davidoff, R.: Malignant mesenchymoma as a primary cardiac tumor. Am. Heart J., *123*: 1071, 1992.

103. Farooki, Z.Q., Henry, J.G., Arciniegas, E., and Green, EX.W.: Ultrasonic pattern of ventricular rhabdomyoma in two infants. Am. J. Cardiol., *34*:842, 1974.

104. Fischer, D.R., Beerman, L.B., Park, S.C., Bahnson, H.T., Fricker, F.J., and Mathews, R.A.: Diagnosis of intracardiac rhabdomyoma by two dimensional echocardiography. Am. J. Cardiol., *53*:978, 1984.

105. Colloridi, V., Gallo, P., Pizzuto, F., Toscano, M., and Ruvolo, G.: Rhabdomyoma of the left atrium. A rare case of mitral valve congenital obstruction simulating hypoplastic left heart syndrome. Echocardiographic diagnosis. G. Ital. Cardiol., *12*:442, 1982.

106. Riggs, T.W., Ilbawi, M., DeLeon, S., and Paul, M.H.: Echocardiographic diagnosis of right ventricular rhabdomyoma in two infants. Pediatr. Cardiol., *3*:31, 1982.

107. Takahashi, K., Imamura, Y., Ochi, T., Hamada, M., Ito, T., Hiwada, K., and Kokubu, T.: Echocardiographic demonstration of an asymptomatic patient with left ventricular fibroma. Am. J. Cardiol., *53*:981, 1984.

108. Villasenor, H.R., Fuentes, F., and Walker, W.E.: Left atrial rhabdomyosarcoma mimicking mitral valve stenosis. Texas Heart Institute J., *12*:107, 1985.

109. Bass, J.L., Breningstall, G.N., and Swaiman, K.F.: Echocardiographic incidence of cardiac rhabdomyoma in tuberous sclerosis. Am. J. Cardiol., *55*:1379, 1985.

110. Pillai, R., Kharma, N., Brom, A.G., and Becker, A.E.: Mitral valve origin of pedunculated rhabdomyomas causing subaortic stenosis. Am. J. Cardiol., *67*:663, 1991.

111. Bar-El, Y., Adar, R., Schneiderman, Y., and Motro, M.: Echocardiography in diagnostic assessment of peripheral arterial embolization. Am. Heart J., *119*:1090, 1990.

112. Smythe, J.F., Dyck, J.D., Smallhorn, J.F., and Freedom, R.M.: Natural history of cardiac rhabdomyoma in infancy and childhood. Am. J. Cardiol., *66*:1247, 1990.

113. Awad, M., Dunn, B., Al Halees, Z., Mercer, E., Akhtar, M., Hainau, B., and Duran, C.: Intracardiac rhabdomyosarcoma: Transesophageal echocardiographic findings and diagnosis. J. Am. Soc. Echocardiogr., *5*:199, 1992.

114. Domanski, M.J., Delaney, T.F., Kleiner, D.E., Goswitz, M., Agatston, A., Tucker, E., Johnson, M., and Roberts, W.C.: Primary sarcoma of the heart causing mitral stenosis. Am. J. Cardiol., *66*:893, 1990.

115. Reece, I.J., Houston, A.B., and Pollock, J.C.S.: Interventricular fibroma. Echocardiographic diagnosis and successful surgical removal in infancy. Br. Heart J., *50*: 590, 1983.

116. Behnam, R., Williams, G., Gerlis, L., and Walker, D.: Lipoma of the mitral valve and papillary muscle. Am. J. Cardiol., *51*:1459, 1983.

117. Harada, K., Seki, I., Kobayashi, H., Okuni, M., and Sakurai, L.: Lipoma of the heart in a child. Clinical echocardiographic, angiographic and pathological features. Jpn. Heart J. *21*:903, 1980.

118. Moore, J.A., DeRan, B.P., Minor, R., Arthur, J., Fraker, Jr., T.D.: Transesophageal echocardiographic evaluation of intracardiac lymphoma. Am. Heart J., *124*:514, 1992.

119. Van Veldhuisen, D.J., Hamer, H.P.M., Van Imhoff, G.W., Hollema, H., and Lie, KI: Role of echocardiography in the diagnosis of cardiac lymphoma. Am. Heart J., *119*:973, 1990.

120. Armstrong, W.F., Buck, J.D., Hoffman, R., and Waller, B.F.: Cardiac involvement by lymphoma: Detection and follow-up by two-dimensional echocardiography. Am. Heart J., *112*:627, 1986.

121. Proctor, M.S., Tracy, G.P., and Von Koch, L.: Primary cardiac B-cell lymphoma. Am. Heart J., *118*:179, 1989.

122. Frumin, H., O'Donnell, L., Kerin, N.Z., Levine, F., Nathan, L.E., and Klein, S.P.: Two dimensional echocardiographic detection and diagnostic features of tricuspid papillary fibroelastoma. J. Am. Coll. Cardiol., *2*:1016, 1983.

123. Almagro, U.A., Perry, L.S., Choi, H., and Pintar, K.: Papillary fibroelastoma of the heart. Report of six cases. Arch. Pathol. Lab. Med., *106*:318, 1982.

124. Shub, C., Tajik, A.J., Seward, J.B., Edwards, W.D., Pruitt, R.D., Orszulak, T.A., and Pluth, J.R.: Cardiac papillary fibroelastomas. Two dimensional echocardiographic recognition. Mayo Clin. Proc., *56*:629, 1981.

125. Ong, L.S., Nanda, N.C., and Barold, S.S.: Two dimensional echocardiographic detection and diagnostic features of left ventricular papillary fibroelastoma. Am. Heart J., *103*:917, 1982.

126. Schwinger, M.E., Katz, E., Rotterdam, H., Slater, J., Weiss, E.C., and Kronzon, I.: Right atrial papillary fibroelastoma: Diagnosis by transthoracic and transesophageal echocardiography and percutaneous transvenous biopsy. Am. Heart J., *118*:1047, 1989.

127. Lewis, N.P., Williams, G.T., and Fraser, A.G.: Unusual and intraoperative epicardial echocardiographic features of a papillary tumour of the aortic valve. Br. Heart J., *62*:470, 1989.

128. Fowles, R.E., Miller, D.C., Egbert, B.M., Fitzgerald, J.W., and Popp, R.L.: Systemic embolization from mitral valve papillary endocardial fibroma detected by two dimensional echocardiography. Am. Heart J., *102*:128, 1981.

129. Politzer, F., Kronzon, I., Wieczorek, R., Feiner, H., DeMarco, L.E.G., Weintraub, P.R., Schlossman, R.E., and Hisler, S.: Intracardiac leiomyomatosis: Diagnosis and treatment. J. Am. Coll. Cardiol., *4*:629, 1984.

130. Martin, J.L. and Boak, J.G.: Cardiac metastasis from uterine leiomyosarcoma. J. Am. Coll. Cardiol., *2*:383, 1983.

131. Maurer, G. and Nanda, M.C.: Two dimensional echocardiographic identification of intracardiac leiomyomatosis. Am. Heart J., *103*:915, 1982.

132. Kaku, K., Kawashima, Y., Kitamura, S., Nakano, S., Mori, T., Beppu, S.U., Kozuka, T., Sakurai, M., Katayama, S., Tanizawa, O., and Sonoda, T.: Resection of leiomyosarcoma originating in internal iliac vein and extending into heart via inferior vena cava. Surgery, *89*:604, 1981.

133. Gonzalez-Lavin, L., Lee, R.H., Falk, L., Gradman, M.D., McFadden, P.M., Basso, L.V., and Scholer, J.F.: Tricuspid valve obstruction due to intravenous leiomyomatosis. Am. Heart J., *108*:1544, 1984.

134. Gindea, A.J., Gentin, B., Naidich, D.P., Freedberg, R.S., McCauley, D., and Kronzon, I.: Unusual cardiac metastasis in hypernephroma: The complementary role

of echocardiography and magnetic resonance imaging. Am. Heart J., *116*:1359, 1988.

135. Henuzet, C., Franken, P., Polis, O., and Fievez, M.: Cardiac metastasis of rectal adenocarcinoma diagnosed by two dimensional echocardiography. Am. Heart J., *104*:637, 1982.

136. Grenadier, E., Lima, C.O., Barron, J.V., Allen, H.D., Sahn, D.J., Valdes-Cruz, L.M., Hutter, J.J., and Goldberg, S.J.: Two dimensional echocardiography for evaluation of metastatic cardiac tumors in pediatric patients. Am. Heart J., *107*:122, 1984.

137. Johnson, M.H. and Soulen, R.L.: Echocardiography of cardiac metastases. AJR Am. J. Roentgenol., *141*:677, 1983.

138. Koiwaya, Y., Kawachi, Y., Orita, Y., Nakamura, M., Mirata, T., Yamamoto, K., and Omae, T.: Echocardiographic detection of metastatic cardiac mural tumor. JCU, *8*:443, 1980.

139. Kubac, G., Doris, I., Ondro, M., and Davey, P.W.: Malignant granular cell myoblastoma with metastatic cardiac involvement: Case report and echocardiogram. Am. Heart J., *100*:227, 1980.

140. Steffens, T.G., Mayer, H.S., and Das, S.K.: Echocardiographic diagnosis of a right ventricular metastatic tumor. Arch. Intern. Med., *140*:122, 1980.

141. Itoh, K., Matsubara, T., Yanagisawa, K., Hibi, N., Nishimura, K., Kambe, T., Sakamoto, N., Tanaka, M., and Abe, T.: Right ventricular metastasis of cervical squamous cell carcinoma. Am. Heart J., *108*:1369, 1984.

142. Schrem, S.S., Colvin, S.B., Weinreb, J.C., Glassman, E., and Kronzon, I.: Metastatic cardiac liposarcoma: Diagnosis by transesophageal echocardiography and magnetic resonance imaging. J. Am. Soc. Echocardiogr., *3*:149, 1990.

143. Cheek, G.A., Bansal, R.C., Bouland, D., and Vyhmeister, E.: Embryonal carcinoma of the testis presenting as a left heart mass. J. Am. Soc. Echocardiogr., *4*:76, 1991.

144. Popovic, A.D., Harrigan, P., Sanfilippo, A.J., and Weyman, A.E.: Echocardiographic diagnosis of cardiac metastases secondary to breast malignancy. Echocardiography, *6*:283, 1989.

145. Lestuzzi, C., Biasi, S., Nicolosi, G.L., Lodeville, D., Pavan, D., Collazzo, R., Guindani, A., and Zanuttini, D.: Secondary neoplastic infiltration of the myocardium diagnosed by two-dimensional echocardiography in seven cases with anatomic confirmation. J. Am. Coll. Cardiol., *9*:439, 1987.

146. Norell, M.S., Sarvasvaran, R., and Sutton, G.C.: Solitary tumor metastasis: A rare cause of right ventricular outflow tract obstruction and sudden death. Eur. Heart J., *5*:684, 1984.

147. Moosa, Y.A. and Lewis, J.F.: Rare metastatic tumors of the right ventricular cavity: Detection by two-dimensional echocardiography. Echocardiography, *6*:289, 1989.

148. Rey, M., Alfonso, F., Torrecilla, E., Ramirez, J.A., Berjon, J., and Renedo, G.: Right heart metastatic endocardial implants: Echocardiographic and pathologic correlation. Am. Heart J., *119*:1217, 1990.

149. Schmidt, D.R., Johns, J.P., and Linville, K.W.: Detection of intracavitary right ventricular polypoid masses due to metastatic lymphoma using contrast echocardiography. Am. Heart J., *120*:446, 1990.

150. Schaefer, S., Shohet, R.V., Nixon, J.V., and Peshock, R.M.: Right ventricular obstruction from cervical carcinoma: A rare, single metastatic site. Am. Heart J., *113*:397, 1987.

151. Miller, D.L., Katz, N.M., and Pallas, R.S.: Hepatoma presenting as a right atrial mass. Am. Heart J., *114*:906, 1987.

152. Mohan, J.C., Agarwala, R., and Khanna, S.K.: Dissecting intramyocardial hematoma presenting as a massive pseudotumor of the right ventricle. Am. Heart J., *124*:1641, 1992.

153. Koch, P.C., Kronzon, I., Winer, H.E., Adams, P., and Trubek, M.: Displacement of the heart by a giant mediastinal cyst. Am. J. Cardiol., *40*:445, 1977.

154. Tingelstad, J.B., McWilliams, N.B., and Thomas, C.E.: Confirmation of a retrosternal mass by echocardiogram. JCU, *4*:129, 1976.

155. Canedo, M.I., Otken, L., and Stefadouros, M.A.: Echocardiographic features of cardiac compression by a thymoma simulating cardiac tamponade and obstruction of the superior vena cava. Br. Heart J., *39*:1038, 1977.

156. Farooki, Z.Q., Hakimi, N., Arciniegas, E., and Green, E.W.: Echocardiographic features in a case of intrapericardial teratoma. JCU, *6*:108, 1978.

157. Yoshikawa, J., Sabah, I., Yanagihara, K., Owaki, T., Kato, H., and Tanemoto, K.: Cross-sectional echocardiographic diagnosis of large left atrial tumor and extracardiac tumor compressing the left atrium. Am. J. Cardiol., *42*:853, 1978.

158. Lin, T.K., Stech, J.M., Eckert, W.G., Lin, J.J., Farha, S.J., and Hagan, C.T.: Pericardial angiosarcoma simulating pericardial effusion by echocardiography. Chest. *73*:881, 1978.

159. Chandraratna, P.A.N., Littman, B.B., Serafini, A., Whayne, T., and Robinson, H.: Echocardiographic evaluation of extracardiac masses. Br. Heart J., *40*:741, 1978.

160. Lestuzzi, C., Nicolosi, G.L., Mimo, R., Pavan, D., and Zanuttini, D.: Usefulness of transesophageal echocardiography in evaluation of paracardiac neoplastic masses. Am. J. Cardiol., *70*:247, 1992.

161. Breall, J.A., Goldberger, A.L., Warren, S.E., Diver, D.J., and Ellke, F.W.: Posterior mediastinal masses: Rare causes of cardiac compression. Am. Heart J., *124*:523, 1992.

162. D'Cruz, I.A., Hoffman, P.K., and Ewald, F.W.: Echocardiography of the posterior mediastinal masses encroaching on the left atrium. Echocardiography, *6*:485, 1989.

163. D'Cruz, I.A.: The echocardiographic diagnosis of space-occupying lesions anterior to the heart. Pract. Cardiol., *12*:63, 1986.

164. Shah, A. and Schwartz, H.: Echocardiographic features of cardiac compression by mediastinal pancreatic pseudocyst. Chest, *77*:440, 1980.

165. Gondi, B. and Nanda, N.C.: Two-dimensional echocardiographic diagnosis of mediastinal hematoma causing cardiac tamponade. Am. J. Cardiol., *53*:974, 1984.

166. Hsiung, M.C., Chen, C.C., Wang, D.J., Shieh, S.M., and Chiang, B.N.: Two dimensional echocardiographic diagnosis of acquired right ventricular outflow obstruction due to external cardiac compression. Am. J. Cardiol., *53*:973, 1984.

167. Baduini, G., Paolillo, V., and Di Summa, M.: Echocardiographic findings in a case of acquired pulmonic stenosis from extrinsic compression by a mediastinal cyst. Chest, *80*:507, 1981.

168. Dawkins, P.R., Stoddard, M.F., Liddell, N.E., Longaker, R., Keedy, D., and Kupersmith, J.: Utility of transesophageal echocardiography in the assessment of mediastinal masses and superior vena cava obstruction. Am. Heart J., *122*:1469, 1991.

169. Iwase, M., Nagura, E., Miyahara, T., Goto, J., Kajita, M., and Yamada, H.: Malignant lymphoma compressing the heart and causing acute left-sided heart failure. Am. Heart J., *119*:968, 1990.

170. Coplan, N.L., Kennish, A.J., Burgess, N.L., Deligdish, L., and Goldman, M.E.: Pericardial mesothelioma masquerading as a benign pericardial effusion. J. Am. Coll. Cardiol., *4*:1307, 1984.

171. Farooki, Z.Q., Arciniegas, E., Hakimi, M., Clapp, S., Jackson, W., and Green E.W.: Real-time echocardiographic features of intrapericardial teratoma. JCU, *10*: 125, 1982.

172. Seguin, J.R., Coulon, P.L., Perez, M., Grolleau-Raoux, R., and Chaptal, P.A.: Echocardiographic diagnosis of an intrapericardial teratoma in infancy. Am. Heart J., *113*:1239, 1987.

173. Rosamond, T.L., Hamburg, M.S., Vacek, J.L., and Borkon, A.M.: Intrapericardial pheochromocytoma. Am. J. Cardiol., *70*:700, 1992.

174. Nishimura, T., Kondo, M., Miyazaki, S., Michizuki, T., Umadome, H., and Shimono, Y.: Two dimensional echocardiographic findings of cardiovascular involvement by invasive thymoma. Chest, *81*:7512, 1982.

175. Hynes, J.K., Tajik, A.J., Osborn, M.J., Orszulak, T.A., and Seward, J.B.: Two dimensional echocardiographic diagnosis of pericardial cyst. Mayo Clin. Proc., *58*:60, 1983.

176. Percy, R.F., Conetta, D.A., and Miller, A.B.: Esophageal compression of the heart presenting as an extracardiac mass on echocardiography. Chest, *85*:826, 1984.

177. Hoit, B.D. and Eppert, D.: Presbyesophagus masquerading as an extracardiac mass on echocardiography. Am. Heart J., *118*:419, 1989.

178. D'Cruz, I.A., Holman, M., and Battu, P.: Echocardiographic manifestations of esophageal carcinoma. Am. Heart J., *123*:1703, 1992.

179. Frohwein, S.C., Karalis, D.G., McQuillan, J.M., Ross, J.J., Mintz, G.S., and Chandrasekaran, K.: Preoperative detection of pericardial angiosarcoma by transesophageal echocardiography. Am. Heart J., *122*:874, 1991.

180. Maze, S.S., Kotler, M.N., and Parry, W.R.: The contribution of color Doppler flow imaging to the assessment of a left ventricular thrombus. Am. Heart J., *115*:479, 1988.

181. Falk, R.H., Foster, E., and Coats, M.H.: Ventricular thrombi and thromboembolism in dilated cardiomyopathy: A prospective follow-up study. Am. Heart J., *123*: 136, 1992.

182. Stratton, J.R., Nemanich, J.W., Johannessen, K-A., and Resnick, A.D.: Fate of left ventricular thrombi in patients with remote myocardial infarction or idiopathic cardiomyopathy. Circulation, *78*:1388, 1988.

183. Keren, A., Goldberg, S., Gottlieb, S., Klein, J., Schuger, C., Medina, A., Tzivoni, D., and Stern, S.: Natural history of left ventricular thrombi: Their appearance and resolution in the posthospitalization period of acute myocardial infarction. J. Am. Coll. Cardiol., *15*:790, 1990.

184. Jugdutt, B.I., Sivaram, C.A., Wortman, C., Trudell, C., and Penner, P.: Prospective two-dimensional echocardiographic evaluation of left ventricular thrombus and embolism after acute myocardial infarction. J. Am. Coll. Cardiol., *13*:554, 1989.

185. Mikell, F.L., et al.: Regional stasis of blood in the dysfunctional left ventricle: Echocardiographic detection and differentiation from early thrombosis. Circulation, *66*:755, 1982.

186. Maze, S.S., Kotler, M.N., and Parry, W.R.: Flow characteristics in the dilated left ventricle with thrombus: Qualitative and quantitative Doppler analysis. J. Am. Coll. Cardiol., *13*:873, 1989.

187. Chin, W.W., VanTosh, A., Hecht, S.R., and Berger, M.: Left ventricular thrombus with normal left ventricular function in ulcerative colitis. Am. Heart J., *116*:562, 1988.

188. Bansal, R.C., Heywood, J.T., Applegate, P.M., and Jutzy, K.R.: Detection of left atrial thrombi by two-dimensional echocardiography and surgical correlation in 148 patients with mitral valve disease. Am. J. Cardiol., *64*:243, 1989.

189. Okun, M., Plotnick, G.D., Salmon, D., and Lee, Y-C.: Two-dimensional echocardiographic detection of biatrial thrombi. Am. Heart J., *114*:184, 1987.

190. Hwang, J-J., Kuan, P., Lin, S-C., Chen, W-J., Lei, M-H., Ko, Y-L., Cheng, J-J., Lin, J-L., Chen, J-J., and Lien, W-P.: Reappraisal by transesophageal echocardiography of the significance of left atrial thrombi in the prediction of systemic arterial embolization in rheumatic mitral valve disease. Am. J. Cardiol., *70*:769, 1992.

191. Herzog, C.A., Bass, D., Kane, M., and Asinger, R.: Two dimensional echocardiographic imaging of left atrial appendage thrombi. J. Am. Coll. Cardiol., *3*:1340, 1984.

192. Olson, J.D., Goldenberg, I.F., Pedersen, W., Brandt, D., Kane, M., Daniel, J.A., Nelson, R.R., Mooney, M.R., and Lange, H.W.: Exclusion of atrial thrombus by transesophageal echocardiography. J. Am. Soc. Echocardiogr., *5*:52, 1992.

193. Manning, W.J., Reis, G.J., and Douglas, P.S.: Use of transesophageal echocardiography to detect left atrial thrombi before percutaneous balloon dilatation of the mitral valve: A prospective study. Br. Heart J., *67*:170, 1992.

194. Vigna C., Russo A., DeRito V., Perna G.P., Villella A., Testa M., Sollazzo V., Fanelli R., Loperfido F.: Frequency of left atrial thrombi by transesophageal echocardiography in idiopathic and in ischemic dilated cardiomyopathy. *70*:1500–1501, 1992. Dec. No. 18 Am. J. Cardiol.

195. Kuo, C-T., Chiang, C-W., Lee, Y-S., Ho, Y-S., and Chang, C-H.: Left atrial ball thrombus in nonrheumatic atrial fibrillation diagnosed by transesophageal echocardiography. Am. Heart J., *123*:1394, 1992.

196. Furukawa, K., Katsume, H., Matsukubo, H., and Inoue, D.: Echocardiographic findings of floating thrombus in left atrium. Br. Heart J., *44*:599, 1980.

197. Gottdiener, J.S., Temeck, B.K., Patterson, R.H., and Fletcher, R.D.: Transient ("hole-in-one") occlusion of the mitral valve orifice by a free-floating left atrial ball thrombus: Identification by two dimensional echocardiography. Am. J. Cardiol., *53*:1730, 1984.

198. Chen, C.C., Hsiung, M., and Chiang, B.N.: Variable diastolic rumbling murmur caused by floating left atrial thrombus. Br. Heart J., *50*:190, 1983.

199. Wrisley, D., Giambartolomei, A., Lee, T., and Brownlee, W.: Left atrial ball thrombus: Review of clinical and echocardiographic manifestations with suggestions for management. Am. Heart J., *121*:1784, 1991.

200. Wrisley, D., Giambartolomei, A., Levy, I., Brownlee, W., Lee, I., and Erickson, J.: Left atrial ball thrombus: Apparent detachment following initiation of anticoagulant therapy. Am. Heart J., *116*:1351, 1988.

201. Rey, M., Tunon, J., Vinolas, X., Compres, H., Criado, A., and Rabago, R.: Free-floating left atrial thrombus and its mechanical interaction with mitral regurgitant jet assessed by color Doppler echocardiography. Am. Heart J., *123*:1067, 1992.

202. Samdarshi, T.E., Morrow, W.R., Helmcke, F.R.,

Nanda, N.C., Bargeron, L.M., and Pacificio, A.D.: Assessment of pulmonary vein stenosis by transesophageal echocardiography. Am. Heart J., *122*:1495, 1991.

202a. Chen, C., Koschyk, D., Hamm, C., Sievers, B., Kupper, W., and Bleifeld, W.: Usefulness of transesophageal echocardiography in identifying small left ventricular apical thrombus. J. Am. Coll. Cardiol., *21*:208, 1993.

203. Tsai, L-M., Chen, J-H., Fang, C-J., Lin, L-J., and Kwan, C-M.: Clinical implications of left atrial spontaneous echo contrast in nonrheumatic atrial fibrillation. Am. J. Cardiol., *70*:327, 1992.

204. Black, I.W., Hopkins, A.P., Lee, L.C.L., Walsh, W.F., and Jacobson, B.M.: Left atrial spontaneous echo contrast: A clinical and echocardiographic analysis. J. Am. Coll. Cardiol., *18*:398, 1991.

205. Obarski, T.P., Salcedo, E.E., Castle, L.W., and Stewart, W.J.: Spontaneous echo contrast in the left atrium during paroxysmal atrial fibrillation. Am. Heart J., *120*:988, 1990.

206. Daniel, W.G., Nellessen, U., Schroder, E., Nonnast-Daniel, B., Bednarski, P., Nikutta, P., and Lichtlen, P.R.: Left atrial spontaneous echo contrast in mitral valve disease: An indicator for an increased thromboembolic risk. J. Am. Coll. Cardiol., *11*:1204, 1988.

207. Erbel, R., Stern, H., Ehrenthal, W., Schreiner, G., Treese, N., Kramer, G., Thelen, M., Schweizer, P., and Meyer, J.: Detection of spontaneous echocardiographic contrast within the left atrium by transesophageal echocardiography: Spontaneous echocardiographic contrast. Clin. Cardiol., *9*:245, 1986.

208. Pozzoli, M., Febo, O., Torbicki, A., Tramarin, R., Calsamiglia, G., Cobelli, F., Specchia, G., and Roelandt, J.R.T.C.: Left atrial appendage dysfunction: A cause of thrombosis? Evidence by transesophageal echocardiography—Doppler studies. J. Am. Soc. Echocardiogr., *4*:435, 1991.

209. Pollick, C. and Taylor, D.: Assessment of left atrial appendage function by transesophageal echocardiography. Implications for the development of thrombus. Circulation, *84*:223, 1991.

210. Torrecilla, E.G., Garcia-Fernandez, M.A., San Roman, D., Munoz, R., Palomo, J., and Delcan, J.L.: Left atrial spontaneous echocardiographic contrast after heart transplantation. Am. J. Cardiol., *69*:817, 1992.

211. Nestico, P.F., et al.: Surgical removal of right atrial thromboembolus detected by two dimensional echocardiography in pulmonary embolism. Am. Heart J., *107*:1278, 1984.

212. De Dominicis, E., Ometto, R., Ivic, N., and Vincenzi, M.: Two dimensional echocardiographic diagnosis of a thromboembolic mass in the right atrium. G. Ital. Cardiol., *13*:265, 1983.

213. Quinn, T.J., Plehn, J.F., and Liebson, P.R.: Echocardiographic diagnosis of mobile right atrial thrombus: Early recognition and treatment. Am. Heart J., *108*:1548, 1984.

214. Redberg, R.F., Hecht, S.R., and Berger, M.: Echocardiographic detection of transient right heart thrombus: Now you see it, now you don't. Am. Heart J., *122*:862, 1991.

215. Adamick, R. and Zoneraich, S.: Echocardiographic visualization of a large mobile right atrial thrombus with sudden embolization during real-time scanning. Am. Heart J., *120*:699, 1990.

216. Chiarella, F., Lupi, G., and Vecchio, C.: Early echocardiographic detection of right-sided intracardiac thrombus. Int. J. Cardiol., *11*:121, 1986.

217. Vargas-Barron, J., Lacy-Niebla, M.C., Keirns, C., Attie, F., Gonzalez-Medina, A., Madrid, J.V., and Ferrari, F.Q.: Echocardiographic detection of dynamic intracavitary echoes and right atrial thrombus. Am. Heart J., *113*: 829, 1987.

218. Van Kuyk, M., Mols, P., and Englert, M.: Right atrial thrombus leading to pulmonary embolism. Br. Heart J., *51*:462, 1984.

219. Felner, J.M. Churchwell, A.L., and Murphy, D.A.: Right atrial thromboemboli: Clinical, echocardiographic and pathophysiologic manifestations. J. Am. Coll. Cardiol., *4*:1041, 1984.

220. Starkey, I.R. and DeBono, D.P.: Echocardiographic identification of right-sided cardiac intracavitary thromboembolus in massive pulmonary embolism. Circulation, *66*:1322, 1982.

221. Ouyang, P., Camara, E.J., Jain, A., Richman, P.S., and Shapiro, E.P.: Intracavitary thrombi, in the right heart associated with multiple pulmonary emboli. Report of two patients. Chest, *84*:296, 1983.

222. Saner, H.E., Asinger, R.W., Daniel, J.A., and Elsperger, K.J.: Two dimensional echocardiographic detection of right-sided cardiac intracavitary thromboembolus with pulmonary embolism. J. Am. Coll. Cardiol., *4*:1294, 1984.

223. Lim, S.P., Hakim, S.Z., and van der Bel-Kahn, J.M.: Two dimensional echocardiography for detection of primary right atrial thrombus in pulmonary embolism. Am. Heart J., *108*:1546, 1984.

224. Farfel, Z., Shechter, M., Vered, Z., Rath, S., Goor, D., and Gafni, J.: Review of echocardiographically diagnosed right heart entrapment of pulmonary emboli-intransit with emphasis on management. Am. Heart J., *113*: 171, 1987.

225. Pasierski, T.J., Alton, M.E., Van Fossen, D.B., and Pearson, A.C.: Right atrial mobile thrombus: Improved visualization by transesophageal echocardiography. Am. Heart J., *123*:802, 1992.

226. Kreher, S.K., Ulstad, V.K., Dick, C.D., DeGroff, R., Olivari, T., and Homans, D.C.: Frequent occurrence of occult pulmonary embolism from venous sheaths during endomyocardial biopsy. J. Am. Coll. Cardiol., *19*:581, 1992.

227. Gabrielsen, F., Schmidt, A., Eggeling, T., Hoeher, M., Kochs, M., and Hombach, V.: Massive main pulmonary artery embolism diagnosed with two-dimensional echocardiography. Clin. Cardiol., *15*:545, 1992.

228. Evans, B.H. and Maurer, G.: Echocardiographic diagnosis of pulmonary embolus. Am. Heart J., *120*:1236, 1990.

229. Zaidi, S.J.: Two-dimensional echocardiographic detection of asymptomatic pulmonary thromboembolism. Echocardiography, *9*:17, 1992.

230. Johnson, M.E., Furlong, R., and Schrank, K.: Diagnostic use of emergency department echocardiogram in massive pulmonary emboli. Ann. Emerg. Med., *21*:760, 1992.

231. Klein, A.L., Stewart, W.C., Cosgrove, III, D.M., Mick, M.J., and Salcedo, E.: Visualization of acute pulmonary emboli by transesophageal echocardiography. J. Am. Soc. Echocardiogr., *3*:412, 1990.

232. Nixdorff, U., Erbel, R., Drexler, M., and Meyer, J.: Detection of thromboembolus of the right pulmonary artery by transesophageal two-dimensional echocardiography. Am. J. Cardiol., *61*:488, 1988.

233. Hunter, J.J., Johnson, K.R., Karagianes, T.G., and Dittrich, H.C.: Detection of massive pulmonary embolus-in-transit by transesophageal echocardiography. Chest, *100*:1210, 1991.

234. Popovic, A.D., Milovanovic, B., Neskovic, A.N., and Pavlovski, K.: Detection of massive pulmonary embolism by transesophageal echocardiography. Cardiology, *80*:94, 1992.

235. Gelernt, M.D., Mogtader, A., and Hahn, R.T.: Transesophageal echocardiography to diagnose and demonstrate resolution of an acute massive pulmonary embolus. Chest, *102*:297, 1992.

236. Guindo, J., Montagud, M., Carreras, F., Dominquez, J.M., Bartolucci, J., Martinez-Ruiz, M.D., Sadurni, J., Vinolas, X., Fontcuberta, J., and de Luna, A.B.: Fibrinolytic therapy for superior vena cava and right atrial thrombosis: Diagnosis and follow-up with biplane transesophageal echocardiography. Am. Heart J., *124*:510, 1992.

237. Podolsky, L.A., Manginas, A., Jacobs, L.E., Kotler, M.N., and Ioli, A.W.: Superior vena caval thrombosis detected by transesophageal echocardiography. J. Am. Soc. Echocardiogr., *4*:189, 1991.

238. Gengenbach, S. and Ridker, P.M.: Left ventricular hemangioma in Kasabach-Merritt syndrome. Am. Heart J., *121*:202, 1991.

239. Weir, I., Mills, P., and Lewis, T.: A case of left atrial haemangioma: Echocardiographic, surgical, and morphological features. Br. Heart J., *58*:665, 1987.

240. Desnos, M., Brochet, E., Cristofini, P., Cosnard, G., Keddari, M., Mostefai, M., and Gay, J.: Polyvisceral echinococcosis with cardiac involvement imaged by two-dimensional echocardiography, computed tomography and nuclear magnetic resonance imaging. Am. J. Cardiol., *59*:383, 1987.

241. Limacher, M.C., et al.: Cardiac echinococcal cyst: Diagnosis by two dimensional echocardiography. J. Am. Coll. Cardiol., *2*:574, 1983.

242. Picchio, E., Giovannini, E., Siolari, F., and Lotti, A.: Cardiac echinococcosis. Two dimensional echocardiographic diagnosis. G. Ital. Cardiol., *11*:1327, 1981.

243. Ernst, A., Cikes, I., and Radovanovic, N.: Two dimensional echocardiographic study of a cardiac hydatid cyst. Am. J. Cardiol., *52*:1361, 1983.

244. Green, S.E., Joynt, L.F., Fitzgerald, P.J., Rubenson, D.S., and Popp, R.L.: In vivo ultrasonic tissue characterization of human intracardiac masses. Am. J. Cardiol., *51*:231, 1983.

245. Allan, L.D., Joseph, M.C., and Tynan, M.: Clinical value of echocardiographic colour image processing in two cases of primary cardiac tumor. Br. Heart J., *49*:154, 1983.

246. Mikell, F.L., et al.: Tissue acoustic properties of fresh left ventricular thrombi and visualization by two dimensional echocardiography: Experimental observations. Am. J. Cardiol., *49*:1157, 1982.

247. McPherson, D.D., Knosp, B.M., Kieso, R.A., Bean, J.A., Kerber, R.E., Skorton, D.J., and Collins, S.M.: Ultrasound characterization of acoustic properties of acute intracardiac thrombi: Studies in a new experimental model. J. Am. Soc. Echocardiogr., *1*:254, 1988.

248. Vandenberg, B.F., Kieso, R.A., Fox-Eastham, K., Kerber, R.E., Melton, H.E., Collins, S.M., and Skorton, D.J.: Characterization of acute experimental left ventricular thrombi with quantitative backscatter imaging. Circulation, *81*:1017, 1990.

249. Iliceto, S., DiBiase, M., Antonelli, G., Favale, S., and Rizzon, P.: Two dimensional echocardiographic recognition of a pacing catheter perforation of the interventricular septum. PACE, *5*:934, 1982.

250. Schiavone, W.A., Castle, L.W., Salcedo, E., and Graor, R.: Amaurosis fugax in a patient with a left ventricular endocardial pacemaker. PACE, *7*:288, 1984.

251. Boughner, D.R. and Gulamhusein, S.: Echocardiographic demonstration of a left ventricular endocardial pacemaker wire. JCU, *11*:240, 1983.

252. Chazal, R.A. and Feigenbaum, H.: Two dimensional echocardiographic identification of epicardial pacemaker wire perforation. Am. Heart J., *107*:165, 1984.

253. Tobin, A.M., Grodman, R.S., Fisherkeller, M., and Micolosi, R.: Two dimensional echocardiographic localization of a malpositioned pacing catheter. PACE, *6*:291, 1983.

254. Gondi, B. and Nanda, N.C.: Real-time two dimensional echocardiographic features of pacemaker perforation. Circulation, *64*:97, 1981.

255. Judson, P.L., Moore, T.B., Swank, M., and Ashworth, H.E.: Two dimensional echocardiograms of a transvenous left ventricular pacing catheter. Chest, *80*:228, 1981.

256. Zehender, M., Buchner, C., Geibel, A., Kasper, W., Meinertz, T., and Just, H.: Diagnosis of hidden pacemaker lead sepsis by transesophageal echocardiography and a new technique for lead extraction. Am. Heart J., *118*:1050, 1989.

257. Crie, J.S., Hajar, R., and Folger, G.: Umbilical catheter masquerading at echocardiography as a left atrial mass. Clin. Cardiol., *12*:728, 1989.

258. Reeves, W.C., Movahed, A., Chitwood, R., Williams, M., Jolly, S.R., Jordan, J.C., Webb, S., and Challinor, K.: Utility of precordial, epicardial and transesophageal two-dimensional echocardiography in the detection of intracardiac foreign bodies. Am. J. Cardiol., *64*:406, 1989.

259. Giyanani, V.L., Fertel, D., and Eggerstedt, J.: Use of ultrasound for localization of a foreign object in the heart. JCU, *17*:379, 1989.

260. Fyfe, D.A., Edgerton, J.R., Chaikhouni, A., and Kline, C.H.: Preoperative localization of an intracardiac foreign body by two-dimensional echocardiography. Am. Heart J., *113*:210, 1987.

261. Xie, S.W. and Picard, M.H.: Two-dimensional and color Doppler echocardiographic diagnosis of penetrating missile wounds of the heart. Chronic complications from intracardiac course of a bullet. J. Am. Soc. Echocardiogr., *5*:81, 1992.

262. Drinkovi̇o, N.: Subcostal echocardiography to determine right ventricular pacing catheter position and control advancement of electrode catheters in intracardiac electrophysiologic studies. Am. J. Cardiol., *47*:1260, 1981.

263. Iliceto, S., et al.: Two dimensional echocardiographic recognition of complications of cardiac invasive procedures. Am. J. Cardiol., *53*:846, 1984.

264. Win, A., Pastore, J.O., Coletta, D., and Junda, R.J.: Echocardiographic detection of a retained left atrial catheter. Am. Heart J., *99*:93, 1980.

265. Ross, W.B., Mohiuddin, S.M., Pagano, T., and Hughes, D.: Malposition of a transvenous cardiac electrode associated with amaurosis fugax. PACE, *6*:119, 1983.

266. VanCamp, G. and Vandenbossche, J.L.: Recognition of pacemaker lead infection by transesophageal echocardiography. Br. Heart J., *65*:229, 1991.

267. Villanueva, F.S., Heinsimer, J.A., Burkman, M.H., Fananapazir, L., Halvorsen, R.A., and Chen, J.T.: Echocardiographic detection of perforation of the cardiac ventricular septum by a permanent pacemaker lead. Am. J. Cardiol., *59*:370, 1987.

268. Mugge, A., Gulba, D.C., Jost, S., and Daniel, W.G.: Dissolution of a right atrial thrombus attached to pace-

maker electrodes: Usefulness of recombinant tissue-type plasminogen activator. Am. Heart J., *119*:1437, 1990.

269. Perry, R.A., Clarke, D.B., and Shiu, M.F.: Entanglement of embolised thrombus with an endocardial lead causing pacemaker malfunction and subsequent pulmonary embolism. Br. Heart J., *57*:292, 1987.

270. Cohen, G.I., Klein, A.L., Chan, K-L., Stewart, W.J., and Salcedo, E.E.: Transesophageal echocardiographic diagnosis of right-sided cardiac masses in patients with central lines. Am. J. Cardiol., *70*:925, 1992.

270a.Vilacosta, I., Zamorano, J., Camino, A., San Roman, J.A., Rollan, M.J., and Pinto, A.: Infected transvenous permanent pacemakers: Role of transesophageal echocardiography. Am. Heart J., *125*:904, 1993.

271. Brenner, J.I., Gaines, S., Cordier, J., Reiner, B.I., Haney, P.J., and Gundry, S.R.: Cardiac strangulation: Two-dimensional echo recognition of a rare complication of epicardial pacemaker therapy. Am. J. Cardiol., *61*:654, 1988.

272. Katz, E.S., Tunick, P.A., and Kronzon, I.: Observations of coronary flow augmentation and balloon function during intraaortic balloon counterpulsation using transesophageal echocardiography. Am. J. Cardiol., *69*:1636, 1992.

273. Perry, L.W., et al.: Two dimensional echocardiography for catheter location and placement in infants and children. Pediatrics, *67*:541, 1981.

274. French, J.W., Popp, R.L., and Pitlick, P.T.: Cardiac localization of transvascular bioptome using two dimensional echocardiography. Am. J. Cardiol., *51*:219, 1983.

275. Copeland, J.G., Valdes-Cruz, L., and Sahn, D.J.: Endomyocardial biopsy with fluoroscopic and two dimensional echocardiographic guidance: Case report of a patient suspected of having multiple cardiac tumors. Clin. Cardiol., *7*:449, 1984.

276. Pierard, L., et al.: Two dimensional echocardiographic guiding of endomyocardial biopsy. Chest, *85*:759, 1984.

277. Guttas, J.J., Brent, B.N., and Kersh, E.: Biopsy of a right atrial mass under transesophageal echocardiographic guidance. Echocardiography, *9*:129, 1992.

278. Potek, I.J. and Wright, J.S.: Needle in the heart. Br. Heart J., *45*:325, 1981.

278a.Reeves, W.C., Movahed, A., Chitwood, W.R., Williams, M., Jolly, S.R., Jordan, J.C., Webb, S., and Challinor, K.: Utility of precordial, epicardial and transesophageal two-dimensional echocardiography in the detection of Intracardiac foreign bodies. Am. J. Cardiol., *64*:408, 1989.

278b.Brathwaite, C.E., Weiss, R.L., Baldino, W.A., Hoganson, N., and Ross, S.E.: Multichamber gunshot wounds of the heart. The utility of transesophageal echocardiography. Chest, *101*:187, 1992.

279. Hausmann, D., Mugge, A., Becht, I., and Daniel, W.G.: Diagnosis of patent foramen ovale by transesophageal echocardiography and association with cerebral and peripheral embolic events. Am. J. Cardiol., *70*:668, 1992.

279a.Stollberger, C., Schneider, B., Abzieher, F., Wollner, T., and Meinertz, T.: Diagnosis of patent foramen ovale by transesophageal contrast echocardiography. Am. J. Cardiol. *71*:604, 1993.

280. deBelder, M.A., Tourikis, L., Leech, G., and Camm, A.J.: Risk of patent foramen ovale for thromboembolic events in all age groups. Am. J. Cardiol., *69*:1316, 1992.

280a.Van Camp, G., Schulze, D., Cosyns, B., and Vandenbossche, J-L.: Relation between patent foramen ovale and unexplained stroke. Am. J. Cardiol., *71*:596, 1993.

280b.Louie, E.K., Konstadt, S.N., Rao, T.L., and Scanlon, P.J.: Transesophageal echocardiographic diagnosis of right to left shunting across the foramen ovale in adults without prior stroke. J. Am. Coll. Cardiol., *21*:1231, 1993.

281. Nagelhout, D.A., Pearson, A.C., and Labovitz, A.J.: Diagnosis of paradoxic embolism by transesophageal echocardiography. Am. Heart J., *121*:1552, 1991.

282. Nelson, C.W., Snow, F.R., Barnett, M., Mcroy, L., and Wechsler, A.S.: Impending paradoxical embolism: Echocardiographic diagnosis of an intracardiac thrombus crossing a patent foramen ovale. Am. Heart J., *122*:859, 1991.

282a.Stoddard, M.F., Keedy, D.L., Dawkins, P.R., Harvey, D., and Shepherd, M.: The cough test is superior to the Valsalva maneuver in the delineation of right-to-left shunting through a patent foramen ovale during contrast transesophageal echocardiography. Am. Heart J., *125*: 185, 1993.

283. Kronzon, I., Tunick, P.A., Schrem, S.S., and Yarmush, L.: Fingerlike mass in the left atrium. J. Am. Soc. Echocardiogr., *4*:75, 1991.

284. Black, J.W., Hopkins, A.P., Lee, L.C.L., Jacobson, B.M., and Walsh, W.F.: Role of transesophageal echocardiography in evaluation of cardiogenic embolism. Br. Heart J., *66*:302, 1991.

285. Bar-El, Y., Adar, R., Schneiderman, Y., and Motro, M.: Echocardiography in diagnostic assessment of peripheral arterial embolization. Am. Heart J., *119*:1090, 1990.

286. DeBelder, M.A., Lovat, L.B., Tourikis, L., Leech, G., and Camm, A.J.: Limitations of transesophageal echocardiography in patients with focal cerebral ischaemic events. Br. Heart J., *67*:297, 1992.

286a.Vandenbogaerde, J., DeBleecker, J., Decoo, D., Francois, K., Cambier, B., Bergen, J.M., Vandermersch, C., DeReuck, J., and Clement, D.L.: Transesophageal echo-Doppler in patients suspected of a cardiac source of peripheral emboli. Eur. Heart J., *13*:88, 1992.

287. Ciaccheri, M., Castelli, G., Cecchi, F., Nannini, M., Santoro, G., Troiani, V., Zuppiroli, A., and Dolara, A.: Lack of correlation between intracavitary thrombosis detected by cross sectional echocardiography and systemic emboli in patients with dilated cardiomyopathy. Br. Heart J., *62*:26, 1989.

288. Alam, M.: Pitfalls in the echocardiographic diagnosis of intracardiac and extracardiac masses. Echocardiography, *10*:181, 1993.

# 12

# Diseases of the Aorta

Transesophageal echocardiography has revolutionized the sonographic examination of the aorta. Transthoracic two-dimensional echocardiography and M-mode echocardiography provided limited access for detecting aortic disease. With the availability of transesophageal echocardiography, especially with biplane or multiplane capability, virtually the entire thoracic aorta is now easily accessible to ultrasonic visualization. Figure 12–1 is a reminder of how transesophageal echocardiography can evaluate the thoracic aorta in both horizontal (transverse) and longitudinal (sagittal) views. From a technical viewpoint, only a small area of the arch of the aorta remains difficult to examine echocardiographically.

With the multiple examining planes now available and the enhanced resolution that comes with an unobstructed window and higher frequency transducers, transesophageal echocardiography is literally rewriting the textbook on the in vivo examination of the aorta. Transthoracic echocardiography is less invasive and is still preferred as an initial examination. In many situations, however, a definitive sonographic examination of aortic disease will require a transesophageal study. Intravascular ultrasound is emerging as a tool that may also play a major role in detecting aortic disease.

## AORTIC DILATATION AND ANEURYSMS

Dilatation of the aortic root produces fairly characteristic two-dimensional echocardiograms.[1] Figure 12–2 represents a recording of a patient with a dilated aortic root. The increased echogenicity of the anterior and posterior walls is most likely a result of atherosclerotic disease of the aorta. Fuzzy echoes in the anterior half of the aortic root are also seen in Figure 12–2. These echoes are probably secondary to abnormal blood flow within the aorta.

Marfan's syndrome, or annuloaortic ectasia, can produce fairly characteristic two-dimensional echocardiograms.[2–8] A typical example of such a patient is shown in Figure 12–3. The dilated aorta involves the annulus as well as the aorta past the aortic leaflets. Figure 12–4 shows pre- and postoperative echocardiograms of a patient with Marfan's syndrome. The dilated aortic root can be readily appreciated in the preoperative study. After surgical repair, the aorta is considerably smaller.

A mass of echoes is still evident anterior to the functional aorta. The source of these echoes depends on the manner in which the aneurysm has been repaired. In this case, the original aorta is still present and a conduit is introduced from the root of the aorta to the normal section of aorta more distally. Acoustic shadowing does not permit one to see the full extent of the remaining posterior aorta. Only faint visualization is seen posteriorly.

Patients with Marfan's syndrome frequently have aortic regurgitation,[9,10] because the aortic annulus is dilated and the aortic valve tissue is insufficient to close the orifice. Figure 12–5 shows long-axis and short-axis views of another patient with Marfan's aortic dilatation. The short-axis view shows how the aortic valve leaflets are insufficient to close the orifice completely (arrows).

As might be expected, transesophageal echocardiography offers an excellent opportunity to visualize these massively dilated aortic roots.[10a] Figure 12–6 shows two views of a patient with annuloaortic ectasia. The aortic root is dilated (arrows) compared with the opening of the aortic valve (AV). In Figure 12–6B, one can appreciate how the aortic root expands immediately from the aortic annulus.

Transesophageal echocardiography also permits greater definition of pathologic change within the aorta. With aortic aneurysms, stagnant blood frequently produces spontaneous contrast and/or thrombus formation.[11] Figure 12–7 shows a patient with a massively dilated descending aorta.[12] The transesophageal examination shows spontaneous contrast (SC) and clot (arrows) along the wall of the aneurysm. The thrombus is so echogenic that acoustic shadowing prevents clear delineation of the true aortic wall.

M-mode echocardiography may still be useful in judging the motion of a dilated aorta. Figure 12–8 demonstrates an M-mode recording of a patient with a dilated aorta. In addition, one sees early systolic closure of the aortic valve, which is somewhat similar to that seen with subaortic stenosis or mitral regurgitation. A possible explanation for this early systolic closure is that the dilated root produces eddy currents beyond the aortic annulus that partially close the valve in early systole. In Figure 12–9, the M-mode echocardiogram of the aorta shows systolic expansion at the aortic valve level (arrow). The left atrium, posterior to the aorta, is so distorted by the dilated aorta that hardly any left atrial cavity is seen.

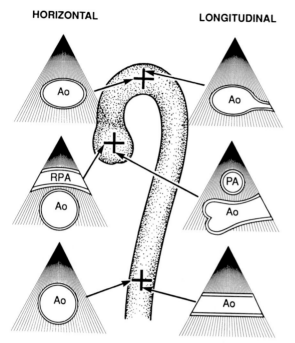

**HORIZONTAL**     **LONGITUDINAL**

**Fig. 12–1.** Diagram demonstrating how biplane transesophageal echocardiography can visualize the entire thoracic aorta. Ao = aorta; RPA = right pulmonary artery; PA = pulmonary artery.

## AORTIC DISSECTION

Transesophageal echocardiography is becoming the procedure of choice for the diagnosis and evaluation of aortic dissection.[13–20a] The hallmark of the echocardiographic diagnosis of aortic dissection is identifying an intimal flap that divides the true aortic lumen from the false lumen.[21–25] Figure 12–10 shows a transthoracic two-dimensional echocardiogram of the thoracic aorta of a patient with dissection demonstrating the intimal flap (IF) running through the aorta (AO).[26] Color flow Doppler assists in establishing the fact that the aorta is divided into two compartments.[27,28] The flow characteristics within the two chambers are now altered. The

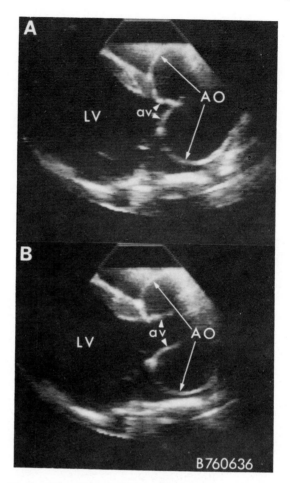

**Fig. 12–3.** Diastolic, *A*, and systolic, *B*, long-axis, parasternal two-dimensional echocardiograms of a patient with Marfan's syndrome. The aorta (AO) is markedly dilated. Note the marked discrepancy between the aortic valve (av) opening and the size of the aorta. LV = left ventricle.

higher velocity systolic flow is recorded in the true lumen (Fig. 12–9B). Figure 12–11 shows a biplane transesophageal color flow Doppler study in a patient with aortic dissection. Blood flow in the true lumen is recorded in blue in the longitudinal view *(A)* and in red in the transverse plane *(B)*. The false lumen (FL) is below the intimal flap (IF). No flow is recorded in systole. Instead, one sees spontaneous contrast (SC). Flow in the opposite direction, however, is seen in the false lumen in diastole (Fig. 12–12B).

Several important echocardiographic techniques are used to distinguish the true lumen from the false lumen. Seeing systolic flow with color flow Doppler is one of the principle techniques. In addition, one can note the pulsatile nature of the true lumen. Figure 12–13 illustrates how the true lumen increases in size in systole and collapses in diastole. This particular patient has a large false lumen. The true lumen opens in systole (Fig. 12–13A) and is virtually closed in diastole (Fig. 12–13B).

Another way of identifying the true lumen is to record the entry site of the dissection. Figure 12–14 shows an-

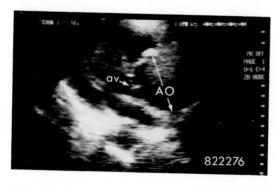

**Fig. 12–2.** Parasternal long-axis two-dimensional echocardiogram of a patient with a dilated aorta (AO). The walls of the aorta are also very echogenic. av = aortic valve.

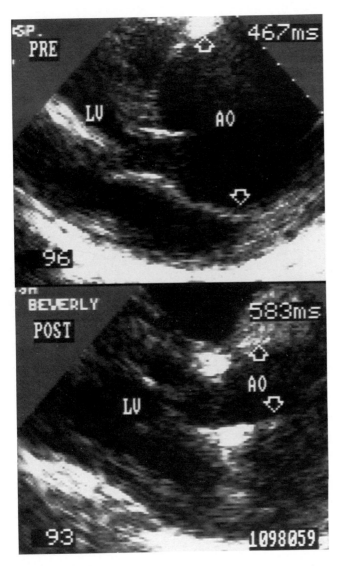

**Fig. 12–4.** Parasternal long-axis echocardiogram of a patient with Marfan's syndrome before (PRE) and after (POST) surgical correction of the abnormality. The preoperative echogram shows a dilated *(arrows)* aorta (AO). In the postoperative recording, the functional aorta, which is made up of a graft, is considerably smaller *(arrows)*. One can faintly see the residual dilated aorta anterior and posterior to the graft. LV = left ventricle.

other patient with aortic dissection whereby the true lumen (TL), false lumen (FL), and entry site are identified. In this biplane transesophageal examination, one can see high-velocity flow passing through the entry site into the false lumen in systole. This patient also has thrombus (TH) within the false lumen.

Figure 12–15 shows another example of an entry site using Doppler flow imaging. In this recording, the Doppler flow imaging is in black and white rather than in color. One can easily see the small high-velocity jet (Fig. 12–15B, *arrow*) passing from the true lumen to the false lumen.

The M-mode examination may still be helpful in showing the oscillations of the intimal flap.[29–33] Figure 12–16

shows a subcostal echocardiographic examination of the descending aorta in a patient with dissection. The false and true lumens can be seen in the descending aorta. The M-mode examination demonstrates the wildly undulating motion of the intimal flap.

Intravascular ultrasound has been used for the detection of aortic dissection.[34–36] In Figure 12–17 an intravascular sonographic image shows the dissection in both the ascending aorta (Fig. 12–17A) and the distal portion of the descending aorta (Fig. 12–17B). Intravascular sonography has the advantage of visualizing the entire aorta, including the abdominal aorta. To date, experience with this technique is limited.

Many important clinical questions about aortic dissection can be answered with echocardiography. One of the key issues is the type of dissection. Figure 12–18 shows a diagram and transesophageal echocardiograms of a patient with a DeBakey type I aortic dissection. This dissection begins at the root of the aorta and involves the

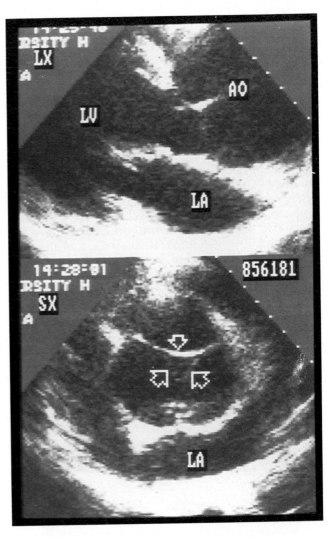

**Fig. 12–5.** Long-axis (LX) and short-axis (SX) views of another patient with Marfan's syndrome demonstrating incomplete closure of the aortic valve. In the short-axis view, one can see how the three cusps *(arrows)* fail to completely seal off the aortic orifice.

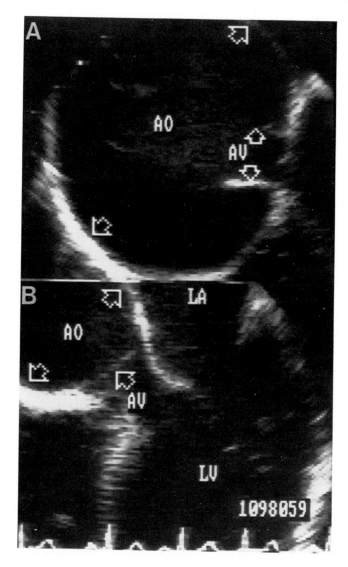

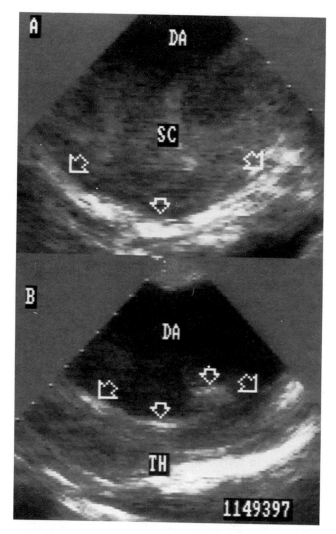

**Fig. 12–6.** Transesophageal echocardiogram of a patient with Marfan's syndrome demonstrating a tremendously dilated aortic root (AO, *arrows, A*) compared to the orifice indicated by the separation of the aortic valve leaflets (AV). The left ventricular outflow tract examination *(B)* shows how the aorta dilates immediately from the origin of the aortic valve and annulus. LA = left atrium; LV = left ventricle.

**Fig. 12–7.** Horizontal *(A)* and longitudinal *(B)* biplane transesophageal echocardiograms of a patient with a massively dilated descending aorta (DA). The aorta is filled with spontaneous contrast (SC) and thrombus (TH, *arrows*). The thrombus is so echogenic that the true wall of the aorta is not clearly defined because of shadowing.

entire length of the transthoracic aorta. Thus, one can find evidence of dissection in the root, the arch, and the descending aorta. Figure 12–19 is a transthoracic echocardiogram demonstrating a type I aortic dissection. The dissection with its false channel (FC) can be seen in the aortic root (Fig. 12–19*A* and *B*), the arch (Fig. 12–19*C*), and the descending aorta (Fig. 12–19*D*).

A type II dissection is limited only to the ascending aorta. A type III dissection is illustrated in Figure 12–20. This aortic problem begins with a dissection beyond the arch of the aorta, usually at the origin of the left subclavian artery. The dissection then proceeds distally to involve the rest of the aorta. As noted in Figure 12–20, the transverse and sagittal views of the root and aortic arch show no evidence of dissection. In the descending

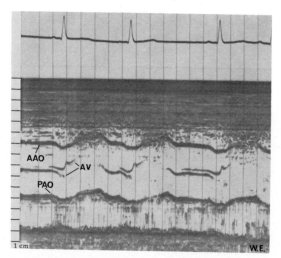

**Fig. 12–8.** Echocardiogram of a patient with a dilated aorta. AAO = anterior aortic wall; PAO = posterior aortic wall; AV = aortic valve.

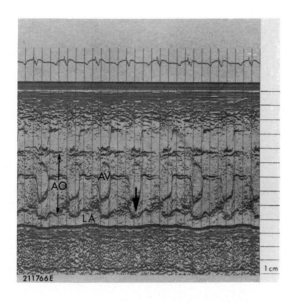

**Fig. 12–9.** M-mode echocardiogram of a dilated aorta (AO) at the level of the aortic valve (AV). Note systolic expansion *(arrow)* of the posterior aortic wall and the markedly diminished size of the left atrium (LA).

aorta, however, one sees the true and false lumens separated by an intimal flap. Thrombus within the false lumen can also be noted in this transesophageal examination. Figure 12–21 shows another example of a type III aortic dissection using transesophageal echocardiography. Figure 12–21A shows a longitudinal examination of the ascending aorta, with no evidence of dissection. The left coronary artery is well visualized coming off the aorta. It is important to know whether or not the coronary arteries are involved in a dissection. Obviously, in a type III dissection, the coronary arteries are not an issue, but with a type I dissection, whether or not the coronary arteries are coming off the true or false lumen is a major issue from a management point of view. In Figure 12–21, the descending aorta shows the dissection. The black and white, Doppler flow imaging demonstrates systolic flow in the true lumen.

Transesophageal echocardiography is proving to be helpful in following the natural history of dissecting aneurysms.[37,38] Because of enhanced resolution, this examination is improving our understanding of the etiology and outcome of this aortic abnormality. Figure 12–22 shows what appears to be an initiating event with an aortic dissection.[39] Figure 12–22A shows a biplane transesophageal examination of a patient who has an aneurysm with a thickened aortic wall and a small intra-

mural hematoma in the ascending aorta. A follow-up echocardiogram 5 days later (Fig. 12–22B) shows a well-formed intimal flap that separates the aorta into true and false lumens. The natural history of an established aortic dissection is shown in Figure 12–23. In this serial study, one can see how the false lumen develops spontaneous contrast, and then solid thrombus forms and effectively closes the false lumen. Filling a false lumen with clot is one means of hemodynamically correcting a dissection.[40]

Although echocardiography has become an extremely powerful tool for the diagnosis and management of aortic dissection, many technical details must be known to avoid diagnostic errors.[41,42,42a] In several situations, one may falsely identify an intimal flap. One possible artifact is side lobes, which can produce a simulated intimal flap. Figure 12–24 shows a patient with a dilated ascending aorta (AO), as well as a thickened aortic valve and aortic annulus. These thickened structures produce side lobes *(arrows)* within the relatively echo-free aorta in the long-axis view (LX). In the short-axis view, another more discrete side lobe can produce echocardiographic findings that initially simulate an intimal flap. Figure 12–25 shows another example of a transesophageal echocardiogram in which echoes resemble intimal flaps. In this biplane transesophageal study, the artifactual linear

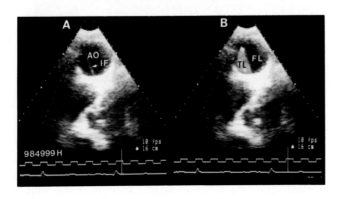

**Fig. 12–10.** Suprasternal two-dimensional echocardiograms of a patient with aortic dissection. The intimal flap (IF) is visible in *A* between the true lumen and the false lumen. Color flow Doppler *(B)* shows flow within the true lumen (TL) and no flow within the false lumen (FL). (From Feigenbaum, H.: Doppler color flow imaging. *In* Heart Disease: A Textbook of Cardiovascular Medicine, 3rd Ed. Update Two. Edited by E. Braunwald. Philadelphia, W.B. Saunders Co., 1988.)

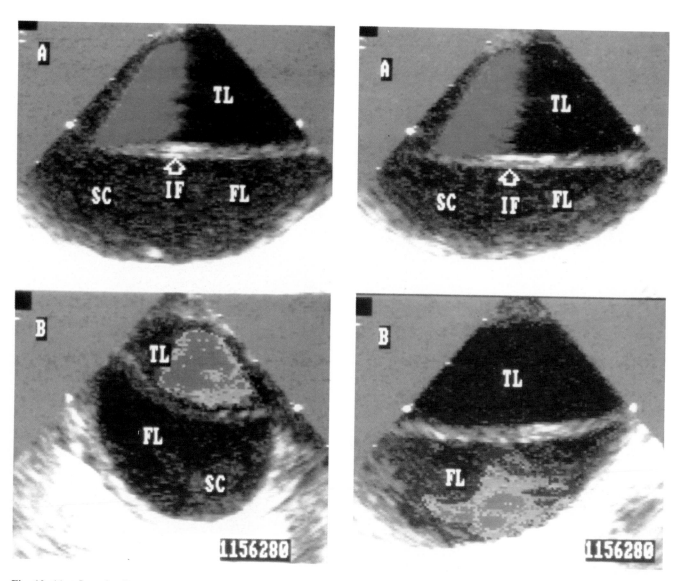

**Fig. 12–11.** Longitudinal *(A)* and horizontal *(B)* transesophageal echocardiograms of a patient with aortic dissection. The intimal flap (IF), true lumen (TL), and false lumen (FL) can be identified. Color flow Doppler shows flow within the true lumen. The false lumen contains spontaneous contrast (SC).

**Fig. 12–12.** Systolic *(A)* and diastolic *(B)* transesophageal echocardiographic views of the same patient noted in Figure 12–11. Color flow Doppler shows flow within the true lumen (TL) in systole and flow in the opposite direction in the false lumen (FL) in diastole. IF = intimal flap; SC = spontaneous contrast.

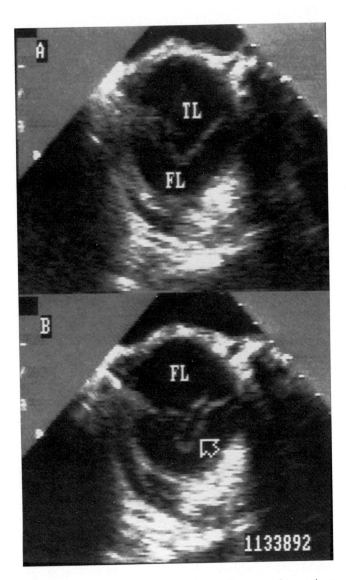

**Fig. 12–13.** Transesophageal echocardiogram of a patient with aortic dissection shows the true lumen (TL) is larger in systole *(A)* than in diastole *(arrow, B)*. FL = false lumen.

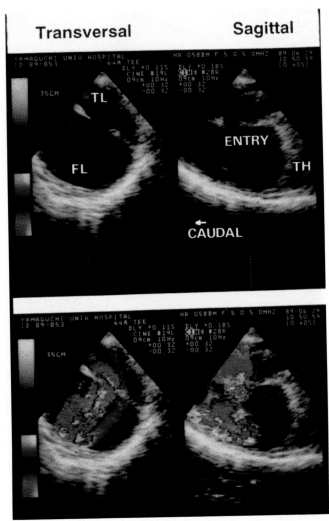

**Fig. 12–14.** Biplane transesophageal echocardiographic examinations and color flow images demonstrating the entry site of aortic dissection. Blood flows from the true lumen (TL) into the false lumen (FL). TH = thrombus. (From Matsuzaki, M., et al.: Clinical applications of transesophageal echocardiography. Circulation, *82*:713, 1990, by permission of the American Heart Association, Inc.)

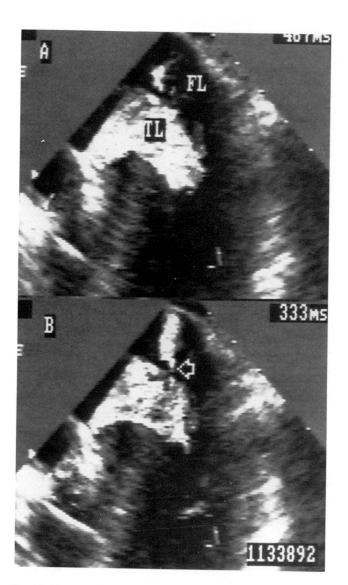

**Fig. 12–15.** Doppler flow imaging in black and white showing an entry jet *(arrow)* passing from the true lumen (TL) into the false lumen (FL) of a patient with aortic dissection.

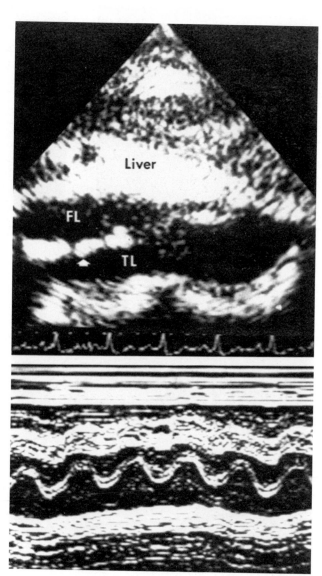

**Fig. 12–16.** Subcostal two-dimensional and M-mode echocardiograms of a patient with aortic dissection. The M-mode recording shows oscillations of the intimal flap between the false lumen (FL) and the true lumen (TL). (From Khandheria, B.K., et al.: Aortic dissection: Review of value and limitations of two-dimensional echocardiography in a six-year experience. J. Am. Soc. Echocardiogr., *2*:17, 1989.)

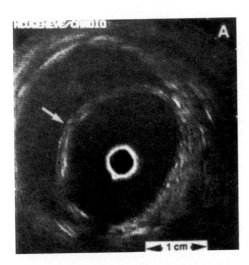

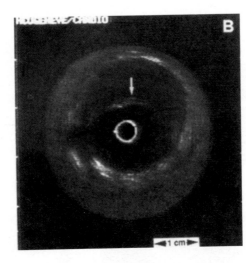

**Fig. 12–17.** Intravascular ultrasonic examination of a patient with aortic dissection. The circular structure in the center is the transducer. The intimal flap *(arrow)* is identified with this invasive ultrasonic examination. (From Pande, A., et al.: Intravascular ultrasound for diagnosis of aortic dissection. Am. J. Cardiol., *67*:663, 1991.)

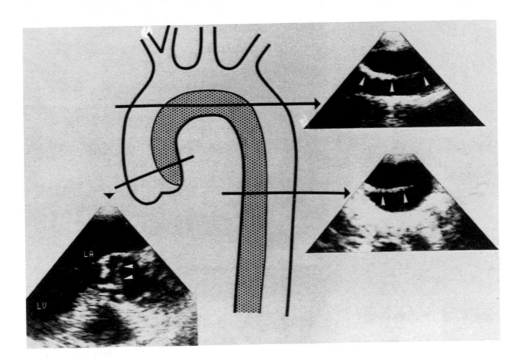

**Fig. 12–18.** Diagram and transesophageal echocardiograms of a patient with a DeBakey type I aortic dissection. The dissection begins at the root of the aorta and extends the entire length of the vessel. The intimal flap *(arrows)* can be identified at all levels of the aorta. LA = left atrium; LV = left ventricle. (From Erbel, R., et al.: Detection of aortic dissection by transesophageal echocardiography. Br. Heart J., *58*:48, 1987.)

**Fig. 12–20.** Biplane transesophageal echocardiogram and diagram of a patient with a DeBakey type III aortic dissection. The dissection begins just beyond the arch of the aorta and extends distally. Echocardiograms at the ascending aorta and arch fail to find evidence of an intimal flap. The dissection with true lumen (TL) and false lumen (FL) are seen in the descending aorta. TH = thrombus; RPA = right pulmonary artery; PA = pulmonary artery; AO = aorta; AV = aortic valve; FE = spontaneous echo contrast. (From Matsuzaki, M., et al.: Clinical applications of transesophageal echocardiography. Circulation, *82*:712, 1990, by permission of the American Heart Association, Inc.)

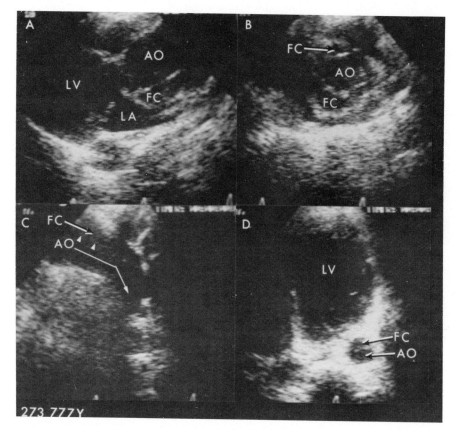

**Fig. 12–19.** Parasternal long-axis *(A)*, short-axis *(B)*, suprasternal *(C)* and apical *(D)* views of a patient with a dissecting aortic aneurysm. The false channel (FC) can be seen in every view. The intimal flap *(arrowheads)* is only faintly seen in the suprasternal examination *(C)*. AO = true aortic lumen; LV = left ventricle; LA = left atrium.

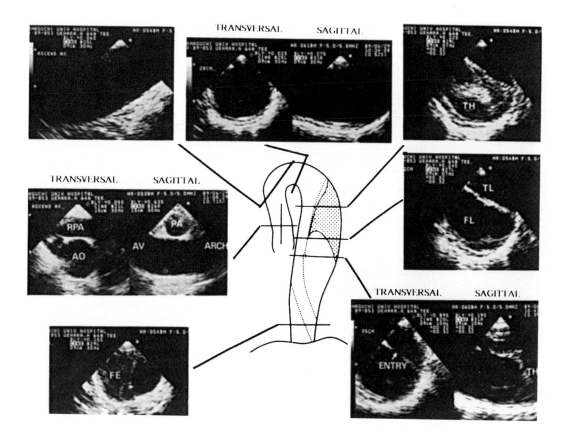

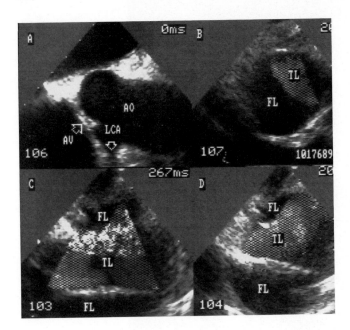

**Fig. 12–21.** Transesophageal echocardiogram of another type III aortic dissection. Longitudinal scan of the aortic root *(A)* shows only a dilated aorta and no evidence of the dissection. Examinations of the descending aorta *(B, C,* and *D)* show systolic flow (black and white Doppler flow imaging) in the true lumen (TL). *C* and *D* demonstrate that the false lumen (FL) surrounds the true lumen. AV = aortic valve; AO = aorta; LCA = left coronary artery.

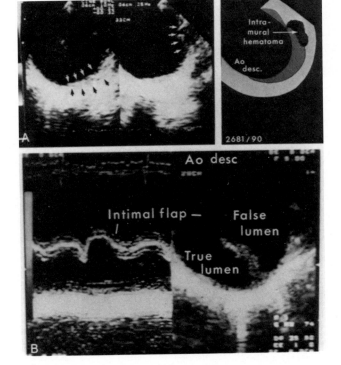

**Fig. 12–22.** Transesophageal biplane echocardiogram immediately after the onset of an aortic dissection *(A)* reveals a thickened aortic wall *(arrows,* left) and an intramural hematoma *(arrows,* right). Five days later *(B),* a clear intimal flap divides the aorta into a true lumen and a false lumen. (From Zotz, R.J., et al.: Non-communicating intramural hematoma: An indication of developing aortic dissection? J. Am. Soc. Echocardiogr., *4:*637, 1991.)

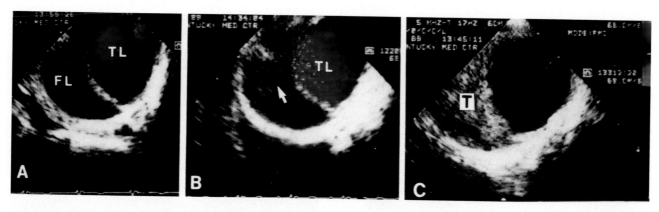

**Fig. 12–23.** Serial transesophageal echocardiograms of a patient with aortic dissection. The initial examination *(A)* demonstrates a double lumen with pulsatile flow in both the true (TL) and false (FL) lumens of the aorta. A repeat examination 4 days later *(B)* reveals spontaneous contrast within the false lumen *(arrow).* At 8 weeks *(C),* the spontaneous contrast previously noted in the false lumen is replaced by thrombus (T). (From Hixson, C.S., Cater, A., and Smith, M.D.: Diagnosis and documentation of healing in descending thoracic aortic dissection by transesophageal echocardiography and Doppler color flow imaging. Am. Heart J., *119*:1434, 1990.)

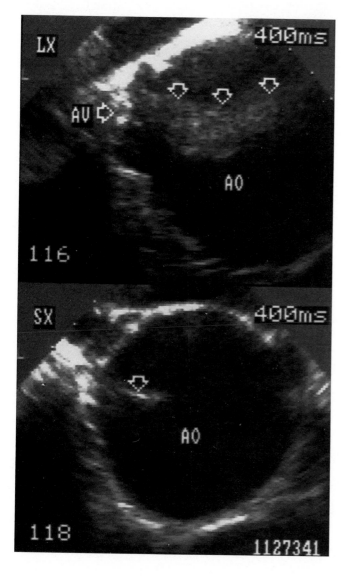

**Fig. 12–24.** Long-axis (LX) and short-axis (SX) transesophageal echocardiograms of a patient with a dilated ascending aorta (AO). The aortic valve is thickened and produces a side lobe *(arrows)* that may be confused with aortic dissection.

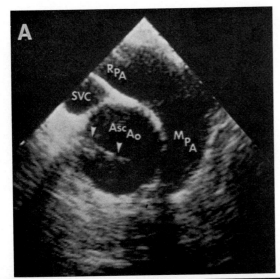

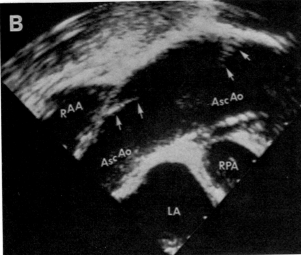

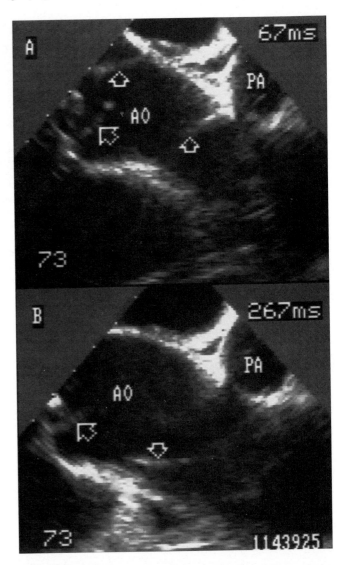

**Fig. 12–25.** Horizontal *(A)* and longitudinal *(B)* biplane transesophageal echocardiograms of a patient who demonstrates linear reverberations *(arrows)*, which can be confused with aortic dissection. Change in transducer frequency, alternating the depth of the image, nonanatomic appearance, and nondisturbed color flow signal can identify the artifactual nature of this observation in most situations. Occasionally, linear artifacts cannot be adequately distinguished from aortic dissection. RPA = right pulmonary artery; SVC = superior vena cava; Asc Ao = ascending aorta; MPA = main pulmonary artery; RAA = right atrial appendage; LA = left atrium. (From Seward, J.B., et al.: Critical appraisal of transesophageal echocardiography: Limitations, pitfalls, and complications. J. Am. Soc. Echocardiogr., 5:288, 1992.)

**Fig. 12–26.** Transesophageal echocardiogram demonstrating multiple linear echoes *(arrows)* that could not be adequately distinguished from aortic dissection. The etiology of the echoes was not totally resolved. Aortography and CT scanning showed no evidence of dissection. AO = aorta; PA = pulmonary artery.

echoes are thought to be reverberations originating from overlying lung. Yet another potentially confusing transesophageal echocardiogram is shown in Figure 12–26. In this example of a patient with a dilated aorta, multiple linear echoes *(arrows)* are noted throughout the recording. There was considerable confusion with regard to possible dissection. In this case, follow-up study with aortography and CT scanning showed no evidence of dissection. The etiology of all of these echoes is not totally understood. The echoes could be a combination of reverberations and side lobe artifacts. A left brachiocephalic vein may mimic aortic dissection.[42b]

True dissections may also produce confusing echocardiograms. Figure 12–27 shows diagrams and transesophageal echocardiograms of a patient who had a complex dissection whereby the intimal flap coiled into a mass-like structure.[43] Under these circumstances, the intimal flap appeared more as a mobile mass than as a true dissection.

Even transthoracic echocardiograms, which are frequently used as a screening device for possible dissection, must be carefully scrutinized to make certain that a false-negative result does not lead to mismanagement of a patient.[44–46] In Figure 12–28, the parasternal long-

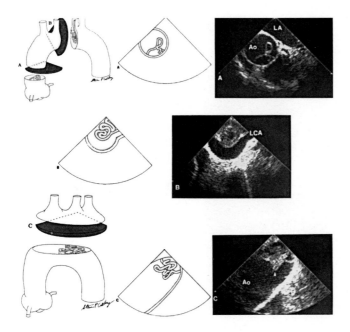

**Fig. 12–27.** Diagrams and transesophageal echocardiograms of a patient with a complex intimal flap in a patient with aortic dissection. *A* is the transverse view demonstrating the circumferential intimal tear within the aorta (Ao). In the aortic arch longitudinal view *(B)*, the intimal flap appears as a mass extending into the left carotid artery (LCA). In the transverse view of the arch *(C)*, the intimal flap again appears as a mass *(arrowhead)*. LA = left atrium. (From Lourie, J.K., Appelbe, A., and Martin, R.P.: Detection of complex intimal flaps in aortic dissection by transesophageal echocardiography. Am. J. Cardiol., 69:1362, 1992.)

axis examination shows a dilated aortic root with little evidence of dissection; however, with the short-axis examination, one sees that the dilated aorta is primarily a false lumen. The relatively small aorta and the intimal flap are seen in the short-axis but not the long-axis examination.

Several important complications of aortic dissection were discussed in previous chapters. Aortic regurgitation occurs when the dissection involves the aortic valve or support of the valve.[47,48] Doppler echocardiography, both spectral and flow imaging, is the procedure of choice for determining the presence and severity of aortic regurgitation. The Doppler study can be done either with transthoracic or transesophageal echocardiography. A second important complication is when the dissection involves the pericardial sac producing bloody pericardial effusion and possible tamponade. Again, echocardiography is ideal for making this determination either with a transthoracic or transesophageal technique. Rare complications, such as dissection into the right ventricle, has also been detected with echocardiography.[49] An aorta-to-right atrium fistula is another possible complication of aortic dissection.[50–52] Thus, the value of echocardiography in the management of patients with aortic dissection is not only in making the diagnosis but also in noting the extent of the dissection and any cardiac involvement.[53]

## AORTIC FALSE ANEURYSMS

An aortic false aneurysm or pseudoaneurysm is a situation whereby there is perforation of the entire aortic wall, and the blood is trapped by clot and surrounding soft tissue to prevent exsanguination of the patient.[54,55]

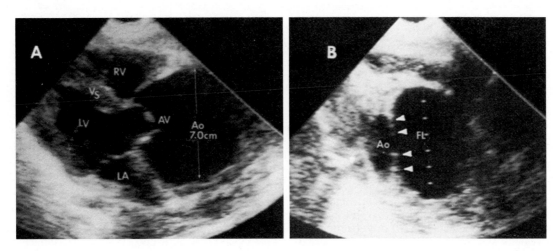

**Fig. 12–28.** Long-axis *(A)* and short-axis *(B)* transthoracic echocardiograms of a patient with a type I aortic dissection. The long-axis view shows only an abnormally dilated aortic root (7.0 cm). The short-axis examination reveals an aortic dissection. The false lumen (FL) is considerably larger and is what was visualized in the long-axis examination. The true aortic lumen (Ao) is small and is separated from the false lumen by an intimal flap *(arrowheads)*. RV = right ventricle; VS = ventricular septum; LV = left ventricle; LA = left atrium; AV = aortic valve. (From Khandheria, B.K., et al.: Aortic dissection: Review of value and limitations of two-dimensional echocardiography in a six-year experience. J. Am. Soc. Echocardiogr., 2:117, 1989.)

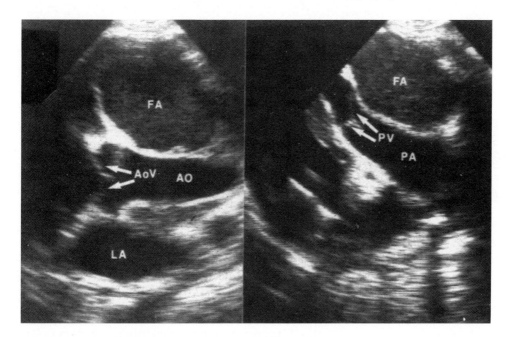

**Fig. 12–29.** Transthoracic echocardiograms of a patient with a false aneurysm (FA) anterior to the aorta (AO) and pulmonary artery (PA). The false aneurysm is filled with spontaneous contrast echoes. AoV = aortic valve; LA = left atrium; PV = pulmonary valve. (From Come, P.C., et al.: Aortic false aneurysm: Recognition by non-invasive techniques four years after mitral valve replacement. Am. J. Cardiol., *58*:1137, 1986.)

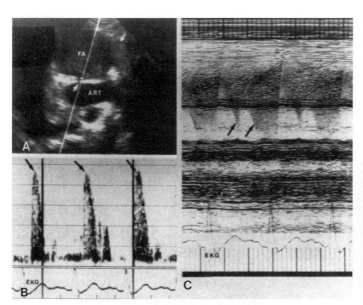

**Fig. 12–30.** Two-dimensional pulsed Doppler and M-mode recordings of the same patient as in Figure 12–29. The two-dimensional examination *(A)* shows an apparent communication *(arrow)* between the false aneurysm (FA) and the aorta (ART). A pulsed Doppler examination *(B)* from that location reveals high-velocity systolic flow. An M-mode echocardiogram *(C)* shows spontaneous contrast *(arrows)* communicating between the upper false aneurysm and the lower aorta. (From Come, P.C., et al.: Aortic false aneurysm: Recognition by non-invasive techniques four years after mitral valve replacement. Am. J. Cardiol., *58*:1138, 1986.)

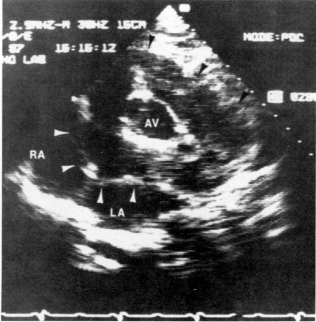

**Fig. 12–31.** Another transthoracic echocardiogram at the base of the heart demonstrating a large pseudoaneurysm *(arrowheads)* that completely surrounds the aorta. The pseudoaneurysm was a result of coronary artery dehiscence after surgical repair of an aortic aneurysm in a Marfan's patient. AV = aortic valve; RA = right atrium; LA = left atrium. (From Rice, M.J., McDonald, R.W., and Reller, M.D.: Diagnosis of coronary artery dehiscence and pseudoaneurysm formation in post-operative Marfan patient by color flow Doppler echocardiography. JCU, *17*:361 1989.)

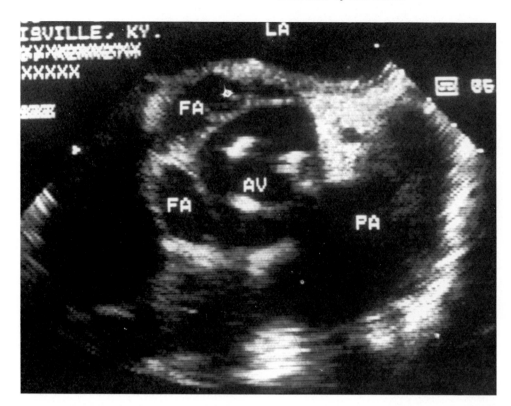

**Fig. 12–32.** Transesophageal echocardiogram at the level of an aortic valve bioprosthesis (AV) demonstrating a multichambered, periaortic false aneurysm (FA). The outermost wall of the false aneurysm is a pericardial patch and the inner wall is the aorta. LA = left atrium; PA = pulmonary artery. (From Liddell, N.E., et al.: Transesophageal echocardiographic diagnosis of complex false aneurysm with aorta-left atrial communication complicating aortic valve and root replacement. Am. Heart J., *123*:544, 1992.)

False aneurysms may occur after cardiac surgery.[56–59] During aortic cross clamping and canulation of the aorta, a postoperative leak can be responsible for a false aneurysm. Figure 12–29 shows an example of a patient with a huge false aneurysm anterior to the ascending aorta. This echo-free space can be extremely large and can compress surrounding structures, including the aorta attached to an aortic graft.[59a] The Doppler study (Fig. 12–30) shows that a communication remains between the aorta and the false aneurysm.

Figure 12–31 illustrates another patient with an aortic pseudoaneurysm in the short-axis presentation. The huge pseudoaneurysm *(arrowheads)* totally surrounds the aorta and aortic valve. The pseudoaneurysm resulted from coronary artery dehiscence following repair of a Marfan's aortic aneurysm. Figure 12–32 shows a transesophageal echocardiographic study of another patient who developed a false aneurysm after aortic valve replacement. In this instance, the periaortic false aneurysm is multichambered. The outermost wall of the aneurysm is a pericardial patch and the inner wall is the aorta. The intent of the surgery in this particular patient was to correct a subannular abscess. Pericardium was used to patch the area of the abscess. Color flow Doppler can be used to identify a residual leak into the false aneurysm. Figure 12–33 shows a transesophageal echocardiographic study in a patient with a false aneurysm.[60] Doppler imaging demonstrates a communication between the aortic root and the pseudoaneurysm. False aneurysms can also be a result of aortic dissection.[61] Figure 12–34 shows an aortic dissection in which there

is rupture of the free wall of the false lumen *(arrow)*. The resultant hematoma becomes the false aneurysm. False aneurysms can also occur because of traumatic rupture of the aorta. An example of such a false aneurysm is described in the section on traumatic damage to the aorta.

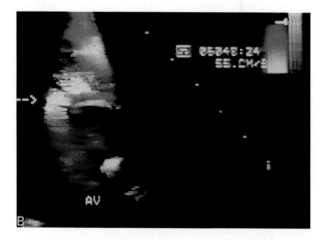

**Fig. 12–33.** Color flow Doppler study of the same patient as in Figure 12–32. The Doppler examination demonstrates turbulent flow entering the false aneurysm *(arrow)* from the aorta at the level of the prosthetic aortic valve (AV) during diastole. (From Liddell, N.E., et al.: Transesophageal echocardiographic diagnosis of complex false aneurysm with aorta-left atrial communication complicating aortic valve and root replacement. Am. Heart J., *123*:544, 1992.)

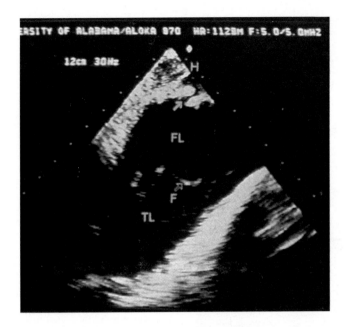

**Fig. 12–34.** Transesophageal echocardiogram of a patient with aortic dissection whose false lumen (FL) ruptures *(arrow)* and communicates with a false aneurysm that contains a hematoma (H). F = intimal flap; TL = true lumen. (From Ballal, R.S.: Usefulness of transesophageal echocardiography in assessment of aortic dissection. Circulation, *84*:1910, by permission of the American Heart Association, Inc.)

## SINUS OF VALSALVA ANEURYSMS

The echocardiographic findings for sinus of Valsalva aneurysm have been described in numerous reports.[62–73] Figure 12–35 shows long-axis and short-axis views of a patient with an intact sinus of Valsalva aneurysm. As is usually the case, the aneurysm extends anteriorly and to the right. When the aneurysms rupture, they frequently rupture into the right side of the heart.[74–76] Figure 12–36 shows such an aneurysm with rupture into the right atrium. The aneurysm is best seen in the short-axis view in diastole. One can actually see the defect in the aneurysm *(double arrow)*. In this patient, the defect and resultant shunt are demonstrated by the use of contrast echocardiography.[77,78] In diastole, one sees a jet of negative contrast from the aorta to the right atrium *(double arrow)*. Multiple sinus of Valsalva aneurysms have been reported. The aneurysmal formation can involve any of the coronary sinuses.

Doppler[79] and particularly Doppler flow imaging is the procedure of choice for identifying a ruptured sinus of Valsalva aneurysm.[80–82] Figure 12–37 shows apical four-chamber and short-axis views of a patient with a sinus of Valsalva aneurysm. In the four-chamber view, one sees a Doppler jet going from the vicinity of the left ventricular outflow tract into the right atrium (Fig. 12–37, *1B*). In the short-axis view, one can faintly see an outpouching of the noncoronary sinus *(arrow, 2A)*. Color flow imaging demonstrates a diastolic jet passing from the aorta into the right atrium *(2B)*.

The sinus of Valsalva aneurysm occasionally ruptures into the interventricular septum.[83–88] When this occurs, bizarre echocardiograms may be recorded. Figure 12–38 is an M-mode echocardiogram of such a patient. One sees an abrupt downward motion of the interventricular septum into the left ventricular outflow tract. The unusual echoes *(arrows)* are actually from the aneurysm and the left side of the dissected interventricular septum,

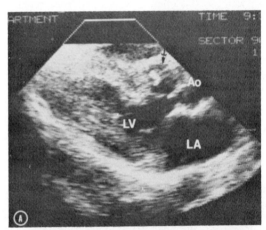

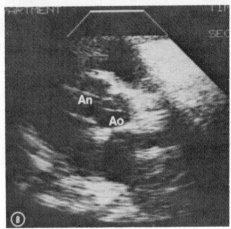

**Fig. 12–35.**   Long-axis *(A)* and short-axis *(B)* two-dimensional echocardiograms of a patient with an intact sinus of Valsalva aneurysm. The aneurysm *(arrow* in *A* and *An* in *B)* can be seen adjacent to the aorta (Ao). LV = left ventricle; LA = left atrium.

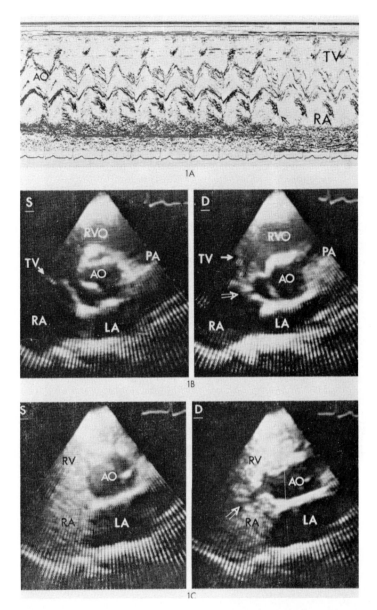

**Fig. 12–36.** M-mode echocardiogram and short-axis two-dimensional echocardiograms of a patient with a sinus of Valsalva aneurysm that ruptured into the right atrium (RA). The aneurysm is best seen in the short-axis view in diastole *(1B D)*. The defect communicating with the right atrium is seen in that view *(arrow)*. The defect also can be noted with contrast echocardiography *(1C D)* as a negative contrast jet *(arrow)*. TV = tricuspid valve; AO = aorta; RVO = right ventricular outflow tract; PA = pulmonary artery; LA = left atrium. (From Nakamura, K., et al.: Detection of ruptured aneurysm of sinus of Valsalva by contrast two-dimensional echocardiography. Br. Heart J., *45*:219, 1981).

both of which fill with blood in diastole and empty during systole.

A sinus of Valsalva aneurysm can dissect into a variety of places. Besides the right atrium and interventricular septum, these aneurysms can dissect into the left ventricle and mimic aortic regurgitation.[89] The aneurysm can communicate with the right ventricle. At times, such a communication can increase the right ventricular diastolic pressure to the point that premature opening of the pulmonary valve occurs.[90] Rupture into the left atrium has also been reported.[90a]

Transesophageal echocardiography can again define a sinus of Valsalva aneurysm with great clarity. Figure 12–39 shows a transesophageal study of a patient with a sinus of Valsalva aneurysm. The aneurysm bulges into the left atrium in diastole (Fig. 12–39A) and collapses in systole (Fig. 12–39B). Most sinus of Valsalva aneurysms can be detected with transthoracic echocardiography because the aortic root is the site of the aneurysms and this area is well seen with the transthoracic examination. However, the transesophageal study may identify resultant fistulas with greater clarity.[90b]

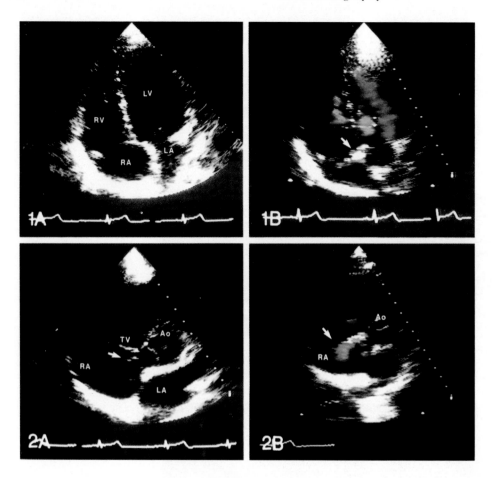

**Fig. 12–37.** Four-chamber (*1A* and *1B*) and short-axis (*2A* and *2B*) views of a patient with a ruptured sinus of Valsalva aneurysm. The aneurysm can be faintly seen in the short-axis view *(arrow, 2A)*. The abnormality, however, is better appreciated by seeing the abnormal communicating blood *(arrows, 1B* and *2B)* flowing from the aorta (Ao) to the right atrium (RA). (From Peters, P., et al.: Doppler color flow mapping detection of ruptured sinus of Valsalva aneurysm. J. Am. Soc. Echocardiogr., *2:* 196, 1989.)

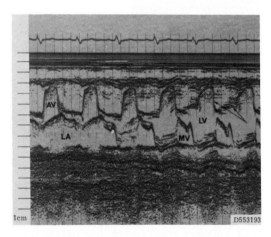

**Fig. 12–38.** Echocardiogram of a patient with a sinus of Valsalva aneurysm that ruptured into the interventricular septum. The abnormal echoes *(arrows)* represent the aneurysm and the dissected interventricular septum. In diastole, the aneurysm and the dissected septum fill with blood and expand into the left ventricular outflow tract. AV = distorted aortic valve; LA = left atrium; LV = left ventricle; MV = mitral valve. (From Rothbaum, D.A., et al.: Echocardiographic manifestations of right sinus of Valsalva aneurysm. Circulation, *49:*768, 1974 by permission of the American Heart Association, Inc.)

## TRAUMATIC DAMAGE TO THE AORTA

A variety of abnormalities of the aorta can occur as a result of trauma.[91] Blunt chest trauma can produce a fistula between the aorta and other parts of the cardiovascular system. A fistula between the sinus of Valsalva and right atrium have been reported by several investigators.[92] A post-traumatic fistula between the abdominal aorta and the inferior vena cava has also been detected.[93] Doppler echocardiography using flow imaging is the sonographic procedure of choice for detecting these fistulas. Figure 12–40 shows a transthoracic echocardiogram of a small traumatic aneurysm arising from the arch of the aorta.[94] A larger traumatic aneurysm is noted in Figure 12–41. This aneurysm originated just past the origin of the subclavian artery.

Trauma can produce aortic transsection.[95] When this occurs, the patient usually dies unless the bleeding is trapped by soft tissue and a false aneurysm is produced (Fig. 12–42). Trauma to the aorta can also produce aortic thrombosis. Figure 12–43 shows a patient who developed a huge thrombus in the descending aorta after sustaining a gunshot wound.[96] Such a thrombus has the potential for peripheral embolization.

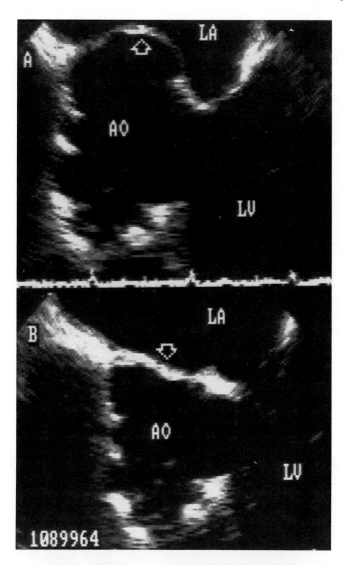

Fig. 12–39. Transesophageal echocardiogram of a patient with a sinus of Valsalva aneurysm. One can appreciate how the aneurysm bulges during systole *(A)* into the left atrium *(arrow)*. With diastole *(B)*, the aneurysm moves toward the aorta *(arrow)*. LA = left atrium; AO = aorta; LV = left ventricle.

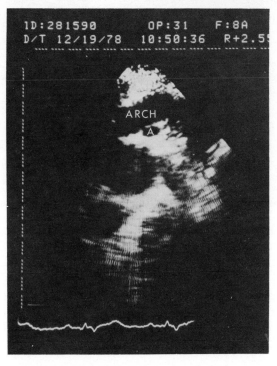

Fig. 12–40. Suprasternal two-dimensional echocardiogram showing a small aneurysm (A) arising from the arch of the aorta. The aneurysm was apparently traumatic in origin.

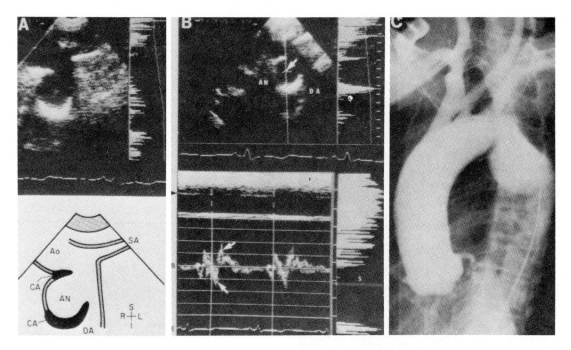

**Fig. 12–41.** Two-dimensional echocardiograms, aortogram, and Doppler echocardiogram of a patient with a traumatic aneurysm (AN) in the descending aorta (DA) just past the origin of the subclavian artery (SA). The Doppler study shows flow both away and toward the transducer *(arrows)*. Ao = aorta; CA = calcium. (From Doenhoff, L.J. and Nanda, N.C.: Chronic traumatic thoracic aneurysm: Demonstration by two-dimensional echocardiography. Am. J. Cardiol., *54*:692, 1984.)

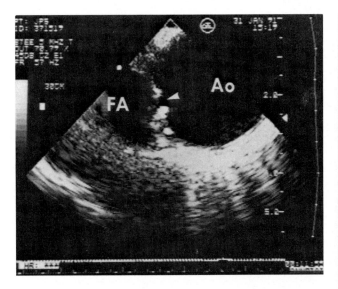

**Fig. 12–42.** Transesophageal echocardiogram of a patient with trans-section of the aorta. A communication *(arrowhead)* can be seen between the aorta (Ao) and a thrombus-filled false aneurysm (FA). (From Snow, C.C., et al.: Diagnosis of aortic transection by transesophageal echocardiography. J. Am. Soc. Echocardiogr., *5*:101, 1992.)

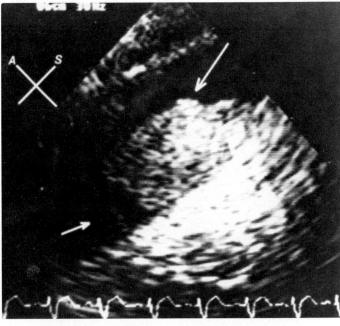

**Fig. 12–43.** Longitudinal transesophageal echocardiographic examination of the descending aorta of a patient who developed a large thrombus *(arrows)* after a gunshot wound. (From Bergin, B.J.: Aortic thrombosis and peripheral embolization after thoracic gun shot wound diagnosed by transesophageal echocardiography. Am. Heart J., *119*:688, 1990.)

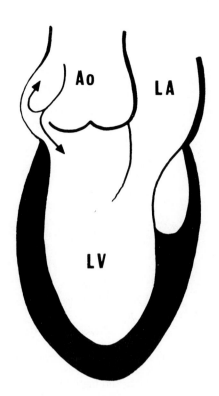

**Fig. 12–44.** Diagram illustrating an aorto-left ventricular communication. Ao = aorta; LA = left atrium; LV = left ventricle. (From Serino, W., et al.: Aorto-left ventricular communication after closure: Late postoperative problems. Br. Heart J., *49*:501, 1983.)

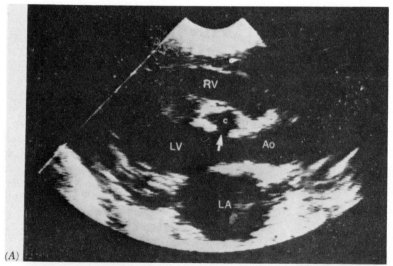

*(A)*

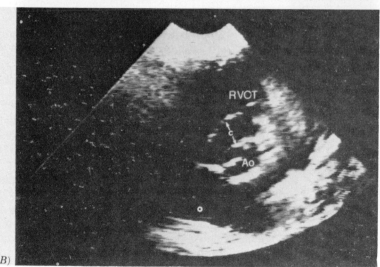

*(B)*

**Fig. 12–45.** Long-axis *(A)* and short-axis *(B)* two-dimensional echocardiograms of a patient with an aorto-left ventricular communication (c). The connection *(arrow)* between the abnormal communication and the left ventricle (LV) can be seen in the long-axis view. The short-axis view illustrates the relationship of the communication (c) to the aorta (Ao). RV = right ventricle; LA = left atrium; RVOT = right ventricular outflow tract. (From Serino, W., et al.: Aorto-left ventricular communication after closure: Late postoperative problems. Br. Heart J., *49*:501, 1983.)

## INFECTIONS OF THE AORTA

Infections of the aortic valve can extend into the aortic root and produce abscesses or aneurysms. Such complications of bacterial endocarditis can be devastating. This topic has been discussed in the section on endocarditis in the chapter on valvular heart disease.[97-101] Infections of the aorta can also produce a false aneurysm of the mitral aortic intervalvular fibrosa.[102]

## AORTO-LEFT VENTRICULAR TUNNEL

Congenital aorto-left ventricular communication or tunnel represents a severe form of aortic regurgitation in the neonate or infant. Figure 12–44 is a diagram demonstrating the pathologic communication between the aorta and the left ventricle in these patients. The two-dimensional echocardiogram in Figure 12–45 illustrates the abnormal communication. In the long-axis view, one sees the tunnel communicating with the left ventricle below the level of the aorta. The tunnel at the level of the aorta is best seen in the short-axis view.[103,104] Doppler echocardiography may assist in the detection of the aorto-left ventricular tunnel.[105]

## AORTIC ATHEROSCLEROSIS

Transesophageal echocardiography has provided an opportunity to study atherosclerosis of the thoracic aorta.[106-109] Figure 12–46 demonstrates a longitudinal

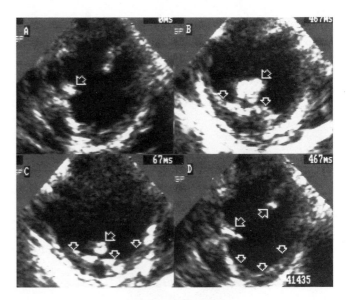

**Fig. 12–47.** Horizontal transesophageal echocardiograms of a patient with extensive atherosclerosis. The atherosclerotic material *(arrows)* is variable and highly mobile.

view of the descending aorta in a patient with extensive atherosclerotic plaque. The irregular, multiple echoes *(arrows)* are readily appreciated in this examination. Figure 12–47 shows horizontal transesophageal echocardiograms of another patient with extensive aortic atherosclerosis. One can appreciate the variability in the echogenic material. Much of the atheroma is mobile. In this illustration, the moving large plaques are indicated by the larger arrows and the more stable intimal atherosclerosis is noted by the smaller arrows. Figure 12–48 attempts to show the variability in the degree of atherosclerosis that can be detected with transesophageal echocardiography.[110] Figure 12–48A shows mild plaque with a smooth surface and no ulceration. In Figure 12–48B, one sees complex debris with plaque protruding well into the aortic lumen. The echogram in Figure 12–48C again shows complex debris with an ulcerated cavity, and Figure 12–48D again reveals extensive debris with adherent mobile thrombus.

The ability of transesophageal echocardiography to detect atherosclerosis has shed new light on this entity in vivo. Angiography has never had the resolution to detect this abnormality with clarity. Aortic atherosclerosis is better appreciated now that one can see the highly mobile, striking atheromata with a transesophageal examination. Studying the wall of the aorta has become a major part of the esophageal examination and is a strong reason for doing such an examination in a patient in whom a source of embolus is sought.[111-114]

Despite the fact that these atheromatous plaques can be mobile and are striking and are probably the cause of some peripheral embolization (Fig. 12–49),[115-122] the proper management of these atheromata is unclear. The fact remains, however, that the transesophageal echocardiographic demonstration of extensive aortic atherosclerosis has provided new insight into this problem and

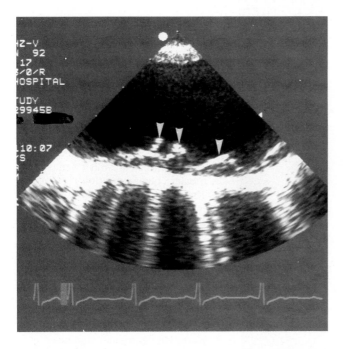

**Fig. 12–46.** Longitudinal transesophageal echocardiogram of the descending aorta of a patient with extensive atherosclerosis *(arrowheads)* within the descending aorta.

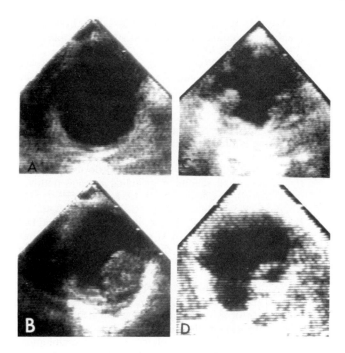

**Fig. 12–48.** Transesophageal echocardiograms of the descending aorta in four patients with varying degrees of atherosclerosis. A mild plaque is noted in *A*. The surface is smooth, with no protrusion or ulceration. A protruding plaque is identified in *B*. The examination in *C* shows complex debris with ulceration. *D* also shows complex debris with an adherent mobile thrombus. (From Rubin, D.C., Plotnick, G.D., and Hawke, M.W.: Intraaortic debris as a potential source of embolic stroke. Am. J. Cardiol., *69*:819, 1992.)

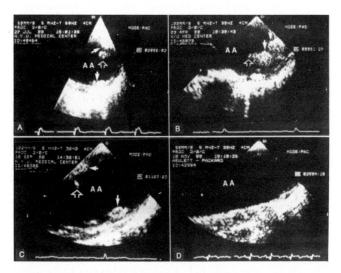

**Fig. 12–49.** Transesophageal echocardiograms of patients with protruding atherosclerotic plaques (*A*, *B*, and *C*) compared with a normal aorta (*D*). The solid arrows identify stable atherosclerotic plaque layered against the aorta. The open arrows indicate mobile projections from the plaques. AA = aortic arch. (From Tunick, P.A. and Kronzon, I.: Protruding atherosclerotic plaque in the aortic arch of patients with systemic embolization: A new finding seen by transesophageal echocardiography. Am. Heart J., *120*:659, 1990.)

raises new questions about the risk of spontaneous embolization or embolization through diagnostic or therapeutic maneuvers involving the aorta.[118]

The excellent visualization of the aorta with transesophageal echocardiography provides an opportunity to measure aortic stiffness, which may be an early sign of atherosclerosis.[123,124]

## REFERENCES

1. DeMaria, A.N., Bommer, W., Neumann, A., Weinert, L., Bogren, H., and Mason, D.T.: Identification and localization of aneurysms of the ascending aorta by cross-sectional echocardiography. Circulation, *59*:755, 1979.
2. Kronzon, I., Weisinger, B., and Glassman, E.: Illustrative echocardiogram: cystic medial necrosis with severe aortic root dilatation. Chest, *66*:79, 1974.
3. D'Cruz, I.A., Jain, D.P., Hirsch, L., Levinsky, R., Cohen, H.C., and Glick, G.: Echocardiographic diagnosis of dilatation of the ascending aorta using right parasternal scanning. Radiology, *129*:465, 1978.
4. Fox, R., Ren, J.-F., Panidis, I.P., Kotler, M.N., Mintz, G.S., and Ross, J.: Anuloaortic ectasia: A clinical and echocardiographic study. Am. J. Cardiol., *54*:177, 1984.
5. Schneeweiss, A., Feigl, A., Motro, M., Blieden, L.C., and Neufeld, H.N.: Unusual echocardiographic findings in the Marfan syndrome. Eur. Heart J., *3*:88, 1982.
6. Come, P.C., Fortuin, N.J., White, R.I., Jr., and McKusick, V.A.: Echocardiographic assessment of cardiovascular abnormalities in the Marfan syndrome. Am. J. Med., *74*:465, 1983.
7. Geva, T., Sanders, S.P., Diogenes, M.S., Rockenmacher, S., and Van Praagh, R.: Two-dimensional and Doppler echocardiographic and pathologic characteristics of the infantile Marfan syndrome. Am. J. Cardiol., *65*:1230, 1990.
8. Aldrich, H.R., Labarre, R.L., Roman, M.J., Rosen, S.E., Spitzer, M.C., and Devereux, R.B.: Color flow and conventional echocardiography of the Marfan syndrome. Echocardiography, *9*:627, 1992.
9. Matsuo, T., Ikushima, I., Hanada, Y., Nakagawa, S., Koiwaya, Y., and Tanaka, K.: Aortic regurgitation secondary to diastolic prolapse of a tubular intimal flap into the left ventricle in a patient with anuloaortic ectasia. Clin. Cardiol., *11*:719, 1988.
10. Liu, M.W., Louie, E.K., and Levitsky, S.: Color flow Doppler assessment of aortic regurgitation complicated by aneurysmal dilation and dissection of the ascending aorta in the Marfan syndrome. Am. Heart J., *115*:1118, 1988.
10a. Simpson, I.A., de Belder, M.A., Treasure, T., Camm, A.J., and Pumphrey, C.W.: Cardiovascular manifestations of Marfan's syndrome: Improved evaluation by transesophageal echocardiography. Br. Heart J., *69*:104, 1992.
11. Tunick, P.A., Lackner, H., Katz, E.S., Culliford, A.T., Giangola, G., and Kronzon, I.: Multiple emboli from a large aortic arch thrombus in a patient with thrombotic diathesis. Am. Heart J., *124*:239, 1992.
12. Castello, R., Pearson, A.C., Fagan, L., and Labovitz, A.J.: Spontaneous echocardiographic contrast in the descending aorta. Am. Heart J., *120*:915, 1990.
13. Neinaber, C.A., Spielmann, R.P., von Kodolitsch, Y., Siglow, V., Piepho, A., Jaup, T., Nicolas, V., Weber, P., Triebel H-J., and Bleifeld, W.: Diagnosis of thoracic aortic dissection. Circulation, *85*:434, 1992.

14. Om, A., Porter, T., and Mohanty, P.K.: Transesophageal echocardiographic diagnosis of acute aortic dissection complicating cocaine abuse. Am. Heart J., *123*:532, 1992.

15. Barbant, S.D., Eisenberg, M.J., and Schiller, N.B.: The diagnostic value of imaging techniques for aortic dissection. Am. Heart J., *124*:541, 1992.

16. Adachi, H., Omoto, R., Kyo, S., Matsumura, M., Kimura, S., Takamoto, S., and Yokote, Y.: Emergency surgical intervention of acute aortic dissection with the rapid diagnosis by transesophageal echocardiography. Circulation, *84*:III–14, 1991.

17. Hashimoto, S., Kumada, T., Osakada, G., Kubo, S., Tokunaga, S., Tamaki, S., Yamazato, A., Nishimura, K., Ban, T., and Kawai, C.: Assessment of transesophageal Doppler echography in dissecting aortic aneurysm. J. Am. Coll. Cardiol., *14*:1252, 1989.

18. Erbel, R., Borner, N. Steller, D., Brunier, J., Thelen, M., Pfeiffer, C., Mohr-Kahaly, S., Iversen, S., Oelert, H., and Meyer, J.: Detection of aortic dissection by transesophageal echocardiography. Br. Heart J., *58*:45, 1987.

19. Takamoto, S. and Omoto, R.: Visualization of thoracic dissecting aortic aneurysm by transesophageal Doppler color flow mapping. Herz, *12*:187, 1987.

20. Engberding, R., Bender, F., Grosse-Heitmeyer, W., Most, E., Muller, U.S., Bramann, H.U., and Schneider, D.: Identification of dissection or aneurysm of the descending thoracic aorta by conventional and transesophageal two-dimensional echocardiography. Am. J. Cardiol., *59*:717, 1987.

20a. Simon, P., Owen, A.N., Havel, M., Moidl, R., Hiesmayr, M., Wolner, E., and Mohl, W.: Transesophageal echocardiography in the emergency surgical management of patients with aortic dissection. J. Thorac. Cardiovasc. Surg., *103*:1113, 1992.

21. Wilansky, S., Burns, R.J., David, T.E., and Pollick, C.: Valve-like intimal flap: A new echocardiographic finding of aortic dissection. Am. Heart J., *111*:1204, 1986.

22. Rubenson, D.S., Fowles, R.E., Miller, D.C., Guthaner, D.F., and Popp, R.L.: Spontaneous dissection of the ascending aorta diagnosed by two dimensional echocardiography. Chest, *80*:587, 1981.

23. Victor, M.F., Mintz, G.S., Kotler, M.N., Wilson, A.R., and Segal, B.L.: Two dimensional echocardiographic diagnosis of aortic dissection. Am. J. Cardiol., *48*:1155, 1981.

24. Smuckler, A.L., Nomeir, A.M., Watts, L.E., and Hackshaw, B.T.: Echocardiographic diagnosis of aortic root dissection by M-mode and two dimensional techniques. Am. Heart J., *103*:897, 1982.

25. Come, P.C.: Improved cross-sectional echocardiographic technique for visualization of the retrocardiac descending aorta in its long axis. Am. J. Cardiol., *51*:1029, 1983.

26. Mattleman, S., Oanidis, I., Kotler, M.N., Mintz, G., Victor, M., and Ross, H.: Dissecting aneurysm in a patient with Marfan's syndrome: Recognition of extensive involvement of the aorta by two dimensional echocardiography. JCU, *12*:219, 1984.

27. Iliceto, S., Nanda, N.C., Rizzon, P., Hsuing, M., Goyal, R.G., Amico, A., and Sorino, M.: Color Doppler evaluation of aortic dissection. Circulation, *75*:748, 1987.

28. Chia, B.L., Yan, P.C., Ee, B.K., Choo, M.H., Tay, M.B., and Lee, C-N.: Two-dimensional echocardiography and Doppler color flow abnormalities in aortic root dissection. Am. Heart J., *116*:192, 1988.

29. Nicholson, W.J. and Cobbs, B.W., Jr.: Echocardiographic oscillating flap in aortic root dissecting aneurysm. Chest, *70*:305, 1976.

30. Krueger, S.K., Wilson, C.S., Weaver, W.F., Reese, H.E., Caudill, C.C., and Rourke, T.: Aortic root disection: Echocardiographic demonstration of torn intimal flap. JCU, *4*:35, 1976.

31. Kounis, N.B. and Chrysanthopoulos, C.: Aortic root dissection: M-mode echocardiographic appearance of the dissecting intima. J. Ultrasound Med., *2*:329, 1983.

32. D'Cruz, I.A., Jain, M., Campbell, C., and Goldberg, A.N.: Ultrasound visualization of aortic dissection by right parasternal scanning, including systolic flutter of the intimal flap. Chest, *80*:239, 1981.

33. Roudaut, R.P., Billes, M.A., Gosse, P., Deville, C., Baudet, E., Fontan, F., Besse, P., Bricaud, H., and Dallocchio, M.: Accuracy of M-mode and two-dimensional echocardiography in the diagnosis of aortic dissection: An experience with 128 cases. Clin. Cardiol., *11*:553, 1988.

34. Cavaye, D.M., White, R.A., Lerman, R.D., Kopchok, G.E., Tabbara, M.R., Cormier, F., and French, W.J.: Usefulness of intravascular ultrasound imaging for detecting experimentally induced aortic dissection in dogs and for determining the effectiveness of endoluminal stenting. Am. J. Cardiol., *69*:705, 1992.

35. Pande, A., Meier, B., Fleisch, M., Kammerlander, R., Simonet, F., and Lerch, R.: Intravascular ultrasound for diagnosis of aortic dissection. Am. Heart J., *122*:495, 1991.

36. Pandian, N.G., Kreis, A., Brockway, B., Sacharoff, A., and Caro, R.: Intravascular high frequency two-dimensional ultrasound detection of arterial dissection and intimal flaps. Am. J. Cardiol., *65*:1278, 1990.

37. Porter, T., Lenhart, M., Arrowood, J., Moskowitz, W., Paulsen, W., Lofland, G., and Nixon, J.V.: Dissecting aortic aneurysm eight years after aortic commissurotomy for congenital aortic stenosis: Detailed identification by transesophageal echocardiography. Am. Heart J., *120*:716, 1990.

38. Mohr-Kahaly, S., Erbel, R., Rennollet, H., Wittlich, N., Drexler, M., Oelert, H., and Meyer, J.: Ambulatory follow-up of aortic dissection by transesophageal two-dimensional and color-coded Doppler echocardiography. Circulation, *80*:24, 1989.

39. Zotz, R.J., Erbel, R., and Meyer, J.: Noncommunicating intramural hematoma: An indication of developing aortic dissection? J. Am. Soc. Echocardiogr., *4*:636, 1991.

40. Hixson, C.S., Cater, A., and Smith, M.D.: Diagnosis and documentation of healing in descending thoracic aortic dissection by transesophageal echocardiography and Doppler color flow imaging. Am. Heart J., *119*:1432, 1990.

41. Chan, K-L.: Usefulness of transesophageal echocardiography in the diagnosis of conditions mimicking aortic dissection. Am. Heart J., *122*:495, 1991.

42. Seward, J.B., Khanheria, B.K., Oh, J.K., Freeman, W.K., and Tajik, A.J.: Critical appraisal of transesophageal echocardiography: Limitations, pitfalls, and complications. J. Am. Soc. Echocardiogr., *5*:288, 1992.

42a. Appelbe, A.F., Walker, Yeoh, J.K., Bonitatibus, A., Yoganathan, A.P., and Martin, R.P.: Clinical significance and origin of artifacts in transesophageal echocardiography of the thoracic aorta. J. Am. Coll. Cardiol., *21*:754, 1993.

42b. Appelbe, A.F., Olson, S., Biby, L.D., Curling, P.E., and

Martin, R.P.: Left brachiocephalic vein mimicking an aortic dissection on transesophageal echocardiography. Echocardiography, *10*:67, 1993.

43. Lourie, J.K., Appelbe, A., and Martin, R.P.: Detection of complex intimal flaps in aortic dissection by transesophageal echocardiography. Am. J. Cardiol., *69*:1361, 1992.
44. Nestico, P., et al.: Atherosclerotic plaque simulating aortic dissection by echocardiography and angiography. Am. Heart J., *109*:607, 1985.
45. Come, P.C., Bivas, N.K., Sacks, B., Thurer, R.L., Weintraub, R.M., and Axelrod, P.: Unusual echographic findings in aortic dissection: Diastolic prolapse of intimal flap into left ventricle. Am. Heart J., *107*:790, 1984.
46. Khandheria, B.K., Tajik, A.J., Taylor, C.L., Safford, R.E., Miller, Jr., F.A., Stanson, A.W., Sinak, L.J., Oh, J.K., and Seward, J.B.: Aortic dissection: Review of value and limitations of two-dimensional echocardiography in a six-year experience. J. Am. Soc. Echocardiogr., *2*:17, 1989.
47. Chappell, J.H., Nassef, L.A., Pharr, W.F., and Menapace, Jr., F.J.: Abbreviated aortic insufficiency in aortic dissection caused by prolapse of the intimal flap. J. Am. Soc. Echocardiogr., *3*:72, 1990.
48. Nakatani, S., Beppu, S., Miyatake, F., Matsuo, H., Nagata, S., and Nimura, Y.: Interruption of aortic regurgitation by the intimal flap of an aortic dissection: Doppler echocardiographic observations. Am. Heart J., *117*:486, 1989.
49. Davies, N.J., Butany, J., Yock, P.G., and Rakowski, H.: Aortic dissection and rupture that produce right ventricular perforation: Detection by echocardiography and color flow mapping. J. Am. Soc. Echocardiogr., *3*:140, 1990.
50. Millward, D.K., Robinson, N.J., and Craige, E.: Dissecting aortic aneurysm diagnosed by echocardiography in a patient with rupture of the aneurysm into the right atrium. Am. J. Cardiol., *30*:427, 1972.
51. Nicod, P., Firth, B.G., Peshock, R.M., Gaffney, F.A., and Hillis, L.D.: Rupture of dissecting aortic aneurysm into the right atrium: Clinical and echocardiographic recognition. Am. Heart J., *107*:1276, 1984.
52. Berman, A.D., Come, P.C., Riley, M.F., Weintraub, R.M., Johnson, R.G., and Aroesty, J.M.: Two-dimensional and Doppler echocardiographic diagnosis of an aortic to right atrial fistula complicating aortic dissection. J. Am. Coll. Cardiol., *9*:228, 1987.
53. Ballal, R.S., Nanda, J.C., Gatewood, R., D'Arcy, B., Samdarshi, T.E., Holman, W.L., Kirklin, J.K., and Pacifico, A.D.: Usefulness of transesophageal echocardiography in assessment of aortic dissection. Circulation, *84*:1903, 1991.
54. Perrella, M.A., Smith, H.C., and Khandheria, B.K.: Pseudoaneurysm of the aortic root diagnosed by noninvasive imaging: Report of a case. J. Am. Soc. Echocardiogr., *4*:499, 1991.
55. Hoadley, S.D. and Hartshore, M.F.: Noninvasive diagnosis of pseudoaneurysm of the ascending aorta. JCU, *15*:325, 1987.
56. Barbetseas, J., Crawford, E.S., Safi, H.J., Coselli, J.S., Quinones, M.A., and Zoghbi, W.A.: Doppler echocardiographic evaluation of pseudoaneurysms complicating composite grafts of the ascending aorta. Circulation, *85*:212, 1992.
57. Liddell, N.E., Stoddard, M.F., Prince, C., Johnstone, J., Perkins, D., and Kupersmith, J.: Transesophageal echocardiographic diagnosis of complex false aneurysm

with aorto-left atrial communication complicating aortic valve and root replacement. Am. Heart J., *123*:543, 1992.
58. Rice, M.J., McDonald, R.W., and Reller, M.D.: Diagnosis of coronary artery dehiscence and pseudoaneurysm formation in postoperative Marfan patient by color flow Doppler echocardiography. JCU, *17*:359, 1989.
59. Come, P.C., Riley, M.F., Kaufman, H., Parker, J.A., Morgan, J.P., Lorell, B., Thurer, R., Weintraub, R., and Axelrod, P.: Aortic false aneurysm: Recognition by noninvasive techniques four years after mitral valve replacement. Am. J. Cardiol., *58*:1137, 1986.
59a. Vilacosta, I., Camino, A., San Roman, J.A., Rollan, M.J., delaLlana, R., Gil, M., and Harguinday, L.S.: Supravalvular aortic stenosis after replacement of the ascending aorta. Am. J. Cardiol., *70*:1505, 1992.
60. Dorsa, F.B., Tunick, P.A., Culliford, A., and Kronzon, I.: Pseudoaneurysm of the thoracic aorta due to cardiopulmonary resuscitation: Diagnosis by transesophageal echocardiography. Am. Heart J., *123*:1398, 1992.
61. Silvey, S.V., Stoughton, T.L., Pearl, W., Collazo, W.A., and Belbel, R.J.: Rupture of the outer partition of aortic dissection during transesophageal echocardiography. Am. J. Cardiol., *68*:286, 1991.
62. Lewis, B.S.: Echocardiographic diagnosis of unruptured sinus of Valsalva aneurysm. Am. Heart J., *107*:1025, 1984.
63. Nakamura, K., Suzuki, S., and Satomi, G.: Detection of ruptured aneurysm of sinus of Valsalva by contrast two dimensional echocardiography. Br. Heart J., *45*:219, 1981.
64. Schatz, R.A., Schiller, N.B., Tri, T.B., Bowen, T.E., Ports, T.A., and Silverman, N.H.: Two dimensional echocardiographic diagnosis of a ruptured right sinus of Valsalva aneurysm. Chest, *79*:584, 1981.
65. McKenney, P.A., Shemin, R.J., and Wiegers, S.E.: Role of transesophageal echocardiography in sinus of Valsalva aneurysm. Am. Heart J., *123*:228, 1992.
66. Abdelkhirane, C., Roudaut, R., and Dallocchio, M.: Diagnosis of ruptured sinus of Valsalva aneurysms: Potential value of transesophageal echocardiography. Echocardiography, 7:555, 1990.
67. Blackshear, J.L., Safford, R.E., Lane, G.E., Freeman, W.K., and Schaff, H.V.: Unruptured noncoronary sinus of Valsalva aneurysm: Preoperative characterization by transesophageal echocardiography. J. Am. Soc. Echocardiogr., *4*:485, 1991.
68. Katz, E.S., Cziner, D.G., Rosenzweig, B.P., Attubato, M., Feit, F., and Kronzon, I.: Multifaceted echocardiographic approach to the diagnosis of a ruptured sinus of Valsalva aneurysm. J. Am. Soc. Echocardiogr., *4*:494, 1991.
69. Sahasakul, Y., Panchavinnin, P., Chaithiraphan, S., and Sakiyalak, P.: Echocardiographic diagnosis of a ruptured aneurysm of the sinus of Valsalva: Operation without catheterization in seven patients. Br. Heart J., *64*:195, 1990.
70. Chamsi-Pasha, H., Musgrove, C., and Morton, R.: Echocardiographic diagnosis of multiple congenital aneurysms of the sinus of Valsalva. Br. Heart J., *59*:724, 1988.
71. Chiang, C-W., Lin, F-C., Fang, B-R., Kuo, C-T., Lee, Y-S., and Chang, C-H.: Doppler and two-dimensional echocardiographic features of sinus of Valsalva aneurysm. Am. Heart J., *116*:1283, 1988.
72. Atay, A.E., Alpert, M.A., Bertuso, J.R., and Lawson, D.L.: Right sinus of Valsalva aneurysm presenting as an

echocardiographic right atrial mass. Am. Heart J., *112*:
169, 1986.

73. Rubin, D.C., Carliner, N.H., Salter, D.R., Plotnick, G.D., and Hawke, M.W.: Unruptured sinus of Valsalva aneurysm diagnosed by transesophageal echocardiography. Am. Heart J., *124*:225, 1992.

74. Purcaro, A., Ciampani, N., Blandini, A., Breccia Fratadocchi, G., Massacci, C., Piva, R., and Brugnami, R.: Echocardiographic diagnosis of aneurysm of Valsalva's sinus with fistulization into the right atrium. G. Ital. Cardiol., *12*:302, 1982.

75. Terdjman, N., Bourdarias, J.-P., Farcot, J.-C., Gueret, P., Dubourg, O., Ferrier, A., and Hanania, G.: Aneurysms of sinus of Valsalva: Two dimensional echocardiographic diagnosis and recognition of rupture into the right heart cavities. J. Am. Coll. Cardiol., *3*:1227, 1984.

76. Hangying, L. and Zhisheng, L.: Echocardiographic manifestations of ruptured aneurysm of right sinus of Valsalva into right ventricle. Chin. J. Cardiol., *8*:10, 1980.

77. Vered, Z., Rath, S., Benjamin, P., Motro, M., and Neufeld, H.N.: Ruptured sinus of Valsalva: Demonstration by contrast echocardiography during cardiac catheterization. Am. Heart J., *109*:365, 1985.

78. Cooper, M.J., Silverman, N.H., and Huey, E.: Group A β-hemolytic streptococcal endocarditis precipitating rupture of sinus of Valsalva aneurysm: Evaluation by two-dimensional, Doppler, and contrast echocardiography. Am. Heart J., *115*:1132, 1988.

79. Ryan, T., Markel, M.L., Waller, B.F., Armstrong, W.F., and Feigenbaum, H.: Doppler echocardiographic detection of a ruptured acquired aneurysm of the sinus of Valsalva. Chest, *91*:626, 1987.

80. Jain, S.P., Mahan, III, E.F., Nanda, N.C., Barold, S.S., Willis, J.E., and Pinheiro, L.: Doppler color flow mapping in the diagnosis of sinus of Valsalva aneurysm. Echocardiography, *6*:533, 1989.

81. Peters, P., Juziuk, E., and Gunther, S.: Doppler color flow mapping detection of ruptured sinus of Valsalva aneurysm. J. Am. Soc. Echocardiogr., *2*:195, 1989.

82. Chia, B.L., Ee, B.K., Choo, M.H., and Yan, P.C.: Ruptured aneurysm of Valsalva: Recognition by Doppler color flow mapping. Am. Heart J., *115*:686, 1988.

83. Rothbaum, D.A., Dillon, J.C., Chang, S., and Feigenbaum, H.: Echocardiographic manifestation of right sinus of Valsalva aneurysm. Circulation, *49*:768, 1974.

84. Liss, G.B., Pechacek, L.W., Garcia, E., and DeCastro, C.M.: Echocardiographic demonstration of an aneurysm of the right coronary sinus of Valsalva with dissection into the interventricular septum. J. Ultrasound Med., *3*: 477, 1984.

85. Chen, W.W.C. and Tai, Y.T.: Dissection of interventricular septum by aneurysm of sinus of Valsalva. Br. Heart J., *50*:293, 1983.

86. Engel, P.J., Held, J.S. Van der Bel-Kahn, J., and Spitz, H.: Echocardiographic diagnosis of congenital sinus of Valsalva aneurysm with dissection of the interventricular septum. Circulation, *63*:705, 1981.

87. Yuksel, H., Yazicioglu, N., Sarioglu, T., Celiker, C., Paker, T., Enar, R., Aytac, A., and Demiroglu, C.: Dissection of the interventricular septum by unruptured right and left sinus of Valsalva aneurysms. Am. Heart J., *122*: 1777, 1991.

88. Dev, V. and Shrivastava, S.: Echocardiographic diagnosis of unruptured aneurysm of the sinus of Valsalva dissecting into the ventricular septum. Am. J. Cardiol., *66*: 502, 1990.

89. Rothbart, R.M. and Chahine, R.A.: Left sinus of Valsalva aneurysm with rupture into the left ventricular outflow tract: Diagnosis by color-encoded Doppler imaging. Am. Heart J., *120*:224, 1990.

90. Weyman, A.E., Dillon, J.C., Feigenbaum, H., and Chang, S.: Premature pulmonic valve opening following sinus of Valsalva aneurysm rupture into the right atrium. Circulation, *51*:556, 1975.

90a. Cabanes, L., Garcia, E., VanDamme, C., Berrebi, A., Conzeau-Gouge, P., Fouchard, J., and Guerin, F.: Aneurysm of the noncoronary sinus of Valsalva ruptured into the left atrium. Am. Heart J., *124*:1659, 1992.

90b. Thomas, M.R., Monaghan, M.J., Michalis, L.K., and Jewitt, D.E.: Aortoatrial fistulae diagnosed by transthoracic and transesophageal echocardiography: Advantages of the transesophageal approach. J. Am. Soc. Echocardiogr., *6*:21, 1993.

91. Davis, G.A., Sauerisen, S., Chandrasekaran, K., Karalis, D.G., Ross, Jr., J., and Mintz, G.S.: Subclinical traumatic aortic injury diagnosed by transesophageal echocardiography. Am. Heart J., *123*:534, 1992.

92. Kamiya, H., Hanaki, Y., Kojima, S., Ohsugi, S., Ohno, M., Ina, H., Hayase, S., Hiramatsu, H., and Horiba, M.: Fistula between noncoronary sinus of Valsalva and right atrium after blunt chest trauma. Am. Heart J., *114*:429, 1987.

93. Daxini, B.V., Desai, A.G., and Sharma, S.: Echo-Doppler diagnosis of aortocaval fistula following blunt to abdomen. Am. Heart J., *118*:843, 1989.

94. VonDoenhoff, L.J. and Nanda, N.C.: Chronic traumatic thoracic aneurysm: Demonstration by two dimensional echocardiography. Am. J. Cardiol., *54*:692, 1984.

95. Snow, C.C., Appelbe, A.F., Martin, T.D., and Martin, R.P.: Diagnosis of aortic transection by transesophageal echocardiography. J. Am. Soc. Echocardiogr., *5*:100, 1992.

96. Bergin, P.J.: Aortic thrombosis and peripheral embolization after thoracic gunshot wound diagnosed by transesophageal echocardiography. Am. Heart J., *119*:688, 1990.

97. Griffiths, B.E., Petch, M.C., and English, T.A.H.: Echocardiographic detection of subvalvular aortic root aneurysm extending to mitral valve annulus as complication of aortic valve endocarditis. Br. Heart J., *47*:392, 1982.

98. Wong, C.M., Oldershaw, P., and Gibson, D.G.: Echocardiographic demonstration of aortic root abscess after infective endocarditis. Br. Heart J., *46*:584, 1981.

99. Agatston, A.S., Asnani, H., Ozner, M., and Kinney, E.L.: Aortic valve ring abscess: Two-dimensional echocardiographic features leading to valve replacement. Am. Heart J., *109*:171, 1985.

100. Chow, W.H., Leung, W.H., Tai, Y.T., Lee, W.T., and Cheung, K.L.: Echocardiographic diagnosis of an aortic root abscess after mycobacterium fortuitum prosthetic valve endocarditis. Clin. Cardiol., *14*:273, 1991.

101. Saner, H.E., Asinger, R.W., Homans, D.C., Helseth, H.K., and Elsperger, K.J.: Two-dimensional echocardiographic identification of complicated aortic root endocarditis: Implications for surgery. J. Am. Coll. Cardiol., *10*: 859, 1987.

102. Reid, C.L., McKay, C., Kawanishi, D.T., Edwards, C., Rahimtoola, S.H., and Chandraratna, P.A.N.: False aneurysm of mitral-aortic intervalvular fibrosa: Diagnosis by two dimensional contrast echocardiography at cardiac catheterization. Am. J. Cardiol., *51*:1801, 1983.

103. Perry, J.C., Nanda, N.C., Hicks, D.G., and Harris, J.P.: Two dimensional echocardiographic identification of

aorto-left ventricular tunnel. Am. J. Cardiol., *52*:913, 1983.

104. Serino, W., Andrade, J.L., Ross, D., DeLeval, M., and Somerville, J.: Aorto-left ventricular communication after closure. Late postoperative problems. Br. Heart J., *49*:501, 1983.

105. Bash, S.E., Huhta, J.C., Nihill, M.R., Vargo, T.A., and Hallman, G.L.: Aortico-left ventricular tunnel with ventricular septal defect: Two-dimensional Doppler echocardiographic diagnosis. J. Am. Coll. Cardiol., *5*:757, 1985.

106. Lanza, G.M., Zabalgoitia-Reyes, M., Frazin, L., Meyers, S.N., Spitzzeri, C.L., Vonesh, M.J., Mehlman, D.J., Talano, J.V., and McPherson, D.D.: Plaque and structural characteristics of the descending thoracic aorta using transesophageal echocardiography. J. Am. Soc. Echocardiogr., *4*:19, 1991.

107. Ono, S., Matsuzaki, M., Michishige, H., Wasaki, Y., Tomochika, Y., Murata, K., Tokisawa, I., Nishimura, Y., Okuda, F., and Kusukawa, R.: Estimation of atherosclerotic lesions in the thoracic aorta by transesophageal echocardiography. J. Cardiol., *21*:57, 1991.

108. Tunick, P.A. and Kronzon, I.: Protruding atherosclerotic plaque in the aortic arch of patients with systemic embolization: A new finding seen by transesophageal echocardiography. Am. Heart J., *120*:658, 1990.

109. Tomochika, Y., Matsuzaki, M., Okuda, F., Tohma, Y., Michishige, H., Ono, S., Wasaki, Y., Tokisawa, I., Fujino, H., and Kusukawa, R.: Assessment of atherosclerotic lesions and distensibility of the thoracic aorta in familial hypercholesterolemia by biplane transesophageal echocardiography. J. Cardiol., *21*:463, 1991.

109a. Matsuzaki, M., Ono, S., Tomochika, Y., Michishige, H., Tanaka, N., Okuda, F., and Kusukawa, R.: Advances in transesophageal echocardiography for the evaluation of atherosclerotic lesions in thoracic aorta—the effects of hypertension, hypercholesterolemia, and aging on atherosclerotic lesions. Jpn. Circ. J., *56*:592, 1992.

110. Yoshida, S., Hirata, K., and Fukuda, M.: Semi-quantitative evaluation of atherosclerotic lesions of the thoracic aorta with high resolution transesophageal ultrasound. J. Cardiol., *21*:37, 1991.

111. Simons, A.J., Carlson, R., Hare, C.L., Obeid, A.I., and Smulyan, H.: The use of transesophageal echocardiography in detecting aortic atherosclerosis in patients with embolic disease. Am. Heart J., *123*:224, 1992.

112. Karalis, D.G., Chandrasekaran, K., Victor, M.F., Ross, J.J., and Mintz, G.S.: Recognition and embolic potential of intraaortic atherosclerotic debris. J. Am. Coll. Cardiol., *17*:73, 1991.

113. Mitchell, M.M., Frankville, D.D., Weinger, M.B., and Dittrich, H.C.: Detection of thoracic aortic atheroma with transesophageal echocardiography in patients without symptoms of embolism. Am. Heart J., *122*:1768, 1991.

114. Coy, K.M., Maurer, G., Goodman, D., and Siegel, R.J.: Transesophageal echocardiographic detection of aortic atheromatosis may provide clues to occult renal dysfunction in the elderly. Am. Heart J., *123*:1684, 1992.

115. Koppang, J.R., Nanda, N.C., Coghlan, H.C., and Sanyal, R.: Histologically confirmed cholesterol atheroemboli with identification of the source by transesophageal echocardiography. Echocardiography, *9*:379, 1992.

116. Rubin, D.C., Plotnick, G.D., and Hawke, M.W.: Intraaortic debris as a potential source of embolic stroke. Am. J. Cardiol., *69*:819, 1992.

117. Tunick, P.A., Perez, J.L., and Kronzon, I.: Protruding atheromas in the thoracic aorta and systemic embolization. Ann. Intern. Med., *115*:423, 1991.

118. Katz, E.S., Tunick, P.A., Rusinek, H., Ribakove, G., Spener, F.C., and Kronzon, I.: Protruding aortic atheromas predict stroke in elderly patients undergoing cardiopulmonary bypass: Experience with intraoperative transesophageal echocardiography. J. Am. Coll. Cardiol., *20*: 70, 1992.

119. DeRook, F.A., Comess, K.A., Albers, G.W., and Popp, R.L.: Transesophageal echocardiography in the evaluation of stroke. Ann. Intern. Med., *117*:922, 1992.

120. Toyoda, K., Yasaka, M., Nagata, S., and Yamaguchi, T.: Aortogenic embolic stroke: A transesophageal echocardiographic approach. Stroke, *23*:1056, 1992.

121. Amarenco, P., Cohen, A., Baudrimont, M., and Bousser, M.G.: Transesophageal echocardiographic detection of aortic arch disease in patients with cerebral infarction. Stroke, *23*:1005, 1992.

122. Horowitz, D.R., Tuhrim, S., Budd, J., and Goldman, M.E.: Aortic plaque in patients with brain ischemia: Diagnosis by transesophageal echocardiography. Neurology, *42*:1602, 1992.

123. Mugge, A., Daniel, W.G., Niedermeyer, J., Hausmann, D., Nikutta, P., and Lichtlen, P.R.: Usefulness of a new automatic boundary detection system acoustic (quantification) for assessing stiffness of the descending thoracic aorta by transesophageal echocardiography. Am. J. Cardiol., *70*:1629, 1992.

124. Lacombe, F., Dart, A., Dewar, E., Jennings, G., Cameron, J., and Laufer, E.: Arterial elastic properties in man: A comparison of echo-Doppler indices of aortic stiffness. Eur. Heart J., *13*:1040, 1992.

# Appendix

## Echocardiographic Measurements and Normal Values

### APPENDICES A TO D: M-MODE MEASUREMENTS

Appendices A through D provide normal values for M-mode echocardiographic measurements. The four sets of values were derived at different institutions at different times during the course of the development of echocardiography.

### Appendix A: Traditional Normal Echocardiographic Values

Appendix A presents data obtained in 1972 that represent the oldest normal values. These measurements do not utilize current American Society of Echocardiography recommendations. Most measurements are from trailing edge to leading edge.

*Definition of Echocardiographic Measurements. Right ventricular dimension (RVD)* represents the distance between the trailing echoes of the anterior right ventricular wall and the leading echo of the right side of the interventricular septum at the R wave of the electrocardiogram. *Left ventricular internal dimension (LVID)* is measured from the trailing edge of the left side of the septum to the leading edge of the posterior endocardium at the R wave of the electrocardiogram. *Posterior left ventricular wall thickness* represents the distance be-

tween the leading edge of the posterior left ventricular endocardium and the leading edge of the epicardium at the R wave of the electrocardiogram. *Posterior left ventricular wall amplitude* is the maximum amplitude of the posterior left ventricular endocardial echo. *Interventricular septal (IVS) wall thickness* is the distance between the leading edge of the left septal echo and the trailing edge of the right septal echo at the R wave of the electrocardiogram. *Midinterventricular septal (mid IVS) amplitude* is the amplitude of motion of the left septal echo with the ultrasonic beam traversing the midportion of the left ventricle. *Apical interventricular septal (apical IVS) amplitude* is the systolic amplitude of motion of the left septal echo with the ultrasonic beam directed toward the apex in the vicinity of the papillary muscles. *Left atrial dimension (LAD)* represents the distance between the trailing edge of the posterior aortic wall echo and the leading edge of the posterior left atrial wall echo at the level of the aortic valve at end-systole. *Aortic root dimension* is the distance between the leading edge of the anterior aortic wall and the leading edge of the posterior aortic wall at the R wave of the electrocardiogram. *Aortic cusp separation* represents the distance between the trailing edge of the anterior aortic valve leaflet and the leading edge of the posterior aortic valve leaflet in early systole.

**Table A–1**
Adult Normal Values

|  | Range (cm) | Mean (cm) | Number |
|---|---|---|---|
| Age (years) | 13 −54 | 26 | 134 |
| Body surface area (M²) | 1.45– 2.22 | 1.8 | 130 |
| RVD-flat | 0.7 − 2.3 | 1.5 | 84 |
| RVD-left lateral | 0.9 − 2.6 | 1.7 | 83 |
| LVID-flat | 3.7 − 5.6 | 4.7 | 82 |
| LVID-left lateral | 3.5 − 5.7 | 4.7 | 81 |
| Post. LV wall thickness | 0.6 − 1.1 | 0.9 | 137 |
| Post. LV wall amplitude | 0.9 − 1.4 | 1.2 | 48 |
| IVS wall thickness | 0.6 − 1.1 | 0.9 | 137 |
| Mid IVS amplitude | 0.3 − 0.8 | 0.5 | 10 |
| Apical IVS amplitude | 0.5 − 1.2 | 0.7 | 38 |
| Left atrial dimension | 1.9 − 4.0 | 2.9 | 133 |
| Aortic root dimension | 2.0 − 3.7 | 2.7 | 121 |
| Aortic cusps separation | 1.5 − 2.6 | 1.9 | 93 |
| Mean rate of circumferential shortening (Vcf) | 1.02– 1.94 circ./sec. | 1.3 circ./sec. | 38 |

## Table A–2
### Adult Normal Values, Corrected for Body Surface Area

|  | Range (cm) | Mean (cm) | Number |
|---|---|---|---|
| RVD/M²—flat | 0.4–1.4 | 0.9 | 76 |
| RVD/M²—left lateral | 0.4–1.4 | 0.9 | 79 |
| LVID/M²—flat | 2.1–3.2 | 2.6 | 77 |
| LVID/M²—left lateral | 1.9–3.2 | 2.6 | 81 |
| LAD/M² | 1.2–2.2 | 1.6 | 127 |
| Aortic root/M² | 1.2–2.2 | 1.5 | 115 |

## Table A–3
### Normal Values for Children Arranged by Weight

|  | Weight (lbs) | Mean (cm) | Range (cm) | Number of Subjects |
|---|---|---|---|---|
| RVD | 0– 25 | .9 | .3–1.5 | 26 |
|  | 26– 50 | 1.0 | .4–1.5 | 26 |
|  | 51– 75 | 1.1 | .7–1.8 | 20 |
|  | 76–100 | 1.2 | .7–1.6 | 15 |
|  | 101–125 | 1.3 | .8–1.7 | 11 |
|  | 126–200 | 1.3 | 1.2–1.7 | 5 |
| LVID | 0– 25 | 2.4 | 1.3–3.2 | 26 |
|  | 26– 50 | 3.4 | 2.4–3.8 | 26 |
|  | 51– 75 | 3.8 | 3.3–4.5 | 20 |
|  | 76–100 | 4.1 | 3.5–4.7 | 15 |
|  | 101–125 | 4.3 | 3.7–4.9 | 11 |
|  | 126–200 | 4.9 | 4.4–5.2 | 5 |
| LV and IV septal wall thickness | 0– 25 | .5 | .4– .6 | 26 |
|  | 26– 50 | .6 | .5– .7 | 26 |
|  | 51– 75 | .7 | .6– .7 | 20 |
|  | 76–100 | .7 | .7– .8 | 15 |
|  | 101–125 | .7 | .7– .8 | 11 |
|  | 126–200 | .8 | .7– .8 | 5 |
| LA dimension | 0– 25 | 1.7 | .7–2.3 | 26 |
|  | 26– 50 | 2.2 | 1.7–2.7 | 26 |
|  | 51– 75 | 2.3 | 1.9–2.8 | 20 |
|  | 76–100 | 2.4 | 2.0–3.0 | 15 |
|  | 101–125 | 2.7 | 2.1–3.0 | 11 |
|  | 126–200 | 2.8 | 2.1–3.7 | 5 |
| Aortic root | 0– 25 | 1.3 | .7–1.7 | 26 |
|  | 26– 50 | 1.7 | 1.3–2.2 | 26 |
|  | 51– 75 | 2.0 | 1.7–2.3 | 20 |
|  | 76–100 | 2.2 | 1.9–2.7 | 15 |
|  | 101–125 | 2.3 | 1.7–2.7 | 11 |
|  | 126–200 | 2.4 | 2.2–2.8 | 5 |
| Aortic valve opening | 0– 25 | .9 | .5–1.2 | 26 |
|  | 26– 75 | 1.2 | .9–1.6 | 26 |
|  | 76–100 | 1.4 | 1.2–1.7 | 20 |
|  | 101–125 | 1.6 | 1.3–1.9 | 15 |
|  | 126–200 | 1.7 | 1.4–2.0 | 11 |
|  |  | 1.8 | 1.6–2.0 | 5 |

## Table A–4
### Normal Values for Children Arranged by Body Surface Area

|  | BSA (M²) | Mean (cm) | Range (cm) | Number of Subjects |
|---|---|---|---|---|
| RVD | .5 or less | .8 | .3–1.3 | 24 |
|  | .6 to 1.0 | 1.0 | .4–1.8 | 39 |
|  | 1.1 to 1.5 | 1.2 | .7–1.7 | 29 |
|  | over 1.5 | 1.3 | .8–1.7 | 11 |
| LVID | .5 or less | 2.4 | 1.3–3.2 | 24 |
|  | .6 to 1.0 | 3.4 | 2.4–4.2 | 39 |
|  | 1.1 to 1.5 | 4.0 | 3.3–4.7 | 29 |
|  | over 1.5 | 4.7 | 4.2–5.2 | 11 |
| LV and IV septal wall thickness | .5 or less | .5 | .4– .6 | 24 |
|  | .6 to 1.0 | .6 | .5– .7 | 39 |
|  | 1.1 to 1.5 | .7 | .6– .8 | 29 |
|  | over 1.5 | .8 | .7– .8 | 11 |
| LA dimension | .5 or less | 1.7 | .7–2.4 | 24 |
|  | .6 to 1.0 | 2.1 | 1.8–2.8 | 39 |
|  | 1.1 to 1.5 | 2.4 | 2.0–3.0 | 29 |
|  | over 1.5 | 2.8 | 2.1–3.7 | 11 |
| Aortic root | .5 or less | 1.2 | .7–1.5 | 24 |
|  | .6 to 1.0 | 1.8 | 1.4–2.2 | 39 |
|  | 1.1 to 1.5 | 2.2 | 1.7–2.7 | 29 |
|  | over 1.5 | 2.4 | 2.0–2.8 | 11 |
| Aortic valve opening | .5 or less | .8 | .5–1.0 | 24 |
|  | .6 to 1.0 | 1.3 | .9–1.6 | 39 |
|  | 1.1 to 1.5 | 1.6 | 1.3–1.9 | 29 |
|  | over 1.5 | 1.8 | 1.5–2.0 | 11 |

### Appendix B: Normal Echocardiographic Measurements from Infancy to Old Age

Appendix B is provided by Henry et al.[1,2] He and his associates developed new normal measurements in 1978 that account for changes in age and are based on the American Society of Echocardiography's recommendations.

Methods of measurement are shown in Figure B–1. The method for using the normal data graphs is exemplified in Figure B–2A and B.

The 387 subjects initially screened were between 21 and 97 years of age. Subjects were excluded if they had (1) history of heart disease or hypertension, (2) abnormal EKG or chest radiographic findings, (3) obesity, (4) abnormal physical examination of the heart, or (5) abnormal or otherwise unsatisfactory echocardiograms. Of the 387 subjects initially screened, 251 were excluded. The remaining 136 subjects were included in the study (Table B–1).

Echocardiographic parameters related to age and body surface area are (1) left ventricular internal dimensions (Figs. B–3 and B–4), (2) ventricular septal thickness (Fig. B–5), (3) left ventricular free wall thickness (Fig. B–6), (4) estimated left ventricular mass (Fig. B–7), (5) aortic root dimension (Fig. B–8), (6) left atrial dimension (Fig. B–9), and (7) mitral valve E-F slope (Fig. B–10). Except for mitral valve E-F slope, all parameters were derived from measurements that were ob-

**NORMAL DATA**

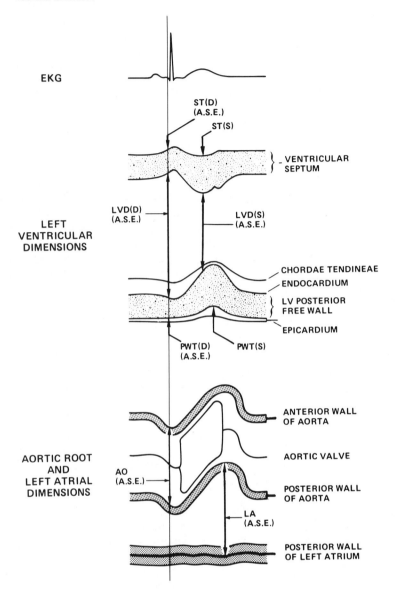

EKG

ST(D)
(A.S.E.)

ST(S)

—VENTRICULAR
SEPTUM

LEFT
VENTRICULAR
DIMENSIONS

LVD(D)
(A.S.E.)

LVD(S)
(A.S.E.)

CHORDAE TENDINEAE
ENDOCARDIUM

LV POSTERIOR
FREE WALL

EPICARDIUM

PWT(D)
(A.S.E.)

PWT(S)

AORTIC ROOT
AND
LEFT ATRIAL
DIMENSIONS

AO
(A.S.E.)

ANTERIOR WALL
OF AORTA

AORTIC VALVE

POSTERIOR WALL
OF AORTA

LA
(A.S.E.)

POSTERIOR WALL
OF LEFT ATRIUM

**Fig. B–1.**  Methods of measurement.

---

Abbreviations:

| | |
|---|---|
| LVD (D)—(A.S.E.)* | Left ventricular internal dimension at end diastole measured at onset of QRS complex |
| LVD (D)—(MAX) | Maximum left ventricular internal dimension at end diastole |
| LVD (S) (A.S.E.* and MIN) | Left ventricular internal dimension at end systole measured at peak posterior motion of ventricular septum (also corresponds to minimum internal dimension) |
| ST (D)—(A.S.E.)* | Ventricular septal thickness at end diastole measured at onset of QRS complex |
| ST (D) | Ventricular septal thickness in late diastole measured immediately before atrial systole |
| ST (S) | Ventricular septal thickness at end systole measured at maximum thickness |
| PWT (D) (A.S.E.)* | Left ventricular posterobasal free wall thickness at end diastole measured at onset of QRS complex |
| PWT (D) | Left ventricular posterobasal free wall thickness in late diastole measured immediately before atrial systole |
| PWT (S) | Left ventricular posterobasal free wall thickness at end systole measured at maximum thickness |
| AO—(A.S.E.)* | Aortic root dimension at end diastole measured at onset of QRS complex from leading edge of anterior wall of aorta to leading edge of posterior wall of aorta |
| LA—(A.S.E.)* | Left atrial dimension at end systole measured at the maximum dimension from the leading edge of the posterior wall of aorta to the dominant line representing the posterior wall of the left atrium (identified by the switched-gain circuit or by manual damping) |

---

* Measurement obtained by way of standards recommended by the American Society of Echocardiography

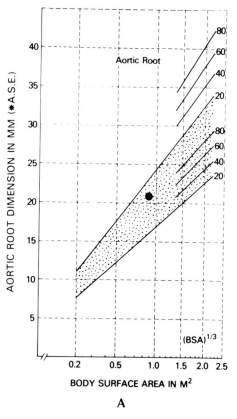

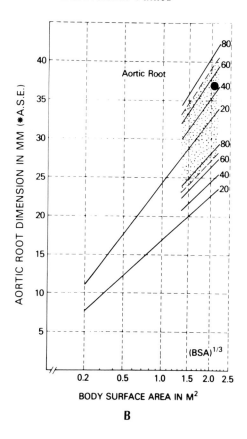

A                                         B

**Fig. B–2.** Method for using normal data graphs.

*A,* An example of a normal data graph for subjects aged one month to 20 years. The graph was prepared for an 8-year-old child with a body surface area of 0.9 m² and an aortic root dimension of 21 mm. Since the child is less than 20 years of age, the two lines that extend from 0.2 to 2.2 m² (labeled 20) are used as the upper and lower limits of normal. In this example, an aortic root dimension of 21 mm is within the 95% prediction limits of normal for an 8-year-old child with a body surface area of 0.9 m².

*B,* An example of a normal graph for subjects more than 20 years of age. This graph was prepared for a 70-year-old man with a body surface area of 2.2 m² and an aortic root dimension of 37 mm. For this subject, the upper limit of normal is determined by extrapolating a line midway between the upper limits for ages 60 and 80 (labeled 60 and 80). The lower limit of normal is extrapolated in the same way. In this example, an aortic root dimension of 37 mm is within the 95% prediction limits of normal for a 70-year-old patient with a body surface of 2.2 m².

tained by way of standards recommended by the American Society of Echocardiography.

Normal echocardiographic parameters unrelated to age and body surface area are as follows:

### Table B–1
Newer Normal Data

| Age | Males | Females | Total |
|---|---|---|---|
| 1–5 days | 7 | 6 | 13 |
| 1 month–20 years | 45 | 47 | 92 |
| 21–30 years | 15 | 10 | 25 |
| 31–40 years | 9 | 15 | 24 |
| 41–50 years | 16 | 13 | 29 |
| 51–60 years | 19 | 10 | 29 |
| 61–70 years | 9 | 8 | 17 |
| 71–97 years | 10 | 2 | 12 |
| Total | 130 | 111 | 241 |

1. Left ventricular fractional shortening
   Mean: 36% 95% prediction limits: 28–44%*
   (Mean: 37% 95% prediction limits: 29–45%)†
2. Left ventricular ejection fraction (cubed)
   Mean: 74% 95% prediction limits: 64–83%*
   (Mean: 75% 95% prediction limits: 65–84%)†
3. Ventricular septal thickening (younger normal data)
   Mean: 35% 95% prediction limits: 18–53%*
4. Left ventricular free wall thickening (younger normal data)
   Mean: 60% 95% prediction limits: 39–82%*

* Derived from measurements that were obtained by way of standards recommended by the American Society of Echocardiography.
† Derived from measurement of left ventricular internal dimension at end diastole at point of maximum dimension.

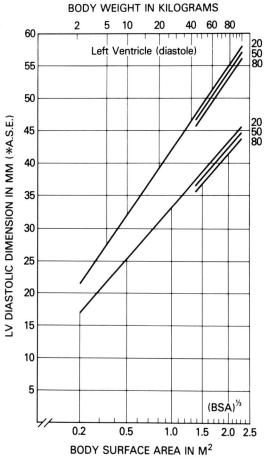

Fig. B–3.

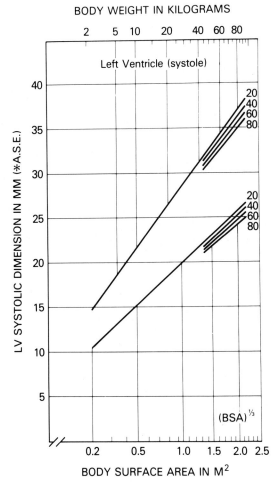

Fig. B–4.

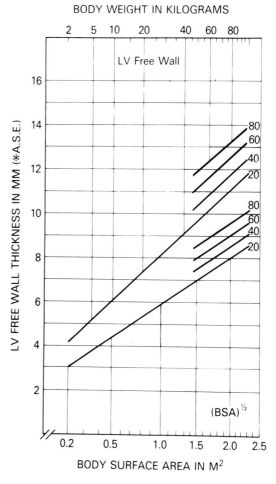

Fig. B–6.

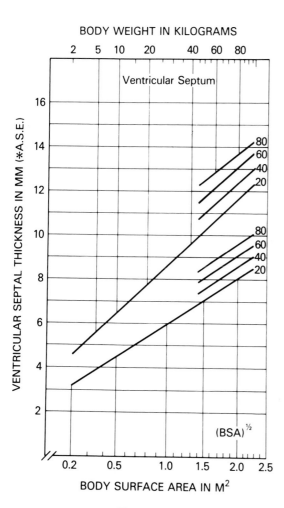

Fig. B–5.

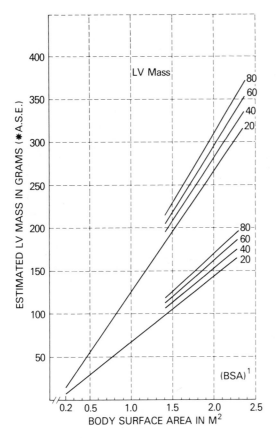

**Fig. B–7.**

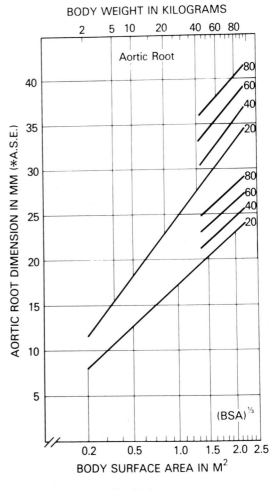

**Fig. B–8.**

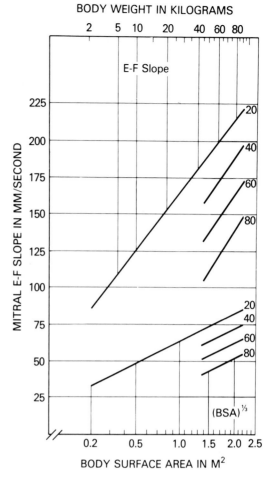

Fig. B–10.

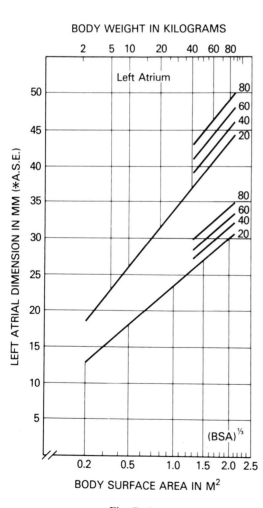

Fig. B–9.

## Appendix C: Echocardiographic Measurements Plotted Against Body Surface Area in Children

Appendix C presents graphs that plot echocardiographic measurements against body surface area in a series of children (Figs. C–1 through C–10). The data are obtained from research performed by Goldberg, Allen, and Sahn.[3]

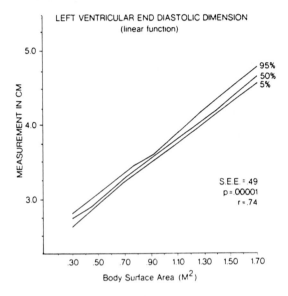

Fig. C–1.

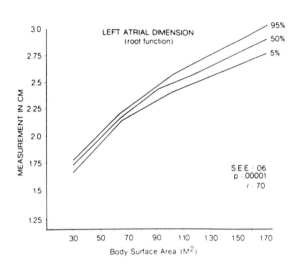

Fig. C–2.

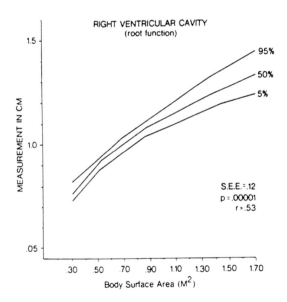

Fig. C–3.

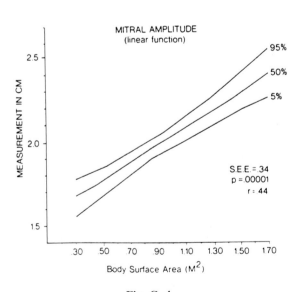

Fig. C–4.

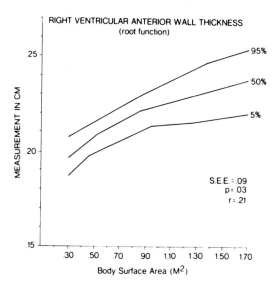

Fig. C–5.

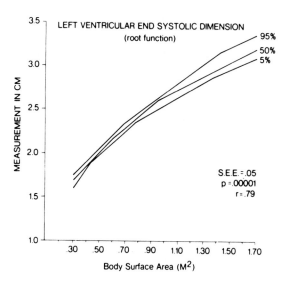

Fig. C–6.

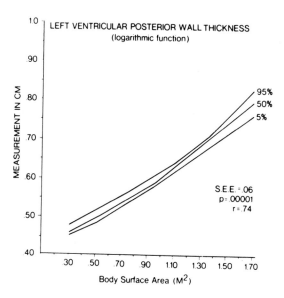

Fig. C–7.

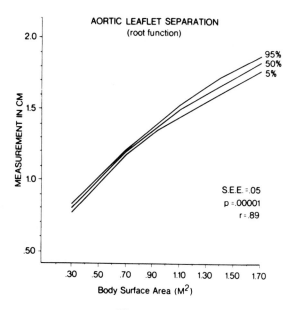

Fig. C–8.

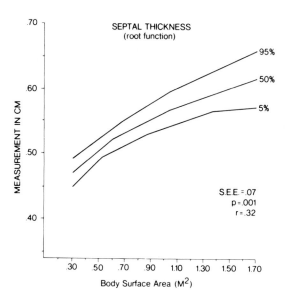

Fig. C–9.

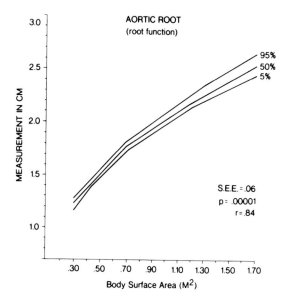

Fig. C–10.

## Appendix D: Normal Echocardiographic Values in Newborns

Table D–1, reprinted from an article by Moss et al.,[4] lists from the literature some normal echocardiographic values for newborns.

**Table D–1**
Normal Echocardiographic Values in Newborns

| Reference<br>Age of Patient<br>Weight | Hagan,<br>et al.[5]<br>10–72 hr<br>2.7–4.5 kg | Meyer and<br>Kaplan[6]<br>1½–192 hr<br>2.3–4.9 kg | Solinger,<br>et al.[7]<br>6 hr–4 wk<br>2.2–4.5 kg | Godman,<br>et al.[8]<br>1 wk–1 mo<br>1.9–4.3 kg | Lundstrom[9]<br>1 wk–1 mo<br>? | Winsberg[10]<br>12–120 hr<br>2.8–4.5 kg | Sahn,<br>et al.[11]<br>12–120 hr<br>2.7–4.5 kg | All Cases<br>1½ hr–1 mo<br>1.9–4.9 kg | |
|---|---|---|---|---|---|---|---|---|---|
| No. of Cases | (200) | (50) | (240) | (50) | (10) | (11) | (72) | (633) | |
| MVD | . . . . . . . | 31–47 | 22–32 | . . . . . . | . . . . . . | . . . . . . | . . . . . . | (290) | 22–47 mm |
| MVTE | . . . . . . . | | 8.5–13.1 | 6.5–12.4 | 10–14 | . . . . . . | . . . . . . | (300) | 6.5–1.4 mm |
| MVDE | 6–12 | 6–12 | . . . . . . | | 7–9 | | . . . . . . | (210) | 6–12 mm |
| MVVS | 60–130 | 36–80 | | . . . . . . | | | . . . . . . | (250) | 36–130 mm/sec |
| TVD | . . . . . . . | 24–32 | 13–19 | . . . . . . | | | . . . . . . | (290) | 13–32 mm |
| TVTE | . . . . . . . | 8–14 | 8.8–14.2 | 8–13 | 12 | | . . . . . . | (300) | 8–14.2 mm |
| TVDE | 7–14 | | . . . . . . | | | | . . . . . . | (200) | 7–14 mm |
| TVVS | 60–116 | 34–56 | . . . . . . | | | | . . . . . . | (250) | 34–11 mm/sec |
| ARD | 8.1–12 | 7–12(S) | 9.2–13.6(S) | 8–11(S) | | | . . . . . . | (540) | 7–13.6 mm |
| AVO | . . . . . . . | | 4–6.8 | | | | . . . . . . | (240) | 4–6.8 mm |
| PRD | 9.4–13 | . . . . . . | 10.7–15.8(S) | | | | | (490) | 9.2–15.8 mm |
| PVO | . . . . . . . | | 5.8–9.9 | . . . . . . | | | . . . . . . | (240) | 5.8–9.9 mm |
| LAD | 5–10 | 6–13(S) | 6.8–13.5(S) | 4–10.5(S) | | | . . . . . . | (540) | 4–13.5 mm |
| IST | 1.8–4 | . . . . . . | 2.1–4.5 (D) | | | | . . . . . . | (440) | 1.8–4.5 mm |
| LVPW(S) | 2.5–6 | . . . . . . | | . . . . . . | | | . . . . . . | (200) | 2.5–6 mm |
| LVPW(D) | 1.6–3.7 | | 2–4.6 | . . . . . . | | 6 | . . . . . . | (440) | 1.6–4.6 mm |
| LVD(S) | 8–18.6 | . . . . . . | | | | 8–12 | . . . . . . | (211) | 8–18.6 mm |
| LVD(D) | 12.23–3 | 12–20 | 16.1–24.1 | 12–20.4 | | 16–20 | . . . . . . | (351) | 12–24.1 mm |
| RVAW(S) | 3.3–7.3 | . . . . . . | | | | | . . . . . . | (200) | 3.3–7.3 mm |
| RVAW(D) | 2–4.7 | | 1.1–4.1 | | | | . . . . . . | (440) | 1.1–4.7 mm |
| RVD(S) | 5.5–11.4 | . . . . . . | | | | | . . . . . . | (200) | 5.5–11.4 mm |
| RVD(D) | 6.1–15 | 10–17 | 10.4–17.7 | 10–17.5 | . . . . . . | | . . . . . . | (540) | 6.1–17.7 mm |
| MVCF | . . . . . . . | | | | | | 0.92–2.2 | ( 72) | 0.92–2.2 circ/sec |

| | | |
|---|---|---|
| MDV = mitral valve depth | ARD = aortic root diameter | RVAW = right ventricular anterior wall |
| MVTE = mitral valve total excursion | AVO = aortic valve opening | RVD = right ventricular dimension |
| MVDE = mitral valve diastolic excursion | PRD = pulmonary root diameter | MVCF = mean velocity circumferential fiber |
| MVVS = mitral valve velocity slope | PVO = pulmonary valve opening | shortening |
| TVD = tricuspid valve depth | LAD = left atrial dimension | (S) = systole |
| TVTE = tricuspid valve total excursion | IST = interventricular septal thickness | (D) = diastole |
| TVDE = tricuspid valve diastolic excursion | LVPW = left ventricular posterior wall | |
| TVVS = tricuspid valve velocity slope | LVD = left ventricular dimension | |

### Appendix E: Two-Dimensional Echocardiographic Measurements

Numerous measurements utilizing two-dimensional echocardiography have been mentioned in the literature. Many of these measurements are discussed in detail in Chapter 3, "Echocardiographic Evaluation of Cardiac Chambers." There has been no generalized agreement among echocardiographers regarding which two-dimensional echocardiographic measurements should be included in the routine examination. Almost all agree that some quantitative assessment of left ventricular function should be part of most two-dimensional echocardiographic examinations. Figure E–1 demonstrates some of the measurements that are being obtained routinely in some laboratories. The parasternal long-axis and short-

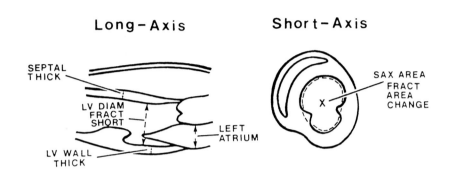

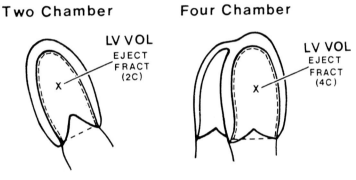

**Fig. E–1.** Diagram demonstrating some of the measurements that can be obtained from two-dimensional echocardiograms. The dimensions obtained in the parasternal long-axis view are modifications of the M-mode measurements noted in Figure B–1. The left ventricular diameters and fractional shortening provide an assessment of the size and systolic function of the base of the left ventricle. The short-axis (SAX) areas and fractional area change at the papillary muscle level give similar information of the midportion of the left ventricle. Left ventricular volumes (LV VOL) and ejection fraction can be determined from two-chamber and four-chamber echocardiograms utilizing prolate ellipse or Simpson's rule formulas for calculating volumes.

### Table E–1
Normal Values, Two-dimensional Echocardiography (50 Subjects; Age 19–63 Years—Mean, 31.2 ± 10.0)

| | Range | Range Corrected For B.S.A. | Number |
|---|---|---|---|
| Body surface area (B.S.A.) | | | |
|   1.44–2.48 (mean = 1.84 ± 0.18) | | | 50 |
| LV diameter-diastole | 3.6–5.2 cm | 2.0–2.8 cm/M$^2$ | 49 |
| LV diameter-systole | 2.3–3.9 cm | 1.3–2.1 cm/M$^2$ | 49 |
| Fractional shortening | 0.18–0.42 | | 49 |
| LV Sax area-diastole | 9.5–22.3 cm$^2$ | 5.5–11.9 cm/M$^2$ | 44 |
| LV Sax area-systole | 4.0–11.6 cm$^2$ | 2.4–6.4 cm/M$^2$ | 44 |
| Fractional area change | 0.36–0.64 | | 44 |
| Left atrial diameter | 2.1–3.7 cm | 1.2–2.0 cm/M$^2$ | 49 |

**Table E–2**

Normal Left Ventricular Volumes, Two-dimensional Echocardiography (21 Subjects—13 Females, 8 Males; Age 21–61 Years—Mean, 33)

|  | Diastole | Systole | Ejection Fraction |
|---|---|---|---|
| Volume | 95.5 ml | 38.6 ml | 60% |
| Standard deviation | ±19.4 ml | ±9.5 ml | ±6.2% |
| Volume index | 54.5 ml/M² | 22.1 ml/M² | |
| Standard deviation | ±8.7 ml/M² | ±4.9 ml/M² | |

(From Gordon, E.P., Schmittger, I., Fitzgerald, P.J., Williams, P., and Popp, R.L.: Reproducibility of left ventricular volumes by two-dimensional echocardiography. J. Am. Coll. Cardiol., *2*:506, 1983.)

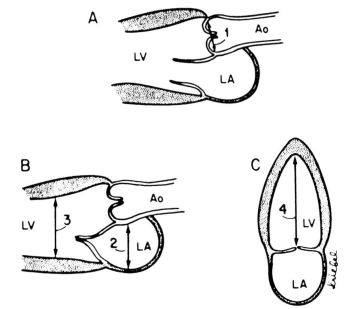

**Fig. E–2.** Linear dimensions from two-dimensional echocardiograms of the diameter of the aortic annulus (1), the left atrium (2), and the left ventricle (3). The length of the left ventricle (4) is obtained from an apical two-chamber view. LV = left ventricle; Ao = aorta; LA = left atrium. (From Nidorf, S.M., et al.: New perspectives in the assessment of cardiac chamber dimensions during development and adulthood. J. Am. Coll. Cardiol., *19*:983, 1992.)

axis measurements are essentially modifications of the M-mode dimensions that have been part of the routine examination for many years. The apical four-chamber and two-chamber views are used to calculate ventricular volumes using modifications of angiographic formulas used to calculate volumes.

Table E–1 demonstrates normal values using the parasternal long-axis and short-axis measurements from two-dimensional echocardiograms. These data were obtained by Dr. Richard Chazal at the Indiana University echocardiographic laboratories. The septal and left ventricular free-wall thicknesses are not listed because they proved to be identical to the M-mode normal values for wall thickness. The normal range for the left ventricular diameters and the left atrial systolic diameter are slightly different from those used with M-mode echocardiography.

Tables E–2 and E–3 give normal values for left ventricular volumes from two different echocardiographic laboratories.[12,13] The volumes from the Stanford University echocardiographic laboratory are slightly smaller than those derived by Erbel et al. The ejection fractions, however, are almost identical.

Figure E–2 illustrates additional linear measurements derived from two-dimensional echocardiograms.[14] The authors measured the diameters of the aortic root, the left atrium, and the left ventricle, and the left ventricular length. Figure E–3 demonstrates the four dimensions plotted against age. These investigators found that the measurements correlated best with body height (Fig. E–4).

Figures E–5 through E–8 demonstrate some two-dimensional measurements obtained from transesophageal echocardiograms.[15] These measurements include

**Table E–3**

Normal Left Ventricular Volumes, Two-dimensional Echocardiography

|  | Diastole | Systole | Stroke Volume | Ejection Fraction |
|---|---|---|---|---|
| *35 Males; Mean Age 30.2 Years* | | | | |
| Volume index | 66.8 ml/M² | 26.9 ml/M² | 39.9 ml/M² | 59.2% |
| Standard deviation | ±8.8 ml/M² | ±5.2 ml/M² | ±7.0 ml/M² | ±6.0% |
| 95% Confidence | 82 ml/M² | 35.9 ml/M² | 27.8 ml/M² | 48.8% |
| *20 Females; Mean Age 26.2 Years* | | | | |
| Volume index | 60.7 ml/M² | 25.7 ml/M² | 35.9 ml/M² | 58.1% |
| Standard deviation | ±12.5 ml/M² | ±7.4 ml/M² | ±10.6 ml/M² | ±6.5% |
| 95% Confidence | 85.0 ml/M² | 40.1 ml/M² | 56.5 ml/M² | 45.5% |

(From Erbel, R., Schweizer, P., Herrn, G., Mayer, J., and Effert, S.: Apical two-dimensional echocardiography: Normal values for single and bi-plane determination of left ventricular volume and ejection fraction. Dtsch. Med. Wochenschr., *107*:1872, 1982.)

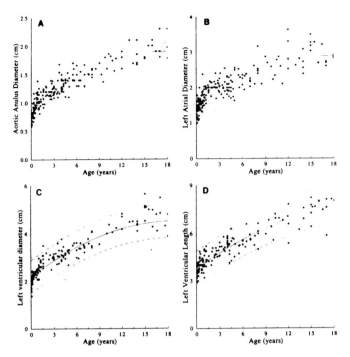

**Fig. E–3.** Graph plotting the aortic annulus diameter (*A*), the left atrial diameter (*B*), the left ventricular diameter (*C*), and the left ventricular length (*D*), against age. (From Nidorf, S.M., et al.: New perspectives in the assessment of cardiac chamber dimensions during development and adulthood. J. Am. Coll. Cardiol., *19*:983, 1992.)

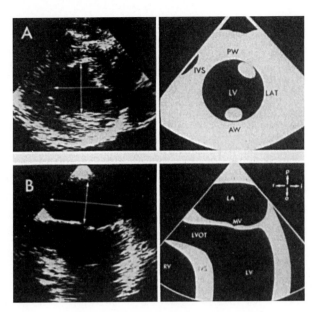

**Fig. E–5.** Transesophageal echocardiograms and diagrams showing the linear dimensions derived from a short-axis view of the left ventricle (*A*) and the four-chamber view of the left atrium (*B*). PW = posterior left ventricular wall; IVS = interventricular septum; LV = left ventricle; AW = anterior ventricular wall; LAT = lateral wall; LA = left atrium; MV = mitral valve; LVOT = left ventricular outflow tract; RV = right ventricle. (From Drexler, M., et al.: Measurement of intracardiac dimensions and structures in normal young adult subjects by transesophageal echocardiography. Am. J. Cardiol., *65*:1491, 1990.)

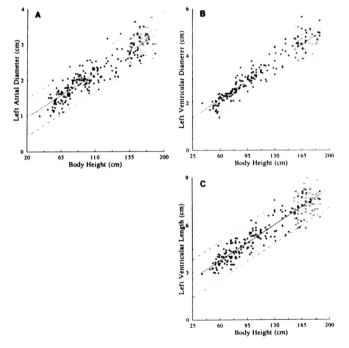

**Fig. E–4.** Graph plotting left atrial diameter (*A*), left ventricular diameter (*B*), and left ventricular length (*C*) against body height. (From Nidorf, S.M., et al.: New perspectives in the assessment of cardiac chamber dimensions during development and adulthood. J. Am. Coll. Cardiol., *19*:983, 1992.)

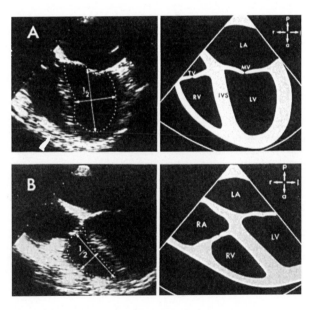

**Fig. E–6.** Long-axis and minor axis measurements of the left ventricle (LV) (*A*) and the right ventricle (RV) (*B*) from a transesophageal four-chamber examination. LA = left atrium; TV = tricuspid valve; MV = mitral valve; IVS = interventricular septum; RA = right atrium. (From Drexler, M., et al.: Measurement of intracardiac dimensions and structures in normal young adult subjects by transesophageal echocardiography. Am. J. Cardiol., *65*:1491, 1990.)

**Table E–4**

Measurements in Normal Young Adult Subjects by Transesophageal Echocardiography

| Patient | Age (yrs) | Body Surface (M²) | Left Ventricular Short Axis (cm/M²) D ↔ | D ↕ | S ↔ | S ↕ | Fractional Shortening D(%) ↔ | D(%) ↕ | Left Ventricular Long Axis (cm/M²) D ↔ | D ↕ | S ↔ | S ↕ | Left Atrium (cm/M²) D ↕ | D ↔ | S ↕ | S ↔ | Right Ventricular Long Axis (cm/M²) D ↕ | D ↔ | S ↕ | S ↔ |
|---|---|---|---|---|---|---|---|---|---|---|---|---|---|---|---|---|---|---|---|---|
| 1 | 24 | 2.09 | 2.5 | 2.6 | 1.5 | 1.7 | 40 | 34 | — | — | — | — | 1.0 | 2.0 | 1.7 | 2.5 | — | — | — | — |
| 2 | 29 | 2.12 | — | — | — | — | — | — | 2.6 | 3.6 | 1.8 | 2.7 | 0.8 | 1.7 | 1.1 | 2.4 | — | — | — | — |
| 3 | 24 | 1.65 | 2.5 | 2.6 | 1.6 | 1.6 | 37 | 37 | — | — | — | — | 0.8 | 1.7 | 1.4 | 2.5 | — | — | — | — |
| 4 | 23 | 1.91 | — | — | — | — | — | — | 2.8 | 3.9 | 2.0 | 3.3 | 1.4 | 1.4 | 1.9 | 2.1 | 2.5 | 1.5 | 2.0 | 1.0 |
| 5 | 26 | 2.22 | — | — | — | — | — | — | 2.4 | 3.1 | 1.6 | 2.4 | — | — | — | — | 2.7 | 1.7 | 2.3 | 1.2 |
| 6 | 22 | 1.79 | 2.4 | 2.4 | 1.6 | 1.6 | 35 | 34 | 2.5 | 3.1 | 1.6 | 2.4 | 0.7 | 1.7 | 1.4 | 2.3 | 2.6 | 1.3 | 2.2 | 1.0 |
| 7 | 30 | 2.08 | 3.0 | 2.7 | 1.8 | 1.7 | 42 | 36 | 2.4 | 3.4 | 1.6 | 2.7 | 1.3 | 1.8 | 1.9 | 2.6 | 2.7 | 1.6 | 2.2 | 1.2 |
| 8 | 22 | 2.05 | — | — | — | — | — | — | — | — | — | — | — | — | — | — | — | — | — | — |
| 9 | 22 | 1.67 | — | — | — | — | — | — | 2.8 | 3.5 | 2.2 | 3.0 | 0.4 | 1.1 | 1.1 | 2.2 | 2.8 | 1.8 | 2.5 | 1.2 |
| 10 | 22 | 1.89 | — | — | — | — | — | — | 2.7 | 3.1 | 1.8 | 2.7 | — | — | — | — | 2.5 | 1.3 | 2.0 | 1.0 |
| 11 | 19 | 1.67 | 2.5 | 2.5 | 1.5 | 1.5 | 41 | 38 | 2.3 | 3.0 | 1.7 | 2.4 | 0.8 | 1.7 | 1.4 | 2.3 | 2.7 | 1.2 | 2.4 | 0.8 |
| 12 | 27 | 1.55 | 2.9 | 2.9 | 1.8 | 1.9 | 38 | 34 | 2.9 | 3.4 | 2.0 | 2.5 | 0.4 | 1.5 | 1.4 | 2.8 | — | — | — | — |
| 13 | 24 | 1.87 | 2.5 | 2.6 | 1.7 | 1.9 | 31 | 27 | — | — | — | — | — | — | — | — | 2.8 | 1.6 | 2.3 | 0.9 |
| 14 | 23 | 2.00 | — | — | — | — | — | — | — | — | — | — | — | — | — | — | 3.1 | 1.6 | 2.6 | 1.1 |
| 15 | 26 | 2.06 | 2.8 | 2.6 | 1.8 | 1.9 | 35 | 27 | — | — | — | — | 0.6 | 1.3 | 1.2 | 2.1 | 2.8 | 1.5 | 2.2 | 0.9 |
| 16 | 22 | 1.84 | 2.7 | 2.6 | 1.7 | 1.7 | 35 | 36 | — | — | — | — | — | — | — | — | — | — | — | — |
| 17 | 22 | 1.83 | 2.4 | 2.4 | 1.6 | 1.6 | 34 | 31 | — | — | — | — | — | — | — | — | 2.7 | 1.3 | 2.3 | 1.1 |
| 18 | 22 | 1.73 | 2.6 | 2.6 | 1.9 | 1.8 | 28 | 30 | — | — | — | — | — | — | — | — | 2.4 | 1.3 | 2.1 | 0.9 |
| 19 | 23 | 1.82 | 2.5 | 2.5 | 1.6 | 1.7 | 35 | 33 | 2.6 | 2.9 | 1.9 | 2.5 | 0.5 | 1.7 | 1.2 | 2.3 | 2.9 | 1.6 | 2.2 | 1.0 |
| 20 | 25 | 1.61 | — | — | — | — | — | — | 2.4 | 3.7 | 1.7 | 2.8 | 0.9 | 1.4 | 1.8 | 2.5 | 2.9 | 1.6 | 2.3 | 1.0 |
| 21 | 23 | 1.86 | — | — | — | — | — | — | 2.5 | 3.1 | 1.7 | 2.6 | 0.8 | 1.5 | 1.4 | 2.1 | 3.0 | 1.4 | 2.6 | 1.1 |
| 22 | 22 | 1.53 | 2.5 | 2.3 | 1.7 | 1.6 | 29 | 42 | 2.6 | 3.7 | 1.9 | 2.8 | 1.2 | 1.8 | 2.0 | 2.7 | 3.0 | 1.3 | 2.4 | 1.0 |
| 23 | 20 | 1.55 | 2.6 | 2.5 | 1.5 | 1.7 | 38 | 37 | — | — | — | — | — | — | — | — | — | — | — | — |
| 24 | 23 | 2.07 | 2.6 | 2.4 | 1.8 | 1.6 | 30 | 31 | 2.5 | 3.0 | 2.0 | 2.3 | — | — | — | — | 2.6 | 1.3 | 1.9 | 0.8 |
| 25 | 22 | 1.83 | 2.3 | 2.2 | 1.5 | 1.5 | 39 | 31 | 2.5 | 3.7 | 1.9 | 2.9 | 1.4 | 1.5 | 2.1 | 2.8 | 2.9 | 2.0 | 2.4 | 1.2 |
| Mean | | | 2.6 | 2.5 | 1.7 | 1.7 | 35 | 34 | 2.6 | 3.4 | 1.8 | 2.7 | 0.9 | 1.6 | 1.5 | 2.4 | 2.8 | 1.6 | 2.3 | 1.0 |
| ± 2 SD | | | 0.4 | 0.3 | 0.3 | 0.3 | 8 | 8 | 0.4 | 0.6 | 0.4 | 0.5 | 0.7 | 0.4 | 0.6 | 0.5 | 0.4 | 0.3 | 0.4 | 0.2 |
| Tolerance | | | 2.1– | 2.1– | 1.3– | 1.3– | 25– | 23– | 2.1– | 2.7– | 1.3– | 2.1– | 0.1– | 1.1– | 0.9– | 1.8– | 2.3– | 1.2 | 1.8 | 0.8– |
| | | | 3.1 | 2.9 | 2.1 | 2.1 | 45 | 43 | 3.1 | 4.1 | 2.3 | 3.3 | 1.8 | 2.1 | 2.1 | 3.0 | 3.3 | 2.0 | 2.8 | 1.2 |

Mean values and double standard deviation (x ± 2 SD) and tolerance limits for all cardiac and extracardiac structures and dimensions measured by transesophageal echocardiography. D = end-diastole; S = end-systole; ↔, ↗ = lateral axes; ↕, ↘ = sagittal axes; ↔ = lateral axes; ● = cross-sectional area. (From Drexler M., Erbel, R., Muller, U., Wittlich, N., Mohr-Kahly, S., and Meyer, J.: Measurement of intracardiac dimensions and structures in normal young adult subjects by transesophageal echocardiography. Am. J. Cardiol., *65*:1491, 1990.)

| Right Atrium (cm/M²) | | | | Aortic Valve cm/M² | cm/M² | | Asc Aorta cm²/M² | | | Desc Aorta cm²/M² | cm/M² | | Tricuspid Ring (cm/M²) | | Mitral Ring | Atrial Septum (cm) | | Right Main Pulmonary Artery (cm) | |
|---|---|---|---|---|---|---|---|---|---|---|---|---|---|---|---|---|---|---|---|
| D ↙ | D ↘ | S ↗ | S ↘ | D ↕ | D ↔ | cm²/M² ● | D ↕ | D ↔ | cm²/M² ● | D ↕ | D ↔ | cm²/M² ● | D | S | cm/M² ○ | D | S | ○ | ○ |
| — | — | — | — | 1.6 | 1.8 | 4.5 | 1.3 | 1.8 | 3.7 | 0.8 | 1.3 | 1.8 | — | — | 1.8 | — | — | — | — |
| — | — | — | — | 1.3 | 1.7 | 3.3 | 1.3 | 1.7 | 3.7 | 0.8 | 1.1 | 1.6 | — | — | 1.8 | — | — | — | — |
| — | — | — | — | 1.7 | 2.0 | 4.8 | 1.6 | 1.9 | 4.1 | — | — | — | — | — | 2.2 | — | — | — | — |
| 1.8 | 2.4 | 2.4 | 2.6 | 1.3 | 1.7 | 3.4 | — | — | — | 1.0 | 1.3 | 2.1 | 1.8 | 1.4 | 1.9 | 1.6 | 2.1 | 1.2 | 1.8 |
| — | — | — | — | 1.4 | 1.7 | 4.1 | 1.5 | 1.9 | 5.1 | 1.0 | 1.2 | 2.3 | 1.7 | 1.4 | 1.5 | — | — | — | — |
| 1.9 | 1.8 | 2.5 | 1.9 | 1.3 | 1.7 | 2.8 | 1.5 | 1.7 | 3.5 | 0.9 | 1.4 | 1.8 | 1.6 | 1.0 | 1.5 | 1.6 | 2.1 | 1.2 | 2.1 |
| 2.2 | 2.2 | 2.4 | 2.4 | 1.5 | 1.9 | 4.5 | — | — | — | 0.9 | 1.4 | 2.1 | 1.8 | 1.3 | 1.8 | 1.6 | 2.1 | 1.4 | 2.1 |
| — | — | — | — | 1.4 | 1.8 | 4.0 | 1.3 | 1.7 | 3.6 | 0.9 | 1.2 | 1.7 | — | — | 1.8 | — | — | — | — |
| 1.8 | 1.9 | 2.5 | 1.8 | 1.5 | 1.7 | 3.4 | — | — | — | — | — | — | 1.7 | 1.2 | 1.7 | 1.4 | 1.8 | 1.2 | 1.8 |
| 1.8 | 1.8 | 2.0 | 2.0 | — | — | — | 1.3 | 1.8 | 3.8 | — | — | — | 1.5 | 1.5 | 1.5 | 1.6 | 2.2 | 1.1 | 1.6 |
| 1.9 | 1.7 | 2.4 | 1.8 | 1.5 | 2.0 | 3.9 | 1.6 | 1.8 | 4.0 | 0.8 | 1.3 | 1.5 | 1.3 | 1.2 | 1.5 | 1.7 | 2.2 | 1.4 | — |
| — | — | — | — | 1.3 | 1.9 | 3.3 | 1.3 | 1.8 | 3.1 | 1.0 | 1.3 | 1.6 | — | — | 1.9 | — | — | — | — |
| — | — | — | — | 1.5 | 1.7 | 4.6 | — | — | — | 1.0 | 1.4 | 2.2 | — | — | — | — | — | — | — |
| 1.9 | 2.4 | 2.8 | 2.3 | 1.3 | 1.8 | 3.5 | 1.3 | 1.6 | 3.3 | 0.9 | 1.5 | 2.2 | 1.7 | 1.5 | 1.9 | 1.6 | 2.1 | 1.0 | 2.0 |
| — | — | — | — | 1.5 | 1.8 | 4.4 | 1.2 | 1.5 | 3.1 | 0.9 | 1.3 | 1.9 | 2.0 | 1.5 | 1.9 | — | — | — | — |
| 1.7 | 2.2 | 2.3 | 2.1 | 1.4 | 2.0 | 4.1 | — | — | — | 1.0 | 1.5 | 2.6 | — | — | — | 1.6 | 1.7 | 1.1 | 2.1 |
| 1.7 | 2.0 | 2.3 | 2.2 | 1.6 | 2.1 | 4.8 | — | — | — | 0.9 | 1.4 | 1.4 | 1.7 | 1.4 | — | 1.4 | 1.7 | 1.2 | 2.2 |
| 1.7 | 1.9 | 2.3 | 2.0 | 1.4 | 1.9 | 3.7 | 1.4 | 1.7 | 3.7 | 0.8 | 1.4 | 1.7 | 1.5 | 1.3 | — | 1.6 | 2.0 | 1.1 | 2.3 |
| 1.9 | 2.4 | 2.7 | 2.7 | 1.5 | 2.1 | 4.7 | 1.3 | 1.6 | 3.1 | 0.9 | 1.2 | 1.6 | 1.8 | 1.4 | 1.7 | 1.2 | 1.8 | 1.2 | 2.0 |
| 1.8 | 2.1 | 2.7 | 1.9 | 1.5 | 2.2 | 5.1 | 1.5 | 1.9 | 3.7 | 0.9 | 1.4 | 2.3 | 1.7 | 1.5 | 2.0 | 1.9 | 2.6 | 1.0 | 2.0 |
| 1.4 | 1.7 | 2.2 | 1.9 | — | — | — | 1.3 | 1.6 | 3.3 | 0.8 | 1.2 | 1.3 | 1.6 | 1.2 | 1.7 | 1.5 | 2.0 | 1.3 | — |
| 2.2 | 1.9 | 3.0 | 2.0 | 1.6 | 2.1 | 4.8 | 1.7 | 1.9 | 4.2 | 0.8 | 1.3 | 1.8 | 1.5 | 1.4 | 2.1 | 1.9 | 2.7 | 1.0 | — |
| — | — | — | — | 1.4 | 1.9 | 3.4 | 1.5 | 1.7 | 3.3 | 0.9 | 1.6 | 1.9 | — | — | — | — | — | — | — |
| 1.9 | 2.4 | 2.2 | 2.4 | — | — | — | — | — | — | 1.1 | 1.5 | 2.7 | 1.8 | 1.4 | — | 1.4 | 1.7 | — | — |
| 1.7 | 2.1 | 2.3 | 2.0 | 1.7 | 1.9 | 3.6 | 1.4 | 1.6 | 3.4 | 0.9 | 1.5 | 2.0 | 1.8 | 1.3 | 2.0 | 1.6 | 2.5 | 1.3 | — |
| 1.8 | 2.1 | 2.4 | 2.1 | 1.5 | 1.9 | 4.0 | 1.4 | 1.7 | 3.6 | 0.9 | 1.3 | 1.9 | 1.7 | 1.4 | 1.8 | 1.6 | 2.1 | 1.2 | 2.0 |
| 0.4 | 0.5 | 0.4 | 0.6 | 0.3 | 0.3 | 1.2 | 0.3 | 0.3 | 1.0 | 0.2 | 0.3 | 0.8 | 0.3 | 0.3 | 0.4 | 0.4 | 0.7 | 0.2 | 0.4 |
| 1.3 | 1.6 | 1.9 | 1.5 | 1.2– | 1.6– | 2.8– | 1.0– | 1.4– | 2.4– | 0.7– | 1.0– | 1.1– | 1.3– | 1.0– | 1.3– | 1.1– | 1.2– | 0.9– | 1.5– |
| 2.3 | 2.6 | 2.9 | 2.7 | 1.8 | 2.2 | 5.2 | 1.8 | 2.1 | 4.8 | 1.1 | 1.6 | 2.7 | 2.1 | 1.8 | 2.3 | 2.1 | 3.0 | 1.3 | 2.5 |

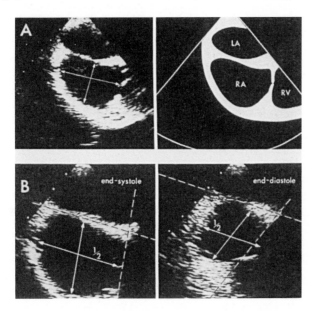

**Fig. E–7.**   End-systolic and end-diastolic measurements (*B*) of the right atrium (RA). LA = left atrium; RV = right ventricle. (From Drexler, M., et al.: Measurement of intracardiac dimensions and structures in normal young adult subjects by transesophageal echocardiography. Am. J. Cardiol., *65*:1491, 1990.)

linear dimensions of the left ventricle in the short-axis (Fig. E–5*A*) and four-chamber views (Fig. E–6*A*), left atrial dimensions from the four-chamber view (Fig. E–5*B*), right ventricular dimensions (Fig. E–6*B*), and right atrial measurements (Fig. E–7). A short-axis study through the base of the heart provides dimensions of the ascending aorta (Fig. E–8*A*) and pulmonary artery (Fig. E–8*B*). Normal values for these dimensions are listed in Table E–4.

Other studies that also provide normal ranges of two-dimensional echocardiographic measurements are listed in the references.[16–20]

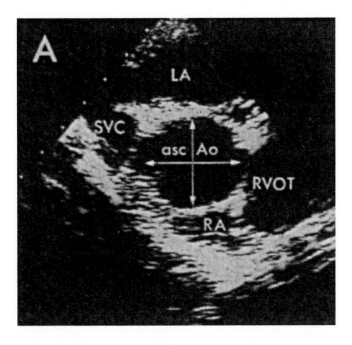

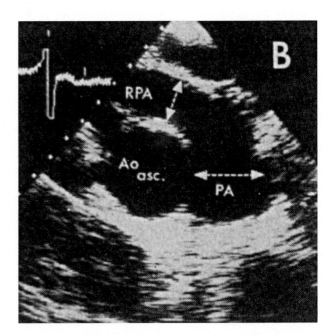

**Fig. E–8.**   Transesophageal examination of the base of the heart showing measurements of the ascending aorta (Asc AO), the right pulmonary artery (RPA), and the main pulmonary artery (PA). SVC = superior vena cava; LA = left atrium; RVOT = right ventricular outflow tract; RA = right atrium. (From Drexler, M., et al.: Measurement of intracardiac dimensions and structures in normal young adult subjects by transesophageal echocardiography. Am. J. Cardiol., *65*:1491, 1990.)

**Table F–1**
Normal Maximal Velocities, Doppler Measurements

| | Children | | Adults | |
| --- | --- | --- | --- | --- |
| | Mean | Range | Mean | Range |
| Mitral flow | 1.00 m/sec | 0.8–1.3 m/sec | 0.90 m/sec | 0.6–1.3 m/sec |
| Tricuspid flow | 0.60 m/sec | 0.5–0.8 m/sec | 0.50 m/sec | 0.3–0.7 m/sec |
| Pulmonary artery | 0.90 m/sec | 0.7–1.1 m/sec | 0.75 m/sec | 0.6–0.9 m/sec |
| Left ventricle | 1.00 m/sec | 0.7–1.2 m/sec | 0.90 m/sec | 0.7–1.1 m/sec |
| Aorta | 1.50 m/sec | 1.2–1.8 m/sec | 1.35 m/sec | 1.0–1.7 m/sec |

(From Hatle, L. and Angelsen, B.: Doppler Ultrasound in Cardiology, Second Edition. Philadelphia, Lea & Febiger, 1985.)

## Appendix F: Doppler Echocardiographic Measurements

Measurements of flow using Doppler echocardiography play an important role in the cardiovascular examination. Table F–1 lists the normal peak flows through the four cardiac valves in adults.[21] More detailed analysis of flow through the aorta and pulmonary artery in adults is noted in Table F–2.[22] Figure F–1 illustrates how the measurements are obtained for the aortic and pulmonary artery flow measurements. Normal Doppler flow velocities in children are listed in Table F–3.[23]

Another study listing Doppler measurements of normal aortic valve and left ventricular outflow tract is listed in the references.[24]

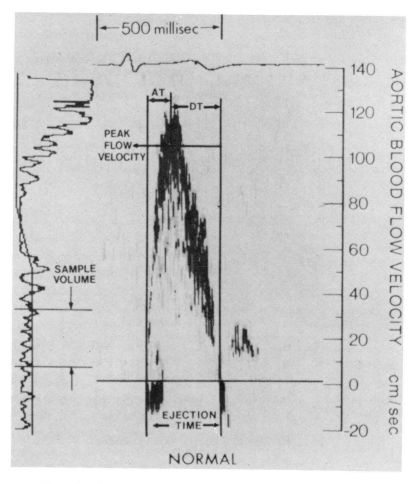

**Fig. F–1.** Pulsed Doppler recording of aortic blood flow velocity demonstrating how ejection time, peak flow velocity, acceleration time (AT) and deceleration time (DT) are measured. (From Gardin, J.M., Burn, C.S., Childs, W.J., and Henry, W.L.: Evaluation of blood flow velocity in the ascending aorta and main pulmonary artery of normal subjects by Doppler echocardiography. Am. Heart J., *107*:310, 1984.)

**Table F–2**

Normal Aortic and Pulmonary Artery Flow Doppler Measurements (20 Subjects—12 Males, 8 Females; Age 21–46 Years—Mean, 28)

|  | Aorta | Pulmonary Artery |
|---|---|---|
| *Peak Velocity* | | |
| Mean | 92 cm/sec | 63 cm/sec |
|  |  | ±9.0 cm/sec |
| Standard deviation | ±11 cm/sec | |
| Range | 72–120 cm/sec | 44–78 cm/sec |
| *Ejection Time* | | |
| Mean | 294 cm/sec | 331 msec |
| Standard deviation | ±19 msec | ±23 msec |
| Range | 265–325 msec | 280–380 msec |
| *Acceleration Time* | | |
| Mean | 98 msec | 159 msec |
| Standard deviation | ±10 msec | ±18 msec |
| Range | 83–118 msec | 130–185 msec |
| *Average Acceleration* | | |
| Mean | 940 cm/sec² | 396 cm/sec² |
| Standard deviation | ±161 cm/sec² | ±70 cm/sec² |
| Range | 735–1318 cm/sec² | 270–515 cm/sec² |
| *Average Deceleration* | | |
| Mean | 473 cm/sec² | 356 cm/sec² |
| Standard deviation | ±73 cm/sec² | ±54 cm/sec² |
| Range | 390–630 cm/sec² | 257–460 cm/sec² |

(From: Gardin, J.M., Burn, C.S., Childs, W.J., and Henry, W.L.: Evaluation of blood flow velocity in the ascending aorta and main pulmonary artery of normal subjects by Doppler echocardiography. Am. Heart J., *107*:310, 1984.)

**Table F–3**

Normal Doppler Velocities in Children

| Site | Mean | Range |
|---|---|---|
| SVC | 51 cm/sec | 28–80 cm/sec |
| RA (peak) | 47 | 38–74 |
| RV inflow | 62 | 41–84 |
| MPA | 76 | 50–105 |
| LA (peak) | 58 | 45–80 |
| LV inflow | 78 | 44–128 |
| AA | 97 | 60–154 |

SVC = superior vena cava; RA = right atrium; RV = right ventricle; MPA = main pulmonary artery; LA = left atrium; LV = left ventricle; AA = ascending aorta. (From: Goldberg, S.J., Allen, H.D., Marx, G.R., and Flinn, C.J.: Doppler Echocardiography. Philadelphia, Lea & Febiger, 1985.)

Figure F–2 demonstrates venous and ventricular inflow velocity measurements. Tables F–4 and F–5 give normal values for these measurements.[25] Normal Doppler left ventricular inflow velocities tabulated by age are listed in Table F–6.[26] Other studies examining normal venous and ventricular inflow Doppler velocities are described in the references.[27–30]

**Table F–4**

Left Ventricular Filling Dynamics in Normal Subjects

|  | <50 Years (n = 61) | ≥50 Years (n = 56) | P Value |
|---|---|---|---|
| Left ventricular inflow | | | |
| Peak E (cm/sec) | 72 ± 14 | 62 ± 14 | <0.01 |
| Peak A (cm/sec) | 40 ± 10 | 59 ± 14 | <0.01 |
| E/A | 1.9 ± 0.6 | 1.1 ± 0.3 | <0.01 |
| DT (msec) | 179 ± 20 | 210 ± 36 | <0.01 |
| IVRT (msec) | 76 ± 11 | 90 ± 17 | <0.01 |
| Pulmonary vein | (n = 44) | (n = 41) | |
| Peak S (cm/sec) | 48 ± 9 | 71 ± 9 | <0.01 |
| Peak D (cm/sec) | 50 ± 10 | 38 ± 9 | <0.01 |
| Peak AR (cm/sec) | 19 ± 4 | 23 ± 14 | <0.01 |

See Figure F–2 for abbreviations. (From Klein A.L. and Cohen, G.I.: Doppler echocardiographic assessment of constrictive pericarditis, cardiac amyloidosis, and cardiac tamponade. Cleve. Clin. J. Med., *59*:281, 1992.)

**Table F–5**

Right Ventricular Filling Dynamics in Normal Subjects

|  | <50 Years (n = 61) | ≥50 Years (n = 56) | P Value |
|---|---|---|---|
| Right ventricular inflow | | | |
| Peak E (cm/sec) | 51 ± 7 | 41 ± 8 | <0.01 |
| Peak A (cm/sec) | 27 ± 8 | 33 ± 8 | <0.01 |
| E/A | 2.0 ± 0.5 | 1.34 ± 0.4 | <0.01 |
| DT (msec) | 188 ± 22 | 198 ± 23 | <0.01 |
| IVRT (msec) | 76 ± 11 | 90 ± 17 | <0.01 |
| Superior vena cava | (n = 59) | (n = 53) | |
| Peak S (cm/sec) | 41 ± 9 | 42 ± 12 | Not significant |
| Peak D (cm/sec) | 22 ± 5 | 22 ± 5 | Not significant |
| Peak AR (cm/sec) | 13 ± 3 | 16 ± 3 | <0.01 |

See Figure F–2 for abbreviations. (From Klein A.L. and Cohen, G.I.: Doppler echocardiographic assessment of constrictive pericarditis, cardiac amyloidosis, and cardiac tamponade. Cleve. Clin. J. Med., *59*:281, 1992.)

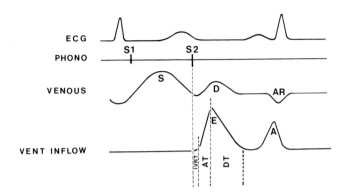

**Fig. F–2.** Diagram showing the relationship between the electrocardiogram (ECG), phonocardiogram (PHONO), and venous and ventricular inflow Doppler recordings. S1 = first heart sound; S2 = second heart sound; S = systolic venous velocity; D = diastolic venous velocity; AR = atrial reversal; E = early diastolic velocity; A = velocity with atrial contraction; IVRT = isovolumic relaxation time; AT = acceleration time; DT = deceleration time.

**Table F–6**
Doppler Left Ventricular Diastolic Function Indexes by Age (Years)

| | 20–29 (n = 21) | 30–39 (n = 20) | 40–49 (n = 22) | 50–59 (n = 21) | 60–69 (n = 22) | ≥70 (n = 21) | All Ages (n = 127) |
|---|---|---|---|---|---|---|---|
| **Peak velocity E (m/sec)** | | | | | | | |
| Mean | 0.71 | 0.66 | 0.63 | 0.61 | 0.55 | 0.53 | 0.61 |
| SD | 0.14 | 0.14 | 0.10 | 0.11 | 0.11 | 0.17 | 0.14 |
| **Peak velocity A (m/sec)** | | | | | | | |
| Mean | 0.35 | 0.38 | 0.45 | 0.49 | 0.55 | 0.64 | 0.48 |
| SD | 0.06 | 0.06 | 0.08 | 0.11 | 0.10 | 0.14 | 0.14 |
| **Peak velocity E/A** | | | | | | | |
| Mean | 2.08 | 1.75 | 1.44 | 1.29 | 1.03 | 0.84 | 1.40 |
| SD | 0.55 | 0.40 | 0.26 | 0.28 | 0.26 | 0.29 | 0.54 |
| **Time velocity integral E (m)** | | | | | | | |
| Mean | 0.093 | 0.085 | 0.086 | 0.086 | 0.076 | 0.072 | 0.083 |
| SD | 0.022 | 0.018 | 0.016 | 0.017 | 0.015 | 0.023 | 0.019 |
| **Time velocity integral A (m)** | | | | | | | |
| Mean | 0.030 | 0.029 | 0.0397 | 0.040 | 0.042 | 0.052 | 0.038 |
| SD | 0.005 | 0.006 | 0.007 | 0.009 | 0.009 | 0.014 | 0.012 |
| **Time velocity integral E/A** | | | | | | | |
| Mean | 3.24 | 3.02 | 2.35 | 2.23 | 1.89 | 1.45 | 2.35 |
| SD | 0.85 | 0.69 | 0.39 | 0.41 | 0.50 | 0.47 | 0.83 |
| **Atrial filling fraction** | | | | | | | |
| Mean | 0.24 | 0.25 | 0.29 | 0.30 | 0.35 | 0.42 | 0.31 |
| SD | 0.05 | 0.05 | 0.03 | 0.04 | 0.06 | 0.06 | 0.08 |

SD = ± standard deviation. (From Benjamin, E.J., Levy, D., Anderson, K.M., Wolf, P.A., Plehn, J.F., Evans, J.C., Comai, K., Fuller, D.L., and St. John Sutton, M.: Determinants of Doppler indexes of left ventricular diastolic function in normal subjects (the Framingham Heart Study). Am. J. Cardiol., *70:*508, 1992.)

**Table G–1**
Normal Values for Mechanical Prostheses in Mitral Position

| Prosthesis | References | No. of Patients | Peak Velocity | Peak Gradient | Mean Velocity | Mean Gradient | Half-Time | MVA | Regurgitant Valves No. | % |
|---|---|---|---|---|---|---|---|---|---|---|
| Starr-Edwards | 32 | 3 | 1.80 ± 0.20 | 13.00 ± 5.00 | 1.12 ± 0.22 | 5.00 ± 2.00 | 105 ± 32.5 | 2.10 ± 0.50 | 1 | 33 |
| | 33 | 12 | 2.00 | 17.00 | NI | NI | 105 | 2.10 | 5 | 42 |
| | 34 | 10 | 1.58 | 10.00 | NI | NI | 110 ± 19.4 | 2.00 ± 0.30 | 3 | 30 |
| | 35 | 18 | 1.97 ± 0.42 | 15.50 ± 5.80 | 1.06 ± 0.29 | 4.47 ± 2.42 | 113 ± 29 | 1.95 ± 0.50 | NI | NI |
| **Total** | | 43 | 1.88 ± 0.40 | 14.56 ± 5.50 | 1.07 ± 0.28 | 4.55 ± 2.40 | 109.5 ± 26.6 | 2.01 ± 0.49 | 9 | 36 |
| St. Jude | 36 | 13 | 1.38 ± 0.33 | 7.62 ± 0.64 | 0.73 ± 0.16 | 2.30 ± 0.90 | 61.2 ± 16.9 | 3.60 ± 0.99 | NI | NI |
| | 32 | 44 | 1.60 ± 0.30 | 11 00 ± 4.00 | 1.12 ± 0.22 | 5.00 ± 2.00 | 73.3 ± 14.7 | 3.00 ± 0.60 | 14 | 32 |
| | 35 | 56 | 1.63 ± 0.27 | 10.63 ± 3.52 | 0.76 ± 0.18 | 2.32 ± 1.10 | 78.0 ± 16.0 | 2.93 ± 0.60 | NI | NI |
| | 37 | 10 | 1.73 ± 0.32 | 12.00 ± 4.40 | 1.18 ± 0.22 | 5.60 ± 2.10 | 71.0 ± 18.3 | 3.10 ± 0.80 | 2 | 20 |
| | 38 | 33 | 1.40 ± 0.30 | 7.84 ± 3.36 | 0.80 ± 0.10 | 3.30 ± 1.10 | 86.0 ± 21.0 | 2.56 ± 0.62 | NI | NI |
| **Total** | | 156 | 1.56 ± 0.29 | 9.98 ± 3.62 | 0.88 ± 0.19 | 3.49 ± 1.34 | 76.5 ± 17.1 | 2.88 ± 0.64 | 16 | 30 |
| Bjork-Shiley | 39 | 9 | NI | NI | NI | NI | 13.3 ± 32.7 | 2.13 ± 0.72 | NI | NI |
| | 32 | 8 | 1.60 ± 0.30 | 10.00 ± 3.00 | 1.12 ± 0.22 | 5.00 ± 2.00 | 100.0 ± 18.8 | 2.20 ± 0.40 | 3 | 38 |
| | 34 | 36 | 1.58 | 10.00 | NI | NI | 88.0 ± 28.2 | 2.50 ± 0.80 | 4 | 11 |
| | 40 | 17 | 1.27 ± 0.39 | 6.41 ± 3.30 | 0.71 ± 0.28 | 2.00 ± 1.56 | 102.8 ± 12.5 | 2.14 ± 0.26 | 3 | 19 |
| | 35 | 40 | 1.57 ± 0.24 | 9.86 ± 2.78 | 0.79 ± 0.22 | 2.47 ± 1.36 | 82.0 ± 17.0 | 2.68 ± 0.56 | NI | NI |
| | 41 | 6 | NI | NI | 1.17 ± 0.28 | 5.50 ± 2.65 | NI | NI | NI | NI |
| | 42 | 12 | 2.36 ± 0.33 | 22.30 ± 5.82 | NI | NI | NI | NI | NI | NI |
| **Total** | | 128 | 1.61 ± 0.30 | 10.72 ± 2.74 | 0.84 ± 0.24 | 2.90 ± 1.61 | 90.2 ± 22.4 | 2.44 ± 0.62 | 10 | 16 |
| Lillehei-Kaster | 35 | 10 | 1.84 | 13.54 | 0.92 | 3.35 | 125.0 ± 29.0 | 1.88 ± 0.56 | NI | NI |
| Beall | 32 | 13 | 1.80 ± 0.2 | 13.40 ± 4.0 | 1.22 ± 0.20 | 6.00 ± 2.00 | 129.4 ± 15.2 | 1.70 ± 0.20 | NI | NI |

MVA = mitral valve area; NI = no information. (From Reisner, S.A. and Meltzer, R.S.: Normal values of prosthetic valve Doppler echocardiographic parameters: A review. J. Am. Soc. Echocardiogr., *1*:201, 1988.)

**Table G–2**
Normal Values for Tissue Prostheses in Mitral Position

| Prosthesis | References | No. of Patients | Peak Velocity | Peak Gradient | Mean Velocity | Mean Gradient | Half-Time | MVA | Regurgitant Valves No. | % |
|---|---|---|---|---|---|---|---|---|---|---|
| Ionescu-Shiley | 43 | 17 | 1.39 ± 0.20 | 7.73 ± 2.00 | 0.94 ± 0.11 | 3.54 ± 0.80 | 93.5 ± 23.0 | 2.35 ± 0.77 | NI | NI |
| | 35 | 12 | 1.56 ± 0.35 | 9.73 ± 3.87 | 0.84 ± 0.27 | 2.90 ± 1.60 | 93.0 ± 28.0 | 2.37 ± 0.71 | NI | NI |
| **Total** | | 29 | 1.46 ± 0.27 | 8.53 ± 2.91 | 0.90 ± 0.19 | 3.28 ± 1.19 | 93.3 ± 25.0 | 2.36 ± 0.75 | NI | NI |
| Carpentier-Edwards | 44 | 38 | 1.60 ± 0.20 | 10.24 ± 2.40 | NI | NI | 90.0 ± 23.0 | 2.44 ± 0.84 | NI | NI |
| | 37 | 25 | 2.10 ± 0.37 | 17.30 ± 5.30 | 1.37 ± 0.22 | 7.50 ± 0.20 | 84.6 ± 31.2 | 2.60 ± 0.70 | NI | NI |
| | 43 | 12 | 1.55 ± 0.24 | 9.63 ± 2.74 | 1.04 ± 0.26 | 4.36 ± 1.93 | 100.0 ± 16.7 | 2.20 ± 0.44 | NI | NI |
| **Total** | | 75 | 1.76 ± 0.24 | 12.49 ± 3.64 | 1.26 ± 0.23 | 6.48 ± 2.12 | 89.8 ± 25.4 | 2.45 ± 0.74 | NI | NI |
| Hancock | 39 | 8 | NI | NI | NI | NI | 157.0 ± 76.3 | 1.40 ± 0.68 | NI | NI |
| | 45 | 14 | NI | NI | 1.54 ± 0.3 | 6.50 ± 1.4 | 142.9 ± 27.9 | 1.54 ± 0.30 | NI | NI |
| | 33 | 29 | 1.90 | 14.00 | NI | NI | 91.7 | 2.40 ± 0.80 | 12 | 42 |
| | 40 | 23 | 1.21 ± 0.27 | 5.83 ± 2.48 | 0.77 ± 0.19 | 2.39 ± 1.16 | 141.0 ± 30.8 | 1.56 ± 0.34 | 3 | 14 |
| | 46 | 28 | 1.38 ± 0.24 | 7.62 ± 2.65 | NI | NI | 136.0 ± 18.0 | 1.62 ± 0.27 | 1 | 4 |
| | 47 | 5 | NI | NI | 10.70 | 4.60 | NI | NI | NI | NI |
| | 7 | 7 | 1.80 ± 0.30 | 12.96 ± 4.32 | 1.10 ± 0.30 | 5.90 ± 3.00 | 150.0 ± 80.0 | 1.47 ± 0.78 | NI | NI |
| **Total** | | 114 | 1.54 ± 0.26 | 9.70 ± 3.20 | 1.07 ± 0.25 | 4.29 ± 2.14 | 128.6 ± 30.9 | 1.71 ± 0.41 | 16 | 20 |

MVA = mitral valve area; NI = no information. (From Reisner, S.A. and Meltzer, R.S.: Normal values of prosthetic valve Doppler echocardiographic parameters: A review. J. Am. Soc. Echocardiogr., *1*:201, 1988.)

## Appendix G: Doppler Measurements of Prosthetic Valves

Tables G–1 to G–7 give Doppler measurements from a variety of normally functioning prosthetic valves.[31] The data in the tables are derived from multiple studies and multiple authors.[32–49] Additional studies listing Doppler measurements of normally performing prosthetic valves are listed in the references.[50–52]

### Table G–3
Normal Values for the St. Jude Medical Prosthesis (27 to 31 mm)

| Size (mm) | References | No. of Patients | Peak Velocity | Peak Gradient | Mean Velocity | Mean Gradient | Half-Time | Mitral Valve Area |
|---|---|---|---|---|---|---|---|---|
| 27 | 38,32 | 18 | 1.54 ± 0.20 | 9.69 ± 3.06 | | | | |
| | 32 | 8 | | | 1.12 ± 0.22 | 5.00 ± 2.00 | | |
| | 39 | 1 | | | | | 137.5 | 1.60 |
| | 35,38,32 | 86 | 1.59 ± 0.27 | 10.11 ± 3.43 | | | | |
| 29 | 35,32 | 79 | | | 0.82 ± 0.21 | 2.71 ± 1.36 | | |
| | 35 | 56 | | | | | 78.0 ± 16.0 | 2.93 ± 0.60 |
| | 38,32 | 25 | 1.54 ± 0.36 | 9.90 ± 4.49 | | | | |
| 31 | 32 | 15 | | | 1.12 ± 0.34 | 5.00 ± 3.00 | | |
| | 37 | 3 | | | | | 57.9 ± 6.10 | 3.80 ± 0.40 |

(From Reisner, S.A. and Meltzer, R.S.: Normal values of prosthetic valve Doppler echocardiographic parameters: A review. J. Am. Soc. Echocardiogr., *1*:201, 1988.)

### Table G–4
Normal Values for Mechanical Prostheses in Aortic Position

| Prosthesis | References | No. of Patients | Peak Velocity | Peak Gradient | Mean Velocity | Mean Gradient | Regurgitant Valves No. | Regurgitant Valves % |
|---|---|---|---|---|---|---|---|---|
| St. Jude | 32 | 38 | 2.30 ± 0.60 | 22.0 ± 12.0 | 1.73 ± 0.57 | 12.0 ± 7.00 | 22 | 58 |
| | 36 | 7 | 1.97 ± 0.52 | 15.5 ± 8.2 | 1.23 ± 0.25 | 6.0 ± 2.50 | NI | NI |
| | 48 | 12 | 2.70 ± 0.40 | 30.0 ± 9.0 | 1.80 ± 0.30 | 16.0 ± 5.60 | NI | NI |
| | 37 | 13 | 2.50 ± 0.50 | 26.5 ± 9.1 | 2.00 ± 0.35 | 16.0 ± 5.60 | 4 | 30 |
| **Total** | | 70 | 2.37 ± 0.27 | 25.5 ± 5.12 | 1.69 ± 0.47 | 12.5 ± 6.35 | 26 | 51 |
| Bjork-Shiley | 32 | 8 | 2.60 ± 0.50 | 17.0 ± 9.00 | 1.87 ± 0.40 | 1.48 ± 6.00 | 5 | 62 |
| | 40 | 20 | 2.35 ± 0.28 | 22.0 ± 5.31 | 1.80 ± 0.36 | 13.0 ± 5.20 | 3 | 17 |
| | 49 | 20 | 2.17 ± 0.40 | 18.8 ± 6.94 | NI | NI | 2 | 10 |
| | 34 | 33 | 3.29 ± 0.50 | 21.5 ± 10.0 | NI | NI | 8 | 26 |
| | 48 | 21 | 2.70 ± 0.40 | 30.0 ± 9.00 | 1.80 ± 0.30 | 16.0 ± 5.00 | NI | NI |
| **Total** | | 102 | 2.62 ± 0.42 | 23.8 ± 8.80 | 1.82 ± 0.34 | 14.3 ± 5.25 | 18 | 22 |
| Starr-Edwards | 32 | 4 | 3.20 ± 0.20 | 40.0 ± 3.0 | 2.45 ± 0.20 | 24.0 ± 4.0 | 3 | 75 |
| | 49 | 12 | 3.35 ± 0.45 | 45.0 ± 12.0 | NI | NI | 6 | 50 |
| | 33 | 34 | 3.10 | 40.0 | NI | NI | 18 | 53 |
| | 34 | 6 | 2.71 ± 0.61 | 29.3 ± 13.3 | NI | NI | 2 | 33 |
| **Total** | | 56 | 3.10 ± 0.47 | 38.6 ± 11.7 | 2.45 ± 0.20 | 24.0 ± 4.0 | 29 | 52 |

NI = no information. (From Reisner, S.A. and Meltzer, R.S.: Normal values of prosthetic valve Doppler echocardiographic parameters: A review. J. Am. Soc. Echocardiogr., *1*:201, 1988.)

**Table G–5**
Normal Values for Tissue Prostheses in Aortic Position

| Prosthesis | References | No. of Patients | Peak Velocity | Peak Gradient | Mean Velocity | Mean Gradient | Regurgitant Valves No. | % |
|---|---|---|---|---|---|---|---|---|
| Carpentier-Edwards | 44 | 24 | 2.44 ± 0.48 | 23.81 ± 9.37 | NI | NI | 2 | 8 |
| | 49 | 43 | 2.17 ± 0.49 | 18.84 ± 8.51 | NI | NI | 9 | 22 |
| | 48 | 7 | 2.70 ± 0.70 | 31.00 ± 15.0 | 1.90 ± 0.5 | 18.0 ± 9.0 | NI | NI |
| | 37 | 41 | 2.50 ± 0.40 | 26.10 ± 7.70 | 1.95 ± 0.31 | 15.2 ± 4.8 | 11 | 26 |
| | 43 | 28 | 2.34 ± 0.40 | 23.10 ± 8.20 | 1.75 ± 0.42 | 12.3 ± 5.9 | NI | NI |
| **Total** | | 143 | 2.37 ± 0.46 | 23.18 ± 8.72 | 1.87 ± 0.37 | 14.4 ± 5.7 | 22 | 20 |
| Hancock | 40 | 22 | 2.00 ± 0.19 | 16.0 ± 2.97 | 1.66 ± 0.17 | 11.40 ± 2.29 | 5 | 22 |
| | 49 | 32 | 2.56 ± 02.3 | 26.2 ± 4.71 | NI | NI | 7 | 22 |
| | 33 | 10 | 2.70 | 30.0 | NI | NI | 5 | 50 |
| | 34 | 27 | 2.37 ± 0.53 | 22.4 ± 10.1 | NI | NI | 8 | 26 |
| **Total** | | 91 | 2.38 ± 0.35 | 23.0 ± 6.71 | 1.66 ± 0.17 | 11.0 ± 2.29 | 25 | 27 |
| Ionescu-Shiley | 37 | 16 | 2.60 ± 0.50 | 27.0 ± 9.10 | 2.00 ± 0.33 | 16.40 ± 5.3 | NI | NI |
| | 43 | 16 | 3.37 ± 0.31 | 21.96 ± 5.86 | 1.70 ± 0.21 | 11.57 ± 2.9 | NI | NI |
| **Total** | | 32 | 2.49 ± 1.71 | 24.68 ± 7.65 | 1.85 ± 0.29 | 13.99 ± 4.3 | NI | NI |

NI = no information. (From Reisner, S.A. and Meltzer, R.S.: Normal values of prosthetic valve Doppler echocardiographic parameters: A review. J. Am. Soc. Echocardiogr., *1*:201, 1988.)

**Table G–6**
Normal Values for Mechanical Prostheses in the Aortic Position According to Size

| Prosthesis | Size (mm) | References | No. of Patients | Peak Velocity | Peak Gradient | Mean Velocity | Mean Gradient |
|---|---|---|---|---|---|---|---|
| St. Jude Medical | 19 | 37,32 | 6 | 3.00 ± 0.77 | 31.2 ± 17.3 | | |
| | | 48,32 | 5 | | | 2.36 ± 0.58 | 22.2 ± 11.0 |
| | 21 | 37,48,32 | 14 | 2.70 ± 0.26 | 30.0 ± 5.7 | | |
| | | 41,32 | 11 | | | 1.89 ± 0.33 | 14.4 ± 5.0 |
| | 23 | 37,32 | 17 | 2.32 ± 0.60 | 23.2 ± 11.5 | | |
| | | 48,32 | 19 | | | 1.64 ± 0.48 | 10.8 ± 6.3 |
| | 25 | 37,32 | 12 | 2.20 ± 0.46 | 19.8 ± 8.2 | | |
| | | 32 | 9 | | | 1.24 ± 0.45 | 11.0 ± 6.0 |
| Bjork-Shiley | 19 | 48 | 3 | | | 2.29 ± 0.38 | 21.0 ± 7.00 |
| | 21 | 49 | 4 | 2.76 ± 0.90 | 30.5 ± 19.87 | | |
| | | 48 | 1 | | | 2.0 | 16.0 |
| | 23 | 40,49 | 11 | 2.59 ± 0.42 | 27.29 ± 8.70 | | |
| | | 40,48 | 20 | | | 18.7 ± 0.33 | 14.0 ± 5.00 |
| | 25 | 40,49 | 13 | 2.14 ± 0.31 | 18.38 ± 5.31 | | |
| | | 40,48 | 13 | | | 1.82 ± 0.17 | 13.3 ± 2.53 |
| | 27 | 40,49 | 10 | 1.91 ± 0.20 | 14.55 ± 3.06 | | |
| | | 40,48 | 7 | | | 1.56 ± 0.20 | 9.7 ± 2.53 |
| | 29 | 49 | 2 | 1.87 ± 0.20 | 13.99 ± 2.54 | 1.32 ± 0.57 | 7.0 ± 6.00 |

(From Reisner, S.A. and Meltzer, R.S.: Normal values of prosthetic valve Doppler echocardiographic parameters: A review. J. Am. Soc. Echocardiogr., *1*:201, 1988.)

**Table G–7**
Normal Values for Tissue Prostheses in the Aortic Position According to Size

| Prosthesis | Size (mm) | References | No. of Patients | Peak Velocity | Peak Gradient | Mean Velocity | Mean Gradient |
|---|---|---|---|---|---|---|---|
| Hancock | 21 | 49 | 1 | 3.50 | 49.00 | | |
| | 23 | 40,49 | 10 | 2.37 ± 0.24 | 22.97 ± 4.55 | | |
| | | 40 | 7 | | | 1.73 ± 0.14 | 12.0 ± 2.0 |
| | 25 | 40,49 | 22 | 2.26 ± 0.25 | 20.69 ± 4.57 | | |
| | | 40 | 10 | | | 1.66 ± 0.15 | 11.0 ± 2.00 |
| | 27 | 40,49 | 18 | 2.12 ± 0.35 | 20.53 ± 5.69 | | |
| | | 40 | 5 | | | 1.58 ± 0.24 | 10.0 ± 3.0 |
| | 29 | 49 | 2 | 2.23 ± 0.40 | 19.89 ± 7.14 | | |
| Carpentier-Edwards | 19 | 37,43 | 11 | 2.80 ± 0.66 | 31.55 ± 14.88 | | |
| | | 43 | 3 | | | 2.03 ± 0.12 | 16.47 ± 1.40 |
| | 21 | 43 | 7 | 27.31 ± 0.40 | 27.31 ± 9.90 | 1.90 ± 0.39 | 14.50 ± 6.00 |
| | 23 | 37,43,49 | 28 | 2.56 ± 0.44 | 26.61 ± 8.93 | | |
| | | 38,43 | 13 | | | 1.78 ± 0.40 | 12.67 ± 5.69 |
| | 25 | 37,43,49 | 27 | 2.54 ± 0.40 | 24.37 ± 7.88 | | |
| | | 48,43 | 6 | | | 1.60 ± 0.18 | 10.37 ± 2.27 |
| | 27 | 37,43,49 | 28 | 2.41 ± 0.37 | 23.57 ± 7.24 | | |
| | | 48,43 | 3 | | | 1.55 ± 0.08 | 9.87 ± 1.00 |
| | 29 | 43,49 | 12 | 2.38 ± 0.44 | 22.76 ± 8.38 | | |
| | | 43 | 1 | | | 1.70 | 11.60 |
| | 31 | 49 | 5 | 2.36 ± 0.43 | 22.29 ± 8.12 | | |

(From Reisner, S.A. and Meltzer, R.S.: Normal values of prosthetic valve Doppler echocardiographic parameters: A review. J. Am. Soc. Echocardiogr., *1*:201, 1988.)

## REFERENCES

1. Henry, W.L., Ware, J., Gardin, J.M., Hepner, S.I., McKay, J., and Weiner, M.: Echocardiographic measurements in normal subjects: Growth-related changes that occur between infancy and early adulthood. Circulation, *57*:278, 1978.
2. Gardin, J.M., Henry, W.L., Savage, D.D., Ware, J.H., Burn, C., and Borer, J.S.: Echocardiographic measurements in normal subjects: Evaluation of an adult population without clinically apparent heart disease. JCU, *7*:439, 1979.
3. Goldberg, S.J., Allen, H.D., and Sahn, D.J.: Pediatric and Adolescent Echocardiography. Chicago, Yearbook Medical Publishers, 1975.
4. Moss, A.J., Gussoni, C.C., and Isabel-Jones, J.: Echocardiography in congenital heart disease. West. J. Med., *124*:102, 1976.
5. Hagan, A.D., Deely, W.J., Sahn, D.J., Karliner, J., Friedman, W.F., and O'Rourke, R.: Ultrasound evaluation of systolic anterior septal motion in patients with and without right ventricular volume overload. Circulation, *50*:1221, 1973.
6. Meyer, R.A. and Kaplan, S.: Echocardiography in the diagnosis of hypoplasia of the left or right ventricle in the neonate. Circulation, *46*:55, 1972.
7. Solinger, R., Elbl, F., and Minhas, K.: Echocardiography in the normal neonate. Circulation, *47*:108, 1973.
8. Godman, M.J., Tham, P., and Kidd, B.S.L.: Echocardiography in the evaluation of the cyanotic newborn infant. Br. Heart J., *36*:154, 1974.
9. Lundstrom, N.R. and Elder, I.: Ultrasound cardiography in infants and children. Acta Paediatr. Scand., *60*:117, 1971.
10. Winsberg, F.: Echocardiography of the fetal and newborn heart. Invest. Radiol., *7*:152, 1972.
11. Sahn, D.J., Deely, W.J., Hagan. A.D., and Friedman, W.F.: Echocardiographic assessment of left ventricular performance in normal newborns. Circulation, *49*:232, 1974.
12. Gordon, E.P., Schnittger, I., Fitzgerald, P.J., Williams, P., and Popp, R.L.: Reproducibility of left ventricular volumes by two-dimensional echocardiography. J. Am. Coll. Cardiol., *2*:506, 1983.
13. Erbel, R., Schweizer, P., Herrn, G., Mayer, J., and Effert, S.: Apical two-dimensional echocardiography: Normal values for single and bi-plane determination of left ventricular volume and ejection fraction. Dtsch. Med. Wochenschr., *107*:1872, 1982.
14. Nidorf, S.M., Picard, M.H., Triulizi, M.O., Thomas, J.D., Newell, J., King, M.E., and Weyman, A.E.: New perspectives in the assessment of cardiac chamber dimensions during development and adulthood. J. Am. Coll. Cardiol., *19*:983, 1992.
15. Drexler, M., Erbel, R., Muller, U., Wittlich, N., Mohr-Kahaly, S., and Meyer, J.: Measurement of intracardiac dimensions and structures in normal young subjects by transesophageal echocardiography. Am. J. Cardiol., *65*:1491, 1990.
16. Rijsterborgh, H., Romdoni, R., Vletter, W., Bom, N., and Roelandt, J.: Reference ranges of left ventricular cross-sectional echocardiographic measurements in adult men. J. Am. Soc. Echocardiogr., *2*:415, 1989.
17. Pearlman, J.D., Triulzi, M.O., King, M.E., Abascal, V.M., Newell, J., and Weyman, A.E.: Left atrial dimensions in growth and development: Normal limits for two-dimensional echocardiography. J. Am. Coll. Cardiol., *16*:1168, 1990.

18. Foale, R., Nihoyannopoulos, P., McKenna, W., Kliene-benne, A., Nadazdin, A., Rowland, E., and Smith, G.: Echocardiographic measurement of the normal adult right ventricle. Br. Heart J., *56*:33, 1986.

19. Ichida, F., Aubert, A., Denef, B., Dumoulin, M., and Van Der Hauwaert, L.G.: Cross sectional echocardiographic assessment of great artery diameters in infants and children. Br. Heart J., *58*:627, 1987.

20. Daniels, S.R., Meyer, R.A., Liang, Y., and Bove, K.E.: Echocardiographically determined left ventricular mass index in normal children, adolescents and young adults. J. Am. Coll. Cardiol., *12*:703, 1988.

21. Hatle, L. and Angelsen, B.: Doppler Ultrasound in Cardiology, Second edition. Philadelphia, Lea & Febiger, 1985.

22. Gardin, J.M., Burn, C.S., Childs, W.J., and Henry, W.L.: Evaluation of blood flow velocity in the ascending aorta and main pulmonary artery of normal subjects by Doppler echocardiography. Am. Heart J., *107*:310, 1984.

23. Goldberg, S.J., Allen, H.D., Marx, G.R., and Flinn, C.J.: Doppler Echocardiography. Philadelphia, Lea & Febiger, 1985.

24. Davidson, W.R., Pasquale, M.J., and Fanelli, C.: A Doppler echocardiographic examination of the normal aortic valve and left ventricular outflow tract. Am. J. Cardiol., *67*:547, 1991.

25. Klein, A.C. and Cohen, G.I.: Doppler echocardiographic assessment of constrictive pericarditis, cardiac amyloidosis, and cardiac tamponade. Cleve. Clin. J. Med., *59*:281, 1992.

26. Benjamin, E.J., Levy, D., Anderson, K.M., Wolf, P.A., Plehn, J.F., Evans, J.C., Comai, K., Fuller, D.L., and St. John Sutton, M.: Determinants of Doppler indexes of left ventricular diastolic function in normal subjects (the Framingham Heart Study). Am. J. Cardiol., *70*:508, 1992.

27. Meijburg, H.W.J., Visser, C.A., Westerhof, P.W., Kasteleyn, I., van der Twell, I., and deMedina, E.O.R.: Normal pulmonary venous flow characteristics as assessed by transesophageal pulsed Doppler echocardiography. J. Am. Soc. Echocardiogr., *5*:588, 1992.

28. Kitzman, D.W., Sheikh, K.H., Beere, P.A., Philips, J.L., and Higginbotham, M.B.: Age-related alterations of Doppler left ventricular filling indexes in normal subjects are independent of left ventricular mass, heart rate, contractility and loading conditions. J. Am. Coll. Cardiol., *18*:1243, 1991.

29. Lernfelt, B., Wikstrand, J., Svanborg, A., and Landahl, S.: Aging and left ventricular function in elderly healthy people. Am. J. Cardiol., *68*:547, 1991.

30. Pye, M.P., Pringle, S.D., and Cobbe, S.M.: Reference values and reproducibility of Doppler echocardiography in the assessment of the tricuspid valve and right ventricular diastolic function in normal subjects. Am. J. Cardiol., *67*:269, 1991.

31. Reisner, S.A. and Meltzer, R.S.: Normal values of prosthetic valve Doppler echocardiographic parameters: A review. J. Am. Soc. Echocardiogr., *1*:201, 1988.

32. Panidis, I.P., Ross, J., and Mintz, G.S.: Normal and abnormal prosthetic valve function as assessed by Doppler echocardiography. J. Am. Coll. Cardiol., *8*:317, 1986.

33. Rothbart, R.M., Smucker, M.L., and Gibson, R.S.: Overestimation by Doppler echocardiography of pressure gradients across Starr-Edwards prosthetic valves in the aortic position. Am. J. Cardiol., *61*:475, 1988.

34. Williams, G.A. and Labovitz, A.J.: Doppler hemodynamic evaluation of prosthetic (Starr-Edwards and Bjork-Shiley) and bioprosthetic (Hancock and Carpentier-Edwards) cardiac valves. Am. J. Cardiol., *56*:325, 1985.

35. Cruitus, J.M., Pawelzik, H., Mittmann, B., Breuer, H.W., and Loogen, F.: Doppler echocardiography normal values in various types of mitral valve prostheses. Z. Kardiol., *76*:25, 1987.

36. Weinstein, I.R., Marbarger, J.P., and Perez, J.E.: Ultrasonic assessment of the St. Jude prosthetic valve: M-mode two-dimensional and Doppler echocardiography. Circulation, *68*:897, 1983.

37. Cooper, D.M., Stewart, W.J., Schiavone, W.A., Lombardo, H.P., Lytle, B.W., Loop, F.O., and Salcedo, E.E.: Evaluation of normal prosthetic valve function by Doppler echocardiography. Am. Heart J., *114*:576, 1987.

38. Kisanuki, A., Tei, C., Arikawa, K., Natsugoe, K., Otsuji, Y., Kawazoe, Y., Tanaka, H., Morishita, Y., Maruko, M., and Taira, A.: Continuous wave Doppler assessment of prosthetic valves in the mitral position: Comparison of the St. Jude medical mechanical valve and the porcine xenograft valve. J. Cardiogr., *15*:1119, 1985.

39. Holen, J., Joie, J., and Semb, B.: Obstructive characteristics of Bjork-Shiley, Hancock, and Lillehei-Kaster prosthetic mitral valves in the immediate postoperative period. Acta Med. Scand., *204*:5, 1978.

40. Sagar, K.B., Wann, S., Paulsen, W.H.J., and Romhilt, D.W.: Doppler echocardiographic evaluation of Hancock and Bjork-Shiley prosthetic valves. J. Am. Coll. Cardiol., *7*:681, 1986.

41. Holen, J., Simonsen, S., and Froysaker, T.: An ultrasound Doppler technique for the noninvasive determination of the pressure gradient in the Bjork-Shiley mitral valve. Circulation, *59*:436, 1979.

42. Dubach-Reber, P.A. and Vargus-Barron, J.: Velocidad maxima del flujo en la prostesis mitrale de Bjork-Shiley normofuncion-ante. Arch. Inst. Cardiol. Mex., *56*:57, 1986.

43. Lesbre, J.P., Chassat, C., Lesperance, J., Petitclerc, R., Bonan, R., Dyrda, I., Pasternac, A., and Bourassa, M.: Evaluation of new pericardial bioprostheses by pulsed and continuous Doppler ultrasound. Arch. Mal. Coeur, *79*:1439, 1986.

44. Gibbs, J.C., Wharton, G.A., and Williams, G.J.: Doppler echocardiographic characteristics of the Carpentier-Edwards xenograft. Eur. Heart J., *7*:353, 1986.

45. Fawzy, M.E., Halim, M., Ziady, G., Mercer, E., Phillips, R., and Andaya, W.: Hemodynamic evaluation of porcine bioprostheses in the mitral position by Doppler echocardiography. Am. J. Cardiol., *59*:643, 1987.

46. Ryan, T., Armstrong, W.F., Dillon, J.C., and Feigenbaum, H.: Doppler echocardiographic evaluation of patients with porcine mitral valves. Am. Heart J., *111*:237, 1986.

47. Holen, J., Simonsen, S., and Froysaker, T.: Determination of pressure gradient in the Hancock mitral valve from noninvasive ultrasound Doppler data. Scand. J. Clin. Lab. Invest., *41*:177, 1981.

48. Kisanuki, A., Tei, C., Arikawa, K., Otsuji, Y., Kawazoe, Y., Natsugoe, K., Tanaka, H., Morishita, Y., and Taira, A.: Continuous wave Doppler echocardiographic assessment of prosthetic aortic valves. J. Cardiogr., *16*:121, 1986.

49. Ramirez, M.L., Wong, M., Sadler, N., and Shah, P.M.: Doppler evaluation of bioprosthetic and mechanical aortic valves: Data from four models in 107 stable, ambulatory patients. Am. Heart J., *115*:418, 1988.

50. Nihoyannopoulos, P., Kambouroglou, D., Athanasso-poulos, G., Nadazdin, A., Smith, P., and Oakley, C.M.: Doppler hemodynamic profiles of clinically and echocardiographically normal mitral and aortic valve prostheses. Eur. Heart J., *13*:348, 1992.

51. Heldman, D. and Gardin, J.M.: Evaluation of prosthetic valves by Doppler echocardiography. Echocardiography, 6:63, 1989.

52. Goldrath, N., Zimes, R., and Vered, Z.: Analysis of Doppler-obtained velocity curves in functional evaluation of mechanical prosthetic valves in the mitral and aortic positions. J. Am. Soc. Echocardiogr., *1*:211, 1988.

# Index

Page numbers in *italics* refer to illustrations; numbers followed by "t" indicate tables.